Advances of Membrane Vesicles in Drug Delivery Systems

Advances of Membrane Vesicles in Drug Delivery Systems

Guest Editor

Yong Chen

MDPI

Basel • Beijing • Wuhan • Barcelona • Belgrade • Novi Sad • Cluj • Manchester

Guest Editor
Yong Chen
School of Pharmacy
Nanchang University
Nanchang
China

Editorial Office
MDPI AG
Grosspeteranlage 5
4052 Basel, Switzerland

This is a reprint of the Special Issue, published open access by the journal *Pharmaceutics* (ISSN 1999-4923), freely accessible at: https://www.mdpi.com/journal/pharmaceutics/special_issues/Vesicles.

For citation purposes, cite each article independently as indicated on the article page online and as indicated below:

Lastname, A.A.; Lastname, B.B. Article Title. *Journal Name* **Year**, *Volume Number*, Page Range.

ISBN 978-3-7258-2983-5 (Hbk)
ISBN 978-3-7258-2984-2 (PDF)
https://doi.org/10.3390/books978-3-7258-2984-2

Contents

About the Editor

Yong Chen

Yong Chen obtained a bachelor's degree in Biology from Nanchang University, Nanchang, China, in 1997; a Master's degree in Biology from Jinan University, Guangzhou, China, in 2000; and a PhD in Optics from the Chinese Academy of Sciences in 2003. Then, he worked as a teaching assistant and lecturer at the Department of Chemistry of Jinan University, Guangzhou, China, from 2003 to 2004, followed by acting as a visiting postdoc and research assistant professor at the Department of Microbiology and Immunology of the University of Illinois at Chicago, Chicago, IL, from 2004 to 2009. He was a full professor at the Institute for Advanced Study of Nanchang University between 2009 and 2024. Since July 2024, Yong Chen has been a full professor at the School of Pharmacy of Nanchang University, Nanchang, China. He also visited the Department of Cell Biology of SUNY Downstate Medical Center, New York, NY, between 2017 and 2019. Yong Chen has been the principle investigator of more than 20 scientific projects and has participated in more than 10 other projects. To date, he has co-authored more than 120 publications in scientific journals and is serving as an Editorial Board Member for more than 10 international journals including *Pharmaceutics, BMC Mol. Cell Biol., Current Drug Delivery, Cardiovascular Innovations and Applications,* etc. or as a Guest Editor for some international journals including *Pharmaceut. Biol., Int. J. Mol. Sci., Front. Pharmacol.*, etc. He has been an expert of project-peer reviewing for the European Research Council, the NKFIH of Hungary, and organizations in China. He has also served as a reviewer for more than 70 international journals. His current research interests include bio-inspired drug delivery systems, plasma lipoproteins and apolipoproteins, atherosclerotic cardiovascular diseases, cell biology (particularly cellular biomechanics), pharmaceutics or pharmacology, fluorescent probes or biosensors, and others.

pharmaceutics

Editorial

Membrane Vesicles as Drug Delivery Systems: Source, Preparation, Modification, Drug Loading, In Vivo Administration and Biodistribution, and Application in Various Diseases

Chenhan Sun, Ying Qin, Hongda Zhuang, Yuan Zhang, Zhiwen Wu and Yong Chen *

Jiangxi Key Laboratory for Microscale Interdisciplinary Study, Institute for Advanced Study, Nanchang University, Nanchang 330031, China; sunchenhan0708@126.com (C.S.); qinying1013@hotmail.com (Y.Q.); hongdadazhuang@gmail.com (H.Z.); 15279115010@163.com (Y.Z.); 15179658052@163.com (Z.W.)

* Correspondence: tychen@ncu.edu.cn or dr_yongchen@hotmail.com

Abstract: Bioinspired (or biologically inspired) drug delivery systems (DDSs) have been intensively studied in the last decades. As bioinspired DDSs, membrane vesicles, including extracellular vesicles (EVs) released from eukaryotic cells, outer membrane vesicles (OMVs) from bacteria, cell-bound membrane vesicles (CBMVs) isolated in situ from cell surfaces, membrane vesicles reorganized after the isolation of the plasma membrane of cells, and others have been rapidly developed and are attracting more and more attention. Most recently, a collection of 25 papers on the advances in membrane vesicle-based drug delivery systems was published in a Special Issue of *Pharmaceutics* entitled "Advances of membrane vesicles in drug delivery systems". These papers cover many related topics including the source, preparation, modification, drug loading, and in vivo administration and biodistribution of membrane vesicles (mainly extracellular vesicles or exosomes and bacterial outer membrane vesicles), as well as application of membrane vesicles as DDSs in the treatment of various diseases.

Keywords: drug delivery systems (DDSs); membrane vesicles; extracellular vesicles (EVs); exosomes; bacterial outer membrane vesicles (OMVs)

Citation: Sun, C.; Qin, Y.; Zhuang, H.; Zhang, Y.; Wu, Z.; Chen, Y. Membrane Vesicles as Drug Delivery Systems: Source, Preparation, Modification, Drug Loading, In Vivo Administration and Biodistribution, and Application in Various Diseases. *Pharmaceutics* **2023**, *15*, 1903. https://doi.org/10.3390/pharmaceutics15071903

Received: 30 June 2023
Accepted: 4 July 2023
Published: 7 July 2023

1. Introduction

Drug delivery systems (DDSs) are defined as formulations or devices that deliver therapeutic substances specifically to their sites of action without reaching nontarget sites (cells, tissues, or even organs). Many benefits to drugs can be achieved by drug delivery systems, including an elevated stability, higher water solubility, prolonged circulation time, better sustained drug release, stronger tissue/cell targetability, lower drug dosage, impaired side effects, enhanced efficacy, etc. Over the latest two decades, bioinspired (or biologically inspired) drug delivery systems have been intensively studied. Compared with traditional DDSs, the advantages of bioinspired DDSs include lower/no immunogenicity, biocompatibility, biodegradability, better safety, among others. By mimicking (or being prepared from) natural components inside the body, many bioinspired DDSs have been tested, including biomolecule (e.g., peptides)-, lipid-protein complex (e.g., reconstituted high-density lipoprotein [1,2]), membrane vesicles-, virus-, and even whole cell (e.g., bacterium, red blood cell, platelet, stem cell)-inspired DDSs (Figure 1a shows 27 types of bioinspired DDSs frequently studied in recent decades).

As one specific type of bioinspired DDSs, membrane vesicles have a membranous structure derived from natural cells. Several types of membrane vesicles have been reported including well-known extracellular vesicles (EVs) released from eukaryotic cells, outer membrane vesicles (OMVs) from bacteria, cell-bound membrane vesicles (CBMVs) isolated in situ from cell surfaces [3–5], membrane vesicles reorganized after the isolation of the plasma membrane of cells, etc. Extracellular vesicles are generally divided into three categories: exosomes, microvesicles or microparticles, and apoptotic bodies among which the research on exosomes predominates in the research field of extracellular vesicles (Figure 1b). The bearing of some specific molecules, which originally exists on/in the source cells enables membrane vesicles to have specific functions (e.g., making the target cells have some properties of the source cells). In recent decade, membrane vesicles, particularly extracellular vesicles and bacterial outer membrane vesicles, have been rapidly developed as inspired DDSs (Figure 2 displays the EV-/OMV-related publications by year). In the Special Issue "Advances of membrane vesicles in drug delivery systems" of the Journal *Pharmaceutics* which belongs to the section "Drug Delivery and Controlled Release", 25 papers on the recent advances in membrane vesicle-based drug delivery systems have been collected and arranged in this Editorial article in the following order: the source, preparation, modification, drug loading, and in vivo administration and biodistribution of membrane vesicles (mainly extracellular vesicles or exosomes and bacterial outer membrane vesicles), as well as application of membrane vesicles as DDSs in the treatment of various diseases.

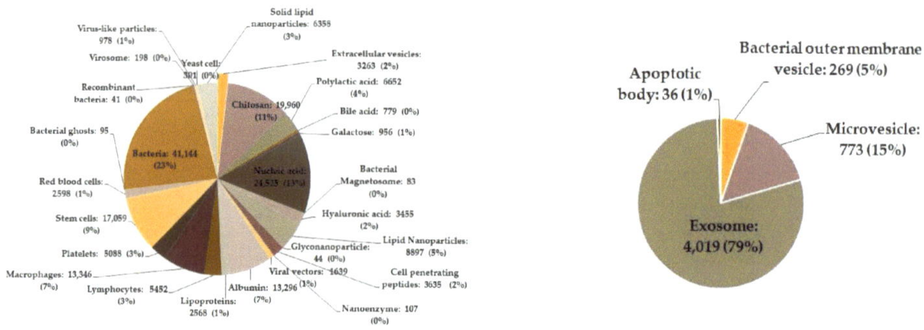

(a) (b)

Figure 1. Publications of different types of bioinspired drug delivery systems (DDSs). (**a**) 27 types of bioinspired DDSs; (**b**) Main types of membrane vesicles as DDSs including extracellular vesicles (EVs which are divided into three subtypes: Exosome, microvesicle or microparticle, and apoptotic body) and bacterial outer membrane vesicles. The data were obtained from the Web of Science database by searching for article title or the abstract field using the following keywords: 'Drug delivery' or 'drug carrier' and 'the name of a drug delivery system' (publication data is as of 18 June 2023).

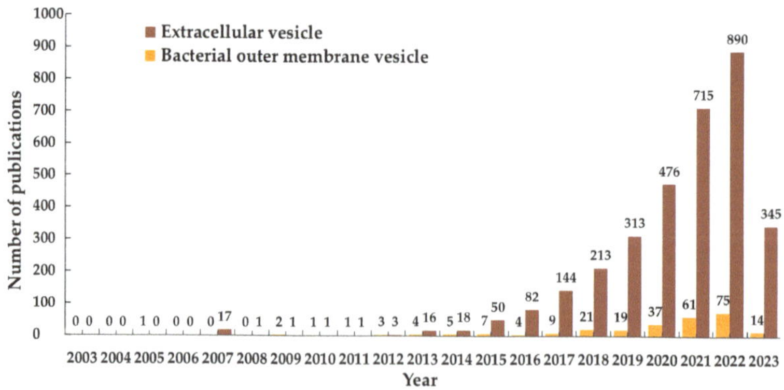

Figure 2. Publications by year of extracellular vesicles (EVs) and bacterial outer membrane vesicles (OMVs). The data were obtained from the Web of Science database by searching for article title or the abstract field using the following keywords: 'Drug delivery' or 'drug carrier' and 'the name of a drug delivery system' (the timespan is from 1 January 2003 to 18 June 2023).

2. Sources of Membrane Vesicles for DDSs

The selection of the sources for membrane vesicle production is crucial and needs to be prioritized during studies since it determines the composition and biological activity of membrane vesicles and influences the functional state of membrane vesicles as DDSs. Some studies have shown that extracellular vesicles exerted a better therapeutic efficacy than the cells releasing the EVs [6]. At present, abundant sources of membrane vesicles have been developed, including various biological fluids (e.g., blood, milk [7,8], orange juice [9]), animal cells (e.g., mesenchymal stem/stromal cells (MSCs) [7,10,11], dendritic cells [12], macrophages [13], tumor cells [14], red blood cells [15], different animal cell lines [16], and others), plant cells (e.g., grapes, conifers, ginger, garlic, tea, etc.) [17], bacteria (e.g., intestinal flora and probiotics) [18–20], and others [21,22]. Among the abovementioned sources, MSCs are widely used because of their pluripotency and the ability of differentiation into a variety of cell types; cell sources, e.g., $\gamma\delta$ T cells and macrophages, are also the best sources for EVs targeting cancer cells [23]; Recently, researchers are paying more attention to developing new natural membrane vesicle sources and engineered EVs [16].

3. Preparation and Modification of Membrane Vesicles as DDSs

The preparation of membrane vesicles is important for the following characterizations and applications of membrane vesicles as DDSs, and high vesicle yield and separation efficiency are required for practical production of membrane vesicles. The methods for membrane vesicle preparation should have the characteristics of robustness, ease of use, economy, repeatability, time-saving, and high throughput, and sometimes depend on the sources of membrane vesicles to a certain degree. The frequently used methods include differential ultrafiltration centrifugation (dUC), density gradient centrifugation, ultrafiltration (UF), precipitation, dimensional exclusion chromatography (SEC), and immunoaffinity capture, as well as emerging technologies (e.g., microfluidic) [6]. In this Special Issue, commercial ExoQuick-Tc^{TM} Exosome Precipitation Solution was used for the isolation of dendritic cell-derived exosomes [12] and of human cell-secreted EVs [16]; differential ultracentrifugation method was used to separate EVs from mesenchymal/stromal stem cells [7] or from orange (*Citrus sinensis*) juice [9]; and density gradient centrifugation method was also utilized to prepare milk EVs [7].

Physiochemical or biological modification can improve the targeting, bioactivity, kinetics, and biodistribution of membrane vesicles. At present, multiple methods have been applied for membrane vesicle modification, including modification of donor cells (e.g., genetic engineering modification), direct modification of isolated vesicles (e.g., chemical modification), combination strategy, and others [10,20]. In this Special Issue, modification of donor cells by regulating the expressions of CP05 [24], TRAIL [23], CD81 [16], CCR7 [12], etc., direct modifications of isolated EVs by using iRGD, hyaluronic acid, and folic acid [8], and combination modifications with $\alpha v\beta 3$ integrin subunit and iRGD [23] were applied. Akbari et al. reviewed the genetic and chemical functionalization of exosomes for tumor-targeted drug delivery [25].

4. Drug Loading of Membrane Vesicles as DDSs

It has been proved that membrane vesicles of various origins contain specific biomolecules. For example, extracellular vesicles can carry proteins, lipids, nucleic acids, and other signaling molecules to neighboring and distant cells, affecting various physiological and pathological functions of the recipient and parental cells, and participating in the development of various diseases. Not only can membrane vesicles be used as a "messenger" to modulate cells, but also as a "shooter" to target diseases. As a promising tool for drug delivery, membrane vesicles have been recruited to load different types of drugs. In this Special Issue, curcumin was loaded in extracellular vesicles for neuroinflammation [13]; peroxidase and dopamine for Parkinson's disease [26]; lncRNA H19 for osteoporosis [14]; miRNA-210 and miRNA-132 for cardiac repair [10]; paclitaxel for head and neck squamous cell carcinoma [23]; and even CRISPR/Cas9 for gene editing [27]. Similarly, different drugs were loaded by bacterial membrane vesicles as DDSs for disease treatment. For example, CuS and levofloxacin were loaded into OMV secreted by *E. coli* and *A. baumannii*, respectively [18]. Moreover, the potential of membrane vesicles derived from probiotics as DDSs is reviewed by Krzyzek et al. [19].

5. Characterization of Membrane Vesicles as DDSs

With the rapid development of membrane vesicles, corresponding characterization methods have been developed. The characterization methods can be utilized according to the physical properties of membrane vesicles including vesicle structure, size, buoyancy density, optical property, zeta potential, among others [28]. A survey shows that western blotting, single particle tracking, and electron microscopy are the three most widely used techniques for the characterization of extracellular vesicles [29]. The current guidance recommendations on extracellular vesicles or Minimal Information for Studies of Extracellular Vesicles ("MISEV") have been proposed first in 2014 ("MISEV2014") and updated in 2018 ("MISEV2018") by the International Society for Extracellular Vesicles (ISEV) [30] and widely recognized. According to the guidance recommendations, characterization of extracellular vesicles is mainly divided into three categories: Quantification, General characterization, and Characterization of individual extracellular vesicles based on which various techniques are required (Table 1 [30]). There is also the MISEV revision and update of the MISEV2018 in 2022, and the newest recommendations are expected to be released in 2023, whose draft ("MISEV2022 Draft") has been shown to the public. Compared to "MISEV2018", it is added in the characterization aspect of the draft that researchers should provide their assay's limit of detection when EVs are being characterized with quantitative metrics. In this Special Issue, Tolomeo et al. used tunable resistive pulse sensing (TRPS) to measure EV particle size [11]; Zhang et al. utilized single particle interferometric reflectance imaging sensing (SP-IRIS) technique for capturing EVs and recording their particle size [16].

Table 1. A brief summary of the characterization recommendations by the International Society for Extracellular Vesicles (ISEV) which is extracted from "MISEV2014" and "MISEV2018" (see the reference [30] for detailed information).

Category	MISEV2014	MISEV2018
Quantification	No recommendations	**Both the source of EV and the preparation of EV must be described quantitatively.** **Sourse:** Number of cultured cells, total starting volume of biofluid, or weight/volume/size of tissue. **Preparation:** Total protein amount, total particle number, total lipid quantification and the ratios among these.
General characterization	Analysis of the protein composition of EVs requires "three positives and one negative", with at least three positive protein markers containing at least one transmembrane/lipid bound protein, and one cytoplasmic protein; at least one negative protein marker.	Still valid but the categories of EV proteins to characterize have evolved. Mainly used for property identification, assessment of EV purity, subtype differentiation.
Characterization of individual EV	Use of 2 different but complementary techniques, such as electron microscopy and single particle analysis instruments (not electron microscope-based)	Still valid but techniques used to analyze EVs have envolved.
Additional characterization	---	The topology of EV associated components should be assessed

6. In Vivo Administration and Biodistribution of Membrane Vesicles as DDSs

Studying the in vivo drug administration and biodistribution of DDSs has a constructive role for membrane vesicles. In this Special Issue, Tolomeo et al. explored the biodistribution patterns of membrane vesicles derived from human mesenchymal stromal cells (MSCs) following different administration routes, including intratracheal, intranasal, and intravenous injections [11]. Using fluorescently labeled MSC-derived EVs in a mouse model, they revealed that regardless of the administration route, EVs exhibit widespread distribution in various organs such as the lungs, spleen, liver, and kidneys. However, the biodistribution patterns differ among the administration routes. The findings will contribute to our understanding of the administration strategies and biodistribution of membrane vesicles as DDSs, paving the way for further optimization and clinical translation of these promising drug carriers.

7. Applications of Membrane Vesicles as DDSs for Treating Different Diseases

With the development of different types of membrane vesicles, almost all types of membrane vesicles were tested to serve as DDSs or drug carriers for treating various diseases, shedding light on the therapeutic potential of membrane vesicle-based drug delivery systems across various medical conditions. A lot of related studies have been reported and summarized in many review articles. In this Special Issue, the applications of membrane vesicles as DDSs in bone-related diseases [14], anticancer and antimicrobial therapies [15,18,21,25,27], gastrointestinal diseases [17,19], organ transplant related diseases [31], cardiovascular diseases [10,12,32], neurodegenerative disorders [13,26,33], neurological anomalies associated with multidrug-resistant superbugs [20], and others were reviewed (Figure 3). Since the application of probiotics in myocardial infarction has been reported [34], it seems also potential that the membrane vesicles derived from probiotics can be recruited as DDSs to treat cardiovascular diseases (e.g., myocardial infarction). The potential impact of membrane vesicle-based therapies in these diseases is significant, as demonstrated by the studies reviewed.

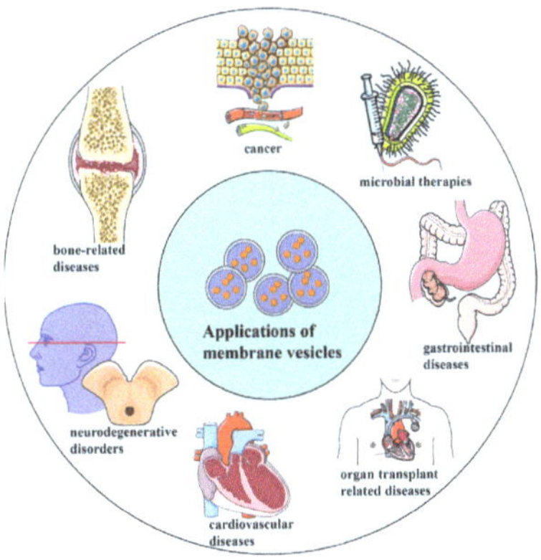

Figure 3. Membrane vesicles as DDSs in the treatment of different diseases.

Membrane vesicles (particularly extracellular vesicles and bacterial membrane vesicles) serve as effective carriers for delivering specific cell-derived molecules or therapeutic molecules or drugs, leveraging their targeted nature and intercellular communication properties [9,11,25]. The advances in recent years including those in this Special Issue will pave the way for the clinical translation of membrane vesicle-based drug delivery systems, promising improved treatment outcomes for patients. However, further studies are necessary to refine membrane vesicle production and purification methods, optimal drug loading approaches, more advanced characterization techniques, and in-depth applications in more diseases.

Author Contributions: Conceptualization, Y.C.; writing—original draft preparation, C.S., Y.Q., H.Z., Y.Z., Z.W., and Y.C.; writing—review and editing, C.S. and Y.C.; supervision, Y.C.; funding acquisition, Y.C. All authors have read and agreed to the published version of the manuscript.

Funding: This research was funded by the National Natural Science Foundation of China (grant numbers: 31760320 and 81970386), the Natural Science Foundation of Jiangxi Province of China (grant number: 20212ACB206035), and the Interdisciplinary Innovation Fund of Nanchang University (grant number: 9167-28220007-ZD2101).

Institutional Review Board Statement: Not applicable.

Informed Consent Statement: Not applicable.

Data Availability Statement: All data generated or analyzed are included in this article.

Conflicts of Interest: The authors declare no conflict of interest.

References

1. Wei, B.; Li, Y.; Ao, M.; Shao, W.; Wang, K.; Rong, T.; Zhou, Y.; Chen, Y. Ganglioside GM3-functionalized reconstituted high-density lipoprotein (GM3-rHDL) as a novel nanocarrier enhances antiatherosclerotic efficacy of statins in apoE$^{-/-}$ C57BL/6 mice. *Pharmaceutics* **2022**, *14*, 2534. [CrossRef] [PubMed]
2. Rong, T.; Wei, B.; Ao, M.; Zhao, H.; Li, Y.; Zhang, Y.; Qin, Y.; Zhou, J.; Zhou, F.; Chen, Y. Enhanced anti-atherosclerotic efficacy of pH-responsively releasable ganglioside GM3 delivered by reconstituted high-density lipoprotein. *Int. J. Mol. Sci.* **2021**, *22*, 13624. [CrossRef] [PubMed]
3. Tang, Q.S.; Zhang, X.J.; Zhang, W.D.A.; Zhao, S.Y.; Chen, Y. Identification and characterization of cell-bound membrane vesicles. *BBA-Biomembr.* **2017**, *1859*, 756–766. [CrossRef] [PubMed]
4. Zhang, Y.; Liu, Y.; Zhang, W.D.; Tang, Q.S.; Zhou, Y.; Li, Y.F.; Rong, T.; Wang, H.Y.; Chen, Y. Isolated cell-bound membrane vesicles (CBMVs) as a novel class of drug nanocarriers. *J. Nanobiotechnol* **2020**, *18*, 69. [CrossRef]
5. Zhou, Y.; Qin, Y.; Sun, C.H.; Liu, K.F.; Zhang, W.D.; Gaman, M.A.; Chen, Y. Cell-bound membrane vesicles contain antioxidative proteins and probably have an antioxidative function in cells or a therapeutic potential. *J. Drug Deliv. Sci. Technol.* **2023**, *81*, 104240. [CrossRef]
6. Ester, M.C.; Day, R.M. Production and Utility of Extracellular Vesicles with 3D Culture Methods. *Pharmaceutics* **2023**, *15*, 663. [CrossRef]
7. Mukhopadhya, A.; Tsiapalis, D.; McNamee, N.; Talbot, B.; O'Driscoll, L. Doxorubicin Loading into Milk and Mesenchymal Stem Cells' Extracellular Vesicles as Drug Delivery Vehicles. *Pharmaceutics* **2023**, *15*, 718. [CrossRef]
8. Zhong, Y.X.; Wang, X.D.; Zhao, X.; Shen, J.H.; Wu, X.; Gao, P.F.; Yang, P.; Chen, J.g.; An, W.L. Multifunctional Milk-Derived Small Extracellular Vesicles and Their Biomedical Applications. *Pharmaceutics* **2023**, *15*, 1418. [CrossRef]
9. Pomatto, M.A.C.; Gai, C.R.; Negro, F.; Massari, L.; Deregibus, M.C.; Grange, C.; De Rosa, F.G.; Camussi, G. Plant-Derived Extracellular Vesicles as a Delivery Platform for RNA-Based Vaccine: Feasibility Study of an Oral and Intranasal SARS-CoV-2 Vaccine. *Pharmaceutics* **2023**, *15*, 974. [CrossRef]
10. You, B.S.; Yang, Y.; Zhou, Z.X.; Yan, Y.M.; Zhang, L.L.; Jin, J.H.; Qian, H. Extracellular Vesicles: A New Frontier for Cardiac Repair. *Pharmaceutics* **2022**, *14*, 1848. [CrossRef]
11. Tolomeo, A.M.; Zuccolotto, G.; Malvicini, R.; De Lazzari, G.; Penna, A.; Franco, C.; Caicci, F.; Magarotto, F.; Quarta, S.; Pozzobon, M.; et al. Biodistribution of Intratracheal, Intranasal, and Intravenous Injections of Human Mesenchymal Stromal Cell-Derived Extracellular Vesicles in a Mouse Model for Drug Delivery Studies. *Pharmaceutics* **2023**, *15*, 548. [CrossRef]
12. Zhang, Y.M.; Gao, W.; Yuan, J.; Zhong, X.; Yao, K.; Luo, R.; Liu, H.B. CCR7 Mediates Dendritic-Cell-Derived Exosome Migration and Improves Cardiac Function after Myocardial Infarction. *Pharmaceutics* **2023**, *15*, 461. [CrossRef]
13. Yuan, Y.W.; Sun, J.; You, T.Y.; Shen, W.W.; Xu, W.Q.; Dong, Q.; Cui, M. Extracellular Vesicle-Based Therapeutics in Neurological Disorders. *Pharmaceutics* **2022**, *14*, 2652. [CrossRef]
14. Huang, J.W.; Xu, Y.; Wang, Y.X.; Su, Z.; Li, T.T.; Wu, S.S.; Mao, Y.H.; Zhang, S.H.; Weng, X.Q.; Yuan, Y. Advances in the Study of Exosomes as Drug Delivery Systems for Bone-Related Diseases. *Pharmaceutics* **2023**, *15*, 220. [CrossRef]
15. Biagiotti, S.; Abbas, F.; Montanari, M.; Barattini, C.; Rossi, L.; Magnani, M.; Papa, S.; Canonico, B. Extracellular Vesicles as New Players in Drug Delivery: A Focus on Red Blood Cells-Derived EVs. *Pharmaceutics* **2023**, *15*, 365. [CrossRef]
16. Zhang, J.Y.; Brown, A.; Johnson, B.; Diebold, D.; Asano, K.; Marriott, G.; Lu, B. Genetically Engineered Extracellular Vesicles Harboring Transmembrane Scaffolds Exhibit Differences in Their Size, Expression Levels of Specific Surface Markers and Cell-Uptake. *Pharmaceutics* **2022**, *14*, 2564. [CrossRef]
17. Donoso-Meneses, D.; Figueroa-Valdes, A.I.; Khoury, M.; Alcayaga-Miranda, F. Oral Administration as a Potential Alternative for the Delivery of Small Extracellular Vesicles. *Pharmaceutics* **2023**, *15*, 716. [CrossRef]
18. Celik, P.A.; Erdogan-Gover, K.; Barut, D.; Enuh, B.M.; Amasya, G.; Sengel-Turk, C.T.; Derkus, B.; Cabuk, A. Bacterial Membrane Vesicles as Smart Drug Delivery and Carrier Systems: A New Nanosystems Tool for Current Anticancer and Antimicrobial Therapy. *Pharmaceutics* **2023**, *15*, 1052. [CrossRef]

19. Krzyzek, P.; Marinacci, B.; Vitale, I.; Grande, R. Extracellular Vesicles of Probiotics: Shedding Light on the Biological Activity and Future Applications. *Pharmaceutics* **2023**, *15*, 522. [CrossRef]
20. Srivastava, P.; Kim, K.S. Membrane Vesicles Derived from Gut Microbiota and Probiotics: Cutting-Edge Therapeutic Approaches for Multidrug-Resistant Superbugs Linked to Neurological Anomalies. *Pharmaceutics* **2022**, *14*, 2370. [CrossRef]
21. Chen, W.J.; Wu, Y.L.; Deng, J.J.; Yang, Z.M.; Chen, J.B.; Tan, Q.; Guo, M.F.; Jin, Y. Phospholipid-Membrane-Based Nanovesicles Acting as Vaccines for Tumor Immunotherapy: Classification, Mechanisms and Applications. *Pharmaceutics* **2022**, *14*, 2446. [CrossRef] [PubMed]
22. Zhang, Y.; Lu, Y.M.; Xu, Y.X.; Zhou, Z.K.; Li, Y.C.; Ling, W.; Song, W.L. Bio-Inspired Drug Delivery Systems: From Synthetic Polypeptide Vesicles to Outer Membrane Vesicles. *Pharmaceutics* **2023**, *15*, 368. [CrossRef] [PubMed]
23. Dzaman, K.; Czerwaty, K. Extracellular Vesicle-Based Drug Delivery Systems for Head and Neck Squamous Cell Carcinoma: A Systematic Review. *Pharmaceutics* **2023**, *15*, 1327. [CrossRef] [PubMed]
24. Li, T.W.; Li, X.Q.; Han, G.P.; Liang, M.; Yang, Z.R.; Zhang, C.Y.; Huang, S.Z.; Tai, S.; Yu, S. The Therapeutic Potential and Clinical Significance of Exosomes as Carriers of Drug Delivery System. *Pharmaceutics* **2023**, *15*, 21. [CrossRef] [PubMed]
25. Akbari, A.; Nazari-Khanamiri, F.; Ahmadi, M.; Shoaran, M.; Rezaie, J. Engineered Exosomes for Tumor-Targeted Drug Delivery: A Focus on Genetic and Chemical Functionalization. *Pharmaceutics* **2023**, *15*, 66. [CrossRef]
26. Sun, K.; Zheng, X.; Jin, H.Z.; Yu, F.; Zhao, W. Exosomes as CNS Drug Delivery Tools and Their Applications. *Pharmaceutics* **2022**, *14*, 2252. [CrossRef]
27. Zhu, X.L.; Gao, M.Y.; Yang, Y.F.; Li, W.M.; Bao, J.; Li, Y. The CRISPR/Cas9 System Delivered by Extracellular Vesicles. *Pharmaceutics* **2023**, *15*, 984. [CrossRef]
28. Rupert, D.L.M.; Claudio, V.; Lasser, C.; Bally, M. Methods for the physical characterization and quantification of extracellular vesicles in biological samples. *BBA-Gen. Subj.* **2017**, *1861*, 3164–3179. [CrossRef]
29. Gardiner, C.; Di Vizio, D.; Sahoo, S.; Thery, C.; Witwer, K.W.; Wauben, M.; Hill, A.F. Techniques used for the isolation and characterization of extracellular vesicles: Results of a worldwide survey. *J. Extracell. Vesicles* **2016**, *5*, 32945. [CrossRef]
30. Thery, C.; Witwer, K.W.; Aikawa, E.; Alcaraz, M.J.; Anderson, J.D.; Andriantsitohaina, R.; Antoniou, A.; Arab, T.; Archer, F.; Atkin-Smith, G.K.; et al. Minimal information for studies of extracellular vesicles 2018 (MISEV2018): A position statement of the International Society for Extracellular Vesicles and update of the MISEV2014 guidelines. *J. Extracell. Vesicles* **2018**, *7*, 1535750. [CrossRef]
31. Spiers, H.V.M.; Stadler, L.K.J.; Smith, H.; Kosmoliaptsis, V. Extracellular Vesicles as Drug Delivery Systems in Organ Transplantation: The Next Frontier. *Pharmaceutics* **2023**, *15*, 891. [CrossRef]
32. Jiapaer, Z.; Li, C.Y.; Yang, X.Y.; Sun, L.F.; Chatterjee, E.; Zhang, L.Y.; Lei, J.; Li, G.P. Extracellular Non-Coding RNAs in Cardiovascular Diseases. *Pharmaceutics* **2023**, *15*, 155. [CrossRef]
33. Lim, W.Q.; Luk, K.H.M.; Lee, K.Y.; Nurul, N.; Loh, S.J.; Yeow, Z.X.; Wong, Q.X.; Looi, Q.H.D.; Chong, P.P.; How, C.W.; et al. Small Extracellular Vesicles' miRNAs: Biomarkers and Therapeutics for Neurodegenerative Diseases. *Pharmaceutics* **2023**, *15*, 1216. [CrossRef]
34. Cai, J.; Jiang, H. Application potential of probiotics in acute myocardial infarction. *Cardiovasc. Innov. Appl.* **2022**, *7*, 1–9. [CrossRef]

pharmaceutics

Review

Bio-Inspired Drug Delivery Systems: From Synthetic Polypeptide Vesicles to Outer Membrane Vesicles

Yu Zhang [1], Yiming Lu [1], Yixin Xu [1], Zunkang Zhou [2], Yichong Li [2], Wei Ling [2] and Wenliang Song [2,*]

[1] School of Pharmacy, Shanghai University of Medicine & Health Sciences, Shanghai 201318, China
[2] School of Materials and Chemistry, University of Shanghai for Science and Technology, Shanghai 200093, China
* Correspondence: wenliang@usst.edu.cn

Abstract: Nanomedicine is a broad field that focuses on the development of nanocarriers to deliver specific drugs to targeted sites. A synthetic polypeptide is a kind of biomaterial composed of repeating amino acid units that are linked by peptide bonds. The multiplied amphiphilicity segment of the polypeptide could assemble to form polypeptide vesicles (PVs) under suitable conditions. Different from polypeptide vesicles, outer membrane vesicles (OMVs) are spherical buds of the outer membrane filled with periplasmic content, which commonly originate from Gram-negative bacteria. Owing to their biodegradability and excellent biocompatibility, both PVs and OMVs have been utilized as carriers in delivering drugs. In this review, we discuss the recent drug delivery research based on PVs and OMVs. These related topics are presented: (1) a brief introduction to the production methods for PVs and OMVs; (2) a thorough explanation of PV- and OMV-related applications in drug delivery including the vesicle design and biological assessment; (3) finally, we conclude with a discussion on perspectives and future challenges related to the drug delivery systems of PVs and OMVs.

Keywords: drug delivery; polypeptides vesicles; outer membrane vesicles; biological properties

Citation: Zhang, Y.; Lu, Y.; Xu, Y.; Zhou, Z.; Li, Y.; Ling, W.; Song, W. Bio-Inspired Drug Delivery Systems: From Synthetic Polypeptide Vesicles to Outer Membrane Vesicles. *Pharmaceutics* **2023**, *15*, 368. https://doi.org/10.3390/pharmaceutics15020368

Academic Editors: Anna Angela Barba and Anne Marie Healy

Received: 4 December 2022
Revised: 10 January 2023
Accepted: 19 January 2023
Published: 21 January 2023

1. Introduction

Pharmacologically active agents (also known as therapeutics or drugs) are used in medicine to control or stop the progression of disease [1,2]. Improved delivery methods and a better understanding of how drug administration affects safety and efficacy have been thoroughly discussed [3,4]. Drug delivery systems (DDSs) are technological systems that comprehensively regulate the distribution of drugs in the organism in terms of space, time, and dose [5–10]. The goal is to deliver the right amount of drug to the right place at the right time, thus increasing the efficiency of drug utilization, improving efficacy, reducing costs, and reducing toxic side effects [11,12]. To date, DDS usage has seen widespread integration in synthetic chemistry, materials science, biology, and medical sciences and is becoming increasingly prevalent in clinical practice. However, drug delivery targeting is not easily controlled because the release rate, the targeted sites, and the stability of the carrier and drug are inconsistent in different environments. Understanding the drug delivery characteristics of specific vesicles is a significant basis for their future application.

Polypeptides are crucial, artificially prepared biomaterials [13,14]. Their outstanding biocompatibility, appropriate biodegradability, and biological chain design abilities allow polypeptides to be employed in a variety of applications, such as drug delivery, antibacterial applications, and gene delivery [14,15]. In addition, unique secondary structures of polypeptides, such as α-helices and β-sheets, endow them with interesting self-assembly behavior and biological properties. Generally, three approaches can be applied to the synthesis of polypeptide materials, including solid-phase synthesis, α-amino acid N-carboxyanhydride (NCA) polymerization, and microbial fermentation [16]. Among these, the ring-opening polymerization (ROP) of NCAs represents a facile route to obtain high-molecular-weight polymers with the desired functionality. Due to the variety of ROP chemical and synthetic strategies, a polypeptide not only can be conjugated with multiple polypeptide segments, but it can also be blocked with non-peptidic materials. The peptides mentioned in this review are mainly synthetic polypeptides, which are biomaterials composed of repeating amino acid units linked by peptide bonds. In particular, amphiphilic polypeptides, which are composed of hydrophobic and hydrophilic chains, can easily self-assemble into micelles under suitable conditions. The vesicle is the most interesting assembled morphology of micelles. Further, the designed pH-responsive residues could be used as candidates to load hydrophilic cargos and be released upon appropriate stimulation. A subtle tactic to reduce unintended toxicity and increase effectiveness is the design of smart chemistry methods for programmed release in DDSs. Polymers with a variety of specific functionalities that react to internal or external stimuli and cause payloads to be released at the target site are needed. As a result, controlled release using vesicles, which is otherwise challenging to achieve in delivery systems based on other biopolymers, can be made possible by tuning the built-in molecular structures of polypeptide segments.

Different from artificially assembled polypeptide vesicles, vesicles derived from the outer membrane of Gram-negative bacteria are called OMVs [17–20]. OMVs are widely produced, vary in size and composition, and contain soluble periplasmic content. Given the diversity of OMV-producing pathways, species-dependent differences in the envelope architecture, and environmental influences on envelope composition, it is difficult to identify a single molecular or genetic basis for OMV production. OMVs were first reported more than 50 years ago in research on bacterial growth and were described to be able to release vesicles with diameters of 20 to 300 nm [21]. Since the outer membrane of the original bacteria was studied, several bacteria have been reported to be capable of producing OMVs, such as *Pseudomonas aeruginosa*, *Helicobacter pylori*, *Escherichia coli*, *Shigella* sp., *Borrelia burgdorferi*, *Vibrio* sp., *Neisseria* sp., etc. [22–26]. As they are derived from the membrane, OMVs mainly contain phospholipids, lipopolysaccharides, outer membrane proteins, and periplasm, along with different cytoplasmic components. These vesicles have been connected to several physiological activities because of their composition, including protein transport, nutrition acquisition, cell-to-cell communication, antibacterial activity, toxin delivery, and host immune response regulation. In addition, differently from the clear ROP polymerization and self-assembly mechanism, the mechanism of OMVs remains a mystery. Recently, owing to some gene and biochemistry studies, some clues about this complex process have been reported. In recent years, it has been found that OMVs could be used in antigens for vaccines, drug delivery, bioimaging, nanogenerators, and new adjuvants. Studies have also revealed that OMVs have great potential in the transport of small-molecule drugs. Further, it has been demonstrated how to electroporate medications into the OMV lumen. Finally, passive diffusion can be employed for tiny molecules that are generally hydrophobic and positively charged, so that they can easily interact with lipophilic membranes (Table 1).

Table 1. Comparison of characteristics of PVs and OMVs.

Classification	PVs	OMVs	Reference
Origin	Synthetic polymers	Gram-negative bacteria	[13,17]
Production	Solution self-assembly	Biogenesis	[15,21]
Size	Several nanometers~micrometers	20~300 nm	[14,27]
Biomedical applications	Antibacterial Mineralization Drug delivery Imaging and sensing Therapeutic	Bacterial vaccines Adjuvants Cancer immunotherapy Drug delivery Anti-bacteria adhesion	[14,28]

In this review, first, we highlight recent achievements in research on artificial PVs and natural OMVs (Figure 1). The production methods of PVs and OMVs are summarized. Then, the comparison of the fabrication of PV- and OMV-based DDSs and especially their biological evaluation are extensively discussed. In the end, the current challenges regarding PVs and OMVs are also presented.

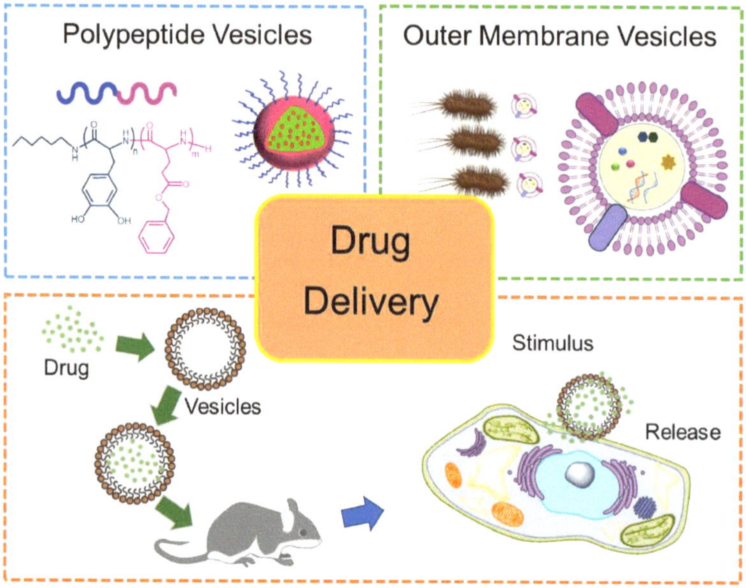

Figure 1. Schematic illustration of PVs and OMVs, along with their drug delivery properties.

2. Production and Characterization of PVs and OMVs

2.1. Production of PVs

In polypeptide clinical transformation, the precise control of chemical structures and the polydispersity index (PDI) is very important for polymer vesicle formation. In recent decades, continued efforts have been made to produce polypeptides with controlled molecular weight, narrow PDI, peptide segments, and physical–chemical biological effects [13,29]. However, solid-phase peptide synthesis and microbial fermentation have been characterized by low yield, high costs, and limited achievable chain length. Herein, we mainly focus on the polymerization method for obtaining polypeptides via the ROP of α-amino acid NCAs and the vesicles subsequently assembled in solution.

In 1921, Curtius, Wessel, and their coworkers used NCAs to produce polypeptides using ROP methods [30]. The "normal amine mechanism" (NAM) (Figure 2a) and the "active monomer mechanism" (AMM) (Figure 2b) are the two typical routes via which nucleophiles or bases initiate the ROP of NCAs [31]. The NAM not only includes primary and secondary amines but also alcohols and thiols as initiators. Initiation often occurs due to the nucleophilic attack of the carbonyl group of the NCA ring. The intermediate product, carbamic acid, is subsequently formed due to proton transfer and ring opening. Further, the decarboxylation of carbamic acid eliminates CO_2 and promotes the propagation of the polymer chain. It has been reported that the NAM can control the molecular weight of polypeptides and the adjustable end groups well. However, due to the side reaction that often occurs along with this process, cyclic polymers and terminated active end groups derived from the impurities in the reactions (water, reaction solvent, or contaminants in NCAs) can be found in the resulting polymers. On the other hand, the AMM mainly involves tertiary amines and alkoxides. It might occur that the resultant NCA anions catch the proton from the nitrogen group of NCAs (3-N). NCA anions can initiate further reactions with other NCAs, as propagation could further involve the attacking of the 5-CO group of other NCAs. In this case, polymerization is untraceable, generating ill-defined polypeptides [32]. It is worth pointing out that these two mechanisms often co-exist in one polymerization process, so the precise control of the reaction conditions is the main issue that needs addressing.

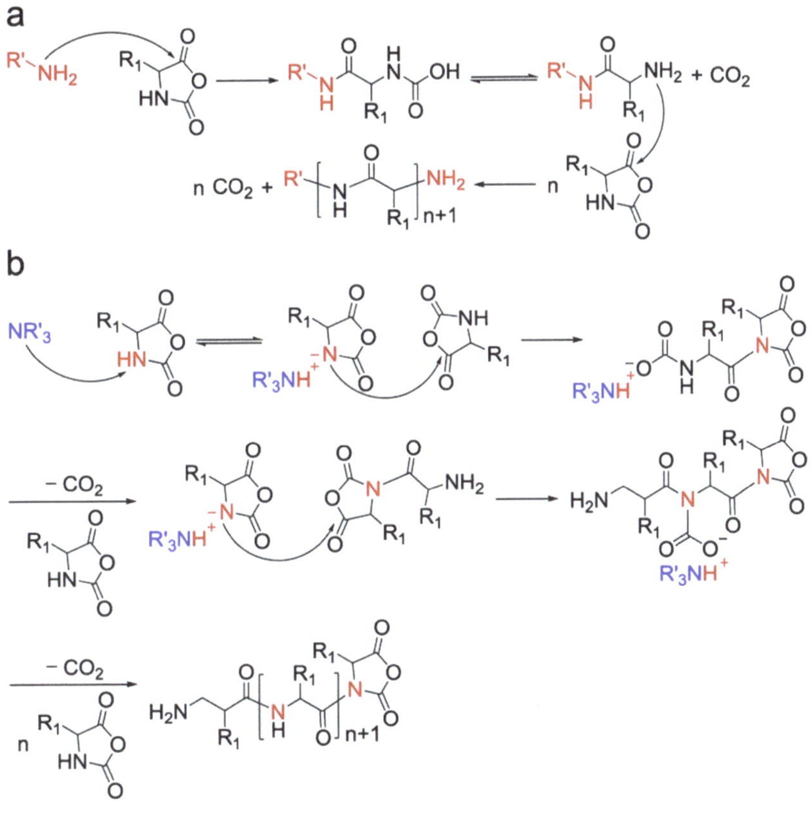

Figure 2. Schematic illustration of polypeptide formation mechanism, (**a**) normal amine mechanism and (**b**) active monomer mechanism. Reprinted with permission from Ref. [32]. Copyright: 1997, John Wiley & Sons, Inc.

By considering this reported mechanism, various polymerization methods with different initiators, catalysts, and pre-designed NCAs have been reported for polypeptide design over the years. Living polymer methods can greatly enhance the speed of NCA polymerization, and the reaction time can even be minimized to a few minutes. Moreover, "Click chemistry" can be used for the post-conjugation of various groups on the polypeptide chain, thus giving the resulting polypeptide unique stimulus responsiveness. In this method, firstly, various initiators can be used, such as metal-based complexes, amine salts, silane derivatives, etc. Even without any initiators, photo-based chemistry can lead to a polypeptide with tunable molecular weight. Secondly, the catalyst has an important role in controlling the ROP of NCAs. Metallic catalysts and organic catalysts are the two main types of catalysts for controlling the speed of reaction by shortening the propagation time. Metal-based catalysts often result in metal residues on the resulting polypeptide. As organic catalysts do not have this problem, leaving no traces of metal, they offer the most freedom to control the fabrication of polymers that are suitable for various applications, especially in the biomedical area. Additionally, the conditions of high vacuum, low reaction temperatures, N_2 flow, and UV can all be applied to polypeptide synthesis and have the ability to accelerate the reaction speed and reduce the side reaction. These improved polymerization technologies are significant, as they give researchers the chance to obtain polypeptide-based polymers with different topologies and interesting structures. Not only can linear, hinged, cyclic, and branched polypeptides be quickly obtained, but also random, alternating, block, and grafted copolypeptides can be obtained by applying sophisticated chemical synthesis skills. These copolymerized polypeptides with different topologies also greatly improve vesicle formation.

PVs are hollow spheres in shape with a bilayer wall of polymers. Commonly, they are formed through the self-assembly of amphiphilic polymers (Figure 3). These vesicles have various advantages over common polymer micelles: (1) the inner aqueous cavity can be loaded with hydrophilic cargo; (2) hydrophobic cargo can be loaded on the membrane of the vesicles; and (3) vesicles can easily disassemble to achieve suitable drug release properties. Thus, stimulus responsiveness is very important in PV formation; for instance, PV nano-assemblies can disassemble or reassemble under the simulation of pH, ROS, enzymes, or infrared light. Thus, in drug delivery, nano-assemblies can easily carry the drug compound to suitable sites and release it with the disassembly of the vesicles.

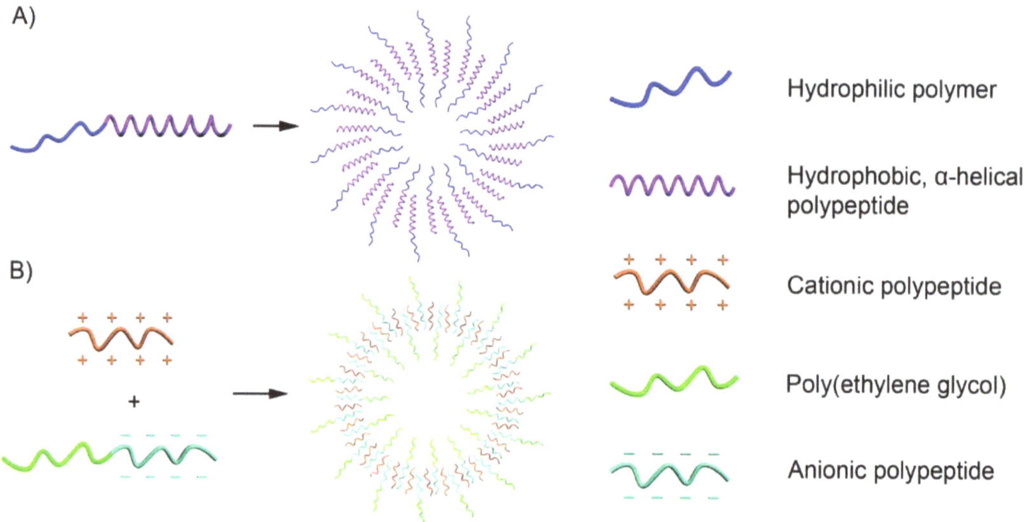

Figure 3. Schematic illustration of polypeptide vesicle formation. (**A**) a-helical polypeptide segments and (**B**) PVs from two polymers containing charged polypeptide segments with opposite charges. Reprinted with permission from Ref. [14]. Copyright: 2017, The Royal Society of Chemistry.

2.1.1. Anisotropic Packing of α-Helical, Hydrophobic Polypeptides

The α-helical conformation can be observed in a variety of polypeptides with rigid rods, such as polyleucine and polyphenylalanine. This is attributed to the hydrophobic polypeptide segment, even at a high hydrophilic-to-hydrophobic ratio. Moreover, research also shows that randomly coiled copolymers can only form micelles, even with finely controlled components. The hydrophobic block becomes the essential component for assembling hydrophobic polypeptides (Figure 3A). For example, as early as 2005, Timothy J. Deming already reported on the charged polypeptides of poly(l-lysine)-b-poly(l-leucine) block copolypeptides, which could be assembled into vesicular assemblies [33]. Afterwards, cationic polypeptides and anionic polypeptides were both reported to be able to form vesicles under suitable conditions [34–36]. Polypeptides with carbohydrate moieties can be covalently linked to the side chains of amino acids and form glycopeptides, with this segment as the hydrophilic chain, and polypeptide vesicles can also be formed. Andreas Heise et al. showed that poly(γ-benzyl-l-glutamate) (PBLG)-b-poly (galactosylated propargylglycine) can also form stable vesicles, in which hydrophobic PBLG plays a decisive role [37]. Since hydrophobic polypeptide segments are limited, the hydrophilic chain can be varied. Not only peptide materials but also biodegradable polymers, such as polyethylene glycol (PEG) and hyaluronan (HYA), have been reported in research studies on vesicle preparation.

2.1.2. Oppositely Charged Polymers

Amphiphilic polypeptides can be used to form vesicles using the traditional self-assembly methods introduced by Eisenberg [38] (Figure 3B). First, a solvent dissolves the amphiphilic polypeptides; after that, a solvent specific to one segment is added to the system to induce the formation of vesicles. On the other hand, Kataoka's group further showed that oppositely charged polypeptides can be assembled into vesicles in aqueous solution. Even without any trace of organic solvent, water can induce vesicle formation.

2.1.3. Others

Recently, reports have also shown that poly(ε-caprolactone)-block-poly(lysine-stat-phenylalanine) [PCL-b-P(Lys-stat-Phe)] and poly(ε-caprolactone)-block-poly(tryptophan)-block-poly(lysine-stat-phenylalanine) might also be able to assemble into vesicles, where PCLs are the resulting hydrophobic membranes [39,40]. Specifically, these are dual corona vesicles, which are induced using solvent-switch methods. In addition, poly (L-glutamic acid) have good solubility at neutral pH; in fact, it was reported that poly (trimethylene carbonate)-b-poly(l-glutamic acid) materials could also assemble into vesicles with altered sizes of 60 nm and 130 nm at pH values of 7.4 and 10.5, respectively [41].

2.2. *Production of OMVs*

Cells create and release membrane-bound material, which is sometimes referred to as membrane vesicles, microvesicles, exosomes, tolerasomes, agrosomes, and virus-like particles, in all domains of life (Figure 4). The first time OMVs were observed dates to the 1960s, when Chatterjee and Das studied the cell-wall structures of *Vibrio cholera* (*V. cholera*) in vitro. Moreover, K. W. Knox et al. firstly found changes in the lysine-limited culture of Escherichia coli, characterized by cell growth with surrounding "globules" and "hollow spheres" [42]. Recently, the biosynthesis field has achieved great advances, and the physiological roles of OMVs have also been found. Moreover, related reports have shown that released vesicles contain lipids, proteins, DNA, RNA, and lipopolysaccharides [43]. In general, OMVs are vesicle structures ranging from about 20 to 300 nm and are produced by almost all Gram-negative bacteria, though a similar phenomenon has also been detected in Gram-positive bacteria. The production of OMVs is still unclear, and why all bacterial cargo can be detected in OMVs remains unknown. However, a growing body of biological evidence is being collected to explain these complex processes. The ability of OMVs to transport a significant amount of the biological materials present in the parent bacterium to distant sites in the host, thus facilitating bacterial communication, the transmission of virulence factors, and the maintenance of bacterial communities, is ultimately due to their capacity to carry cargo [44]. To date, although the mechanism of OMV production remains unclear, three models of OMV biogenesis have been proposed.

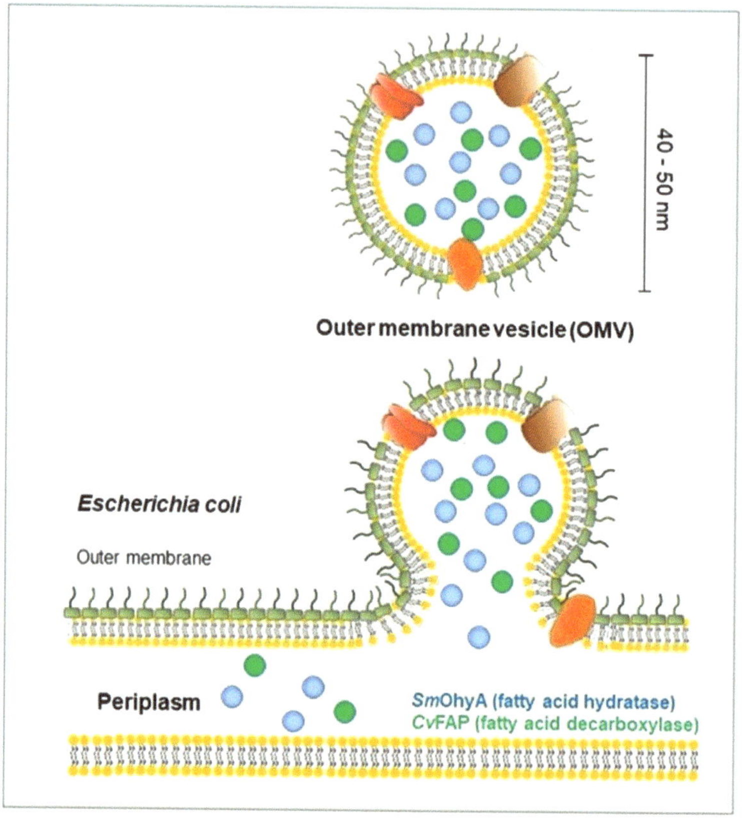

Figure 4. Biogenesis of OMV production in bacteria. Reprinted with permission from Ref. [44]. Copyright: 2021, John Wiley & Sons, Inc.

2.2.1. Reduced Lipoprotein Linkages

Hypervesiculation is often observed in the case of reduced crosslinking between the outer membrane and the underlying peptidoglycan layer. The reduced number of linkages can lead to the bulging of the outer membrane, thus resulting in the production of vesicles. Dick Hoekstra already showed that vesicles may be easily formed in areas with a low number of outer membrane–murein linkages [45]. Similar results can also be found in the reports by Meta J. Kuehn and Maria Kaparakis-Liaskos [46,47]. Both *Acinetobacter baumannii* and *Escherichia coli* have similar OMV production tendencies with reduced crosslinking.

2.2.2. Peptidoglycan Residues

According to this hypothesis, there are locations where the concentration of peptidoglycans is greater during the production of the peptidoglycan layer, which causes protrusions in the outer membrane, signaling the start of vesicle formation. OMVs are released when peptidoglycan residue accumulation causes the outer membrane to bulge even more. For example, Meta J. Kuehn et al. reported that periplasmic peptidoglycan components could increase OMV biogenesis [48].

2.2.3. Electrically Charged Lipopolysaccharides (LPSs)

Electrically charged LPSs are the subject of the third and final OMV production model. Positively charged LPSs and neutrally charged LPSs are the two forms of LPSs that *Pseudomonas aeruginosa* produce. OMVs are predominantly made of negatively charged LPSs when produced by *Pseudomonas aeruginosa* under oxidative stress. Due to the repelling effect of the negatively charged outer membrane, an increase in negatively charged LPSs within the cell envelope might facilitate the release of OMVs [49].

2.2.4. Other Mechanisms

OMV biogenesis appears to be a diverse multi-factorial process stimulated or regulated by a variety of pathways/mechanisms that may function simultaneously. For example, the environment has been found to have an important role in OMV production. Kuehn et al. reported that OMV production is a stress-responsive process and that temperature could have an effect on Serratia marcescens and *E.coli* [48,50]. Wael Elhenawy et al. reported in the *Salmonella enterica serovar Typhimurium* model that a lipid is necessary for OMV biogenesis [51], that is, deacylation happens within a multifactorial procedure, including planned modification of the outer membrane. Lynne Turnbull et al. used super-resolution microscopy to observe the OMV production process in *Pseudomonas aeruginosa* biofilms [52]. The release of cytosolic material in *Pseudomonas aeruginosa* biofilms was found to result from the explosive cell lysis of a subpopulation of cells. Explosive cell lysis also generates broken membrane fragments that form OMVs quickly. Sandro Roier et al. showed that VacJ/Yrb ABC (ATP-binding cassette) is also involved in OMV formation [53]. VacJ/Yrb ABC is a phospholipid transporter. The accumulation of phospholipids in the outer leaflet of the outer membrane causes this general mechanism of OMV generation.

3. Drug Delivery Performance of PVs and OMVs

Recently, it has been found that both PVs and OMVs can be employed in a variety of bio-applications, such as drug delivery [15,29,54–56], vaccination [57–59], cancer therapy [60–62], bioimaging [63,64], biosensing [65,66], and antibacterial applications [39,66–72]. PVs are generally obtained with amphiphilic block copolymers; thus, hydrophobic membranes can very easily carry hydrophobic drugs. In addition, delivering biomolecules from the parent bacterium to specific distant sites is one of the important functions of OMVs in nature. Further, the stimulus-responsive ability of PVs and OMVs offers the best way to release the loaded drug. Under specific stimuli, such as physical (heat or light), chemical (pH and reducing agents), and biomarker (e.g., ATP or RNA) agents, PVs and OMVs can also respond in a certain way to achieve targeted drug release. Both PVs and OMVs have natural advantages in terms of drug delivery (Table 2).

Table 2. Comparison of drug loading and releasing by PVs and OMVs.

DDS	PVs	References	OMVs	References
Drug loading	Hydrophobic interaction Electrostatic interactions Metal coordination	[73,74] [75] [77]	Electroporation Passive diffusion Biogenesis	[55] [76] [78,79]
Drug releasing	Change peptide assembly behavior	[80,81]	Degradation of OMVs	[55]
	Change drug–polypeptide interaction	[82]	Coating on polymer Bioengineering	[83] [84]

3.1. *Advantages of PVs and OMVs in DDSs*

Due to multiple advantages, both PVs and OMVs can be used as platforms in DDSs [15]. The first advantage is the suitable size. PVs can be assembled in vesicles of suitable size by changing the nanoprecipitation conditions. The solvent and injection rate are the main impact factors when water is added to the polymer solvent. Furthermore, pH, polymer concentration, and temperature are important factors in the design of the size of vesicles. Moreover, the size can be altered from several nanometers to micrometers. OMVs commonly have sizes of 50 nm~250 nm. The size of both PVs and OMVs can allow them to pass through the tumor cell membrane owing to the enhanced permeability and retention effect [27]. Secondly, they are biocompatible and biodegradable. Due to the fact that they are derived from natural compounds, both PVs and OMVs are biocompatible and enzyme biodegradable. For example, Sofroniew and Deming showed that amphiphilic polypeptides can be used for the sustainable release of cargo; these polypeptides were detected to have no detectable toxicity to normal cells and could be fully degraded over several weeks [85,86]. OMVs have also been shown to be environmentally inert and biodegradable. Using electron microscopy to analyze OMV morphology, Schulz et al. also discovered that OMVs are biocompatible with differentiated macrophages and epithelial cells [87]. Thirdly, both PVs and OMVs can easily be loaded with the drug compound and protect it [88,89]. Fourthly, both PVs and OMVs can easily deliver drugs to target sites. For example, folic acid can be conjugated with a polypeptide chain and be used as the targeted group [9,90–92]. By genetically modifying the parent bacterium, targeting ligands can be added to OMVs. Targeting ligands make it easier for medications to build up at the desired sites. Lastly, PVs can be designed and conjugated with fluorescence groups, such as pyrene or NIR-II, which makes superior fluorescence imaging possible [93,94]. OMVs are produced from bacteria and contain a variety of pathogen-associated molecular patterns; because neutrophils and macrophages can recognize and internalize them, OMVs can also be employed to deliver specific cargoes to these cells [95,96].

Additionally, they each have their own advantages. For example, the chemical synthetic approaches designed so far allow polypeptide-based vesicles to be more easily designed. The stimulus properties of PVs can be engineered with various responsive groups. poly(N-isopropylacrylamide) (PNIPAM) has been found to undergo thermally responsive transformation in water at 32 °C [97]. After conjugating with PNIPAM, PVs become sensitive to temperature, thus achieving selective release. Furthermore, amino acids can be altered depending on the tumor environment. By selecting poly(L-histidine), pH-responsive vehicles were designed based on the closed pKa $\approx$ 6.0 of the tumor environment [98,99]. In addition, polypeptides can be obtained in just a few minutes depending on the development of the catalysts. Thus, PVs have a bright future in mass production. OMVs trigger an immunological response that is advantageous for the treatment of tumors. This, however, also presents disadvantages, as the immunological response might harm the host if proper measures are not taken to control it.

3.2. Techniques for Drug Loading in PVs and OMVs

3.2.1. Drug Loading in PVs

In PV drug loading, drugs can be divided into hydrophobic drugs, hydrophilic drugs, and metal-based drugs [100,101]. Hydrophobic interaction is the main approach for loading hydrophobic drugs. For example, Sebastien Lecommandoux et al. reported that PEO-b-PBLG diblock and PBLG-b-PEO-b-PBLG triblock copolymers could be loaded with the hydrophobic drug doxorubicin (DOX) [73]. DOX could encapsulate as much as 18 wt.%. Kim et al. showed that poly(ethylene glycol) methyl ether acrylate-block-poly(l-lysine)-block-poly(l-histidine) [$p(PEGA)_{30}$-b-$p(Lys)_{25}$-b-$p(His)_n$] can be used for the design of and assembly into the vesicles [74] (Figure 5a). These vesicles, with suitable sizes of 200~372 nm and hydrophobic chains of p(His), were used as a loading site for DOX. The content of DOX was as high as 21 $\pm$ 2% and the loading efficiency was 68%.

Besides hydrophobic drugs, hydrophilic drugs can be loaded into PVs through electrostatic interactions, and metallic coordination can easily encapsulate metal-based drugs. For instance, Chen's group developed PEG-b-poly(l-glutamic acid) (PEG-b-PLG) through the ROP of NCAs using $PEG\text{-}NH_2$ as the initiator [75]. Having a portable amino group in the sugar moiety, DOX·HCl is a positively charged and amphiphilic drug. The carboxylate of the glutamic acid units is then electrostatically loaded with DOX-HCl, creating mPEG-b-PLG-DOX·HCl through intermolecular hydrophobic stacking. Kazunori Kataoka's group prepared oxaliplatin and (1,2-diaminocyclohexane)platinum(II) (DACHPt)-loaded PEG-b-PLG copolymers [77] (Figure 5b). This stable polymer metal complex could be formed to induce drug-loaded PVs.

3.2.2. Drug Loading in OMVs

The in vitro and in vivo loading methods are the two main techniques for drug loading in OMVs. The lipid bilayer of OMVs endows them with the potential to be loaded with both hydrophobic and hydrophilic drugs. For example, Sangyong Jon et al. showed that electroporation can be used for loading siRNA into $Affi_{HER2}$OMVs [55] (Figure 6a). This method was well tolerated by OMVs as evidenced by the integrity of OMVs following siRNA loading and the preserved circular shape. Li Ye's group also showed that DOX could be loaded into OMVs via passive diffusion [76] (Figure 6b). OMVs from *Klebsiella pneumonia* were loaded with DOX via passive diffusion in 12 h. DOX fluorescence was observed, which might have concentrated in the nucleus due to the preferential DNA-binding property of DOX. Besides these approaches, incubation, ultrasonication, and extrusion have been reported to be effective methods for in vitro drug loading.

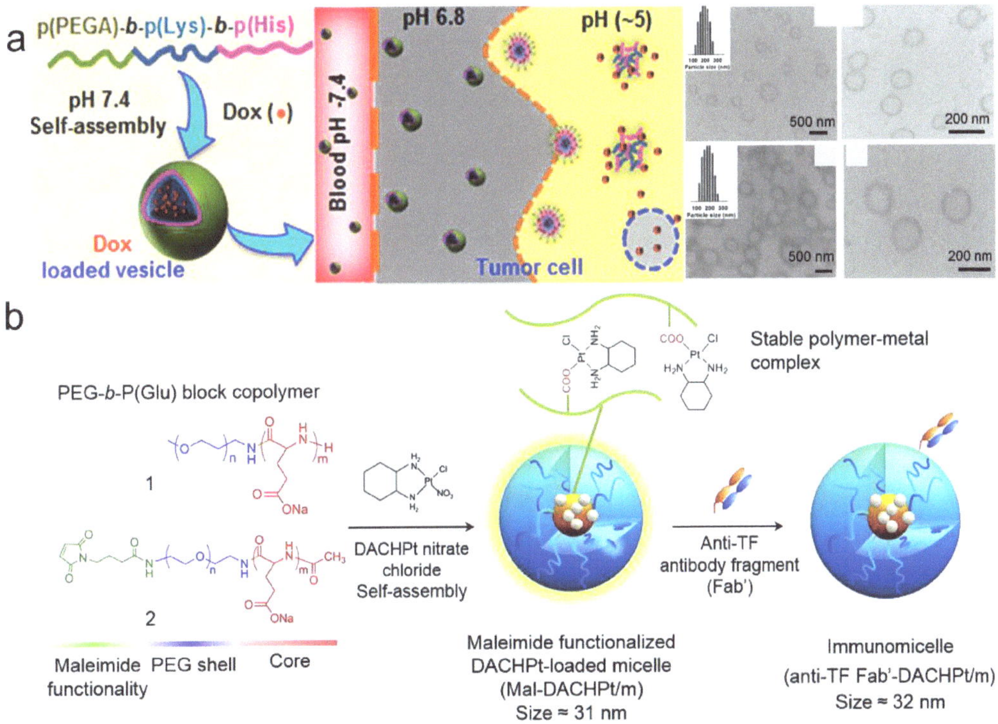

Figure 5. Drug loading in PVs. (**a**) $p(PEGA)_{30}$-b-$p(Lys)_{25}$-b-$p(His)_n$ assembled into vesicles with DOX loading. Reprinted with permission from Ref. [74]. Copyright: 2015, American Chemical Society. (**b**) DACHPt loading into PEG-b-PLG copolymers. Reprinted with permission from Ref. [77]. Copyright: 2015, Elsevier.

The uniqueness of drug loading in OMVs is that the drug loading process can also be designed during their biogenesis. With such a bioengineering process, it is possible to load cancer treatment drugs. During the generation of OMVs, the incorporation of the drug compound within their parental bacterium is possible. Terry J. Beveridge's group reported on the treatment of *Pseudomonas aeruginosa* PAO1 with gentamicin; the released OMVs were found to have the gentamicin [102]. Moreover, gentamicin effects that could arrest cancer cell growth were observed. Ana L. Carvalho et al. showed that OMVs could produce keratinocyte growth factor-2 (KGF-2), a human therapeutic protein, in a stable form [78]. It decreased disease severity when given orally and encouraged intestinal epithelium repair and recovery in animals given colitis-inducing dextran sodium sulfate. Vasilis

Ntziachristos' group also showed that the engineered *E. coli* could express rate-limiting enzymes in melanin biosynthesis [79]. Thus, the resulting OMVs could kill melanin in vivo. These reports suggest that OMVs could induce cytokine-mediated antitumor activity.

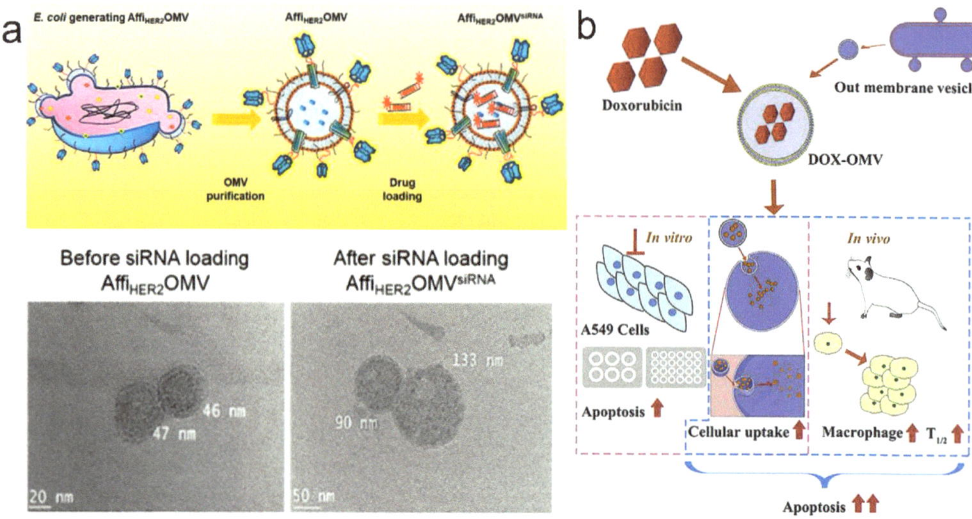

Figure 6. Drug loading in OMVs. (**a**) Loading of siRNA into Affi$_{HER2}$OMVs. Reprinted with permission from Ref. [55]. Copyright: 2014, American Chemical Society. (**b**) DOX can be loaded into OMVs via passive diffusion. Reprinted with permission from Ref. [76]. Copyright: 2020, Elsevier.

3.3. Targeted Drug Delivery via PVs and OMVs

3.3.1. Targeted Drug Delivery via PVs

After loading the drug compound, its programmed delivery and release at the targeted site are significant. In PVs, changes in the polypeptide assembly behavior and drug–polypeptide interactions are the two main approaches to releasing the drug compound. Since PVs can be easily destroyed due to changes in pH, light, glucose, and reactive oxygen species (ROS) [104] and due to the acidic environment of the tumor, pH responsiveness is the most common stimulus used to release the drug compound. For instance, the sensitivity of poly(L-histidine) could allow the released DOX load to kill cancers [105]. Ding et al. reported that the micelle-to-vesicle transition could be observed on a cholesterol-decorated polypeptide [80]. Due to ROS changes, the conformation of the polypeptide could change from β-sheet to α-helix and further induce on-demand drug release at the targeted sites. The advantage of synthesized polypeptides is that the various environmentally sensitive nonpeptide groups can be conjugated on light polymer chains. Light- and glucose-responsive groups such as phenylboronic acid, spiropyran, and coumarin can change the assembly behavior upon environmental changes such as UV irradiation and insulin delivery systems. For instance, Dong's group showed that it is possible to first design S-(o-nitrobenzyl)-l-cysteine and then block it with PEG via ROP [81]. The o-nitrobenzyl groups can be leveled off with UV irradiation. Moreover, the release of the drug compound can be controlled using the irradiation time.

Another important approach is destroying the interactions between the drug compound and the polypeptides. As mentioned above, the drug compound can be covalently or non-covalently conjugated with the polypeptides. Metal complexation and covalently linked drugs bearing polypeptides are mainly used in this release method. Kazunori Kataoka et al. designed hydrazide groups as the linkages between polypeptide chains and the drug DOX [82]. The hydrazide group can be disrupted as the pH changes and further release free DOX. Greg G. Qiao's group showed that ligand exchange could be used for metal-based drug delivery [103] (Figure 7a). Cisplatin complexed with PEG-B-PLG could be released in the presence of chloride ions. However, it was found that the metal–ligand exchange could only lead to a relatively slow release of the drug compound. This release rate was enhanced when mimicking the endosomal/lysosomal environment (pH 5.2/35 mM [Cl^-]).

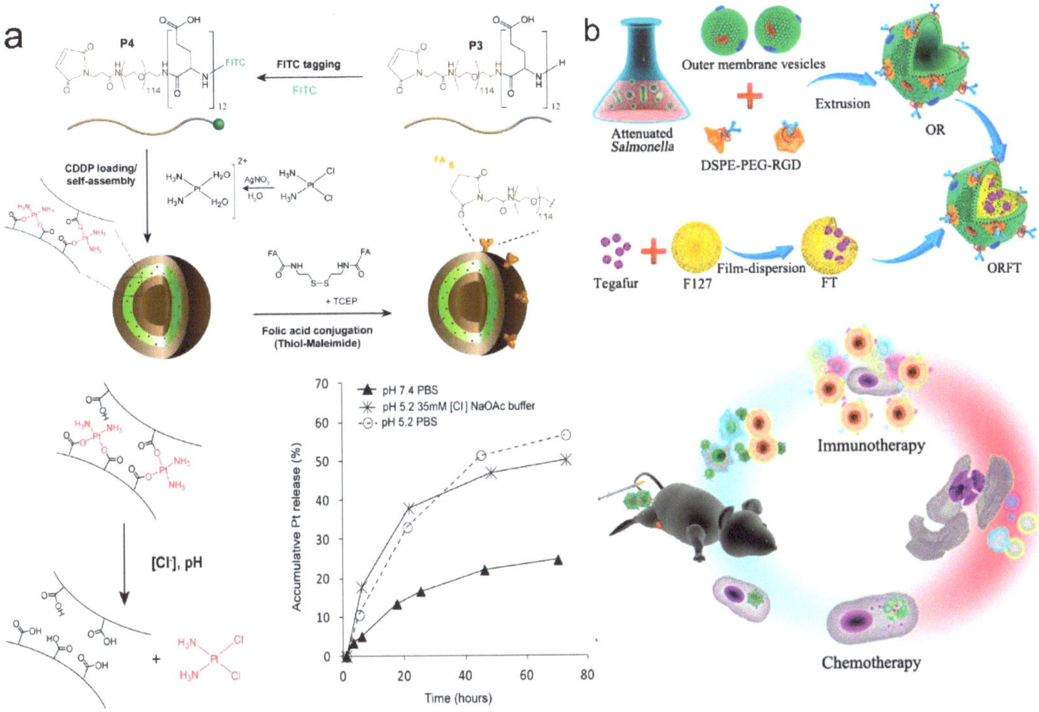

Figure 7. Targeted drug delivery via PVs and OMVs. (**a**) Drug release ability of cisplatin complexed with the PEG-b-PLG. Reprinted with permission from Ref. [103]. Copyright: 2015, American Chemical Society. (**b**) Schematic diagram of bioengineered OMV-coated polymeric nanomedicine. Reprinted with permission from Ref. [83]. Copyright: 2020, American Chemical Society.

3.3.2. Targeted Drug Delivery via OMVs

Compared with the scalable and chemically designable PVs, the use of OMVs in targeted drug delivery has only been sporadically reported in recent years and is still an emerging area requiring urgent research [28]. Sangyong Jon's study is recognized as the first report on using OMVs for targeted drug delivery [55]. After the electroporation of the siRNA drug compound (~15%) into OMVs, the anticancer activity of the drug-containing OMVs was found to be able to inhibit cancer cell proliferation. The detailed mechanism was observed with a confocal microscope as follows: the acidic environment could enhance the degradation of OMVs, and free siRNA was gradually detected along with dead cancer cells. Further, an in vivo study also suggested that the EPR effect is the drug force necessary for targeted drug delivery. Recently, Ping et al. showed that *Salmonella*-based OMVs could be even coated on polymer F127 nanoparticles [83] (Figure 7b). In this case, the drug compound was loaded on polymer micelles, whereas the OMVs only triggered the host immune response to cancer immunotherapy. This OMV-coated type of DDS provides a new combined system for potential targeted drug delivery. In addition, some recently emerged research also showed that bioengineered OMVs could induce specific CD8 T cell response, and this cell could control tumor growth via viral replication [84]. These recent findings open further possibilities for OMV drug delivery studies.

4. Conclusions and Outlook

This review mainly describes PVs and OMVs in drug delivery applications. PVs are obtained with the artificial synthesis of polypeptides, where the NMM and AMM are the two major mechanisms for polypeptide synthesis via the ROP of NCAs. Polymer vesicles are then obtained via self-assembly. The anisotropic packing of α-helical, hydrophobic polypeptides and the use of oppositely charged polymers are methods for the preparation of PVs. Compared with PVs, OMV biogenesis remains a mystery; however, three models, i.e., reduced lipoprotein linkages, peptidoglycan residues, and electrically charged lipopolysaccharides, are recognized as the major influencing factors. In addition, other factors, such as the environment and lipids, are important for OMV biogenesis in certain bacteria. Finally, the similarities and differences between these two vesicle types in drug delivery applications are elaborately compared. Specifically, we compare their applications in DDSs in the following aspects: general advantages, drug loading techniques, and targeted drug delivery performance. Based on state-of-the-art PVs and OMVs, we believe that future research should address the following issues to advance toward further DDS applications:

(1) Mass production of OMVs and PVs: Currently, the production of OMVs and PVs is still in the laboratory research stage. Although, recently, the production efficiency of polypeptide materials has been rapidly improved, technical solutions for assembling vesicles still lack specific standards, and large-scale production of PVs is not yet possible. OMV sizes are difficult to regulate, and there is significant variance among batches. In addition, low particle programmability is caused by our lack of knowledge regarding the precise OMV assembly mechanism. Enhancing safety and reducing costs are also still problems that need to be addressed.

(2) Universality of drug loading and delivery targeting: The drug loading mechanism in the process of production and post-treatment is inefficient and is in urgent need of optimization. Given the relevance of various cancer types and given that there are various PV and OMV types, consistent tumor cell targeting standards still need to be achieved and further improved. Individual PVs and OMVs may be effective for certain cancers.

(3) Other specific issues: The immunotoxicity of OMVs is a problem that cannot be ignored in DDSs. Moreover, the artificial production of OMVs also deserves more in-depth study on its potential. In PVs, the deprotection process in the production of specific polypeptides (such as polyhistidine, polylysine, and polycysteine) is tedious. Finally, programmed drug release and the benefits of the unique secondary structure of PVs are also worthy of more in-depth research.

Author Contributions: Y.Z. and W.S. wrote the original draft; Y.L. (Yiming Lu) and Z.Z. reviewed and edited the manuscript; Y.X., Y.L. (Yichong Li) and W.L. critically reviewed and revised the manuscript. All authors have read and agreed to the published version of the manuscript.

Funding: The following financial supports are appreciated: Scientific Research Foundation of the Shanghai University of Medicine and Health Sciences (SSF-22-07-02) and Shanghai Sailing Program (22YF1417700).

Institutional Review Board Statement: Not applicable.

Informed Consent Statement: Not applicable.

Data Availability Statement: Data supporting this publication are available from the corresponding authors.

Conflicts of Interest: The authors declare no conflict of interest.

References

1. Li, J.; Yu, F.; Chen, Y.; Oupický, D. Polymeric drugs: Advances in the development of pharmacologically active polymers. *J. Control. Release* **2015**, *219*, 369–382. [CrossRef] [PubMed]
2. Gale, G.R.; Morris, C.R.; Atkins, L.M.; Smith, A.B. Binding of an antitumor platinum compound to cells as influenced by physical factors and pharmacologically active agents. *Cancer Res.* **1973**, *33*, 813–818. [PubMed]
3. Xian, C.; Chen, H.; Xiong, F.; Fang, Y.; Huang, H.; Wu, J. Platinum-based chemotherapy via nanocarriers and co-delivery of multiple drugs. *Biomater. Sci.* **2021**, *9*, 6023–6036. [CrossRef] [PubMed]
4. Tabakoglu, S.; Kołbuk, D.; Sajkiewicz, P. Multifluid electrospinning for multi-drug delivery systems: Pros and cons, challenges, and future directions. *Biomater. Sci.* **2022**, *11*, 37–61. [CrossRef] [PubMed]
5. Tibbitt, M.W.; Dahlman, J.E.; Langer, R. Emerging frontiers in drug delivery. *J. Am. Chem. Soc.* **2016**, *138*, 704–717. [CrossRef] [PubMed]
6. Wang, S.; Gao, J.; Wang, Z. Outer membrane vesicles for vaccination and targeted drug delivery. *Wiley Interdiscip. Rev. Nanomed. Nanobiotechnol.* **2019**, *11*, e1523. [CrossRef] [PubMed]
7. Loo, Y.S.; Bose, R.J.; McCarthy, J.R.; Azmi, I.D.M.; Madheswaran, T. Biomimetic bacterial and viral-based nanovesicles for drug delivery, theranostics, and vaccine applications. *Drug Discov. Today* **2021**, *26*, 902–915. [CrossRef]
8. Al-Dossary, A.A.; Isichei, A.C.; Zhang, S.; Li, J.; Errachid, A.; Elaissari, A. Outer membrane vesicles (OMVs) as a platform for vaccination and targeted drug delivery. In *Pharmaceutical Nanobiotechnology for Targeted Therapy*; Springer: Berlin/Heidelberg, Germany, 2022; pp. 1–25.
9. Tang, Y.; Varyambath, A.; Ding, Y.; Chen, B.; Huang, X.; Zhang, Y.; Yu, D.-g.; Kim, I.; Song, W. Porous organic polymers for drug delivery: Hierarchical pore structures, variable morphologies, and biological properties. *Biomater. Sci.* **2022**, *10*, 5369–5390. [CrossRef]
10. Wang, Y.; Lu, X.; Wu, X.; Li, Y.; Tang, W.; Yang, C.; Ding, B. Chemically modified DNA nanostructures for drug delivery. *Innovation* **2022**, *3*, 100217. [CrossRef]
11. Song, W.; Zhang, M.; Huang, X.; Chen, B.; Ding, Y.; Zhang, Y.; Yu, D.G.; Kim, I. Smart l-borneol-loaded hierarchical hollow polymer nanospheres with antipollution and antibacterial capabilities. *Mater. Today Chem.* **2022**, *26*, 101252. [CrossRef]
12. Zhou, Y.; Wang, M.; Yan, C.; Liu, H.; Yu, D.-G. Advances in the application of electrospun drug-loaded nanofibers in the treatment of oral ulcers. *Biomolecules* **2022**, *12*, 1254. [CrossRef] [PubMed]
13. Zhang, Y.; Liu, R.; Jin, H.; Song, W.; Augustine, R.; Kim, I. Straightforward access to linear and cyclic polypeptides. *Commun. Chem.* **2018**, *1*, 40. [CrossRef]
14. Song, Z.; Han, Z.; Lv, S.; Chen, C.; Chen, L.; Yin, L.; Cheng, J. Synthetic polypeptides: From polymer design to supramolecular assembly and biomedical application. *Chem. Soc. Rev.* **2017**, *46*, 6570–6599. [CrossRef] [PubMed]
15. Wang, X.; Song, Z.; Wei, S.; Ji, G.; Zheng, X.; Fu, Z.; Cheng, J. Polypeptide-based drug delivery systems for programmed release. *Biomaterials* **2021**, *275*, 120913. [CrossRef] [PubMed]
16. Malonis, R.J.; Lai, J.R.; Vergnolle, O. Peptide-based vaccines: Current progress and future challenges. *Chem. Rev.* **2019**, *120*, 3210–3229. [CrossRef]
17. Li, R.; Liu, Q. Engineered bacterial outer membrane vesicles as multifunctional delivery platforms. *Front. Mater.* **2020**, *7*, 202. [CrossRef]
18. Chen, W.; Wu, Y.; Deng, J.; Yang, Z.; Chen, J.; Tan, Q.; Guo, M.; Jin, Y. Phospholipid-membrane-based nanovesicles acting as vaccines for tumor immunotherapy: Classification, mechanisms and applications. *Pharmaceutics* **2022**, *14*, 2446. [CrossRef]
19. Srivastava, P.; Kim, K.-S. Membrane vesicles derived from gut microbiota and probiotics: Cutting-edge therapeutic approaches for multidrug-resistant superbugs linked to neurological anomalies. *Pharmaceutics* **2022**, *14*, 2370. [CrossRef]
20. Chen, Y.; Liu, L.; Fu, H.; Wei, C.; Jin, Q. Comparative proteomic analysis of outer membrane vesicles from Shigella flexneri under different culture conditions. *Biochem. Biophys. Res. Commun.* **2014**, *453*, 696–702. [CrossRef]
21. Avila-Calderón, E.D.; Ruiz-Palma, M.D.S.; Aguilera-Arreola, M.G.; Velázquez-Guadarrama, N.; Ruiz, E.A.; Gomez-Lunar, Z.; Witonsky, S.; Contreras-Rodríguez, A. Outer membrane vesicles of gram-negative bacteria: An outlook on biogenesis. *Front. Microbiol.* **2021**, *12*, 557902. [CrossRef]
22. Gao, W.; Fang, R.H.; Thamphiwatana, S.; Luk, B.T.; Li, J.; Angsantikul, P.; Zhang, Q.; Hu, C.-M.J.; Zhang, L. Modulating antibacterial immunity via bacterial membrane-coated nanoparticles. *Nano Lett.* **2015**, *15*, 1403–1409. [CrossRef] [PubMed]
23. Turner, L.; Praszkier, J.; Hutton, M.L.; Steer, D.; Ramm, G.; Kaparakis-Liaskos, M.; Ferrero, R.L. Increased outer membrane vesicle formation in a Helicobacter pylori tolB mutant. *Helicobacter* **2015**, *20*, 269–283. [CrossRef] [PubMed]
24. Tsai, S.-L.; Oh, J.; Singh, S.; Chen, R.; Chen, W. Functional assembly of minicellulosomes on the Saccharomyces cerevisiae cell surface for cellulose hydrolysis and ethanol production. *Appl. Environ. Microbiol.* **2009**, *75*, 6087–6093. [CrossRef] [PubMed]
25. Bauman, S.J.; Kuehn, M.J. Purification of outer membrane vesicles from Pseudomonas aeruginosa and their activation of an IL-8 response. *Microbes Infect.* **2006**, *8*, 2400–2408. [CrossRef] [PubMed]
26. Chatterjee, D.; Chaudhuri, K. Association of cholera toxin with Vibrio cholerae outer membrane vesicles which are internalized by human intestinal epithelial cells. *FEBS Lett.* **2011**, *585*, 1357–1362. [CrossRef] [PubMed]

27. Li, M.; Zhou, H.; Yang, C.; Wu, Y.; Zhou, X.; Liu, H.; Wang, Y. Bacterial outer membrane vesicles as a platform for biomedical applications: An update. *J. Control. Release* **2020**, *323*, 253–268. [CrossRef]
28. Huang, Y.; Nieh, M.P.; Chen, W.; Lei, Y. Outer membrane vesicles (OMVs) enabled bio-applications: A critical review. *Biotechnol. Bioeng.* **2022**, *119*, 34–47. [CrossRef]
29. Zhang, Y.; Kim, I.; Lu, Y.; Xu, Y.; Yu, D.-G.; Song, W. Intelligent poly(l-histidine)-based nanovehicles for controlled drug delivery. *J. Control. Release* **2022**, *349*, 963–982. [CrossRef]
30. Leuchs, H.; Geiger, W. The anhydrides of alpha-amino-N-carboxylic and alpha-amino acids. *Ber. Dtsch. Chem. Ges.* **1908**, *41*, 1721–1726. [CrossRef]
31. Liu, Y.; Li, D.; Ding, J.; Chen, X. Controlled synthesis of polypeptides. *Chin. Chem. Lett.* **2020**, *31*, 3001–3014. [CrossRef]
32. Deming, T.J. Polypeptide Materials: New synthetic methods and applications. *Adv. Mater.* **1997**, *9*, 299–311. [CrossRef]
33. Holowka, E.P.; Pochan, D.J.; Deming, T.J. Charged Polypeptide vesicles with controllable diameter. *J. Am. Chem. Soc.* **2005**, *127*, 12423–12428. [CrossRef] [PubMed]
34. Sun, V.Z.; Choe, U.J.; Rodriguez, A.R.; Dai, H.; Deming, T.J.; Kamei, D.T. Transfection of mammalian cells using block copolypeptide vesicles. *Macromol. Biosci.* **2013**, *13*, 539–550. [CrossRef] [PubMed]
35. Choe, U.-J.; Rodriguez, A.R.; Lee, B.S.; Knowles, S.M.; Wu, A.M.; Deming, T.J.; Kamei, D.T. Endocytosis and intracellular trafficking properties of transferrin-conjugated block copolypeptide vesicles. *Biomacromolecules* **2013**, *14*, 1458–1464. [CrossRef] [PubMed]
36. Rodriguez, A.R.; Choe, U.-J.; Kamei, D.T.; Deming, T.J. Blending of diblock and triblock copolypeptide amphiphiles yields cell penetrating vesicles with low toxicity. *Macromol. Biosci.* **2015**, *15*, 90–97. [CrossRef] [PubMed]
37. Huang, J.; Bonduelle, C.; Thévenot, J.; Lecommandoux, S.; Heise, A. Biologically active polymersomes from amphiphilic glycopeptides. *J. Am. Chem. Soc.* **2012**, *134*, 119–122. [CrossRef]
38. Yu, K.; Eisenberg, A. Bilayer morphologies of self-assembled crew-cut aggregates of amphiphilic PS-b-PEO diblock copolymers in solution. *Macromolecules* **1998**, *31*, 3509–3518. [CrossRef]
39. Yang, Y.-Y.; Chen, L.-S.; Sun, M.; Wang, C.-Y.; Fan, Z.; Du, J.-Z. Biodegradable polypeptide-based vesicles with intrinsic blue fluorescence for antibacterial visualization. *Chin. J. Polym. Sci.* **2021**, *39*, 1412–1420. [CrossRef]
40. Xi, Y.; Wang, Y.; Gao, J.; Xiao, Y.; Du, J. Dual Corona vesicles with intrinsic antibacterial and enhanced antibiotic delivery capabilities for effective treatment of biofilm-induced periodontitis. *ACS Nano* **2019**, *13*, 13645–13657. [CrossRef]
41. Sanson, C.; Schatz, C.; Le Meins, J.-F.; Soum, A.; Thévenot, J.; Garanger, E.; Lecommandoux, S. A simple method to achieve high doxorubicin loading in biodegradable polymersomes. *J. Control. Release* **2010**, *147*, 428–435. [CrossRef]
42. Knox, K.; Vesk, M.; Work, E. Relation between excreted lipopolysaccharide complexes and surface structures of a lysine-limited culture of Escherichia coli. *J. Bacteriol.* **1966**, *92*, 1206–1217. [CrossRef] [PubMed]
43. Katsui, N.; Tsuchido, T.; Hiramatsu, R.; Fujikawa, S.; Takano, M.; Shibasaki, I. Heat-induced blebbing and vesiculation of the outer membrane of Escherichia coli. *J. Bacteriol.* **1982**, *151*, 1523–1531. [CrossRef] [PubMed]
44. Song, J.-W.; Baeg, Y.; Jeong, H.-Y.; Lee, J.; Oh, D.-K.; Hollmann, F.; Park, J.-B. Bacterial outer membrane vesicles as nano-scale bioreactors: A fatty acid conversion case study. *ChemCatChem* **2021**, *13*, 4080–4086. [CrossRef]
45. Hoekstra, D.; van der Laan, J.W.; de Leij, L.; Witholt, B. Release of outer membrane fragments from normally growing *Escherichia coli. Biochim. Biophys. Acta (BBA) Biomembr.* **1976**, *455*, 889–899. [CrossRef]
46. Schwechheimer, C.; Rodriguez, D.L.; Kuehn, M.J. NlpI-mediated modulation of outer membrane vesicle production through peptidoglycan dynamics in Escherichia coli. *MicrobiologyOpen* **2015**, *4*, 375–389. [CrossRef]
47. Pathirana, R.D.; Kaparakis-Liaskos, M. Bacterial membrane vesicles: Biogenesis, immune regulation and pathogenesis. *Cell. Microbiol.* **2016**, *18*, 1518–1524. [CrossRef]
48. McBroom, A.J.; Kuehn, M.J. Release of outer membrane vesicles by gram-negative bacteria is a novel envelope stress response. *Mol. Microbiol.* **2007**, *63*, 545–558. [CrossRef]
49. Kadurugamuwa, J.L.; Beveridge, T.J. Virulence factors are released from Pseudomonas aeruginosa in association with membrane vesicles during normal growth and exposure to gentamicin: A novel mechanism of enzyme secretion. *J. Bacteriol.* **1995**, *177*, 3998–4008. [CrossRef]
50. McMahon, K.J.; Castelli, M.E.; Vescovi, E.G.; Feldman, M.F. Biogenesis of outer membrane vesicles in Serratia marcescens is thermoregulated and can be induced by activation of the Rcs phosphorelay system. *J. Bacteriol.* **2012**, *194*, 3241–3249. [CrossRef]
51. Elhenawy, W.; Bording-Jorgensen, M.; Valguarnera, E.; Haurat, M.F.; Wine, E.; Feldman, M.F. LPS remodeling triggers formation of outer membrane vesicles in Salmonella. *mBio* **2016**, *7*, e00940-16. [CrossRef]
52. Turnbull, L.; Toyofuku, M.; Hynen, A.L.; Kurosawa, M.; Pessi, G.; Petty, N.K.; Osvath, S.R.; Cárcamo-Oyarce, G.; Gloag, E.S.; Shimoni, R.; et al. Explosive cell lysis as a mechanism for the biogenesis of bacterial membrane vesicles and biofilms. *Nat. Commun.* **2016**, *7*, 11220. [CrossRef] [PubMed]
53. Roier, S.; Zingl, F.G.; Cakar, F.; Durakovic, S.; Kohl, P.; Eichmann, T.O.; Klug, L.; Gadermaier, B.; Weinzerl, K.; Prassl, R.; et al. A novel mechanism for the biogenesis of outer membrane vesicles in Gram-negative bacteria. *Nat. Commun.* **2016**, *7*, 10515. [CrossRef] [PubMed]

54. Zhang, Y.; Song, W.; Lu, Y.; Xu, Y.; Wang, C.; Yu, D.-G.; Kim, I. Recent advances in poly(alpha-L-glutamic acid)-based nanomaterials for drug delivery. *Biomolecules* **2022**, *12*, 636. [CrossRef] [PubMed]
55. Gujrati, V.; Kim, S.; Kim, S.-H.; Min, J.J.; Choy, H.E.; Kim, S.C.; Jon, S. Bioengineered bacterial outer membrane vesicles as cell-specific drug-delivery vehicles for cancer therapy. *ACS Nano* **2014**, *8*, 1525–1537. [CrossRef]
56. Yin, L.; Cheng, J.; Deming, T.J.; Vicent, M.J. Synthetic polypeptides for drug and gene delivery, and tissue engineering. *Adv. Drug Delivery Rev.* **2021**, *178*, 113995. [CrossRef] [PubMed]
57. Lv, S.; Song, K.; Yen, A.; Peeler, D.J.; Nguyen, D.C.; Olshefsky, A.; Sylvestre, M.; Srinivasan, S.; Stayton, P.S.; Pun, S.H. Well-defined mannosylated polymer for peptide vaccine delivery with enhanced antitumor immunity. *Adv. Healthc. Mater.* **2022**, *11*, 2101651. [CrossRef] [PubMed]
58. O'Neill, C.L.; Shrimali, P.C.; Clapacs, Z.P.; Files, M.A.; Rudra, J.S. Peptide-based supramolecular vaccine systems. *Acta Biomater.* **2021**, *133*, 153–167. [CrossRef]
59. van der Pol, L.; Stork, M.; van der Ley, P. Outer membrane vesicles as platform vaccine technology. *Biotechnol. J.* **2015**, *10*, 1689–1706. [CrossRef]
60. Kim, O.Y.; Park, H.T.; Dinh, N.T.H.; Choi, S.J.; Lee, J.; Kim, J.H.; Lee, S.-W.; Gho, Y.S. Bacterial outer membrane vesicles suppress tumor by interferon-γ-mediated antitumor response. *Nat. Commun.* **2017**, *8*, 626. [CrossRef]
61. Ding, Y.; Ma, Y.; Du, C.; Wang, C.; Chen, T.; Wang, Y.; Wang, J.; Yao, Y.; Dong, C.-M. NO-releasing polypeptide nanocomposites reverse cancer multidrug resistance via triple therapies. *Acta Biomater.* **2021**, *123*, 335–345. [CrossRef]
62. Wang, Q.; Jiang, N.; Fu, B.; Huang, F.; Liu, J. Self-assembling peptide-based nanodrug delivery systems. *Biomater. Sci.* **2019**, *7*, 4888–4911. [CrossRef] [PubMed]
63. Qi, G.B.; Gao, Y.J.; Wang, L.; Wang, H. Self-assembled peptide-based nanomaterials for biomedical imaging and therapy. *Adv. Mater.* **2018**, *30*, 1703444. [CrossRef] [PubMed]
64. Li, H.; Huang, H.; Feng, J.-J.; Luo, X.; Fang, K.-M.; Wang, Z.-G.; Wang, A.-J. A polypeptide-mediated synthesis of green fluorescent gold nanoclusters for Fe^{3+} sensing and bioimaging. *J. Colloid Interface Sci.* **2017**, *506*, 386–392. [CrossRef] [PubMed]
65. Wang, J.; Wang, D.; Hui, N. A low fouling electrochemical biosensor based on the zwitterionic polypeptide doped conducting polymer PEDOT for breast cancer marker BRCA1 detection. *Bioelectrochemistry* **2020**, *136*, 107595. [CrossRef] [PubMed]
66. Oh, K.J.; Cash, K.J.; Hugenberg, V.; Plaxco, K.W. Peptide Beacons: A new design for polypeptide-based optical biosensors. *Bioconjug. Chem.* **2007**, *18*, 607–609. [CrossRef] [PubMed]
67. Zhang, Y.; Song, W.; Li, S.; Kim, D.-K.; Kim, J.H.; Kim, J.R.; Kim, I. Facile and scalable synthesis of topologically nanoengineered polypeptides with excellent antimicrobial activities. *Chem. Commun.* **2020**, *56*, 356–359. [CrossRef]
68. Lu, Z.; Wu, Y.; Cong, Z.; Qian, Y.; Wu, X.; Shao, N.; Qiao, Z.; Zhang, H.; She, Y.; Chen, K. Effective and biocompatible antibacterial surfaces via facile synthesis and surface modification of peptide polymers. *Bioact. Mater.* **2021**, *6*, 4531–4541. [CrossRef] [PubMed]
69. Wu, Y.; Chen, K.; Wu, X.; Liu, L.; Zhang, W.; Ding, Y.; Liu, S.; Zhou, M.; Shao, N.; Ji, Z.; et al. Superfast and Water-Insensitive Polymerization on α-amino acid N-carboxyanhydrides to prepare polypeptides using tetraalkylammonium carboxylate as the initiator. *Angew. Chem. Int. Ed.* **2021**, *60*, 26063–26071. [CrossRef]
70. Ding, X.; Duan, S.; Ding, X.; Liu, R.; Xu, F.-J. Versatile antibacterial materials: An emerging arsenal for combatting bacterial pathogens. *Adv. Funct. Mater.* **2018**, *28*, 1802140. [CrossRef]
71. Pizarro-Cerdá, J.; Cossart, P. Bacterial adhesion and entry into host cells. *Cell* **2006**, *124*, 715–727. [CrossRef]
72. Asadi, A.; Razavi, S.; Talebi, M.; Gholami, M. A review on anti-adhesion therapies of bacterial diseases. *Infection* **2019**, *47*, 13–23. [CrossRef] [PubMed]
73. Kakkar, D.; Mazzaferro, S.; Thevenot, J.; Schatz, C.; Bhatt, A.; Dwarakanath, B.S.; Singh, H.; Mishra, A.K.; Lecommandoux, S. Amphiphilic PEO-b-PBLG diblock and PBLG-b-PEO-b-PBLG triblock copolymer based nanoparticles: Doxorubicin loading and in vitro evaluation. *Macromol. Biosci.* **2015**, *15*, 124–137. [CrossRef] [PubMed]
74. Johnson, R.P.; Uthaman, S.; John, J.V.; Lee, H.R.; Lee, S.J.; Park, H.; Park, I.-K.; Suh, H.; Kim, I. Poly(PEGA)-b-poly(l-lysine)-b-poly(l-histidine) hybrid vesicles for tumoral pH-triggered intracellular delivery of doxorubicin hydrochloride. *ACS Appl. Mater. Interfaces* **2015**, *7*, 21770–21779. [CrossRef] [PubMed]
75. Li, M.; Song, W.; Tang, Z.; Lv, S.; Lin, L.; Sun, H.; Li, Q.; Yang, Y.; Hong, H.; Chen, X. Nanoscaled poly(l-glutamic acid)/doxorubicin-amphiphile complex as pH-responsive drug delivery system for effective treatment of nonsmall cell lung cancer. *ACS Appl. Mater. Interfaces* **2013**, *5*, 1781–1792. [CrossRef]
76. Kuerban, K.; Gao, X.; Zhang, H.; Liu, J.; Dong, M.; Wu, L.; Ye, R.; Feng, M.; Ye, L. Doxorubicin-loaded bacterial outer-membrane vesicles exert enhanced anti-tumor efficacy in non-small-cell lung cancer. *Acta Pharm. Sin. B* **2020**, *10*, 1534–1548. [CrossRef]
77. Ahn, J.; Miura, Y.; Yamada, N.; Chida, T.; Liu, X.; Kim, A.; Sato, R.; Tsumura, R.; Koga, Y.; Yasunaga, M.; et al. Antibody fragment-conjugated polymeric micelles incorporating platinum drugs for targeted therapy of pancreatic cancer. *Biomaterials* **2015**, *39*, 23–30. [CrossRef] [PubMed]
78. Carvalho, A.L.; Fonseca, S.; Miquel-Clopés, A.; Cross, K.; Kok, K.-S.; Wegmann, U.; Gil-Cardoso, K.; Bentley, E.G.; Al Katy, S.H.; Coombes, J.L. Bioengineering commensal bacteria-derived outer membrane vesicles for delivery of biologics to the gastrointestinal and respiratory tract. *J. Extracell. Vesicles* **2019**, *8*, 1632100. [CrossRef]

79. Gujrati, V.; Prakash, J.; Malekzadeh-Najafabadi, J.; Stiel, A.; Klemm, U.; Mettenleiter, G.; Aichler, M.; Walch, A.; Ntziachristos, V. Bioengineered bacterial vesicles as biological nano-heaters for optoacoustic imaging. *Nat. Commun.* **2019**, *10*, 1114. [CrossRef]
80. Liu, H.; Wang, R.; Wei, J.; Cheng, C.; Zheng, Y.; Pan, Y.; He, X.; Ding, M.; Tan, H.; Fu, Q. Conformation-directed micelle-to-vesicle transition of cholesterol-decorated polypeptide triggered by oxidation. *J. Am. Chem. Soc.* **2018**, *140*, 6604–6610. [CrossRef]
81. Liu, G.; Dong, C.-M. Photoresponsive Poly(S-(o-nitrobenzyl)-l-cysteine)-b-PEO from a l-cysteine N-carboxyanhydride monomer: Synthesis, self-assembly, and phototriggered drug release. *Biomacromolecules* **2012**, *13*, 1573–1583. [CrossRef]
82. Bae, Y.; Fukushima, S.; Harada, A.; Kataoka, K. Design of Environment-Sensitive Supramolecular assemblies for intracellular drug delivery: Polymeric micelles that are responsive to intracellular pH change. *Angew. Chem. Int. Ed.* **2003**, *42*, 4640–4643. [CrossRef] [PubMed]
83. Chen, Q.; Bai, H.; Wu, W.; Huang, G.; Li, Y.; Wu, M.; Tang, G.; Ping, Y. Bioengineering bacterial vesicle-coated polymeric nanomedicine for enhanced cancer immunotherapy and metastasis prevention. *Nano Lett.* **2020**, *20*, 11–21. [CrossRef] [PubMed]
84. Schetters, S.T.T.; Jong, W.S.P.; Horrevorts, S.K.; Kruijssen, L.J.W.; Engels, S.; Stolk, D.; Daleke-Schermerhorn, M.H.; Garcia-Vallejo, J.; Houben, D.; Unger, W.W.J. Outer membrane vesicles engineered to express membrane-bound antigen program dendritic cells for cross-presentation to CD8+ T cells. *Acta Biomater.* **2019**, *91*, 248–257. [CrossRef] [PubMed]
85. Song, B.; Song, J.; Zhang, S.; Anderson, M.A.; Ao, Y.; Yang, C.-Y.; Deming, T.J.; Sofroniew, M.V. Sustained local delivery of bioactive nerve growth factor in the central nervous system via tunable diblock copolypeptide hydrogel depots. *Biomaterials* **2012**, *33*, 9105–9116. [CrossRef]
86. Zhang, S.; Anderson, M.A.; Ao, Y.; Khakh, B.S.; Fan, J.; Deming, T.J.; Sofroniew, M.V. Tunable diblock copolypeptide hydrogel depots for local delivery of hydrophobic molecules in healthy and injured central nervous system. *Biomaterials* **2014**, *35*, 1989–2000. [CrossRef]
87. Schulz, E.; Goes, A.; Garcia, R.; Panter, F.; Koch, M.; Müller, R.; Fuhrmann, K.; Fuhrmann, G. Biocompatible bacteria-derived vesicles show inherent antimicrobial activity. *J. Control. Release* **2018**, *290*, 46–55. [CrossRef]
88. Liu, Y.; Xie, J.; Zhao, X.; Zhang, Y.; Zhong, Z.; Deng, C. A polymeric IDO inhibitor based on poly(ethylene glycol)-b-poly(l-tyrosine-co-1-methyl-d-tryptophan) enables facile trident cancer immunotherapy. *Biomater. Sci.* **2022**, *10*, 5731–5743. [CrossRef]
89. Mohammadi, M.; Taghavi, S.; Abnous, K.; Taghdisi, S.M.; Ramezani, M.; Alibolandi, M. Hybrid vesicular drug delivery systems for cancer therapeutics. *Adv. Funct. Mater.* **2018**, *28*, 1802136. [CrossRef]
90. Song, W.; Zhang, Y.; Yu, D.-G.; Tran, C.H.; Wang, M.; Varyambath, A.; Kim, J.; Kim, I. Efficient synthesis of folate-conjugated hollow polymeric capsules for accurate drug delivery to cancer cells. *Biomacromolecules* **2021**, *22*, 732–742. [CrossRef]
91. Cui, Y.; Deng, R.; Li, X.; Wang, X.; Jia, Q.; Bertrand, E.; Meguellati, K.; Yang, Y.-W. Temperature-sensitive polypeptide brushes-coated mesoporous silica nanoparticles for dual-responsive drug release. *Chin. Chem. Lett.* **2019**, *30*, 2291–2294. [CrossRef]
92. Lin, B.; Wu, J.; Wang, Y.; Sun, S.; Yuan, Y.; Tao, X.; Lv, R. Peptide functionalized upconversion/NIR II luminescent nanoparticles for targeted imaging and therapy of oral squamous cell carcinoma. *Biomater. Sci.* **2021**, *9*, 1000–1007. [CrossRef] [PubMed]
93. Li, T.; Li, C.; Ruan, Z.; Xu, P.; Yang, X.; Yuan, P.; Wang, Q.; Yan, L. Polypeptide-conjugated second near-infrared organic fluorophore for image-guided photothermal therapy. *ACS Nano* **2019**, *13*, 3691–3702. [CrossRef] [PubMed]
94. Duhamel, J.; Kanagalingam, S.; O'Brie, T.J.; Ingratta, M.W. Side-chain dynamics of an α-helical polypeptide monitored by fluorescence. *J. Am. Chem. Soc.* **2003**, *125*, 12810–12822. [CrossRef]
95. Tan, K.; Li, R.; Huang, X.; Liu, Q. Outer membrane vesicles: Current status and future direction of these novel vaccine adjuvants. *Front. Microbiol.* **2018**, *9*, 783. [CrossRef]
96. Bielig, H.; Rompikuntal, P.; Dongre, M.; Zurek, B.; Lindmark, B.; Ramstedt, M.; Wai, S.; Kufer, T. NOD-like receptor activation by outer membrane vesicles from Vibrio cholerae non-O1 non-O139 strains is modulated by the quorum-sensing regulator HapR. *Infect. Immun.* **2011**, *79*, 1418–1427. [CrossRef]
97. Johnson, R.P.; Jeong, Y.I.; John, J.V.; Chung, C.-W.; Kang, D.H.; Selvaraj, M.; Suh, H.; Kim, I. Dual stimuli-responsive poly(N-isopropylacrylamide)-b-poly(l-histidine) chimeric materials for the controlled delivery of doxorubicin into liver carcinoma. *Biomacromolecules* **2013**, *14*, 1434–1443. [CrossRef]
98. Liu, J.; Huang, Y.; Kumar, A.; Tan, A.; Jin, S.; Mozhi, A.; Liang, X.-J. pH-Sensitive nano-systems for drug delivery in cancer therapy. *Biotechnol. Adv.* **2014**, *32*, 693–710. [CrossRef] [PubMed]
99. Bazban-Shotorbani, S.; Hasani-Sadrabadi, M.M.; Karkhaneh, A.; Serpooshan, V.; Jacob, K.I.; Moshaverinia, A.; Mahmoudi, M. Revisiting structure-property relationship of pH-responsive polymers for drug delivery applications. *J. Control. Release* **2017**, *253*, 46–63. [CrossRef]
100. He, T.; Li, D.; Yang, Y.; Ding, J.; Jin, F.; Zhuang, X.; Chen, X. Mesomeric configuration makes polyleucine micelle an optimal nanocarrier. *Biomater. Sci.* **2016**, *4*, 814–818. [CrossRef]
101. Zhang, Y.; Uthaman, S.; Song, W.; Eom, K.H.; Jeon, S.H.; Huh, K.M.; Babu, A.; Park, I.-K.; Kim, I. Multistimuli-responsive polymeric vesicles for accelerated drug release in chemo-photothermal therapy. *ACS Biomater. Sci. Eng.* **2020**, *6*, 5012–5023. [CrossRef]
102. Allan, N.D.; Beveridge, T.J. Gentamicin delivery to burkholderia cepacia group IIIa strains via membrane vesicles from pseudomonas aeruginosa PAO1. *Antimicrob. Agents Chemother.* **2003**, *47*, 2962–2965. [CrossRef] [PubMed]
103. Shirbin, S.J.; Ladewig, K.; Fu, Q.; Klimak, M.; Zhang, X.; Duan, W.; Qiao, G.G. Cisplatin-induced formation of biocompatible and biodegradable polypeptide-based vesicles for targeted anticancer drug delivery. *Biomacromolecules* **2015**, *16*, 2463–2474. [CrossRef] [PubMed]

104. Lee, S.H.; Gupta, M.K.; Bang, J.B.; Bae, H.; Sung, H.J. Current progress in reactive oxygen species (ROS)-responsive materials for biomedical applications. *Adv. Healthc. Mater.* **2013**, *2*, 908–915. [CrossRef] [PubMed]
105. Johnson, R.P.; Jeong, Y.-I.; Choi, E.; Chung, C.-W.; Kang, D.H.; Oh, S.-O.; Suh, H.; Kim, I. Biocompatible poly(2-hydroxyethyl methacrylate)-b-poly(L-histidine) hybrid materials for pH-sensitive intracellular anticancer drug delivery. *Adv. Funct. Mater.* **2012**, *22*, 1058–1068. [CrossRef]

pharmaceutics

MDPI

Review

Phospholipid-Membrane-Based Nanovesicles Acting as Vaccines for Tumor Immunotherapy: Classification, Mechanisms and Applications

Wenjuan Chen [1,2,†], Yali Wu [1,2,†], Jingjing Deng [1,2], Zimo Yang [1,2], Jiangbin Chen [1,2], Qi Tan [1,2], Mengfei Guo [1,2] and Yang Jin [1,2,*]

1 Department of Respiratory and Critical Care Medicine, Hubei Province Clinical Research Center for Major Respiratory Diseases, NHC Key Laboratory of Pulmonary Diseases, Wuhan Union Hospital, Tongji Medical College, Huazhong University of Science and Technology, 1277 Jiefang Avenue, Wuhan 430022, China
2 Hubei Province Engineering Research Center for Tumor-Targeted Biochemotherapy, MOE Key Laboratory of Biological Targeted Therapy, Wuhan Union Hospital, Tongji Medical College, Huazhong University of Science and Technology, 1277 Jiefang Avenue, Wuhan 430022, China
* Correspondence: whuhjy@126.com; Tel.: +86-135-5436-1146
† These authors contributed equally to this work.

Abstract: Membrane vesicles, a group of nano- or microsized vesicles, can be internalized or interact with the recipient cells, depending on their parental cells, size, structure and content. Membrane vesicles fuse with the target cell membrane, or they bind to the receptors on the cell surface, to transfer special effects. Based on versatile features, they can modulate the functions of immune cells and therefore influence immune responses. In the field of tumor therapeutic applications, phospholipid-membrane-based nanovesicles attract increased interest. Academic institutions and industrial companies are putting in effort to design, modify and apply membrane vesicles as potential tumor vaccines contributing to tumor immunotherapy. This review focuses on the currently most-used types of membrane vesicles (including liposomes, bacterial membrane vesicles, tumor- and dendritic-cell-derived extracellular vesicles) acting as tumor vaccines, and describes the classification, mechanism and application of these nanovesicles.

Keywords: liposomes; bacterial membrane vesicles; tumor-derived extracellular vesicles; dendritic-cell-derived extracellular vesicles; vaccine; tumor immunotherapy

Citation: Chen, W.; Wu, Y.; Deng, J.; Yang, Z.; Chen, J.; Tan, Q.; Guo, M.; Jin, Y. Phospholipid-Membrane-Based Nanovesicles Acting as Vaccines for Tumor Immunotherapy: Classification, Mechanisms and Applications. *Pharmaceutics* **2022**, *14*, 2446. https://doi.org/10.3390/pharmaceutics14112446

Academic Editor: Tania Limongi

Received: 26 October 2022
Accepted: 10 November 2022
Published: 11 November 2022

1. Introduction

Nanovesicles composed of lipid bilayers have aroused considerable interest and attention for fundamental study and practical applications. There are two types of phospholipid-membrane-based nanovesicles: pure lipid and/or protein vesicles and comparatively complex cell-membrane-derived vesicles (also called extracellular vesicles (EVs)) [1]. Natural or synthetic lipid and/or protein ingredients make nanovesicles, involving liposomes or proteoliposomes, an ideal model of the membrane system with the advantages of an easy and low-cost production [2]. Furthermore, cell-derived membrane vesicles are regarded as nano- to micrometer-sized containers comprising components such as cellular proteins, nucleic acids and lipids, for the reason that cell plasma or cytosol membranes can enclose these contents while membrane vesicles are secreted [3].

Increasing studies have noticed that EVs are versatile communication tools to establish a link between tumor and host, contributing to tumor development, progression and metastasis. Both tumor and nontumor cells secrete lots of EVs, having a local impact on tumor cells, or traveling through blood vessels to bring about distant influence [4]. Furthermore, bacterial membrane vesicles (BMVs), a type of cell-membrane-based EVs, which are derived from bacteria membrane architecture, own nanoscale vesicle structures containing biomembrane elements of phospholipids. Additionally, BMVs consist of considerable proteins, for example, original bacterial antigens and pathogen-associated molecular pattern components [5]. Therefore, antigen-presenting cells (APCs) are able to recognize and absorb BMVs, and subsequently signaling pathways in immune cells are activated followed by specific immune responses. The molecular components and biological activity of BMVs or further-modified ones render them possible to be a potent vaccine to treat infectious or noninfectious diseases, including cancer [6].

As membrane vesicles have a general characteristic, they contain a lipid bilayer structure that can package hydrophobic and hydrophilic compounds. Despite the practical condition that they are loaded with compounds from the parental cells, a further modification, transformation and fabrication could be conducted as needed to achieve expected goals, such as an enhanced output level, toxicity reduction, targeting improvement, etc. [7]. So far, how membrane vesicles take a part in tumor vaccines is a hot topic. For instance, membrane vesicles conjugated with antitumor immunomodulators have been studied to prevent and treat tumors. The potential of these membrane vesicles as tumor vaccines will be described and discussed in the following section.

Herein, we review the categorization in existence, mechanisms to date and preclinical and clinical applications so far regarding the use of phospholipid-membrane-based nanovesicles as tumor vaccines in the field of tumor immunotherapy.

2. Different Origins of Membrane-Based Nanovesicles Are Likely to Act as Tumor Vaccines

There are two primary types of phospholipid-membrane-based nanoparticles, including liposomes and extracellular vesicles (EVs). As EVs are a complex group of biomembrane-based nanostructures, based on their size, biogenesis and function, diverse classification methods have been used. According to the diameter of EVs, they could be roughly classified into small EVs (~100 nm) or large EVs (~100–1000 nm and/or >1000 nm) [8]. Moreover, in terms of biogenesis, EVs can be precisely categorized into exosomes (30–100 nm) produced from the perinuclear luminal membrane and released through multivesicular fusion with the cell membrane, microvesicles (namely microparticles, 100–1000 nm) generated from the cell membrane budding and apoptotic bodies (500–2000 nm) produced through the protrusion of apoptotic cell membrane by dying cells [3,9–11]. On the basis of modification or not, natural EVs and engineered ones are included in the family of EVs. Furthermore, EVs have various origins, for example, generated from prokaryotic or eukaryotic cells, or from cell or plasma membranes, since a number of cells are able to secret EVs and subsequently EVs are filled with original components [1].

We then focus on the use of biomembrane-based nanoparticles as a kind of tumor vaccine in the field of tumor immunotherapy or precaution. The classification, structure and composition of four major types of these nanoparticles are going to be exemplified in the following sections, involving liposomes, BMVs, tumor-derived EVs (TEVs) and dendritic-cell-derived EVs (DEVs) (Figure 1).

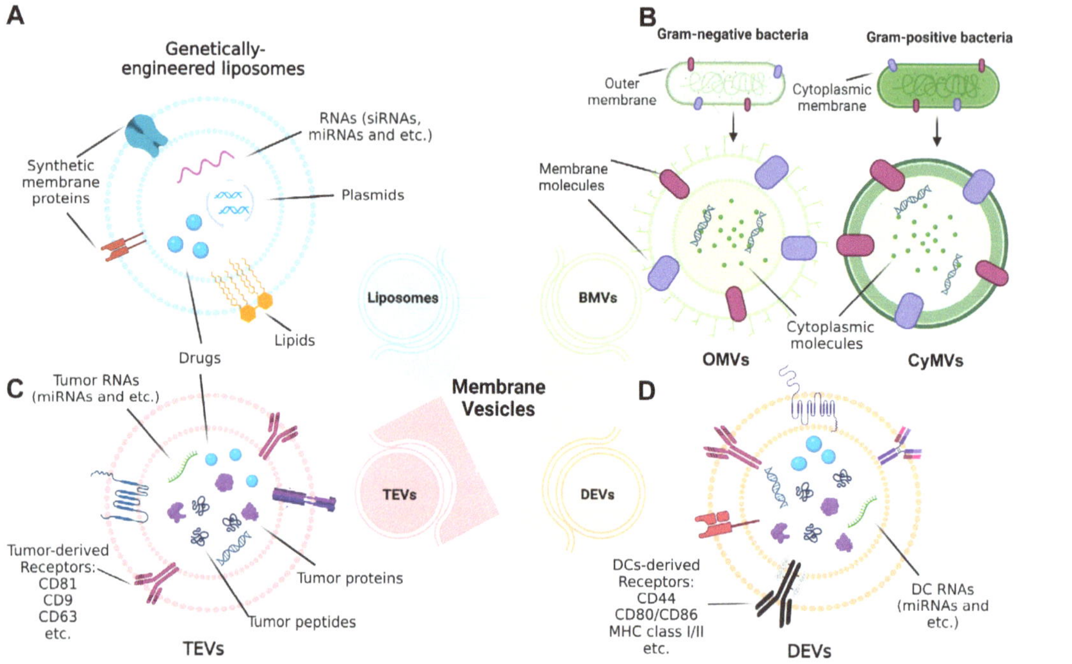

Figure 1. Structure of nanoscale vesicles standing for tumor vaccines in the range of biomembrane-based nanovesicles. (**A**) Liposomes are genetically engineered with genes (including RNAs and plasmids) and proteins or modified with drugs or other small molecules. (**B**) For bacteria membrane vesicles (BMVs), outer membrane vesicles (OMVs) and cytoplasmic membrane vesicles (CyMVs) are, respectively, representatives of Gram-negative and Gram-positive bacteria-generated membrane vesicles, whose structures separately rely on the origins of bacteria. (**C**) Extracellular vesicles (EVs) derived from tumor cells (TEVs) and (**D**) Evs secreted by dendritic cells (DCs); namely, DEVs are typical cell-membrane-based vesicles widely used for tumor immunotherapy, and their composition depending on parental cells presents different forms, for example, types of membrane receptors.

2.1. Liposomes

From a biological point of view, since a cornucopia of lipids and proteins are combined together to naturally form cell membranes, in vitro natural lipids (for example phospholipids) or synthetic components are able to self-assemble into spherical bilayer nanoparticles, namely liposomes. Depending on the preparation methods, the size of the liposomes varies from each other ranging from small (3–5 nm) to giant vesicles (>1 μm) [12].

In terms of the biomedical application of liposomes as a tumor vaccine, it is not surprising that simplified membrane vesicle liposomes alone could not perform effective vaccination in various diseases, since the structure and composition are limited and blood circulation times and stability lack satisfaction when they are applied. Thanks to its versatility, scientists take advantage of the properties of phospholipid membranes including chemical (amphiphilicity) and mechanical (stability, permeability and bending and stretching elasticity) peculiarity [13,14]. Therefore, the modification and functionalization of liposomes are necessary and available. Based on seminal reconstitution protocols, liposomes can achieve characteristics and be smart. For instance, liposomes could be stabilized by covering them with densely packed coats such as biocompatible PEG chains (poly (ethylene glycol)) and a crystalline bacterial cell surface layer [15,16]. In addition, according to the charge and specific membrane structure, reconstructed and engineered liposomes are present to mitigate drug delivery problems (safety, efficiency, internalization and targeting ability) [2,17]. Then, the liposome capacity of the efficiently delivering and suitably releasing cargoes (drugs, antigens, siRNA, etc.) can be improved. Taking some construction means as an example, Lian, Shu et al. designed cationic liposomes containing si-CD47 and si-PD-L1 and modified them with EpCAM (epithelial cell adhesion molecule), so they not only enhanced the immune therapeutic efficacy of liposomes, but also improved the targeting ability owing to the overexpression of EpCAM proteins in tumor cells [18].

2.2. Bacterial Membrane Vesicles

BMVs are capable of transporting a variety of molecules (proteins, nucleic acids and toxins), and to some extent, the structure of the vesicles and composition of the cargoes differ between Gram-positive and -negative bacteria [19,20]. Both of them exhibit significant effects on innate and adaptive responses. For example, BMVs have been demonstrated to have protective characters against exogenous pathogens or endogenous mutants and have been applied for vaccine exploration [21,22].

For Gram-negative bacteria-derived BMVs, it is widely regarded that the vesicle structure is formed from three stratified layers of the fluid phospholipid bilayer, peptidoglycan cell wall and phospholipid membrane characteristically carrying lipopolysaccharide (LPS) in turn from inside to outside [23]. As a critical participant in bacterial communication and homeostasis, outer membrane vesicles (OMVs) are naturally generated from Gram-negative bacteria, and thus contain pathogen-associated molecular patterns (PAMPs). Therefore, these vesicles, such as pathogen mimetic adjuvants, possess intrinsic immunostimulatory properties acting as a vaccine. Moreover, since membrane vesicles are capable of drug delivery, their natural composition could be enriched by modifying these vesicles with other immunomodulatory agents [24–26].

In the aspect of the structure of Gram-positive bacteria-derived BMVs, depending on their own construction, these BMVs lack the package of the outer membrane, while they are coated with rigid peptidoglycan cell walls from the cytoplasmic membrane layer [27]. Hence, these cytoplasmic membrane-generated BMVs are named CyMVs. Although the biological processes of Gram-positive BMVs are less understood than Gram-negative BMVs, they are still being taken into consideration for vaccine applications. The vaccination efficacy of BMVs from certain bacterial strains has been estimated as a strategy to fight against Gram-positive bacteria, and vaccine safety has been detected as well through monitoring toxin-specific antibodies. For the purpose of controlling and decreasing toxicity, approaches to producing genetically engineered BMVs emerge one after another. For instance, Wang, Xiaogang et al. purified BMVs from Staphylococcus aureus to establish an *S. aureus* vaccine platform which could package cytosolic and secreted proteins, such as cytolysins and phenol-soluble modulins, contributing to BMVs biogenesis and detoxification [28].

2.3. Tumor-Cell-Derived EVs

As EVs play a crucial role in cell–cell communication, tumor-cell-derived EVs (TEVs) take part in tumorous progression, tumor microenvironment modulation and distant metastasis, and even accelerate these processes [29,30].

Compared with liposomes, the contents and structure of EVs are relatively complicated. Meanwhile, the innate composition of TEVs inherited from parental tumor cells has gained a lot of attention. Considerable evidence from recent studies has demonstrated that there are lots of oncoproteins (such as phosphorylated epidermal growth factor receptor (EGFR), vascular endothelial growth factor (VEGF), stromal-cell-derived factor 1 (SDF1), etc.) and oncogenic RNA (in particular miRNAs) in TEVs, making a contribution to tumor growth, invasion, migration and angiogenesis [31–34]. For these TEVs carrying parent-cell-specific signatures, they permit an interaction between the targeting cells and are potentially used to be explored or confirmed as biomarkers in liquid biopsies for distinctive diseases [35]. Due to the existing biological qualities of TEVs, development for them acting as potential therapeutic strategies becomes suitable and overwhelming. For example, approaches inhibiting the preparation and secretion of native EVs or loading TEVs with antitumor drugs or RNAs which encode information of disrupting tumor progression are emerging rapidly [36].

Since TEVs are assembled and packaged in a tumor-cell-specific manner, the components (in particular, the tumor antigens) are distinct from the EVs from mesenchymal stem cells or blood cells. Peptides in antigen-rich TEVs could be presented by major histocompatibility class (MHC) receptors and then cause the following interaction with immune cells ($CD8^+$, $CD4^+$ T cells or natural killer cells (NKs)) to help enhance cancer immunotherapy [22,37]. Additionally, to maintain biocompatibility and elevate the immunogenicity of TEVs, the formulation should be well designed, in order not only to guarantee biosecurity, but also to positively regulate antitumor immune responses and deliver therapeutics to tumor sites. In numerous basic or clinical studies, engineered or nonengineered, autologous or nonautologous TEVs have been fabricated and administrated to biomedical model species or human subjects [38].

2.4. Dendritic-Cell-Derived EVs

Cell-membrane-based EVs are also secreted by immune cells in tumor tissues to contact the rest of the immune cells and tumor cells [39]. Immune-cell-derived EVs play a crucial role in cell–cell communication for tumor cells to escape from immunological surveillance and for further studies to design potential tumor vaccines [40]. Among these EVs, a relatively large focus has been put on dendritic cells (DCs)-derived EVs (DEVs or dexosomes) as a tumor vaccine, and thus DEVs have become an attractive candidate for tumor immunotherapies.

In a typical immune loop, antigen-presenting cells (APCs), among which DCs are the most potent APCs, prime the immune responses when the immune system defends against tumorous, viral or bacterial diseases [41]. It is commonly believed that DCs expressing MHC class I or II molecules on the cell surface interact with other immune cells such as $CD8^+$ or $CD4^+$ T lymphocytes and natural killer cells to initiate an immune reaction [42,43]. During EVs secretion from DCs, it has been found that EVs also encapsulate peptide-MHC complexes (p-MHC) together with costimulatory molecules such as CD40 and CD86 [44–46]. Additionally, it could carry abundant immunoregulatory cargos, including cytokines, complement factors and immunosuppressive or active molecular mediators [47]. It has been verified that in the absence of APCs, DEVs own the ability to activate T cells since they can directly interact with T-cell receptor (TCR) complexes [48]. Flourishing evidence proves that the capability of modified or engineered DEVs to elicit antigen-specific antitumor immune responses could be enhanced when costimulatory factors are upregulated and immunoregulatory/immunosuppressive signals are reduced [49]. It is no wonder that DEVs continue to be a promising nanomaterial for further research on vaccination in tumor immunotherapy.

3. Membrane Vesicles Work to Bring a Stone to the Building of Tumor Immunotherapy from the Perspective of Basic Mechanisms

The potential role of membrane vesicles as tumor vaccines in tumorous immune responses has been extensively documented and exploited. In most cases, the membrane vesicles listed above have been well designed, engineered and modified, before they are used to treat cancer or other diseases. The function of membrane vesicles acting in immune regulation is likely due to diverse reasons, including their presentation or transfer of antigenic peptides (tumor-specific antigens (TSAs) or tumor-associated antigens (TAAs)), delivery of adjuvants, immunomodulatory molecules or cytosolic DNA, gene-expression manipulation by miRNA or plasmids and induction of favorable signaling pathways by ligands expressed on the surface of the vesicles [11]. Generally speaking, in terms of mechanisms based on immunity, membrane vesicle vaccines induce the activation and maturation of DCs, provoke T cells and arouse immune memory, to play a role in tumor-suppressive efficacy and prolonged survival of multiple tumor biological models. In the following review portion, we discuss the key mechanisms primarily focusing on the change in immune responses under the administration of these four types of potential membrane vesicle vaccines at the level of basic medicine (Figure 2).

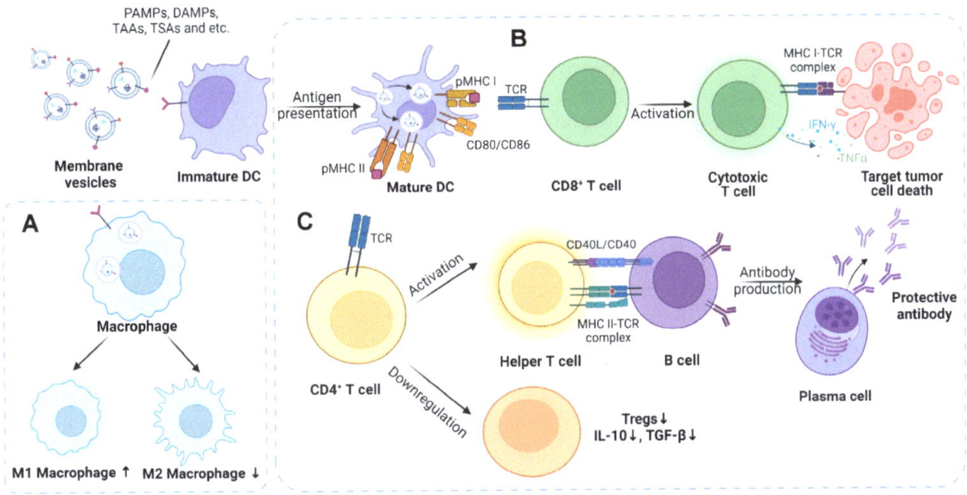

Figure 2. Role of membrane vesicles as tumor vaccines in immune modulation. Membrane vesicles carrying stimulators (such as tumor antigens/peptides, adjuvants, RNAs, etc.) have potentials to arouse antitumor innate and acquired immune responses. (**A**) The modified vesicles interact with macrophages and induce polarization of M2 (a protumor type) to M1 (an antitumor type) phenotype. (**B**) The vesicles containing specific antigens or peptides can be presented by DCs to further stimulate $CD8^+$ T cells, causing cytotoxic T-lymphocyte (CTL) antitumor response. (**C**) In addition, during the process of antigen presentation, $CD4^+$ T cells could be activated as well, leading to long-term memory immunity and downregulation of Tregs, a predominant type of immunosuppressive T cells in tumor microenvironment. ↑ means upregulation, while ↓ stands for downregulation.

3.1. The Mechanisms of Liposomes as a Tumor Vaccine

As typical synthetic phospholipid-based vectors, liposomes have outstanding properties, such as flexible characteristics (including excellent elasticity and changeable degrees of liquidity), ideal biocompatibility and low toxicity [50,51]. Although it is tough for simple and hollow lipid-membrane-based nanovesicles to be directly used as a vaccine, the versatile features make it possible for them to achieve functions of tumor vaccines via adventurous artificial liposome modification.

Currently, increasing studies have exploited or are developing liposomes encapsulated with antigens, antibodies, adjuvants or chemical drugs depending on their hydrophilic and hydrophobic moieties. To conduct feasible applications of liposomes in tumor immunotherapy, cationic liposomes containing synthetic tumor long peptides have been designed and prepared, and such nanoparticle vaccines have been demonstrated to stimulate both $CD4^+$ and $CD8^+$ T cells and enhance the efficacy of a checkpoint inhibitor for lung cancer [52]. Apart from the combination of liposomes and checkpoint inhibitors, liposomes can carry some inhibitors to improve the therapeutic effects of a checkpoint blockade. For example, Tu, Kun et al. verified that liposomes codelivering BMS-202 (one of the PD-L1 inhibitors) and chidamide (CHI, an epigenetic modulator inducing immunogenic cell death) boosted antitumor immune responses through CHI-related increased immunogenicity and a BMS-202-mediated PD-L1 intercept [53]. In addition to carrying tumor antigens, liposomes could be firstly modified with cholesterol cationic peptide DP7, which makes liposomes successfully transfer mRNA into DCs, and then the production of the DCs antigen presentation activity and secretion of proinflammatory cytokines were found to elevate, further contributing to antigen-specific lymphocyte reactions and tumor inhibition [54]. Additionally, many more complex modifications to improve the antitumor effects of liposomes has also drawn lots of attention. For example, Liang, Ruijing et al. fabricated a gold nanoplatform coated with liposomes and meanwhile tethered aCD11c (a ligand to target DCs), monophosphoryl lipid A (a strong adjuvant to induce immune responses) and peptides from tyrosinase-related protein 2 (a melanoma antigen to stimulate specific immune activity) [55]. The researchers have taken the superiorities of liposomes and endowed them with immunogenic functions, so as to activate a complete antitumor immune response involving DCs maturation, cytotoxic $CD8^+$ T lymphocytes (CTLs) activation and other routes of the immune system.

3.2. The Immunologic Mechanisms Triggered by Bacterial Membrane Vesicles

Owing to the microbe-associated molecular patterns (MAMPs) and nanoscale structure, BMVs have a high immunogenicity. They are developed into vaccines against infectious or noninfectious diseases through chemical, physical and genetic modifications. Thanks to the evolution of these modifications, BMVs can be endowed with more appropriate and ideal functions or properties to fight against certain diseases, for instance, increased safety and efficacious therapeutic ability.

Speaking of activating the influence of BMVs on immunity, it is essential to mention that vesicle contents, including lipoproteins, nucleic acids and other immunostimulatory MAMPs, may be recognized by the relevant receptors such as pattern recognition receptors (PRR), which are detected to express on the surface of epithelial cells and immune cells (in particular DCs) [56]. The ligand–receptor combination triggers the immune responses, whereas the form and intensity of these responses vary from each other, relying on the composition and structure of the BMVs to some extent [25]. As extensively reported, Toll-like receptor 4 (TLR4), one of the PRR, has been verified to interact with BMVs containing MAMPs such as LPS via the induction of PRR signaling, for example TLR4-dependent CXCL8 (CXC-chemokine ligand 8, also known as IL-8) production, MAPK (mitogen-activated protein kinase) -AP1 (activator protein 1) signaling, etc. [57,58]. Moreover, when peptidoglycan (PG) existing on the membrane wall of BMVs dominates the ligand–receptor communication, the NOD1 (nucleotide binding oligomerization domain 1), known for an intracellular sensor, could be activated via recognizing PG, and the ascent of the cytokines CXCL2 expression level has been found [59].

In addition to the innate immune system of which MAMPs in BMVs can drive the generation, BMVs can effectively incite cellular and mucosal immunity. For instance, engineered BMVs with the expression of IL-10 on the surface and the encapsulation of HPV16 E17 protein into them have been demonstrated to prevent the exhaustion of T cells, presentation of p-MHC I complexes and activation of $CD8^+$ T cells transforming into CTLs, causing the inhibition of tumor growth and metastasis and implying a novel tumor immunotherapeutic strategy [60].

Among components of bacterial nanosized vaccine platforms, outer membrane vesicles (OMVs) produced by Gram-negative bacteria are the most overlooked [21]. Numerous studies have employed OMVs as therapeutic agents to treat cancer by means of the induction of antitumor immune responses. In an interesting study, bacterial OMVs were loaded with polymeric micelles (a kind of liposome) which are responsible for chemotherapeutic function and even help achieve the stimulation of T cells, and such modified OMVs elicited stronger immune responses, resulting in an increased survival rate and decreased tumor growth and metastasis in rodents [49]. OMVs can carry abundant quantities of LPS or other immunomodulatory factors, whose capacity for immune activation and modulation has been used to reduce tumor growth [61]. However, LPS is a double-edged sword, because it is a kind of strong inducer of inflammation and thus is the main reason that OMVs have biotoxicity [62]. Therefore, the biosecurity of OMVs should be taken into much consideration. Hopefully, incomplete LPS structures in genetically engineered OMVs cause toxicity to decline and keep the immunogenicity at the same time [63]. In the study conducted by Kim, Oh Youn et al., OMVs, extracted from genetically modified Escherichia coli (E. coli) whose genes encoding the lipid component of LPS were dampened ahead of time, exhibited biosafety, a targeting ability and ideal tumor attenuation after systematical administration, and induced the production of CXCL10 and IFN-γ (interferon-γ) in colon cancer cell-bearing mice [64]. Although the immune-associated mechanisms involved are not completely understood, the potential of OMVs as a classical tool for tumor vaccine design is worth being highlighted.

3.3. The Mechanisms of Tumor-Cell-Derived EVs Designed to Be Tumor Vaccines

TEVs have emerged as a booming drug- or compound-delivery system for the development of tumor treatment, including chemotherapy and immunotherapy.

Generally speaking, TEVs suppress innate and/or adaptive antitumor immune responses. In the aspect of innate immunity, natural TEVs have been found to influence macrophage polarization and inhibit the activation and proliferation of NK cells. Bardi, Gina T et al. demonstrated that melanoma exosomes could upregulate the cytokine secretion of the M2 phenotype and thus induce a protumor macrophage activation phenotype mixture [65]. In addition, as Liu, Cunren et al. have studied the impact of carcinoma exosomes on NK cell function, TEVs could suppress NK cell cytotoxic activity by inhibiting the release of perforin and the expression of cyclin D3 [66]. Referring to adaptive immunity, TEVs are loaded with a composition similar to the parental cells and it is well known that tumor cells express the surface-protein-programmed death-ligand 1 (PD-L1) to evade immune detection. TEVs have the same topology of PD-L1 as that on the cell membrane, and TEVs could dumb the function of $CD8^+$ T cells to facilitate tumor development [67]. Chen, Zhenzhen et al. demonstrated that TEVs from diffuse large B cell lymphoma were detected to elevate the expression of PD-1 on the surface of T cells, hence acting as an immunosuppressive mediator [68].

Conversely, in certain situations, TEVs could exert a tumor-inhibiting role through the activation of the antitumor immune system. Interestingly, the formation of TEVs may influence their behavior in promoting or suppressing tumor cells. It has been revealed that TEVs derived from radiation-irritated lung cancer cells have antitumor therapeutic effects via tumor microenvironment (TME) remodeling [69]. Furthermore, tumor antigen profiles in TEVs endow them with the potential to be tumor vaccines. TEVs carry damage-associated molecular patterns (DAMPs) such as heat shock proteins (HSP) and subsequently activate the immune cells, specifically DCs [70]. As Ma, Jingwei et al. have reported, TEVs can increase lysosomal pH and drive lysosomal centripetal migration, promoting the formation of p-MHC I complexes by DCs, which present antigen peptides to $CD8^+$ T cells [71]. In addition, HSP70-overexpressing tumor cells could release EVs rich in HSP70 proteins, and these EVs become a reservoir of extracellular HSP70 to activate and augment the cytotoxic activity of NK cells, or to play an immunostimulatory role in antigen presentation and T cell priming [72,73]. Not surprisingly, TEVs, especially batch-to-batch engineered or modified vesicles, exhibit a splendid character for tumor antigen delivery. The goals to engineer or modify TEVs are various, including the enhancement of pharmacokinetic and/or pharmacodynamic characteristics, maintenance of biocompatibility, decrease in biotoxicity or improvement of immunogenicity [22]. These tumorous antigens or peptides that TEVs possess can be presented by APCs forming p-MHC compounds to incite interactions with other immune cells. In addition to antigens associated with the activation of DCs, the DNA components in TEVs can also activate DCs in some signaling pathways. In the recent few years, increasing amounts of researchers have revealed the connection between epigenetic mechanisms and immunoregulation within a tumorous niche, aiming to boost antitumor immune responses under the impact of epigenetic therapy [74]. Some strategies have been conducted to genetically modify TEVs or other membrane nanovesicles with epigenetic agents performing gene silencing through various signaling pathways, for example, altered micro RNAs, histones and abnormal DNA methylation [75,76]. In addition, the stimulator of interferon genes (STING) is an important signaling pathway because it plays a vital part in the differentiation and manipulation of myeloid-derived suppressor cells (MDSCs) and EVs generate specific T-cell responses via the aforementioned pathway to perform anticancer effects [77,78]. Y. Kitai et al. treated breast cancer cells with an inhibitor of topoisomerase I before they collected and extracted cancer-derived EVs which could contain a larger volume of DNA, and then DCs were activated to elicit antitumor immunity by the TEVs via the cGAS-STING pathway [79]. Moreover, our previous study concluded that TEVs packaging the metabolism-relevant inhibitor Fluvastatin can suppress cancer cells via reversing immunosuppressive TME by increasing the infiltration of CTLs, M1-macrophages and activated NK cells and downregulating immunosuppressive cells including M2-macrophages, Tregs and MDSCs [80]. Therefore, not spontaneous TEVs, but these processed ones have the potential to become an ideal tumor vaccine.

3.4. The Potential Mechanisms of Dendritic-Cell-Derived EVs Acting as a Tumor Vaccine

As described ahead, cell-free vectors DEVs also show therapeutic promise, since they directly present the specific antigen to T cells and the activation of these effector cells is stimulated. DEVs bear peptide-MHC complexes and inherit the properties that parental DCs have. A number of fundamental and clinical studies load tumor antigen peptides to DEVs, in a bid to suppress tumor growth by evoking helpful antitumor immunity. Zuo, Bingfeng et al. painted DEVs with hepatocellular carcinoma peptides, α-fetoprotein epitope and an immunoadjuvant (which was nucleosome-binding protein 1) to promote the recruitment and activation of DCs in tumor sites, achieving the cross-presentation of tumor neoantigens and causing tumor eradication [81]. Except containing peptides of a signal tumor, DEVs could be engineered to carry tumor antigens from multiple tumors. From the perspective of Tian, Xin and his colleagues, DEVs bearing dual antigens from melanoma and lung adenocarcinoma were generated to induce specific tumor-rejected immune responses owing to the upregulation and stimulation of CTLs [82]. Alternatively, antigens in DEVs could be ingested by other APCs, and then APCs deliver such antigenic EVs to the specific sites to elicit the priming of T cell and/or B cell crosstalk [83]. In some in vitro studies, it has been shown that DEVs have to be recaptured by DCs and then transfer antigen information so as to accomplish the interaction with T cells [84].

Despite the fact that the type of antigens carried by DEVs is crucial for them to specifically initiate an immune response, the size of EVs should also be considered. Wahlund, Casper J E et al. unraveled the divergence of DC-derived exosomes and microvesicles. They found that exosomes carried much more ovalbumin (OVA), whereas the OVA in microvesicles was hardly detectable [85]. Hence DC-derived exosomes show a stronger capacity to induce antigen-specific T cell responses or antibody production, indicating that exosomes own much more obvious immunogenicity, and more importantly implying that subpopulations of EVs need be carefully concerned before design, manipulation and application. In addition to antigen peptides and the size of DEVs, the origin of DEVs is also important, for the reason that there are diverse developmental stages during the maturation of DCs. Admyre, Charlotte et al. evaluated the T cell stimulatory capacity with exosomes from lipopolysaccharide-matured DCs in advance and found an enhanced level of the activated function of T cells compared with exosomes from immature DCs [86].

4. The Current Advances of Representative Membrane Vesicles as Tumor Vaccines in Preclinical Studies

Owing to the unceasing and evolving processes of understanding how immune cells interact with each other and communicate with tumor cells or other cells, continuously developing membrane vesicles are emerging as tumor vaccines and are utilized for immunotherapy. Phospholipid-membrane-based nanovesicles can be loaded with antigenic payloads, immunomodulatory factors or therapeutic drugs, or receive epigenetically/genetically engineered reprogramming to overexpress or downregulate the expression of certain molecules for the antitumor purpose. These nanomaterials have curative and tumor-killing effects in different types of tumors through stimulating antitumor immune responses and reversing the immunosuppressive microenvironment. Additionally, to generate an effective, qualified or even excellent tumor vaccine, it is critical to evoke the specific, robust and long-term immunity and induce the attenuating of immunosuppressive factors. Here, an overview of the multiple vaccines from modified and/or engineered membrane vesicles against tumors in the recent decade is provided.

4.1. Synthetic Liposomes Used as a Tumor Vaccine

Through the versatile and operational characteristics of liposomes, there is no doubt that liposomes are widely applied in antitumor treatment. Existing material design strategies for liposomes acting as tumor vaccines are generally to functionalize them with immunogenicity, targeting ability and immunomodulatory capacity by carrying adjuvants, tumor-specific antigens/peptides, molecules specifically recognizing certain receptors or different RNA types (Table 1). In addition, during fabrication processes, emphasis should be put on internalization efficiency, circulation traffic, biocompatibility and security. We list some representative studies about liposomes used for tumor immunotherapy in recent years (Table 1). The design approaches, application in tumors and immune-associated mechanisms are briefly described in Table 1.

Table 1. Fundamental applications of liposomes as tumor vaccines.

Modification Strategy	Targeting Tumor Types	Mechanisms and Outcomes	Year, Reference
Cationic liposome encapsulated with mRNA encoding cytokeratin 19	Lung caner	DC maturation (CD86 ↑; MHCII ↑); cytokine elevation (IL-12 ↑, TNF-α ↑, IL-2 ↑, IL-4 ↑). Induction of an antitumor immune response.	2020, [87]
Liposomes enveloped with ErbB-2 and OVA peptide	Lung carcinoma cells; breast cancer	ErbB-2 (known as Her-2) activates B cells to generate antibodies targeted by Pertuzumab; OVA provides T cell support.	2020, [88]
Liposomes carrying tumor antigens Gangliosides	Pancreatic cancer	Ganglioside liposomes bind to CD169 and are internalized by $CD169^+$ DCs and macrophages causing cytokine production, robust cross-presentation and specific activation of $CD8^+$ T cells.	2020, [89]
pH-sensitive liposomes containing OVA and α-GalCer	T lymphoma	Induction of OVA-specific IgG1 and IgG2b antibody responses; increased production of IFN-γ and IL-4; prophylactic vaccination efficacy.	2018, [90]
Liposomes containing HPV16 E7 peptide and CpG oligodeoxynucleotides and modified with DC-targeting mannose	Cervical cancer	Increased proportions of $CD4^+$ and $CD8^+$ T cells and CTL; reducing numbers of inhibitory immune cells such as MDSCs.	2020, [91]
Liposomes conjugated with adjuvant cRGD	Lung cancer; melanoma; breast cancer; liver cancer	cRGD promotes immunogenic cell death; cRGD-liposomes increase cellular accumulation of thymidine conjugate and enhance cytotoxicity following UVA activation.	2019, [92]
Liposomes admixed with HPV-16 E7 epitope	Cervical cancer	Induction of antigen-specific $CD8^+$ T cells and production of relevant cytokines (TNF-α and IL-2); increased percentages of central and effector memory T cells.	2021, [93]

Table 1. *Cont.*

Modification Strategy	Targeting Tumor Types	Mechanisms and Outcomes	Year, Reference
Liposomes modified with the adjuvant system including CoPoP, PHAD and immunostimulatory molecules QS-21	Colon cancer	CoPoP induces particle formation of peptides; particle-based peptides are better taken up by APCs and are represented on an MHC-I surface; generation of antigen-specific $CD8^+$ T cells.	2021, [94]
Liposomes modified with ICG and pardaxin peptide	Melanoma	Under NIR, the liposomes induce the release of DAMPs and TAAs with high immunogenicity.	2022, [95]
RNA-loaded magnetic liposomes	Glioblastoma	Iron oxide enhances DCs transfection and enables tracking of DCs migration with MRI, thus predicting individual treatment effects	2019, [96]
Liposomal nanoparticles composed of mRNA (containing Ψ and 5meC) and α-GalCer	Melanoma; lymphoma	The nanosystem leads to the activation of iNKT after presented by APCs, and then cytokines (IFN-γ, IL-4, etc.) secreted by iNKT activate DCs and CTL.	2019, [97]
Liposome-decorated cancer cell membrane enveloping a plasmid encoding shRNA against Pvt1	Colorectal cancer	The biolipid nanoparticles strengthen Oxa-induced ICD; activation of DCs; inhibition of MDSCs; generation of immune memory responses for tumor ectopic rechallenging and metastasis.	2022, [98]
Cationic liposome encapsulated with tumor-derived mRNA	Melanoma; lung cancer	Increased coexpression of CD11c and PD-L1 in host-myeloid cells sensitize immunologically "cold" tumor; $PD\text{-}L1^+$ APCs elicit IFN-γ production causing expansion of specific $CD8^+$ T cells; combination with ICIs enhances T cell activity and synergistic antitumor efficacy.	2018, [99]
MMP2 responsive folate-modified liposome carrying doxorubicin	Breast cancer	Elimination of M2-TAMs resulting in a decrease in immunosuppressive cytokines and Treg cells, ensuring antitumor effector T cells; promotion of DCs maturation and immunostimulatory cytokines secretion.	2019, [100]

Abbreviations: CpG, cytosine–phosphate–guanine; OVA, ovalbumin; α-GalCer, α-galactosylceramide; CoPoP, cobalt–porphyrin; PHAD, monophosphoryl lipid A; ICG, indocyanine green; MRI, magnetic resonance imaging; NIR, near-infrared irradiation; Ψ, pseudouridine; 5meC, 5-methylcytidine; iNKT, invariant natural killer T cells; shRNA, short hair-pinned RNA; Pvt1, plasmacytoma variant translocation 1; ICIs, immune checkpoint inhibitors; Oxa, Oxaliplatin; ICD, immunogenic cell death; MMP2, matrix metalloprotease 2; TAMs, tumor-associated macrophages; TAAs, tumor-associated antigens; BMDCs, bone-marrow-derived DCs. ↑: Upregulation of certain subpopulations of DCs or cytokines.

4.2. The Design and Engineering Modification of Bacterial Membrane Vesicles

BMVs are designed not only to target tumor sites and provoke effective immune reactions, but also to reduce inflammatory toxicity and specifically kill tumor cells. Comprehensive studies revealing various fabrications of BMVs as tumor vaccines are documented in Table 2.

BMVs have been reported to induce the production of antitumor-associated cytokines such as IFN-γ, TNF-α and IL-12 [25,101]. Except the immunological functions of BMVs, BMVs have a rigid membrane structure which makes nanoplatforms stabilized. Moreover, it is easy to produce BMVs by fermentation and purification procedures, and it is workable to acquire genetically engineered BMVs [102]. Owing to theses intrinsic properties, it is not surprising that integrating BMVs into tumor vaccines is appealing. BMVs can be originated from various types of bacteria, while nanosized OMVs secreted by Gram-negative bacteria, especially E. coli, are mostly developed to be a tumor vaccine. Before collecting BMVs, original bacteria can be genetically engineered by being transfected with RNA interference, miRNAs, etc., for some purpose, such as detoxification. Additionally, a modification is commonly applied after BMVs are ultracentrifuged and purified, for example, binding them with tumor antigens or immunoadjuvants (Table 2).

Table 2. Fundamental applications of BMVs as tumor vaccines.

Parent Bacteria	Modification Strategy	Targeting Tumor Types	Mechanisms and Outcomes	Year, Reference
Escherichia coli (*E. coli*)	Bacteria and liposome biohybrid vaccine combined with tumor antigen and adjuvant	Colorectal cancer	Increased expression of CD40, CD80 and CD86 on BMDCs and enhanced infiltration of $CD8^+$ T cell	2021, [103]
E. coli	Genetically engineered OMVs binding with L7Ae (RNA binding protein) and listeriolysin O (lysosomal escape protein)	Melanoma; colon cancer	Listeriolysin O-mediated endosomal escape contributes to cross-presentation of DCs; induction of a long-term immune memory.	2022, [104]
E. coli	OMVs fused with thylakoid membranes from spinach	Colon cancer; breast cancer	Photodynamic effects from thylakoid cause tumor destruction, resulting in release of TAAs and DAMPs presented by DCs and inducing tumor-specific $CD8^+$ T cell responses.	2022, [105]
E. coli	OMVs fused with protein cytolysin A	Pulmonary metastatic melanoma; colon cancer	The antigen-bearing OMVs stimulate DCs maturation and protect animals against tumorous rechallenge.	2022, [106]
E. coli	Conjunctive products of OMVs, Mal and 1-MT (IDO inhibitor)	Colon cancer	The nanoparticles bind to tumor antigens and overcome the immune inhibition of IDO on effector T cells.	2022, [107]
E. coli	OMVs fused with ClyA protein and decorated with tag/catcher protein pairs	Lung melanoma metastasis; colorectal cancer	The vaccine platform "Plug-and-Display" technology displays the tumor antigens and induces innate and specific T-cell-mediated immune responses.	2021, [108]
E. coli	Synthetic OMVs combined with TEVs	Melanoma	Synthetic OMVs have barely any systemic proinflammatory responses; The combined membrane vesicles activate BMDCs, Th-1 T cells and balance antibody production; efficacy of antiPD-1 inhibitor is improved.	2021, [61]
Salmonella Typhimurium	A eukaryotic–prokaryotic vesicle (EPV) nanoplatform containing TEVs and OMVs	Melanoma	It is verified to be a prevention vaccine to trigger antitumor memory immune responses; photothermal effects are motivated by combination with EPV through DCs maturation and production of TNF-α and IL-12.	2020, [109]

Table 2. *Cont.*

Parent Bacteria	Modification Strategy	Targeting Tumor Types	Mechanisms and Outcomes	Year, Reference
E. coli	OMVs modified by insertion of the ectodomain of PD1	Colon cancer; melanoma	OMVs bind to PD-L1 on the tumor cell surface and thus protect T cells from PD1/PD-L1 axis; OMVs induce the accumulation of effector T cells in TME.	2020, [110]
Salmonella Typhimurium	OMVs from *Salmonella Typhimurium*	Colorectal carcinoma; hepatocellular carcinoma; breast cancer	OMVs enhance recruitment of NK cells through upregulation of caspase-3, Beclin-1 and CD49b.	2021, [111]

Abbreviations: Mal, maleimide; 1-MT, 1-methyl-tryptophan; IDO, indoleamine 2, 3-dioxygenase.

4.3. The Proper and Multiple Strategies for Producing Tumor Vaccines from Tumor-Cell-Derived EVs

As TEVs play a crucial biological role in tumorous biogenesis, development and metastasis, it cannot be denied that antitumor strategies vary from each other depending on the distinctive mechanisms, for example, suppressing TEV secretion, interrupting TEV uptake by recipient cells or delivering functional cargoes [4]. Apart from these approaches, the applications of TEVs as tumor vaccines in the last few years are summarized below (Table 3).

Table 3. Fundamental applications of TEVs as tumor vaccines.

Modification Strategy	Targeting Tumor Types	Mechanisms and Outcomes	Year, Reference
Tumor-derived antigenic microparticles (T-MPs) carrying nanoFe_3O_4 and adjuvant CpG	Melanoma; colon cancer	Nanomaterials absorbed by APCs elicit antigen-specific host immune responses; reversion of tumor-associated macrophages into a tumor-suppressive M1 phenotype; increased infiltration of CTL.	2019, [112]
Irradiated tumor-cell-derived EVs	Hepatoma; breast cancer	Radiation endows TEVs with tumor antigens (for example, CDCP1) and HSP; enhanced infiltration of $CD8^+$ and $CD4^+$ T cells and activation of CTL.	2020, [113]
TEV surface modification with glycocalyx and removal of sialic acids	Glioblastoma	Increased internalization by DCs via receptor-mediated glycan-depending targeting to DCs.	2019, [114]
α-LA-engineered cancer exosomes loaded with ICD stimulators (ELANE and TLR3 agonist Hiltonol)	Breast cancer	Homing to the tumor sites and induction of ICD in cancer cells; activation of cDC1s and tumor-reactive $CD8^+$ T cells.	2022, [115]
TEVs mixed with an oligonucleotide duplex and assembled with CpG-DNA	Melanoma	TEVs prolong residence in tumor tissue and activate DCs more efficiently than tumor or fibroblast cells.	2019, [116]
Exosomes derived from immunogenically dying tumor cells and modified with MART-1 and CCL22 siRNA	Pancreatic cancer	MART-1 peptide can expand T-cell-related responses; CCL22 siRNA inhibits the communication between DCs and Tregs via the CCR4/CCL22 axis.	2022, [117]
irradiated C6 (malignant glioma-cell-derived EVs	Glioblastoma	Increased percentages of apoptotic tumor cells and helper, cytotoxic and regulatory T cells.	2019, [118]

Table 3. *Cont.*

Modification Strategy	Targeting Tumor Types	Mechanisms and Outcomes	Year, Reference
TEVs derived from irradiated cancer cells	Breast cancer	TEVs transfer dsDNA to promote production of IFN-γ via cGAS/STING pathway; TEVs evoke specific antitumor responses of $CD8^+$ T cells and perform prophylactic vaccination.	2018, [119]
TEVs carrying adjuvant HMGN1	Hepatocellular carcinoma	TEVs potentiate immunogenicity and activate DCs; TEVs promote DCs homing to lymphoid tissues and augment memory lymphocytes.	2020, [120]
TEVs modified with microRNA (miR-155, miR-142 and let-7i)	Breast cancer	Induction of DCs maturation by detecting expression of MHCII, CD80 and CD40; microRNA-targeting genes (IL-6, TGFβ, IFN-γ, TLR4, SOCS1, etc.) are confirmed to mature DCs.	2019, [121]
TEVs derived from leukemia cells whose PD-L1 have been downregulated by PD-L1 shRNA	Leukemia	Modified TEVs evoke DCs maturation, T-cell activation and release of Th1 cytokine.	2022, [122]

Abbreviations: HSP, heat-shock proteins; CDCP1, CUB domain-containing protein 1; α-LA, α-lactalbumin; ELANE, neutrophil elastase; cDC1s, type one conventional DCs; HMGN1, high mobility group nucleosome-binding protein 1.

Notably, compared with the composition of liposomes or BMVs, TEVs innately contain a plethora of bioactive molecules, especially tumor antigens (TAAs and TSAs), which are critical when TEVs are involved in immunity modulation. Nevertheless, naturally autosecreted TEVs cannot be directly applied in tumor immunotherapy, since they have an important part in tumor biogenesis and progress as we have mentioned above. Therefore, engineering or modification methods are essential to fully obtain their advantages and potentials as a tumor vaccine. Before isolation is conducted, tumor-cell-related genetic engineering can be performed, including gene/protein-encoding interference (miRNAs, mRNA, siRNAs and others) and genome editing (plasmid DNAs) [1]. Furthermore, therapeutic drugs, adjuvants or antigen peptides can also be attached to TEVs before or after isolation so as to improve their capacity to be a feasible tumor vaccine.

4.4. Transforming Dendritic-Cell-Derived EVs into an Ideal Tumor Vaccine

Since DEVs partially similar to DCs participate in the initiation of proper antitumor immune responses of T cells consisting of antigen recognition (p-MHC complexes-TCR communication performs an important role), costimulation and/or production of T-cell stimulatory cytokines, it is inevitable to further consider the DEVs used in tumor immunotherapy [22]. Additionally, DEVs are able to trigger or modulate innate antitumor immune responses, for example, the activation of NK cells [123]. Rather than the direct use of naked EVs generated from different types of DCs in tumor immunotherapy, DEVs also undergo multiple design means. Similar to the approaches described in the previous section, DEVs can be loaded with therapeutic sensitizers, immunomodulators, adjuvants, tumor-specific peptides or small molecules targeting some signaling pathway. It is noted that not only do TEVs carry tumor-associated antigens (TAAs), but DEVs can also be pulsed with TAAs when they are generated from patient tissues [4].

We document representative preclinical studies in recent years about DEVs modified to be a tumor vaccine and give a brief description of immune-related mechanisms and how DEVs evoke potent antitumor immunity (Table 4).

Table 4. Fundamental applications of DEVs as tumor vaccines.

Modification Strategy	Targeting Tumor Types	Mechanisms and Outcomes	Year, Reference
DEVs loaded with MBPN-TCyP (an AIE-photosensitizer)	Breast cancer; colon cancer	The modified DEVs induce ICD and immune-modulation function like parental DCs; DEVs synergize photodynamic immunotherapy.	2022, [124]
DEVs derived from A-Pas chiRNA-transfected DCs	Esophagus cancer	DEXs induce DC maturation (upregulation of CD83, CD86, MHC-I and MHC-II) and $CD8^+$ T-cell-mediated antitumor responses.	2022, [125]
DEVs assembled with tumor peptide P47-P, AFP and immunomodulators N1ND-N	Hepatocellular carcinoma	DEVs promote DCs recruitment, activation, cross-presentation of antigens; DEVs induce antitumor responses by increasing IFN-$\gamma^+$$CD8^+$ effector T cells.	2022, [81]
Exosomes derived from AFP-expressing DCs	Hepatocellular carcinoma	DEVs remodel TME by increasing IFN-$\gamma^+$$CD8^+$ T cells and cytokines (IFN-γ and IL-2) and by decreasing $CD25^+$$Foxp3^+$ Treg and cytokines (IL-2 and TGF-β).	2017, [126]
DEVs conjugated with MUC1 glycopeptide antigen	Melanoma	Induction of MUC1-specific IgG antibody; activation of CTL against MUC1-positive tumor cells.	2022, [127]
DEVs derived from OVA-pulsed and activated dendritic cells modified with antiCTLA-4 antibody	Melanoma	DEVs target to T cells and activate tumor-specific T-cell responses; CTLA-4 in DEVs block inhibitory immunity and enhance the specific responses by T cells.	2020, [128]
DEVs loaded with antigen E749-57 peptide and inducer poly(I:C)	Cervical cancer	Activation of CTL; Promoted immunity of vaccinated mice splenocytes.	2018, [129]
DEVs derived from tumor cell lysate-pulsed DCs	Lung cancer	Induced proliferation of allogeneic T cell, including the subpopulation of $CD3^+V\gamma9$ T and $CD8^+$ T cells; Activated cytotoxicity of alloPBMCs against tumor cells.	2020, [130]

Abbreviations: AIE, aggregation-induced emission; A-Pas chiRNA, a cancer-specific aberrant transcription-induced chimeric RNA; AFP, α-fetoprotein; N1ND-N, nucleosome-binding protein 1; TME, tumor microenvironment; Treg, regulatory T cells; TGF-β, transforming growth factor-β; alloPBMCs, allogeneic peripheral blood mononuclear cells.

5. The Clinical Applications Relevant to Tumor Vaccines of Biomembrane-Based Nanovesicles Are Developing

The aforementioned applications of membrane vesicles as potential tumor vaccines are mainly focused on the fundamental level, that is to say, applied in vitro or in animal models. Due to the preponderance of drug/molecule-delivery efficiency, internalization ability, ease of modifying and biocompatibility, these membrane-based nanovesicles (liposomes, BMVs, TEVs and DEVs) exhibit potential for clinical and biomedical translation. For the purpose of the clinical evaluation of tumor vaccine efficacy, tumor status (tumor growth, invasion and metastasis), survival indexes (overall survival and progression-free survival) and systemic and local immunity (implying how vaccines work and influence the human body) are involved in the assessment system. In addition to therapeutic effect appraisals, adverse effects caused by vaccines are always crucial and need careful observation [131]. Since membrane vesicles act as vaccines potentially influencing patient immunity, monitoring immune responses is essential for the sake of security during the clinical trials, not just for the evaluation of curative effects. On account of the fact that a wide range of clinical trials has been undertaken, the advances and meanings of complete or developing clinical studies to date are going to be reviewed in the following section. Additionally, the brief synopsis of these representative clinical trials appearing in the context can be seen in Table 5.

Table 5. Representative clinical trials applying tumor vaccines.

Trial ID	Phase	Status	Intervention	Applied Conditions
NCT04163094	Phase 1	Active, not recruiting	A liposome-based mRNA vaccine combined with chemotherapy.	Ovarian cancer
NCT01915524	Phase 1	Terminated	RNActive®-derived cancer vaccine coding for tumor antigens.	Nonsmall cell lung carcinoma
NCT01052142	Phase 1	Completed	A liposomal vaccine.	Melanoma
NCT01095848	Phase 1	Completed	DPX-0907 consists of seven tumor-specific HLA-A2-restricted peptides, a universal T-Helper peptide, a polynucleotide adjuvant, a liposome, etc.	Ovarian, breast and prostatic neoplasms
NCT00623831	Phase 1	Completed; has Results	Mixed bacterial vaccine.	Melanoma, sarcoma, gastrointestinal stromal tumor, etc.
NCT02010203	Phase 1/2	Terminated; has Results	HS-410: a vaccine derived from irradiated cancer cells genetically engineered to continually secrete gp96; BCG: a vaccine derived from a live bacterium.	Bladder cancer
NCT03762291	Phase 1	Recruiting	CVD908ssb-TXSV: Salmonella-based survivin vaccine.	Multiple myeloma
NCT02657460	Phase 2	Unknown	Tumor-derived microparticles packaging chemotherapy drugs.	Malignant pleural effusion
NCT01550523	Phase 1	Completed	Exosomes from autologous glioma cells combined with an antisense molecule.	Malignant glioma of brain
NCT00020462	Phase 1	Completed	Autologous tumor cell vaccine plus interleukin-2.	Lymphoma
NCT05559177	Early Phase 1	Recruiting	Personalized chimeric exosome tumor vaccines.	Recurrent or metastatic bladder cancer
NCT00065442	Phase 3	Completed; has Results	Sipuleucel-T: Autologous antigen presenting cells loading with PA2024.	Prostate Cancer
NCT02693236	Phase1/2	Unknown	Monocyte-derived dendritic cells (moDCs) combined with cytokine-induced killer cells.	Squamous cell carcinoma of esophagus
NCT01159288	Phase 2	Completed	Dex2: tumor antigen-loaded dendritic-cell-derived exosomes.	Nonsmall cell lung carcinoma

Liposomes, amongst membrane vesicles having a relatively long history, are used for tumor vaccines in a number of clinical trials. In the Netherlands, eligible ovarian cancer patients are treated with a liposome-formulated mRNA vaccine that can encode TAAs and later peripheral blood mononuclear cells, and the intratumoral accumulation of immune cells are used to determine immune responses (NCT04163094). Additionally, liposome-based mRNA vaccines exhibit fewer side effects, a higher stability and stronger efficacy than the sole mRNA vaccines in cancer treatment, including lung cancer and colon cancer (NCT01915524) [132,133]. Furthermore, a liposomal vaccine called Lipovaxin-MM in a completed phase I trial has been demonstrated to be safe and effective in metastatic melanoma participants (NCT01052142). Despite the potentially effective vaccines of simple-ingredient liposomal systems, liposomes can be designed to be encapsulated with several components performing their special duties. In a phase I trial, a complex nanovesicle vaccine named DPX-0907 based on IVT's DepoVax™ (DPX) formulation was applied to ovarian, breast and prostatic cancers, which consisted of tumor and T helper peptides, a polynucleotide adjuvant and lipid components, respectively (NCT01095848). Although the safety was confirmed in the phase I study, a subsequent study to determine the treatment effects need to be carefully planned and the results remain unknown.

There have been a batch of clinical studies that used bacteria or modified ones as potent tumor vaccines to inherently modulate and stimulate antitumor immune responses or reverse immunosuppressive immunity. In spite of some clinical studies using bacteria for tumor vaccines (NCT00623831, NCT02010203, NCT03762291, etc.), bacteria may pose a risk for infection during the treatment, so applying bacteria-derived vesicles that contain concise components seems to be safer [134]. Bacteria contain lots of unnecessary or even toxic components, so it is welcomed through discarding the "dross" and meanwhile selecting the "essence". Despite the current condition that lots of clinical trials about BMVs emerge to cure infectious diseases, the existing registered clinical trials about BMVs acting as a tumor vaccine are limited, indicating that there are many challenges setting obstacles for tumor vaccines in clinical translation [135]. Meanwhile, lots of concerns have been raised about the biosafety of BMVs. For example, the introduction of LPS or other proinflammatory factors in BMVs may potentially cause an inflammatory storm. Therefore, a variety of methods have been introduced to diminish the component toxicity of BMVs to decrease the incidence of systemic inflammatory responses [136,137].

The parental materials for TEV fabrication applied in patients are various, for example using autologous tumor cells or synthesizing tumor neoantigens loaded in TEVs. In 2019, we published our clinical data about autologous tumor-cell-derived microparticles encapsulated with methotrexate (aTMPs-MTX) used in advanced lung cancer patients with malignant pleural effusion [138]. The clinical results showed that aTMPs-MTX not only decreased the pleural effusion volume but also activated patient antitumor immunity (for example, the upregulation of CTLs) (NCT02657460). Furthermore, TEVs can carry other bioactive byproducts to play a role in the modulation of antitumor immunity in clinical studies. For instance, in a phase I clinical trial, exosomes from patient glioma tissues encapsulated in small diffusion chambers can gently release tumor antigens and perform the activation of immune cells (NCT01550523). Despite the fact that some synthetic TEVs as tumor vaccines seem to be effective in prolonging survival, combination therapy in clinical trials is not unusual. In a phase I trial (NCT00020462), patients with follicular lymphoma receive the therapy strategy combining the autologous tumor cell vaccine and IL-2. Additionally, hybrid or chimeric EVs vaccines exist in clinical studies. Currently, an early phase 1 trial is being conducted, referring to the membrane vesicle combination of chimeric exosomal tumor vaccines prepared from bladder tumor tissues and peripheral blood immune cells (DCs or macrophages) (NCT05559177). However, the treatment effects of incomplete trials remain to be detected.

A decade ago, the FDA approved monocyte-derived DCs pulsed with the antigen prostatic acid phosphatase and the immunomodulatory factor GM-CSF as a form of cellular immunotherapy against prostate cancer, which was demonstrated to be effective in phase III trials (NCT00065442) [139]. In consideration of the functions of DCs being potent tumor vaccines and the novel promising cell-free EVs from DCs, Narita, Miwako et al. performed and reported phase I/II clinical trials (NCT02693236) for patients diagnosed with esophageal cancer, in which DEVs were isolated from antigen peptide-pulsed DCs, and then CTLs were found activated later after the administration of DEVs in patients, while the efficacy of DEVs remained unknown [140]. Another phase II clinical trial in France focused on the immunotherapeutic effects of metronomic cyclophosphamide followed by tumor antigen-loaded DEVs, whose safety and feasibility on unresectable nonsmall cell lung cancer was verified in a phase I trial (NCT01159288). It is notable that not all the trials showed the desired efficacy, which was mainly attributed to the low immune stimulatory capacities of these synthetic membrane vesicles. To relieve or solve the obstacles occurring in the clinical application of membrane vesicle vaccines, the design of the vaccine itself, timing and frequency of vaccination, routes and sites of injection and vaccine doses should be gradually and rigorously established.

6. Outlooks

Phospholipid-membrane-based vesicles own evident features making them attractive for basic or clinical applications. With the membrane properties, membrane vesicles are born to be flexible and easy-to-carry cargoes or internalized by recipient cells. As a result, they have inevitably become a promising drug/molecule-delivery platform. Nevertheless, due to the different sources of membrane vesicles, the function and capacities are distinctive from each other, so researchers should properly design strategies according to the actual situations so as to take full advantage of nanosized tumor vaccines, rather than applying them mechanically. There are several approaches concluded as follows to improve the therapeutic successfulness of tumor vaccines: 1. standardized preparation techniques in order to improve the uniformity of nanovesicles including their size and contents; 2. detoxicating toxic components and purifying vesicles to wipe off impurities; 3. selecting a specific and conducive cargo, including antigen peptides (such as hot-discussed personalized neoantigens), immunomodulatory factors, chemical drugs and nucleic acids (such as mRNA, miRNA and siRNA encoding with specific functions); 4. The appropriate modification of vesicle surface or intercellular compartments. It is believed that the advances of membrane vesicles used in tumor immunotherapy are endless.

Although a number of preclinical studies contribute to exploiting developing methods in order to design membrane vesicles as ideal tumor vaccines, several reasons as follows may set obstacles to the clinical translation of membrane vesicles. 1. in the aspect of biosafety, complex contents in vesicles may not only cause side effects (for example, impaired glucose tolerance and fasting hyperglycemia) but may also be difficult to metabolize, thus prolonging in vivo residence, indicating that the toxicology and pharmacokinetics should be further carefully concerned during the intervention [51,141,142]; 2. despite ongoing efforts to improve the procedures associated with the isolation and storage of membrane nanovesicles, the homogeneity of extraction is hard to ensure and the quality control still remains problematic [143]; 3. the technique causes the therapeutic membrane vesicles to be expensive and such curative approaches may raise the cost burden to patients [22]; 4. due to the physiological uniqueness of each patient and/or low immunogenicity of nanoscale tumor vaccines, the precision medicine and/or therapeutic effects are difficult to be determined and guaranteed; 5. ethical issues may hinder the clinical application, for the reason of the potential adverse impact of genetically modified membrane vesicles, such as uncomfortable feelings (fatigue, fever, etc.) or even continuous tumor development probably caused by the cargoes in the membrane nanovesicles [131,144]; 6. the retention in the systemic circulation is not durable and nanovesicles may be rapidly cleared by the mononuclear phagocytic system, resulting in a low efficiency and high frequency of vaccination, so novel therapeutic systems such as nanovesicles camouflaged with red blood cell or platelet membranes are being studied [141,145]. Taken together, uniform and definite criteria are difficult to accomplish, and researchers have to be faced with and overcome existing hindrances. In summary, although there is still an arduous and long road to go for the development of membrane-vesicle-based tumor vaccines, it does not keep membrane vesicles from being promising tumor vaccines.

Author Contributions: Conceptualization, W.C. and Y.W.; writing—original draft preparation, W.C.; writing—review and editing, W.C., Y.W., J.D., Z.Y. and Y.J.; visualization, J.C. and Q.T.; funding acquisition, M.G. and Y.J. All authors have read and agreed to the published version of the manuscript.

Funding: Our study was supported by grants from the National Natural Science Foundation of China (No.: 82070099, 81900095, 82001988, 82100112, 82270110).

Institutional Review Board Statement: Not applicable.

Informed Consent Statement: Not applicable.

Acknowledgments: We appreciate the contribution that undergraduate student Jingwei Chen from Shanghai Jian Qiao University and the online tool BioRender (https://biorender.com/ (accessed on 18 October 2020)) made to the excellent drawings.

Conflicts of Interest: The authors declare no conflict of interest. The funders had no role in the design of the study; in the writing of the manuscript; or in the decision to publish the study.

References

1. Wang, J.; Zhu, M.; Nie, G. Biomembrane-Based Nanostructures for Cancer Targeting and Therapy: From Synthetic Liposomes to Natural Biomembranes and Membrane-Vesicles. *Adv. Drug Deliv. Rev.* **2021**, *178*, 113974. [CrossRef] [PubMed]
2. Pick, H.; Alves, A.C.; Vogel, H. Single-Vesicle Assays Using Liposomes and Cell-Derived Vesicles: From Modeling Complex Membrane Processes to Synthetic Biology and Biomedical Applications. *Chem. Rev.* **2018**, *118*, 8598–8654. [CrossRef] [PubMed]
3. Théry, C.; Witwer, K.W.; Aikawa, E.; Alcaraz, M.J.; Anderson, J.D.; Andriantsitohaina, R.; Antoniou, A.; Arab, T.; Archer, F.; Atkin-Smith, G.K.; et al. Minimal Information for Studies of Extracellular Vesicles 2018 (MISEV2018): A Position Statement of the International Society for Extracellular Vesicles and Update of the MISEV2014 Guidelines. *J. Extracell. Vesicles* **2018**, *7*, 1535750. [CrossRef]
4. Wang, S.E. Extracellular Vesicles in Cancer Therapy. *Semin. Cancer Biol.* **2022**, *86*, 296–309. [CrossRef] [PubMed]
5. Toyofuku, M.; Nomura, N.; Eberl, L. Types and Origins of Bacterial Membrane Vesicles. *Nat. Rev. Microbiol.* **2019**, *17*, 13–24. [CrossRef] [PubMed]
6. Brahmbhatt, H.; MacDiarmid, J.A. Bacterial Minicells to the Rescue: Cyto-Immunotherapy for the Treatment of Late Stage Cancers with Minimal to No Toxicity. *Microb. Biotechnol.* **2022**, *15*, 91–94. [CrossRef]
7. Kim, S.-H.; Kim, K.-S.; Lee, S.-R.; Kim, E.; Kim, M.-S.; Lee, E.-Y.; Gho, Y.S.; Kim, J.-W.; Bishop, R.E.; Chang, K.-T. Structural Modifications of Outer Membrane Vesicles to Refine Them as Vaccine Delivery Vehicles. *Biochim. Biophys. Acta* **2009**, *1788*, 2150–2159. [CrossRef]
8. Luo, P.; Mao, K.; Xu, J.; Wu, F.; Wang, X.; Wang, S.; Zhou, M.; Duan, L.; Tan, Q.; Ma, G.; et al. Metabolic Characteristics of Large and Small Extracellular Vesicles from Pleural Effusion Reveal Biomarker Candidates for the Diagnosis of Tuberculosis and Malignancy. *J. Extracell. Vesicles* **2020**, *9*, 1790158. [CrossRef]
9. Cheng, L.; Hill, A.F. Therapeutically Harnessing Extracellular Vesicles. *Nat. Rev. Drug Discov.* **2022**, *21*, 379–399. [CrossRef]
10. Zhang, X.; Zhang, H.; Gu, J.; Zhang, J.; Shi, H.; Qian, H.; Wang, D.; Xu, W.; Pan, J.; Santos, H.A. Engineered Extracellular Vesicles for Cancer Therapy. *Adv. Mater.* **2021**, *33*, 2005709. [CrossRef]
11. Kalluri, R.; LeBleu, V.S. The Biology, Function, and Biomedical Applications of Exosomes. *Science* **2020**, *367*, eaau6977. [CrossRef] [PubMed]
12. Kita-Tokarczyk, K.; Itel, F.; Grzelakowski, M.; Egli, S.; Rossbach, P.; Meier, W. Monolayer Interactions between Lipids and Amphiphilic Block Copolymers. *Langmuir ACS J. Surf. Colloids* **2009**, *25*, 9847–9856. [CrossRef]
13. Dimova, R. Recent Developments in the Field of Bending Rigidity Measurements on Membranes. *Adv. Colloid Interface Sci.* **2014**, *208*, 225–234. [CrossRef] [PubMed]
14. Bayer, A.M.; Alam, S.; Mattern-Schain, S.I.; Best, M.D. Triggered Liposomal Release through a Synthetic Phosphatidylcholine Analogue Bearing a Photocleavable Moiety Embedded within the Sn-2 Acyl Chain. *Chem. Weinh. Bergstr. Ger.* **2014**, *20*, 3350–3357. [CrossRef]
15. Immordino, M.L.; Dosio, F.; Cattel, L. Stealth Liposomes: Review of the Basic Science, Rationale, and Clinical Applications, Existing and Potential. *Int. J. Nanomed.* **2006**, *1*, 297–315.
16. Mader, C.; Küpcü, S.; Sleytr, U.B.; Sára, M. S-Layer-Coated Liposomes as a Versatile System for Entrapping and Binding Target Molecules. *Biochim. Biophys. Acta* **2000**, *1463*, 142–150. [CrossRef]
17. Ho, N.T.; Siggel, M.; Camacho, K.V.; Bhaskara, R.M.; Hicks, J.M.; Yao, Y.-C.; Zhang, Y.; Köfinger, J.; Hummer, G.; Noy, A. Membrane Fusion and Drug Delivery with Carbon Nanotube Porins. *Proc. Natl. Acad. Sci. USA* **2021**, *118*, e2016974118. [CrossRef]
18. Lian, S.; Xie, R.; Ye, Y.; Xie, X.; Li, S.; Lu, Y.; Li, B.; Cheng, Y.; Katanaev, V.L.; Jia, L. Simultaneous Blocking of CD47 and PD-L1 Increases Innate and Adaptive Cancer Immune Responses and Cytokine Release. *EBioMedicine* **2019**, *42*, 281–295. [CrossRef]
19. Krishnan, N.; Kubiatowicz, L.J.; Holay, M.; Zhou, J.; Fang, R.H.; Zhang, L. Bacterial Membrane Vesicles for Vaccine Applications. *Adv. Drug Deliv. Rev.* **2022**, *185*, 114294. [CrossRef]
20. Silhavy, T.J.; Kahne, D.; Walker, S. The Bacterial Cell Envelope. *Cold Spring Harb. Perspect. Biol.* **2010**, *2*, a000414. [CrossRef]
21. Gerritzen, M.J.H.; Martens, D.E.; Wijffels, R.H.; van der Pol, L.; Stork, M. Bioengineering Bacterial Outer Membrane Vesicles as Vaccine Platform. *Biotechnol. Adv.* **2017**, *35*, 565–574. [CrossRef] [PubMed]
22. Mehanny, M.; Lehr, C.-M.; Fuhrmann, G. Extracellular Vesicles as Antigen Carriers for Novel Vaccination Avenues. *Adv. Drug Deliv. Rev.* **2021**, *173*, 164–180. [CrossRef] [PubMed]
23. Jan, A.T. Outer Membrane Vesicles (OMVs) of Gram-Negative Bacteria: A Perspective Update. *Front. Microbiol.* **2017**, *8*, 1053. [CrossRef] [PubMed]

24. Gnopo, Y.M.D.; Watkins, H.C.; Stevenson, T.C.; DeLisa, M.P.; Putnam, D. Designer Outer Membrane Vesicles as Immunomodulatory Systems—Reprogramming Bacteria for Vaccine Delivery. *Adv. Drug Deliv. Rev.* **2017**, *114*, 132–142. [CrossRef]
25. Kaparakis-Liaskos, M.; Ferrero, R.L. Immune Modulation by Bacterial Outer Membrane Vesicles. *Nat. Rev. Immunol.* **2015**, *15*, 375–387. [CrossRef]
26. Bachmann, M.F.; Jennings, G.T. Vaccine Delivery: A Matter of Size, Geometry, Kinetics and Molecular Patterns. *Nat. Rev. Immunol.* **2010**, *10*, 787–796. [CrossRef]
27. Brown, L.; Wolf, J.M.; Prados-Rosales, R.; Casadevall, A. Through the Wall: Extracellular Vesicles in Gram-Positive Bacteria, Mycobacteria and Fungi. *Nat. Rev. Microbiol.* **2015**, *13*, 620–630. [CrossRef]
28. Wang, X.; Thompson, C.D.; Weidenmaier, C.; Lee, J.C. Release of Staphylococcus Aureus Extracellular Vesicles and Their Application as a Vaccine Platform. *Nat. Commun.* **2018**, *9*, 1379. [CrossRef]
29. Hoshino, A.; Costa-Silva, B.; Shen, T.-L.; Rodrigues, G.; Hashimoto, A.; Tesic Mark, M.; Molina, H.; Kohsaka, S.; Di Giannatale, A.; Ceder, S.; et al. Tumour Exosome Integrins Determine Organotropic Metastasis. *Nature* **2015**, *527*, 329–335. [CrossRef]
30. Willms, E.; Cabañas, C.; Mäger, I.; Wood, M.J.A.; Vader, P. Extracellular Vesicle Heterogeneity: Subpopulations, Isolation Techniques, and Diverse Functions in Cancer Progression. *Front. Immunol.* **2018**, *9*, 738. [CrossRef]
31. Raulf, N.; Lucarelli, P.; Thavaraj, S.; Brown, S.; Vicencio, J.M.; Sauter, T.; Tavassoli, M. Annexin A1 Regulates EGFR Activity and Alters EGFR-Containing Tumour-Derived Exosomes in Head and Neck Cancers. *Eur. J. Cancer Oxf. Engl. 1990* **2018**, *102*, 52–68. [CrossRef] [PubMed]
32. Demory Beckler, M.; Higginbotham, J.N.; Franklin, J.L.; Ham, A.-J.; Halvey, P.J.; Imasuen, I.E.; Whitwell, C.; Li, M.; Liebler, D.C.; Coffey, R.J. Proteomic Analysis of Exosomes from Mutant KRAS Colon Cancer Cells Identifies Intercellular Transfer of Mutant KRAS. *Mol. Cell. Proteom. MCP* **2013**, *12*, 343–355. [CrossRef] [PubMed]
33. Cho, J.A.; Park, H.; Lim, E.H.; Lee, K.W. Exosomes from Breast Cancer Cells Can Convert Adipose Tissue-Derived Mesenchymal Stem Cells into Myofibroblast-like Cells. *Int. J. Oncol.* **2012**, *40*, 130–138. [CrossRef] [PubMed]
34. Al-Nedawi, K.; Meehan, B.; Kerbel, R.S.; Allison, A.C.; Rak, J. Endothelial Expression of Autocrine VEGF upon the Uptake of Tumor-Derived Microvesicles Containing Oncogenic EGFR. *Proc. Natl. Acad. Sci. USA* **2009**, *106*, 3794–3799. [CrossRef]
35. Tkach, M.; Kowal, J.; Théry, C. Why the Need and How to Approach the Functional Diversity of Extracellular Vesicles. *Philos. Trans. R. Soc. Lond. B. Biol. Sci.* **2018**, *373*, 20160479. [CrossRef]
36. Herrmann, I.K.; Wood, M.J.A.; Fuhrmann, G. Extracellular Vesicles as a Next-Generation Drug Delivery Platform. *Nat. Nanotechnol.* **2021**, *16*, 748–759. [CrossRef]
37. Robbins, P.D.; Morelli, A.E. Regulation of Immune Responses by Extracellular Vesicles. *Nat. Rev. Immunol.* **2014**, *14*, 195–208. [CrossRef]
38. Villa, A.; Garofalo, M.; Crescenti, D.; Rizzi, N.; Brunialti, E.; Vingiani, A.; Belotti, P.; Sposito, C.; Franzè, S.; Cilurzo, F.; et al. Transplantation of Autologous Extracellular Vesicles for Cancer-Specific Targeting. *Theranostics* **2021**, *11*, 2034–2047. [CrossRef]
39. Pelissier Vatter, F.A.; Cioffi, M.; Hanna, S.J.; Castarede, I.; Caielli, S.; Pascual, V.; Matei, I.; Lyden, D. Extracellular Vesicle- and Particle-Mediated Communication Shapes Innate and Adaptive Immune Responses. *J. Exp. Med.* **2021**, *218*, e20202579. [CrossRef]
40. Okoye, I.S.; Coomes, S.M.; Pelly, V.S.; Czieso, S.; Papayannopoulos, V.; Tolmachova, T.; Seabra, M.C.; Wilson, M.S. MicroRNA-Containing T-Regulatory-Cell-Derived Exosomes Suppress Pathogenic T Helper 1 Cells. *Immunity* **2014**, *41*, 89–103. [CrossRef]
41. Banchereau, J.; Briere, F.; Caux, C.; Davoust, J.; Lebecque, S.; Liu, Y.J.; Pulendran, B.; Palucka, K. Immunobiology of Dendritic Cells. *Annu. Rev. Immunol.* **2000**, *18*, 767–811. [CrossRef] [PubMed]
42. Kambayashi, T.; Laufer, T.M. Atypical MHC Class II-Expressing Antigen-Presenting Cells: Can Anything Replace a Dendritic Cell? *Nat. Rev. Immunol.* **2014**, *14*, 719–730. [CrossRef] [PubMed]
43. Wculek, S.K.; Cueto, F.J.; Mujal, A.M.; Melero, I.; Krummel, M.F.; Sancho, D. Dendritic Cells in Cancer Immunology and Immunotherapy. *Nat. Rev. Immunol.* **2020**, *20*, 7–24. [CrossRef] [PubMed]
44. Sheng, K.-C.; Day, S.; Wright, M.D.; Stojanovska, L.; Apostolopoulos, V. Enhanced Dendritic Cell-Mediated Antigen-Specific CD4+ T Cell Responses: IFN-Gamma Aids TLR Stimulation. *J. Drug Deliv.* **2013**, *2013*, 516749. [CrossRef]
45. Segura, E.; Nicco, C.; Lombard, B.; Véron, P.; Raposo, G.; Batteux, F.; Amigorena, S.; Théry, C. ICAM-1 on Exosomes from Mature Dendritic Cells Is Critical for Efficient Naive T-Cell Priming. *Blood* **2005**, *106*, 216–223. [CrossRef]
46. Leone, D.A.; Rees, A.J.; Kain, R. Dendritic Cells and Routing Cargo into Exosomes. *Immunol. Cell Biol.* **2018**, *96*, 683–693. [CrossRef]
47. Mardpour, S.; Hamidieh, A.A.; Taleahmad, S.; Sharifzad, F.; Taghikhani, A.; Baharvand, H. Interaction between Mesenchymal Stromal Cell-Derived Extracellular Vesicles and Immune Cells by Distinct Protein Content. *J. Cell. Physiol.* **2019**, *234*, 8249–8258. [CrossRef]
48. Sprent, J. Direct Stimulation of Naïve T Cells by Antigen-Presenting Cell Vesicles. *Blood Cells. Mol. Dis.* **2005**, *35*, 17–20. [CrossRef]
49. Damo, M.; Wilson, D.S.; Simeoni, E.; Hubbell, J.A. TLR-3 Stimulation Improves Anti-Tumor Immunity Elicited by Dendritic Cell Exosome-Based Vaccines in a Murine Model of Melanoma. *Sci. Rep.* **2015**, *5*, 17622. [CrossRef]
50. Kiaie, S.H.; Mojarad-Jabali, S.; Khaleseh, F.; Allahyari, S.; Taheri, E.; Zakeri-Milani, P.; Valizadeh, H. Axial Pharmaceutical Properties of Liposome in Cancer Therapy: Recent Advances and Perspectives. *Int. J. Pharm.* **2020**, *581*, 119269. [CrossRef]
51. Ye, T.; Li, F.; Ma, G.; Wei, W. Enhancing Therapeutic Performance of Personalized Cancer Vaccine via Delivery Vectors. *Adv. Drug Deliv. Rev.* **2021**, *177*, 113927. [CrossRef] [PubMed]

52. Arbelaez, C.A.; Estrada, J.; Gessner, M.A.; Glaus, C.; Morales, A.B.; Mohn, D.; Phee, H.; Lipford, J.R.; Johnston, J.A. A Nanoparticle Vaccine That Targets Neoantigen Peptides to Lymphoid Tissues Elicits Robust Antitumor T Cell Responses. *Npj Vaccines* **2020**, *5*, 106. [CrossRef] [PubMed]
53. Tu, K.; Yu, Y.; Wang, Y.; Yang, T.; Hu, Q.; Qin, X.; Tu, J.; Yang, C.; Kong, L.; Zhang, Z. Combination of Chidamide-Mediated Epigenetic Modulation with Immunotherapy: Boosting Tumor Immunogenicity and Response to PD-1/PD-L1 Blockade. *ACS Appl. Mater. Interfaces* **2021**, *13*, 39003–39017. [CrossRef] [PubMed]
54. Zhang, R.; Tang, L.; Tian, Y.; Ji, X.; Hu, Q.; Zhou, B.; Ding, Z.; Xu, H.; Yang, L. DP7-C-Modified Liposomes Enhance Immune Responses and the Antitumor Effect of a Neoantigen-Based MRNA Vaccine. *J. Control. Release Off. J. Control. Release Soc.* **2020**, *328*, 210–221. [CrossRef] [PubMed]
55. Liang, R.; Xie, J.; Li, J.; Wang, K.; Liu, L.; Gao, Y.; Hussain, M.; Shen, G.; Zhu, J.; Tao, J. Liposomes-Coated Gold Nanocages with Antigens and Adjuvants Targeted Delivery to Dendritic Cells for Enhancing Antitumor Immune Response. *Biomaterials* **2017**, *149*, 41–50. [CrossRef]
56. Long, Q.; Zheng, P.; Zheng, X.; Li, W.; Hua, L.; Yang, Z.; Huang, W.; Ma, Y. Engineered Bacterial Membrane Vesicles Are Promising Carriers for Vaccine Design and Tumor Immunotherapy. *Adv. Drug Deliv. Rev.* **2022**, *186*, 114321. [CrossRef]
57. Allison, C.C.; Kufer, T.A.; Kremmer, E.; Kaparakis, M.; Ferrero, R.L. Helicobacter Pylori Induces MAPK Phosphorylation and AP-1 Activation via a NOD1-Dependent Mechanism. *J. Immunol. Baltim. Md. 1950* **2009**, *183*, 8099–8109. [CrossRef]
58. Söderblom, T.; Oxhamre, C.; Wai, S.N.; Uhlén, P.; Aperia, A.; Uhlin, B.E.; Richter-Dahlfors, A. Effects of the Escherichia Coli Toxin Cytolysin A on Mucosal Immunostimulation via Epithelial Ca^{2+} Signalling and Toll-like Receptor 4. *Cell. Microbiol.* **2005**, *7*, 779–788. [CrossRef]
59. Kaparakis, M.; Turnbull, L.; Carneiro, L.; Firth, S.; Coleman, H.A.; Parkington, H.C.; Le Bourhis, L.; Karrar, A.; Viala, J.; Mak, J.; et al. Bacterial Membrane Vesicles Deliver Peptidoglycan to NOD1 in Epithelial Cells. *Cell. Microbiol.* **2010**, *12*, 372–385. [CrossRef]
60. Hua, L.; Yang, Z.; Li, W.; Zhang, Q.; Ren, Z.; Ye, C.; Zheng, X.; Li, D.; Long, Q.; Bai, H.; et al. A Novel Immunomodulator Delivery Platform Based on Bacterial Biomimetic Vesicles for Enhanced Antitumor Immunity. *Adv. Mater. Deerfield Beach Fla.* **2021**, *33*, e2103923. [CrossRef]
61. Park, K.; Svennerholm, K.; Crescitelli, R.; Lässer, C.; Gribonika, I.; Lötvall, J. Synthetic Bacterial Vesicles Combined with Tumour Extracellular Vesicles as Cancer Immunotherapy. *J. Extracell. Vesicles* **2021**, *10*, e12120. [CrossRef] [PubMed]
62. Kim, J.H.; Lee, J.; Park, J.; Gho, Y.S. Gram-Negative and Gram-Positive Bacterial Extracellular Vesicles. *Semin. Cell Dev. Biol.* **2015**, *40*, 97–104. [CrossRef] [PubMed]
63. Liu, Q.; Liu, Q.; Yi, J.; Liang, K.; Liu, T.; Roland, K.L.; Jiang, Y.; Kong, Q. Outer Membrane Vesicles Derived from Salmonella Typhimurium Mutants with Truncated LPS Induce Cross-Protective Immune Responses against Infection of Salmonella Enterica Serovars in the Mouse Model. *Int. J. Med. Microbiol.* **2016**, *306*, 697–706. [CrossRef] [PubMed]
64. Kim, O.Y.; Park, H.T.; Dinh, N.T.H.; Choi, S.J.; Lee, J.; Kim, J.H.; Lee, S.-W.; Gho, Y.S. Bacterial Outer Membrane Vesicles Suppress Tumor by Interferon-γ-Mediated Antitumor Response. *Nat. Commun.* **2017**, *8*, 626. [CrossRef]
65. Bardi, G.T.; Smith, M.A.; Hood, J.L. Melanoma Exosomes Promote Mixed M1 and M2 Macrophage Polarization. *Cytokine* **2018**, *105*, 63–72. [CrossRef]
66. Liu, C.; Yu, S.; Zinn, K.; Wang, J.; Zhang, L.; Jia, Y.; Kappes, J.C.; Barnes, S.; Kimberly, R.P.; Grizzle, W.E.; et al. Murine Mammary Carcinoma Exosomes Promote Tumor Growth by Suppression of NK Cell Function. *J. Immunol. Baltim. Md. 1950* **2006**, *176*, 1375–1385. [CrossRef]
67. Chen, G.; Huang, A.C.; Zhang, W.; Zhang, G.; Wu, M.; Xu, W.; Yu, Z.; Yang, J.; Wang, B.; Sun, H.; et al. Exosomal PD-L1 Contributes to Immunosuppression and Is Associated with Anti-PD-1 Response. *Nature* **2018**, *560*, 382–386. [CrossRef]
68. Chen, Z.; You, L.; Wang, L.; Huang, X.; Liu, H.; Wei, J.Y.; Zhu, L.; Qian, W. Dual Effect of DLBCL-Derived EXOs in Lymphoma to Improve DC Vaccine Efficacy in Vitro While Favor Tumorgenesis in Vivo. *J. Exp. Clin. Cancer Res. CR* **2018**, *37*, 190. [CrossRef]
69. Wan, C.; Sun, Y.; Tian, Y.; Lu, L.; Dai, X.; Meng, J.; Huang, J.; He, Q.; Wu, B.; Zhang, Z.; et al. Irradiated Tumor Cell–Derived Microparticles Mediate Tumor Eradication via Cell Killing and Immune Reprogramming. *Sci. Adv.* **2020**, *6*, eaay9789. [CrossRef]
70. Veerman, R.E.; Güçlüler Akpinar, G.; Eldh, M.; Gabrielsson, S. Immune Cell-Derived Extracellular Vesicles—Functions and Therapeutic Applications. *Trends Mol. Med.* **2019**, *25*, 382–394. [CrossRef]
71. Ma, J.; Wei, K.; Zhang, H.; Tang, K.; Li, F.; Zhang, T.; Liu, J.; Xu, P.; Yu, Y.; Sun, W.; et al. Mechanisms by Which Dendritic Cells Present Tumor Microparticle Antigens to CD8(+) T Cells. *Cancer Immunol. Res.* **2018**, *6*, 1057–1068. [CrossRef] [PubMed]
72. Elsner, L.; Muppala, V.; Gehrmann, M.; Lozano, J.; Malzahn, D.; Bickeböller, H.; Brunner, E.; Zientkowska, M.; Herrmann, T.; Walter, L.; et al. The Heat Shock Protein HSP70 Promotes Mouse NK Cell Activity against Tumors That Express Inducible NKG2D Ligands. *J. Immunol. Baltim. Md. 1950* **2007**, *179*, 5523–5533. [CrossRef] [PubMed]
73. Taha, E.A.; Ono, K.; Eguchi, T. Roles of Extracellular HSPs as Biomarkers in Immune Surveillance and Immune Evasion. *Int. J. Mol. Sci.* **2019**, *20*, 4588. [CrossRef] [PubMed]
74. Gougousis, S.; Petanidis, S.; Poutoglidis, A.; Tsetsos, N.; Vrochidis, P.; Skoumpas, I.; Argyriou, N.; Katopodi, T.; Domvri, K. Epigenetic Editing and Tumor-dependent Immunosuppressive Signaling in Head and Neck Malignancies (Review). *Oncol. Lett.* **2022**, *23*, 196. [CrossRef] [PubMed]

75. Yin, Y.; Liu, B.; Cao, Y.; Yao, S.; Liu, Y.; Jin, G.; Qin, Y.; Chen, Y.; Cui, K.; Zhou, L.; et al. Colorectal Cancer-Derived Small Extracellular Vesicles Promote Tumor Immune Evasion by Upregulating PD-L1 Expression in Tumor-Associated Macrophages. *Adv. Sci. Weinh. Baden-Wurtt. Ger.* **2022**, *9*, 2102620. [CrossRef] [PubMed]
76. Mannavola, F.; D'Oronzo, S.; Cives, M.; Stucci, L.S.; Ranieri, G.; Silvestris, F.; Tucci, M. Extracellular Vesicles and Epigenetic Modifications Are Hallmarks of Melanoma Progression. *Int. J. Mol. Sci.* **2019**, *21*, 52. [CrossRef] [PubMed]
77. Jang, S.C.; Economides, K.D.; Moniz, R.J.; Sia, C.L.; Lewis, N.; McCoy, C.; Zi, T.; Zhang, K.; Harrison, R.A.; Lim, J.; et al. ExoSTING, an Extracellular Vesicle Loaded with STING Agonists, Promotes Tumor Immune Surveillance. *Commun. Biol.* **2021**, *4*, 497. [CrossRef]
78. Zhang, C.-X.; Ye, S.-B.; Ni, J.-J.; Cai, T.-T.; Liu, Y.-N.; Huang, D.-J.; Mai, H.-Q.; Chen, Q.-Y.; He, J.; Zhang, X.-S.; et al. STING Signaling Remodels the Tumor Microenvironment by Antagonizing Myeloid-Derived Suppressor Cell Expansion. *Cell Death Differ.* **2019**, *26*, 2314–2328. [CrossRef]
79. Kitai, Y.; Kawasaki, T.; Sueyoshi, T.; Kobiyama, K.; Ishii, K.J.; Zou, J.; Akira, S.; Matsuda, T.; Kawai, T. DNA-Containing Exosomes Derived from Cancer Cells Treated with Topotecan Activate a STING-Dependent Pathway and Reinforce Antitumor Immunity. *J. Immunol. Baltim. Md 1950* **2017**, *198*, 1649–1659. [CrossRef]
80. Chen, W.; Tan, Q.; Guo, M.; Liao, T.; Li, Y.; Yin, Z.; Zhou, E.; Deng, J.; Li, M.; Yang, Z.; et al. Tumor Cell-Derived Microparticles Packaging Monocarboxylate Transporter4 Inhibitor Fluvastatin Suppress Lung Adenocarcinoma via Tumor Microenvironment Remodeling and Improve Chemotherapy. *Chem. Eng. J.* **2023**, *451*, 138972. [CrossRef]
81. Zuo, B.; Zhang, Y.; Zhao, K.; Wu, L.; Qi, H.; Yang, R.; Gao, X.; Geng, M.; Wu, Y.; Jing, R.; et al. Universal Immunotherapeutic Strategy for Hepatocellular Carcinoma with Exosome Vaccines That Engage Adaptive and Innate Immune Responses. *J. Hematol. Oncol.* **2022**, *15*, 46. [CrossRef] [PubMed]
82. Tian, X.; Zhu, M.; Tian, Y.; Ramm, G.A.; Zhao, Y.; Nie, G. A Membrane Vesicle-Based Dual Vaccine against Melanoma and Lewis Lung Carcinoma. *Biomaterials* **2012**, *33*, 6147–6154. [CrossRef] [PubMed]
83. Zitvogel, L.; Regnault, A.; Lozier, A.; Wolfers, J.; Flament, C.; Tenza, D.; Ricciardi-Castagnoli, P.; Raposo, G.; Amigorena, S. Eradication of Established Murine Tumors Using a Novel Cell-Free Vaccine: Dendritic Cell-Derived Exosomes. *Nat. Med.* **1998**, *4*, 594–600. [CrossRef] [PubMed]
84. Théry, C.; Duban, L.; Segura, E.; Véron, P.; Lantz, O.; Amigorena, S. Indirect Activation of Naïve CD4+ T Cells by Dendritic Cell-Derived Exosomes. *Nat. Immunol.* **2002**, *3*, 1156–1162. [CrossRef] [PubMed]
85. Wahlund, C.J.E.; Güclüler, G.; Hiltbrunner, S.; Veerman, R.E.; Näslund, T.I.; Gabrielsson, S. Exosomes from Antigen-Pulsed Dendritic Cells Induce Stronger Antigen-Specific Immune Responses than Microvesicles in Vivo. *Sci. Rep.* **2017**, *7*, 17095. [CrossRef]
86. Admyre, C.; Johansson, S.M.; Paulie, S.; Gabrielsson, S. Direct Exosome Stimulation of Peripheral Human T Cells Detected by ELISPOT. *Eur. J. Immunol.* **2006**, *36*, 1772–1781. [CrossRef]
87. Mai, Y.; Guo, J.; Zhao, Y.; Ma, S.; Hou, Y.; Yang, J. Intranasal Delivery of Cationic Liposome-Protamine Complex MRNA Vaccine Elicits Effective Anti-Tumor Immunity. *Cell. Immunol.* **2020**, *354*, 104143. [CrossRef] [PubMed]
88. Wallis, J.; Katti, P.; Martin, A.M.; Hills, T.; Seymour, L.W.; Shenton, D.P.; Carlisle, R.C. A Liposome-Based Cancer Vaccine for a Rapid and High-Titre Anti-ErbB-2 Antibody Response. *Eur. J. Pharm. Sci. Off. J. Eur. Fed. Pharm. Sci.* **2020**, *152*, 105456. [CrossRef]
89. Affandi, A.J.; Grabowska, J.; Olesek, K.; Lopez Venegas, M.; Barbaria, A.; Rodríguez, E.; Mulder, P.P.G.; Pijffers, H.J.; Ambrosini, M.; Kalay, H.; et al. Selective Tumor Antigen Vaccine Delivery to Human CD169(+) Antigen-Presenting Cells Using Ganglioside-Liposomes. *Proc. Natl. Acad. Sci. USA* **2020**, *117*, 27528–27539. [CrossRef]
90. Okazaki, S.; Iwasaki, T.; Yuba, E.; Watarai, S. Evaluation of PH-Sensitive Fusogenic Polymer-Modified Liposomes Co-Loaded with Antigen and α-Galactosylceramide as an Anti-Tumor Vaccine. *J. Vet. Med. Sci.* **2018**, *80*, 197–204. [CrossRef]
91. Zhao, Y.; Wang, H.; Yang, Y.; Jia, W.; Su, T.; Che, Y.; Feng, Y.; Yuan, X.; Wang, X. Mannose-Modified Liposome Co-Delivery of Human Papillomavirus Type 16 E7 Peptide and CpG Oligodeoxynucleotide Adjuvant Enhances Antitumor Activity Against Established Large TC-1 Grafted Tumors in Mice. *Int. J. Nanomed.* **2020**, *15*, 9571–9586. [CrossRef] [PubMed]
92. Yang, R.; Wang, Z.; Yuan, Y.; Qian, T.; Zhou, Q. CRGD Target Liposome Delivery System Promoted Immunogenic Cell Death through Enhanced Anticancer Potency of a Thymidine Conjugate under UVA Activation as a Cancer Vaccine. *Eur. J. Med. Chem.* **2019**, *167*, 499–509. [CrossRef] [PubMed]
93. He, X.; Zhou, S.; Quinn, B.; Jahagirdar, D.; Ortega, J.; Abrams, S.I.; Lovell, J.F. HPV-Associated Tumor Eradication by Vaccination with Synthetic Short Peptides and Particle-Forming Liposomes. *Small Weinh. Bergstr. Ger.* **2021**, *17*, e2007165. [CrossRef] [PubMed]
94. He, X.; Zhou, S.; Huang, W.-C.; Seffouh, A.; Mabrouk, M.T.; Morgan, M.T.; Ortega, J.; Abrams, S.I.; Lovell, J.F. A Potent Cancer Vaccine Adjuvant System for Particleization of Short, Synthetic CD8(+) T Cell Epitopes. *ACS Nano* **2021**, *15*, 4357–4371. [CrossRef]
95. Liu, X.; Liu, Y.; Li, X.; Huang, J.; Guo, X.; Zhang, J.; Luo, Z.; Shi, Y.; Jiang, M.; Qin, B.; et al. ER-Targeting PDT Converts Tumors into In Situ Therapeutic Tumor Vaccines. *ACS Nano* **2022**, *16*, 9240–9253. [CrossRef]
96. Grippin, A.J.; Wummer, B.; Wildes, T.; Dyson, K.; Trivedi, V.; Yang, C.; Sebastian, M.; Mendez-Gomez, H.R.; Padala, S.; Grubb, M.; et al. Dendritic Cell-Activating Magnetic Nanoparticles Enable Early Prediction of Antitumor Response with Magnetic Resonance Imaging. *ACS Nano* **2019**, *13*, 13884–13898. [CrossRef]
97. Verbeke, R.; Lentacker, I.; Breckpot, K.; Janssens, J.; Van Calenbergh, S.; De Smedt, S.C.; Dewitte, H. Broadening the Message: A Nanovaccine Co-Loaded with Messenger RNA and α-GalCer Induces Antitumor Immunity through Conventional and Natural Killer T Cells. *ACS Nano* **2019**, *13*, 1655–1669. [CrossRef]

98. Liu, F.; Dai, Z.; Cheng, Q.; Xu, L.; Huang, L.; Liu, Z.; Li, X.; Wang, N.; Wang, G.; Wang, L.; et al. LncRNA-Targeting Bio-Scaffold Mediates Triple Immune Effects for Postoperative Colorectal Cancer Immunotherapy. *Biomaterials* **2022**, *284*, 121485. [CrossRef]
99. Sayour, E.J.; Grippin, A.; De Leon, G.; Stover, B.; Rahman, M.; Karachi, A.; Wummer, B.; Moore, G.; Castillo-Caro, P.; Fredenburg, K.; et al. Personalized Tumor RNA Loaded Lipid-Nanoparticles Prime the Systemic and Intratumoral Milieu for Response to Cancer Immunotherapy. *Nano Lett.* **2018**, *18*, 6195–6206. [CrossRef]
100. Deng, C.; Zhang, Q.; Jia, M.; Zhao, J.; Sun, X.; Gong, T.; Zhang, Z. Tumors and Their Microenvironment Dual-Targeting Chemotherapy with Local Immune Adjuvant Therapy for Effective Antitumor Immunity against Breast Cancer. *Adv. Sci.* **2019**, *6*, 1801868. [CrossRef]
101. Kim, O.Y.; Choi, S.J.; Jang, S.C.; Park, K.-S.; Kim, S.R.; Choi, J.P.; Lim, J.H.; Lee, S.-W.; Park, J.; Di Vizio, D.; et al. Bacterial Protoplast-Derived Nanovesicles as Vaccine Delivery System against Bacterial Infection. *Nano Lett.* **2015**, *15*, 266–274. [CrossRef] [PubMed]
102. Klimentová, J.; Stulík, J. Methods of Isolation and Purification of Outer Membrane Vesicles from Gram-Negative Bacteria. *Microbiol. Res.* **2015**, *170*, 1–9. [CrossRef] [PubMed]
103. Naciute, M.; Kiwitt, T.; Kemp, R.A.; Hook, S. Bacteria Biohybrid Oral Vaccines for Colorectal Cancer Treatment Reduce Tumor Growth and Increase Immune Infiltration. *Vaccine* **2021**, *39*, 5589–5599. [CrossRef] [PubMed]
104. Li, Y.; Ma, X.; Yue, Y.; Zhang, K.; Cheng, K.; Feng, Q.; Ma, N.; Liang, J.; Zhang, T.; Zhang, L.; et al. Rapid Surface Display of MRNA Antigens by Bacteria-Derived Outer Membrane Vesicles for a Personalized Tumor Vaccine. *Adv. Mater. Deerfield Beach Fla.* **2022**, *34*, e2109984. [CrossRef] [PubMed]
105. Zhuang, W.-R.; Wang, Y.; Lei, Y.; Zuo, L.; Jiang, A.; Wu, G.; Nie, W.; Huang, L.-L.; Xie, H.-Y. Phytochemical Engineered Bacterial Outer Membrane Vesicles for Photodynamic Effects Promoted Immunotherapy. *Nano Lett.* **2022**, *22*, 4491–4500. [CrossRef] [PubMed]
106. Yue, Y.; Xu, J.; Li, Y.; Cheng, K.; Feng, Q.; Ma, X.; Ma, N.; Zhang, T.; Wang, X.; Zhao, X.; et al. Antigen-Bearing Outer Membrane Vesicles as Tumour Vaccines Produced in Situ by Ingested Genetically Engineered Bacteria. *Nat. Biomed. Eng.* **2022**, *6*, 898–909. [CrossRef]
107. Li, Y.; Zhang, K.; Wu, Y.; Yue, Y.; Cheng, K.; Feng, Q.; Ma, X.; Liang, J.; Ma, N.; Liu, G.; et al. Antigen Capture and Immune Modulation by Bacterial Outer Membrane Vesicles as In Situ Vaccine for Cancer Immunotherapy Post-Photothermal Therapy. *Small Weinh. Bergstr. Ger.* **2022**, *18*, e2107461. [CrossRef] [PubMed]
108. Cheng, K.; Zhao, R.; Li, Y.; Qi, Y.; Wang, Y.; Zhang, Y.; Qin, H.; Qin, Y.; Chen, L.; Li, C.; et al. Bioengineered Bacteria-Derived Outer Membrane Vesicles as a Versatile Antigen Display Platform for Tumor Vaccination via Plug-and-Display Technology. *Nat. Commun.* **2021**, *12*, 2041. [CrossRef]
109. Chen, Q.; Huang, G.; Wu, W.; Wang, J.; Hu, J.; Mao, J.; Chu, P.K.; Bai, H.; Tang, G. A Hybrid Eukaryotic-Prokaryotic Nanoplatform with Photothermal Modality for Enhanced Antitumor Vaccination. *Adv. Mater. Deerfield Beach Fla.* **2020**, *32*, e1908185. [CrossRef]
110. Li, Y.; Zhao, R.; Cheng, K.; Zhang, K.; Wang, Y.; Zhang, Y.; Li, Y.; Liu, G.; Xu, J.; Xu, J.; et al. Bacterial Outer Membrane Vesicles Presenting Programmed Death 1 for Improved Cancer Immunotherapy via Immune Activation and Checkpoint Inhibition. *ACS Nano* **2020**, *14*, 16698–16711. [CrossRef]
111. Aly, R.G.; El-Enbaawy, M.I.; Abd El-Rahman, S.S.; Ata, N.S. Antineoplastic Activity of Salmonella Typhimurium Outer Membrane Nanovesicles. *Exp. Cell Res.* **2021**, *399*, 112423. [CrossRef] [PubMed]
112. Zhao, H.; Zhao, B.; Wu, L.; Xiao, H.; Ding, K.; Zheng, C.; Song, Q.; Sun, L.; Wang, L.; Zhang, Z. Amplified Cancer Immunotherapy of a Surface-Engineered Antigenic Microparticle Vaccine by Synergistically Modulating Tumor Microenvironment. *ACS Nano* **2019**, *13*, 12553–12566. [CrossRef] [PubMed]
113. Lin, W.; Xu, Y.; Chen, X.; Liu, J.; Weng, Y.; Zhuang, Q.; Lin, F.; Huang, Z.; Wu, S.; Ding, J.; et al. Radiation-Induced Small Extracellular Vesicles as "Carriages" Promote Tumor Antigen Release and Trigger Antitumor Immunity. *Theranostics* **2020**, *10*, 4871–4884. [CrossRef] [PubMed]
114. Dusoswa, S.A.; Horrevorts, S.K.; Ambrosini, M.; Kalay, H.; Paauw, N.J.; Nieuwland, R.; Pegtel, M.D.; Würdinger, T.; Van Kooyk, Y.; Garcia-Vallejo, J.J. Glycan Modification of Glioblastoma-Derived Extracellular Vesicles Enhances Receptor-Mediated Targeting of Dendritic Cells. *J. Extracell. Vesicles* **2019**, *8*, 1648995. [CrossRef] [PubMed]
115. Huang, L.; Rong, Y.; Tang, X.; Yi, K.; Qi, P.; Hou, J.; Liu, W.; He, Y.; Gao, X.; Yuan, C.; et al. Engineered Exosomes as an in Situ DC-Primed Vaccine to Boost Antitumor Immunity in Breast Cancer. *Mol. Cancer* **2022**, *21*, 45. [CrossRef]
116. Matsumoto, A.; Takahashi, Y.; Ariizumi, R.; Nishikawa, M.; Takakura, Y. Development of DNA-Anchored Assembly of Small Extracellular Vesicle for Efficient Antigen Delivery to Antigen Presenting Cells. *Biomaterials* **2019**, *225*, 119518. [CrossRef]
117. Zhou, W.; Chen, X.; Zhou, Y.; Shi, S.; Liang, C.; Yu, X.; Chen, H.; Guo, Q.; Zhang, Y.; Liu, P.; et al. Exosomes Derived from Immunogenically Dying Tumor Cells as a Versatile Tool for Vaccination against Pancreatic Cancer. *Biomaterials* **2022**, *280*, 121306. [CrossRef]
118. Pineda, B.; Sánchez García, F.J.; Olascoaga, N.K.; Pérez de la Cruz, V.; Salazar, A.; Moreno-Jiménez, S.; Hernández Pedro, N.; Márquez-Navarro, A.; Ortiz Plata, A.; Sotelo, J. Malignant Glioma Therapy by Vaccination with Irradiated C6 Cell-Derived Microvesicles Promotes an Antitumoral Immune Response. *Mol. Ther. J. Am. Soc. Gene Ther.* **2019**, *27*, 1612–1620. [CrossRef]
119. Diamond, J.M.; Vanpouille-Box, C.; Spada, S.; Rudqvist, N.-P.; Chapman, J.R.; Ueberheide, B.M.; Pilones, K.A.; Sarfraz, Y.; Formenti, S.C.; Demaria, S. Exosomes Shuttle TREX1-Sensitive IFN-Stimulatory DsDNA from Irradiated Cancer Cells to DCs. *Cancer Immunol. Res.* **2018**, *6*, 910–920. [CrossRef]

120. Zuo, B.; Qi, H.; Lu, Z.; Chen, L.; Sun, B.; Yang, R.; Zhang, Y.; Liu, Z.; Gao, X.; You, A.; et al. Alarmin-Painted Exosomes Elicit Persistent Antitumor Immunity in Large Established Tumors in Mice. *Nat. Commun.* **2020**, *11*, 1790. [CrossRef]
121. Taghikhani, A.; Hassan, Z.M.; Ebrahimi, M.; Moazzeni, S.-M. MicroRNA Modified Tumor-Derived Exosomes as Novel Tools for Maturation of Dendritic Cells. *J. Cell. Physiol.* **2019**, *234*, 9417–9427. [CrossRef] [PubMed]
122. Huang, F.; Li, Z.; Zhang, W.; Li, J.; Hao, S. Enhancing the Anti-Leukemia Immunity of Acute Lymphocytic Leukemia-Derived Exosome-Based Vaccine by Downregulation of PD-L1 Expression. *Cancer Immunol. Immunother. CII* **2022**, *71*, 2197–2212. [CrossRef] [PubMed]
123. Viaud, S.; Théry, C.; Ploix, S.; Tursz, T.; Lapierre, V.; Lantz, O.; Zitvogel, L.; Chaput, N. Dendritic Cell-Derived Exosomes for Cancer Immunotherapy: What's Next? *Cancer Res.* **2010**, *70*, 1281–1285. [CrossRef] [PubMed]
124. Cao, H.; Gao, H.; Wang, L.; Cheng, Y.; Wu, X.; Shen, X.; Wang, H.; Wang, Z.; Zhan, P.; Liu, J.; et al. Biosynthetic Dendritic Cell-Exocytosed Aggregation-Induced Emission Nanoparticles for Synergistic Photodynamic Immunotherapy. *ACS Nano* **2022**, *16*, 13992–14006. [CrossRef]
125. Xiong, X.; Ke, X.; Wang, L.; Lin, Y.; Wang, S.; Yao, Z.; Li, K.; Luo, Y.; Liu, F.; Pan, Y.; et al. Neoantigen-Based Cancer Vaccination Using Chimeric RNA-Loaded Dendritic Cell-Derived Extracellular Vesicles. *J. Extracell. Vesicles* **2022**, *11*, e12243. [CrossRef]
126. Lu, Z.; Zuo, B.; Jing, R.; Gao, X.; Rao, Q.; Liu, Z.; Qi, H.; Guo, H.; Yin, H. Dendritic Cell-Derived Exosomes Elicit Tumor Regression in Autochthonous Hepatocellular Carcinoma Mouse Models. *J. Hepatol.* **2017**, *67*, 739–748. [CrossRef]
127. Zhu, H.; Wang, K.; Wang, Z.; Wang, D.; Yin, X.; Liu, Y.; Yu, F.; Zhao, W. An Efficient and Safe MUC1-Dendritic Cell-Derived Exosome Conjugate Vaccine Elicits Potent Cellular and Humoral Immunity and Tumor Inhibition in Vivo. *Acta Biomater.* **2022**, *138*, 491–504. [CrossRef]
128. Phung, C.D.; Pham, T.T.; Nguyen, H.T.; Nguyen, T.T.; Ou, W.; Jeong, J.-H.; Choi, H.-G.; Ku, S.K.; Yong, C.S.; Kim, J.O. Anti-CTLA-4 Antibody-Functionalized Dendritic Cell-Derived Exosomes Targeting Tumor-Draining Lymph Nodes for Effective Induction of Antitumor T-Cell Responses. *Acta Biomater.* **2020**, *115*, 371–382. [CrossRef]
129. Chen, S.; Lv, M.; Fang, S.; Ye, W.; Gao, Y.; Xu, Y. Poly(I:C) Enhanced Anti-Cervical Cancer Immunities Induced by Dendritic Cells-Derived Exosomes. *Int. J. Biol. Macromol.* **2018**, *113*, 1182–1187. [CrossRef]
130. Than, U.T.T.; Le, H.T.; Hoang, D.H.; Nguyen, X.-H.; Pham, C.T.; Bui, K.T.V.; Bui, H.T.H.; Nguyen, P.V.; Nguyen, T.D.; Do, T.T.H.; et al. Induction of Antitumor Immunity by Exosomes Isolated from Cryopreserved Cord Blood Monocyte-Derived Dendritic Cells. *Int. J. Mol. Sci.* **2020**, *21*, 1834. [CrossRef]
131. Wadman, M. Public Needs to Prep for Vaccine Side Effects. *Science* **2020**, *370*, 1022. [CrossRef] [PubMed]
132. Papachristofilou, A.; Hipp, M.M.; Klinkhardt, U.; Früh, M.; Sebastian, M.; Weiss, C.; Pless, M.; Cathomas, R.; Hilbe, W.; Pall, G.; et al. Phase Ib Evaluation of a Self-Adjuvanted Protamine Formulated MRNA-Based Active Cancer Immunotherapy, BI1361849 (CV9202), Combined with Local Radiation Treatment in Patients with Stage IV Non-Small Cell Lung Cancer. *J. Immunother. Cancer* **2019**, *7*, 38. [CrossRef] [PubMed]
133. Huang, T.; Peng, L.; Han, Y.; Wang, D.; He, X.; Wang, J.; Ou, C. Lipid Nanoparticle-Based MRNA Vaccines in Cancers: Current Advances and Future Prospects. *Front. Immunol.* **2022**, *13*, 922301. [CrossRef] [PubMed]
134. Xie, J.; Li, Q.; Haesebrouck, F.; Van Hoecke, L.; Vandenbroucke, R.E. The Tremendous Biomedical Potential of Bacterial Extracellular Vesicles. *Trends Biotechnol.* **2022**, *40*, 1173–1194. [CrossRef] [PubMed]
135. Johnson, P.V.; Blair, B.M.; Zeller, S.; Kotton, C.N.; Hohmann, E.L. Attenuated Listeria Monocytogenes Vaccine Vectors Expressing Influenza A Nucleoprotein: Preclinical Evaluation and Oral Inoculation of Volunteers. *Microbiol. Immunol.* **2011**, *55*, 304–317. [CrossRef]
136. Li, M.; Zhou, H.; Yang, C.; Wu, Y.; Zhou, X.; Liu, H.; Wang, Y. Bacterial Outer Membrane Vesicles as a Platform for Biomedical Applications: An Update. *J. Control. Release Off. J. Control. Release Soc.* **2020**, *323*, 253–268. [CrossRef]
137. Cheng, K.; Kang, Q.; Zhao, X. Biogenic Nanoparticles as Immunomodulator for Tumor Treatment. *Wiley Interdiscip. Rev. Nanomed. Nanobiotechnol.* **2020**, *12*, e1646. [CrossRef]
138. Guo, M.; Wu, F.; Hu, G.; Chen, L.; Xu, J.; Xu, P.; Wang, X.; Li, Y.; Liu, S.; Zhang, S.; et al. Autologous Tumor Cell–Derived Microparticle-Based Targeted Chemotherapy in Lung Cancer Patients with Malignant Pleural Effusion. *Sci. Transl. Med.* **2019**, *11*, eaat5690. [CrossRef]
139. Kantoff, P.W.; Higano, C.S.; Shore, N.D.; Berger, E.R.; Small, E.J.; Penson, D.F.; Redfern, C.H.; Ferrari, A.C.; Dreicer, R.; Sims, R.B.; et al. Sipuleucel-T Immunotherapy for Castration-Resistant Prostate Cancer. *N. Engl. J. Med.* **2010**, *363*, 411–422. [CrossRef]
140. Narita, M.; Kanda, T.; Abe, T.; Uchiyama, T.; Iwafuchi, M.; Zheng, Z.; Liu, A.; Kaifu, T.; Kosugi, S.; Minagawa, M.; et al. Immune Responses in Patients with Esophageal Cancer Treated with SART1 Peptide-Pulsed Dendritic Cell Vaccine. *Int. J. Oncol.* **2015**, *46*, 1699–1709. [CrossRef]
141. Zhou, J.; Kroll, A.V.; Holay, M.; Fang, R.H.; Zhang, L. Biomimetic Nanotechnology toward Personalized Vaccines. *Adv. Mater. Deerfield Beach Fla.* **2020**, *32*, e1901255. [CrossRef] [PubMed]
142. Cao, M.; Isaac, R.; Yan, W.; Ruan, X.; Jiang, L.; Wan, Y.; Wang, J.; Wang, E.; Caron, C.; Neben, S.; et al. Cancer-Cell-Secreted Extracellular Vesicles Suppress Insulin Secretion through MiR-122 to Impair Systemic Glucose Homeostasis and Contribute to Tumour Growth. *Nat. Cell Biol.* **2022**, *24*, 954–967. [CrossRef] [PubMed]
143. Görgens, A.; Corso, G.; Hagey, D.W.; Jawad Wiklander, R.; Gustafsson, M.O.; Felldin, U.; Lee, Y.; Bostancioglu, R.B.; Sork, H.; Liang, X.; et al. Identification of Storage Conditions Stabilizing Extracellular Vesicles Preparations. *J. Extracell. Vesicles* **2022**, *11*, e12238. [CrossRef]

144. Kudo, K.; Miki, Y.; Carreras, J.; Nakayama, S.; Nakamoto, Y.; Ito, M.; Nagashima, E.; Yamamoto, K.; Higuchi, H.; Morita, S.-Y.; et al. Secreted Phospholipase A(2) Modifies Extracellular Vesicles and Accelerates B Cell Lymphoma. *Cell Metab.* **2022**, *34*, 615–633.e8. [CrossRef]
145. Xiao, Y.; Tian, J.; Wu, W.-C.; Gao, Y.-H.; Guo, Y.-X.; Song, S.-J.; Gao, R.; Wang, L.-B.; Wu, X.-Y.; Zhang, Y.; et al. Targeting Central Nervous System Extracellular Vesicles Enhanced Triiodothyronine Remyelination Effect on Experimental Autoimmune Encephalomyelitis. *Bioact. Mater.* **2022**, *9*, 373–384. [CrossRef] [PubMed]

pharmaceutics

MDPI

Review

Multifunctional Milk-Derived Small Extracellular Vesicles and Their Biomedical Applications

Youxiu Zhong [1], Xudong Wang [1], Xian Zhao [1], Jiuheng Shen [1], Xue Wu [1], Peifen Gao [1], Peng Yang [1], Junge Chen [2,*] and Wenlin An [1,*]

1 Wenlin An's Laboratory, National Vaccine & Serum Institute (NVSI), China National Biotech Group (CNBG), Sinopharm Group, No. 38 Jing Hai Second Road, Beijing 101111, China
2 Beijing Advanced Innovation Center for Biomedical Engineering, School of Engineering Medicine & Shenzhen Institute of Beihang University, Beihang University, Beijing 100083, China
* Correspondence: chenjg19@buaa.edu.cn (J.C.); anwenlin@sinopharm.com (W.A.)

Abstract: In recent years, small extracellular vesicles (sEVs) have been regarded as the next generation of novel delivery systems after lipid nanoparticles because of their advantages and huge prospects in drug delivery. Studies have shown that sEVs are abundant in milk and therefore can be a large and economical source of sEVs. Natural milk-derived small extracellular vesicles (msEVs) have important functions such as immune regulation, anti-bacterial infection, anti-oxidative, etc., and play a beneficial role in human health at multiple levels, including intestinal health, bone/muscle metabolism, and microbiota regulation. In addition, because they can pass the gastrointestinal barrier and have low immunogenicity, good biocompatibility, and stability, msEVs are considered a crucial oral drug delivery vehicle. Moreover, msEVs can be further engineered for targeted delivery to prolong the circulation time or enhance local drug concentrations. However, msEVs separation and purification, complex contents, and quality control hinder their application in drug delivery. This paper provides a comprehensive review of the biogenesis and characteristics, isolation and purification, composition, loading methods, and function of msEVs, based on which their applications in biomedical fields are further explored.

Keywords: milk-derived small extracellular vesicles (msEVs); small extracellular vesicles (sEVs) engineering; isolation and purification; drug delivery; biopharmaceutical applications

Citation: Zhong, Y.; Wang, X.; Zhao, X.; Shen, J.; Wu, X.; Gao, P.; Yang, P.; Chen, J.; An, W. Multifunctional Milk-Derived Small Extracellular Vesicles and Their Biomedical Applications. *Pharmaceutics* **2023**, *15*, 1418. https://doi.org/10.3390/pharmaceutics15051418

Academic Editor: Dong Keun Han

Received: 27 February 2023
Revised: 25 April 2023
Accepted: 3 May 2023
Published: 6 May 2023

1. Introduction

sEVs are biological nanovesicles that range in size from 30 to 150 nm, and cells continuously secrete or accept sEV from other cell sources [1]. Almost all cells are capable of secreting sEVs in normal or abnormal physiological states [2], which are present in the fluids of the eukaryotic body (e.g., saliva, blood, urine, amniotic fluid, etc.), plant juices, and supernatants of cultured cells, and different environmental factors and health conditions can affect the composition of sEVs [3–5]. Among these sources, milk is utilized with great interest due to its large yield, easy availability, and high sEVs content, which endow it with great potential in clinical applications. In milk, sEVs play significant roles in immune defense, growth, and physiological regulation via nucleic acids, proteins, sugars, etc. [6–9]. Being different from the other sEVs from body fluids, milk sEVs stay the same upon subjecting them to highly acidic conditions as well as digestive enzymes in gastroenteric environments.

Nowadays, sEV biomarkers include CD9, CD63, CD81, TSG101, HSP70, etc. [10–13]. sEVs are regarded as a crucial communication intermediary for cells [14]. Donor cells are capable of transferring important information or functional substances (e.g., proteins, nucleic acids, and lipids) to responsive cells through sEVs. Information and substance delivery by sEVs play a crucial role in several biological activities [15,16]. Thus, sEVs can be utilized to assess normal physiological changes or mechanisms of disease onset and progression. In addition, sEVs can be used as biomarkers of a variety of diseases for disease detection.

Over the past decades, nano-drug delivery systems have made significant progress, including various formulations for biomolecular and chemical drugs [17–19]. Nevertheless, two challenges, such as poor biocompatibility and short blood circulation, need to be overcome for these delivery systems before practical applications [20]. Due to their unique natural properties, sEVs are considered the next generation of highly promising delivery vehicles after lipid nanoparticles [21]. CD47, which is present on the surface of sEVs, prevents recognition by macrophages, therefore facilitating the prolongation of sEV circulation in the blood. It is demonstrated that the integrity of msEVs bilayers can be sustained in vitro for a long time, even under strong acid in the stomach and degradation in the intestine. Furthermore, they can reach the target tissue through the biological barrier. As a member of the sEVs family, msEVs are considered potentially excellent drug vehicles, especially the oral route, in terms of stability, toxicity, and cost [22].

This review summarizes the important and advantageous implications of msEVs on human health from several perspectives. A comprehensive outlook on the future functional and application development of msEVs is provided by summarizing the strategies related to the purification and drug loading of msEVs. Moreover, new forms of sEV applications, such as engineering modifications, are also reviewed. On this basis, we analyze the challenges faced in the application development of msEVs. The outline of the review is shown in Figure 1.

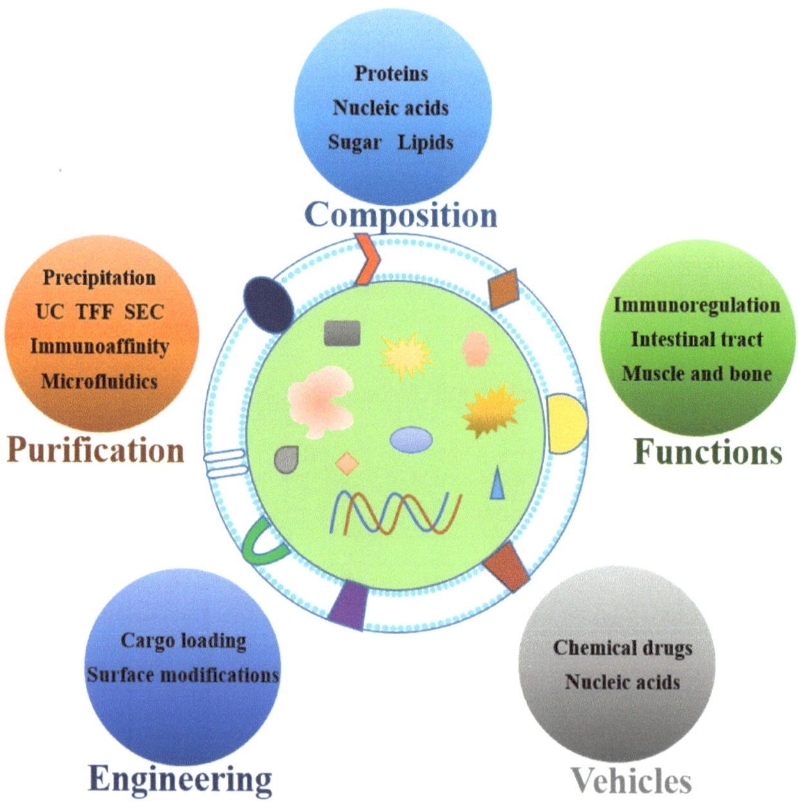

Figure 1. Overall framework of the full text.

2. Biogenesis and Characteristics of sEVs

Extracellular vesicles are categorized according to the biosynthesis or release pathway: sEVs have a diameter of 30–150 nm and are generated from the endocytic pathway; from the plasma membrane, particulate/micro-vesicles are released immediately and are about 100–1000 nm in diameter; apoptotic vesicles are about 50 nm–2 μm in diameter and are generated by apoptosis. The current most hotly studied subgroup is the sEVs.

sEV biogenesis is a strictly controlled procedure consisting of three distinct stages: endocytic vesicle formation through plasma membrane invagination, multivesicular body formation through endosomal growth, and plasma membrane fusion, which results in the release of vesicles from multivesicular bodies, as shown in Figure 2. sEVs formation relies upon the endosomal sorting complex required for transport (ESCRT) and some GTP-binding protein-directed mechanisms [23–25]. In the early stage, the plasma membrane develops inward to give rise to the early endosomes, which change into mature late endosomes by degrees. In this process, material from the cell is selectively absorbed into luminal vesicles in the endosome, controlled by the ESCRT mechanism [26]. However, it has been demonstrated that sEVs can form in the absence of important components of four ESCRT complexes, suggesting that there are other modes of sEV formation [27]. In addition to the ESCRT protein family, lipids and several other proteins, such as lactadherins, platelet-derived growth factor receptors, membrane associates, microsomal proteins, GTPases, HSP, and quadruple transmembrane proteins, also participate in the biological process that produces sEVs [28–30]. It has been proven that lipids play a crucial role in vesicle biogenesis and transport, such as membrane deformation, fission, and fusion [31].

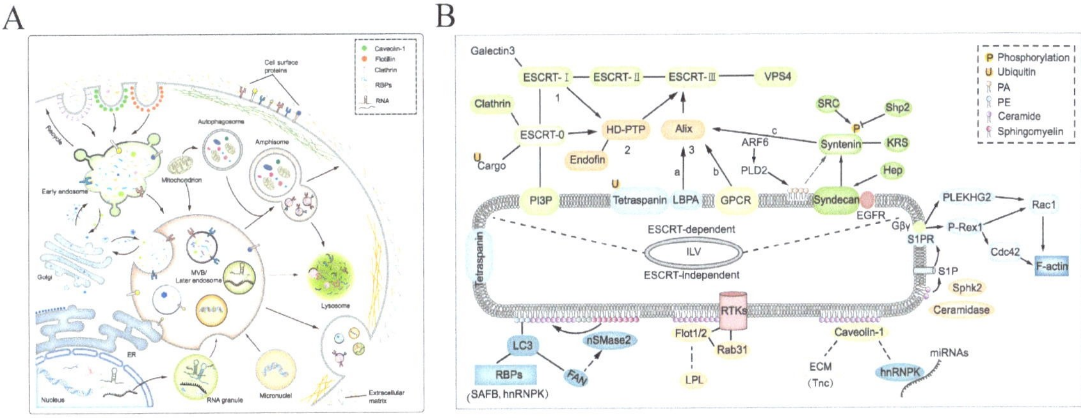

Figure 2. Overview of the process for sEV biogenesis (**A**) and multiple mechanisms (**B**); Copyright 2022, Springer Nature [32].

SEVs protein composition is inextricably linked to the type of cell or tissue from which they come. sEVs typically contain fusion proteins and membrane transport, and most sEVs have integrins, HSP, ALIX, members of the transmembrane 4 superfamily, and the Ras-associated protein GTPases Rab. The surfaces of both colostrum and msEVs contain surface markers: four transmembrane proteins (including CD63, CD9, CD81, and TM4SF), milk fat globule epidermal growth factor 8, raft-associated proteins, and internal signature proteins such as TSG101, ALIX, and HSP70 [33,34]. The endosomal sorting complexes or additional related factors such as TSG101 and ALIX participate in sEV genesis and can therefore be detected. All of these can be utilized as trustworthy sEVs identification markers, as shown in Table 1. sEVs do not contain p-selectin, integrin-β1, CD40, or calnexin, which are thought to be markers of vesicles of other origin. Differences in sEV compositions, especially in surface proteins, have a great influence on the recipient cells. sEVs surface expression of specific markers makes it possible to purify and identify specific groups of sEVs.

sEVs often require uptake by receptor cells to exert their function. MsEV trafficking in Caco-2 cells, human vascular endothelial cells, and IEC-6 cells is mediated by endocytosis [35,36]. This endocytosis-mediated msEVs uptake is dependent on cellular and msEVs surface glycoproteins in the rat and human intestines [35]. Due to the metabolic function of the liver, sEVs or msEVs accumulate mainly in the liver.

Table 1. sEVs common protein markers.

sEVs Proteins	MW (kDa)	Classification	Function	Specimen Source
CD63	63	Four transmembrane proteins	It is a lysosomal membrane protein with the activity of activating platelet surface antigens;	Bovine milk [34,36,37], mesenchymal stromal cells [38], and plasma [39,40];
CD9	24–27	Four transmembrane proteins	Participate in the interaction between cells and the outside world;	Bovine milk [36], mesenchymal stem cells [41,42], and saliva [43,44];
CD81	81	Four transmembrane proteins	Key structural sites for perceiving external signals in cells;	Bovine milk [37,45], synovial fluid [46], and cerebrospinal fluid [47];
TSG101	44	Internal signature proteins	A component of the functional ESCRT-I complex that regulates vesicular transport;	Bovine milk [34,48], rat serum [40], and bile [49];
ALIX	95	Internal signature proteins	A phylogenetically conserved cytosolic scaffold protein;	Bovine milk [34,36,48], brain [50], and fibroblast [51];
HSP70	70	Internal signature proteins	It is an important member of the heat shock protein family.	Bovine milk [34,45], plasma [39,44], and urine [52,53].

3. Isolation and Purification of msEVs

How to obtain large amounts of high-purity sEVs is the primary problem to be solved to expand their application. Although many easy-to-use commercial kits have been developed, the generation of sEVs produced from milk on a huge scale for clinical use cannot be fundamentally solved by kits. The common purification methods for msEVs are comparable to traditional sEV purification techniques, including polyethylene glycol (PEG) precipitation, ultracentrifugation, density gradient centrifugation, ultrafiltration centrifugation, immunoaffinity capture, size-exclusion chromatography (SEC), and microfluidic techniques [54–56], as shown in Table 2.

Table 2. Common methods of sEV separation.

Separation Method	Principle	Purity	Production	Time Consuming	References
PEG precipitation purification	Macromolecule aggregation precipitation;	+	+++	+	[57]
Ultracentrifugation	Difference of sedimentation coefficient;	++	++	++	[53,58,59]
Density gradient centrifugation	Density gradient difference;	+++	+	+++	[60]
Ultrafiltration centrifugation	Specific molecular weight cutoff;	++	+++	+	[61]
Tangential Flow Filtration	Tangential filtering;	++	+++	+	[62]
Size exclusion chromatography	Particle size difference;	+++	++	++	[63–65]
Affinity purification	Intermolecular specific binding.	++++	+	++	[66]

Note: The "+" in the table represents different degrees, and the more "+", the higher the degree.

3.1. Common Methods for sEV Purification

PEG precipitation purification is a method of coagulation and precipitation of large molecules of solutes caused by the addition of very hydrophilic PEG at specific salt concentration conditions and is commonly used for the isolation of proteins, nucleic acids, viruses, etc. sEVs have similar size and physicochemical properties to viruses. Therefore, PEG co-precipitation can be used to isolate sEVs, and PEG precipitation is also a commonly used method for commercial kits [57]. By employing this strategy, sEVs could be obtained with filtration or low-speed centrifugation without the need for special equipment. However, the purity of sEVs is low on account of coprecipitation proteins and polymers.

Currently, the most commonly used approach for purifying sEVs is ultracentrifugation [53]. The steps of low-speed centrifugation and high-speed centrifugation are mainly used in sequence: low-speed centrifugation can be used to separate milk's floating fat and some free proteins, while ultracentrifugation is used to separate the majority of the cell waste and free proteins. Finally, clear jelly-like sEV aggregates can be observed in the centrifuge tube's bottom, and sEVs of uniform size are gradually separated [58,59]. The current gold standard for sEV purification is ultracentrifugation. However, the purity of sEVs obtained by ultracentrifugation is still not guaranteed, and the sEV structure may be disrupted by repeated centrifugation. In order to improve their purity, density gradient centrifugation is carried out by layering a decreasing concentration of sucrose solution or iodixanol solution. sEVs are enriched mostly in the density range of 1.13–1.21 g/mL when subjected to a particular centrifugal force. Using this method, sEVs can be separated with high purity. Izumi et al. separated bovine msEVs by ultracentrifugation [58]. In order to improve their purity, the msEVs were washed twice to remove impurities such as proteins and lipids. By ultracentrifugation, proteins and lipoproteins in msEVs can be removed. In addition, Linares et al. pointed out that high-speed centrifugation leads to sEV aggregation, which can affect subsequent data processing [50]. Furthermore, the collection time is relatively high and the process is tedious, which limits the practical application of isolating sEVs on a large scale [44].

With a specific molecular weight cutoff, sEVs are separated by ultrafiltration centrifugation through an ultrafiltration membrane. sEVs relative molecular weight differs significantly from other impurities, and the use of membranes with appropriate molecular mass cutoffs allows the separation of sEVs from other biomolecules. Lobb and his colleagues have compared ultracentrifugation and ultrafiltration for sEV isolation, demonstrating that the isolation time of ultrafiltration (20 min) was much less than that of ultracentrifugation (180 min) [46]. Additionally, the above strategy has no influence on the biological activity of sEVs [61]. Nevertheless, clogging is observed on the membrane surface during the ultrafiltration separation process, leading to a reduction in the lifetime of membranes and low isolation efficiency. The clogging of the membrane surface is solved by tangential flow filtration (TFF). The flowing liquid is oriented perpendicular to the filtered liquid in a manner that is less likely to cause impurities or target product buildup on the membrane surface. Commonly used in the form of hollow fiber tubes and membrane packages, it is capable of separating and purifying biomolecules quickly and efficiently and can be used in many biological applications. Tangential flow devices have a number of drawbacks, such as high cost, significant shear stress, and difficulties working with small quantities [62].

The sEVs obtained by the above methods still have some room for improvement [61]. Kun Huang et al. found that increasing size exclusion chromatography (SEC) after superionization can further improve the purity of sEVs [67]. SEC isolates solutes due to the correlation between the sample's particle radius and the pore size in the particles of the purification column. When impurities with smaller particle sizes enter the purification column, they will be temporarily intercepted, and the overall moving distance is longer. The sEVs do not enter the pores and are able to travel faster through the purification column; thus, they can be isolated and purified. The sEVs enriched by SEC technology are structurally intact, highly pure, retain strong functional activity, are simple to operate, and have good reproducibility [63–65].

Affinity purification is a purification method that uses specific binding interactions between molecules, such as specific binding between antigen and antibody. sEVs have several specific marker proteins on their surface, and magnetic beads with specific antibodies can be used for their capture. Surface markers vary between different sEV types and allow the isolation of different sEV isoforms. Immunoaffinity capture ensures the sEVs morphological integrity. It is highly specific, simple to perform, and does not require expensive instrumentation. However, this method is largely marker dependent and requires specific immunomagnetic beads, resulting in high cost and low benefit [66].

3.2. Large-Scale Purification of High-Purity msEVs

While the above methods for purification of sEVs are largely adequate for research applications of sEVs, higher purity is often required for commercialization and clinical use of sEVs. It is more difficult to scale up sEV extraction from milk than from cell supernatants.

Various types of extracellular vesicles and proteins are present in milk, making it a complex fluid. There is a high concentration of proteins in milk (about 3.5%), and most of them exist in aggregated form [68]. sEVs separation can be interfered with by some proteins mixing with them. sEVs separation may be hampered by the mixing of some proteins with sEVs. Casein forms micelles that are comparable in size to sEVs and can be co-separated with sEVs. Moreover, protein phosphorylation is one of the most important interference factors. The majority of the casein in milk has undergone phosphorylation and has a surface charge state resembling the phospholipid bilayer structure of sEVs [69]. Consequently, initial pre-treatment of milk is critical for sEV extraction and affects the purity and quantity of the separated sEVs.

Therefore, individual purification methods often fail to completely isolate high purity sEVs. The use of tandem methods for advantageous complementary purification of sEVs in milk becomes the preferred option. The general purification process is divided into three steps: pre-treatment of precipitated milk using acids, salts, and PEG, combined with techniques such as centrifugation, ultrafiltration, and tangential flow to remove a large number of heteroproteins such as casein, and further using size exclusion, well-established commercial Core700, qEV, and other methods to obtain high-purity msEVs [70–75], as shown in Figure 2. The combination of the above methods and the introduction of other new technologies make it possible to produce high-purity msEVs on a large scale and to achieve good batch stability and reproducibility.

4. Composition and Functions of msEVs

Although the substances contained in sEVs from different sources have some commonalities, they are more often highly individual. Similar to sEVs isolated from other sources, sEVs from milk are rich in proteins, nucleic acids, sugars, lipids, etc., and many components are often unique to them [59,76], as shown in Figure 3.

A

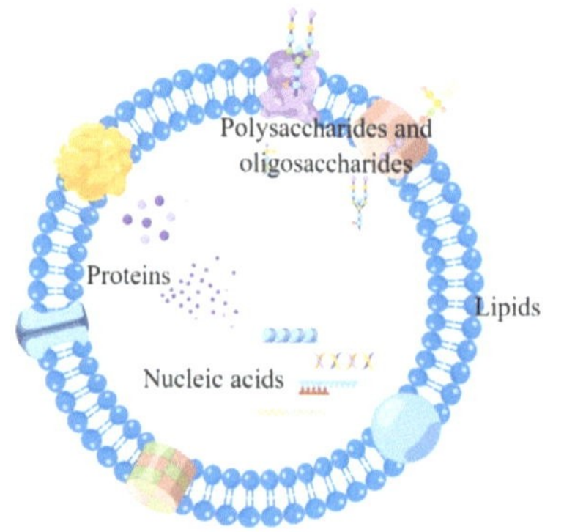

Figure 3. *Cont.*

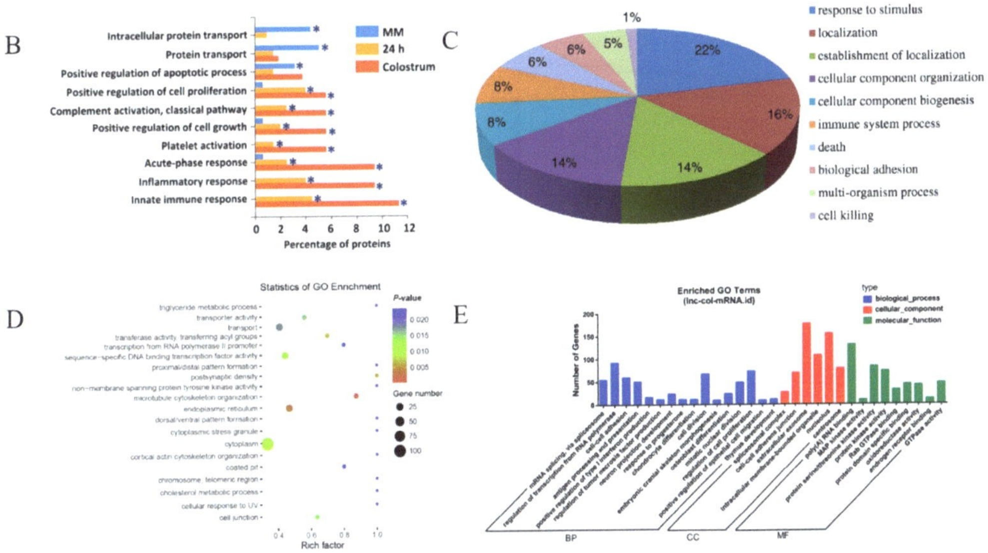

Figure 3. Composition and functions of msEVs. (**A**) Schematic of the composition of msEVs (by Figdraw, www.figdraw.com (accessed on 10 April 2023)) (**B**) Functional enrichment analysis using FunRich revealed msEVs from colostrum are enriched with proteins implicated in immune response. * $p < 0.05$; Copyright 2017, Springer Nature [48]. (**C**) GO annotation for msEV proteins in biological processes; Copyright 2017, Elsevier [77]. (**D**) The 20 most enriched GO terms for the circular RNA host gene; Copyright 2019, Elsevier [78]. (**E**) Gene ontology (GO) annotation analysis of bovine msEV long noncoding RNA (lncRNA); Copyright 2019, Elsevier [79].

4.1. Composition of msEVs

4.1.1. Proteins

Proteins are important substances for the physiological functions of living organisms, and msEV proteins are essential for physiology and pathology. To date, the composition of bovine milk proteins has been reported to have changed in more than 300 articles depending on season, lactation period, breed, and health status, and it is inferred that the composition of msEVs varies accordingly.

The physiology and immunology of the host are revealed by sEVs proteins in milk, and between uninfected and infected cattle, there are 118 proteins that are expressed differentially and are engaged in many biological processes, including cellular processes, metabolic processes, and catalytic activities [80]. Using quantitative proteomic analysis, it has been demonstrated that the sEV load and that sEVs made from colostrum contain more proteins related to immune response, antimicrobial peptides, inflammatory response factors, cell growth, and complement activators than mature msEVs, which are rich in transport and apoptosis-related proteins [48].

The main milk lipoglobulin membrane proteins (Xanthine oxidase, Butyrophilin, Lactadherin, and Adipophilin) are the most prevalent proteins present in msEVs [81]. msEVs proteins are involved in multiple KEGG pathways, including leukocyte transendothelial migration, glycolysis/gluconeogenesis, amino acid-tRNA biosynthesis, galactose metabolism, the pentose phosphate pathway, and fatty acid biosynthesis [77]. Four abundant milk proteins, lactose anhydride, butyryl protein, periplasmin-2, and xanthine dehydrogenase/oxygenase, occur in the top 20 sEVs generated from cow's and human's milk [82]. The proteomes of BMEC-sEVs demonstrate their participation in the production of milk, suggesting that they may be one of the sources of msEVs [83]. The literature-based manual management online open database BoMiProt (http://bomiprot.org (accessed on

10 April 2023)) of the bovine milk proteome covers more than 3100 proteins from fat globule membranes, whey, and sEVs [84].

MsEV protein profiles provide important information in the area of newborn nutrition and health, providing novel insights into the composition of human and cow's milk. The above information provides us with knowledge of bovine and human msEVs and may point to potential directions for the development of neonatal formulas, functional foods, and biomarkers.

4.1.2. Nucleic Acids

Nucleic acids are among the most basic substances that constitute life and perform genetic information delivery and other physiological functions, containing miRNA, mRNA, and lncRNA that play crucial roles in the development of both physiological and pathological processes. Despite the high RNase activity in milk, there are roughly 1000 ng and 1700 ng of total RNA in the microvesicles that were extracted from 6 mL of mature and colostrum milk, respectively, and the majority of this RNA is miRNA [85]. The results showed that msEVs had higher levels of RNA under 200 nt than separated sEVs' supernatant [85]. Numerous immune-related miRNAs can be found in msEVs. Colostrum had higher levels of immune-related miRNA expression compared to mature milk [86,87]. One study discovered 245 miRNAs in raw milk, and each miRNA can be dramatically changed at various lactational stages [88]. It is interesting that the expression of seven miRNAs remained relatively stable over the course of lactation [88].

In sEVs generated from milk, a substantial number of mRNAs were discovered. Most of the whey's mRNAs were discovered in sEVs, according to a microarray study, while miRNAs in whey were found in supernatant and sEVs [58,85]. In the sEVs of milk and colostrum, mRNAs coding for CD36, FAS, Ea1, MHC-II, and MFG-E8 were proven to be present by RT-PCR [33].

A large number of lncRNAs are also present in bovine msEVs. lncRNAs regulate immune function, cell-cell communication, neurodevelopment, cell proliferation, reproduction, and osteoblastogenesis. lncRNAs are differentially expressed during different stages of lactation [79]. Digestion experiments have shown that bovine msEV lncRNAs are resistant to decomposition with several digestive fluids, such as pancreatic juice, gastric juice, bile, and saliva, in vitro [79]. Since they are packaged in membranes and the msEVs are extremely stable, the RNAs in them can be absorbed by the receptors to continue their functional effects [58].

The processing of milk also affects the content of nucleic acids in sEVs. The presence of ncRNA (non-coding RNA) in sEVs from seven commercial dairy products obtained at various processing phases was examined in one study, which demonstrated that processing had a substantial impact on ncRNA expression values [89]. Ultrasound treatment of milk also reduced the content of sEVs and miRNAs in milk [90].

4.1.3. Polysaccharides and Oligosaccharides

Milk oligosaccharides are thought to provide a natural way to alter key aspects of innate immunity in newborns. Studying oligosaccharides in msEVs provides greater insight into the interactions between breastfeeding and mucosal immune system development in infants. msEVs transport is a very important way for oligosaccharides from milk to reach the recipient cells [91]. Yet, little has been known about the oligosaccharides in msEVs, or "free sugars".

The sEVs protein glycosylation study is a comprehensive tool for understanding the targeted delivery mechanism. One study analyzed the O-glycans, N-glycans, and free oligosaccharides of msEVs and whey by multiple derivatization strategies and identified 114 glycoproteins, most of which were located in sEVs [92]. These studies have contributed to our understanding of the biological and functional roles played by glycans in sEVs.

4.1.4. Lipids

Although many dairy products are skimmed, the lipids in milk are still considered to be of great nutritional value. For example, milk phospholipids have a significant impact on infant intestinal and brain development [93]. MsEVs, like other sEV sources, are vesicles enveloped by double-layer lipids that secrete into milk through a different secretion mechanism from fat globules. Lipids are mainly composed of a unique mixture of polar lipids. Although there are different mechanisms involved in the formation and release of EV, they all need to be driven by the cooperation between lipids and proteins [94].

sEVs are rich in sphingolipids, cholesterol, and phosphatidylserine, and their content is two to three times that of donor cells [95]. Research has shown that the cholesterol content in msEVs accounts for 43.6% of the total lipid extract, which can increase membrane rigidity. There is an interaction between cholesterol and phospholipids in the sEV membrane, which causes the bilayer lipid membrane to be in a liquid-phase ordered state. The membrane fluidity of msEVs is slightly higher than that of liposomes composed of similar components [96]. Lipidomic analysis of msEVs would be more useful to understand the reasons for the superior stability of msEVs compared to other sources of sEVs.

4.2. Function of msEVs

After oral administration, the msEVs pass through the gastrointestinal barrier and reach the whole body through the circulation of blood and other bodily fluids. Macrophages, intestinal cells, and vascular endothelial cells all take up msEVs, which are then transferred to surrounding organs [36]. After the sEVs reach the receptor cells, some bind to the cell surface through protein-protein or receptor-ligand interactions to start the signal cascade and activate the endocytosis pathway. Some cells ingest sEVs through phagocytosis, phagocytosis, and fusion [97,98]. In vitro cell experiments or in vivo animal experiments have exhibited that msEVs can enter the cytoplasm through endocytosis and release their contents, such as miRNAs [76,99]. These studies indicate that sEVs in milk can be absorbed in vitro and in vivo, thus performing physiological functions. The physiological function of the sEVs in milk is multifaceted, as shown in Figure 4 and Table 3.

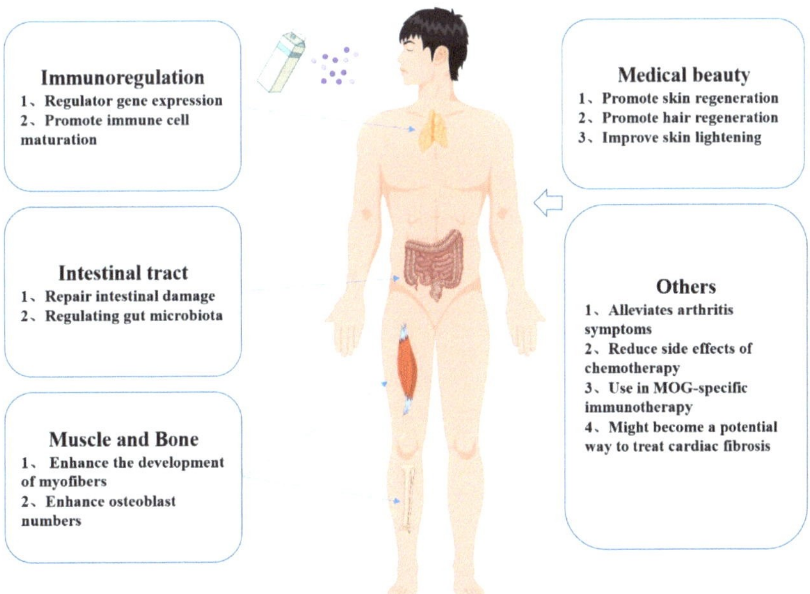

Figure 4. Functions and applications of msEVs (by Figdraw, www.figdraw.com).

Table 3. Functions of msEVs.

Function	Therapeutic Agent	Effect	Mechanism	References
Immunoregulation	TGF-β and miRNA-30b	Play a crucial role in the biogenesis and improvement of infant immune function.	Regulation of immune-related factors (such as miRNAs and antibodies).	[100–106]
Regulation of intestinal tract function	bta-miR-34a, miR-155, and miR-146a	Antioxidant stress; Resistance to hypoxic injury; Reduce the inflammatory response induced by LPS, DSS, and other factors in the mouse intestinal model.	Enhance cell activity, inhibit inflammation, regulate intestinal flora, etc.	[107–123]
Development of muscle and bone	miR-21 and miR-29a	The growth and development of muscle and bone can be altered by miRNAs from msEVs.	Increase the number of osteoblasts, promote bone formation and osteoblast differentiation, and encourage myofiber formation in myotube cells.	[124–127]
Promote skin regeneration	TGF-β and miRNA-21	Promote the transformation of inflammation into tissue and further promote the healing of skin wounds.	Induce ECM deposition and regulate tissue regeneration by regulating the phosphorylation of the Smad pathway.	[128]
Detection of bovine diseases		Bovines can be monitored for infection with pathogenic bacteria such as Staphylococcus aureus or their health status.	Examining the nucleic acids, proteins, and lipids in msEVs to identify illness signs.	[129–134]
Alleviates arthritis symptoms	immunoregulatory microRNAs (miR-30a, miR-223, miR-92a), beta-lactoglobulin mRNA, and milk-specific beta-casein	Delayed the onset of arthritis, and histology showed diminished cartilage pathology and bone marrow inflammation in both models.	Decreased MCP-1 and IL-6 production by splenic cells in serum; Decreased splenic Th1 (Tbet) and Th17 (RORT) mRNA levels, which were also associated with decreased anticollagen IgG2a levels.	[135]
Reduce the side effects of chemotherapy		Protect cells from chemotherapeutic drug-induced cytotoxicity.	Affect the cell cycle of RAW 264.7 with and without cisplatin.	[136]
Use in MOG-specific immunotherapy	butyrophilin (BTN)	Could be thought of as an attractive method to help patients with multiple sclerosis develop MOG-specific tolerance.	The BTN content of these vesicles can pass past the skin's epidermis and other biological barriers, serving as Trojan horses for the body.	[137]
Can be a useful medicinal ingredient for improving skin lightening	miR-2478	Inhibit melanin production.	Through the Akt-GSK3 signaling pathway, Rap1a expression inhibition reduced melanogenesis.	[138]
Might become a potential way to treat cardiac fibrosis		Improved heart performance in cardiac fibrosis rats.	Significant improvements were made to the proangiogenic growth factors.	[139]
Have the potential to promote hair regeneration.		Promote hair regeneration.	Promote dermal papillary cell (DP) proliferation and rescue dihydrotestosterone (DHT)-induced follicular development arrest.	[140]

4.2.1. Immunoregulation

MsEVs have significant impacts on metabolism and immune processes. Milk is rich in a variety of immune-related factors, and sEVs affect intercellular communication by binding to target cell receptors through surface antigens or by delivering sEVs RNA and proteins to target cells [100].

An enzyme called DNA methyltransferase 1 (DNMT1) is important in controlling epigenetic processes. MiRNA-148a, found in msEVs and milk fat globules, attenuates DNMT1 expression [106]. Kosaka and coworkers have reported that miRNA delivered by sEVs in breast milk could facilitate the immune system's development in infants [141]. The number of Foxp3+ CD4+ CD25+ regulatory T cells in infants was increased in the presence of both miRNA-181a and miRNA-17, which are transported by sEVs. Inducing regulatory T cells is beneficial not only for healthy individuals but also for infants. Furthermore, T-cell-regulating miRNAs such as miR-181 and miR-155 were also rich in msEVs, which were beneficial for the differentiation of B-cells. As genetic material, miRNA could be transferred from mother to infant, supporting the development of an infant's immune system and preventing a lot of infections. Similarly, Pieters et al. have demonstrated that sEVs in commercial milk have immunoregulatory cargo, including miRNAs and TGF-β, which could induce the differentiation of Th17 cells [104]. The results confirmed that the milk recipient's immune system could be regulated by msEVs.

4.2.2. Regulation of Intestinal Tract Function

MsEVs have been validated to exert vital roles in the digestive tract [107,108]. Bovine msEVs possess protection against H_2O_2-induced oxidative stress. Evidence revealed that IEC-6 pretreatment with msEVs could enhance viability, increase GPX and SOD activity, reduce H_2O_2-induced LDH, ROS, and MDA accumulation, increase the amount of intracellular miR-155 and miR-146a, and inhibit H_2O_2-induced elevated Nrf2 and Ho1 gene expression [109]. In IEC-6 cells, msEVs can attenuate H_2O_2-induced alterations in purine metabolism and energy state and reduce purine nucleotide catabolism so as to exert their protective effects against oxidative stress [110].

The intestinal epithelial cell is an essential intestinal barrier, and its function will be impaired by hypoxia induction. Damage to the intestinal barrier can be prevented by msEV miRNAs in lactation. Among those miRNAs, bta-miR-34a is a potent regulator of mitigating hypoxic damage in IEC-6 [111]. sEVs made from yak milk have been shown to promote the growth of intestinal epithelial cells under hypoxia and activate protective signaling pathways, thus strengthening IEC-6 cell survival, and the protective effect is better than that of bovine msEVs [86]. As observed, IEC-6 cells ingested more msEVs generated from yak milk, which may be due to higher membrane protein expression [86].

The function of intestinal epithelial cells can also be impaired by other damaging factors, such as lipopolysaccharides. TLR4, which contributes to the occurrence of intestinal inflammation and necrotizing enterocolitis (NEC), can be inhibited by msEVs [112]. In a mouse genetically engineered to have ulcerative colitis, msEVs could prevent severe ulcerative phenotypes and intestinal inflammation [113]. Oral administration of msEVs can prevent NEC as approved by reducing morphological damage and injury to the ileum and reducing the number of MUC2+ and GRP94+ cells [114]. MsEVs enhanced the activity of gastric goblet cells and prevented experimental necrotizing small bowel colitis [115]. MsEVs can prevent dextran sulfate sodium-induced enterocolitis by inhibiting inflammation and oxidative stress, especially in colostrum-derived msEVs [116], as shown in Figure 5A. MsEVs altered the characteristic cuboidal form of normal colonic epithelial cells into a mesenchymal-like morphology and induced proliferation, which had not been seen in tumor cells [117]. The mechanism was attributed to the fact that msEVs up-regulated type I collagen expression and down-regulated Twist1 gene expression and PTEN proteins. sEVs derived from yak milk attenuate LPS-induced intestinal inflammation by suppressing activation of the PI3K/AKT/C3 signal pathway [118]. Severe acute malnutrition (SAM) is usually caused by epithelial atrophy and intestinal barrier disruption, and sEVs isolated from milk ameliorate malnutrition-induced intestinal barrier dysfunction [119].

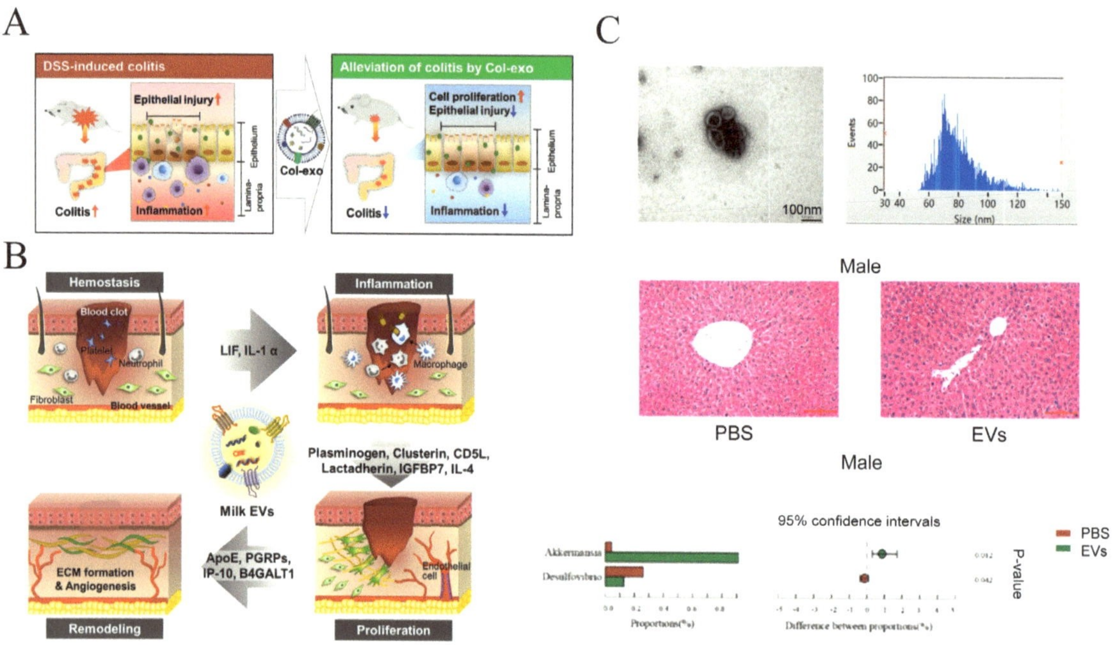

Figure 5. MsEVs have protective functions in the intestinal tract and promote skin regeneration. (**A**) Overall schematic diagram and characterization of the colostrum-derived sEVs; Copyright 2022, Royal Society of Chemistry [116]. (**B**) Schematic diagram of milk EVs-mediated cutaneous wound healing; Copyright 2021, John Wiley and Sons [128]. (**C**) Oral msEVs have positive effects on the intestinal microbiome and serum metabolism in mice; Copyright 2021, Royal Society of Chemistry [142].

Furthermore, msEV proteins and miRNAs were capable of preventing colitis through attenuating inflammation [123]. Upon subjecting cells to msEVs, TLR4-NF-κB as well as the NLRP3 signaling pathway in cells were inhibited, resulting in a reduction of the inflammatory response. In the inflamed colon, the disorder of cytokine production was corrected, and the balance between Th17 and Treg cells was also balanced. Additionally, msEVs could restore gut microbiota in ulcerative colitis, thereby modulating intestinal immunity. Therefore, the supplementation of milk sEVs in the daily diet was essential to maintaining the normal physiological function of the gut. Studies have demonstrated that dietary sEV deficiency leads to changes in the bacterial community of young rats and damages their intestinal health. sEVs generated from milk administered orally boosted the expression of GATA4, Muc2, MyD88, and RegII-g, all of which are associated with intestinal immunity [120]. Changes in the cecal bacterial community in C57BL/6 mice induced by consumption of msEVs [121]. Oral msEVs have positive effects on the intestinal microbiome and serum metabolism in mice [142], as shown in Figure 5C. The intestine is closely related to many inflammatory diseases. Systemic inflammatory illnesses like lupus erythematosus, multiple sclerosis, and rheumatoid arthritis can cause increased intestinal permeability, an unbalanced microbiota in the gut, and intestinal inflammation. Intervention of the intestinal tract, particularly the microbiome, by msEVs is expected to be a therapeutic measure for these diseases [122].

4.2.3. Regulation of Muscle and Bone Development

MiRNAs from msEVs can alter the growth and development of muscle and bone, such as miR-21 and miR-29a, which can amplify mTOR signaling [124]. In mice, it has been noted that msEVs enhance osteoblast numbers and promote bone formation and osteoblast differentiation [125]. MsEVs enhance the development of myofibers in mouse C2C12 myotubular cells and have a moderate effect on grip strength, amino acid profile, and gene expression in C57BL/6 mouse skeletal muscle [126]. In an osteoporosis-induced mouse model, sEVs from dietary bovine milk enhanced bone health [127]. After incubating Raw264.7 cells with msEVs, tartaric acid phosphatase-resistant staining was significantly inhibited, indicating reduced differentiation of osteoclasts. The group of mice given sEVs had considerably higher bone mineral density. sEVs isolated from bovine milk may be potential candidates for preventing osteoporosis, improving bone remodeling, and inhibiting bone resorption.

4.2.4. Promote Skin Regeneration

SEVs derived from stem cells usually have the function of tissue regeneration. More and more clinical studies use them as tissue regeneration materials to promote wound healing and reduce scar formation. Studies have shown that bovine colostrum also has excellent natural healing power, and its msEVs can promote the transformation of inflammation into tissue and further promote the healing of skin wounds [128], as shown in Figure 5B. msEVs can promote fibroblast proliferation, migration, and endothelial tube formation. In the mouse model of the excised wound, the msEVs can promote re-epithelialization, activate angiogenesis, and promote the maturation of the extracellular matrix. The mechanism may be that bovine msEVs can induce ECM deposition and regulate tissue regeneration by regulating the phosphorylation of the Smad pathway, and their miRNA-21 also plays a key regulatory role. It shows that they are very promising to be developed into anti-inflammatory drugs, especially for the treatment of skin wounds.

4.2.5. Detection of Bovine Diseases

SEVs composition is finely controlled by the parental cells. Therefore, the analysis of sEV components can be used to infer the functional state of the parental cells or even the organism as a whole [1,129]. The analysis of multi-omics profiles or disease markers, including nucleic acids, proteins, and lipids, in msEVs can be used to determine the health of donor cows, laying the foundation for a non-invasive body fluid biopsy approach to detect disease [130]. In addition, msEVs also perform epigenetic modification functions. A profound understanding of sEV's epigenetic modification functions is essential to improving breeding success and the profitability of dairy farms [131].

Staphylococcus aureus infection is a common disease in cattle. The variations in the sEV composition of cattle infected with S. aureus are more intensively studied. MiRNA content in msEVs is regulated by many variables, including the health status of the host and the stage of lactation. Analysis of staphylococcus aureus-infected bovine msEVs genomic broad miRNA profiling revealed significant expression differences between healthy and infected animals for at least 18 miRNAs, with up-regulation of miR-142-5p, miR-183, and miR-223 and down-regulation of miR-99a-5p, miR-101, and miR-2285-3p. Changes in miR-223, miR-142-5p, miR-378, and miR-185 are particularly thought of as promising possibilities for mastitis screening indicators [9,132]. Proteomic analysis can likewise provide much relevant information. Quantitative data revealed that among the 2971 proteins identified in msEVs, over 300 were associated with host defense. Additionally, compared to uninfected controls, 94 proteins were significantly differently regulated in cow's msEVs from S. aureus-infected animals [133]. Western blotting data demonstrate that in msEVs from BLV-infected cows, the structural proteins gp51 and p24 of the bovine leukemia virus (BLV) were discovered [134].

4.2.6. Other Functions

sEVs from milk taken orally reduce the signs and symptoms of arthritis in IL-1 Ra-deficient spontaneous polyarthritis mice and arthritis animal models generated by collagen [135]. In response to chemotherapeutic side effects, msEVs protect macrophages from cisplatin-induced cytotoxicity [136]. A protein known as butyryl protein (BTN), which shares an epitope with the myelin oligodendrocyte glycoprotein (MOG), was identified in milk, and transdermal administration of msEVs to patients with multiple sclerosis induced the development of MOG-specific tolerance for use in MOG-specific immunotherapy [137]. MsEVs can be an effective medicinal ingredient to improve skin lightening. MiR-2478 insEVs inhibits melanogenesis by the Akt-GSK3β signal pathway and is able to reduce melanin content, tyrosinase activity, and melanogenesis-related gene expression in melanoma cells and melanocytes [138]. The use of msEVs might become a potential way to treat cardiac fibrosis. MsEVs attenuate the effects of cardiac fibrosis by enhancing angiogenesis and improving cardiac function in rats with cardiac fibrosis [139]. Colostrum-derived sEVs have the potential to promote hair regeneration. It was reported that colostrum sEVs could promote dermal papillary cell (DP) cell proliferation, rescue dihydrotestosterone (DHT)-induced follicular development arrest, and induce dorsal hair regrowth in mice at levels similar to minoxidil therapies without related side effects, such as rash [140].

4.3. Potential Health Risks Associated with msEVs

There is a general belief that excessive intake of nutrients is extremely detrimental to health. Milk is popular for its excellent taste and nutritional content, but excessive intake is considered to be one of the contributing factors to adverse consequences such as diabetes, obesity, and cardiovascular disease. sEVs' function in milk has also received a lot of interest. Epidemiological studies have linked msEV intake to a higher risk of type 2 diabetes, obesity, Parkinson's disease, and cardiovascular disease [141,143–145]. The reason why msEVs may increase the risk of these diseases is often believed to be caused by the miRNAs they contain. For example, miR-148a is a biomarker of obesity in human subjects and mouse models and can inhibit Wnt1 and promote adipocyte differentiation [141]. Furthermore, miRNA-148a and miRNA-21 can enhance miRNA-148a/DNMT1 dependency. The α-Synuclein may further aggravate type 2 diabetes and Parkinson's disease [143]. These concerns are warranted, but until more systematic studies or studies that can corroborate each other are available, remain positive about their use.

5. MsEVs as Drug Delivery Vehicles

Advancements in medication delivery technology are gaining momentum as lipid nanoparticles (LNPs) delivering mRNA are widely recognized as vaccines against COVID-19 outbreaks. The emergence of novel delivery systems may offer opportunities for diseases that are difficult to cure with existing drugs or methods. However, viral vectors and manufactured nanoparticles have obvious disadvantages as exogenous delivery vehicles, such as high toxicity, high immunogenicity, low targeting, a short half-life, easy clearance, and the production of antibodies after multiple doses that affect the delivery effect.

sEVs as a natural drug delivery system inherently perform functions such as signal delivery in vivo, do not cause the problems described above, and have much superior potential. These advantages include the small size of sEVs, their ability to penetrate deeper tissues, their slightly negative surface charge that contributes to long circulation, their similarity to cell membranes, and their deformable cytoskeleton [146–148]. Additionally, some sEVs show improved resistance to immune system destruction or clearance [149]. sEVs are not only highly biocompatible and less toxic and immunogenic, but also have a targeted "homing" effect. The ability of sEVs to reach all organs of the body after entering by intramuscular or intravenous routes is largely due to their capacity to penetrate past physiological barriers such as the placental, gastric, and blood-brain barriers. Drug resistance can be reduced by sEVs-mediated delivery because it can avoid the P-glycoprotein drug efflux pathway. sEVs have "do not swallow me" signaling molecules like CD47 on their surface, which resist macrophage phagocytosis and lengthen in vivo half-lives.

Oral administration is the preferred method of drug delivery compared to intramuscular, subcutaneous, and intravenous administration. However, the challenges of oral drug delivery are enormous, which is attributed to the gastrointestinal tract's hostile environment rich in gastric acid and digestive enzymes, which makes it challenging for medications to enter the body through the stomach, resulting in low bioavailability. Therefore, the search for delivery systems that can be used for oral drug delivery is a relentless pursuit for researchers.

Due to their unique evolutionary advantages over other sources of sEVs, msEVs are expected to be a new vehicle for oral drug delivery. The resistant glycoproteins (XDH, BTN, and MUC1) and surface proteins (FLOT1, ICAM1, ALIX, and EpCAM) of msEVs make them resistant to pepsin and have good stability [150]. Some studies have also shown that msEVs are absorbed by the intestine in the form of intact particles under the protection of Fc receptors (FcRn) [98].

5.1. Biosafety of msEVs

The safety of sEVs generated from milk as medicine delivery systems is the primary concern. Milk provides a large number of nutrients to the body, and humans have a long history of milk consumption, so it is widely believed that it is very safe to drink milk from cows. Due to the complexity of the raw material, it remains difficult to isolate pure sEVs from milk. Some proteins in milk are important allergens. Therefore, as an important component of milk, the biosafety and biocompatibility assessment of msEVs is indispensable.

Studies have revealed that high-purity msEVs are readily absorbed by macrophages without cytotoxic effects [45]. In addition, msEV injection into the tail vein did not result in systemic toxicity [45]. MsEVs did not produce any by-effects or immunogenicity in mice, and no anaphylactic shock effect was observed after continuous administration in mice [151]. All the mice survived the experiment in good health. Both single and repeated oral administrations of msEVs at a 25 mg/kg dosage led to no discernible changes in the clinical symptoms, indicating the safety of msEVs. Additionally, compared with the control group, oral administration of msEVs had no discernible effects on aspartate aminotransferase or creatinine levels in the serum [33]. This indicates that msEVs did not exert detrimental impacts on liver and kidney performance and were well tolerated.

5.2. Engineering of msEVs

Engineering sEVs is an important tool to expand their applications. sEVs are highly engineerable, and engineered sEVs are endowed with tissue or cell specificity, such as targeting. sEVs can be engineered in a manner that includes genetic approaches, biological manipulation, chemical and physical modifications, and other methods to engineer the surface and interior of sEVs [152].

5.2.1. Cargo Loading

Drug delivery in sEVs can be achieved by direct or indirect loading: (1) drugs with small molecules can be loaded directly into sEVs through passive incubation methods or active strategies like electroporation, saponification, repeated freeze-thawing, ultrasonication, extrusion, etc. These are the common methods for loading msEVs with drugs, followed by further purification to remove the unencapsulated small molecules; (2) indirect methods by modifying the sEV-derived cells, e.g., using transfection or transduction expression vectors, so that the sEV donor cells secrete sEVs containing functional drug molecules. In contrast, msEVs are mainly isolated and purified before being engineered and are currently focused on loading drugs into them for functional applications.

Co-incubation, the simplest method of sEV drug loading, is appropriate for loading hydrophobic small compounds like curcumin and paclitaxel. The co-incubation of hydrophobic drugs with sEVs was loaded in a passive diffusion manner, but the co-incubation method of drug loading is less efficient. In contrast, loading of such substances as hydrophilic molecules and macromolecules requires transient perforation or disruption of the membrane because the sEVs are blocked by lipid membranes, and the methods that can be used include freeze-thaw cycles, electroporation, extrusion, ultrasound, and surfactant treatment.

The freeze-thaw cycling method is based on co-incubation and takes advantage of the process of disruption and remodeling of the membrane structure of sEVs in buffer for loading. The sEVs membrane is momentarily disrupted by the production of ice crystals during freezing, thus permitting hydrophilic substances to penetrate the interior before membrane reconstruction, and after thawing, the ice crystals disappear and the sEVs membrane undergoes remodeling and encapsulates the drug. The extrusion method involves mixing the sEVs with the free drug and passing it through channels containing nanoscale pores, where shear breaks the lipid membrane and permits the exogenous drug to enter the sEVs. Electroporation can form pores on the surface of the sEV membrane, and the pore can be closed, and the lipid layer can be formed again when the electric field is removed. Electroporation can be used to aid the entry of hydrophilic small molecules into sEVs and improve the loading efficiency of siRNA [30]. The development of continuous flow electroporation is expected to increase the scale of application of this method. Ultrasonication is another method for loading drugs into sEVs [153,154]. Ultrasound-based drug loading methods use an ultrasound probe to apply ultrasound energy, which reduces the rigidity of the sEV membrane and enables drug diffusion. However, ultrasound treatment may cause the cleavage of sEVs. Cargoes such as nucleic acids and chemicals can be penetrated into sEVs by ultrasound ultrasonication, but the cargoes may mostly only adhere to the surface of sEVs.

Recently, a team developed the "ENP" drug delivery system, a nanofluidic device containing 30,000 modules working in parallel and capable of high-throughput loading a variety of cargoes into sEVs. The sEVs pass through nanochannels that are similar in size to them, and mechanical compression and fluid penetration have the ability to shear the sEV membrane, allowing cargo molecules to enter the sEVs while preserving their integrity. The sEVs nanopuncturer uses an array of 30,000 nanochannels, the highest number of channels available for a single chip. sEVs treated with the sEVs nanopuncturer can deliver drugs to human non-small cell lung cancer cells and can lead to their apoptosis [155].

The drug can also be loaded into sEVs using $CaCl_2$. This method was carried out by sEVs and cargo in 100 mm $CaCl_2$ and subjected to ice incubation and thermal excitation treatment [156]. The load efficiency of this method is close to that of electroporation. Saponin is a kind of decontaminant that can open the pores of the lipid membrane by removing membrane cholesterol. The disadvantage of saponins is their potential cytotoxic effect.

Cationic lipids can also be used to deliver mRNA into sEVs, and the method has been shown to be safe and has been applied to create the SARS-CoV-2 vaccine [157]. In this method, the mRNA was mixed with cationic lipids to form polymers, and then sEVs were added for further fusion to achieve the purpose of loading. Lipofectamine uses cationic substances to facilitate the interaction with the lipid membrane and subsequent internalization, which can effectively load nucleic acids into the sEV's interior [158]. Exogenous hsa-mir148a-3p could be loaded into msEVs by Lipofectamine 2000, and its biological function was evaluated [70].

5.2.2. Modification of msEVs

SEVs of different origins are often targeted with similar "homing" effects. sEVs have high engineering ability, and surface-engineered sEVs can achieve cell and tissue specificity and similar "homing" effects. For example, synthetic biology can be used to add biomolecules (targeting ligands, immune evasion molecules, and stimuli-responsive molecules) to the sEV surface.

Targeted delivery of drugs through sEVs raises the medicinal agent's local concentration and reduces adverse effects. The surface-modified msEVs can achieve the purpose of specific drug delivery to tumor cells. Loading the iRGD tumor-targeting peptide on the sEVs surface could change the organ aggregation rate of sEVs [98]. Hyaluronic acid-modified sEVs could target delivering doxorubicin (DOX) to tumor cells with high expression of CD44, thus triggering significant tumor cell death [159]. The approach involves functionalizing hyaluronic acid (HA) with the amphiphilic molecule DSPE-PEG2000, which allows Dox-loaded msEVs to be spontaneously decorated with HA on a phospholipid bilayer. Folic acid (FA), a tumor-targeting ligand, was linked to msEVs and loaded with paclitaxel (PAC), which increased the cancer cell targeting ability of sEVs, thereby enhancing the tumor-killing effect. Subcutaneous tumor xenografts were significantly inhibited by oral FA-ExoPAC, but a similar dose of PAC has no obvious effect [160]. The HA-msEVs-FA system constructed with msEVs modified by FA-encapsulated CD44 specific ligand HA could fight against liver fibrosis by regulating NLRP3-mediated apoptosis [161].

MsEVs with environmentally responsive functions are also being developed. The modified msEVs were used to target the transport of Adriamycin to triple-negative breast cancer cells and were able to respond intelligently to oxygen concentration [162]. The peptide-targeted hypoxia-responsive msEVs were created in this experiment using Neurofibrillin receptor agonist peptide (iRGD) and hypoxia-responsive liposomes. These doxorubicin-encapsulated sEVs in a model of triple-negative breast cancer cell monolayers and three-dimensional (3D) spheres demonstrated their environmentally responsive tumor-killing ability.

Surface modification of sEVs can improve the half-life of msEVs in vivo. In one study, msEVs were hydrophobically coated with a hydrophilic polyethylene glycol (PEG) layer, which greatly decreased the breakdown of sEVs in an acidic stomach environment and increased the permeability by more than 3-fold [72]. CD47 is a "do not swallow me" signal, an immune escape indicator abundant on the surface of cancer cells. By attaching to SIRP, CD47 reduces macrophages' capacity to phagocytose tumor cells [163]. Many sEVs also contain CD47 signaling proteins, which prolong the half-life of sEVs circulating in vivo. Engineering donor cells or directly modifying sEVs to increase the abundance of CD47 signaling on their surface is becoming an important direction for engineering sEVs.

5.3. MsEVs for Drug Delivery

MsEVs can be utilized as efficient drugs and gene carriers, as shown in Figure 6. Due to their distinct evolutionary capacity and distinctive characteristics, sEVs obtained through acid administration and ultracentrifugation are tolerable in vivo, and msEVs may travel through the gastrointestinal tract and be completely absorbed as entire particles. The drugs are encapsulated in sEVs and avoid decomposition by the gastrointestinal environment [58,151,164]. Bioluminescence experiments in mice by the oral route confirmed that sEVs have high bioavailability [98]. sEVs therefore have a significant potential for being efficient medication carriers.

5.3.1. Delivery of Chemical Drugs

Several chemotherapeutic agents exhibiting various functions, such as superior antioxidant, antiproliferative, anti-inflammatory, and pro-apoptotic, are being developed. However, their development is limited by their low permeability, low solubility, and poor oral bioavailability. Hence, it is necessary to develop efficient delivery systems and systems with robust bioavailability. MsEVs are widely recognized as chemotherapeutic agent carriers and have many advantages in oral administration. Using the proper solvents, a variety of chemotherapy drugs were loaded into msEVs, including curcumin, anthocyanins, paclitaxel, celastrol, rotenone, and doxorubicin [33,154,165–167]. Due to the differences in molecular weight, lipophilicity, and functional groups of these small molecules, the efficiency of sEV loading is between 10% and 40%.

When loaded into sEVs, curcumin could increase intestinal permeability and withstand breakdown by human digestive enzymes [166]. sEVs are agents of anthocyanins that are able to fight against many cancer types. Compared to free Anthos, Anthos-loaded sEVs have enhanced anti-inflammatory and anti-proliferative functions on a variety of cancer cells in vitro and showed significant enhancement of lung cancer xenograft therapy. In wild-type mice, anthos-loaded sEVs exhibited no obvious or systemic toxicity symptoms [168]. MsEVs loaded with anthocyanins can prevent colorectal cancer and alleviate symptoms caused by an intestinal microbiota imbalance [169]. Paclitaxel is traditionally administered by intravenous injection. Due to the poor solubility of paclitaxel in water, oral administration cannot reach the therapeutic dose. MsEVs encapsulated with paclitaxel could overcome these problems by oral administration [165]. It was demonstrated that msEVs carrying paclitaxel showed good and stable antitumor efficacy [165]. Furthermore, msEVs carrying paclitaxel reduced hepatic, renal, and systemic toxicity [165]. sEVs offer an effective alternative to oral administration of chemotherapeutic agents with high efficacy, low cost, and high safety.

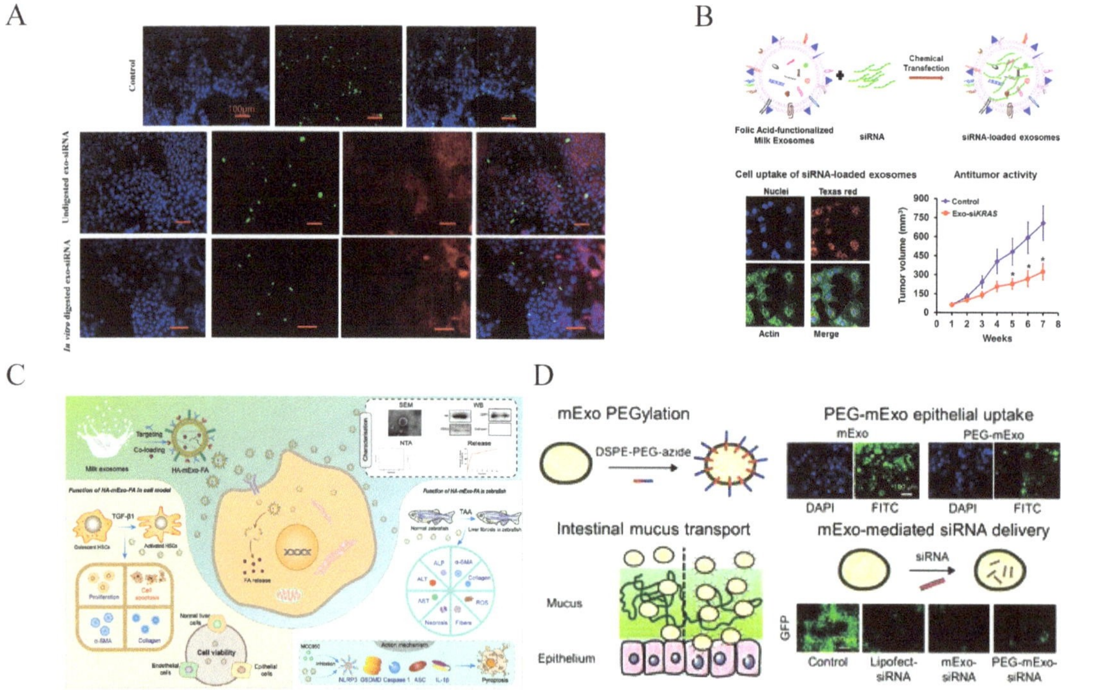

Figure 6. MsEVs are developed as a drug delivery system. (**A**) Delivery of AF-488 siRNA in Caco-2 cells via msEVs in vitro; Copyright 2017, American Chemical Society [170]. (**B**) MsEVs deliver siRNA for the treatment of cancer; Copyright 2019, Elsevier [171]. * $p < 0.05$. (**C**) CD44 targeting the drug delivery system of sEVs loading FA for treatment of liver fibrosis; Copyright 2023, John Wiley and Sons [161]. (**D**) MsEVs with enhanced mucus penetrability for oral delivery of siRNA; Copyright 2020, Royal Society of Chemistry [72].

5.3.2. Delivery of Nucleic Acids

MsEVs are attracting delivery vectors for small interfering RNA (siRNA) [72,170,171], as shown in Figure 6A,B,D. SiRNA has gene silencing functions and can treat various diseases, including cancer. However, there are many bottlenecks in siRNA development, including stable intracellular delivery and targeted delivery. sEVs can stably and efficiently deliver siRNA to specific receptor cells. Encapsulating siRNA in msEVs can resist harsh digestive processes, including saliva, gastric juice, and bile, improve intestinal permeability, and enhance payload protection [170–172]. β-Catenin siRNA was packed into msEVs by using lipofectamine, and these sEVs showed good target gene knockdown efficiency [172]. Using msEVs loaded with siRNAs targeting VEGF, EGF, AKT, MAPK, and KRAS, it showed a 2- to 10-fold decrease in the expression levels of the corresponding targets in various cancers [171], as shown in Figure 6B. When Bcl-2 siRNA was loaded into msEVs using an ultrasonic technique, both in vitro and in vivo cancer cell migration and the formation of gastrointestinal tumors were significantly suppressed [173].

MsEVs are also good miRNA carriers. The miRNA hsa-mir148a-3p, which was exogenously loaded into msEVs, could be ingested by HepG2 and Caco-2 cell lines, and its biological function was explored by microarray gene expression [70]. Therefore, msEVs can be an important source of functional miRNA nanocarriers and help develop new methods of nucleic acid therapy.

5.3.3. Delivery of Other Small Molecules

MsEVs-encapsulated epigallocatechin gallate (ECG) enhances neuroprotection against Parkinson's disease [154]. MsEVs were successfully delivered to SHSY5Y cells and inhibited rotenone-induced SHSY5Y cell injury through anti-apoptotic and anti-phagocytosis [154]. Evidence showed that the anti-diabetic drug liraglutide, loaded into msEVs, could reduce blood glucose levels when administered sublingually [174].

6. MsEVs and Nutritional Supplements

Mammalian breast milk itself has great nutritional value and is capable of performing physiological functions such as immune enhancement, resistance to bacterial infection, and resistance to oxidative stress. A large part of these functions may be a direct function of the proteins, nucleic acids, lipids, and sugars carried by their sEVs. Breastfeeding is associated with a lower risk of infection, immune-mediated disorders, obesity, and even cancer during the first six months of life and can satisfy all of an infant's nutritional demands at various stages of growth [175]. Infants who are breastfed have higher Preschool Language Measure Scores, the Psychomotor Developmental Index, and the Mental Developmental Index than infants who are fed different formulas, according to phenotypes seen in infant feeding studies [59].

The physiological functions performed by sEVs provide strong evidence to promote breastfeeding in infants. However, a large number of infants and children require the use of deeply processed infant formula or other dairy products as nutritional supplies due to the deficiency of maternal breast milk. Key elements such as sEVs are often lacking in infant formula or commercially available deeply processed dairy products, or functional factors are disrupted during production. EVs structural integrity and molecular makeup are impacted by conventional industrial processing of milk [176]. Commercial milk heated by pasteurization or ultra-high-temperature sterilization contains fewer or no intact sEVs [177]. Initial evidence suggested that msEVs were bound by the lectins in the infant soy formula, resulting in reduced absorption [178]. Compared to breast milk, the amount of sEVs and miRNAs in infant formula is negligible. Some highly conserved miRNAs exist in human, bovine, and goat milk but cannot be detected in infant formula [179].

sEVs can be added to infant formula or other health foods for the development of new clinical therapies. MsEVs exhibit good cross-species tolerance and do not cause unfavorable immunological or inflammatory reactions. The development of msEVs as an important functional component in this field is still in its infancy. It is also possible that the msEVs miRNA concentration is not sufficient to produce gene regulation [180]. Large amounts of exogenous miRNAs or other regulatory molecules can be engineered to be loaded into msEVs, and the oral msEV-loaded cargo can reach tissues in the body. There may be great efficacy and market prospects for adding msEVs to infant formulas or nutraceuticals targeting the elderly population.

7. Conclusions and Prospects

The phospholipid bilayer, proteins, and nucleic acids of msEV are very similar to those of their parent cells, and their compositions are finely controlled by parent cells. Thus, msEVs can be employed as biomarkers to detect diseases. Furthermore, msEVs are involved in regulating multiple biological processes, including immunoregulation, anti-bacterial infection, and antioxidants, which play a beneficial role in human health at multiple levels, such as intestinal health, bone and muscle metabolism, and microbiota regulation. In addition to directly utilizing the natural functions of msEV, due to its superior biological activity over LNP, msEV can also serve as an important carrier for delivering exogenous substances. Although the application prospect of msEVs is promising, there is still much work to be done in the commercial application of biopharmaceuticals.

Before the practical application of msEVs, it is necessary to overcome the challenge of large-scale purification. In the biological products industry, utilizing raw materials from animal sources is usually restricted. In daily life, many people are allergic to dairy products. This puts forward higher requirements for the development of msEVs. Improving the level of purification and reducing the residue of allergic substances are two important solutions to this problem. The recent emergence of new technologies such as microfluidics has provided new ideas for the purification of msEV. However, for the large-scale application of msEVs, microfluidic methods still require some optimization.

Through histological analysis, it was confirmed that msEVs are rich in active substances such as nucleic acids, proteins, carbohydrates, lipids, etc. Their content varies depending on season, species, physiological conditions, and other factors and has a significant impact on physiology and pathophysiology. There may also be significant heterogeneity in msEVs from different production batches. In order to obtain a unified-quality msEV, the following issues may need to be considered: 1. A stable and reliable milk source supply is required; 2. the establishment of a raw milk quality control system; 3. the establishment of standardized production operation processes; and 4. the establishment of strict quality standards for MSEV, for example, using several key proteins or miRNAs to establish product release standards.

The main application pathway for msEVs is oral administration. After passing through the gastrointestinal barrier, they mainly accumulate in the liver, and some of them carry miRNAs and other substances through the blood circulation to other organs for action. There is relatively little research on the natural targeting of msEVs, and most of it focuses on engineering modifications to improve their targeting. In addition to the engineering modification of msEVs for loading exogenous substances and improving targeting, it can also achieve an extension of their half-life. In addition, the application of msEVs in nasal sprays or injection preparations can be discussed. In order to address these issues, it is necessary to cultivate more msEVs professionals, improve and develop large-scale purification and engineering technologies, and establish industry standards to promote the commercialization of products. In the near future, it is believed that both natural msEV functional products and engineered products will be clinically transformed.

Author Contributions: Y.Z. and W.A. developed the review outline, drafted it, and wrote the manuscript. X.W. (Xudong Wang) developed the figures. Y.Z., X.Z. and W.A. conceived the idea and supervised the content and writing. X.Z., J.S., X.W. (Xue Wu), P.G., J.C. and P.Y. critically contributed to the content and reviewed the manuscript to ensure accuracy and completeness. J.C. contributed to the revision of the manuscript. All authors have read and agreed to the published version of the manuscript.

Funding: This work was supported by the National Natural Science Foundation of China (grant no. 82202336) and the Guangdong Basic and Applied Basic Research Foundation (grant no. 2021A1515110619).

Institutional Review Board Statement: Not applicable.

Informed Consent Statement: Not applicable.

Data Availability Statement: No additional data are available.

Conflicts of Interest: The authors declare no conflict of interest.

Abbreviations

BLV	Bovine leukemia virus
BTN	Butyrophilin
DAI	Disease activity index
DNMT1	DNA methyltransferase 1
DSS	Dextran sulfate sodium salt
DOX	Delivering doxorubicin
DOX	Delivering doxorubicin
DSPE	1,2-distearoyl-sn-glycero-3-phosphoethanolamine
DP	Dermal papillary cell
DHT	Dihydrotestosterone
ECG	Epigallocatechin gallate
ENP	Exosome nanopuncturer
ESCRT	Endosomal sorting complex required for transport
FA	Folic acid
HA	Hyaluronic acid
LNPs	Lipid nanoparticles
lncRNA	Long non-coding RNA
LPS	Lipopolysaccharide
msEVs	Milk-derived small extracellular vesicles
miRNA	MicroRNA
mRNA	Messenger RNA
ncRNA	Non-coding RNA
NEC	Necrotizing enterocolitis
PAC	Paclitaxel
PEG	Polyethylene glycol
sEVs	Small extracellular vesicles
SEC	Size-exclusion chromatography
siRNA	Interfering RNA
SAM	Severe acute malnutrition
TFF	Tangential flow filtration
TLR4	Toll-like receptor 4

References

1. Théry, C.; Zitvogel, L.; Amigorena, S. Exosomes: Composition, biogenesis and function reviews. *Nat. Rev. Immunol.* **2002**, *2*, 569. [CrossRef]
2. Kalluri, R. The biology and function of exosomes in cancer. *J. Clin. Investig.* **2016**, *126*, 1208–1215. [CrossRef]
3. Keller, S.; Sanderson, M.P.; Stoeck, A.; Altevogt, P. Exosomes: From biogenesis and secretion to biological function. *Immunol. Lett.* **2006**, *107*, 102–108. [CrossRef]
4. An, Q.; van Bel, A.J.; Hückelhoven, R. Do plant cells secrete exosomes derived from multivesicular bodies? *Plant Signal. Behav.* **2007**, *2*, 4–7. [CrossRef] [PubMed]
5. Xia, X.; Shi, B.; Wang, L.; Liu, Y.; Zou, Y.; Zhou, Y.; Chen, Y.; Zheng, M.; Zhu, Y.; Duan, J. From mouse to mouse-ear cress: Nanomaterials as vehicles in plant biotechnology. In *Exploration*; Wiley Online Library: New York, NY, USA, 2021.
6. Haug, A.; Høstmark, A.T.; Harstad, O.M. Bovine milk in human nutrition—A review. *Lipids Health Dis.* **2007**, *6*, 1–16. [CrossRef]
7. Zhou, Q.; Li, M.; Wang, X.; Li, Q.; Wang, T.; Zhu, Q.; Zhou, X.; Wang, X.; Gao, X.; Li, X. Immune-related microRNAs are abundant in breast milk exosomes. *Int. J. Biol. Sci.* **2012**, *8*, 118. [CrossRef] [PubMed]
8. Chen, T.; Xie, M.-Y.; Sun, J.-J.; Ye, R.-S.; Cheng, X.; Sun, R.-P.; Wei, L.-M.; Li, M.; Lin, D.-L.; Jiang, Q.-Y. Porcine milk-derived exosomes promote proliferation of intestinal epithelial cells. *Sci. Rep.* **2016**, *6*, 33862. [CrossRef] [PubMed]
9. Sun, J.; Aswath, K.; Schroeder, S.G.; Lippolis, J.D.; Reinhardt, T.A.; Sonstegard, T.S. MicroRNA expression profiles of bovine milk exosomes in response to Staphylococcus aureus infection. *BMC Genom.* **2015**, *16*, 806. [CrossRef]
10. Kalluri, R.; LeBleu, V.S. The biology, function, and biomedical applications of exosomes. *Science* **2020**, *367*, eaau6977. [CrossRef]
11. Yoshioka, Y.; Konishi, Y.; Kosaka, N.; Katsuda, T.; Kato, T.; Ochiya, T. Comparative marker analysis of extracellular vesicles in different human cancer types. *J. Extracell. Vesicles* **2013**, *2*, 20424. [CrossRef] [PubMed]
12. Gobbo, J.; Marcion, G.; Cordonnier, M.; Dias, A.M.; Pernet, N.; Hammann, A.; Richaud, S.; Mjahed, H.; Isambert, N.; Clausse, V. Restoring anticancer immune response by targeting tumor-derived exosomes with a HSP70 peptide aptamer. *J. Natl. Cancer Inst.* **2016**, *108*, djv330. [CrossRef]

13. Villarroya-Beltri, C.; Baixauli, F.; Mittelbrunn, M.; Fernández-Delgado, I.; Torralba, D.; Moreno-Gonzalo, O.; Baldanta, S.; Enrich, C.; Guerra, S.; Sánchez-Madrid, F. ISGylation controls exosome secretion by promoting lysosomal degradation of MVB proteins. *Nat. Commun.* **2016**, *7*, 13588. [CrossRef] [PubMed]
14. Zitvogel, L.; Regnault, A.; Lozier, A.; Wolfers, J.; Flament, C.; Tenza, D.; Ricciardi-Castagnoli, P.; Raposo, G.; Amigorena, S. Eradication of established murine tumors using a novel cell-free vaccine: Dendritic cell derived exosomes. *Nat. Med.* **1998**, *4*, 594–600. [CrossRef]
15. Konala, V.B.R.; Mamidi, M.K.; Bhonde, R.; Das, A.K.; Pochampally, R.; Pal, R. The current landscape of the mesenchymal stromal cell secretome: A new paradigm for cell-free regeneration. *Cytotherapy* **2016**, *18*, 13–24. [CrossRef]
16. Raposo, G.; Stoorvogel, W. Extracellular vesicles: Exosomes, microvesicles, and friends. *J. Cell Biol.* **2013**, *200*, 373–383. [CrossRef] [PubMed]
17. Hinde, E.; Thammasiraphop, K.; Duong, H.T.; Yeow, J.; Karagoz, B.; Boyer, C.; Gooding, J.J.; Gaus, K. Pair correlation microscopy reveals the role of nanoparticle shape in intracellular transport and site of drug release. *Nat. Nanotechnol.* **2017**, *12*, 81–89. [CrossRef] [PubMed]
18. Sharma, A.K.; Gothwal, A.; Kesharwani, P.; Alsaab, H.; Iyer, A.K.; Gupta, U. Dendrimer nanoarchitectures for cancer diagnosis and anticancer drug delivery. *Drug Discov. Today* **2017**, *22*, 314–326. [CrossRef]
19. Luan, X.; Guan, Y.-Y.; Lovell, J.F.; Zhao, M.; Lu, Q.; Liu, Y.-R.; Liu, H.-J.; Gao, Y.-G.; Dong, X.; Yang, S.-C. Tumor priming using metronomic chemotherapy with neovasculature-targeted, nanoparticulate paclitaxel. *Biomaterials* **2016**, *95*, 60–73. [CrossRef]
20. Haque, S.; Whittaker, M.R.; McIntosh, M.P.; Pouton, C.W.; Kaminskas, L.M. Disposition and safety of inhaled biodegradable nanomedicines: Opportunities and challenges. *Nanomed. Nanotechnol. Biol. Med.* **2016**, *12*, 1703–1724. [CrossRef]
21. Shan, S.; Chen, J.; Sun, Y.; Wang, Y.; Xia, B.; Tan, H.; Pan, C.; Gu, G.; Zhong, J.; Qing, G. Functionalized macrophage exosomes with panobinostat and PPM1D-siRNA for diffuse intrinsic pontine gliomas therapy. *Adv. Sci.* **2022**, *9*, 2200353. [CrossRef]
22. Zhong, J.; Xia, B.; Shan, S.; Zheng, A.; Zhang, S.; Chen, J.; Liang, X.-J. High-quality milk exosomes as oral drug delivery system. *Biomaterials* **2021**, *277*, 121126. [CrossRef] [PubMed]
23. Babst, M.; Katzmann, D.J.; Estepa-Sabal, E.J.; Meerloo, T.; Emr, S.D. Escrt-III: An endosome-associated heterooligomeric protein complex required for mvb sorting. *Dev. Cell* **2002**, *3*, 271–282. [CrossRef] [PubMed]
24. Ostrowski, M.; Carmo, N.B.; Krumeich, S.; Fanget, I.; Raposo, G.; Savina, A.; Moita, C.F.; Schauer, K.; Hume, A.N.; Freitas, R.P. Rab27a and Rab27b control different steps of the exosome secretion pathway. *Nat. Cell Biol.* **2010**, *12*, 19–30. [CrossRef]
25. Hyenne, V.; Apaydin, A.; Rodriguez, D.; Spiegelhalter, C.; Hoff-Yoessle, S.; Diem, M.; Tak, S.; Lefebvre, O.; Schwab, Y.; Goetz, J.G. RAL-1 controls multivesicular body biogenesis and exosome secretion. *J. Cell Biol.* **2015**, *211*, 27–37. [CrossRef]
26. Futter, C.E.; Pearse, A.; Hewlett, L.J.; Hopkins, C.R. Multivesicular endosomes containing internalized EGF-EGF receptor complexes mature and then fuse directly with lysosomes. *J. Cell Biol.* **1996**, *132*, 1011–1023. [CrossRef] [PubMed]
27. Stuffers, S.; Sem Wegner, C.; Stenmark, H.; Brech, A. Multivesicular endosome biogenesis in the absence of ESCRTs. *Traffic* **2009**, *10*, 925–937. [CrossRef]
28. Conde-Vancells, J.; Rodriguez-Suarez, E.; Embade, N.; Gil, D.; Matthiesen, R.; Valle, M.; Elortza, F.; Lu, S.C.; Mato, J.M.; Falcon-Perez, J.M. Characterization and comprehensive proteome profiling of exosomes secreted by hepatocytes. *J. Proteome Res.* **2008**, *7*, 5157–5166. [CrossRef]
29. Subra, C.; Grand, D.; Laulagnier, K.; Stella, A.; Lambeau, G.; Paillasse, M.; De Medina, P.; Monsarrat, B.; Perret, B.; Silvente-Poirot, S. Exosomes account for vesicle-mediated transcellular transport of activatable phospholipases and prostaglandins. *J. Lipid Res.* **2010**, *51*, 2105–2120. [CrossRef] [PubMed]
30. Alvarez-Erviti, L.; Seow, Y.; Yin, H.; Betts, C.; Lakhal, S.; Wood, M.J. Delivery of siRNA to the mouse brain by systemic injection of targeted exosomes. *Nat. Biotechnol.* **2011**, *29*, 341–345. [CrossRef] [PubMed]
31. McMahon, H.T.; Boucrot, E. Membrane curvature at a glance. *J. Cell Sci.* **2015**, *128*, 1065–1070. [CrossRef]
32. Han, Q.-F.; Li, W.-J.; Hu, K.-S.; Gao, J.; Zhai, W.-L.; Yang, J.-H.; Zhang, S.-J. Exosome biogenesis: Machinery, regulation, and therapeutic implications in cancer. *Mol. Cancer* **2022**, *21*, 1–26. [CrossRef]
33. Munagala, R.; Aqil, F.; Jeyabalan, J.; Gupta, R.C. Bovine milk-derived exosomes for drug delivery. *Cancer Lett.* **2016**, *371*, 48–61. [CrossRef]
34. Benmoussa, A.; Ly, S.; Shan, S.T.; Laugier, J.; Boilard, E.; Gilbert, C.; Provost, P. A subset of extracellular vesicles carries the bulk of microRNAs in commercial dairy cow's milk. *J. Extracell. Vesicles* **2017**, *6*, 1401897. [CrossRef]
35. Wolf, T.; Baier, S.R.; Zempleni, J. The intestinal transport of bovine milk exosomes is mediated by endocytosis in human colon carcinoma Caco-2 cells and rat small intestinal IEC-6 cells. *J. Nutr.* **2015**, *145*, 2201–2206. [CrossRef] [PubMed]
36. Kusuma, R.J.; Manca, S.; Friemel, T.; Sukreet, S.; Nguyen, C.; Zempleni, J. Human vascular endothelial cells transport foreign exosomes from cow's milk by endocytosis. *Am. J. Physiol.-Cell Physiol.* **2016**, *310*, C800–C807. [CrossRef] [PubMed]
37. Blans, K.; Hansen, M.S.; Sørensen, L.V.; Hvam, M.L.; Howard, K.A.; Möller, A.; Wiking, L.; Larsen, L.B.; Rasmussen, J.T. Pellet-free isolation of human and bovine milk extracellular vesicles by size-exclusion chromatography. *J. Extracell. Vesicles* **2017**, *6*, 1294340. [CrossRef] [PubMed]
38. Lee, C.; Mitsialis, S.A.; Aslam, M.; Vitali, S.H.; Vergadi, E.; Konstantinou, G.; Sdrimas, K.; Fernandez-Gonzalez, A.; Kourembanas, S. Exosomes mediate the cytoprotective action of mesenchymal stromal cells on hypoxia-induced pulmonary hypertension. *Circulation* **2012**, *126*, 2601–2611. [CrossRef]

39. Fernando, M.R.; Jiang, C.; Krzyzanowski, G.D.; Ryan, W.L. New evidence that a large proportion of human blood plasma cell-free DNA is localized in exosomes. *PLoS ONE* **2017**, *12*, e0183915. [CrossRef]
40. Baranyai, T.; Herczeg, K.; Onódi, Z.; Voszka, I.; Módos, K.; Marton, N.; Nagy, G.; Maeger, I.; Wood, M.J.; El Andaloussi, S. Isolation of exosomes from blood plasma: Qualitative and quantitative comparison of ultracentrifugation and size exclusion chromatography methods. *PLoS ONE* **2015**, *10*, e0145686. [CrossRef]
41. Cheng, X.; Zhang, G.; Zhang, L.; Hu, Y.; Zhang, K.; Sun, X.; Zhao, C.; Li, H.; Li, Y.M.; Zhao, J. Mesenchymal stem cells deliver exogenous miR-21 via exosomes to inhibit nucleus pulposus cell apoptosis and reduce intervertebral disc degeneration. *J. Cell. Mol. Med.* **2018**, *22*, 261–276. [CrossRef]
42. Ferreira, A.D.F.; Cunha, P.D.S.; Carregal, V.M.; Silva, P.D.C.D.; Miranda, M.C.D.; Kunrath-Lima, M.; de Melo, M.I.A.; Faraco, C.C.F.; Barbosa, J.L.; Frezard, F.; et al. Extracellular vesicles from adipose-derived mesenchymal stem/stromal cells accelerate migration and activate AKT pathway in human keratinocytes and fibroblasts independently of miR-205 activity. *Stem Cells Int.* **2017**, *2017*, 9841035. [CrossRef] [PubMed]
43. Keller, S.; Ridinger, J.; Rupp, A.-K.; Janssen, J.W.; Altevogt, P. Body fluid derived exosomes as a novel template for clinical diagnostics. *J. Transl. Med.* **2011**, *9*, 86. [CrossRef]
44. Lässer, C.; Seyed Alikhani, V.; Ekström, K.; Eldh, M.; Torregrosa Paredes, P.; Bossios, A.; Sjöstrand, M.; Gabrielsson, S.; Lötvall, J.; Valadi, H. Human saliva, plasma and breast milk exosomes contain RNA: Uptake by macrophages. *J. Transl. Med.* **2011**, *9*, 1–8. [CrossRef]
45. Somiya, M.; Yoshioka, Y.; Ochiya, T. Biocompatibility of highly purified bovine milk-derived extracellular vesicles. *J. Extracell. Vesicles* **2018**, *7*, 1440132. [CrossRef]
46. Domenis, R.; Zanutel, R.; Caponnetto, F.; Toffoletto, B.; Cifù, A.; Pistis, C.; Di Benedetto, P.; Causero, A.; Pozzi, M.; Bassini, F. Characterization of the proinflammatory profile of synovial fluid-derived exosomes of patients with osteoarthritis. *Mediat. Inflamm.* **2017**, *2017*, 4814987. [CrossRef]
47. Coulter, M.E.; Dorobantu, C.M.; Lodewijk, G.A.; Delalande, F.; Cianferani, S.; Ganesh, V.S.; Smith, R.S.; Lim, E.T.; Xu, C.S.; Pang, S. The ESCRT-III protein CHMP1A mediates secretion of sonic hedgehog on a distinctive subtype of extracellular vesicles. *Cell Rep.* **2018**, *24*, 973–986.e978. [CrossRef]
48. Samuel, M.; Chisanga, D.; Liem, M.; Keerthikumar, S.; Anand, S.; Ang, C.-S.; Adda, C.G.; Versteegen, E.; Jois, M.; Mathivanan, S. Bovine milk-derived exosomes from colostrum are enriched with proteins implicated in immune response and growth. *Sci. Rep.* **2017**, *7*, 5933. [CrossRef] [PubMed]
49. Masyuk, A.I.; Huang, B.Q.; Ward, C.J.; Gradilone, S.A.; Banales, J.M.; Masyuk, T.V.; Radtke, B.; Splinter, P.L.; LaRusso, N.F. Biliary exosomes influence cholangiocyte regulatory mechanisms and proliferation through interaction with primary cilia. *Am. J. Physiol.-Gastrointest. Liver Physiol.* **2010**, *299*, G990–G999. [CrossRef] [PubMed]
50. Polanco, J.C.; Scicluna, B.J.; Hill, A.F.; Götz, J. Extracellular vesicles isolated from the brains of rTg4510 mice seed tau protein aggregation in a threshold-dependent manner. *J. Biol. Chem.* **2016**, *291*, 12445–12466. [CrossRef]
51. Wang, J.; Wu, Y.; Guo, J.; Fei, X.; Yu, L.; Ma, S. Adipocyte-derived exosomes promote lung cancer metastasis by increasing MMP9 activity via transferring MMP3 to lung cancer cells. *Oncotarget* **2017**, *8*, 81880. [CrossRef]
52. Keller, S.; Rupp, C.; Stoeck, A.; Runz, S.; Fogel, M.; Lugert, S.; Hager, H.-D.; Abdel-Bakky, M.; Gutwein, P.; Altevogt, P. CD24 is a marker of exosomes secreted into urine and amniotic fluid. *Kidney Int.* **2007**, *72*, 1095–1102. [CrossRef]
53. Théry, C.; Amigorena, S.; Raposo, G.; Clayton, A. Isolation and characterization of exosomes from cell culture supernatants and biological fluids. *Curr. Protoc. Cell Biol.* **2006**, *30*, 3–22. [CrossRef] [PubMed]
54. Witwer, K.W.; Buzás, E.I.; Bemis, L.T.; Bora, A.; Lässer, C.; Lötvall, J.; Nolte-'t Hoen, E.N.; Piper, M.G.; Sivaraman, S.; Skog, J. Standardization of sample collection, isolation and analysis methods in extracellular vesicle research. *J. Extracell. Vesicles* **2013**, *2*, 20360. [CrossRef]
55. Buschmann, D.; Mussack, V.; Byrd, J.B. Separation, characterization, and standardization of extracellular vesicles for drug delivery applications. *Adv. Drug Deliv. Rev.* **2021**, *174*, 348–368. [CrossRef] [PubMed]
56. Yamada, T.; Inoshima, Y.; Matsuda, T.; Ishiguro, N. Comparison of methods for isolating exosomes from bovine milk. *J. Vet. Med. Sci.* **2012**, *74*, 1523–1525. [CrossRef] [PubMed]
57. Tangwattanachuleeporn, M.; Muanwien, P.; Teethaisong, Y.; Somparn, P. Optimizing Concentration of Polyethelene Glycol for Exosome Isolation from Plasma for Downstream Application. *Medicina* **2022**, *58*, 1600. [CrossRef]
58. Izumi, H.; Tsuda, M.; Sato, Y.; Kosaka, N.; Ochiya, T.; Iwamoto, H.; Namba, K.; Takeda, Y. Bovine milk exosomes contain microRNA and mRNA and are taken up by human macrophages. *J. Dairy Sci.* **2015**, *98*, 2920–2933. [CrossRef]
59. Lobb, R.J.; Becker, M.; Wen Wen, S.; Wong, C.S.; Wiegmans, A.P.; Leimgruber, A.; Möller, A. Optimized exosome isolation protocol for cell culture supernatant and human plasma. *J. Extracell. Vesicles* **2015**, *4*, 27031. [CrossRef]
60. Szatanek, R.; Baran, J.; Siedlar, M.; Baj-Krzyworzeka, M. Isolation of extracellular vesicles: Determining the correct approach. *Int. J. Mol. Med.* **2015**, *36*, 11–17. [CrossRef]
61. Li, P.; Kaslan, M.; Lee, S.H.; Yao, J.; Gao, Z. Progress in exosome isolation techniques. *Theranostics* **2017**, *7*, 789. [CrossRef]
62. Kim, J.Y.; Rhim, W.-K.; Yoo, Y.-I.; Kim, D.-S.; Ko, K.-W.; Heo, Y.; Park, C.G.; Han, D.K. Defined MSC exosome with high yield and purity to improve regenerative activity. *J. Tissue Eng.* **2021**, *12*, 20417314211008626. [CrossRef] [PubMed]
63. Linares, R.; Tan, S.; Gounou, C.; Arraud, N.; Brisson, A. High-speed centrifugation induces aggregation of extracellular vesicles. *J. Extracell. Vesicles* **2015**, *4*, 29509. [CrossRef] [PubMed]

64. Watson, D.C.; Yung, B.C.; Bergamaschi, C.; Chowdhury, B.; Bear, J.; Stellas, D.; Morales-Kastresana, A.; Jones, J.C.; Felber, B.K.; Chen, X. Scalable, cGMP-compatible purification of extracellular vesicles carrying bioactive human heterodimeric IL-15/lactadherin complexes. *J. Extracell. Vesicles* **2018**, *7*, 1442088. [CrossRef] [PubMed]
65. Foers, A.D.; Chatfield, S.; Dagley, L.F.; Scicluna, B.J.; Webb, A.I.; Cheng, L.; Hill, A.F.; Wicks, I.P.; Pang, K.C. Enrichment of extracellular vesicles from human synovial fluid using size exclusion chromatography. *J. Extracell. Vesicles* **2018**, *7*, 1490145. [CrossRef] [PubMed]
66. Monguió-Tortajada, M.; Gálvez-Montón, C.; Bayes-Genis, A.; Roura, S.; Borràs, F.E. Extracellular vesicle isolation methods: Rising impact of size-exclusion chromatography. *Cell. Mol. Life Sci.* **2019**, *76*, 2369–2382. [CrossRef]
67. Huang, K.; Garimella, S.; Clay-Gilmour, A.; Vojtech, L.; Armstrong, B.; Bessonny, M.; Stamatikos, A. Comparison of Human Urinary Exosomes Isolated via Ultracentrifugation Alone versus Ultracentrifugation Followed by SEC Column-Purification. *J. Pers. Med.* **2022**, *12*, 340. [CrossRef]
68. Dalgleish, D.G.; Corredig, M. The structure of the casein micelle of milk and its changes during processing. *Annu. Rev. Food Sci. Technol.* **2012**, *3*, 449–467. [CrossRef]
69. Obeid, S.; Guyomarc'h, F.; David-Briand, E.; Gaucheron, F.; Riaublanc, A.; Lopez, C. The phase and charge of milk polar lipid membrane bilayers govern their selective interactions with proteins as demonstrated with casein micelles. *J. Colloid Interface Sci.* **2019**, *534*, 279–290. [CrossRef]
70. del Pozo-Acebo, L.; López de las Hazas, M.; Tomé-Carneiro, J.; Gil-Cabrerizo, P.; San-Cristobal, R.; Busto, R.; García-Ruiz, A.; Dávalos, A. Bovine milk-derived exosomes as a drug delivery vehicle for miRNA-based therapy. *Int. J. Mol. Sci.* **2021**, *22*, 1105. [CrossRef]
71. Vaswani, K.; Koh, Y.Q.; Almughlliq, F.B.; Peiris, H.N.; Mitchell, M.D. A method for the isolation and enrichment of purified bovine milk exosomes. *Reprod. Biol.* **2017**, *17*, 341–348. [CrossRef]
72. Warren, M.R.; Zhang, C.; Vedadghavami, A.; Bokvist, K.; Dhal, P.K.; Bajpayee, A.G. Milk exosomes with enhanced mucus penetrability for oral delivery of siRNA. *Biomater. Sci.* **2021**, *9*, 4260–4277. [CrossRef]
73. Benmoussa, A.; Michel, S.; Gilbert, C.; Provost, P. Isolating multiple extracellular vesicles subsets, including exosomes and membrane vesicles, from bovine milk using sodium citrate and differential ultracentrifugation. *Bio-Protocol* **2020**, *10*, e3636. [CrossRef] [PubMed]
74. Chen, J.; Xu, Y.; Lu, Y.; Xing, W. Isolation and visible detection of tumor-derived exosomes from plasma. *Anal. Chem.* **2018**, *90*, 14207–14215. [CrossRef] [PubMed]
75. Chen, J.; Xu, Y.; Wang, X.; Liu, D.; Yang, F.; Zhu, X.; Lu, Y.; Xing, W. Rapid and efficient isolation and detection of extracellular vesicles from plasma for lung cancer diagnosis. *Lab Chip* **2019**, *19*, 432–443. [CrossRef]
76. Zempleni, J.; Aguilar-Lozano, A.; Sadri, M.; Sukreet, S.; Manca, S.; Wu, D.; Zhou, F.; Mutai, E. Biological activities of extracellular vesicles and their cargos from bovine and human milk in humans and implications for infants. *J. Nutr.* **2017**, *147*, 3–10. [CrossRef] [PubMed]
77. Yang, M.; Song, D.; Cao, X.; Wu, R.; Liu, B.; Ye, W.; Wu, J.; Yue, X. Comparative proteomic analysis of milk-derived exosomes in human and bovine colostrum and mature milk samples by iTRAQ-coupled LC-MS/MS. *Food Res. Int.* **2017**, *92*, 17–25. [CrossRef] [PubMed]
78. Wang, Y.; Li, D.; Wang, Y.; Li, M.; Fang, X.; Chen, H.; Zhang, C. The landscape of circular RNAs and mRNAs in bovine milk exosomes. *J. Food Compos. Anal.* **2019**, *76*, 33–38. [CrossRef]
79. Zeng, B.; Chen, T.; Xie, M.-Y.; Luo, J.-Y.; He, J.-J.; Xi, Q.-Y.; Sun, J.-J.; Zhang, Y.-L. Exploration of long noncoding RNA in bovine milk exosomes and their stability during digestion in vitro. *J. Dairy Sci.* **2019**, *102*, 6726–6737. [CrossRef]
80. Rahman, M.; Takashima, S.; Kamatari, Y.O.; Badr, Y.; Kitamura, Y.; Shimizu, K.; Okada, A.; Inoshima, Y. Proteomic profiling of milk small extracellular vesicles from bovine leukemia virus-infected cattle. *Sci. Rep.* **2021**, *11*, 2951. [CrossRef]
81. Reinhardt, T.A.; Lippolis, J.D.; Nonnecke, B.J.; Sacco, R.E. Bovine milk exosome proteome. *J. Proteom.* **2012**, *75*, 1486–1492. [CrossRef]
82. Vaswani, K.M.; Peiris, H.; Qin Koh, Y.; Hill, R.J.; Harb, T.; Arachchige, B.J.; Logan, J.; Reed, S.; Davies, P.S.; Mitchell, M.D. A complete proteomic profile of human and bovine milk exosomes by liquid chromatography mass spectrometry. *Expert Rev. Proteom.* **2021**, *18*, 719–735. [CrossRef] [PubMed]
83. Zhang, M.; Ma, Z.; Li, R.; Guo, S.; Qiu, Y.; Gao, X. Proteomic analysis reveals proteins and pathways associated with lactation in bovine mammary epithelial cell-derived exosomes. *J. Proteome Res.* **2020**, *19*, 3211–3219. [CrossRef]
84. Maity, S.; Bhat, A.H.; Giri, K.; Ambatipudi, K. BoMiProt: A database of bovine milk proteins. *J. Proteom.* **2020**, *215*, 103648. [CrossRef] [PubMed]
85. Hata, T.; Murakami, K.; Nakatani, H.; Yamamoto, Y.; Matsuda, T.; Aoki, N. Isolation of bovine milk-derived microvesicles carrying mRNAs and microRNAs. *Biochem. Biophys. Res. Commun.* **2010**, *396*, 528–533. [CrossRef] [PubMed]
86. Gao, H.; Guo, H.; Zhang, H.; Xie, X.; Wen, P.; Ren, F. Yak-milk-derived exosomes promote proliferation of intestinal epithelial cells in an hypoxic environment. *J. Dairy Sci.* **2019**, *102*, 985–996. [CrossRef]
87. Martin, C.; Patel, M.; Williams, S.; Arora, H.; Sims, B. Human breast milk-derived exosomes attenuate cell death in intestinal epithelial cells. *Innate Immun.* **2018**, *24*, 278–284. [CrossRef]

88. Chen, X.; Gao, C.; Li, H.; Huang, L.; Sun, Q.; Dong, Y.; Tian, C.; Gao, S.; Dong, H.; Guan, D. Identification and characterization of microRNAs in raw milk during different periods of lactation, commercial fluid, and powdered milk products. *Cell Res.* **2010**, *20*, 1128–1137. [CrossRef]
89. Shome, S.; Jernigan, R.; Beitz, D.C.; Clark, S.; Testroet, E. Non-coding RNA in raw and commercially processed milk and putative targets related to growth and immune-response. *BMC Genom.* **2021**, *22*, 749. [CrossRef]
90. Sukreet, S.; Braga, C.P.; An, T.T.; Adamec, J.; Cui, J.; Zempleni, J. Ultrasonication of Milk Decreases the Content of Exosomes and MicroRNAs in an Exosome-defined Rodent Diet. *J. Nutr.* **2022**, *152*, 961–970. [CrossRef]
91. He, Y.; He, Z.; Leone, S.; Liu, S. Milk Exosomes Transfer Oligosaccharides into Macrophages to Modulate Immunity and Attenuate Adherent-Invasive *E. coli* (AIEC) Infection. *Nutrients* **2021**, *13*, 3198. [CrossRef]
92. Chen, W.; Wang, R.; Li, D.; Zuo, C.; Wen, P.; Liu, H.; Chen, Y.; Fujita, M.; Wu, Z.; Yang, G. Comprehensive analysis of the glycome and glycoproteome of bovine milk-derived exosomes. *J. Agric. Food Chem.* **2020**, *68*, 12692–12701. [CrossRef] [PubMed]
93. Ortega-Anaya, J.; Jiménez-Flores, R. Symposium review: The relevance of bovine milk phospholipids in human nutrition—Evidence of the effect on infant gut and brain development. *J. Dairy Sci.* **2019**, *102*, 2738–2748. [CrossRef] [PubMed]
94. Hullin-Matsuda, F.; Colosetti, P.; Rabia, M.; Luquain-Costaz, C.; Delton, I. Exosomal lipids from membrane organization to biomarkers: Focus on an endolysosomal-specific lipid. *Biochimie* **2022**, *203*, 77–92. [CrossRef]
95. Skotland, T.; Hessvik, N.P.; Sandvig, K.; Llorente, A. Exosomal lipid composition and the role of ether lipids and phosphoinositides in exosome biology. *J. Lipid Res.* **2019**, *60*, 9–18. [CrossRef]
96. Suga, K.; Matsui, D.; Watanabe, N.; Okamoto, Y.; Umakoshi, H. Insight into the Exosomal Membrane: From Viewpoints of Membrane Fluidity and Polarity. *Langmuir* **2021**, *37*, 11195–11202. [CrossRef] [PubMed]
97. Isaac, R.; Reis, F.C.G.; Ying, W.; Olefsky, J.M. Exosomes as mediators of intercellular crosstalk in metabolism. *Cell Metab.* **2021**, *33*, 1744–1762. [CrossRef]
98. Betker, J.L.; Angle, B.M.; Graner, M.W.; Anchordoquy, T.J. The potential of exosomes from cow milk for oral delivery. *J. Pharm. Sci.* **2019**, *108*, 1496–1505. [CrossRef]
99. Vella, L.J.; Hill, A.F.; Cheng, L. Focus on extracellular vesicles: Exosomes and their role in protein trafficking and biomarker potential in Alzheimer's and Parkinson's disease. *Int. J. Mol. Sci.* **2016**, *17*, 173. [CrossRef]
100. Camussi, G.; Deregibus, M.C.; Bruno, S.; Cantaluppi, V.; Biancone, L. Exosomes/microvesicles as a mechanism of cell-to-cell communication. *Kidney Int.* **2010**, *78*, 838–848. [CrossRef]
101. Pieters, B.C.; Arntz, O.J.; Bennink, M.B.; Broeren, M.G.; van Caam, A.P.; Koenders, M.I.; van Lent, P.L.; van den Berg, W.B.; de Vries, M.; van der Kraan, P.M. Commercial cow milk contains physically stable extracellular vesicles expressing immunoregulatory TGF-β. *PLoS ONE* **2015**, *10*, e0121123. [CrossRef]
102. Yu, S.; Zhao, Z.; Sun, L.; Li, P. Fermentation results in quantitative changes in milk-derived exosomes and different effects on cell growth and survival. *J. Agric. Food Chem.* **2017**, *65*, 1220–1228. [CrossRef]
103. Baier, S.R.; Nguyen, C.; Xie, F.; Wood, J.R.; Zempleni, J. MicroRNAs are absorbed in biologically meaningful amounts from nutritionally relevant doses of cow milk and affect gene expression in peripheral blood mononuclear cells, HEK-293 kidney cell cultures, and mouse livers. *J. Nutr.* **2014**, *144*, 1495–1500. [CrossRef] [PubMed]
104. Naqvi, A.R.; Fordham, J.B.; Nares, S. miR-24, miR-30b, and miR-142-3p regulate phagocytosis in myeloid inflammatory cells. *J. Immunol.* **2015**, *194*, 1916–1927. [CrossRef] [PubMed]
105. Benmoussa, A.; Gotti, C.; Bourassa, S.; Gilbert, C.; Provost, P. Identification of protein markers for extracellular vesicle (EV) subsets in cow's milk. *J. Proteom.* **2019**, *192*, 78–88. [CrossRef] [PubMed]
106. Melnik, B.C.; Schmitz, G. MicroRNAs: Milk's epigenetic regulators. *Best Pract. Res. Clin. Endocrinol. Metab.* **2017**, *31*, 427–442. [CrossRef]
107. Lin, D.; Chen, T.; Xie, M.; Li, M.; Zeng, B.; Sun, R.; Zhu, Y.; Ye, D.; Wu, J.; Sun, J. Oral administration of bovine and porcine milk exosome alter miRNAs profiles in piglet serum. *Sci. Rep.* **2020**, *10*, 6983. [CrossRef]
108. Ross, M.; Atalla, H.; Karrow, N.; Mallard, B.A. The bioactivity of colostrum and milk exosomes of high, average, and low immune responder cows on human intestinal epithelial cells. *J. Dairy Sci.* **2021**, *104*, 2499–2510. [CrossRef]
109. Wang, L.; Shi, Z.; Wang, X.; Mu, S.; Xu, X.; Shen, L.; Li, P. Protective effects of bovine milk exosomes against oxidative stress in IEC-6 cells. *Eur. J. Nutr.* **2021**, *60*, 317–327. [CrossRef]
110. Wang, L.; Wang, X.; Shi, Z.; Shen, L.; Zhang, J.; Zhang, J. Bovine milk exosomes attenuate the alteration of purine metabolism and energy status in IEC-6 cells induced by hydrogen peroxide. *Food Chem.* **2021**, *350*, 129142. [CrossRef]
111. Gao, H.; Ren, F.; Wen, P.; Xie, L.; Wang, R.; Yang, Z.; Li, Y. Yak milk–derived exosomal microRNAs regulate intestinal epithelial cells on proliferation in hypoxic environment. *J. Dairy Sci.* **2021**, *104*, 1291–1303. [CrossRef]
112. Good, M.; Sodhi, C.P.; Egan, C.E.; Afrazi, A.; Jia, H.; Yamaguchi, Y.; Lu, P.; Branca, M.F.; Ma, C.; Prindle, T. Breast milk protects against the development of necrotizing enterocolitis through inhibition of Toll-like receptor 4 in the intestinal epithelium via activation of the epidermal growth factor receptor. *Mucosal Immunol.* **2015**, *8*, 1166–1179. [CrossRef] [PubMed]
113. Stremmel, W.; Weiskirchen, R.; Melnik, B.C. Milk exosomes prevent intestinal inflammation in a genetic mouse model of ulcerative colitis: A pilot experiment. *Inflamm. Intest. Dis.* **2020**, *5*, 117–123. [CrossRef] [PubMed]
114. Wu, D.; Kittana, H.; Shu, J.; Kachman, S.D.; Cui, J.; Ramer-Tait, A.E.; Zempleni, J. Dietary depletion of milk exosomes and their microRNA cargos elicits a depletion of miR-200a-3p and elevated intestinal inflammation and chemokine (CXC motif) ligand 9 expression in Mdr1a$^{-/-}$ mice. *Curr. Dev. Nutr.* **2019**, 3, nzz122. [CrossRef]

115. Li, B.; Hock, A.; Wu, R.Y.; Minich, A.; Botts, S.R.; Lee, C.; Antounians, L.; Miyake, H.; Koike, Y.; Chen, Y. Bovine milk-derived exosomes enhance goblet cell activity and prevent the development of experimental necrotizing enterocolitis. *PLoS ONE* **2019**, *14*, e0211431. [CrossRef]
116. Han, G.; Cho, H.; Kim, H.; Jang, Y.; Jang, H.; Kim, E.S.; Kim, E.H.; Hwang, K.Y.; Kim, K.; Yang, Y. Bovine colostrum derived-exosomes prevent dextran sulfate sodium-induced intestinal colitis via suppression of inflammation and oxidative stress. *Biomater. Sci.* **2022**, *10*, 2076–2087. [CrossRef] [PubMed]
117. Reif, S.; Elbaum Shiff, Y.; Golan-Gerstl, R. Milk-derived exosomes (MDEs) have a different biological effect on normal fetal colon epithelial cells compared to colon tumor cells in a miRNA-dependent manner. *J. Transl. Med.* **2019**, *17*, 1–10. [CrossRef]
118. Gao, H.; Hu, H.; Wen, P.; Lian, S.; Xie, X.; Song, H.; Yang, Z.; Ren, F. Yak milk–derived exosomes alleviate lipopolysaccharide-induced intestinal inflammation by inhibiting PI3K/AKT/C3 pathway activation. *J. Dairy Sci.* **2021**, *104*, 8411–8424. [CrossRef]
119. Maghraby, M.K.; Li, B.; Chi, L.; Ling, C.; Benmoussa, A.; Provost, P.; Postmus, A.C.; Abdi, A.; Pierro, A.; Bourdon, C. Extracellular vesicles isolated from milk can improve gut barrier dysfunction induced by malnutrition. *Sci. Rep.* **2021**, *11*, 7635. [CrossRef]
120. Tong, L.; Hao, H.; Zhang, X.; Zhang, Z.; Lv, Y.; Zhang, L.; Yi, H. Oral Administration of Bovine Milk-Derived Extracellular Vesicles Alters the Gut Microbiota and Enhances Intestinal Immunity in Mice. *Mol. Nutr. Food Res.* **2020**, *64*, 1901251. [CrossRef]
121. Zhou, F.; Paz, H.A.; Sadri, M.; Cui, J.; Kachman, S.D.; Fernando, S.C.; Zempleni, J. Dietary bovine milk exosomes elicit changes in bacterial communities in C57BL/6 mice. *Am. J. Physiol.-Gastrointest. Liver Physiol.* **2019**, *317*, G618–G624. [CrossRef]
122. Aarts, J.; Boleij, A.; Pieters, B.C.; Feitsma, A.L.; van Neerven, R.; Ten Klooster, J.P.; M'Rabet, L.; Arntz, O.J.; Koenders, M.I.; van de Loo, F.A. Flood Control: How Milk-Derived Extracellular Vesicles Can Help to Improve the Intestinal Barrier Function and Break the Gut–Joint Axis in Rheumatoid Arthritis. *Front. Immunol.* **2021**, *12*, 2931. [CrossRef] [PubMed]
123. Tong, L.; Hao, H.; Zhang, Z.; Lv, Y.; Liang, X.; Liu, Q.; Liu, T.; Gong, P.; Zhang, L.; Cao, F. Milk-derived extracellular vesicles alleviate ulcerative colitis by regulating the gut immunity and reshaping the gut microbiota. *Theranostics* **2021**, *11*, 8570. [CrossRef] [PubMed]
124. Melnik, B.C.; John, S.M.; Schmitz, G. Milk is not just food but most likely a genetic transfection system activating mTORC1 signaling for postnatal growth. *Nutr. J.* **2013**, *12*, 103. [CrossRef] [PubMed]
125. Oliveira, M.C.; Arntz, O.J.; Davidson, E.N.B.; van Lent, P.L.; Koenders, M.I.; van der Kraan, P.M.; van den Berg, W.B.; Ferreira, A.V.; van de Loo, F.A. Milk extracellular vesicles accelerate osteoblastogenesis but impair bone matrix formation. *J. Nutr. Biochem.* **2016**, *30*, 74–84. [CrossRef] [PubMed]
126. Leiferman, A.; Shu, J.; Grove, R.; Cui, J.; Adamec, J.; Zempleni, J. A diet defined by its content of bovine milk exosomes and their RNA cargos has moderate effects on gene expression, amino acid profiles and grip strength in skeletal muscle in C57BL/6 mice. *J. Nutr. Biochem.* **2018**, *59*, 123–128. [CrossRef]
127. Yun, B.; Maburutse, B.; Kang, M.; Park, M.; Park, D.; Kim, Y.; Oh, S. Dietary bovine milk–derived exosomes improve bone health in an osteoporosis-induced mouse model. *J. Dairy Sci.* **2020**, *103*, 7752–7760. [CrossRef] [PubMed]
128. Kim, H.; Kim, D.E.; Han, G.; Lim, N.R.; Kim, E.H.; Jang, Y.; Cho, H.; Jang, H.; Kim, K.H.; Kim, S.H. Harnessing the Natural Healing Power of Colostrum: Bovine Milk-Derived Extracellular Vesicles from Colostrum Facilitating the Transition from Inflammation to Tissue Regeneration for Accelerating Cutaneous Wound Healing. *Adv. Healthc. Mater.* **2022**, *11*, 2102027. [CrossRef]
129. Yamamoto, T.; Kosaka, N.; Ochiya, T. Latest advances in extracellular vesicles: From bench to bedside. *Sci. Technol. Adv. Mater.* **2019**, *20*, 746–757. [CrossRef]
130. Colitti, M.; Sgorlon, S.; Stefanon, B. Exosome cargo in milk as a potential marker of cow health. *J. Dairy Res.* **2020**, *87*, 79–83. [CrossRef]
131. Abeysinghe, P.; Turner, N.; Morean Garcia, I.; Mosaad, E.; Peiris, H.N.; Mitchell, M.D. The role of exosomal epigenetic modifiers in cell communication and fertility of dairy cows. *Int. J. Mol. Sci.* **2020**, *21*, 9106. [CrossRef]
132. Ma, S.; Tong, C.; Ibeagha-Awemu, E.M.; Zhao, X. Identification and characterization of differentially expressed exosomal microRNAs in bovine milk infected with Staphylococcus aureus. *BMC Genom.* **2019**, *20*, 934. [CrossRef]
133. Reinhardt, T.A.; Sacco, R.E.; Nonnecke, B.J.; Lippolis, J.D. Bovine milk proteome: Quantitative changes in normal milk exosomes, milk fat globule membranes and whey proteomes resulting from Staphylococcus aureus mastitis. *J. Proteom.* **2013**, *82*, 141–154. [CrossRef] [PubMed]
134. Yamada, T.; Shigemura, H.; Ishiguro, N.; Inoshima, Y. Cell Infectivity in relation to bovine leukemia virus gp51 and p24 in bovine milk exosomes. *PLoS ONE* **2013**, *8*, e77359. [CrossRef] [PubMed]
135. Arntz, O.J.; Pieters, B.C.; Oliveira, M.C.; Broeren, M.G.; Bennink, M.B.; de Vries, M.; van Lent, P.L.; Koenders, M.I.; van den Berg, W.B.; van der Kraan, P.M. Oral administration of bovine milk derived extracellular vesicles attenuates arthritis in two mouse models. *Mol. Nutr. Food Res.* **2015**, *59*, 1701–1712. [CrossRef] [PubMed]
136. Matic, S.; D'Souza, D.H.; Wu, T.; Pangloli, P.; Dia, V.P. Bovine milk exosomes affect proliferation and protect macrophages against cisplatin-induced cytotoxicity. *Immunol. Investig.* **2020**, *49*, 711–725. [CrossRef] [PubMed]
137. Mokarizadeh, A.; Hassanzadeh, K.; Abdi, M.; Soraya, H.; Faryabi, M.R.; Mohammadi, E.; Ahmadi, A. Transdermal delivery of bovine milk vesicles in patients with multiple sclerosis: A novel strategy to induce MOG-specific tolerance. *Med. Hypotheses* **2015**, *85*, 141–144. [CrossRef]
138. Bae, I.-S.; Kim, S.H. Milk Exosome-Derived MicroRNA-2478 Suppresses Melanogenesis through the Akt-GSK3β Pathway. *Cells* **2021**, *10*, 2848. [CrossRef]

139. Zhang, C.; Lu, X.; Hu, J.; Li, P.; Yan, J.; Ling, X.; Xiao, J. Bovine Milk Exosomes Alleviate Cardiac Fibrosis via Enhancing Angiogenesis in Vivo and in Vitro. *J. Cardiovasc. Transl. Res.* **2021**, *15*, 560–570. [CrossRef] [PubMed]
140. Kim, H.; Jang, Y.; Kim, E.; Jang, H.; Cho, H.; Han, G.; Song, H.; Kim, S.; Yang, Y. Potential of Colostrum-Derived Exosomes for Promoting Hair Regeneration through the Transition from Telogen to Anagen Phase. *Front. Cell Dev. Biol.* **2022**, *10*, 815205. [CrossRef]
141. Shi, C.; Zhang, M.; Tong, M.; Yang, L.; Pang, L.; Chen, L.; Xu, G.; Chi, X.; Hong, Q.; Ni, Y. miR-148a is associated with obesity and modulates adipocyte differentiation of mesenchymal stem cells through Wnt signaling. *Sci. Rep.* **2015**, *5*, 9930. [CrossRef]
142. Du, C.; Quan, S.; Nan, X.; Zhao, Y.; Shi, F.; Luo, Q.; Xiong, B. Effects of oral milk extracellular vesicles on the gut microbiome and serum metabolome in mice. *Food Funct.* **2021**, *12*, 10938–10949. [CrossRef] [PubMed]
143. Melnik, B.C. Synergistic effects of milk-derived exosomes and galactose on α-synuclein pathology in Parkinson's disease and type 2 diabetes mellitus. *Int. J. Mol. Sci.* **2021**, *22*, 1059. [CrossRef]
144. Samuel, M.; Fonseka, P.; Sanwlani, R.; Gangoda, L.; Chee, S.H.; Keerthikumar, S.; Spurling, A.; Chitti, S.V.; Zanker, D.; Ang, C.-S. Oral administration of bovine milk-derived extracellular vesicles induces senescence in the primary tumor but accelerates cancer metastasis. *Nat. Commun.* **2021**, *12*, 3950. [CrossRef]
145. Melnik, B.C. Lifetime impact of cow's milk on overactivation of mTORC1: From fetal to childhood overgrowth, acne, diabetes, cancers, and neurodegeneration. *Biomolecules* **2021**, *11*, 404. [CrossRef]
146. Vader, P.; Mol, E.A.; Pasterkamp, G.; Schiffelers, R.M. Extracellular vesicles for drug delivery. *Adv. Drug Deliv. Rev.* **2016**, *106*, 148–156. [CrossRef]
147. Malhotra, H.; Sheokand, N.; Kumar, S.; Chauhan, A.S.; Kumar, M.; Jakhar, P.; Boradia, V.M.; Raje, C.I.; Raje, M. Exosomes: Tunable nano vehicles for macromolecular delivery of transferrin and lactoferrin to specific intracellular compartment. *J. Biomed. Nanotechnol.* **2016**, *12*, 1101–1114. [CrossRef] [PubMed]
148. Rupert, D.L.; Claudio, V.; Lässer, C.; Bally, M. Methods for the physical characterization and quantification of extracellular vesicles in biological samples. *Biochim. Biophys. Acta (BBA)-Gen. Subj.* **2017**, *1861*, 3164–3179. [CrossRef]
149. Hood, J.L. Post isolation modification of exosomes for nanomedicine applications. *Nanomedicine* **2016**, *11*, 1745–1756. [CrossRef] [PubMed]
150. Tian, M.-Y.; Hao, D.-X.; Liu, Y.; He, J.; Zhao, Z.-H.; Guo, T.-Y.; Li, X.; Zhang, Y. Milk exosomes: An oral drug delivery system with great application potential. *Food Funct.* **2023**, *14*, 1320–1337. [CrossRef]
151. Benmoussa, A.; Diallo, I.; Salem, M.; Michel, S.; Gilbert, C.; Sévigny, J.; Provost, P. Concentrates of two subsets of extracellular vesicles from cow's milk modulate symptoms and inflammation in experimental colitis. *Sci. Rep.* **2019**, *9*, 14661. [CrossRef]
152. Liang, Y.; Duan, L.; Lu, J.; Xia, J. Engineering exosomes for targeted drug delivery. *Theranostics* **2021**, *11*, 3183. [CrossRef] [PubMed]
153. Kim, M.S.; Haney, M.J.; Zhao, Y.; Mahajan, V.; Deygen, I.; Klyachko, N.L.; Inskoe, E.; Piroyan, A.; Sokolsky, M.; Okolie, O. Development of exosome-encapsulated paclitaxel to overcome MDR in cancer cells. *Nanomed. Nanotechnol. Biol. Med.* **2016**, *12*, 655–664. [CrossRef] [PubMed]
154. Luo, S.; Sun, X.; Huang, M.; Ma, Q.; Du, L.; Cui, Y. Enhanced neuroprotective effects of epicatechin gallate encapsulated by bovine milk-derived exosomes against parkinson's disease through antiapoptosis and antimitophagy. *J. Agric. Food Chem.* **2021**, *69*, 5134–5143. [CrossRef] [PubMed]
155. Hao, R.; Yu, Z.; Du, J.; Hu, S.; Yuan, C.; Guo, H.; Zhang, Y.; Yang, H. A High-Throughput Nanofluidic Device for Exosome Nanoporation to Develop Cargo Delivery Vehicles. *Small* **2021**, *17*, 2102150. [CrossRef]
156. Zhang, D.; Lee, H.; Zhu, Z.; Minhas, J.K.; Jin, Y. Enrichment of selective miRNAs in exosomes and delivery of exosomal miRNAs in vitro and in vivo. *Am. J. Physiol.-Lung Cell. Mol. Physiol.* **2017**, *312*, L110–L121. [CrossRef]
157. Tsai, S.J.; Atai, N.A.; Cacciottolo, M.; Nice, J.; Salehi, A.; Guo, C.; Sedgwick, A.; Kanagavelu, S.; Gould, S.J. Exosome-mediated mRNA delivery in vivo is safe and can be used to induce SARS-CoV-2 immunity. *J. Biol. Chem.* **2021**, *297*, 101266. [CrossRef]
158. Lin, Y.; Wu, J.; Gu, W.; Huang, Y.; Tong, Z.; Huang, L.; Tan, J. Exosome–liposome hybrid nanoparticles deliver CRISPR/Cas9 system in MSCs. *Adv. Sci.* **2018**, *5*, 1700611. [CrossRef]
159. Li, D.; Yao, S.; Zhou, Z.; Shi, J.; Huang, Z.; Wu, Z. Hyaluronan decoration of milk exosomes directs tumor-specific delivery of doxorubicin. *Carbohydr. Res.* **2020**, *493*, 108032. [CrossRef]
160. Kandimalla, R.; Aqil, F.; Alhakeem, S.S.; Jeyabalan, J.; Tyagi, N.; Agrawal, A.; Yan, J.; Spencer, W.; Bondada, S.; Gupta, R.C. Targeted oral delivery of paclitaxel using colostrum-derived exosomes. *Cancers* **2021**, *13*, 3700. [CrossRef]
161. Gong, L.; Zhou, H.; Zhang, S.; Wang, C.; Fu, K.; Ma, C.; Zhang, Y.; Peng, C.; Li, Y. CD44-targeting Drug Delivery System of Exosomes Loading Forsythiaside A Combats Liver Fibrosis via Regulating NLRP3-mediated Pyroptosis. *Adv. Healthc. Mater.* **2023**, *12*, 2202228. [CrossRef]
162. Pullan, J.; Dailey, K.; Bhallamudi, S.; Feng, L.; Alhalhooly, L.; Froberg, J.; Osborn, J.; Sarkar, K.; Molden, T.; Sathish, V. Modified Bovine Milk Exosomes for Doxorubicin Delivery to Triple-Negative Breast Cancer Cells. *ACS Appl. Bio Mater.* **2022**, *5*, 2163–2175. [CrossRef] [PubMed]
163. Koh, E.; Lee, E.J.; Nam, G.-H.; Hong, Y.; Cho, E.; Yang, Y.; Kim, I.-S. Exosome-SIRPα, a CD47 blockade increases cancer cell phagocytosis. *Biomaterials* **2017**, *121*, 121–129. [CrossRef] [PubMed]
164. Benmoussa, A.; Lee, C.H.C.; Laffont, B.; Savard, P.; Laugier, J.; Boilard, E.; Gilbert, C.; Fliss, I.; Provost, P. Commercial dairy cow milk microRNAs resist digestion under simulated gastrointestinal tract conditions. *J. Nutr.* **2016**, *146*, 2206–2215. [CrossRef]

165. Agrawal, A.K.; Aqil, F.; Jeyabalan, J.; Spencer, W.A.; Beck, J.; Gachuki, B.W.; Alhakeem, S.S.; Oben, K.; Munagala, R.; Bondada, S. Milk-derived exosomes for oral delivery of paclitaxel. *Nanomed. Nanotechnol. Biol. Med.* **2017**, *13*, 1627–1636. [CrossRef] [PubMed]
166. Vashisht, M.; Rani, P.; Onteru, S.K.; Singh, D. Curcumin encapsulated in milk exosomes resists human digestion and possesses enhanced intestinal permeability in vitro. *Appl. Biochem. Biotechnol.* **2017**, *183*, 993–1007. [CrossRef]
167. Chen, J.; Cao, F.; Cao, Y.; Wei, S.; Zhu, X.; Xing, W. Targeted Therapy of Lung Adenocarcinoma by the Nanoplatform Based on Milk Exosomes Loaded with Paclitaxel. *J. Biomed. Nanotechnol.* **2022**, *18*, 1075–1083. [CrossRef]
168. Munagala, R.; Aqil, F.; Jeyabalan, J.; Agrawal, A.K.; Mudd, A.M.; Kyakulaga, A.H.; Singh, I.P.; Vadhanam, M.V.; Gupta, R.C. Exosomal formulation of anthocyanidins against multiple cancer types. *Cancer Lett.* **2017**, *393*, 94–102. [CrossRef]
169. Mudd, A.M.; Gu, T.; Munagala, R.; Jeyabalan, J.; Egilmez, N.K.; Gupta, R.C. Chemoprevention of colorectal cancer by Anthocyanidins and mitigation of metabolic shifts induced by dysbiosis of the gut microbiome. *Cancer Prev. Res.* **2020**, *13*, 41–52. [CrossRef]
170. Shandilya, S.; Rani, P.; Onteru, S.K.; Singh, D. Small interfering RNA in milk exosomes is resistant to digestion and crosses the intestinal barrier in vitro. *J. Agric. Food Chem.* **2017**, *65*, 9506–9513. [CrossRef]
171. Aqil, F.; Munagala, R.; Jeyabalan, J.; Agrawal, A.K.; Kyakulaga, A.-H.; Wilcher, S.A.; Gupta, R.C. Milk exosomes-Natural nanoparticles for siRNA delivery. *Cancer Lett.* **2019**, *449*, 186–195. [CrossRef]
172. Matsuda, A.; Patel, T. Milk-derived extracellular vesicles for therapeutic delivery of small interfering RNAs. In *Extracellular RNA*; Springer: Berlin/Heidelberg, Germany, 2018; pp. 187–197.
173. Tao, H.; Xu, H.; Zuo, L.; Li, C.; Qiao, G.; Guo, M.; Zheng, L.; Leitgeb, M.; Lin, X. Exosomes-coated bcl-2 siRNA inhibits the growth of digestive system tumors both in vitro and in vivo. *Int. J. Biol. Macromol.* **2020**, *161*, 470–480. [CrossRef]
174. Xu, M.; Chen, G.; Dong, Y.; Yang, J.; Liu, Y.; Song, H.; Song, H.; Wang, Y. Liraglutide-Loaded Milk Exosomes Lower Blood Glucose When Given by Sublingual Route. *ChemMedChem* **2022**, *17*, e202100758. [CrossRef]
175. Sánchez, C.; Franco, L.; Regal, P.; Lamas, A.; Cepeda, A.; Fente, C. Breast milk: A source of functional compounds with potential application in nutrition and therapy. *Nutrients* **2021**, *13*, 1026. [CrossRef] [PubMed]
176. Kleinjan, M.; Van Herwijnen, M.J.; Libregts, S.F.; van Neerven, R.J.; Feitsma, A.L.; Wauben, M.H. Regular industrial processing of bovine milk impacts the integrity and molecular composition of extracellular vesicles. *J. Nutr.* **2021**, *151*, 1416–1425. [CrossRef] [PubMed]
177. Reis, M.G.; Harris, P.; Berry, C.; Nguyen, H.; Maclean, P.; Weeks, M. Tracking changes in volatile components and lipids after homogenisation and thermal processing of milk. *Int. Dairy J.* **2020**, *103*, 104624. [CrossRef]
178. Mutai, E.; Ngu, A.K.H.; Zempleni, J. Preliminary evidence that lectins in infant soy formula apparently bind bovine milk exosomes and prevent their absorption in healthy adults. *BMC Nutr.* **2022**, *8*, 7. [CrossRef] [PubMed]
179. Golan-Gerstl, R.; Elbaum Shiff, Y.; Moshayoff, V.; Schecter, D.; Leshkowitz, D.; Reif, S. Characterization and biological function of milk-derived miRNAs. *Mol. Nutr. Food Res.* **2017**, *61*, 1700009. [CrossRef]
180. López de las Hazas, M.-C.; del Pozo-Acebo, L.; Hansen, M.S.; Gil-Zamorano, J.; Mantilla-Escalante, D.C.; Gómez-Coronado, D.; Marín, F.; Garcia-Ruiz, A.; Rasmussen, J.T.; Dávalos, A. Dietary bovine milk miRNAs transported in extracellular vesicles are partially stable during GI digestion, are bioavailable and reach target tissues but need a minimum dose to impact on gene expression. *Eur. J. Nutr.* **2022**, *61*, 1043–1056. [CrossRef] [PubMed]

pharmaceutics

Review

Extracellular Vesicles as New Players in Drug Delivery: A Focus on Red Blood Cells-Derived EVs

Sara Biagiotti [1], Faiza Abbas [1], Mariele Montanari [1], Chiara Barattini [1,2], Luigia Rossi [1], Mauro Magnani [1], Stefano Papa [1] and Barbara Canonico [1,*]

1 Department of Biomolecular Sciences, University of Urbino Carlo Bo, 61029 Urbino, PU, Italy
2 AcZon s.r.l., 40050 Monte San Pietro, BO, Italy
* Correspondence: barbara.canonico@uniurb.it

Abstract: The article is divided into several sections, focusing on extracellular vesicles' (EVs) nature, features, commonly employed methodologies and strategies for their isolation/preparation, and their characterization/visualization. This work aims to give an overview of advances in EVs' extensive nanomedical-drug delivery applications. Furthermore, considerations for EVs translation to clinical application are summarized here, before focusing the review on a special kind of extracellular vesicles, the ones derived from red blood cells (RBCEVs). Generally, employing EVs as drug carriers means managing entities with advantageous properties over synthetic vehicles or nanoparticles. Besides the fact that certain EVs also reveal intrinsic therapeutic characteristics, in regenerative medicine, EVs nanosize, lipidomic and proteomic profiles enable them to pass biologic barriers and display cell/tissue tropisms; indeed, EVs engineering can further optimize their organ targeting. In the second part of the review, we focus our attention on RBCEVs. First, we describe the biogenesis and composition of those naturally produced by red blood cells (RBCs) under physiological and pathological conditions. Afterwards, we discuss the current procedures to isolate and/or produce RBCEVs in the lab and to load a specific cargo for therapeutic exploitation. Finally, we disclose the most recent applications of RBCEVs at the in vitro and preclinical research level and their potential industrial exploitation. In conclusion, RBCEVs can be, in the near future, a very promising and versatile platform for several clinical applications and pharmaceutical exploitations.

Keywords: extracellular vesicles; red blood cell extracellular vesicles; nanomedical drug delivery; drug delivery systems; cargo loading; therapeutic applications

Citation: Biagiotti, S.; Abbas, F.; Montanari, M.; Barattini, C.; Rossi, L.; Magnani, M.; Papa, S.; Canonico, B. Extracellular Vesicles as New Players in Drug Delivery: A Focus on Red Blood Cells-Derived EVs. *Pharmaceutics* **2023**, *15*, 365. https://doi.org/10.3390/pharmaceutics15020365

Academic Editor: Yong Chen

Received: 15 December 2022
Revised: 12 January 2023
Accepted: 18 January 2023
Published: 21 January 2023

1. Extracellular Vesicles: An Overview of Their Origin and Composition

Although the following paragraphs will provide a general introduction to extracellular vesicles (EVs), hints on their isolation, their characterization, and their journey to the different body districts, the main purpose of the present review is to describe EVs as efficient drug carriers. In fact, pharmacologic molecules are protected by EV membranes from proteases, nucleases, pH and osmolality fluctuations, and other external factors. Specifically, we will frame red blood cells as sources of EVs (RBCEVs) that can address the major requirements for efficient drug-delivery, providing a useful and insightful description of procedures (also patented) to produce RBCEVs, with their advantages and limitations.

EVs are cell-derived membrane vesicles that represent an endogenous mechanism for intercellular communication [1]. The original classification distinguished exosomes (nano-sized vesicles with a diameter in the range of 30 to 120 nm) [2], originating from the formation of multivesicular bodies, microvesicles, which are formed by cell membrane budding, and apoptotic bodies, derived from dying cells. This classification has been recently revised by the International Society of Extracellular Vesicles (ISEV), establishing the need to use the term EVs for all the subtypes of vesicles, given that they overlap in size and this can cause confusion [3]. Therefore, the ISEV entitled EVs smaller than 200 nm as "small EVs" and those larger than 200 nm as "large EVs" [3]. Consequently, in depth characterization has led to better categorize EVs on the basis of size, density, biochemical composition, cellular origin (e.g., oncosomes derived from tumour cells) or treatment condition (e.g., hypoxic EVs) [4,5]. As cited, small EVs (exosomes) range between 50 and 150 nm, whereas large EVs (microvesicles) and apoptotic bodies range between <1 μM and 1–5 μm in diameter, respectively [4].

1.1. EV Biogenesis

The differences in size could represent an indication of the specific biogenesis processes. Biogenesis and secretion of EVs are controlled by specific proteins such as GTPases and lipids, as genetic studies have proven. The Rab family of small GTPases plays an important role in intracellular trafficking, and several Rabs play a significant role in EVs release, particularly Rab27a, Rab27b, Rab35, and Rab11 [6–12]. EVs production and release can be modified or orchestrated by internal cellular processes or external stimuli. For example, the modulation of intracellular calcium levels in cancer cells [13] is a possible factor increasing EVs production. Cargo selection, packaging, and compartmentalization are processes regulated at multiple levels. Briefly, the endosomal sorting complex required for transport (ESCRT)-dependent pathway is involved in the selection and distribution of proteins within exosomes [14]. CD63 is a molecule involved in sorting EVs cargo [15], and it guides cargo selection in MVs [16]. However, despite all the knowledge acquired so far, the biogenesis and sorting mechanisms of extracellular vesicles are still unclear. However, exosomes are well-characterized EVs normally generated by the internal budding of endosomes, thus producing multivesicular bodies (MVBs) and ultimately forming intraluminal vesicles (Figure 1). Such vesicles fuse with the cell membrane, releasing the so-called exosomes into the extracellular environment [17]. Besides the production of MVBs, the biogenesis pathway of EVs can also be associated with secretory autophagy [18–21]. Although the current orientation is dictated by the ISEV, which we shared in the initial part of our review, we must continue to differentiate EVs based on their different origins.

The biogenesis of MVs is entirely derived from the plasma membrane and shares many of the same proteins involved in exosome biogenesis [22–24]. This kind of smaller EVs (exosomes), as well as MVs, can transfer bioactive molecules, including proteins, DNA, mRNA, and miRNA, and these cargoes are able to modify the extracellular milieu and recipient cells, both proximally and distally [25,26]. MVs are generated from sites of high membrane blebbing; indeed, their biogenesis involves the vertical trafficking of loaded molecules to the plasma membrane along with the reorganization of membrane lipids. Furthermore, contractile machinery at the surface allows vesicle budding [27] (Figure 1). The ESCRT complex also plays an important role in MV biogenesis. Moreover, ARF-6 is involved in the trafficking of cargo to the cell surface in MVs [28]. Several proteins such as TSG101, ALIX, and ARRDC1 assisted in MV release, and ESCRT-III and ALIX are involved in cytokinetic abscission [6,29]. A significant role in MV structure is played by the extracellular concentration of calcium; in fact, it was reported [30] that a high level of calcium not only induces membrane phospholipid disarrangement but also increases the level of vesiculation to produce more MVs [31], especially in erythrocytes and platelets [32]. Finally, curving of the plasma membrane at the cell periphery and lateral pressure created by protein–protein interactions also play crucial roles in de novo MV formation [33].

1.2. EVs Benefits: Their Journey to the Different Body Districts

The combination of exosomes and nanotechnology can facilitate the development of next-generation theragnostic nanoplatforms. Extracellular vesicles are highly biocompatible and relatively less toxic due to their natural origin. Indeed, EVs can escape immune clearance, which makes them highly stable in blood circulation. These properties make them preferable drug delivery carriers compared to synthetic vehicles or nanoparticles [34–38]. Moreover, there is a clear indication that EVs can cross multiple biological barriers, as demonstrated by several studies of neuronal EVs in the cerebrospinal fluid, blood, urine, and tears [39]. However, delivery to the specific target mainly depends on the surface marker on specific cells [40,41]. These characteristics amplify their target potential; in fact, among the physiological barriers EVs cross, the blood–brain barrier (BBB) opens the possibility that they may be enriched in a specific neuron population. Moreover, naturally occurring molecules in them can be encapsulated with drugs, thus producing a synergic effect [42,43]. Being a highly stable structure, EVs can circulate systemically and have been identified in blood, urine, cerebrospinal fluid, saliva, milk, and tears [39,44–51]. EVs possess an excellent safety profile in both animal models and clinical trials. Different studies reported data on the immunogenicity of EVs from different sources. For example, administration of EVs derived from human embryonic kidney (HEK) 293 T cells exhibited very little toxicity and immune response in healthy mice [52,53]. EVs cargo remains stable even in the highly acidic environment of the stomach, as illustrated by the reduction in delayed-type hypersensitivity by orally supplemented miRNA-150 EVs [54]. Proteomics analysis of the urinary EVs revealed the presence of specific EVs from glomerular endothelial cells and mesangial cells in healthy individuals [55], which truly indicates that endogenous EVs have glomerular filtration barrier (GFB)-penetrating capacity (Figure 2). More tracing evaluation is still needed to clarify the distribution of exogenous EVs; furthermore, the internalization process of EVs is closely dependent on their origins and the type of recipient cells. Exogenously administered EVs possess and display specific biodistribution profiles, natural cell-targeting abilities, and pharmacokinetics due to their peculiar components. Indeed, certain EVs also reveal intrinsic therapeutic characteristics, in the context of regenerative medicine [56]. Furthermore, some EVs display characteristics of tropism for a particular cell or tissue. This feature could be exploited to deliver drugs to specific targets while avoiding off-target effects [57]. The natural targeting properties of EVs can be modulated by their compositions in lipids, integrins, and tetraspanins. Engineering EVs leads to altering these targeting properties in several ways: by the addition of targeting moieties anchored via the phosphatidylserine-binding C1C2 domains of lactadherin [58], the expression of lysosome-associated membrane protein 2 fusion proteins [40], glycosylphosphatidylinositol-anchored targeting moieties [59], and transferrin-conjugated magnetic particles bound to the transferrin receptor expressed on EVs [60] must reach their activity sites within the cell in adequate amounts [61].

In the next topic, specific details will be added to better understand the mechanisms that mediate the EVs' application as tools for mediated drug delivery.

1.3. Extracellular Vesicles (EVs): A Novel Drug Delivery System

We have profusely described EVs as entities carrying diverse cargo, including lipids, proteins, long non-coding RNA (lncRNA), and microRNA (miRNA), that can be transferred to recipient cells to mediate intercellular communication. These naturally occurring nanovesicles are released by different types of cells, including reticulocytes, mesenchymal stem cells, T cells, B lymphocytes, NK cells, dendritic cells, and some tumors. There is strong evidence that extracellular vesicles are involved in both pathological and physiological processes, including cellular homeostasis, infection propagation, cancer development, and cardiovascular diseases [62–65].

Due to their innate function in cell-to-cell communication, EVs can be used effectively for drug delivery. The biggest advantage of EVs as drug delivery vehicles is probably that EVs can be taken from an organism and returned to the same organism in vivo after being loaded with therapeutic agents, which are thought to be non-immunogenic [66]. Another advantage is that EVs can carry molecules through physiological barriers, such as the blood–brain barrier, which are hard to cross using conventional delivery methods; this is particularly true when using nucleic acids as cargo [67–69]. When exogenous RNAs are directly introduced into the body, they are normally degraded by nucleases or filtered in the kidneys before reaching the target site. Various studies have suggested that both coding and noncoding RNAs can be transported through EVs. In addition, microRNAs can be transferred to different cell types via EVs. Thus, EVs can be considered an efficient

RNA-based drug delivery carrier. Several therapeutic applications include gene therapy, targeted therapy, vaccination, and the treatment of kidney and autoimmune diseases [70].

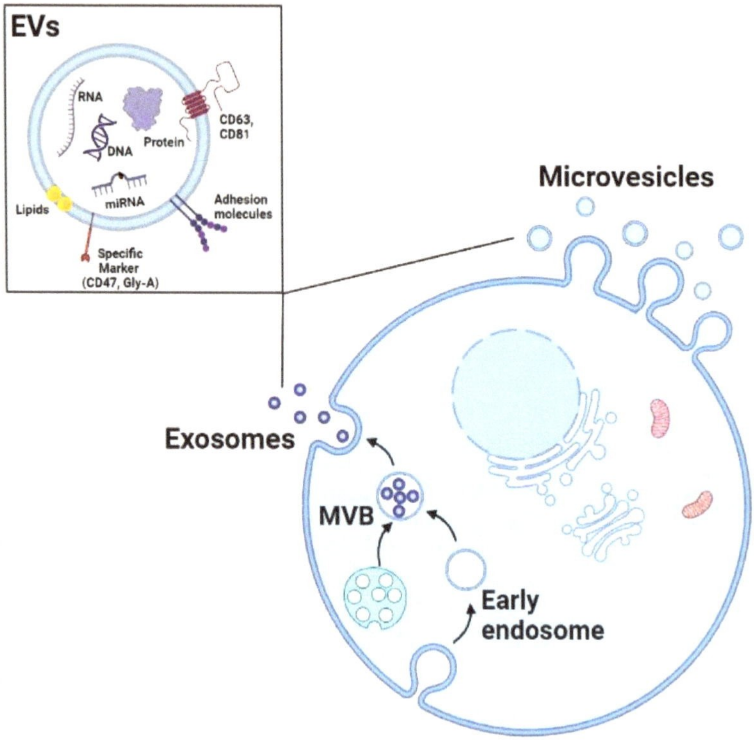

Figure 1. Scheme of biogenesis and typologies of cargoes of extracellular vesicles. Extracellular vesicles (EVs) generated via different mechanisms. Exosomes are produced from inward budding of the endosomal membrane. Microvesicles generated by outward budding of the plasma membrane. The outer EV membrane contains lipids and transmembrane proteins. EVs are also enriched in microRNAs, mRNAs, and proteins that mediate systemic effects. EVs are also known to contain metabolites and mitochondrial DNA. Created in Biorender.com, accessed on 6 December 2022.

1.4. Other Actors in Next Generation Drug Delivery Platforms: Taking a Glance

Although our review is centered on EVs, and in particular, EVs derived from RBCs, we just want to mention other nanosized drug delivery systems (DDS). Liposomes were discovered nearly 55 years ago, and they currently represent a staple in the field of drug delivery. Among nanoDDS, liposomes are small spherical structures [4] that could be modified with different active targeting agents [71]. They displayed proper bioavailability, long half-lives, size-control measures, low risk-to-benefit ratios, and control release features [72]. Our experience [73] with these entities pointed out several advantages of intracellular internalization in triple-negative breast cancer cells (MDA-MB-231) for sucrose-decorated liposomes loaded with berberine hydrochloride. Recently, liposomes demonstrated their significant efficacy in SARS-CoV-2 vaccines [74]. Such formulations are paving the way for future success in several therapeutic applications [74]. The influence of lipid composition and particle size on pharmacokinetics is common to both liposomes and EVs; in addition, EVs are advanced drug delivery entities containing several proteins that may contribute to their pharmacokinetic behavior in vivo [75].

The development of mesoporous materials has prospected their use as drug delivery systems. The well-known textural properties of these materials have inspired their translation to nanoscale constructs, resulting in mesoporous silica nanoparticles (MSNPs) [76]. Our experience is specifically related to fluorescent silica nanoparticles (SiNPs), which appear to be a promising imaging platform and show a specific subcellular localization that is mainly at the mitochondrial level. We conjugated SiNPs to one of the most commonly used anticancer drugs, doxorubicin, and we tested these functionalized SiNPs (DOX-NPs) on the breast cancer cell line MCF-7 [77]. Generally, carrier nanoparticles (NPs) reveal a poor penetration capacity and an inadequate balance between drug retention in the bloodstream and drug release at the specific pathologic body districts [78]. These findings represent an obstacle in drug release that EVs could overcome.

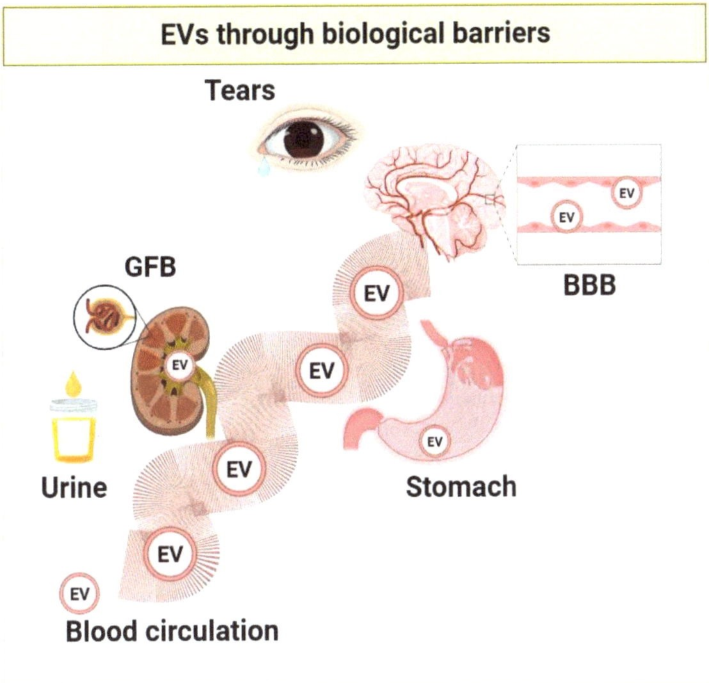

Figure 2. Summary of the different biologic barriers penetrated by EVs. GFB: glomerular filtration barrier; BBB: blood–brain barrier. Created in Biorender.com, accessed on 6 December 2022.

Recently, nanocellulose has attracted considerable attention for its applications in drug delivery platforms; this is mainly due to its biocompatibility, large specific surface area, good mechanical strength, stiffness, and renewability [79]. These characteristics qualify nanocellulose as a material with good drug loading and binding capacities. Khalid and co-workers reported that different types of nanocellulose-based materials such as single, hybrid, or nanocomposite systems have been fabricated for application in drug delivery systems [80]. Nonetheless, it is difficult for the human body to degrade nanocellulose-based materials, and the interaction mechanism between nanocellulose and cells is still unclear. These issues are obviously lacking in EVs, due to their biologic features.

Finally, in the field of cancer immunotherapy and tumor microenvironment remodeling, two different nanostructures will be cited. The first, formulated by Liang et al., represents a novel nanovaccine based on antigen self-presentation and immunosuppression reversal, named ASPIRE. The ASPIRE formulation has a nanoscale size and good stability; its preparation arises from dendritic cells (DCs). Briefly, the nanovaccine is derived from recombinant adenovirus-infected DCs, and anti-PD1 antibodies, MHC-I molecules, and B7 co-stimulatory molecules are concomitantly attached to the membrane of mature DCs through cell reprogramming. Then, Dcnv-rad-ag was separated by multi-step density gradient supercentrifugation. The novel nanovaccine agent ASPIRE greatly improves the efficiency of antigen presentation, activating both naive T cells and exhausted T cells, and improving anti-tumor immunity, finally representing an important progress in tumor immunotherapy [81].

The second nanosized construct, by Cheng and co-workers, is essentially represented by glucose-contained radical micelles for synergistic photoimmunotherapy and aims for dual tumor microenvironment remodeling. They designed a novel amphiphilic copolymer, glucose-PEO-b-PLLA-TEMPO, to encapsulate clinical therapeutics (CUDC101 and photosensitizer IR780), providing a promising strategy to integrate small molecule immune checkpoint inhibition and photodynamic therapy [82].

The above-mentioned issues can by no means exhaust such vast and complex topics, and they do not represent the focus of this review. Nevertheless, this short summary not only highlights other actors (besides EVs) in next-generation drug delivery platforms but also the involvement of our groups in the vast and vital area of drug delivery technologies.

1.5. Different Extracellular Vesicle Preparations/Isolations and Characterization: An Overview

Even if the International Society for Extracellular Vesicles (ISEV) began to publish the Minimal Information for Studies of Extracellular Vesicles (MISEV) guidelines in 2014, with regular updates, nowadays, no general consensus has been reached on the best method for EVs isolation and characterization, and the best option is often related to the starting volume of the EV source and to the processes to be applied downstream [5]. Different techniques have been applied to quantify and characterize EVs: Figure 3 highlights Western blot (WB), flow cytometry (FC), dynamic light scattering (DLS), electron microscopy (TEM and SEM), nanoparticle tracking analysis (NTA), and tunable resistive pulse sensing (TRPS). These methodologies allow analyzing EVs, focusing on different EV features such as: diameters and morphology (TEM), EV dimensions and concentrations (NTA), particle concentration (TRPS), size distribution and polydispersity (DLS), specific EV markers (WB), size, particle concentration, and specific EV marker (FC). Since there are many reviews that deal with methods of EV analysis, in this paragraph we will synthetically focus on the different methodologies for their isolation/obtaining, and subsequent characterization [83–87].

According to the literature, the most employed method to isolate EVs is differential ultracentrifugation, which has been considered the gold standard for a long time [88]. This method includes several centrifugation steps at increasingly longer times and higher speeds (up to 120,000× *g*). Based on Marassi et al.'s work, to pellet large extracellular vesicles, the biological fluid was centrifuged at 10,000× *g* for 30 min and 18,000× *g* for 30 min, then the resulting pellets from both centrifuges were united and resuspended in phosphate buffer followed by ultracentrifugation at 20,000× *g* for 30 min. To collect small extracellular vesicles, large extracellular vesicle-depleted supernatant was ultracentrifuged at 100,000× *g* for 70 min [89]. Among the advantages listed for using this technique are its high versatility due to the possibility of adjusting centrifuge parameters according to a scientist's needs and good final yield. On the other hand, the high centrifuge speed might affect the intactness of the EVs and cause massive aggregation due to the presence of other proteins in the sample [90]. The application of an iodixanol/sucrose density gradient or a sucrose cushion to the high-speed ultracentrifugation significantly improved the quality of the isolated EVs [91]. The iodixanol/sucrose gradient exploits the similarity of exosome density (1.08 to 1.19 g/mL) to that of sucrose and iodixanol, which form a cushion preserving the integrity of EVs and separating high-density contaminant proteins (1.35 g/mL). In this method, the sample is poured onto the density gradient and then centrifuged at high speed. During the centrifugation, vesicles filter through the sucrose/iodixanol gradient until the point at which their density is equal to the gradient. With the employment of the sucrose cushion, vesicles are laid down on a high-density sucrose matrix with lower stress applied to EVs [92].

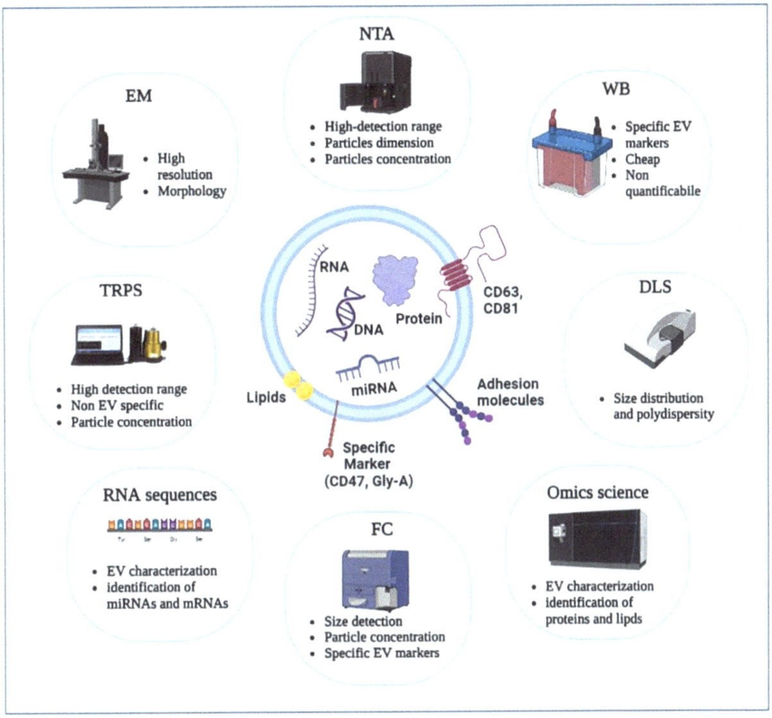

Figure 3. Summary of the different methods for characterization and quantification of EVs. The characterization and quantification of EVs are performed through different techniques such as nanoparticle tracking analysis (NTA), flow cytometry (FC), Western blot (WB), transmission electron microscopy (TEM), and scanning electron microscopy (SEM). TEM analyzes EV diameters and morphology. Dynamic light scattering (DLS) determines EV size distribution and polydispersity by detecting the diffusion coefficient of the scattering EVs. NTA detects EV dimensions and concentrations through scattered light measurement and Brownian motion. RNA sequences and mass spectrometry permit cargo characterization. In particular, FC can be employed for size detection, particle concentration, and EV-specific markers. Tunable resistive pulse sensing (TRPS) only measures particle concentration. Created in Biorender.com, accessed on 6 December 2022.

In recent times, size exclusion chromatography (SEC) has caught on in the multitude of EVs purification protocols. This technique is broadly used for the separation of macromolecules on the basis of their molecular size or hydrodynamic volume. Bigger species are eluted earlier than smaller species, which spend more time crossing the pores typical of the employed resins. Basically, the most widely used protocols include a preliminary ultracentrifugation purification step followed by sample loading on a qEV size exclusion column (Izon Science, New Zealand). To elute EVs from the column, phosphate buffer is used. After protein and particle quantitation, the richest fractions are concentrated using four 10 kDa nominal molecular weight centrifugal filter units [93,94]. Even this technique is not free from drawbacks in terms of purity: species featuring the same size (but different origin) are contemporaneously eluted; in addition, EVs are diluted during the procedure, requiring a supplementary concentration step according to the following activities [1]. Moreover, SEC requires considerable hands-on time for the preparation and maintenance of the isolation column [95–97].

Immuno-capture-based approaches represent an effective alternative to obtaining homogeneous EV samples by exploiting the interactions between proteins, naturally present in EVs, and their respective ligands. Duijvesz and co-workers developed a highly sensitive time-resolved fluorescence immunoassay (TR-FIA) for the capture/detection of EVs using anti-human CD9- or CD63-coated plates [98]. The high specificity of this approach is generally recognized, but, on the other hand, it is limited by the availability of reliable and cost-effective monoclonal antibodies, or aptamers, specific for EV isolation (often targeting tetraspanin proteins) and also by the necessity of a mild elution method that preserves EV integrity [99–102].

Ultrafiltration (UF) uses membranes with a molecular weight cut-off ranging from 10 to 100 kDa to isolate EVs from relatively diluted samples such as urine or blood. It is a quite rapid procedure lasting about 20 min (against several hours spent during ultracentrifugation), in which particles smaller than the membrane cut-off size pass through the membrane itself. This method is affected by a considerable quantity of protein contaminants and EV loss. Near conventional UF, tangential flow filtration (TFF) is utilized for EVs separation. In TFF, the sample moves tangentially across (not directly through) the hollow fiber membrane, which allows smaller molecules to pass while retaining bigger ones. One of the main advantages of using TFF instead of SEC is the higher final concentration of EVs [103,104].

Recently, asymmetrical flow field-flow fractionation (AF4) became one of the most used subcategories of flow field fractionation to separate EVs. In AF4, the separation force is generated by a cross-flow field inside the channel, which is divided from the main parabolic flow pumped through the channel and is directed through a semipermeable membrane that is located at the bottom (the accumulation wall). The membrane pores' size prevents the EVs from passing through but allows smaller contaminants to exit the AF4 channel. The sample fractions are eluted out of the channel in the direction of the detectors by the remaining channel flow. Smaller EVs remain far from the accumulation wall due to their higher diffusion coefficient, in contrast to larger ones. One of the main advantages is due to the absence of stressful forces applied to the sample, on the other side, even in this case, the eluted sample results are diluted and need to be concentrated before being applied in further applications [105,106].

Polyethylene glycol (PEG) is one of the most used compounds present in commercial kits to cause EV precipitation. This isolation method assures a high recovery along with an important concentrative effect, but on the other side, it is highly recommended to isolate EVs before applying the precipitation protocol in order to avoid the massive presence of contaminants [107]. Habitually, an overnight incubation of 4 °C with 10% (w/v) PEG 8000 is used to precipitate EVs [108]. Gallert-Palau used the PRotein Organic Solvent PRecipitation (PROSPR) method to remove soluble proteins from plasma via precipitation in cold acetone with satisfactory results [109].

The analysis of potential showed that EV membrane components are negatively charged. Charge-based isolation techniques exploit this attitude to facilitate the interaction between EVs and positive entities. Ion-exchange chromatography, metal-affinity systems, or positively charged proteins, such as protamine, trap EVs, which can be released from the positively charged matrix by adding a high salt concentration to increase ionic strength [110,111].

In addition to the above-mentioned isolation methods, other techniques, especially those based on the lab-on-chip approach [112], were applied during the last few years, among which were acoustofluidic methods [113], capillary zone electrophoresis [114], conductive polypyrrole nanowire arrays [115], lateral displacement arrays [116], and viscoelasticity-based microfluidic systems [117].

Despite the increase in the development of advanced EV isolation techniques to obtain pure and high-quality EVs, there is currently no consensus on a suitable EV isolation method. This lack of agreement mainly depends on the damages caused by many of these protocols on isolated EVs, making downstream applications difficult. Since different techniques previously described exploit different principles to separate EVs from the rest of the sample macromolecules, the combination of complementary methods is an increasing trend in the literature [118–120].

During the last few decades, even the development of new methods for EVs characterization has increased a lot, but in the same manner as the isolation method, no general consensus has been reached, and the selection of the characterization procedure strongly depends on the EV source, isolation method, and downstream processes.

Electron microscopy can achieve a sufficient resolution (about 1 nm, since the electron wavelength is much shorter than the visible light wavelength) to allow the morphological study of extracellular vesicles, and, for this reason, it has been considered the gold standard for EV characterization for a long time. In transmission electron microscopy (TEM), the samples need to be dehydrated during their preparation to allow fixation with glutaraldehyde and placed in a vacuum environment to focus the electron beam directly on the sample. These requirements often cause artifacts in the analyses. As an alternative, cryo-EM is employed. It is a particular subtype of TEM where samples are rapidly frozen to preserve their morphology. To couple the morphological analysis in EM to EV immunophenotyping, it is possible to employ gold colloidal conjugated antibodies [121,122].

Atomic force microscopy (AFM) is a surface-based imaging technique allowing topographical imaging at sub-nanometer resolution (lateral resolution $\approx$ 3 nm and vertical resolution below 0.1 nm). It is based on the interaction between the probing sharp tip, mounted on a cantilever, and the sample surface. The most used technique for soft objects, such as EVs, characterization is the tapping mode in which the tip directly scans the surface of the sample. Furthermore, using specific antibody-coated surfaces, EV subpopulations can be identified. Unfortunately, even in this case, the preparation of the sample on a highly flat surface, such as mica, might modify the shape of EVs [123,124].

Dynamic light scattering (DLS) analyzes the fluctuation, due to Brownian motion, of the light scattered by nanomaterials and therefore the EVs, when illuminated with a laser beam in solution. The EV size, intended as hydrodynamic radius, and density are obtained using the Stokes–Einstein equation starting from their velocity distribution due to Brownian motion. The sensitivity of DLS ranges from 1 nm to 6 μm and does not require sample pre-treatment, but, in heterogeneous samples, the light scattered by larger particles covers the signal from smaller ones. For this reason, DLS employment in polydisperse samples is limited [125].

Nanoparticle tracking analysis (NTA) exploits the same DLS principle but uses a camera as a detector instead of a photon detector, allowing for the visualization of EVs ranging from 60 to 1000 nm. This feature promotes the use of NTA in place of DLS, especially in highly polydisperse samples. Likewise, DLS or even NTA is a technique requiring a relatively short time (less than one hour) and no sample preparation, but, exploiting the same principle as DLS, even in this case, a few large particles might obscure a multitude of smaller particles [126,127].

Flow cytometry (FC) is a powerful method to detect and characterize surface and/or cytoplasmic protein expression in EVs. In FC particles pass, individually, through a laser beam scattering light and emitting fluorescence signals to different channels. Conventional FC allows the detection of protein on relatively large entities ($\geq$300 nm) and, often, EV scattering intensities are below the background noise. Besides, even the difference in antigen exposed on the surface between cells (>1000) and EVs (<100) needs to be considered before employing this characterization technique. To improve the limit of conventional FC detection, EVs are conjugated to micrometer-sized fluorescent latex beads carrying specific antibodies against membrane EV antigens. Recently, enhanced FC instruments have been developed to detect particles smaller than 300 nm; in particular, in nanoscale FC, thanks to the improvements in optical and fluidic systems, the threshold has been lowered to 100 nm [128,129].

Western blotting is frequently used to detect and quantify the presence of specific proteins in EVs that have been previously purified and disrupted to extract those proteins.

In this method, EVs are lysed, and proteins from the lysate are run on an SDS-PAGE and, subsequently, blotted on a nitrocellulose membrane. The proteins in the membrane are then recognized using primary antibodies against the proteins themselves and secondary antibodies conjugated to revelation enzymes. As EVs are heterogeneous populations, there is no panel of proteins recognized as an exclusive EV marker. According to MISEV, at least one transmembrane protein and one cytosolic protein need to be detected to assess the EV presence in a complex mixture [130].

Near to Western blotting, even enzyme-linked immunosorbent assay (ELISA) is commonly used to detect and quantify EV proteins, in particular in its sandwich variant. In this assay, the plate is coated with capture monoclonal antibodies directed against an EV protein of interest. EV lysates are added to the plate, and the presence of the protein of interest is assessed by a second monoclonal antibody, against a different epitope, conjugated with a revealing enzyme. This assay requires low sample volume and more samples, than in Western blotting, can be contemporary analyzed due to the employment of, at least, 96-well plates. Unfortunately, intra- and inter-assay variability should be considered when employing this kind of test [100,131].

Resistive pulse sensing (RPS) measures the size and concentration of particles in a solution by measuring the change in conductance across a sensing pore upon passage of a particle, exploiting the Coulter principle. This system does not distinguish between EV and non-EV particles, and, in addition, the pore is prone to clogging by aggregates or sticky proteins naturally present in biological samples [132].

It is well known that the specific EV cargo is fundamental for cellular response upon EV delivery. In addition, understanding the specific molecular machinery that regulates the EV cargo intracellularly is necessary to understand the role of EVs in physiology and pathophysiology and their possible therapeutic use [133,134].

High-throughput technologies allow a multifaceted characterization of EVs content by identifying a variety of microRNAs, long non-coding RNAs, and other molecules acting as potential disease biomarkers and putative therapeutic targets [135]. Mass spectroscopy is commonly employed to feature EVs due to the large quantity of information provided. The technique is used to determine EV components in terms of lipids, proteins, and metabolites. Liquid chromatography-electrospray ionization tandem mass spectrometry (LC/ESI-MS/MS) is the most common method for EV characterization. EVs are ionized, and their components are separated according to their mass/charge (m/z) values [136,137].

Cancer cell metabolism is significantly altered due to active cell proliferation. In particular, the alterations of cancer metabolism include faster glycolysis and lactic acid production and upregulation of nucleotide synthesis, which consequently lead to exosomal metabolome changes. Ultra-performance liquid chromatography-tandem mass spectrometer (UPLC-MS/MS) was used by Puhka and co-workers to successfully determine over 100 metabolites in the isolated EVs from prostate cancer patients before and after prostatectomy [138].

Paolino et al., driven by the knowledge of the correlation between psoriasis and the increased amounts of high-density lipoproteins and apolipoprotein A1 and an augmented cardiovascular risk, investigated the lipid content of EVs in psoriasis patients using targeted and untargeted liquid chromatography-mass spectrometry (LC-MS) approaches. Interestingly, they suggest that the determination of lipid changes in patient EVs supports the diagnosis and foresees drug response in psoriatic patients [139].

The analysis of EV RNA seems to be particularly interesting as a non-invasive cancer test with high sensitivity and specificity. Multiple RNA types were identified in EVs, including: microRNA (miRNA), ribosomal RNA (rRNA), transfer RNA (tRNA), long non-coding RNA (lncRNA), piwi-interacting RNA (piRNA), small nuclear RNA, and small nucleolar RNA (snoRNA). Messenger RNA (mRNA) has also been identified in EVs as a functional regulator of target cell behavior [140]. Conley and colleagues used next-generation sequencing to demonstrate that EVs carry tumor-specific alterations and can be analyzed as a sample of cancer cell genetic assets [141]. It is important to underline that the

EV isolation method influences RNA measurements. Furthermore, as it is currently not possible to sequence RNA in single EVs, the RNA copy number must be considered the average RNA copy number of a pool of EVs [134]. A comparison of the pros and cons of each different isolation method is provided in Table 1 below.

Table 1. Pros and cons overview of principal EV isolation methods.

EV Isolation Methods		
Method	**Pros**	**Cons**
Differential ultracentrifugation (dUC)	• Cost-effective [1] • Well established and widely employed [134]	• Lipoprotein contamination [134] • Time consuming [1] • Massive EV aggregation and damaging [1]
Density gradient UC	• EV subpopulations distinction [1]	• Need for operator high training [1] • Low final purity [1] • Small sample volumes can be processed [1]
Size exclusion chromatography (SEC)	• No high-density lipoprotein contamination [111] • Serum albumin removal [111] • Fast and cheap method [134] • EV integrity preservation [1]	• Difficulties in EV subpopulations distinction [111] • Co-isolation of non-EV particles above the cut-off [1,134]
Immuno-capture	• Selective EV isolation from different cell types [111] • Easy method, simple instrumentations [111]	• Expensive ligands [111] • Need for optimization of a mild elution process [111]
Ultrafiltration (UF)	• Simple and cheap method [1,111]	• Protein contamination [111] • Vesicle damaging [1]
Asymmetrial flow field-flow fractionation (AF4)	• Gentle fractionation [111] • Provides a large range of size-based separation [106] • No lipoprotein contamination [111]	• Small sample volumes can be processed [106] • Co-isolation of particles with the same hydrodynamic size [106]

2. RBC-Derived Extracellular Vesicles (RBCEVs): Biogenesis and Composition

Human red blood cells (RBCs) are terminally differentiated, enucleated, and very versatile cells that have been used for drug delivery systems since the end of the last century. Most of their applications as drug delivery systems have been extensively reviewed in [142–144]. RBCs have a flexible biconcave shape with a diameter of 7.5–8.7 μm and thickness of 1.7–2.2 μm, their membrane mainly contains 60% phospholipids, 30% cholesterol, and 10% glycolipids [145]. Moreover, the RBC membrane also contains various proteins, such as peripheral and integral proteins, which can be classified into three groups: cytoskeletal proteins (e.g., spectrin, actin, protein 4.1), integral structural proteins (e.g., band 3, glycophorins), and anchoring proteins (e.g., ankyrin, protein 4.2) [146]. All these features confer on RBCs a high degree of plasticity and elasticity that in vivo allows them to pass across very small capillaries and exert their transporting function, while in vitro they can be exploited for therapeutic purposes. Hemoglobin is the major cytosolic protein in intact RBCs; the cytoplasmic fraction also contains several antioxidant and metabolic enzymes needed for the RBC's own metabolism. These proteins can release adenosine triphosphate (ATP) and NO into the intracellular environment [147]. RBCs are the major vesicle-secreting cells in blood circulation. During their 120-day lifespan, RBCs lose ~20% of their hemoglobin content and membrane integrity during physiological vesiculation [148]. The physiological aging of RBCs accelerates vesicle generation. Indeed, vesiculation is one of the most important mechanisms by which RBCs eliminate harmful substances accumulated throughout their lifespan [149,150]. Under normal physiological conditions, RBC-derived EVs constitute 7.3% of EVs in whole blood, indicating that RBCs are one of the main sources of EVs in peripheral blood [151,152].

RBC membrane vesiculation is a homeostatic process activated in response to impaired signaling machinery; it can be induced by ATP depletion, calcium loading, lysophosphatidic acid exposure, oxidative stress, endotoxins, cytokines, complement, and high shear stress [153]. Red blood cell-derived extracellular vesicles (RBCEVs) can be divided into subpopulations, such as exosomes and microvesicles.

Exosomes can be produced during the reticulocyte or erythroid precursor stage and maintained until the mature RBC stage [4]. Erythropoiesis is a long process that starts with a myeloid precursor and ends with reticulocytes maturing into erythrocytes. This terminal differentiation is accompanied by a cellular remodeling that leads to the disappearance of intracellular organelles, the elimination of membrane and cytoplasmic content, and the acquisition of the typical cellular biconcave form. Blank et al. proposed for the first time that exosome biogenesis and secretion contribute to the net loss of the cell surface membrane via selective vesicular membrane secretion [154]. Exosomes derived from reticulocytes are generated via the typical endosomal pathway of nucleated cells after the plasma membrane has invaginated to form the early endosome. The early endosome subsequently matures into a late endosome that evolves into multivesicular bodies carrying intraluminal vesicles [4].

On the contrary, vesicles may form during the normal aging of circulating erythrocytes due to complement-mediated calcium influx, plasma membrane budding, and subsequent vesicle shedding [155]. The biogenesis and release of microvesicles (MVs), which originate by membrane budding, is an integral part of red blood cell physiology and is linked to their maturation and aging. Indeed, by releasing MVs, the erythrocyte can eliminate damaged components that could also trigger hemostatic and immunological reactions [4]. Primarily, the formation of MVs from red blood cells is triggered by damaged hemoglobin, protein oxidation, degradation caused by senescence, and cytoskeletal binding of ankyrin to band 3. Another mechanism involved in the production of microvesicles is the alteration of phospholipid distribution in the lipid bilayer. Indeed, certain enzymes such as scramblase, calpain, and some proteases can be activated by oxidative stress or an increased influx of calcium ions, thus leading to the inhibition of flippase with the consequent exposure of phosphatidylserine, usually expressed in the inner bilayer layer, or leading to the proteolytic degradation of the cytoskeleton and the consequent aggregation of band 3 [4].

2.1. RBCEVs Composition

RBCEVs are generally visualized as round vesicles of 100–200 nm and comprise phospholipids, proteins, cholesterol, lipid rafts, hemoglobin, and acetylcholinesterase [150]. Although RBCEVs are derived from RBCs, their membrane compositions and internal contents are not exactly the same. Indeed, the final composition of RBCEVs is supposed to be dependent on the resealing and stimulating conditions. Indeed, EVs produced from RBCs are reported to be different when produced naturally in vivo, released ex vivo during blood bag storage, or produced in vitro by chemical treatments [156]. According to Yang et al., RBCEVs lack cytoskeletal components such as spectrin and actin, whereas they are relatively enriched in connexins and lipid raft markers [157]. Thangaraju et al. compared about 30 papers reporting the composition of RBCEVs obtained after different procedures of isolation/production and in different physiological/pathological conditions [4]; while Chiangjong et al. made a deep comparison of the components of the parental cells (RBCs) and those of the derived vesicles (RBCEVs) [150]. Taken together, these data suggest that the different conditions or production methods can affect the final composition; however, some similarities can be found and are reported in the next paragraph.

Extracellular vesicles are highly enriched with proteins with different functions, such as tetraspanins (CD9, CD63, CD81, and CD82), which are involved in cell penetration, invasion, and fusion events; heat shock proteins (HSP70, HSP90), which are involved in antigen anchoring and presentation; and MVB formation proteins (Alix, TSG101), which are involved in exosomal release [158]. Additionally, cytoskeletal proteins (e.g., actin), denatured hemoglobin, proteins 4.1, 4.2, enzymes such as carbonic anhydrase, anion transport proteins (Band 3), glycoproteins (e.g., CD235a), membrane-associated proteins such as stomatin and flotillin, and CD47, which inhibits phagocytosis by interacting with macrophage signal regulatory protein alpha [159]. Whereas, in the membrane lipid part, we find phosphatidylserine (PS), which is often found in the outer membrane layer and has a role in biogenesis (see next paragraphs), phosphatidylethanolamine, phosphatidic acid, diacylglycerol, and cholesterol [4,150]. The most striking and interesting discovery is that these vesicles have different types of miRNAs inside them, which can be harnessed and directed towards a specific target to exert their action as modulators of gene expression [4,160]. Among nucleic acids, DNA is obviously lacking, while miRNAs are present in huge amounts [161]. About 78 different miRNAs were found, with miR-125b-5p, miR-4454, and miR-451a being the most abundant [160,161]. On this basis, Sun et al. proposed that under certain conditions, RBCEVs can send miRNA to recipient cells to exert their function [162].

2.2. RBCEVs Production under Physiological and Pathological Conditions

RBCEVs are naturally produced during the RBC's life and are released into circulation, where they can interact with numerous tissues and/or cells to influence their functions. RBCEVs can play roles both in physiological and pathological conditions, but if the RBCEV level in healthy states is assumed to be normal, their level is supposed to be raised with aging or under other diseased or stressed conditions [157].

The first physiological function that has been discovered is during the maturation of RBCs. Indeed, they remove excess proteins and membranes such as transferrin receptors, acetylcholinesterase, and hemoglobin via vesiculation processes during the passage from reticulocyte to mature RBC [163,164]. RBCEVs can protect RBCs by clearing dangerous molecules and preventing their early clearance from circulation [165,166]. In addition, RBCEVs partly inherit the role of RBCs. RBCEVs are critical for communicating with endothelial cells to regulate NO and O2 homeostasis. Indeed, under storage conditions, RBCEVs react faster with NO than intact red blood cells, causing strong vasoconstriction [147,167]. RBCEVs can affect a variety of immune cells [168–170]. RBCEVs can promote the production of pro-inflammatory cytokines (interleukin (IL)-2, -7, and -15) and tumor necrosis factor-alpha (TNFα) by interacting with macrophages [170]. RBCEVs also increased proliferation in CD4+ and CD8+ T cells by influencing antigen-presenting cells [168]. Finally, RBCEVs may also have a role in coagulopathy [4]. Some authors have suggested that PS exposed to the external membrane layer can contribute to coagulation by triggering the intrinsic pathway. However, other authors reported an anti-coagulant role of RBCEVs mediated by their interaction with protein S, protein C, and fibrinogen [171,172].

As mentioned before, RBCEVs have been known as key regulators of various physiological and pathological processes, including coagulation, inflammation, and also atherosclerosis and thrombosis [173]. Moreover, there is strong evidence that the plasma concentrations of RBCEVs are elevated in the development of cardiovascular-related disease, which can further lead to vascular dysfunction [174]. Furthermore, RBCs infected by *Plasmodium* falciparum are able to transfer DNA (drug resistance and fluorescent protein genes, etc.) through the RBCEVs, helping the parasite survive times of stress [175]. RBCEVs in disease states often have pro-inflammatory and pro-coagulant effects. Different studies have shown that elevated levels of the circulating pro-coagulant RBCEV lead to increased thrombotic and hypercoagulable states in sudden nocturnal hemoglobinuria (PNH) and hemolytic disease [176,177]. RBCEVs can finally interfere with NO homeostasis by increasing ROS production, which can also lead to endothelial dysfunction [178].

2.3. RBCEVs Production and Isolation for Therapeutic Purposes

RBCs are an excellent source for the production of EVs for drug delivery. RBCEVs have several distinct advantages compared with other types of cell-derived and artificially produced EVs [150]. Synthetic nanovesicles created from biomimetic phospholipid bilayers resulted in several improvements, such as increased solubility, prolonged action, reduced toxicity, and lesser adverse effects, by mimicking EV properties [179,180]. However, the issues limiting the utility of those synthetic nanocarriers are immunogenicity and higher clearance by phagocytic cells [181]. Conversely, RBCEVs have been proven extremely safe thanks to their higher biocompatibility compared to synthetic ones. In addition, compared to EVs derived from nucleated cells, RBCEVs have a lower risk of horizontal gene transfer because RBCs lack both nuclear and mitochondrial DNA; thus, RBCEVs are particularly advantageous for delivering genetic material, e.g., RNA molecules and long mRNA molecules [182]. Furthermore, RBCEVs can escape macrophage clearance through the binding of CD47 to inhibitory receptor signal regulatory protein α SIRPα), thus preventing RBCEV clearance via endogenous elimination [159]. Finally, RBCEVs produced by O blood type cells may be used in allogeneic individuals, and the blood cells are easy to obtain from donors. Thus, RBCEVs represent an excellent delivery system for carrying drugs to cellular targets with cost-effectiveness, non-immunogenicity, and high stability and biocompatibility [150].

Nevertheless, the main limitations remain the way of scaling up RBCEVs production to increase the yield and the way to load cargo into EVs. These will be discussed in detail in the following paragraphs.

Methods for Scaling up RBCEVs Yield

Several stimuli have been shown to stimulate RBCEVs; Chiangjong and colleagues summarized them very well in a table reporting a list of chemical reagents, oxidative molecules, and storage conditions for RBCEV production [150]. In the next sub-paragraphs, we will discuss the most used methods for producing high amounts of RBCEVs in vitro or ex vivo; these have been outlined in Figure 4.

Among chemical methods, the most used is the in vitro stimulation with calcium ionophore. Usman and colleagues provided a lab-based approach to treat isolated RBCs with calcium ionophores that can stimulate the release of RBCEVs [182]. The protocol also envisaged the purification by means of several rounds of low-speed centrifugations, filtration, and ultracentrifugation steps. This appeared to be a feasible, cost-effective, and high-yielding approach, thus making it one of the most used in laboratory settings. Large-scale amounts (10^{13}–10^{14}) of RBCEVs can be isolated from RBCs (per unit, 200 mL of blood) when treated with calcium ionophore, which is thus a promising and scalable strategy to obtain EVs in vitro.

Calcium ionophore is supposed to induce vesiculation by activation of PS exposure to the outer surface membrane, thus leading to membrane budding and microvesiculation [150]. Other chemicals can mimic the same process, such as phorbol 12-myristate 13-acetate and lysophosphatidic acid [150].

Another method and/or process that induces vesiculation is the induction of oxidative stress, for example, by means of tert-butyl hydroperoxide, which leads to increased osmotic fragility and Hb oxidation [183].

Finally, it has also been reported that long-term storage, like in blood banking conditions, can stimulate the production of RBCEVs [150,184]. This has obvious consequences in transfusion medicine.

Nowadays, it is not completely understood whether and how different kinds of stimuli can affect RBCEVs' properties and composition, so characterization is an important step at the end of the production.

In addition to chemical methods, there are different so-called "physical" vesiculation methods that encompass several different methods that can mimic "shear stress". One of the most used physical vesiculation methods is extrusion, but recently other methods have been proposed.

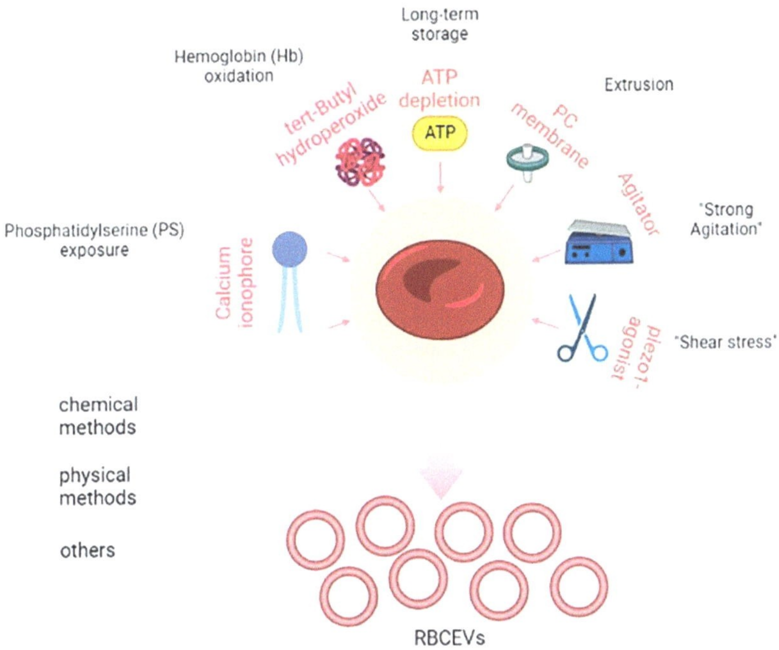

Figure 4. Methods for increasing the yield of RBCEVs production. In the figure, different chemical and physical methods are shown. In particular, molecules and/or mechanical stimuli are depicted together with their effect on the cells that give rise to RBCEVs release. Long-term storage is a particular condition that cannot be included in either the chemical or physical methods. Created in Biorender.com, accessed on 5 December 2022.

Gangadaran and co-workers optimized a scaling-up strategy to produce RBCs exosome mimetics (RBC-EMs) based on extrusion [185]. RBC-EMs produced by this method have similar characteristics as RBC exosomes. To obtain RBC-EMs, RBCs were purified from fresh blood and diluted in phosphate-buffered saline. The diluted RBCs were passed through a 1 μm polycarbonate membrane four times by using an extrusion set. After this physical stress, the obtained samples were purified by ultracentrifugation as before. This seems another promising and scalable strategy to obtain RBCEVs and allowed 130-fold higher production yield in terms of particle numbers compared to native exosome release.

Recently, Erytech Pharma patented a novel vesiculation method to produce large-scale RBCEVs also based on "shear stress". In particular, after the loading procedure (see the next paragraph for a focus on loading procedures), they put loaded RBCs under "strong agitation" for several hours, and this induced the production of RBCEVs. This method will be discussed more deeply in the section dedicated to patents (see "State of the art of the technology from the industrial side").

More recently, other authors proposed another method to induce mechanical stimuli for vesiculation, which is Piezo1 stimulation [186]. Briefly, Sangha and collaborators found that treating 6% hematocrit RBCs with 10 μM piezo1 agonist yoda1 for 30 min maximized RBCEV yield until 10^{12} particles/mL. This paper was available as a pre-print at the time of its writing.

2.4. Methods for Cargo Loading in RBCEVs

Growing evidence shows that RBCEVs can not only deliver biological information but also different kinds of drugs, nucleic acids, and proteins. Nevertheless, another limitation is exactly the way cargo is loaded. Han et al., in 2021, revised the whole methods for loading cargo into different kinds of EVs. He divided the methods between "cell-based" and "non-cell-based" [187]. Cell-based methods, also called pre-loading, are based on the indirect encapsulation of therapeutic cargo into the donor cell before the production of EVs. In this approach, different cargoes can be encapsulated into the donor cells essentially by simple incubation and/or transfection. During vesiculation, cargoes are then packaged into EVs and ultimately delivered to recipient cells for therapeutic use [188]. This method provides a convenient and effective way for loading biological materials and drug therapies into EVs [187]. On the contrary, the non-cell-based loading approach involves the direct loading of chemical or biomolecules into already-produced EVs and can be performed through electroporation, sonication, incubation, and/or transfection [189]. Thus, non-cell-based EV loading methods incorporate therapeutic cargo into EVs after isolation and/or production, and for this reason, it is also known as "post-loading". Different siRNAs, miRNAs, proteins, CRISPR/Cas9, hydrophobic compounds, and anticancer drugs can be loaded into EVs through non-cell-based loading [187]. These loading methods can be further classified into passive loading and active loading [187]. Passive loading involves loading the therapeutic cargo into EVs through diffusion, whereas active loading consists of the disruption of EV membranes through electroporation or sonication, allowing entry into the EVs.

In this review, which is focused on RBCEVs, we prefer to talk about pre-loading and post-loading methods. As mentioned, RBCs have been used longer for drug delivery [143,144,190]; indeed, they possess numerous features that make them ideal candidates for this purpose: (i) are biodegradable; (ii). are available in large quantities; (iii) can circulate for long periods of time (months); (iv) have a large capacity; (v) are not toxic or immunogenic; (vi) have a long in vivo life span; and (vii) several procedures exist to encapsulate a wide range of molecules inside them. Regarding this last point, many loading methods (electroporation, drug-induced endocytosis, osmotic pulsing, and hypotonic hemolysis) have been set up over the years and are mostly based on the transient opening of pores across the cell membrane, as detailed in Rossi et al. and Magnani et al. [190,191].

RBCs possess, in fact, the remarkable capacity for reversible shape change and for reversible deformation, allowing the opening of pores (20–50 nm in diameter) large enough to be crossed by externally placed macromolecules. Among the above-mentioned methods, the hypotonic hemolysis one is what allows for obtaining engineered RBCs with the most suitable characteristics for biomedical applications. In turn, it includes different procedures, such as dilutional, preswell dilutional, and dialysis ones, which can be opportunely selected by the researchers according to them. However, all these procedures are based on the same physical-chemical features of RBCs. When placed in the presence of a hypotonic solution, RBCs increase in volume, and their morphology is converted to spherocytes; since RBCs have little capacity to resist volume increases when placed in solutions of appropriate mOsm/kg, the membranes rupture with the formation of large pores, permitting the influx of molecules of interest. By raising the salt concentration to its original level, the membranes can be resealed and the added substances entrapped in erythrocytes [192,193]. It must be emphasized that when a procedure moves from the laboratory to the clinic, the availability of appropriate equipment based on an appropriate method becomes very important. To date, two companies, ERYtech Pharma S.A. and EryDel S.p.A., have ongoing phase III clinical trials (ClinicalTrials.gov identifiers: NCT03674242 and NCT03563053, respectively) based on engineered RBCs obtained by dialysis or the preswell dilutional method, respectively. Their equipment allows them to carry out fully automated loading procedures in perfect sterility and apirogenicity conditions, as is needed in clinical use.

Regarding the post-loading methods, the most used for RBCEVs are electroporation and transfection. Both of them have been widely used for the encapsulation of nucleic acids. Iconic examples are represented by Usman et al. that used electroporation [182] and Peng et al. that preferred the transfection method [194]. Several other examples are reported in the next paragraph, which focused on the therapeutic applications of RBCEVs.

The different cargo methods are outlined in Figure 5.

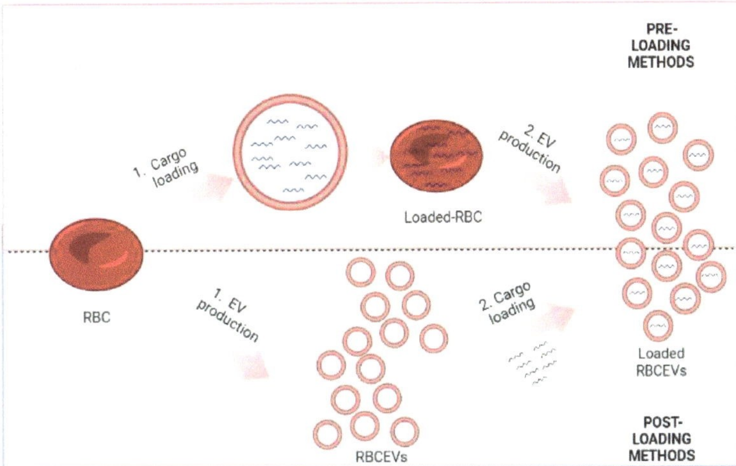

Figure 5. Methods for cargo loading in RBCEVs. Loading methods have been divided into two main classes, namely pre-loading and post-loading methods. In the first, the cargo is loaded into the donor cell before the vesiculation process. While, in the second method, the cargo is loaded into the already produced vesicles. Created in Biorender.com, accessed on 9 January 2023.

2.5. Recent Development in Therapeutic Application of RBCEVs: From the Lab Side to the Industry Side

As discussed, RBCEVs possess several features that make them particularly suitable for therapeutic applications: (i) blood is easily accessible from blood banks, thus RBCs can be produced from blood at large scale and at low cost; (ii) autologous transfusion, from their own donor (or patient), or allogenic transfusion, from a universal 0-donor, of RBCEVs, are possible; (iii) RBCEVs are safer compared with other cell-derived EVs because they lack DNA, minimizing the risk of horizontal gene transfer; (iv) RBCEVs are completely nontoxic and have higher biocompatibility than synthetic EVs; (v) RBCEVs can be frozen and thawed many times without affecting their integrity and efficacy [158]. In this regard, a publication recently investigated different buffers and conditions to allow a longer stability of frozen EVs [195]. The authors demonstrated that EVs, resuspended in suitable buffers, can be stable for up to 2 years. Thus, RBCEVs can be developed into stable pharmaceutical products in the near future (Figure 6). This is probably the main feature that attracted the attention of several biotech and pharma companies.

2.5.1. From the Lab Side

In 2010, Chang and co-workers demonstrated the ability of RBCEVs to efficiently deliver ultra-small superparamagnetic iron oxide particles into human bone marrow mesenchymal stem cells for cellular magnetic resonance imaging in vitro and in vivo [196]. The novel method allowed for higher intracellular labeling efficiency and higher biosafety compared with traditional approaches. RBCEVs were shown for the first time to be biosafe and they can be used as potential delivery vehicles for clinical applications due to their autologous property; this study also gave rise to a patent that is cited in the next section.

But it was in 2018, that the most pioneering study was made by Usman and colleagues, where an efficient delivery system was developed for RNA-based therapeutics using RBCEVs [182]. Small and large RNAs, e.g., antisense oligonucleotides (ASOs), and large RNAs, such as mRNA, were electroporated into RBCEVs and transported to target cells in both solid and liquid tumors. Briefly, microRNA-125b-ASO-loaded RBCEVs significantly reduced both breast tumor growth by intratumoral injection and suppressed acute myeloid leukemia (AML) progression by systemic administration. In addition, genome-editing effects were also observed when RBCEVs were loaded with Cas9 mRNA and guide RNAs. The delivery efficiency was higher, and far less cytotoxicity was observed as compared to other commercial transfection reagents.

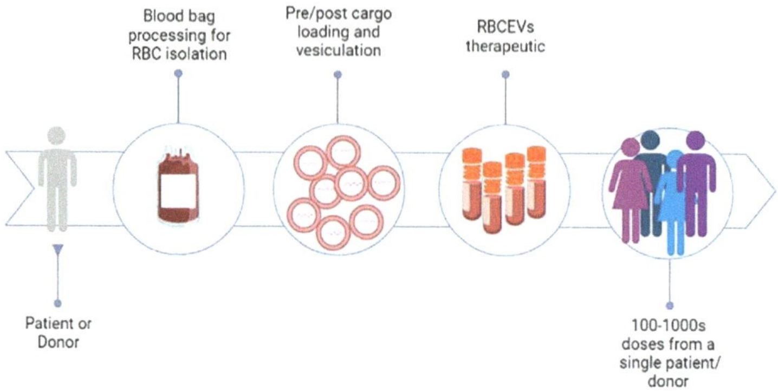

Figure 6. RBCEVs platform for clinical exploitation. The figure represents the road for the clinical exploitation of RBC-derived EVs, which could be achieved in the near future, and shows some of the advantages of this promising strategy. Created in Biorender.com, accessed on 14 December 2022.

Moreover, exosome mimetics (EMs) were produced from red blood cells (RBCs), and the radiolabeling of the RBC-EMs for in vivo imaging was analyzed [185]. Engineered EMs from RBCs were produced on a large scale by a one-step extrusion method and further purified by density gradient centrifugation, the resulting RBC-EMs had a 130-fold greater yield compared to natural nanovesicles generated from RBCs and displayed enhanced in vivo biodistribution. RBC-EMs were labeled with technetium-99m (99mTc). The results demonstrated a simple yet large-scale production method for a novel type of RBC-EMs, which can be effectively labeled with 99mTc, and feasibly monitored in vivo by nuclear imaging. It shows that the RBC-EMs may be used as in vivo drug delivery vehicles [185].

In 2019, RBCEVs were applied in another study in which lipophilic drugs, such as camptothecin, were packaged within RBCEVs and administered to lung carcinoma cells, showing an improvement in targeted delivery when compared with synthetic lipid-based nanocarriers [197].

In 2020, Zhang and colleagues demonstrated that RBC-derived EVs loaded with miR-155 showed an excellent protective effect against acute liver failure, while those loaded with doxorubicin or sorafenib showed significant therapeutic effects against hepatocellular carcinoma without systemic toxicity in mice [198]. In the same year, other authors isolated RBCEVs from subjects infected by *Plasmodium falciparum* and loaded them with the antimalarial drugs atovaquone and tafenoquine [199]. They observed that the free drug was less effective than the RBCEV-loaded one, indicating that RBCEVs can potentially increase the efficacy of several small hydrophobic drugs used for the treatment of malaria.

In 2022, Jayasinghe and co-workers conjugated RBCEVs with several peptides and/or antibodies for targeted delivery of cargoes to cancer cells [200]. They conjugated RBCEVs with a cyclic peptide to specifically target CXCR4 or with a monoclonal antibody anti-CD33 to promote the specific binding and uptake of the conjugated EVs by leukemia cells expressing the corresponding receptors. CXCR4-conjugated RBCEVs were loaded with the pro-apoptotic peptide KLA, demonstrating that these were able to significantly suppress leukemia burden and increase survival in a leukemia xenografted mouse model. Antibody-conjugated RBCEVs were also used to deliver RNA antisense oligonucleotides to knock down FLT3 and miR-125b in cell lines and in patient-derived xenograft models of leukemia [200]. This study demonstrated for the first time that peptide/antibody-conjugated RBCEVs are biocompatible and non-immunogenic and can be used for targeted delivery of therapeutic peptides and RNAs for potential clinical applications. Finally, a novel nanocarrier composed of RBCEVs, surface-linked with doxorubicin using glutaraldehyde, was developed by [7]. The results demonstrated, once again, that drug-loaded RBCEVs could exert superior anticancer activity than free drug, both in vitro and in vivo.

In a very recent study, authors from the same group as Usman et al. [182] re-proposed RNA-loaded RBCEVs for potential immunotherapy [194]. In detail, they loaded the previous 3p-125b-ASO or a novel RIG-I agonist, namely an immunomodulatory RNA. The authors showed that the two agonists stimulated the RIG-I pathway and induced cell death in both mouse and human breast cancer cells. Significant suppression of tumor growth, coupled with increased immune cell infiltration mediated by the activation of the RIG-I cascade, was observed also in vivo after multiple intratumoral injections of RNA-loaded RBCEVs. Finally, they proposed also a targeted delivery using RBCEVs coupled with EGFR-binding nanobody, administrated intrapulmonary to mice, to facilitate the accumulation of RBCEVs in EGFR-positive breast cancer cells.

The main applications reported in the literature have been summarized in Table 2.

Table 2. Main findings on RBCs-based EVs as a drug delivery carrier.

Reference	EV Production Method	Cargo-Loading Method	Cargo	Application	In Vitro	Pre-Clinical	Clinical
[196]	Chemical method, calcium chloride	Incubation under hypo-osmotic conditions	Ultrasmall super-paramagnetic iron oxide (USPIO) particles	Magnetic resonance imaging	X	X	
[182]	Chemical method, calcium ionophore	Post-loading method, electroporation	Antisense oligonucleotides, Cas9 mRNA, and guide RNAs	Cancer therapy	X	X	
[185]	Physical method, extrusion	Post-loading method, incubation	Technetium-99m	In vivo imaging		X	
[197]	Physical method, extrusion	Pre-loading method, hemolysis and incubation	Camptothecin and amphiphilic fluorophore	Cancer therapy	X	X	
[7]	Chemical method, calcium ionophore	Post-loading method, incubation	Doxorubicin	Cancer therapy	X	X	
[194]	Chemical method, calcium ionophore	Post-loading method, transfection and electroporation	Rig-I agonists, small RNAs	Cancer therapy	X	X	
[198]	Chemical method, calcium ionophore	Post-loading method, transfection	Antisense oligonucleotides, doxorubicin and sorafenib	Acute liver failure, cancer therapy	X	X	
[199]	Isolation of naturally produced RBCEVs	Post-loading method, incubation	Antimalarial drug, atovaquone and tafenoquine	Anti-malarial treatment	X		
[200]	Chemical method, calcium ionophore	Post-loading method, transfection	Peptide, Antisense oligonucleotides, siRNA	Cancer therapy	X	X	

2.5.2. To the Industry Side

The first industrial exploitation of RBCEVs-like particles belongs to a researcher at the University of California. In particular, they produced RBC membrane-camouflaged nanoparticles by first producing RBC membrane-derived vesicles by hypotonic treatment and extrusion of RBCs, which were further combined with a polymeric nanoparticle core to produce RBC-derived nanoparticles (Patent Application Publication No. US 2013/0337066A1, Membrane encapsulated nanoparticles and method of use, 2013. Related patent documents:

EP2714017 CN103857387 CA2873404 DK2714017 ES2685333 WO/2013/052167 EP3412282 JP2014518200 US20130337066). The inventive nanoparticle comprises (a) an inner core comprising a non-cellular material and (b) an outer surface comprising a cellular membrane derived from RBCs. These nanoparticles were tested in several applications, such as eliciting an immune response, and treating or preventing diseases or conditions, such as neoplasms or cancer, or diseases or conditions associated with cell membrane insertion of toxins. Later, Cellics Therapeutics invented another application of the aforementioned particles: a biomimetic toxin nanosponge that functions as a toxin decoy in vivo. These nanosponges absorb membrane-damaging toxins and can potentially treat a variety of injuries and diseases caused by pore-forming toxins (US 2017/0095510 A1, use of nanoparticles coated with red blood cell membranes to treat hemolytic diseases and disorders, 2017).

In 2019, Le et al. from the City University of Hong Kong proposed for the first time the use of native RBCEVs for gene therapy (US 2019/0054192 Isolation RBCEVs form RBCs for gene therapy, 2019. Related patent documents US20190054192 CN109402176). The invention comprises the purification and electroporation of the RBCEVs and applying the RNA-loaded EVs to target cells. Briefly, they proposed to stimulate the EVs' production with calcium ionophore, followed by isolation by ultracentrifugation, and finally electroporation to load nucleic acids. Moreover, Minh Le and colleagues from the National University of Singapore and Cornell University developed a method of delivering nucleic acids to immune cells (e.g., T cells) using RBCEVs. These loaded immune cells can be used as immunotherapy to treat cancer (WO 2021/194425 A1, method of delivering nucleic acid to immune cells using RBCEVs, 2021. Related patent documents EP2021777014).

Some years later, researchers at the Imperial College in London proposed the use of targeted delivery of thrombolytic drugs to blood clots using RBCEVs platform WO 2021/123799 A1, red blood cell-derived vesicle, 2021. Related patent documents EP4076481). The invention also extends to a method of: (i) contacting a red blood cell with a hypotonic solution to produce a red blood cell ghost, and (ii) encapsulating an active agent using the red blood cell ghost to thereby produce a red blood cell-derived vesicle comprising an encapsulated active agent. Finally, step (iii) may further comprise extrusion through a filter at least once to produce EVs from ghost RBCs. Using this pre-loading method, RBCEVs have been encapsulated with thrombolytic drugs such as tissue plasminogen activator (tPA), which can further be used to treat ischemic strokes, myocardial infarction, and pulmonary embolism. RBCVs protect thrombolytic agents in the blood circulation, leading to improved stability and prolonged half-life, and temporarily suppress thrombolytic activity, leading to reduced hemorrhagic side effects.

In the same year, Carmine Therapeutics developed next-generation, non-viral based gene therapies to treat a wide range of diseases using RBCEVs (WO 2021/145821 A1, nucleic acid-loaded red blood cells extracellular vesicles 2021. Related patent documents WO/2021/145821 CA3164176 KR1020220127851 CN115151277 EP4090373 NZ789881 JP2022542905). The company proposed a method of isolating calcium ionophore-induced RBCEVs (as before) and further loading these vesicles with nucleic acids (DNA/RNA) by several methods comprising both electroporation and transfection. These platforms showed the ability to carry DNA or RNA payloads ranging from 20 bp to >30 kb and much more. Thus, by using RBCEVs as a drug delivery system, the limitations of viral-based gene therapies, such as immunogenicity, small payload capacity, and manufacturing challenges, can be overcome.

Finally, at the end of the year, Erytech Pharma also filed a patent application for the development of drug delivery RBCEVs from preloaded RBC (WO 2021/228832 A1, red blood cell extracellular vesicles (RCEVS) containing cargoes and methods of use and production thereof, 2021). First, red blood cells were loaded with the desired cargo by "hypotonic encapsulation" and then vesiculated by "strong agitation". The cargo can be comprised of nucleic acids, proteins, small molecules, or components of a gene editing system, including CRISPR/Cas9. These loaded RBCEVs may be used to treat a variety of diseases and disorders, including autoimmune disorders, cancers, cardiovascular diseases, gastrointestinal diseases, genetic disorders, and inflammatory diseases.

To the best of our knowledge, these are the updates at the time of writing.

3. Conclusions and Future Perspectives

Extracellular vesicles, in general, and extracellular vesicles derived from RBCs, are very promising tools in the clinical field. As we mentioned, RBCEVs can act as biological carriers, thus transporting several molecules and cargoes for both therapeutic and diagnostic purposes. The advantages of using EVs over synthetic transport systems are manifold. Indeed, they present greater stability in the bloodstream due to their natural membrane composition, better cargo protection due to their protein–lipid architecture [201], and better biocompatibility, allowing efficient permeability between biological membranes [182]. Especially, RBCEVs present several features that make them particularly suitable for possible clinical applications compared to other types of carriers. RBCEVs are safer when compared to other EVs as RBCs have no nucleus and mitochondria and therefore do not contain genetic material, whereas EVs from other nucleated cell types pose a risk of horizontal gene transfer. Furthermore, RBCEVs are non-toxic and non-immunogenic when transferred to the right blood group, unlike common vectors such as adenoviruses, lentiviruses, nanoparticles, and other synthetic EVs. Finally, blood banks are easily accessible for their production, and the obtained RBCEVs can be frozen and thawed for many cycles without losing their efficacy and integrity [158], thus allowing injectable formulations to be prepared.

A proposed platform for RBCEVs' exploitation has been proposed in Figure 6. On this platform, the blood can be taken from the same patient (autologous) or from a universal or compatible donor (heterologous). Then, the RBCs are purified and processed for vesiculation and cargo loading under GMP conditions. The obtained loaded RBCEVs can be aliquoted, frozen, and stored for the next injection of the patient(s). It can be hypothesized that up to 100–1000 doses can be obtained from a single blood unit.

Despite all these advantages, there are still important limitations regarding: (i) the lack of a standardized method for their isolation; (ii) the limited efficiency in the loading of the drug of interest; and (iii) the large-scale production at a clinical level. To overcome the isolation/production problems, some authors have proposed in vitro chemical methods to stimulate red blood cells to release a large number of RBCEVs, thus providing a possible strategy to obtain EVs [150,182], while other authors have proposed lab-scale production by physical methods, such as extrusion [185] or vesiculation by agitation (WO2021228832A1, red cell extracellular vesicles (RCEVs) containing cargoes and methods of use and production thereof). Regarding vesicle loading, two different approaches have been basically proposed: the molecule of interest can be loaded into the cells before the biogenesis of EVs (pre-loading method) or after their formation by electroporation (post-loading method).

Once these processes are optimized, the applications will be manifold. From gene therapies to RNA-based therapies, from enzyme replacement therapies to the new trends in genome editing. Despite this, there are still many unanswered questions about how they can work in vivo, such as: How are EVs internalized in recipient cells? How is the cargo released in them? How does the vesicular cargo affect the physiology of the recipient cell? What may be the most advantageous routes of administration, and which organs might be possible targets? Finding answers to all these questions will pave the way for the long-awaited transition from the lab to the clinic.

Author Contributions: Conceptualization, C.B. and S.B.; writing—original draft preparation, S.B., F.A., C.B., B.C. and L.R.; writing—review and editing, M.M. (Mariele Montanari), M.M. (Mauro Magnani) and S.P.; supervision, M.M. (Mauro Magnani), C.B., L.R. and S.P. All authors have read and agreed to the published version of the manuscript.

Funding: This paper has been produced with the financial assistance of the European Union POR MARCHE FESR 2014/2020. Asse 1, OS 2, Azione 2.1-Intervento 2.1.1–Sostegno allo sviluppo di una piattaforma di ricerca collaborativa negli ambiti della specializzazione intelligente. Thematic Area:

"Medicina personalizzata, farmaci e nuovi approcci terapeutici". Project acronym: Marche BioBank www.marchebiobank.it. The content of the paper is the sole responsibility of the authors and can under no circumstances be regarded as reflecting the position of the European Union and/or Marche Region authorities.

Data Availability Statement: No new data were created or analyzed in this study. Data sharing is not applicable to this article.

Conflicts of Interest: The authors declare no conflict of interest.

References

1. Villa, F.; Quarto, R.; Tasso, R. Extracellular Vesicles as Natural, Safe and Efficient Drug Delivery Systems. *Pharmaceutics* **2019**, *11*, 557. [CrossRef] [PubMed]
2. Raposo, G.; Stoorvogel, W. Extracellular vesicles: Exosomes, microvesicles, and friends. *J. Cell Biol.* **2013**, *200*, 373–383. [CrossRef]
3. Catitti, G.; De Bellis, D.; Vespa, S.; Simeone, P.; Canonico, B.; Lanuti, P. Extracellular Vesicles as Players in the Anti-Inflammatory Inter-Cellular Crosstalk Induced by Exercise Training. *Int. J. Mol. Sci.* **2022**, *23*, 14098. [CrossRef] [PubMed]
4. Thangaraju, K.; Neerukonda, S.N.; Katneni, U.; Buehler, P.W. Extracellular vesicles from red blood cells and their evolving roles in health, coagulopathy and therapy. *Int. J. Mol. Sci.* **2021**, *22*, 153. [CrossRef] [PubMed]
5. Théry, C.; Witwer, K.W.; Aikawa, E.; Alcaraz, M.J.; Anderson, J.D.; Andriantsitohaina, R.; Antoniou, A.; Arab, T.; Archer, F.; Atkin-Smith, G.K.; et al. Minimal information for studies of extracellular vesicles 2018 (MISEV2018): A position statement of the International Society for Extracellular Vesicles and update of the MISEV2014 guidelines. *J. Extracell. Vesicles* **2018**, *7*, 1535750. [CrossRef] [PubMed]
6. Gurunathan, S.; Kang, M.H.; Qasim, M.; Khan, K.; Kim, J.H. Biogenesis, Membrane Trafficking, Functions, and Next Generation Nanotherapeutics Medicine of Extracellular Vesicles. *Int. J. Nanomed.* **2021**, *16*, 3357–3383. [CrossRef]
7. Wu, S.-H.H.; Hsieh, C.-C.C.; Hsu, S.-C.C.; Yao, M.; Hsiao, J.-K.K.; Wang, S.-W.W.; Lin, C.-P.P.; Huang, D.-M.M. RBC-derived vesicles as a systemic delivery system of doxorubicin for lysosomal-mitochondrial axis-improved cancer therapy. *J. Adv. Res.* **2020**, *30*, 185–196. [CrossRef] [PubMed]
8. Ostrowski, M.; Carmo, N.B.; Krumeich, S.; Fanget, I.; Raposo, G.; Savina, A.; Moita, C.F.; Schauer, K.; Hume, A.N.; Freitas, R.P.; et al. Rab27a and Rab27b control different steps of the exosome secretion pathway. *Nat. Cell Biol.* **2010**, *12*, 19–30. [CrossRef]
9. Hoshino, D.; Kirkbride, K.C.; Costello, K.; Clark, E.S.; Sinha, S.; Grega-Larson, N.; Tyska, M.J.; Weaver, A.M. Exosome secretion is enhanced by invadopodia and drives invasive behavior. *Cell Rep.* **2013**, *5*, 1159–1168. [CrossRef]
10. Colombo, M.; Moita, C.; Van Niel, G.; Kowal, J.; Vigneron, J.; Benaroch, P.; Manel, N.; Moita, L.F.; Théry, C.; Raposo, G. Analysis of ESCRT functions in exosome biogenesis, composition and secretion highlights the heterogeneity of extracellular vesicles. *J. Cell Sci.* **2013**, *126*, 5553–5565. [CrossRef]
11. Lu, A.; Wawro, P.; Morgens, D.W.; Portela, F.; Bassik, M.C.; Pfeffer, S.R. Genome-wide interrogation of extracellular vesicle biology using barcoded miRNAs. *Elife* **2018**, *7*, e41460. [CrossRef]
12. Yeung, V.; Webber, J.P.; Dunlop, E.A.; Morgan, H.; Hutton, J.; Gurney, M.; Jones, E.; Falcon-Perez, J.; Tabi, Z.; Errington, R.; et al. Rab35-dependent extracellular nanovesicles are required for induction of tumour supporting stroma. *Nanoscale* **2018**, *10*, 8547–8559. [CrossRef] [PubMed]
13. Savina, A.; Furlán, M.; Vidal, M.; Colombo, M.I. Exosome release is regulated by a calcium-dependent mechanism in K562 cells. *J. Biol. Chem.* **2003**, *278*, 20083–20090. [CrossRef] [PubMed]
14. Holleman, J.; Marchese, A. The ubiquitin ligase deltex-3l regulates endosomal sorting of the G protein-coupled receptor CXCR4. *Mol. Biol. Cell* **2014**, *25*, 1892–1904. [CrossRef] [PubMed]
15. van Niel, G.; Charrin, S.; Simoes, S.; Romao, M.; Rochin, L.; Saftig, P.; Marks, M.S.; Rubinstein, E.; Raposo, G. The tetraspanin CD63 regulates ESCRT-independent and -dependent endosomal sorting during melanogenesis. *Dev. Cell* **2011**, *21*, 708–721. [CrossRef] [PubMed]
16. Muralidharan-Chari, V.; Clancy, J.; Plou, C.; Romao, M.; Chavrier, P.; Raposo, G.; D'Souza-Schorey, C. ARF6-regulated shedding of tumor cell-derived plasma membrane microvesicles. *Curr. Biol.* **2009**, *19*, 1875–1885. [CrossRef] [PubMed]
17. Hessvik, N.P.; Llorente, A. Current knowledge on exosome biogenesis and release. *Cell. Mol. Life Sci.* **2018**, *75*, 193–208. [CrossRef]
18. Minakaki, G.; Menges, S.; Kittel, A.; Emmanouilidou, E.; Schaeffner, I.; Barkovits, K.; Bergmann, A.; Rockenstein, E.; Adame, A.; Marxreiter, F.; et al. Autophagy inhibition promotes SNCA/alpha-synuclein release and transfer via extracellular vesicles with a hybrid autophagosome-exosome-like phenotype. *Autophagy* **2018**, *14*, 98–119. [CrossRef] [PubMed]
19. Solvik, T.A.; Nguyen, T.A.; Lin, Y.H.T.; Marsh, T.; Huang, E.J.; Wiita, A.P.; Debnath, J.; Leidal, A.M. Secretory autophagy maintains proteostasis upon lysosome inhibition. *J. Cell Biol.* **2022**, *221*, e202110151. [CrossRef]
20. Pleet, M.L.; Branscome, H.; DeMarino, C.; Pinto, D.O.; Zadeh, M.A.; Rodriguez, M.; Sariyer, I.K.; El-Hage, N.; Kashanchi, F. Autophagy, EVs, and infections: A perfect question for a perfect time. *Front. Cell. Infect. Microbiol.* **2018**, *8*, 362. [CrossRef]
21. Buratta, S.; Tancini, B.; Sagini, K.; Delo, F.; Chiaradia, E.; Urbanelli, L.; Emiliani, C. Lysosomal Exocytosis, Exosome Release and Secretory Autophagy: The Autophagic- and Endo-Lysosomal Systems Go Extracellular. *Int. J. Mol. Sci.* **2020**, *21*, 2576. [CrossRef]
22. Mathieu, M.; Martin-Jaular, L.; Lavieu, G.; Théry, C. Specificities of secretion and uptake of exosomes and other extracellular vesicles for cell-to-cell communication. *Nat. Cell Biol.* **2019**, *21*, 9–17. [CrossRef]

23. Zhang, Y.; Liu, Y.; Liu, H.; Tang, W.H. Exosomes: Biogenesis, biologic function and clinical potential. *Cell Biosci.* **2019**, *9*, 19. [CrossRef]
24. Tricarico, C.; Clancy, J.; D'Souza-Schorey, C. Biology and biogenesis of shed microvesicles. *Small GTPases* **2017**, *8*, 220–232. [CrossRef]
25. Balaj, L.; Lessard, R.; Dai, L.; Cho, Y.J.; Pomeroy, S.L.; Breakefield, X.O.; Skog, J. Tumour microvesicles contain retrotransposon elements and amplified oncogene sequences. *Nat. Commun.* **2011**, *2*, 180. [CrossRef] [PubMed]
26. Cocucci, E.; Racchetti, G.; Meldolesi, J. Shedding microvesicles: Artefacts no more. *Trends Cell Biol.* **2009**, *19*, 43–51. [CrossRef] [PubMed]
27. D'Souza-Schorey Crislyn, C.; Clancy, J.W. Tumor-derived microvesicles: Shedding light on novel microenvironment modulators and prospective cancer biomarkers. *Genes Dev.* **2012**, *26*, 1287–1299. [CrossRef]
28. Gulei, D.; Irimie, A.I.; Cojocneanu-Petric, R.; Schultze, J.L.; Berindan-Neagoe, I. Exosomes-Small Players, Big Sound. *Bioconjug. Chem.* **2018**, *29*, 635–648. [CrossRef] [PubMed]
29. Christ, L.; Wenzel, E.M.; Liestøl, K.; Raiborg, C.; Campsteijn, C.; Stenmark, H. ALIX and ESCRT-I/II function as parallel ESCRT-III recruiters in cytokinetic abscission. *J. Cell Biol.* **2016**, *212*, 499–513. [CrossRef] [PubMed]
30. Monteith, G.R.; Prevarskaya, N.; Roberts-Thomson, S.J. The calcium-cancer signalling nexus. *Nat. Rev. Cancer* **2017**, *17*, 367–380. [CrossRef]
31. Crawford, S.; Diamond, D.; Brustolon, L.; Penarreta, R. Effect of increased extracellular ca on microvesicle production and tumor spheroid formation. *Cancer Microenviron.* **2010**, *4*, 93–103. [CrossRef]
32. Bucki, R.; Bachelot-Loza, C.; Zachowski, A.; Giraud, F.; Sulpice, J.C. Calcium induces phospholipid redistribution and microvesicle release in human erythrocyte membranes by independent pathways. *Biochemistry* **1998**, *37*, 15383–15391. [CrossRef]
33. Stachowiak, J.C.; Schmid, E.M.; Ryan, C.J.; Ann, H.S.; Sasaki, D.Y.; Sherman, M.B.; Geissler, P.L.; Fletcher, D.A.; Hayden, C.C. Membrane bending by protein-protein crowding. *Nat. Cell Biol.* **2012**, *14*, 944–949. [CrossRef] [PubMed]
34. Di Bella, M.A. Overview and Update on Extracellular Vesicles: Considerations on Exosomes and Their Application in Modern Medicine. *Biology* **2022**, *11*, 804. [CrossRef] [PubMed]
35. Van Dommelen, S.M.; Vader, P.; Lakhal, S.; Kooijmans, S.A.A.; Van Solinge, W.W.; Wood, M.J.A.; Schiffelers, R.M. Microvesicles and exosomes: Opportunities for cell-derived membrane vesicles in drug delivery. *J. Control. Release* **2012**, *161*, 635–644. [CrossRef] [PubMed]
36. Tan, A.; Rajadas, J.; Seifalian, A.M. Exosomes as nano-theranostic delivery platforms for gene therapy. *Adv. Drug Deliv. Rev.* **2013**, *65*, 357–367. [CrossRef]
37. Batrakova, E.V.; Kim, M.S. Using exosomes, naturally-equipped nanocarriers, for drug delivery. *J. Control. Release* **2015**, *219*, 396–405. [CrossRef]
38. Yang, B.; Chen, Y.; Shi, J. Exosome Biochemistry and Advanced Nanotechnology for Next-Generation Theranostic Platforms. *Adv. Mater.* **2018**, *31*, e1802896. [CrossRef]
39. Pieragostino, D.; Lanuti, P.; Cicalini, I.; Cufaro, M.C.; Ciccocioppo, F.; Ronci, M.; Simeone, P.; Onofrj, M.; van der Pol, E.; Fontana, A.; et al. Proteomics characterization of extracellular vesicles sorted by flow cytometry reveals a disease-specific molecular cross-talk from cerebrospinal fluid and tears in multiple sclerosis. *J. Proteomics* **2019**, *204*, 103403. [CrossRef]
40. Alvarez-Erviti, L.; Seow, Y.; Yin, H.; Betts, C.; Lakhal, S.; Wood, M.J.A. Delivery of siRNA to the mouse brain by systemic injection of targeted exosomes. *Nat. Biotechnol.* **2011**, *29*, 341–345. [CrossRef]
41. Gao, X.; Ran, N.; Dong, X.; Zuo, B.; Yang, R.; Zhou, Q.; Moulton, H.M.; Seow, Y.; Yin, H.F. Anchor peptide captures, targets, and loads exosomes of diverse origins for diagnostics and therapy. *Sci. Transl. Med.* **2018**, *10*, eaat0195. [CrossRef] [PubMed]
42. Ha, D.; Yang, N.; Nadithe, V. Exosomes as therapeutic drug carriers and delivery vehicles across biological membranes: Current perspectives and future challenges. *Acta Pharm. Sin. B* **2016**, *6*, 287–296. [CrossRef]
43. Shi, M.; Sheng, L.; Stewart, T.; Zabetian, C.P.; Zhang, J. New windows into the brain: Central nervous system-derived extracellular vesicles in blood. *Prog. Neurobiol.* **2019**, *175*, 96–106. [CrossRef]
44. Simeone, P.; Celia, C.; Bologna, G.; Ercolino, E.; Pierdomenico, L.; Cilurzo, F.; Grande, R.; Diomede, F.; Vespa, S.; Canonico, B.; et al. Diameters and Fluorescence Calibration for Extracellular Vesicle Analyses by Flow Cytometry. *Int. J. Mol. Sci.* **2020**, *21*, 7885. [CrossRef] [PubMed]
45. Pieragostino, D.; Cicalini, I.; Lanuti, P.; Ercolino, E.; Di Ioia, M.; Zucchelli, M.; Zappacosta, R.; Miscia, S.; Marchisio, M.; Sacchetta, P.; et al. Enhanced release of acid sphingomyelinase-enriched exosomes generates a lipidomics signature in CSF of Multiple Sclerosis patients. *Sci. Rep.* **2018**, *8*, 3071. [CrossRef] [PubMed]
46. Brocco, D.; Lanuti, P.; Simeone, P.; Bologna, G.; Pieragostino, D.; Cufaro, M.C.; Graziano, V.; Peri, M.; Di Marino, P.; De Tursi, M.; et al. Circulating Cancer Stem Cell-Derived Extracellular Vesicles as a Novel Biomarker for Clinical Outcome Evaluation. *J. Oncol.* **2019**, *2019*, 5879616. [CrossRef]
47. Rossi, C.; Cicalini, I.; Cufaro, M.C.; Agnifili, L.; Mastropasqua, L.; Lanuti, P.; Marchisio, M.; De Laurenzi, V.; Del Boccio, P.; Pieragostino, D. Multi-Omics Approach for Studying Tears in Treatment-Naïve Glaucoma Patients. *Int. J. Mol. Sci.* **2019**, *20*, 4029. [CrossRef]
48. Ciccocioppo, F.; Lanuti, P.; Centonze, D.; Miscia, S.; Marchisio, M. The Link Among Neurological Diseases: Extracellular Vesicles as a Possible Brain Injury Footprint. *Neurosignals* **2019**, *27*, 25–39. [CrossRef]

49. Grande, R.; Dovizio, M.; Marcone, S.; Szklanna, P.B.; Bruno, A.; Ebhardt, H.A.; Cassidy, H.; Áinle, F.N.; Caprodossi, A.; Lanuti, P.; et al. Platelet-Derived Microparticles From Obese Individuals: Characterization of Number, Size, Proteomics, and Crosstalk With Cancer and Endothelial Cells. *Front. Pharmacol.* **2019**, *10*, 7. [CrossRef]
50. Lanuti, P.; Santilli, F.; Marchisio, M.; Pierdomenico, L.; Vitacolonna, E.; Santavenere, E.; Iacone, A.; Davì, G.; Romano, M.; Miscia, S. A novel flow cytometric approach to distinguish circulating endothelial cells from endothelial microparticles: Relevance for the evaluation of endothelial dysfunction. *J. Immunol. Methods* **2012**, *380*, 16–22. [CrossRef]
51. Pipino, C.; Mandatori, D.; Buccella, F.; Lanuti, P.; Preziuso, A.; Castellani, F.; Grotta, L.; Di Tomo, P.; Marchetti, S.; Di Pietro, N.; et al. Identification and Characterization of a Stem Cell-Like Population in Bovine Milk: A Potential New Source for Regenerative Medicine in Veterinary. *Stem Cells Dev.* **2018**, *27*, 1587–1597. [CrossRef] [PubMed]
52. Tang, T.T.; Wang, B.; Lv, L.L.; Dong, Z.; Liu, B.C. Extracellular vesicles for renal therapeutics: State of the art and future perspective. *J. Control. Release* **2022**, *349*, 32–50. [CrossRef]
53. Zhu, X.; Badawi, M.; Pomeroy, S.; Sutaria, D.S.; Xie, Z.; Baek, A.; Jiang, J.; Elgamal, O.A.; Mo, X.; Perle, K.L.; et al. Comprehensive toxicity and immunogenicity studies reveal minimal effects in mice following sustained dosing of extracellular vesicles derived from HEK293T cells. *J. Extracell. Vesicles* **2017**, *6*, 1324730. [CrossRef] [PubMed]
54. Wąsik, M.; Nazimek, K.; Nowak, B.; Askenase, P.W.; Bryniarski, K. Delayed-Type Hypersensitivity Underlying Casein Allergy Is Suppressed by Extracellular Vesicles Carrying miRNA-150. *Nutrients* **2019**, *11*, 907. [CrossRef]
55. Hogan, M.C.; Johnson, K.L.; Zenka, R.M.; Cristine Charlesworth, M.; Madden, B.J.; Mahoney, D.W.; Oberg, A.L.; Huang, B.Q.; Leontovich, A.A.; Nesbitt, L.L.; et al. Subfractionation, characterization, and in-depth proteomic analysis of glomerular membrane vesicles in human urine. *Kidney Int.* **2014**, *85*, 1225–1237. [CrossRef]
56. Lai, R.C.; Arslan, F.; Lee, M.M.; Sze, N.S.K.; Choo, A.; Chen, T.S.; Salto-Tellez, M.; Timmers, L.; Lee, C.N.; El Oakley, R.M.; et al. Exosome secreted by MSC reduces myocardial ischemia/reperfusion injury. *Stem Cell Res.* **2010**, *4*, 214–222. [CrossRef] [PubMed]
57. Kooijmans, S.A.A.; Schiffelers, R.M.; Zarovni, N.; Vago, R. Modulation of tissue tropism and biological activity of exosomes and other extracellular vesicles: New nanotools for cancer treatment. *Pharmacol. Res.* **2016**, *111*, 487–500. [CrossRef]
58. Kooijmans, S.A.A.; Gitz-Francois, J.J.J.M.; Schiffelers, R.M.; Vader, P. Recombinant phosphatidylserine-binding nanobodies for targeting of extracellular vesicles to tumor cells: A plug-and-play approach. *Nanoscale* **2018**, *10*, 2413–2426. [CrossRef]
59. Kooijmans, S.A.A.; Aleza, C.G.; Roffler, S.R.; van Solinge, W.W.; Vader, P.; Schiffelers, R.M. Display of GPI-anchored anti-EGFR nanobodies on extracellular vesicles promotes tumour cell targeting. *J. Extracell. Vesicles* **2016**, *5*, 31053. [CrossRef]
60. Qi, H.; Liu, C.; Long, L.; Ren, Y.; Zhang, S.; Chang, X.; Qian, X.; Jia, H.; Zhao, J.; Sun, J.; et al. Blood Exosomes Endowed with Magnetic and Targeting Properties for Cancer Therapy. *ACS Nano* **2016**, *10*, 3323–3333. [CrossRef]
61. Murphy, D.E.; de Jong, O.G.; Brouwer, M.; Wood, M.J.; Lavieu, G.; Schiffelers, R.M.; Vader, P. Extracellular vesicle-based therapeutics: Natural versus engineered targeting and trafficking. *Exp. Mol. Med.* **2019**, *51*, 1–12. [CrossRef]
62. Beck, S.; Hochreiter, B.; Schmid, J.A. Extracellular Vesicles Linking Inflammation, Cancer and Thrombotic Risks. *Front. Cell Dev. Biol.* **2022**, *10*, 859863. [CrossRef] [PubMed]
63. Yáñez-Mó, M.; Siljander, P.R.M.; Andreu, Z.; Zavec, A.B.; Borràs, F.E.; Buzas, E.I.; Buzas, K.; Casal, E.; Cappello, F.; Carvalho, J.; et al. Biological properties of extracellular vesicles and their physiological functions. *J. Extracell. Vesicles* **2015**, *4*, 27066. [CrossRef] [PubMed]
64. Li, S.R.; Man, Q.W.; Gao, X.; Lin, H.; Wang, J.; Su, F.C.; Wang, H.Q.; Bu, L.L.; Liu, B.; Chen, G. Tissue-derived extracellular vesicles in cancers and non-cancer diseases: Present and future. *J. Extracell. Vesicles* **2021**, *10*, e12175. [CrossRef]
65. Kooijmans, S.A.A.; de Jong, O.G.; Schiffelers, R.M. Exploring interactions between extracellular vesicles and cells for innovative drug delivery system design. *Adv. Drug Deliv. Rev.* **2021**, *173*, 252–278. [CrossRef]
66. Kim, S.M.; Kim, H.S. Engineering of extracellular vesicles as drug delivery vehicles. *Stem Cell Investig.* **2017**, *4*, 74. [CrossRef] [PubMed]
67. Saint-Pol, J.; Gosselet, F.; Duban-Deweer, S.; Pottiez, G.; Karamanos, Y. Targeting and Crossing the Blood-Brain Barrier with Extracellular Vesicles. *Cells* **2020**, *9*, 851. [CrossRef]
68. Guo, Y.; Hu, D.; Lian, L.; Zhao, L.; Li, M.; Bao, H.; Xu, S. Stem Cell-derived Extracellular Vesicles: A Promising Nano Delivery Platform to the Brain? *Stem Cell Rev. Rep.* **2022**, *1*, 1–24. [CrossRef]
69. Chen, H.; Sun, T.; Jiang, C. Extracellular vesicle-based macromolecule delivery systems in cancer immunotherapy. *J. Control. Release* **2022**, *348*, 572–589. [CrossRef]
70. György, B.; Hung, M.E.; Breakefield, X.O.; Leonard, J.N. Therapeutic applications of extracellular vesicles: Clinical promise and open questions. *Annu. Rev. Pharmacol. Toxicol.* **2015**, *55*, 439–464. [CrossRef]
71. Costa, C.; Liu, Z.; Simões, S.I.; Correia, A.; Rahikkala, A.; Seitsonen, J.; Ruokolainen, J.; Aguiar-Ricardo, A.; Santos, H.A.; Corvo, M.L. One-step microfluidics production of enzyme-loaded liposomes for the treatment of inflammatory diseases. *Colloids Surf. B Biointerfaces* **2020**, *199*, 111556. [CrossRef] [PubMed]
72. Aghaei, H.; Solaimany Nazar, A.R.; Varshosaz, J. Double flow focusing microfluidic-assisted based preparation of methotrexate–loaded liposomal nanoparticles: Encapsulation efficacy, drug release and stability. *Colloids Surf. A Physicochem. Eng. Asp.* **2021**, *614*, 126166. [CrossRef]
73. Khorshid, S.; Montanari, M.; Benedetti, S.; Moroni, S.; Aluigi, A.; Canonico, B.; Papa, S.; Tiboni, M.; Casettari, L. A microfluidic approach to fabricate sucrose decorated liposomes with increased uptake in breast cancer cells. *Eur. J. Pharm. Biopharm.* **2022**, *178*, 53–64. [CrossRef]

74. Huang, H.; Zhang, C.; Yang, S.; Xiao, W.; Zheng, Q.; Song, X. The investigation of mRNA vaccines formulated in liposomes administrated in multiple routes against SARS-CoV-2. *J. Control. Release* **2021**, *335*, 449–456. [CrossRef] [PubMed]
75. van der Koog, L.; Gandek, T.B.; Nagelkerke, A. Liposomes and Extracellular Vesicles as Drug Delivery Systems: A Comparison of Composition, Pharmacokinetics, and Functionalization. *Adv. Healthc. Mater.* **2022**, *11*, 2100639. [CrossRef]
76. Vallet-Regí, M.; Schüth, F.; Lozano, D.; Colilla, M.; Manzano, M. Engineering mesoporous silica nanoparticles for drug delivery: Where are we after two decades? *Chem. Soc. Rev.* **2022**, *51*, 5365–5451. [CrossRef] [PubMed]
77. Sola, F.; Montanari, M.; Fiorani, M.; Barattini, C.; Ciacci, C.; Burattini, S.; Lopez, D.; Ventola, A.; Zamai, L.; Ortolani, C.; et al. Fluorescent Silica Nanoparticles Targeting Mitochondria: Trafficking in Myeloid Cells and Application as Doxorubicin Delivery System in Breast Cancer Cells. *Int. J. Mol. Sci.* **2022**, *23*, 3069. [CrossRef] [PubMed]
78. Anchordoquy, T.J.; Barenholz, Y.; Boraschi, D.; Chorny, M.; Decuzzi, P.; Dobrovolskaia, M.A.; Farhangrazi, Z.S.; Farrell, D.; Gabizon, A.; Ghandehari, H.; et al. Mechanisms and Barriers in Cancer Nanomedicine: Addressing Challenges, Looking for Solutions. *ACS Nano* **2017**, *11*, 12–18. [CrossRef]
79. Paukkonen, H.; Kunnari, M.; Laurén, P.; Hakkarainen, T.; Auvinen, V.V.; Oksanen, T.; Koivuniemi, R.; Yliperttula, M.; Laaksonen, T. Nanofibrillar cellulose hydrogels and reconstructed hydrogels as matrices for controlled drug release. *Int. J. Pharm.* **2017**, *532*, 269–280. [CrossRef]
80. Khalid, M.Y.; Al Rashid, A.; Arif, Z.U.; Ahmed, W.; Arshad, H. Recent advances in nanocellulose-based different biomaterials: Types, properties, and emerging applications. *J. Mater. Res. Technol.* **2021**, *14*, 2601–2623. [CrossRef]
81. Liang, X.; Cheng, H.; Liu, C.; Liu, G. Antigen self-presenting nanovaccine for cancer immunotherapy. *Sci. Bull.* **2022**, *67*, 1611–1613. [CrossRef]
82. Cheng, H.; Fan, X.; Ye, E.; Chen, H.; Yang, J.; Ke, L.; You, M.; Liu, M.; Zhang, Y.W.; Wu, Y.L.; et al. Dual Tumor Microenvironment Remodeling by Glucose-Contained Radical Copolymer for MRI-Guided Photoimmunotherapy. *Adv. Mater.* **2022**, *34*, 2107674. [CrossRef] [PubMed]
83. Herrmann, I.K.; Wood, M.J.A.; Fuhrmann, G. Extracellular vesicles as a next-generation drug delivery platform. *Nat. Nanotechnol.* **2021**, *16*, 748–759. [CrossRef] [PubMed]
84. Hartjes, T.A.; Mytnyk, S.; Jenster, G.W.; van Steijn, V.; van Royen, M.E. Extracellular Vesicle Quantification and Characterization: Common Methods and Emerging Approaches. *Bioengineering* **2019**, *6*, 7. [CrossRef] [PubMed]
85. Zhang, Y.; Bi, J.; Huang, J.; Tang, Y.; Du, S.; Li, P. Exosome: A Review of Its Classification, Isolation Techniques, Storage, Diagnostic and Targeted Therapy Applications. *Int. J. Nanomed.* **2020**, *15*, 6917–6934. [CrossRef] [PubMed]
86. Holcar, M.; Kandušer, M.; Lenassi, M. Blood Nanoparticles—Influence on Extracellular Vesicle Isolation and Characterization. *Front. Pharmacol.* **2021**, *12*, 3178. [CrossRef]
87. Tiwari, S.; Kumar, V.; Randhawa, S.; Verma, S.K. Preparation and characterization of extracellular vesicles. *Am. J. Reprod. Immunol.* **2021**, *85*, e13367. [CrossRef]
88. Livshts, M.A.; Khomyakova, E.; Evtushenko, E.G.; Lazarev, V.N.; Kulemin, N.A.; Semina, S.E.; Generozov, E.V.; Govorun, V.M. Isolation of exosomes by differential centrifugation: Theoretical analysis of a commonly used protocol. *Sci. Rep.* **2015**, *5*, 17319. [CrossRef]
89. Marassi, V.; Maggio, S.; Battistelli, M.; Stocchi, V.; Zattoni, A.; Reschiglian, P.; Guescini, M.; Roda, B. An ultracentrifugation—Hollow-fiber flow field-flow fractionation orthogonal approach for the purification and mapping of extracellular vesicle subtypes. *J. Chromatogr. A* **2021**, *1638*, 461861. [CrossRef]
90. Linares, R.; Tan, S.; Gounou, C.; Arraud, N.; Brisson, A.R. High-speed centrifugation induces aggregation of extracellular vesicles. *J. Extracell. Vesicles* **2015**, *4*, 29509. [CrossRef]
91. Onódi, Z.; Pelyhe, C.; Nagy, C.T.; Brenner, G.B.; Almási, L.; Kittel, Á.; Mančck-Keber, M.; Ferdinandy, P.; Buzás, E.I.; Giricz, Z. Isolation of high-purity extracellular vesicles by the combination of iodixanol density gradient ultracentrifugation and bind-elute chromatography from blood plasma. *Front. Physiol.* **2018**, *9*, 1479. [CrossRef] [PubMed]
92. Gupta, S.; Rawat, S.; Arora, V.; Kottarath, S.K.; Dinda, A.K.; Vaishnav, P.K.; Nayak, B.; Mohanty, S. An improvised one-step sucrose cushion ultracentrifugation method for exosome isolation from culture supernatants of mesenchymal stem cells. *Stem Cell Res. Ther.* **2018**, *9*, 180. [CrossRef]
93. Brennan, K.; Martin, K.; FitzGerald, S.P.; O'Sullivan, J.; Wu, Y.; Blanco, A.; Richardson, C.; Mc Gee, M.M. A comparison of methods for the isolation and separation of extracellular vesicles from protein and lipid particles in human serum. *Sci. Rep.* **2020**, *10*, 1039. [CrossRef] [PubMed]
94. Gaspar, L.S.; Santana, M.M.; Henriques, C.; Pinto, M.M.; Ribeiro-Rodrigues, T.M.; Girão, H.; Nobre, R.J.; Pereira de Almeida, L. Simple and Fast SEC-Based Protocol to Isolate Human Plasma-Derived Extracellular Vesicles for Transcriptional Research. *Mol. Ther.-Methods Clin. Dev.* **2020**, *18*, 723–737. [CrossRef] [PubMed]
95. Reshi, Q.U.A.; Hasan, M.M.; Dissanayake, K.; Fazeli, A. Isolation of Extracellular Vesicles (EVs) Using Benchtop Size Exclusion Chromatography (SEC) Columns. *Methods Mol. Biol.* **2021**, *2273*, 201–206. [CrossRef]
96. Yang, Y.; Wang, Y.; Wei, S.; Zhou, C.; Yu, J.; Wang, G.; Wang, W.; Zhao, L. Extracellular vesicles isolated by size-exclusion chromatography present suitability for RNomics analysis in plasma. *J. Transl. Med.* **2021**, *19*, 104. [CrossRef]
97. Gámez-Valero, A.; Monguió-Tortajada, M.; Carreras-Planella, L.; Franquesa, M.; Beyer, K.; Borràs, F.E. Size-Exclusion Chromatography-based isolation minimally alters Extracellular Vesicles' characteristics compared to precipitating agents. *Sci. Rep.* **2016**, *6*, 33641. [CrossRef]

98. Duijvesz, D.; Versluis, C.Y.L.; Van Der Fels, C.A.M.; Vredenbregt-Van Den Berg, M.S.; Leivo, J.; Peltola, M.T.; Bangma, C.H.; Pettersson, K.S.I.; Jenster, G. Immuno-based detection of extracellular vesicles in urine as diagnostic marker for prostate cancer. *Int. J. Cancer* **2015**, *137*, 2869–2878. [CrossRef]
99. Stranska, R.; Gysbrechts, L.; Wouters, J.; Vermeersch, P.; Bloch, K.; Dierickx, D.; Andrei, G.; Snoeck, R. Comparison of membrane affinity-based method with size-exclusion chromatography for isolation of exosome-like vesicles from human plasma. *J. Transl. Med.* **2018**, *16*, 1. [CrossRef]
100. Logozzi, M.; Di Raimo, R.; Mizzoni, D.; Fais, S. Immunocapture-based ELISA to characterize and quantify exosomes in both cell culture supernatants and body fluids. *Methods Enzymol.* **2020**, *645*, 155–180. [CrossRef]
101. Beekman, P.; Enciso-Martinez, A.; Rho, H.S.; Pujari, S.P.; Lenferink, A.; Zuilhof, H.; Terstappen, L.W.M.M.; Otto, C.; Le Gac, S. Immuno-capture of extracellular vesicles for individual multi-modal characterization using AFM, SEM and Raman spectroscopy. *Lab Chip* **2019**, *19*, 2526–2536. [CrossRef] [PubMed]
102. Pfeiffer, A.; Petersen, J.D.; Falduto, G.H.; Anderson, D.E.; Zimmerberg, J.; Metcalfe, D.D.; Olivera, A. Selective immunocapture reveals neoplastic human mast cells secrete distinct microvesicle- and exosome-like populations of KIT-containing extracellular vesicles. *J. Extracell. Vesicles* **2022**, *11*, 12272. [CrossRef]
103. Visan, K.S.; Lobb, R.J.; Ham, S.; Lima, L.G.; Palma, C.; Edna, C.P.Z.; Wu, L.Y.; Gowda, H.; Datta, K.K.; Hartel, G.; et al. Comparative analysis of tangential flow filtration and ultracentrifugation, both combined with subsequent size exclusion chromatography, for the isolation of small extracellular vesicles. *J. Extracell. Vesicles* **2022**, *11*, 12266. [CrossRef]
104. Busatto, S.; Vilanilam, G.; Ticer, T.; Lin, W.L.; Dickson, D.W.; Shapiro, S.; Bergese, P.; Wolfram, J. Tangential flow filtration for highly efficient concentration of extracellular vesicles from large volumes of fluid. *Cells* **2018**, *7*, 273. [CrossRef] [PubMed]
105. Wu, B.; Chen, X.; Wang, J.; Qing, X.; Wang, Z.; Ding, X.; Xie, Z.; Niu, L.; Guo, X.; Cai, T.; et al. Separation and characterization of extracellular vesicles from human plasma by asymmetrical flow field-flow fractionation. *Anal. Chim. Acta* **2020**, *1127*, 234–245. [CrossRef] [PubMed]
106. Zhang, H.; Lyden, D. Asymmetric-flow field-flow fractionation technology for exomere and small extracellular vesicle separation and characterization. *Nat. Protoc.* **2019**, *14*, 1027–1053. [CrossRef]
107. Chung, K.Y.; Quek, J.M.; Neo, S.H.; Too, H.P. Polymer-Based Precipitation of Extracellular Vesicular miRNAs from Serum Improve Gastric Cancer miRNA Biomarker Performance. *J. Mol. Diagn.* **2020**, *22*, 610–618. [CrossRef]
108. García-Romero, N.; Madurga, R.; Rackov, G.; Palacín-Aliana, I.; Núñez-Torres, R.; Asensi-Puig, A.; Carrión-Navarro, J.; Esteban-Rubio, S.; Peinado, H.; González-Neira, A.; et al. Polyethylene glycol improves current methods for circulating extracellular vesicle-derived DNA isolation. *J. Transl. Med.* **2019**, *17*, 75. [CrossRef]
109. Gallart-Palau, X.; Serra, A.; Wong, A.S.W.; Sandin, S.; Lai, M.K.P.; Chen, C.P.; Kon, O.L.; Sze, S.K. Extracellular vesicles are rapidly purified from human plasma by PRotein Organic Solvent PRecipitation (PROSPR). *Sci. Rep.* **2015**, *5*, 14664. [CrossRef]
110. Deregibus, M.C.; Figliolini, F.; D'Antico, S.; Manzini, P.M.; Pasquino, C.; De Lena, M.; Tetta, C.; Brizzi, M.F.; Camussi, G. Charge-based precipitation of extracellular vesicles. *Int. J. Mol. Med.* **2016**, *38*, 1359–1366. [CrossRef]
111. Liangsupree, T.; Multia, E.; Riekkola, M.L. Modern isolation and separation techniques for extracellular vesicles. *J. Chromatogr. A* **2021**, *1636*, 461773. [CrossRef] [PubMed]
112. Ko, J.; Carpenter, E.; Issadore, D. Detection and isolation of circulating exosomes and microvesicles for cancer monitoring and diagnostics using micro-/nano-based devices. *Analyst* **2016**, *141*, 450–460. [CrossRef]
113. Wu, M.; Chen, C.; Wang, Z.; Bachman, H.; Ouyang, Y.; Huang, P.H.; Sadovsky, Y.; Huang, T.J. Separating extracellular vesicles and lipoproteins via acoustofluidics. *Lab Chip* **2019**, *19*, 1174–1182. [CrossRef] [PubMed]
114. Piotrowska, M.; Ciura, K.; Zalewska, M.; Dawid, M.; Correia, B.; Sawicka, P.; Lewczuk, B.; Kasprzyk, J.; Sola, L.; Piekoszewski, W.; et al. Capillary zone electrophoresis of bacterial extracellular vesicles: A proof of concept. *J. Chromatogr. A* **2020**, *1621*, 461047. [CrossRef] [PubMed]
115. Lim, J.; Choi, M.; Lee, H.J.; Han, J.Y.; Cho, Y. A novel multifunctional nanowire platform for highly efficient isolation and analysis of circulating tumor-specific markers. *Front. Chem.* **2019**, *7*, 664. [CrossRef]
116. Smith, J.T.; Wunsch, B.H.; Dogra, N.; Ahsen, M.E.; Lee, K.; Yadav, K.K.; Weil, R.; Pereira, M.A.; Patel, J.V.; Duch, E.A.; et al. Integrated nanoscale deterministic lateral displacement arrays for separation of extracellular vesicles from clinically-relevant volumes of biological samples. *Lab Chip* **2018**, *18*, 3913–3925. [CrossRef]
117. Liu, C.; Guo, J.; Tian, F.; Yang, N.; Yan, F.; Ding, Y.; Wei, J.; Hu, G.; Nie, G.; Sun, J. Field-Free Isolation of Exosomes from Extracellular Vesicles by Microfluidic Viscoelastic Flows. *ACS Nano* **2017**, *11*, 6968–6976. [CrossRef]
118. Guerreiro, E.M.; Vestad, B.; Steffensen, L.A.; Aass, H.C.D.; Saeed, M.; Øvstebø, R.; Costea, D.E.; Galtung, H.K.; Søland, T.M. Efficient extracellular vesicle isolation by combining cell media modifications, ultrafiltration, and size-exclusion chromatography. *PLoS ONE* **2018**, *13*, e0204276. [CrossRef]
119. Stam, J.; Bartel, S.; Bischoff, R.; Wolters, J.C. Isolation of extracellular vesicles with combined enrichment methods. *J. Chromatogr. B Anal. Technol. Biomed. Life Sci.* **2021**, *1169*, 122604. [CrossRef]
120. Bellotti, C.; Lang, K.; Kuplennik, N.; Sosnik, A.; Steinfeld, R. High-grade extracellular vesicles preparation by combined size-exclusion and affinity chromatography. *Sci. Rep.* **2021**, *11*, 10550. [CrossRef]
121. Rikkert, L.G.; Nieuwland, R.; Terstappen, L.W.M.M.; Coumans, F.A.W. Quality of extracellular vesicle images by transmission electron microscopy is operator and protocol dependent. *J. Extracell. Vesicles* **2019**, *8*, 1555419. [CrossRef]

122. Emelyanov, A.; Shtam, T.; Kamyshinsky, R.; Garaeva, L.; Verlov, N.; Miliukhina, I.; Kudrevatykh, A.; Gavrilov, G.; Zabrodskaya, Y.; Pchelina, S.; et al. Cryo-electron microscopy of extracellular vesicles from cerebrospinal fluid. *PLoS ONE* **2020**, *15*, e0227949. [CrossRef] [PubMed]
123. Hardij, J.; Cecchet, F.; Berquand, A.; Gheldof, D.; Chatelain, C.; Mullier, F.; Chatelain, B.; Dogné, J.M. Characterisation of tissue factor-bearing extracellular vesicles with AFM: Comparison of air-tapping-mode AFM and liquid peak force AFM. *J. Extracell. Vesicles* **2013**, *2*, 21045. [CrossRef] [PubMed]
124. Parisse, P.; Rago, I.; Ulloa Severino, L.; Perissinotto, F.; Ambrosetti, E.; Paoletti, P.; Ricci, M.; Beltrami, A.P.; Cesselli, D.; Casalis, L. Atomic force microscopy analysis of extracellular vesicles. *Eur. Biophys. J.* **2017**, *46*, 813–820. [CrossRef]
125. Palmieri, V.; Lucchetti, D.; Gatto, I.; Maiorana, A.; Marcantoni, M.; Maulucci, G.; Papi, M.; Pola, R.; De Spirito, M.; Sgambato, A. Dynamic light scattering for the characterization and counting of extracellular vesicles: A powerful noninvasive tool. *J. Nanoparticle Res.* **2014**, *16*, 2583. [CrossRef]
126. Bachurski, D.; Schuldner, M.; Nguyen, P.H.; Malz, A.; Reiners, K.S.; Grenzi, P.C.; Babatz, F.; Schauss, A.C.; Hansen, H.P.; Hallek, M.; et al. Extracellular vesicle measurements with nanoparticle tracking analysis–An accuracy and repeatability comparison between NanoSight NS300 and ZetaView. *J. Extracell. Vesicles* **2019**, *8*, 1596016. [CrossRef]
127. Fortunato, D.; Mladenović, D.; Criscuoli, M.; Loria, F.; Veiman, K.L.; Zocco, D.; Koort, K.; Zarovni, N. Opportunities and pitfalls of fluorescent labeling methodologies for extracellular vesicle profiling on high-resolution single-particle platforms. *Int. J. Mol. Sci.* **2021**, *22*, 10510. [CrossRef]
128. Salmond, N.; Khanna, K.; Owen, G.R.; Williams, K.C. Nanoscale flow cytometry for immunophenotyping and quantitating extracellular vesicles in blood plasma. *Nanoscale* **2021**, *13*, 2012–2025. [CrossRef] [PubMed]
129. Marchisio, M.; Simeone, P.; Bologna, G.; Ercolino, E.; Pierdomenico, L.; Pieragostino, D.; Ventrella, A.; Antonini, F.; Del Zotto, G.; Vergara, D.; et al. Flow cytometry analysis of circulating extracellular vesicle subtypes from fresh peripheral blood samples. *Int. J. Mol. Sci.* **2021**, *22*, 48. [CrossRef]
130. Kowal, E.J.K.; Ter-Ovanesyan, D.; Regev, A.; Church, G.M. Extracellular Vesicle Isolation and Analysis by Western Blotting. *Methods Mol. Biol.* **2017**, *1660*, 143–152. [CrossRef]
131. Iha, K.; Tsurusawa, N.; Tsai, H.Y.; Lin, M.W.; Sonoda, H.; Watabe, S.; Yoshimura, T.; Ito, E. Ultrasensitive ELISA detection of proteins in separated lumen and membrane fractions of cancer cell exosomes. *Anal. Biochem.* **2022**, *654*, 114831. [CrossRef] [PubMed]
132. Maas, S.L.N.; Vrij, J.D.; Broekman, M.L.D. Quantification and size-profiling of extracellular vesicles using tunable resistive pulse sensing. *J. Vis. Exp.* **2014**, *92*, e51623. [CrossRef]
133. Mir, B.; Goettsch, C. Extracellular Vesicles as Delivery Vehicles of Specific Cellular Cargo. *Cells* **2020**, *9*, 1601. [CrossRef]
134. Coumans, F.A.W.; Brisson, A.R.; Buzas, E.I.; Dignat-George, F.; Drees, E.E.E.; El-Andaloussi, S.; Emanueli, C.; Gasecka, A.; Hendrix, A.; Hill, A.F.; et al. Methodological guidelines to study extracellular vesicles. *Circ. Res.* **2017**, *120*, 1632–1648. [CrossRef]
135. Tanasi, I.; Adamo, A.; Kamga, P.T.; Bazzoni, R.; Krampera, M. High-throughput analysis and functional interpretation of extracellular vesicle content in hematological malignancies. *Comput. Struct. Biotechnol. J.* **2020**, *18*, 2670–2677. [CrossRef] [PubMed]
136. Jalaludin, I.; Lubman, D.M.; Kim, J. A guide to mass spectrometric analysis of extracellular vesicle proteins for biomarker discovery. *Mass Spectrom. Rev.* **2021**, e21749. [CrossRef]
137. Bandu, R.; Oh, J.W.; Kim, K.P. Mass spectrometry-based proteome profiling of extracellular vesicles and their roles in cancer biology. *Exp. Mol. Med.* **2019**, *51*, 1–10. [CrossRef] [PubMed]
138. Puhka, M.; Takatalo, M.; Nordberg, M.E.; Valkonen, S.; Nandania, J.; Aatonen, M.; Yliperttula, M.; Laitinen, S.; Velagapudi, V.; Mirtti, T.; et al. Metabolomic profiling of extracellular vesicles and alternative normalization methods reveal enriched metabolites and strategies to study prostate cancer-related changes. *Theranostics* **2017**, *7*, 3824–3841. [CrossRef]
139. Paolino, G.; Buratta, S.; Mercuri, S.R.; Pellegrino, R.M.; Urbanelli, L.; Emiliani, C.; Bertuccini, L.; Iosi, F.; Huber, V.; Brianti, P.; et al. Lipidic Profile Changes in Exosomes and Microvesicles Derived From Plasma of Monoclonal Antibody-Treated Psoriatic Patients. *Front. Cell Dev. Biol.* **2022**, *10*, 1. [CrossRef]
140. Valadi, H.; Ekström, K.; Bossios, A.; Sjöstrand, M.; Lee, J.J.; Lötvall, J.O. Exosome-mediated transfer of mRNAs and microRNAs is a novel mechanism of genetic exchange between cells. *Nat. Cell Biol.* **2007**, *9*, 654–659. [CrossRef]
141. Conley, A.; Minciacchi, V.R.; Lee, D.H.; Knudsen, B.S.; Karlan, B.Y.; Citrigno, L.; Viglietto, G.; Tewari, M.; Freeman, M.R.; Demichelis, F.; et al. High-throughput sequencing of two populations of extracellular vesicles provides an mRNA signature that can be detected in the circulation of breast cancer patients. *RNA Biol.* **2017**, *14*, 305–316. [CrossRef]
142. Biagiotti, S.; Paoletti, M.F.; Fraternale, A.; Rossi, L.; Magnani, M. Drug delivery by red blood cells. *IUBMB Life* **2011**, *63*, 621–631. [CrossRef]
143. Rossi, L.; Fraternale, A.; Bianchi, M.; Magnani, M. Red Blood Cell Membrane Processing for Biomedical Applications. *Front. Physiol.* **2019**, *10*, 1070. [CrossRef] [PubMed]
144. Rossi, L.; Pierigè, F.; Aliano, M.P.; Magnani, M. Ongoing Developments and Clinical Progress in Drug-Loaded Red Blood Cell Technologies. *BioDrugs* **2020**, *34*, 265–272. [CrossRef] [PubMed]
145. Diez-Silva, M.; Dao, M.; Han, J.; Lim, C.T.; Suresh, S. Shape and biomechanics characteristics of human red blood cells in health and disease. *MRS Bull.* **2010**, *35*, 382–388. [CrossRef]
146. De Oliveira, S.; Saldanha, C. An overview about erythrocyte membrane. *Clin. Hemorheol. Microcirc.* **2010**, *44*, 63–74. [CrossRef]

147. Donadee, C.; Raat, N.J.H.; Kanias, T.; Tejero, J.; Lee, J.S.; Kelley, E.E.; Zhao, X.; Liu, C.; Reynolds, H.; Azarov, I.; et al. Nitric oxide scavenging by red blood cell microparticles and cell-free hemoglobin as a mechanism for the red cell storage lesion. *Circulation* **2011**, *124*, 465–476. [CrossRef] [PubMed]
148. Antonelou, M.H.; Seghatchian, J. Update on extracellular vesicles inside red blood cell storage units: Adjust the sails closer to the new wind. *Transfus. Apher. Sci.* **2016**, *55*, 92–104. [CrossRef]
149. Willekens, F.L.A.; Werre, J.M.; Groenen-Döpp, Y.A.M.; Roerdinkholder-Stoelwinder, B.; De Pauw, B.; Bosman, G.J.C.G.M. Erythrocyte vesiculation: A self-protective mechanism? *Br. J. Haematol.* **2008**, *141*, 549–556. [CrossRef]
150. Chiangjong, W.; Netsirisawan, P.; Hongeng, S.; Chutipongtanate, S. Red Blood Cell Extracellular Vesicle-Based Drug Delivery: Challenges and Opportunities. *Front. Med.* **2021**, *8*, 761362. [CrossRef]
151. Shah, M.D.; Bergeron, A.L.; Dong, J.F.; López, J.A. Flow cytometric measurement of microparticles: Pitfalls and protocol modifications. *Platelets* **2008**, *19*, 365–372. [CrossRef]
152. Duan, Z.Y.; Cai, G.Y.; Bu, R.; Lu, Y.; Hou, K.; Chen, X.M. Selection of urinary sediment miRNAs as specific biomarkers of IgA nephropathy. *Sci. Rep.* **2016**, *6*, 23498. [CrossRef] [PubMed]
153. Westerman, M.; Porter, J.B. Red blood cell-derived microparticles: An overview. *Blood Cells. Mol. Dis.* **2016**, *59*, 134–139. [CrossRef] [PubMed]
154. Blanc, L.; De Gassart, A.; Géminard, C.; Bette-Bobillo, P.; Vidal, M. Exosome release by reticulocytes—An integral part of the red blood cell differentiation system. *Blood Cells Mol. Dis.* **2005**, *35*, 21–26. [CrossRef] [PubMed]
155. Kuo, W.P.; Tigges, J.C.; Toxavidis, V.; Ghiran, I. Red Blood Cells: A Source of Extracellular Vesicles. *Methods Mol. Biol.* **2017**, *1660*, 15–22.
156. Zhang, D.X.; Kiomourtzis, T.; Lam, C.K.; Le, M.T.N. The Biology and Therapeutic Applications of Red Blood Cell Extracellular Vesicles. In *Erythrocyte*; IntechOpen: London, UK, 2019; ISBN 978-1-78984-210-4.
157. Yang, L.; Huang, S.; Zhang, Z.; Liu, Z.; Zhang, L. Roles and Applications of Red Blood Cell-Derived Extracellular Vesicles in Health and Diseases. *Int. J. Mol. Sci.* **2022**, *23*, 5927. [CrossRef]
158. Khalyfa, A.; Sanz-Rubio, D. The mystery of red blood cells extracellular vesicles in sleep apnea with metabolic dysfunction. *Int. J. Mol. Sci.* **2021**, *22*, 4301. [CrossRef]
159. Burger, P.; Hilarius-Stokman, P.; De Korte, D.; Van Den Berg, T.K.; Van Bruggen, R. CD47 functions as a molecular switch for erythrocyte phagocytosis. *Blood* **2012**, *119*, 5512–5521. [CrossRef]
160. Doss, J.F.; Corcoran, D.L.; Jima, D.D.; Telen, M.J.; Dave, S.S.; Chi, J.T. A comprehensive joint analysis of the long and short RNA transcriptomes of human erythrocytes. *BMC Genom.* **2015**, *16*, 952. [CrossRef]
161. Huang, H.; Zhu, J.; Fan, L.; Lin, Q.; Fu, D.; Wei, B.; Wei, S. MicroRNA Profiling of Exosomes Derived from Red Blood Cell Units: Implications in Transfusion-Related Immunomodulation. *Biomed Res. Int.* **2019**, *2019*, 2045915. [CrossRef]
162. Sun, L.; Yu, Y.; Niu, B.; Wang, D. Red Blood Cells as Potential Repositories of MicroRNAs in the Circulatory System. *Front. Genet.* **2020**, *11*, 442. [CrossRef] [PubMed]
163. Vidal, M. Exosomes in erythropoiesis. *Transfus. Clin. Biol.* **2010**, *17*, 131–137. [CrossRef] [PubMed]
164. Alaarg, A.; Schiffelers, R.M.; Van Solinge, W.W.; Van Wijk, R. Red blood cell vesiculation in hereditary hemolytic anemia. *Front. Physiol.* **2013**, *4*, 365. [CrossRef]
165. Tissot, J.D.; Canellini, G.; Rubin, O.; Angelillo-Scherrer, A.; Delobel, J.; Prudent, M.; Lion, N. Blood microvesicles: From proteomics to physiology. *Transl. Proteom.* **2013**, *1*, 38–52. [CrossRef]
166. Harisa, G.I.; Badran, M.M.; Alanazi, F.K. Erythrocyte nanovesicles: Biogenesis, biological roles and therapeutic approach: Erythrocyte nanovesicles. *Saudi Pharm. J.* **2017**, *25*, 8–17. [CrossRef] [PubMed]
167. Liu, C.; Zhao, W.; Christ, G.J.; Gladwin, M.T.; Kim-Shapiro, D.B. Nitric oxide scavenging by red cell microparticles. *Free Radic. Biol. Med.* **2013**, *65*, 1164–1173. [CrossRef]
168. Danesh, A.; Inglis, H.C.; Jackman, R.P.; Wu, S.; Deng, X.; Muench, M.O.; Heitman, J.W.; Norris, P.J. Exosomes from red blood cell units bind to monocytes and induce proinflammatory cytokines, boosting T-cell responses in vitro. *Blood* **2014**, *123*, 687–696. [CrossRef]
169. Fischer, D.; Büssow, J.; Meybohm, P.; Weber, C.F.; Zacharowski, K.; Urbschat, A.; Müller, M.M.; Jennewein, C. Microparticles from stored red blood cells enhance procoagulant and proinflammatory activity. *Transfusion* **2017**, *57*, 2701–2711. [CrossRef]
170. Wannez, A.; Devalet, B.; Chatelain, B.; Chatelain, C.; Dogné, J.M.; Mullier, F. Extracellular Vesicles in Red Blood Cell Concentrates: An Overview. *Transfus. Med. Rev.* **2019**, 33, 125–130. [CrossRef]
171. Koshiar, R.L.; Somajo, S.; Norström, E.; Dahlbäck, B. Erythrocyte-derived microparticles supporting activated protein C-mediated regulation of blood coagulation. *PLoS ONE* **2014**, *9*, e104200. [CrossRef]
172. Levin, G.; Sukhareva, E.; Lavrentieva, A. Impact of microparticles derived from erythrocytes on fibrinolysis. *J. Thromb. Thrombolysis* **2016**, *41*, 452–458. [CrossRef] [PubMed]
173. Buttari, B.; Profumo, E.; Riganò, R. Crosstalk between red blood cells and the immune system and its impact on atherosclerosis. *Biomed Res. Int.* **2015**, *2015*, 616834. [CrossRef]
174. Valkov, N.; Das, A.; Tucker, N.R.; Li, G.; Salvador, A.M.; Chaffin, M.D.; De Oliveira, G.P.; Kur, I.; Gokulnath, P.; Ziegler, O.; et al. SnRNA sequencing defines signaling by RBC-derived extracellular vesicles in the murine heart. *Life Sci. Alliance* **2021**, *4*, e202101048. [CrossRef]

175. Regev-Rudzki, N.; Wilson, D.W.; Carvalho, T.G.; Sisquella, X.; Coleman, B.M.; Rug, M.; Bursac, D.; Angrisano, F.; Gee, M.; Hill, A.F.; et al. Cell-cell communication between malaria-infected red blood cells via exosome-like vesicles. *Cell* **2013**, *153*, 1120–1133. [CrossRef] [PubMed]
176. Ataga, K.I. Hypercoagulability and thrombotic complications in hemolytic anemias. *Haematologica* **2009**, *94*, 1481–1484. [CrossRef]
177. Aharon, A.; Rebibo-Sabbah, A.; Tzoran, I.; Levin, C. Extracellular Vesicles in Hematological Disorders. *Rambam Maimonides Med. J.* **2014**, *5*, e0032. [CrossRef]
178. Herring, J.M.; Mcmichael, M.A.; Smith, S.A. Microparticles in health and disease. *J. Vet. Intern. Med.* **2013**, *27*, 1020–1033. [CrossRef] [PubMed]
179. Vázquez-Ríos, A.J.; Molina-Crespo, Á.; Bouzo, B.L.; López-López, R.; Moreno-Bueno, G.; de la Fuente, M. Exosome-mimetic nanoplatforms for targeted cancer drug delivery. *J. Nanobiotechnol.* **2019**, *17*, 85. [CrossRef]
180. Sakai-Kato, K.; Yoshida, K.; Takechi-Haraya, Y.; Izutsu, K.I. Physicochemical Characterization of Liposomes That Mimic the Lipid Composition of Exosomes for Effective Intracellular Trafficking. *Langmuir* **2020**, *36*, 12735–12744. [CrossRef]
181. Lai, R.C.; Yeo, R.W.Y.; Tan, K.H.; Lim, S.K. Exosomes for drug delivery—A novel application for the mesenchymal stem cell. *Biotechnol. Adv.* **2013**, *31*, 543–551. [CrossRef]
182. Usman, W.M.; Pham, T.C.; Kwok, Y.Y.; Vu, L.T.; Ma, V.; Peng, B.; Chan, Y.S.; Wei, L.; Chin, S.M.; Azad, A.; et al. Efficient RNA drug delivery using red blood cell extracellular vesicles. *Nat. Commun.* **2018**, *9*, 2359. [CrossRef]
183. Sudnitsyna, J.; Skverchinskaya, E.; Dobrylko, I.; Nikitina, E.; Gambaryan, S.; Mindukshev, I. Microvesicle Formation Induced by Oxidative Stress in Human Erythrocytes. *Antioxidants* **2020**, *9*, 929. [CrossRef] [PubMed]
184. Prudent, M.; Crettaz, D.; Delobel, J.; Seghatchian, J.; Tissot, J.D.; Lion, N. Differences between calcium-stimulated and storage-induced erythrocyte-derived microvesicles. *Transfus. Apher. Sci.* **2015**, *53*, 153–158. [CrossRef]
185. Gangadaran, P.; Hong, C.M.; Oh, J.M.; Rajendran, R.L.; Kalimuthu, S.; Son, S.H.; Gopal, A.; Zhu, L.; Baek, S.H.; Jeong, S.Y.; et al. In vivo Non-invasive Imaging of Radio-Labeled Exosome-Mimetics Derived From Red Blood Cells in Mice. *Front. Pharmacol.* **2018**, *9*, 817. [CrossRef] [PubMed]
186. Sangha, G.S.; Weber, C.M.; Sapp, R.M.; Setua, S.; Thangaraju, K.; Pettebone, M.; Doctor, A.; Buehler, P.W.; Clyne, A.M. Mechanical Stimuli such as Shear Stress and Piezo1 Stimulation Generate Red Blood Cell Extracellular Vesicles. *bioRxiv* **2022**, *21*, 7885. [CrossRef]
187. Han, Y.; Jones, T.W.; Dutta, S.; Zhu, Y.; Wang, X.; Narayanan, S.P.; Fagan, S.C.; Zhang, D. Overview and update on methods for cargo loading into extracellular vesicles. *Processes* **2021**, *9*, 356. [CrossRef]
188. Kanada, M.; Bachmann, M.H.; Hardy, J.W.; Frimannson, D.O.; Bronsart, L.; Wang, A.; Sylvester, M.D.; Schmidt, T.L.; Kaspar, R.L.; Butte, M.J.; et al. Differential fates of biomolecules delivered to target cells via extracellular vesicles. *Proc. Natl. Acad. Sci. USA* **2015**, *112*, E1433–E1442. [CrossRef]
189. Familtseva, A.; Jeremic, N.; Tyagi, S.C. Exosomes: Cell-created drug delivery systems. *Mol. Cell. Biochem.* **2019**, *459*, 1–6. [CrossRef]
190. Rossi, L.; Serafini, S.; Magnani, M. Red Blood Cell Loading: A Selection of Procedures. In *Erythrocyte Engineering for Drug Delivery and Targeting*; Bioscience, K.A.L., Ed.; Georgetown: New York, NY, USA, 2003; pp. 1–18.
191. Magnani, M.; Serafini, S.; Fraternale, A.; Antonelli, A.; Biagiotti, S.; Pierigè, F.; Sfara, C.; Rossi, L. Red blood cell-based delivery of drugs and nanomaterials for therapeutic and diagnostic applications. In *Encyclopedia of Nanoscience and Nanotechnology*; Nalwa, H.S., Ed.; American Scientific Publishers: Valenciaz, CA, USA, 2011; pp. 309–354. ISBN 1588831876.
192. Baker, R.F. Entry of ferritin into human red cells during hypotonic haemolysis. *Nature* **1967**, *215*, 424–425. [CrossRef] [PubMed]
193. Baker, R.F.; Gillis, N.R. Osmotic hemolysis of chemically modified red blood cells. *Blood* **1969**, *33*, 170–178. [CrossRef]
194. Peng, B.; Nguyen, T.M.; Jayasinghe, M.K.; Gao, C.; Pham, T.T.; Vu, L.T.; Yeo, E.Y.M.; Yap, G.; Wang, L.; Goh, B.C.; et al. Robust delivery of RIG-I agonists using extracellular vesicles for anti-cancer immunotherapy. *J. Extracell. Vesicles* **2022**, *11*, e12187. [CrossRef]
195. Görgens, A.; Corso, G.; Hagey, D.W.; Jawad Wiklander, R.; Gustafsson, M.O.; Felldin, U.; Lee, Y.; Bostancioglu, R.B.; Sork, H.; Liang, X.; et al. Identification of storage conditions stabilizing extracellular vesicles preparations. *J. Extracell. Vesicles* **2022**, *11*, e12238. [CrossRef]
196. Chang, M.; Hsiao, J.K.; Yao, M.; Chien, L.Y.; Hsu, S.C.; Ko, B.S.; Chen, S.T.; Liu, H.M.; Chen, Y.C.; Yang, C.S.; et al. Homologous RBC-derived vesicles as ultrasmall carriers of iron oxide for magnetic resonance imaging of stem cells. *Nanotechnology* **2010**, *21*, 235103. [CrossRef] [PubMed]
197. Malhotra, S.; Dumoga, S.; Sirohi, P.; Singh, N. Red Blood Cells-Derived Vesicles for Delivery of Lipophilic Drug Camptothecin. *ACS Appl. Mater. Interfaces* **2019**, *11*, 22141–22151. [CrossRef] [PubMed]
198. Zhang, G.; Huang, X.; Xiu, H.; Sun, Y.; Chen, J.; Cheng, G.; Song, Z.; Peng, Y.; Shen, Y.; Wang, J.; et al. Extracellular vesicles: Natural liver-accumulating drug delivery vehicles for the treatment of liver diseases. *J. Extracell. Vesicles* **2020**, *10*, e12030. [CrossRef] [PubMed]
199. Borgheti-Cardoso, L.N.; Kooijmans, S.A.A.; Chamorro, L.G.; Biosca, A.; Lantero, E.; Ramírez, M.; Avalos-Padilla, Y.; Crespo, I.; Fernández, I.; Fernandez-Becerra, C.; et al. Extracellular vesicles derived from Plasmodium-infected and non-infected red blood cells as targeted drug delivery vehicles. *Int. J. Pharm.* **2020**, *587*, 119627. [CrossRef] [PubMed]

200. Jayasinghe, M.K.; Pirisinu, M.; Yang, Y.; Peng, B.; Pham, T.T.; Yu Lee, C.; Tan, M.; Vu, L.T.; Dang, X.T.T.; Pham, T.C.; et al. Surface-engineered extracellular vesicles for targeted delivery of therapeutic RNAs and peptides for cancer therapy. *Theranostics* **2022**, *12*, 3288–3315. [CrossRef] [PubMed]
201. Stremersch, S.; Vandenbroucke, R.E.; Van Wonterghem, E.; Hendrix, A.; De Smedt, S.C.; Raemdonck, K. Comparing exosome-like vesicles with liposomes for the functional cellular delivery of small RNAs. *J. Control. Release* **2016**, *232*, 51–61. [CrossRef] [PubMed]

pharmaceutics

MDPI

Review

Extracellular Vesicles of Probiotics: Shedding Light on the Biological Activity and Future Applications

Paweł Krzyżek [1,*], Beatrice Marinacci [2,3], Irene Vitale [2] and Rossella Grande [2]

1 Department of Microbiology, Faculty of Medicine, Wroclaw Medical University, 50-368 Wroclaw, Poland
2 Department of Pharmacy, University "G. d'Annunzio" of Chieti-Pescara, Via dei Vestini, 31, 66100 Chieti, Italy
3 Department of Innovative Technologies in Medicine & Dentistry, University "Gabriele d'Annunzio", Chieti-Pescara, 66100 Chieti, Italy
* Correspondence: krojcerpawel@gmail.com

Abstract: For many decades, the proper functioning of the human body has become a leading scientific topic. In the course of numerous experiments, a striking impact of probiotics on the human body has been documented, including maintaining the physiological balance of endogenous microorganisms, regulating the functioning of the immune system, enhancing the digestive properties of the host, and preventing or alleviating the course of many diseases. Recent research, especially from the last decade, shows that this health-benefiting activity of probiotics is largely conditioned by the production of extracellular vesicles. Although the importance of extracellular vesicles in the virulence of many live-threatening pathogens is widely described in the literature, much less is known with respect to the health-promoting effect of extracellular vesicles secreted by non-pathogenic microorganisms, including probiotics. Based on this, in the current review article, we decided to collect the latest literature data on the health-inducing properties of extracellular vesicles secreted by probiotics. The characteristics of probiotics' extracellular vesicles will be extended by the description of their physicochemical properties and the proteome in connection with the biological activities exhibited by these structures.

Keywords: extracellular vesicles; membrane vesicles; probiotics; probiotic bacteria; postbiotics

Citation: Krzyżek, P.; Marinacci, B.; Vitale, I.; Grande, R. Extracellular Vesicles of Probiotics: Shedding Light on the Biological Activity and Future Applications. *Pharmaceutics* **2023**, *15*, 522. https://doi.org/10.3390/pharmaceutics15020522

Academic Editor: Yong Chen

Received: 22 December 2022
Revised: 20 January 2023
Accepted: 1 February 2023
Published: 4 February 2023

1. Introduction

For time immemorial, the proper functioning of the human body has become a leading topic undertaken by scientists [1]. It quickly became clear that there is a very strong relationship between human health and its resident microbiota [2,3]. As a resultant, the idea of using probiotics was created, i.e., live microorganisms that, when administered in the proper dose, have a beneficial effect on the host [1,4]. One of the first well-documented example of the usefulness of probiotics dates back to 1907, from the observations made by Elie Metchnikoff, who showed the existence of a positive correlation between the consumption of fermented food containing probiotics and the lifespan of the Bulgarian population [1]. This was the starting point for further observations of health-benefiting properties of this microbial group and the development of a powerful trend of research on probiotics in the following years [1,5]. After several decades of experiments, a striking impact of probiotics on the human body has been documented, including maintaining the physiological balance of microbiota, regulating the functioning of the immune system, enhancing the digestive properties of the host, and preventing or alleviating the course of many diseases [1,5,6]. The growing awareness of the benefits of probiotics has contributed to the exponential growth of commercial products containing these microorganisms [4]. The use of probiotics has undoubtedly become very popular, however, their viability in such preparations is often questioned, which is related to their exposure to various unfavorable parameters, such as processing (e.g., dehydration), storage conditions, and physiology of the product's target site (e.g., passage through the physicochemically diverse, harsh environment of the digestive system) [7].

Although probiotics are currently in the center of interest of pharmaceutical concerns, more and more research focuses on searching for alternatives to these classically used products [8,9]. Difficulties in maintaining the viability of probiotics in commercial products and the fact that the viability of these microorganisms is not always necessary to obtain therapeutic effects have led to the concept of postbiotics [5,7,10,11]. Postbiotics are a mixture of metabolic products or non-viable fragments of probiotics that have a beneficial effect on the functioning of the human body [8,12]. Despite the fact that research on postbiotics is still in its infancy, a number of health-promoting properties of these new products have already been demonstrated (maintenance of the proper structure of the resident microbiota, strengthening the host epithelial barrier, modulation of the local and systemic immune response, or increase of the host metabolic activity) [12]. As non-viable elements of probiotics, postbiotics present their strictly defined technological properties and thus represent a promising tool for obtaining therapeutic effects [10,11,13]. These parameters include a favorable level of absorption and distribution of postbiotics [13] and the lack of risk to spread resistance mechanisms, as documented between probiotics and microbiota or pathogens [12]. In 2021, the International Scientific Association of Probiotics and Prebiotics established a new definition of postbiotic as a "preparation of inanimate microorganisms and/or their components that confers a health benefit on the host" [14]. The use of the word 'components' was made because the whole microbial cells are not always required to present health-promoting activity and such an impact may be related to the presence of cellular structures produced by probiotics. The above modification of the meaning of the term 'postbiotic' has opened a new avenue for many new categories of these preparations, including probiotic extracellular vesicles [12].

Extracellular vesicles (EVs) are nanoscale lipid particles secreted by virtually every type of living cell [15]. For this reason, the use of various nomenclature in the description of these structures is frequent. This richness in the nomenclature of the vesicles is related to their physical properties (mostly size), the way they are formed, or the cells that secrete them [15–17]. In order to standardize the nomenclature as much as possible, in accordance with the recommendations of the International Society for Extracellular Vesicles [18], in this review, we will use the term "extracellular vesicles". This is a collective term classically referring to various types of small compartments released from cells, which are surrounded by a lipid bilayer and incapable of spontaneous replication [18]. The main function of EVs is the transport of various classes of macromolecules, including lipids, polysaccharides, proteins, and nucleic acids [9,16,19]. Through this cargo, these structures perform a number of key functions in microorganisms, including long-distance transport of nutrients, protection against environmental stressors, or communication during microorganism–microorganism or microorganism–host interactions [16,17,20]. The importance of EVs in the virulence of many live-threatening pathogens is well known and widely described in the literature [21,22]. Much less is reported with respect to the health-promoting effect of EVs secreted by non-pathogenic microorganisms, including probiotics. For the last few years, however, awareness on probiotic EVs as a very promising therapeutic platform is growing rapidly [15,17,19]. This seems to be strictly related with both the ability of EVs to carry many different bioactive macromolecules and with nanometric dimensions of these structures.

Based on the above facts, in this review article, we decided to collect the latest literature data on the health-promoting properties of extracellular vesicles secreted by probiotics. These characteristics will be extended by the description of physicochemical properties and the proteome of EVs produced by probiotic microorganisms.

2. Review Strategy and Literature Included

To obtain articles comprising the central core of the current review paper, we used the Scopus and PUBMED databases. In that respect, only English-language original articles from the last decade (1 January 2012–30 June 2022) were included. The search terms were "membrane vesicles" or "extracellular vesicles" together with "probiotics". In order to obtain as many records as possible, an additional search phase was performed involving the use of "membrane vesicles" or "extracellular vesicles" together with different genera of the most important probiotic microorganisms, e.g., "*Lactobacillus*" (and all new genera from the Lactobacillaceae family), "*Bifidobacterium*", "*Lactococcus*", "*Pediococcus*", "*Propionibacterium*", etc. As a result of this, we were finally able to obtain 73 original articles, which were subjected to our further analysis and description in subsequent parts of the current review.

3. Discussion

3.1. *Physicochemical Properties of EVs Produced by Probiotics*

Our review of the literature on the ability of probiotic bacteria to produce EVs began with the collection of data describing EVs' physicochemical properties (Table S1). We noticed that this information was available for 60 out of the 73 publications being the central core of this review. Interestingly, in 75% of the cases (45/60), the results concerned Gram-positive bacteria, in particular from the Lactobacillaceae family (Figure 1 and Table S1). The group of Gram-negative bacteria consisted of only two representatives—*Escherichia coli* Nissle 1917 and *Akkermansia muciniphila* ATCC BAA-835 (Figure 1 and Table S1). In our opinion, this situation is the result of frequent interchangeable use of two words with different definitions—'probiotics' and 'lactic acid bacteria (LAB)' [23,24]. The term 'probiotics' is broader and refers to many different groups of microorganisms with beneficial properties for the host, while the term 'LAB' refers only to Gram-positive, lactic acid-producing bacteria for which, many decades ago, numerous health-promoting properties were proved, and, hence, these bacteria were quickly classified as the most important representatives of probiotics [23–26]. In recent years, a strong separation between these two terms is made, contributing to the gradual expansion of research on probiotic properties of Gram-negative bacteria and their EVs. In this context, a mucin-degrading, Gram-negative bacterium *A. muciniphila* deserves special attention, as it was isolated for the first time as lately as in 2004 [27], while, in recent years, there has been an undoubted bloom in interest in this bacterium and its EVs [28]. In our opinion, the above situation has a chance to encourage other researchers focusing on the subject of probiotic microorganisms to expand their search with new, valuable species of probiotics from the group of Gram-negative bacteria.

A careful analysis of the data collected by us showed that, in all 60 articles, the dimensions of probiotics' EVs were determined, while, for this purpose, various research techniques were used (Figure 1 and Table S1). The most frequently applied methods were electron microscopy (21/60; 35%) or nanoparticle tracking analysis (NTA) (19/60; 31.7%). Dynamic light scattering (DLS) (9/60; 15%) was used less commonly for this purpose (Figure 1 and Table S1). In 11 articles, more than one technique was applied to determine the size of EVs, including 6 with microscopy + NTA [29–34], 3 with microscopy + DLS [35–37], and 2 with microscopy + NTA + DLS [38,39] (Figure 1 and Table S1). Among other parameters of EVs measured by researchers, the surface charge/zeta potential and the quantity of EVs can be distinguished. In both cases, the subject was, however, undertaken relatively rarely, i.e., 9/60 (15%) and 18/60 (30%), respectively (Figure 1 and Table S1). The surface charge of EVs was detected most often with the use of DLS (7 of 9 articles) and the quantity of EVs with the use of NTA (14 of 18 articles).

Looking closer at the size analysis of probiotics' EVs, we noticed a large spectrum of results, which depended on both the tested strains/species/genera of bacteria and the analytical techniques used. For Gram-negative bacteria, most of the dimensions were in the range of 20–200 nm (Table S1). On the other hand, for Gram-positive bacteria, the range of the obtained results was greater, although often equal to 50–300 nm (on average, approx. 150 nm) (Table S1). In a comparative context, the articles in which the dimensions of EVs were measured using two or three techniques seem particularly valuable. For example, Hu et al. [29], Liu et al. [30], and Müller et al. [31] showed the convergence of EVs' size values between electron microscopy and NTA, in which the former showed a wider range of detected sizes, while the latter often narrowed this range down to specific values (Table S1). In line with this, electron microscopy might be better than NTA in the analysis of EVs with very low dimensions, as the former suffers from sensitivity and resolution limitations [40,41]. On the other hand, in contrast to NTA, using electron microscopy, it is difficult to precisely determine the mean size of EVs (often being presented as a range of sizes) and it is impossible to determine the concentration of EVs in the sample [40,41]. Nevertheless, the usefulness of both techniques is reflected in the frequency of their use in the articles we analyzed (in total, 51 out of the 60 cases applied one or both of them) (Figure 1 and Table S1). In the context of DLS, according to Shao et al. [40], this method seems also to be quite useful in measuring the dimensions of EVs, but it should be remembered that the critical step during the analysis is to use number distribution, as original size distribution is intensity-weighted and large EVs may over-dominate the obtained results.

As mentioned previously, the parameters of EVs other than dimensions—surface charge/zeta potential and quantity—are of little interest to scientists. In the studies in which this topic was addressed, the zeta potential of EVs had negative values between -0.5 mV [37] and -45 mV [42], with an average ranging from -10 mV to -20 mV (Table S1). The phenomenon of negative charge of EVs is most often related to the presence of extracellular DNA on the surface of these structures, which translates into their important function in supporting adhesion, aggregation, and biofilm formation of microbes [43,44]. Due to this, the electric charge of the EVs of probiotic bacteria can directly affect their colonization capacity of the host [31,39,45]. It seems to us that the low interest in this parameter among the scientific community can be explained by the willingness to administer to patients purified EVs of probiotics, without applying microorganisms secreting them (e.g., in a form of postbiotics) [46]. Although the influence of EVs on the colonization capacity of the probiotics producing them is not widely investigated, it should still be kept in mind that EVs applied in this way could affect the diversity and properties of the host microbiota [47,48].

Taking into account the amount of EVs produced by probiotics, these values were in the range of 10^8–10^{12} per mL when focusing on the most commonly used technique—NTA (14/18; 77.8%) (Table S1). For the other two techniques, tunable resistive pulse sensing (TRPS) [49,50] and flow cytometry [45], these values were equal to approximately 10^{10} and 10^7 per mL, respectively (Table S1). For spectrophotometry [51], the unit used (relative fluorescence units/colony forming units of probiotics) makes it impossible to compare the results with the others (Table S1). Although the frequency in measuring quantity of probiotic EVs was quite low, the high homogeneity of applied research techniques allows for a relatively objective comparison of EVs' production by different probiotics. In our opinion, the lack of universality in measuring the efficiency of production of probiotic EVs is, as stated before, associated with the frequent perception of these EVs as a therapeutic agent with designation to be administered in a purified form to patients (as postbiotics) and not necessarily as structures that would be secreted by the probiotic into the local environment, e.g., the intestines [46].

Other aspects of the biological and physicochemical properties of EVs secreted by probiotics, including the spatial orientation of EVs' membranes or their biological origin (including the participation or lack of cell lysis), were examined extremely rarely—only in the case of single original articles. Therefore, the above properties were not included in the main part of our discussion. The description of the aforementioned problem will be additionally deliberated in Section 3.5. "Challenges and Limitations of Articles Focusing on EVs Produced by Probiotics".

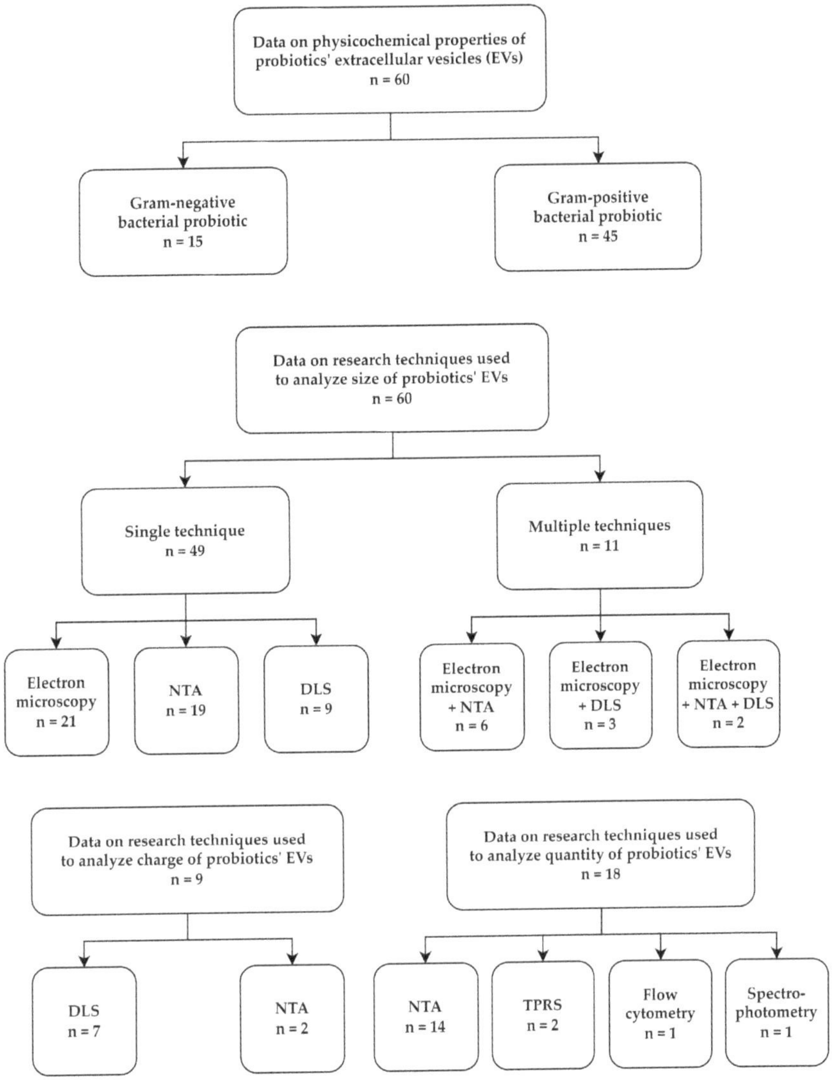

Figure 1. A graph presenting the categorization of articles constituting the core of this review, in which the physicochemical properties of extracellular vesicles (EVs) of probiotics were described. Among the 60 of them, 15 and 45 concerned Gram-negative and Gram-positive bacteria, respectively. All articles assessed the size of the produced EVs, of which 49 determined it using only one technique (21 with electron microscopy [51–71], 19 with NTA [72–90], and 9 with DLS [42,45,49,50,91–95]), while 11 used more than one technique (6 with electron microscopy + NTA [29–34], 3 with electron microscopy + DLS [35–37], and 3 with electron microscopy + NTA + DLS [38,39]). Only 9 papers analyzed the electrical charge of EVs, of which 7 used DLS [31,36–39,42,45] and 2 used NTA [84,85]. The quantity of EVs produced was examined in 18 articles, of which 14 used NTA [31,33,38,39,72–74,76,77,79,83,87–89], 2 used TRSP [49,50], 1 used flow cytometry [45], and 1 used spectrophotometry [51]. Detailed information on the numerical data of the above-presented results can be found in Table S1. Abbreviations: DLS, dynamic light scattering; NTA, nanoparticle tracking analysis; TRSP, tunable resistive pulse sensing.

3.2. Proteomic Profile of EVs Produced by Probiotics

The second aspect analyzed by us was the evaluation of the proteome of EVs produced by probiotic bacteria. Out of 73 articles constituting the core of this review, 17 took up this topic (Table 1). Since the methodology of isolation and purification of EVs or analysis of their proteins may influence the obtained results, we decided to collect this information in Table 1. We noticed that, in both cases, there is a relatively high homogeneity of the research techniques used. Most probiotics' EVs were isolated by ultracentrifugation (14/17; 82.4%), while, in the remaining cases, chemical precipitation (1/17) or size exclusion chromatography (SEC) (2/17) was applied (Table 1). In the analysis of the EVs' proteome, the most frequently used technique was electrophoresis combined with liquid chromatography with tandem mass spectrometry (LC-MS/MS) or matrix-assisted laser desorption/ionization-time of flight (MALDI-TOF) (12/17; 70.6%). Less frequently, chemical (4/17) or magnetic (1/17) precipitation combined with LC-MS/MS was used for this purpose (Table 1).

Despite the relatively high methodological homogeneity, a large discrepancy within the data was noticed. The total number of identified proteins (understood as whole-length gene products) ranged from a dozen [74] to over a thousand (1149 [54] and 1283 [62]), while, in most articles, these values were within the range of several hundred (10/17; 58.8%) (Table 1). In this context, it is also worth highlighting the strong correlation between cellular localization and the number of isolated EVs' proteins. If the protein localization was classified as 'membrane', then the proteome was narrower (11–192 proteins) than when the most abundant protein representation was derived from the cytoplasm (11–1286 proteins; in all cases where the proteome was >300 proteins, 'cytoplasm' dominated) (Table 1). This phenomenon may be caused by two sources—the sensitivity of the research techniques and the level of contamination of the EVs' proteome with proteins derived from bacterial cells producing these structures [40,96,97]. Insufficient level of sensitivity may contribute to the loss of proteins with low representation in the EVs' proteome, the function of which, however, may be of key importance for microorganisms secreting them [98,99]. On the other hand, too high representation of proteins in the EVs' proteome may suggest its contamination and the need to include/improve the purification step of the obtained EVs [96,100]. According to the review by Nagakubo et al. [96], some researchers consider numerous representations of ribosomal proteins (30S and 50S), which are typically of cytoplasmic origin, as an independent indicator of the EVs' proteome contamination. However, there are articles showing that extracellular secretion of ribosomal proteins may have important, extra-ribosomal functions for the physiology of microorganisms, including biofilm formation [101] or resistance against translation-targeting antibiotics [102,103]. Therefore, in our opinion, the detection of ribosomal proteins in the EVs' proteome should not be automatically interpreted as contamination, however, serious consideration for improving the techniques of isolation and analysis of EVs should be made if the proteome of these structures is both too numerous and over-represented by cytoplasmic proteins, including, in particular, the ribosome subunits.

In addition to information about the methodology of isolation of EVs and analysis of their proteome, in Table 1 we also included some details about the most abundant/most important proteins constituting the EVs' proteome of probiotics. To simplify this issue, once again, we have decided to divide the discussion into a part covering Gram-negative and Gram-positive bacteria.

Gram-negative bacteria described in Table 1 were represented only by *E. coli* Nissle 1917, while as many as 4 out of the 17 articles focused on this aspect [29,51,52,72]. It is worth noting that within the most numerous proteins secreted by this bacterium in EVs many adhesive proteins were highlighted, including fimbrial (FocA, Fim1C, FocF, FocG, and FocH) and flagellar (FliC, FliD, FlgA, FlgE, FlgK, and FlgL) subunits, and outer membrane proteins (OmpA, OmpC, OmpF, and NmpC) (Table 1). According to many, the presence of adhesins anchored on the surface of EVs of Gram-negative bacteria is an important element facilitating the colonization of the intestines [104–106]. The second important group of proteins produced by this bacterium within EVs was related to peptidoglycan and cell membrane rearrangement, i.e., murein hydrolases (MltA, MltB, and MltC), murein-interacting protein MipA, and peptidoglycan-associated lipoproteins (Pal, TolB, Sat, LpoA, YbaY, and SlyB) (Table 1). It is indicated that the rearrangement of murein and cell membranes are important steps in the biogenesis of EVs, hence, the presence of proteins related to the above processes within EVs should not come as a surprise [107]. On the other hand, researchers pay attention to the participation of murein hydrolases encased within EVs in the competitive fight against other bacteria [108]. In summary, the main components of the EVs' proteome of *E. coli* Nissle 1917 were adhesins and proteins associated with peptidoglycan rearrangement, which are involved in the effective colonization of the host and its protection against pathogenic microorganisms.

Gram-positive bacteria described in Table 1 were mainly representatives of the Lactobacillaceae family (*Lactiplantibacillus, Lacticaseibacillus, Limosilactobacillus, Ligilactobacillus,* and *Lactobacillus*), and, additionally, by *Bifidobacterium, Propionibacterium, Lactococcus,* and *Pediococcus*. Among the dominant group of proteins located within EVs of these bacteria were metabolic proteins, while, in single cases, peptidoglycan rearrangement proteins (including putative murein hydrolases or lysozyme-like proteins [32,34,36,38]) and proteins related to adhesion or aggregation (including surface proteins, mucus-binding proteins, or aggregation-promoting factors [33,38,78,79]) were also noticed (Table 1). Whereas the function of adhesins and peptidoglycan rearrangement proteins in EVs has been described above and is similar in Gram-positive bacteria, proteins responsible for metabolism deserve special attention. Based on the data collected in Table 1, it can be noticed that this group includes proteins related to the biosynthesis or breakdown of various classes of nutrients, and they are produced by many representatives of probiotics, such as *Lactiplantibacillus* [32,54], *Lacticaseibacillus* [36], *Limosilactobacillus* [34,38], *Ligilactobacillus* [76], *Lactobacillus* [33,74], *Bifidobacterium* [64], *Propionibacterium* [78,79], *Lactococcus* [62], and *Pediococcus* [42]. In addition to this, numerous proteins determining an uptake of glycerol [54], vitamins [54], amino acids and peptides [54,76], phosphates [74,76], inorganic acid ions [76], and iron [64] were detected. All the above-mentioned proteins participate in the transport of nutrients from the local environment and their delivery in an assimilable form. Many scientists point out that this system can provide nutrients not only to the EVs-producing microorganisms, but also to the host, especially in areas with high availability of nutrients, e.g., intestines [109–111]. On this basis, it can be concluded that EVs of Gram-positive probiotic bacteria determine not only their colonization abilities and competition with pathogens, but also may improve digestive processes of the host.

As it can be easily observed, EVs produced by probiotics surely have a different role in the host than those released by pathogens. With regards to probiotics, we speculate that the role of EVs secreted by different probiotics is strain-dependent and, in fact, influenced by the bacterial phenotype, culture conditions (i.e., culture media used or the age of microbial culture), and biogenesis mechanisms by which such EVs are released—including differences between Gram-positive and Gram-negative species [112,113]. For this reason, currently, we cannot state that a "universal molecular mechanism" conditioning benefit of probiotic EVs for the host exists. Unquestionably, further studies based on a deeper proteomic and metabolomic analysis of probiotic EVs, which compares different microbial strains and culture conditions, should be performed to discover microbial components capable of conferring beneficial properties on the host.

3.3. Biological Activities and Properties of EVs Produced by Probiotics

The last aspect considered in our review was the analysis of biological activities and properties of probiotics' EVs. As reported in Table 2, a total amount of 54 articles were considered. In 23 of them, experiments were performed only in in vitro models, and 6 used only in vivo models, while the other 25 analyzed both (amongst these, 5 used ex vivo models). In our opinion, inclusion of both in vitro and in vivo models provides, undoubtedly, a better understanding of EVs' activity. For example, as reported by Chen et al. [76], the use of murine models allows us to assess whether EVs could be transported to the femoral heads of glucocorticoid-treated mice after intragastric administration, thus providing information about EVs' tissue distribution. We can assume that studying EVs' properties addresses the same challenges of characterizing new probiotics. As described by Papadimitriou et al. [114], one of the most important advantage of in vitro assays is the ability to perform different screenings simultaneously, helping to evaluate potential interactions between probiotics and their products with the host. At the same time, these models are affected by some biases since the laboratory conditions only partially reproduce the in vivo situation. As well as probiotics needing to reach the desired body niches alive, EVs' stability needs to be established since it depends on multiple factors. Thus, in vivo assays may be more appropriate because they can reproduce the complexity of the existing interactions. On the other hand, the main weakness of in vivo models is that they cannot be used for high throughput screening due to the increased cost and for ethical issues. For the above-mentioned reasons, a combination of in vitro and in vivo tests could represent an appropriate approach for EVs' study [115].

Table 1. Proteomic data on extracellular vesicles produced by probiotics.

Bacterial Producer	Methodology of Isolation/ Determination	Proteomic Data			Reference
		Total Number of Identified Proteins *	Cellular Localization of Proteins	The Most Abundant Representatives/ Proteins Highlighted by Authors	
Escherichia coli Nissle 1917	Ultracentrifugation (vesicles) Electrophoresis + LC-MS/MS (proteome)	192	Outer membrane ~ 40% Cytoplasm 40% Periplasm 15% Inner membrane < 5 %	- Fimbriae subunits: FocA, FocF, FocG, FocH - Flagellins: FlgK, FlgE, FliD - Murein hydrolase MltB - Metabolic proteins: AnsB, CadA, FbaB, GapA, Icd, Mdh	[52]
	Ultracentrifugation + DGC (vesicles) Electrophoresis + LC-MS/MS (proteome)	189	Outer membrane 28% Cytoplasm 36.5% Periplasm 20% Inner membrane 9.5% Secretory 6%	- Fimbriae subunits: FocA, FocF, FocG, FocH - Flagellins: FlgA, FlgE, FlgK - Outer membrane proteins: OmpA, OmpC, OmpF - Murein hydrolases: MltA, MltC	[29]
	Ultracentrifugation (vesicles) Electrophoresis + LC-MS/MS (proteome)	295	*ND*	- Peptidoglycan-associated lipoproteins: Pal, TolB - Murein-interacting protein MipA - Flagellin subunit FliC - Outer membrane proteins: OmpA, OmpC, OmpF, NmpC	[51]
	Ultracentrifugation + DGC or SEC (vesicles) Chemical precipitation + LC-MS/MS (proteome)	189	Membrane ~ 60% Cytoplasm ~ 40%	- Peptidoglycan-associated lipoproteins: Pal, Sat, LpoA, YbaY, SlyB - Fimbrial protein Fim1C - Flagellin FlgL - Outer membrane proteins: OmpC, NmpC	[72]
Lactiplantibacillus plantarum BGAN8	Ultracentrifugation (vesicles) Electrophoresis + MALDI-TOF (proteome)	1149	Membrane ~ 45% Cytoplasm + ribosomes ~ 52% Secretory < 1%	- Polysaccharide biosynthesis proteins: EpsN, MurJ - Transporters of glycerol (GlpF), niacin (NiaP), oligopeptides (OppC), amino acids (SdaC, CycA) - Translation proteins: 30S and 50S ribosomal subunits (55 different subunits)	[54]

Table 1. *Cont.*

Bacterial Producer	Methodology of Isolation/ Determination	Proteomic Data			Reference
		Total Number of Identified Proteins *	Cellular Localization of Proteins	The Most Abundant Representatives/ Proteins Highlighted by Authors	
Lactiplantibacillus plantarum WCFS1	Chemical precipitation (vesicles) Electrophoresis + LC-MS/MS (proteome)	31	Membrane 42% Cytoplasm 13% Secretory 16%	- Cell wall remodeling proteins: Acm2, DltD, MreC, Lp_2847, Lp_3015, Lp_2162, Lp_3093, Lp_3421 - Metabolic proteins: TpiA, GapB, Pgi, Ldh1	[32]
Lacticaseibacillus casei ATCC 393	Ultracentrifugation (vesicles) Chemical precipitation + LC-MS/MS (proteome)	43	Membrane ~ 20% Cytoplasm 65% Secretory 14%	- Putative family 15 glucoamylase LBCZ_2692 - Lysozyme-like proteins: LBCZ_0210, LCAUW4_1864 - N-acetylmuramoyl-L-alanine amidase LSEI_1536 - Putative cell wall-associated hydrolase LSEI_0281	[38]
Lacticaseibacillus casei BL23	Ultracentrifugation (vesicles) Electrophoresis + LC-MS/MS (proteome)	103	Membrane + secretory 43% Cytoplasm 57%	- Cell wall-associated hydrolases P40 and P75 - Metabolism proteins: GapA, Pgk, LdhL, Fba, AspB, Pyk - Translation proteins: 30S ribosomal subunits (RpsJ, RpsL, RpsS, RpsT, RpsU) and 50S ribosomal subunits (11 different subunits)	[36]
Limosilactobacillus reuteri ATCC 23272	Ultracentrifugation (vesicles) Chemical precipitation + LC-MS/MS (proteome)	17	Membrane 18% Cytoplasm 82%	- Metabolic proteins: Lreu_0426, Lreu_1721, Lreu_1853 - NAD kinase NadK	[38]
Limosilactobacillus reuteri BBC3	Ultracentrifugation + DGC (vesicles) Chemical precipitation + LC-MS/MS (proteome)	92	Membrane 27% Cytoplasm 56.5% Secretory 16%	- Metabolic proteins: GatB, ProS, SerS, IleS, LRI_0925, B5F04_03325, N134_06765 - Cell wall remodeling proteins: Lr1610, MreC - Translation proteins: 30S ribosome subunit (RpsB) and 50S ribosome subunit (RplC)	[34]
Ligilactobacillus animalis ATCC 35046	Ultracentrifugation + DGC (vesicles) Chemical precipitation + nLC-MS/MS (proteome)	340	From the top 74 proteins: Membrane 25.7% Cytoplasm 25.7% Secretory 1.3% Unknown 47.3%	- Sortase SrtA - Transporters of phosphate (PstS), glutamine (GlnP), nitrate/sulfonate/bicarbonate (Lani381_1252) - Metabolism protein Pgi - Antioxidative protein Dsp	[76]
Lactobacillus acidophilus ATCC 53544	Ultracentrifugation (vesicles) Chemical precipitation + LC-MS/MS (proteome)	26	Membrane ~ 30% Cytoplasm 62% Secretory 12%	- Surface proteins: FmtB, SlpX - Mucus binding protein Mub - Transporters of maltose (LBA1864) and glutamine (GlnP) - Bacteriocin LBA1805	[38]

Table 1. *Cont.*

Bacterial Producer	Methodology of Isolation/ Determination	Proteomic Data			Reference
		Total Number of Identified Proteins *	Cellular Localization of Proteins	The Most Abundant Representatives/ Proteins Highlighted by Authors	
Lactobacillus gasseri BC12	Ultracentrifugation (vesicles) Electrophoresis + LC-ESI-MS/MS (proteome)	15	Membrane ~ 44% Cytoplasm ~ 44% Secretory ~ 11%	- Foldase protein PrsA - Enolase 1 (Eno1) and 2 (Eno2) - Translation proteins: elongation factor (EF-Tu) and 30S ribosomal subunit (RpsD) - Metabolism proteins: AtpA, AtpD, AtpF, AtpH, Pyk, TpiA - Phosphonates transporter PhnC	[74]
Lactobacillus crispatus BC5	Ultracentrifugation (vesicles) Electrophoresis + LC-ESI-MS/MS (proteome)	11	Membrane ~ 45% Cytoplasm ~ 45% Secretory ~ 9%	- Enolase Eno1 - Translation proteins: 30S ribosomal subunit (RpsD) and 50S ribosomal subunits (RplB, RplU) - Metabolism proteins: AtpA, AtpD, AtpF - Phosphonates transporter PhnC	[74]
Lactobacillus johnsonii N6.2	Ultracentrifugation (vesicles) Electrophoresis + LC-MS/MS (proteome)	366	Cytoplasm + ribosomes 86% Secretory 14%	- Foldase protein PrsA - Aggregation promoting factors: Apf1, Apf2 - Translation proteins: 30S ribosome subunits (RpsB, RpsC, RpsE) and 50S ribosome subunit (RplA) - Metabolic proteins: PtsP, GalE, InuJ, RfbB, PfkA	[33]
Bifidobacterium longum NCC 2705	Ultracentrifugation (vesicles) Electrophoresis + LC-MS/MS (proteome)	24	Membrane 21% Cytoplasm 75%	- Iron transporter BL1134_04745 - Metabolism proteins: GltX, Pyk, GatA, GapA, SerS, Ppa - Translation proteins: elongation factor (EF-Tu), 30S ribosomal subunits (RpsC, RpsI), 50S ribosomal subunit (RplY)	[64]
Propionibacterium freudenreichii CIRM-BIA 129	SEC (vesicles) Electrophoresis + LC-ESI-MS/MS (proteome)	319	Membrane 16% Cytoplasm 75% Secretory 9%	- Enolase Eno1 - Aconitase Acn - Surface-layer proteins: SlpB, SplE, BopA, InlA - Antioxidative proteins: SodA, AhpC - Metabolic proteins: GlnA1, Gpi, Tpi1	[78]
	SEC (vesicles) Electrophoresis + LC-MS/MS (proteome)	391 (medium-dependent; 358 common for all)	Membrane 16.5% Cytoplasm 74% Secretory 9.5%	- Surface proteins: SlpB, SlpD, BopA, InlA - Metabolism proteins: LacZ, IolC, IolE1, AroH, NirA2 - Translation proteins: 30S ribosomal subunit (RpsG) and 50S ribosomal subunits (RplB, RplC, RplT, RplV) - Antioxidative protein AhpC	[79]

Table 1. *Cont.*

Bacterial Producer	Methodology of Isolation/ Determination	Proteomic Data			Reference
		Total Number of Identified Proteins *	Cellular Localization of Proteins	The Most Abundant Representatives/ Proteins Highlighted by Authors	
Lactococcus lactis FM-YL11	Ultracentrifugation (vesicles) Magnetic precipitation + LC-MS/MS (proteome)	1283	From the top 320 proteins: Membrane 16.5% Cytoplasm 74% Secretory 9.5%	- Translation proteins: elongation factor (EF-Tu), 30S ribosomal subunits (RpsA, RpsB, RpsC, RpsD, RpsE, RpsG, RpsK, RpsM), 50S ribosomal subunits (RplB, RplC, RplD, RplE, RplS, RplT, RplU) - Metabolic proteins: LacB, PyrG, LLT1_01140	[62]
Pediococcus pentosaceus **	Ultracentrifugation (vesicles) Electrophoresis + LC-MS/MS (proteome)	103	Membrane 9% Cytoplasm + ribosomes ~ 83% Secretory 5.5%	- Foldase protein PrsA - Enolase Eno1 - Translation proteins: elongation factors (EF-Tu, EF-G) and 50S ribosome subunits (RplD, RplO, RplQ) - Metabolic proteins: TpiA, ldhL	[42]

Abbreviations: *ND*, no data; DGC, density gradient centrifugation; LC-MS/MS, liquid chromatography with tandem mass spectrometry; nLC-MS/MS, nano-scale liquid chromatographic tandem mass spectrometry; LC-ESI-MS/MS, liquid chromatography electrospray ionization with tandem mass spectrometric; MALDI-TOF, matrix-assisted laser desorption/ionization-time of flight; SEC, size exclusion chromatography. * Total number of whole-length gene products, ** bacterial strain was not reported.

Of the 54 articles considered, a large number of studies focused on the evaluation of EVs' activity on the gastrointestinal system. From them, the most commonly applied models were Caco-2 cells, a model of the intestinal epithelial barrier, and C57BL/6 mice, one of the most adaptable animal models (Table 2). It is widely known that probiotics have a beneficial effect on the intestinal homeostasis, and this is obtained via multifactorial health-promoting activity [1,5,6]. In fact, several authors reported ability of probiotic EVs to enhance the intestinal barrier integrity by increasing the expression of tight junction (TJ) proteins, such as *ocldn*, *zo1*, *zo2*, and *zo3* [68], and by reducing *cldn-2* [67,69] (Table 2). Alterations of TJ barrier function and paracellular permeability are closely associated with the onset of metabolic diseases. All the previously-mentioned proteins aggregate into complexes located at the apical site of the lateral membranes of intestinal epithelial cells and regulate the selective passage of ions, solutes, and water. Occludins, the first identified integral membrane TJ proteins, create a barrier against macromolecules through the hemophilic interactions of their extracellular loops and so they have a crucial role in TJ structure and function [116]. ZO proteins are multi-domain proteins that provide an intracellular scaffold in TJs, creating a direct connection with the actin cytoskeleton and cytoskeleton-associated proteins; it is also recognized that ZO proteins have an important role in the regulation of TJ assembly [116]. Claudins, on the contrary to the two previously-described proteins, confer pore-like properties on TJs and regulate the selective passage of molecules in the paracellular pathways [116]. Of note is that increased claudin-2 expression by intestinal epithelial cells is correlated with colitis and inflammatory bowel disease [117]. As reported in Table 2, EVs produced by *A. muciniphila* can decrease the expression of *cldn-2*, thus regulating the integrity of the intestinal barrier and reducing inflammation [67]. Moreover, in the context of inflammatory bowel diseases (IBD), Hao et al. [93], Tong et al. [94], and Kang et al. [118] detected colitis amelioration in mice treated with EVs. In their studies, these authors used similar models, C57BL/6 and C57BL/6J mice with specific pathogen-free conditions, and colitis was induced by dextran sulfate sodium (DSS). DSS-treated mouse is the most widely used to obtain a good experimental model of ulcerative colitis (UC) since it leads to pathological alternations that are similar to what occurs in human UC [119]. In all three articles [93,94,118], EVs were administered by oral gavage in similar dosage and, despite the difference in the producer strain (*L. plantarum* Q7 [93], *L. rhamnosus* GG (ATCC 53103) [94], and *L. kefirgranum* PRCC-1301 [118]), the results obtained were comparable. They all reported a reversion of colon shortening and a downregulation of pro-inflammatory cytokines, including IL-1β, IL-2, IL-6, and TNF-α. It is worth noting that another common finding was the restoration of the gut microbiota homeostasis [82,93,94,118] (Table 2). Dysbiosis of intestinal microbiota, with reduction of probiotics and rise in pathogenic bacteria, represents a significant feature in UC patients. Consequently, the therapeutic potential of probiotic strains in UC has been examined by several researchers, who have identified different related mechanisms of action [120]. Thus, regarding the articles considered in this review, we can assume that EVs could be considered one of the bacterial products involved. In this context, Ma et al. [81] also highlighted the correlation between EVs treatment and mucus barrier integrity enhancement. This association was widely studied by Petersson et al. [121], who observed that the colonic mucus layer in germ-free mice was very thin compared with that observed in conventionally housed mice. Moreover, the administration of bacterial products (lipopolysaccharide and peptidoglycan) restored the normal mucus levels.

Five studies focused on the correlation between EVs and tumor development (Table 2). Using animal models, Tomasi et al. [122], Luo et al. [92], and Shi et al. [90] tested EVs of *E. coli* Nissle 1917, *A. muciniphila* ATCC BAA-835, and *L. paracasei* PC-H1, respectively. Melanoma, prostate cancer, and colorectal cancer were investigated, and comparable results were obtained despite different routes of administration and dosage; each author reported a reduction in tumor growth. Luo et al. [92] observed an upregulation of M1 macrophages and $CD8^+$ lymphocytes expressing IFN-γ and GZMB, concluding that *A. muciniphila*-EVs stimulate anti-tumor immunity against prostate cancer. Shi et al. [90], instead, found out that the treatment with *L. paracasei*-EVs increased the expression level of Bax and decreased Bcl-2. These results were confirmed in both in vivo and in vitro models, and the authors confirmed that EVs can be taken up by colon cancer cells and inhibit their growth through apoptosis induction. As is well documented, many tumor types induce extensive systemic perturbations in the activity of the immune system, although the microbiome can modulate the systemic immunity and thus influence the outcome of tumor control strategies [123]. Fessler et al. [124] summarized the potential biological mechanisms of microbiome-mediated immune modulation: (1) bacterial translocation to different body districts may stimulate the immune response by providing microbial-derived, conserved antigens; (2) cross-reactive T cells primed against bacterial antigens might exert anti-tumor effects; (3) gut bacteria can release soluble immunomodulatory factors (IL-12, IFN-γ, and TNF-α) that then disseminate systematically and can activate dendritic cells. In this context, given the results obtained by the authors previously mentioned, it can be assumed that EVs could represent one of the effectors of these processes. For the research of Tomasi et al. [122] it is necessary to highlight that they tested *E. coli*-EVs engineered with a cancer-specific epitope and showed that the administration of these EVs, but not of wild type EVs, induced a reduction in tumor growth (Table 2). Given these results, we can assume that, unsurprisingly, not all probiotic strains may have the same health-promoting potential, although engineered EVs could represent a promising tool in cancer therapies. The remaining two articles [56,57] noted the same EVs' properties on HepG2, SW480, and HT29 cells, highlighting an anti-proliferative effect on cancer cell lines (Table 2). According to Behzadi et al. [56], *L. rhamnosus*-EVs can increase the apoptotic index (*bax*/*bcl2* expression ratio) in liver cancer cells in a dose-dependent manner. Keyhani et al. [57], analyzing EVs of the same probiotic strain, reported an inhibitory effect on colon cancer cells too. Otherwise, in the latter article, a specific mechanism of action was not considered.

Other authors frequently reported that EVs have an immunomodulatory effect, which is related to their role in the regulation of different types of cytokines, chemokines, and antibodies [35,37,63,125] (Table 2). The influence of probiotics on the human immune system is not strictly related to pathological conditions, as previously discussed; a large amount of research, in fact, proved that the gut microbiota play a crucial role in the development and regulation of the host immune system and this complex interplay starts already during the birthing process. Under the stimulus of probiotic-derived products, intestinal epithelial cells may release thymic stromal lymphopoietin (TSLP), transforming growth factor-β (TGF-β), IL-25, and B cell activating factor (BAFF) [126]. Furthermore, T_{H17}, T_{Reg}, and IgA-producing cells development is also regulated by gut microbiota [127]. Different strains of probiotics can increase the number of dendritic cells and macrophages, and activate the latter through proinflammatory mediators, such as cytokines, reactive oxygen species or nuclear factor kB, and Toll-like receptor 2 pathways [128]. Fabrega et al. [63] determined that the presence of LPS in *E. coli*-EVs may explain the activation of IL-6, IL-8, and TNF-α, while the upregulation of IL-10 seems to be attributed to the presence of other vesicle factors (Table 2). At the same time, Morishita et al. [84,85] elucidated that EVs-mediated cytokine production is strictly related to their internalization. The release of TNF-α and IL-6 from cells treated with EVs was reduced in the presence of endocytosis and TLR2 inhibitors, with only one exception for RAW264.7 cells, for which no reduction in TNF-α was observed even after blocking clathrin-mediated endocytosis and micropinocytosis (Table 2). This suggests that several pathways could be involved in the EVs–cell interaction, and characterizing the main effectors is the key for the understanding of the immunomodulation in the host.

Interestingly, two articles considered the correlation between gut microbiota and the nervous system when focusing on EVs' activity (Table 2). Choi et al. [129,130] found that EVs treatment reversed the expression of brain-derived neurotrophic factors (BDNFs) in HT22 cells and afforded antidepressant-like effects in C57BL/6 mice with stress-induced depression. In the first study, they examined whether *L. plantarum*-EVs treatment could block stress-induced, depressive-like behaviours in mice during the stress induction phase and during the post-stress phase. In both cases *L. plantarum*-EVs treatment restored the expression levels of BDNFs in the hippocampus and reduced depressive-like behaviors. This correlation was confirmed by their results obtained in vitro using HT22 cells. In the second study, they also considered EVs of *B. subtilis* and *A. muciniphila* and obtained comparable, although not identical, results. These data were also confirmed by several experiments that have proved the existence of the so-called 'gut–brain axis'. Activation of proinflammatory cytokines, such as IL-1 and IL-6, has a certain association with the development of depression, so the impact of probiotics on immune homeostasis could help in the prevention or treatment of depression [128]. However, the detailed mechanisms of the action of EVs and their tissue distribution remain to be explored further.

Considering the influence of microbiota on the host health, two articles evaluated the effect of probiotics on another extraintestinal tissue—the skin [55,87] (Table 2). In this regard, Kim et al. [55] evaluated the therapeutic properties of *L. plantarum*-EVs on *S. aureus*-induced mouse atopic dermatitis model and on keratinocytes. The results showed that *L. plantarum*-EVs decrease skin inflammation by reducing the level of proinflammatory cytokines (IL-4 and IL-6). Since current treatment of atopic dermatitis involves the use of anti-inflammatory drugs and emollients, in order to compensate poor immune tolerance and barrier dysfunction, probiotics and their byproducts could represent an alternative option in the prevention or treatment of this disorder. Another article by Jo et al. [87] evaluated the effect of probiotic EVs on skin aging by using human dermal fibroblasts (CCD986sk) and a clinical trial among Korean women. As reported in Table 2, authors discovered that *L. plantarum*-EVs exert an anti-aging and anti-pigmentation effect and were able to positively regulate multiple pathways in fibroblasts.

Taken together, all the data summarised in Figure 2 and Table 2 suggest a huge variety of applications of probiotic EVs. Most of the studies confirmed their potential in protecting the intestinal barrier integrity and modulating host immune response in both physiological and disease-induced conditions. At the same time, there are many fields that still require further investigations on mechanisms by which probiotic EVs exert their activity. This knowledge could be then used to design innovative approaches in prevention and therapy of difficult-to-treat diseases.

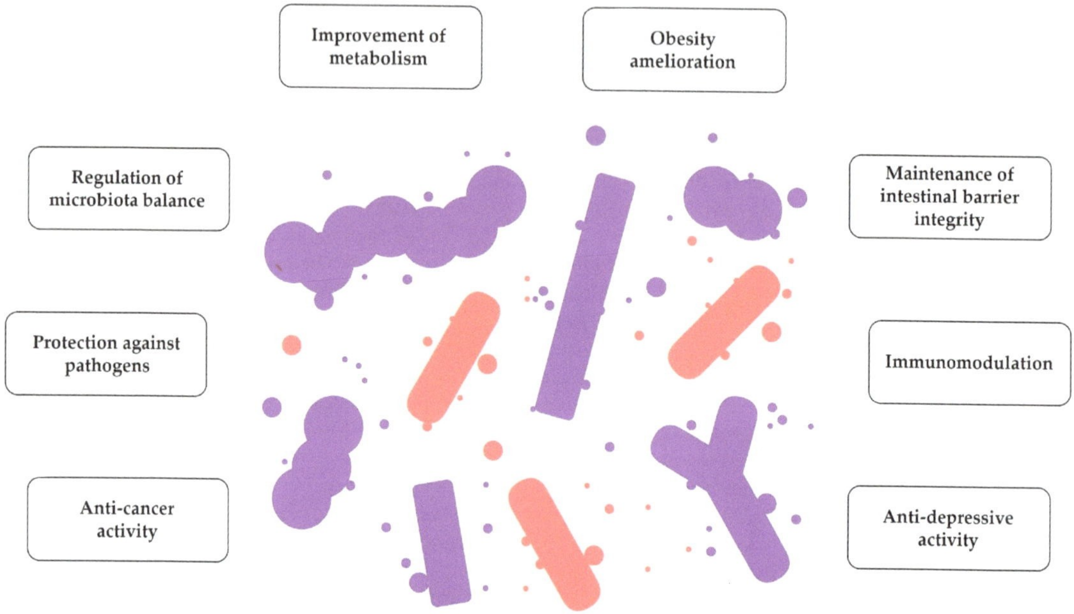

Figure 2. Graphical summary of data on the biological activities of extracellular vesicles secreted by probiotics.

Table 2. Biological activity of extracellular vesicles produced by probiotics reported in in vitro and in vivo models.

Bacterial Producer	In Vitro Model EVs Treatment (Duration)	In Vivo Model EVs Treatment (Duration)	Observations on EVs Activity	EVs Properties	Reference
Escherichia coli Nissle 1917	Caco-2 and T-84 cells (EPEC-infected) 0.1 mg/mL (24 h)	*ND*	- ↑ occludin and claudin-14	- Protection of intestinal barrier integrity against EPEC infection (enhancement of TJ)	[131]
	RAW264.7 murine macrophages 1 μg/mL (16 h)	*ND*	- ↑ IL-4, IL-6, IL-12, and TNF-α - ↑ IL-10	- Anti-inflammatory properties - Enhanced immunomodulatory effect and antimicrobial function	[29]
OVA-*Escherichia coli* Nissle 1917, *Escherichia coli* BL21 Δ*ompA*	*ND*	Tumor in C57BL/6 and BALB/c female 4–8-week-old mice (administration: oral gavage) 10 μg (3–5 times)	- ↑ Tumor-specific T cells in the lamina propria - ↓ Tumor growth	- Protective activity against tumor development	[122]

Table 2. *Cont.*

Bacterial Producer	In Vitro Model EVs Treatment (Duration)	In Vivo Model EVs Treatment (Duration)	Observations on EVs Activity	EVs Properties	Reference
Escherichia coli serotype O6:K5:H1	Caco-2 and HT-29 cells 10 mg/mL (8 h)	*ND*	- Activation of NOD-1 signaling and NF-κB - ↑ IL-6 and IL-8 - ↓ IκBα	- Maintenance of intestinal homeostasis	[132]
	Caco-2 and PMBCs cells 50 μg/mL (5–24 h)	Colon organ culture (ex vivo model) 50 μg/mL (5 h)	- ↑ IL-10, MIP1a, TNF-α, IL-6, and IL-8 by Caco-2/PBMCs co-culture - ↓ IL-12 and TGF-β in ex vivo model	- Modulation of the immune response - Anti-inflammatory properties	[63]
	Human Monocyte-Derived DCs 10 μg/mL (24 h)	*ND*	- ↑ 93 miRNAs and ↓ 64 miRNAs - ↑ miR-155, miR-let7i, and miR-146a - ↑ IFN-γ and IL-12	- Protection against pathogen infections - Anti-inflammatory/tolerogenic action	[133]
Akkermansia muciniphila ATCC BAA-835	Caco-2 cells 0.1, 0.5, and 5 μg (24 h)	*ND*	- ↑ *ocldn*, *zo1*, *zo3*, and *zo2* expression - ↓ *tlr4* and *trl2* expression	- Enhancement of intestinal barrier integrity - Anti-inflammatory properties	[68]
	Caco-2 cells 10 μg (24 h)	HFD induced and ND thirty male C57BL/6 mice (administration: oral gavage) 10 μg (5 weeks)	- ↑ *ZO-1*, *OCLDN*, and *CLDN-1* and ↓ *CLDN-2* expression in HDF mice - ↑ TLR-2 and ↓ TRL-4 expression in cells - ↓ blood glucose, cholesterol levels, and adipocyte dimensions in HDF mice - ↓ TNF-α, IL-6, and TLR-4 expression in HDF mice	- Obesity amelioration and prevention	[67]
Akkermansia muciniphila ATCC BAA-835	*ND*	NFD induced and NF 8-week-old male C57BL/6 mice (administration: oral gavage) 10 μg protein/200 μL (5 weeks)	- ↑ *tlr-2* and IL-10 - ↑ *zo-1* and *ocldn* and ↓ *cldn-2* - ↑ *angptl4* - ↓ *tlr-4*, *tnf-α*, and *tgf-β* - ↓ food intake and glucose level	- Preventive effect on obesity through enhancement of TJ	[69]
	Caco-2 cells (inflammation model) 0.1, 1, and 10 μg (4–8 h)	HFD in 6–8-week-old male C57BL/6 mice (administration: oral gavage) 10 μg (14 days)	- ↑ expression of occludin, zonal occludens, and claudin-5 in mice - ↑ glucose tolerance in mice - ↑ AMPK phosphorylation in cells - ↓ tight junction permeability in cells	- Improvement of gut permeability and metabolic functions (enhancement of tight junctions) - Anti-diabetes properties	[91]
	THP-1 and RAW264.7 10 μg/mL (24 h)	Prostate cancer RM-1 mice model (administration: injection) 40 μg per mouse (13 days)	- ↑ M1 macrophages in cancer in vitro - ↑ proportion of CD8+ and IFN-γ+ T cells in mice - ↓ 60% tumor growth in mice - ↓ proliferation of prostate cells	- Antitumor response and immunotherapy applications for prostate cancer	[92]

Table 2. *Cont.*

Bacterial Producer	In Vitro Model EVs Treatment (Duration)	In Vivo Model EVs Treatment (Duration)	Observations on EVs Activity	EVs Properties	Reference
	LX-2 cells (inflammation model) 1, 10, 50 μg/mL (24 h)	Chronic liver injury in 7–8-week-old male C57BL/6 mice (administration: intraperitoneal injection) 50 μg protein/200 μL (4 weeks)	- ↓ TNF-α and IL-6 and ↑ IL-10 levels in mice - ↓ expression *of a-SMA, pdgf, timp*, and *Col1a1* genes in cells - ↓ *tlr-2* and *tlr-4* gene expression in cells	- Improvement of intestinal permeability - Modulation of inflammatory responses - Prevention of liver injury	[70]
	Caco-2 and Hep-G2 cells 50, 100 μg/mL (24 h)	*ND*	- ↑ mRNA level of FAAH and PPARα gene in both Caco-2 and Hep-G2 cells - ↑ mRNA level of PPARϒ gene in Caco-2 cells - ↑ mRNA level of the CB2R in Hep-G2 cells - ↑ transcription level of the PPARα gene in Hep-G2 cells - ↑ mRNA level of the PPARβ/δ gene in Hep-G2 cells - ↓ mRNA level of CB1R and CB2R in Caco-2 cells	- Prevention of metabolic disorders associated with obesity - Stimulation of fatty acid oxidation and energy metabolism - Control of the activity of ECS compartments (involved in obesity, metabolic disorders, and liver diseases)	[53]
Akkermansia muciniphila ATCC BAA-835	LX-2 cells (inflammation model) 1, 10, 50 μg/mL (24 h)	Livery injury in 8-week-old male C57BL/6 mice (administration: oral gavage) 50 μg protein/200 μL (4 weeks)	- ↑ mRNA level of *ppar-α, ppar-γ*, and *igf* in cells - ↓ *tlr-5* and *tlr-9* gene mRNA level in cells - ↓ TNF-α and IL-6 levels in mouse	- Enhancement of anti-inflammatory responses of the colon, adipose, and liver tissues	[134]
A. muciniphila ATCC BAA-835, *Faecalibacterium prausnitzii* A2-165c	Caco-2 cells 1 and 50 μg/mL (24 h)	*ND*	- ↑ serotonin level - ↑ expression of *Tph1, Htr3B, Htr2B, Slc6a4*, and *Htr4*	- Role in the homeostasis maintenance of the serotonin system	[15]
A. muciniphila ATCC BAA-835, *L. plantarum* KCTC 11401BP, *Bacillus subtilis* *	HT22 cells (stress model) 20 μg (24 h)	Chronic stress in 7-week-old male C57BL6 mice (administration: intraperitoneal injection) 6 μg/100 μL mouse per day (14 days)	- ↑ *Bdnf, Nt3*, and/or *Nt4/5* in mice - ↑ *Bdnf* and *Nt4/5* in cells - ↓ immobility in TST in mice	- Anti-depressive-like effect and restoration of stress levels (especially by *L. plantarum* EVs)	[130]
Lactiplantibacillus plantarum KCTC 11401BP	HT22 cells (stress model) 20 μg/mL (24 h)	Depression in 7-week-old male C57BL/6J mice (administration: intraperitoneal injection) 0.1, 0.18, and 0.27 μg/kg (1–35 days)	- ↑ *tBdnf, Bdnf1, Bdnf4*, and *Ngf* in cells - ↑ *Sirt1* in cells - ↑ *Bdnf1, Bdnf4*, and *Nt4/5* in mouse	- Antidepressant-like effects	[129]
	HaCaT cells and keratinocytes 0.1, 1, and 10 μg/mL (12 h)	*S. aureus* atopic dermatitis-induced mouse model (administration: oral gavage)	- ↓ IL-6 secretion in cells and mice stimulated with *S. aureus* EVs - ↓ epidermal thickening in mice	- Preventive effect on skin inflammation	[55]

Table 2. *Cont.*

Bacterial Producer	In Vitro Model EVs Treatment (Duration)	In Vivo Model EVs Treatment (Duration)	Observations on EVs Activity	EVs Properties	Reference
Lactiplantibacillus plantarum APsulloc 331261	THP1 cells 10 μg/mL (48 h)	Human skin organ culture (ex vivo) 50 μg/mL (2–4 days)	- ↑ IL-10, IL-1β, and GM-CFS - ↑ M2-polarized cell markers	- Anti-inflammatory effect through macrophage polarization	[50]
Lactiplantibacillus plantarum WCFS1	Caco-2 cells 500 μL (24 h)	*C. elegans* Bristol N2 EVs isolated from 10^9 CFU (1–15 days)	- ↑ *CTSB* and *REG3G* expression (cells) - ↑ gene expression of C-type lectin *clec-60* and the gut-specific cysteine protease *cpr-1* - (*C. elegans*)	- Antimicrobial effect - Host defense enhancement against infections	[32]
Lactiplantibacillus plantarum Q7	*ND*	Colitis in 4–5-week-old SPF male C57BL/6J mice (administration: gavage) 10/20 mg Q7-EVs group (0.5/1 mg/kg body weight) (1–18 days)	- ↑ *Bifidobacterium*, *Rikenellaceae*_RC9_gut_group, *Akkermansia*, Muribaculaceae, *Lactobacillus*, and *Alitipes* in gut microbiota - ↓ IL-1β, IL-2, IL-6, and TNF-α - ↓ colon shortening - ↓ spleen index	- Colitis alleviation - Regulation of intestinal microbiota - Anti-inflammatory properties	[93]
Lactiplantibacillus plantarum *	CCD-986Sk cells 0.625%, 1.25%, 5%, and 10% EVs (24 h)	Korean women in their 50s (administration: topically on the skin) (twice a day, 4 weeks)	- ↑ fibroblasts proliferation - ↑ expression of ECM components (Type 1 procollagen, filaggrin, HAS2) - ↑ water content in the skin - ↓ mRNA of MMP-1 - ↓ elastase activity - ↓ distribution and formation of wrinkles - ↓ pigmentation of the lesion sites	- Anti-aging and anti-pigmentation effect	[87]
Lactiplantibacillus plantarum YW11	Primary cortical neurons from C57BL/6 mice (OGD model) Co-culturing with EVs (24 h)	tMCAO (ischemic stroke model) in 10–12-week-old male C57BL/6 mice (administration: injection through the tail vein) 100 μg/day (3 days)	- ↑ miR-101a-3p expression and blocking of c-Fos/TGF-β axis in neurons - ↓ Bax and caspase 3 and ↑ Bcl-2 - ↓ neurological deficits and infarct size in tMCAO mice	- Anti-apoptotic effect on ischemic neurons both in vivo and in vitro	[86]
Lacticaseibacillus casei BL23	T84 and HT-29 cells 20 ng/mL to 10 μg/mL (24 h)	*ND*	- ↑ EGFR phosphorylation caused by P40 and P75 bounds to EVs	- Immunomodulatory effects	[35]
Lacticaseibacillus casei ATCC 393	Caco-2 cells 100 and 150 μg/mL (24 h)	*ND*	- ↑ IL-10, IL-4, IL-6, and GM-CSF - ↓ IFNγ - ↓ *TLR9* expression	- Immunomodulatory effects	[37]
L. casei DSMZ 20011, *L. plantarum* NCIMB 8826	Caco-2 and THP-1 cells (inflammation model) 5×10^{11}–5×10^{12} EVs/mL (24 h)	*ND*	- ↑ IL-10 - ↓ TNF-α and IL-8	- Anti-inflammatory properties	[83]

Table 2. *Cont.*

Bacterial Producer	In Vitro Model EVs Treatment (Duration)	In Vivo Model EVs Treatment (Duration)	Observations on EVs Activity	EVs Properties	Reference
	THP-1 cells (inflammation model) 1:2 EVs per well (48 h)	*ND*	- ↑ IL-10 - ↓ TNF-α	- Anti-inflammatory properties	[31]
Lacticaseibacillus paracasei *	RAW 264.7 cells (inflammation model) 0.1, 1, 10, 50 μg/mL (12 h) HT 29 cells (inflammation model) 500 ng/mL (12 h)	Acute colitis-induced 7-week-old male C57BL/6 mice (administration: oral gavage) 5 mg/day (12 days)	- ↑ ER-stress-associated proteins (CHOP, p-PERK, p-IRE1, and cleaved ATF6) in cells - ↑ IL-10 and TGFβ in both models - ↓ IL-1α, IL-1β, IL-2, TNFα, and NO in cells - ↓ COX-2 and iNOS expression in both models	- Anti-inflammatory effect through the activation of ER stress - Protective properties in an acute colitis-induced mouse model	[58]
Lacticaseibacillus paracasei PC-H1	Colorectal cancer cell line, HCT116, SW1116, and SW620 cells 200 μg/mL (24 h)	4-week-old female BALB/c nude mice (administration with HCT116 and EVs through subcutaneous injection) 200 μg/mL (30 days)	- ↑ apoptosis in cancer cells - ↓ growth of tumor tissue in mice	- Inhibition of colon cancer cell migration and invasion through apoptosis activation	[90]
Lactobacillus crispatus BC3, BC5; *Lactobacillus gasseri* BC12, BC13	Human T-lymphocyte MT-4 and Jurkat-tat cell lines 50 μL (1–72 h)	Human tissue cultures (ex vivo model) 10^8 EVs/mL (12 days)	- ↓ HIV replication	- Anti-viral properties by EVs from *L. gasseri* B12	[74]
Limosilactobacillus reuteri BBC3	HD11 cells 10 μg/mL (6 h or 12 h) Splenic lymphocytes 10 μg/mL (12 h)	Broiler chicks (inflammation model) (administration: oral gavage) 200 μg/bird (21 days) Jejunum explant culture (ex vivo model) (inflammation model) 10 μg/mL (6 h)	- ↑ IL-10 and TGF-β (jejunum and cells) - ↓ TNF-α, IL-1β, IL-6, IL-17, IL-8, and MIP-1β in jejunum and cells	- Anti-inflammatory properties - Immunomodulatory effect	[34]
Lacticaseibacillus rhamnosus GG	HepG2 cells 50, 100, 150, and 200 μg (24 h)	*ND*	- ↑ *bac/bcl-2* gene expression - ↑ apoptosis	- Anti-proliferative effect on liver cancer cells	[56]
	SW480 and HT 29 cells (human colon cancer cell lines) 5–200 μg/mL (24 h)	*ND*	- ↑ expression of *cea* gene and CEA protein synthesis - inhibitory effects on both cell lines	- Anti-proliferative effect on cancer cells	[57]
	ND	Colitis-induced 4–5-week-old C57BL/6J male mice (administration: oral gavage) 1.2 mg/kg of body weight (14 days)	- ↑ the α-diversity of gut microbiota (Firmicutes and Bacteroidetes) - ↓ body weight - ↓ colon shortening - ↓ IL-1β, IL-2, IL-6, and TNF-α	- Anti-inflammatory effect - Colitis amelioration	[94]

Table 2. *Cont.*

Bacterial Producer	In Vitro Model EVs Treatment (Duration)	In Vivo Model EVs Treatment (Duration)	Observations on EVs Activity	EVs Properties	Reference
Lacticaseibacillus rhamnosus JB-1	HT-29 and MODE-K cells 3×10^{10} EVs (2 h)	8- to 10-week-old SPF BALB/c male mice (administration: oral gavage) 3×10^{10} EVs (2 h)	- ↑ Toll-like receptor 2 (TLR2) - ↑ IL-10 - EVs contain immunologically active lipoteichoic acid (LTA)	- Enrollment of LTA on immunoregulatory activity	[88]
L. rhamnosus GG, *L. reuteri* DSM 17938	PBMCs cells 500:1, 100:1, and 20:1 (48 h)	*ND*	- ↑ IL-6, IL-10, IL-17A, and IFN-γ	- Immunomodulatory properties	[135]
Lentilactobacillus kefirgranum PRCC-1301	Caco-2 and HCT116 cells 0, 10, and 100 μg/mL (6–48 h)	Colitis-induced 6-week-old male C57BL/6 mice (administration: oral gavage) 3 mg/kg (3–14 days)	- ↑ ZO-1, claudin, and occludin in cells - ↓ IL-2, IL-8, and TNF-α in cells - ↓ shortening of the colon length in chronic colitis (mice)	- Enhancement of the intestinal barrier integrity (TJ) - Attenuation of chronic colitis - Anti-inflammatory effect	[118]
Lentilactobacillus kefir KCTC 3611, *Lentilactobacillus kefiranofaciens* KCTC 5075, *Lentilactobacillus kefirgranum* KCTC 5086	Caco-2 cells (inflammation model) 1×10^9 EVs/mL (24 h)	IBD-induced 8-week-old male BALB mice (administration: oral gavage) (3×10^8 or 3×10^{10} EVs/head)	- ↓ IL-8 in cells - ↓ TNBS-induced infiltration of transmural leukocyte and loss of goblet cells in mice	- Preventing of enterorrhagia and diarrhea - Reduction of MPO activity - Anti-inflammatory properties	[60]
Latilactobacillus sakei NBRC 15893	PP and BMDCs from BALB/c mice (female, 7–14 weeks old) 30 μg protein/mL (4 days)	*ND*	- ↑ IgA in PP cells - ↑ expression *of IL-6, IL-10, IL-12, TNF-α,* and *NOS2* in BMDCs - ↑ NO and RA production	- Immunomodulatory effect	[125]
	PP cells 37 μg/mL EVs (1–4 days)	*ND*	- ↑ IL-6 production via TLR2 signal - ↑ IgA level	- Activation of the mucosal immune system	[61]
Ligilactobacillus animalis ATCC 35046	HMECs, MLO-Y4, MC3T3-E1, and BMSCs(MPS-treated) 10 μg/mL (6–24 h)	GC-induced ONFH male C57BL/6J mice (administration: oral gavage) 30 μg/200 μL (once a week)	- ↑ tube formation of the MPS-treated HMECs - ↑ BMSCs mineralization in BMSCs - ↑ blood vessel volume and numbers of CD31-positive endothelial cells and OCN-stained osteoblasts in MPS-treated mice - ↓ MPS-induced negative effect on osteogenic differentiation of BMSCs - ↓ MPS-induced apoptosis of HMECs, MLO-Y4, MC3T3-E1, and BMSCs - ↓ apoptotic cell number and serum levels of IL-2 and IFN-γ in MPS-treated mice	- Prevention of GC-induced ONFH	[76]

Table 2. *Cont.*

Bacterial Producer	In Vitro Model EVs Treatment (Duration)	In Vivo Model EVs Treatment (Duration)	Observations on EVs Activity	EVs Properties	Reference
Lactobacillus johnsonii N6.2	Pancreatic cell line βlox5, Caco-2, Jurkat, and THP-1 cells 10^8 or 10^{10} EVs/mL (2–8 h)	Pancreatic islets isolated from human donors(ex vivo model) 6×10^9 EVs/mL (5 h)	- ↑ OAS1, OAS3, AHR pathways, CYP1A1, and CYP1B1 in βlox5 cells - ↑ GLUT6, SREBF1, PRKACA, and mRNA of GLP1R - ↑ MTA2 and STC2 and ↓ SOD1 in pancreatic islets - ↑ CYP1A1 in THP-1 and Caco-2 cells - ↑ TNFα, IL-1β, IL10, TLR2, and TLR7 in THP-1 cells - ↑ T-STAT3/actin and pYSTAT3/T-STAT3 ratio in THP-1 cells	- Dose-dependent protection against apoptosis in pancreatic beta cell line - Stimulation of insulin release in human islets under high glucose stimulation - Regulation of intra-islets environment - Potential protective effect against insulin - resistance and in type 2 diabetes metabolic syndrome	[136]
Lactococcus lactis *	Dendritic cells isolated from asthmatic patients 10 μg/mL (24 h)	Allergic asthma-induced 6-week-old female BALB/c mice (administration: intranasally) 10 μg/20 μL PBS (5 days)	- ↑ IFN-γ in the BALF of mice - ↑ secretion of IL-12p70 from dendritic cells - ↓ IL-5 and IL-13 - ↓ expression of GATA-3 and phosphorylation of STAT6	- Immuno-modulating effect in allergic airway inflammation - Regulation of allergic response by enhancing Th1 immune activation	[95]
Bifidobacterium longum KACC 91563	PP, T cells, B cells, eosinophils, and BMCCs from mice 2 μg/mL (2 h)	Food allergy-induced 6- to 8-week-old BALB/c mice (administration: oral gavage) EVs from 10^9 CFU/mouse (2 weeks)	- ↑ annexin V+ apoptotic cells in mast cells - ↓ mast cell numbers	- Therapeutic effect on food allergy through apoptosis	[137]
Bifidobacterium bifidum LMG 13195	Monocyte-derived DCs and naïve T cells 0.1 μg/mL (48 h)	*ND*	- ↑ IL-10 - ↑ differentiation of $CD25^{high}$ $FOXP3^{high}$ $CD127^{-/low}$ Treg cells	- Immunotherapy application (SIT vaccines)	[138]
B. longum *, *L. plantarum* WCFS1	DC2.4 and RAW264.7 cells 0.01 or 0.1 μg/well (6–24 h)	*ND*	- ↑ TNF-α and IL-6 - ↓ TNF-α and IL-6 from DC2.4 after inhibition of the clathrin-mediated endocytosis or macropinocytosis pathway	- Immunomodulatory effect through clathrin-mediated endocytosis and macropinocytosis	[85]
	DC2.4 and RAW264.7 cells 0.5 μg/well (6 h)	*ND*	- ↑ TNF-α and IL-6 - ↓ TNF-α and IL-6 in the presence of TLR2 inhibition	- Immunomodulatory effect through TLR-2 signaling	[84]

Table 2. *Cont.*

Bacterial Producer	In Vitro Model EVs Treatment (Duration)	In Vivo Model EVs Treatment (Duration)	Observations on EVs Activity	EVs Properties	Reference
Propionibacterium freudenreichii CIRM-BIA 129	HT-29 cells (inflammation model) 10^9 EVs/mL (1 h)	*ND*	- ↓ NF-kB activation - ↓ IL-8	- Anti-inflammatory and immunomodulatory properties through NF-kB pathway	[78]
	HT-29 cells (inflammation model) 10^9 EVs/mL (24 h)	*ND*	- ↓ IL-8 especially with LPS-induced inflammation - ↓ NF-kB activation especially with LPS-induced inflammation	- Anti-inflammatory properties (depending on the media conditions)	[79]
Bacillus subtilis 168	Caco-2 cells 1.3 × 10^9 EVs (0–4 h)	*ND*	- - Uptake of MVs by transcytosis (dose-dependent)	- Immunomodulatory properties through transcytosis	[80]
Clostridium butyricum MIYAIRI 588	*ND*	Ulcerative colitis in 40–60-day-old male C57BL/6 mice (administration: intragastrically) 15 μg/200 μL (once a day, 5 days)	- Inhibition of disease progression and reduction of mortality rate - ↑ MUC2 and ZO-1 - ↑ Bacilli, Bacteroidia, and Verrucomicrobiae - ↑ proportion of M2 cells and ↓ M1 cells in the gut - ↓ inflammation and tissue damage - ↓ Enterobacteriaceae, Helicobacteraceae, and Lachnospiraceae	- Re-establishment of M1/M2 in UC models - Reversing of the gut microbial dysbiosis - Protective effect against UC	[82]
	ND	Ulcerative colitis-induced male C57BL6J mice (administration: oral gavage) 50 μg/day (11 days)	- ↑ expression of *Muc1*, *Muc2*, *Muc3*, *Muc4*, *Claudin1*, *Claudin3*, *Zo-1*, *Svs1*, *Doxl2*, and *Rik* genes - ↑ ERK1 and ERK2 cascades - ↑ *Ruminiclostridium* and Ruminococcaceae in the gut - ↓ LPS, IL-6, and TNF-α - ↓ inflammatory cell infiltration and mucus layer damage in the colon - ↓ expression of *Tlr4*, *Nf-kb*, *TNF-α*, *F4/80*, *Cd11c*, *Mcp1*, and *Ccl5* genes	- Protection of gut barrier function - Modulation of gut microbiota homeostasis - Reduction of ulcerative colitis symptoms - Anti-inflammatory properties	[81]
Leuconostoc holzapfelii GFC1203H, *L. plantarum* *, *B. longum* *, *B. animalis* *, *L. acidophilus* *	Human HFDP cells 1, 2.5, 5, and 10 μg/mL (6 h, 12 h, 24 h)	*ND*	- ↑ cell migration and cell proliferation (7 to 24%) - ↑ Bcl-2 and Bax - ↑ Wnt5A, Wnt10B, β-catenin, VSC, Lef1, BAMBI, and BMP-2 - ↓ sub-G1 phase and ↑ G2/M phase - ↓ Caspase-3 activity	- Anti-apoptotic effect - Induction of cell division, migration, and proliferation - Induction of hair growth	[77]

Table 2. *Cont.*

Bacterial Producer	In Vitro Model EVs Treatment (Duration)	In Vivo Model EVs Treatment (Duration)	Observations on EVs Activity	EVs Properties	Reference
Pediococcus pentosaceus *, *Ligilactobacillus salivarius* *	E.G7–EL4 and HEK-BLUE hTLR2, BMDCsMouse splenocytes (inflammation model) 0.2, 1, and 5 mg/mL (24 h)	Liver-fibrosis in 6- to 8-week-old male C57BL/6 mice (administration: injection) 10 μg/mouse (14 days)	- ↓ aSMA expression - ↑ collagen in the liver - ↑ M2 polarization - ↑ TLR-2 signaling	- Immunomodulatory effect and inflammatory properties	[42]

Abbreviations: *ND*, no data; MVs, membrane vesicles; EPEC, enteropathogenic *Escherichia coli*; TJ, tight junctions; TNF, tumor necrosis factor; IL, interleukin; IκBα, nuclear factor of kappa light polypeptide gene enhancer in B-cells inhibitor; NOD, nucleotide-binding oligomerization domain; TGF, transforming growth factor; TLR. toll-like receptor; HFD, high-fat diet; ND, normal diet; PP, Peyer's Patch; IgA, immunoglobulin A; ZO, zonula occludens; OCLDN, occludin; CLDN, claudin; TLR, toll-like receptor; PPAR, peroxisome proliferator-activated receptors; Angptl4, angiopoietin-like 4; HT-29, human colonic epithelial; MODE-K, mouse duodenal epithelial; GC, glucocorticoid; TST, tail suspension test; BDNF, brain-derived neurotrophic factor; Sirt1, sirtuin 1; GM-CFS, granulocyte-macrophage colony-stimulating factor; *CTSB*, cysteine proteinase; *REG3G*, C-type Lectin; SIT, allergen-specific immunotherapy; LTA, lipoteichoic acid; NFKβ, nuclear factor kappa-light-chain-enhancer of activated B cells; LPS, lipopolysaccharides; CG, glucocorticoid; Sirt1, Sirtuin 1; PMBCs, peripheral blood mononuclear cells; ER, endoplasmatic reticulum; BMCCs, bone marrow-derived mast cells; MPO, myeloperoxidase; HMECs, human microvascular endothelial cells; MLO-Y4, mouse long bone osteocyte-Y4; MC3T3-E1, mouse preosteoblast cells; BMSCs, mouse bone marrow mesenchymal stem cells; ONFH, osteonecrosis of the femoral head; MPS, methylprednisolone; CB1R and CB2R, cannabinoid receptors; FAAH, fatty acid amide hydrolase; PPARs, peroxisome proliferator-activated receptors; ECS, endocannabinoid system; CCD-986Sk, human dermal fibroblasts; MMP-1, matrix metalloproteinase-1; ECM, extracellular matrix; HAS2, hyaluronidase 2; CEA, carcinoembryonic antigen; OVA, ovalbumin; BALF, bronchoalveolar lavage fluid; UC, ulcerative colitis; MUC2, mucin 2; ZO-1, zonula occludens protein 1; M2, M2 macrophages; M1, M1 macrophages; OAS, 2′,5′-oligoadenylate synthetase; AHR, aryl hydrocarbon receptor; CYP1A1 and CYP1B1, cytochrome P450 superfamily enzymes; GLUT6, glucose transporter 6; SREBF1, sterol regulatory element binding transcription factor 1; GLP1R, glucagon-like peptide 1 receptor; PRKACA, protein kinase catalytic subunit α; MTA2, metastasis-associated 1 family member 2; STC2, stanniocalcin-2; SOD1, superoxide dismutase 1; tMCAO, transient middle cerebral artery occlusion; OGD, oxygen-glucose deprivation; HFDPCs, human hair follicle dermal papilla cells. * Bacterial strain was not reported.

3.4. Future Application and Perspectives on EVs Produced by Probiotics

Unquestionably, we consider it very optimistic to find an exponential increase over the last decade in the number of publications on the production of probiotic EVs. For example, in 2012, only a single research article was published, while, in the first half of 2022 alone, as many as 15 original papers were released. Because of such a high dynamic of new articles appearing, during our analysis of the already collected literature and preparation of the central core of the manuscript's discussion, we were unable to include newly-published articles from the second half of 2022. In this regard, however, we would like to point out that seven more original articles appeared during this time. These studies showed the protective effect of probiotic EVs on atopic dermatitis [139] and various intestinal pathologies (chemoresistant colorectal cancer [140] or intestinal infections made by enterotoxigenic *E. coli* [141]). It was also noticed that probiotic EVs have a strong immunomodulatory effect on the human body (including the intestines) [142], and that they can be used in the design of innovative vaccines against infectious diseases [143] and cancers [122]. In the last publication, attention was drawn to the participation of prophages in the secretion of EVs by the tested probiotic bacteria [144].

The latest research, together with the papers already analyzed in this review, lead us to highlight multiple applications of probiotic EVs. As previously mentioned, the close interconnection between probiotics and the gastrointestinal system is of great interest. In this context, EVs could represent a new strategy for the treatment of metabolic diseases, such as diabetes and obesity. There is evidence supporting the role of diet in shaping the host microbiota and the release of gut microbiota EVs, which, in turn, can exert their beneficial effect on human gut homeostasis [145]. In addition, another study showed that probiotic-derived EVs have a protective effect on Caco-2/HT29-MTX co-cultures exposed to enterotoxigenic *E. coli*, confirming the role of this bacterial structure in the maintenance of intestinal barrier integrity [141]. Considering their application in perspective, some authors also suggest that the administration of probiotic EVs alone could be a safer alternative than delivering live probiotics, especially in immunocompromised patients [146–148]. Moreover, in relation to some probiotic strains, the use of EVs alone could also represent an advantage in terms of efficacy. For example, Pang et al. [141] noted that EVs of *L. reuteri* DSM 17938 are more effective in the treatment of infantile colic compared to the bacterial cells of this strain.

Taking into account their biological properties, probiotic EVs could also be used for the treatment of certain neurological diseases. In fact, having the potential to cross the blood–brain barrier, they could represent efficient transporters for the delivery of drugs into the central nervous system [11]. Yuan et al. [149] and Sun et al. [150] extensively reported in their reviews the potential application of EVs-based strategies in the treatment of neurological disorders. Although in those papers only eukaryotic cells-based vesicles were considered, we cannot ignore the fact that they show comparable structure and properties to bacterial ones, which lead us to believe that a similar application of probiotics-derived EVs is reasonable. In a recent work, González-Lozano et al. [148] reported several examples of EVs' applications in neurological disorders, focusing on their ability to transport active bacterial-produced compounds through different body districts. In addition, it is worth highlighting that the possibility to engineer EVs to improve their properties also exists. In this context, the surface modification can improve the EVs' targeting capability and, as a consequence, their therapeutic potential [150]. To sum up, EVs biocompatibility, size, and drug delivering capabilities make them promising tools for future biomedical applications [147].

3.5. Challenges and Limitations of Articles Focusing on EVs Produced by Probiotics

As a summary, below, we would like to draw attention to a few challenges and limitations, the consideration of which may help the scientific community in an even more robust and reliable study of EVs produced by probiotics in the future.

We discovered that most research on the above topic focuses on the properties of EVs produced by Gram-positive bacteria; however, research on *E. coli* or *A. muciniphila* shows that the health-promoting properties of EVs of Gram-negative bacteria can be equally valuable (Table S1 and Table 2). It is also worth mentioning that other probiotic microorganisms, including yeasts of the genus *Saccharomyces*, have many health-benefiting properties [151] and EVs produced by them could possibly constitute very valuable therapeutics. For this reason, we would like to encourage scientists to increase the pool of tested microorganisms not only with new strains of the bacterial species tested so far, but also with novel genera or families of microorganisms [152,153].

The second aspect we would like to discuss is insufficiently low attention paid to characterizing biological and physicochemical properties of EVs produced by probiotics. As we proved in Figure 1 and Table S1, when undertaking such an analysis, it is mostly limited only to estimating the size of EVs. Other parameters were determined either rarely (electric charge and quantity) or extremely rarely (spatial orientation of EVs' membranes or biological origin). Since we have already discussed the subject of electric charge and quantity of probiotic EVs, here, we would like to pay special attention to the second group of parameters. In none of the articles we analyzed, the spatial orientation of EVs (inside-out or right-side-out) was determined. The issue of the biological origin of EVs, and, thus, the precise nomenclature of isolated structures, has also been addressed sporadically. In most of the original articles, the term 'extracellular vesicles' (43) or 'membrane vesicles' (16) was used, while the presence of EVs' subpopulations was included in only one article [51]. It is worth mentioning that cell lysis can be a significant source of EVs, and, hence, determining its intensity is also of importance [96,112]. Again, however, this phenomenon was rarely established (only in two publications [62,66]). In connection to the above description, we would like to sensitize scientists to increase their attention toward characterizing the properties of probiotic EVs and include "minimal information for studies of extracellular vesicles", as recommended by the International Society for Extracellular Vesicles [18].

Another aspect we would like to highlight is the proteomic analysis of probiotic EVs. We noticed that, despite the relatively high methodological homogeneity, consisting of ultracentrifugation followed by electrophoresis combined with LC-MS/MS or MALDI-TOF, a large discrepancy within the data was noticed (Table 1). The total number of identified proteins (understood as whole-length gene products) ranged from as low as a dozen [74] to as high as over a thousand [54,62]. Still, however, in most articles, these values were within the range of several hundred. The phenomenon of under- or over-representation of identified EVs' proteins may be caused by two sources—the sensitivity of the research techniques and the level of contamination of the EVs' proteome with proteins derived from bacterial cells secreting these structures [40,96,97]. In line with this, we propose to make serious considerations for changing the techniques of isolation and analysis of EVs if the proteome of these structures is either too sparse or too numerous (especially when over-represented by cytoplasmic proteins).

Finally, the last issue worth recalling is the scope of the conducted research. In Table 2, we extensively presented the data of original articles describing biological activities of EVs produced by probiotics. As it can be relatively easily observed, a large amount of research on EVs produced by probiotics focuses on the evaluation of the biological effect of these structures only on the gastrointestinal system. For obvious reasons, including the ingestible administration of probiotic EVs, the action of these structures on the digestive system is highly intuitive and justified [154,155]. However, it should still be remembered that EVs, due to their nanometric dimensions, can reach various tissues of the host, and, therefore, their effect on different types of human cells should be discovered [13,156]. As described in this review, a good example of a different approach to evaluating the biological activity of probiotic EVs is the original article aimed at the skin [55,87] or the nervous system [129,130]. Undoubtedly, the health-promoting impact of probiotic EVs on the host should be extended to many other organs untested yet, such as the oral cavity, cardiovascular system, respiratory system, or genitourinary system.

4. Conclusions

Many decades of numerous studies on probiotics have confirmed their health-promoting effect on humans. Despite this, knowledge about the activity of EVs produced by probiotic microorganisms is still in its infancy. As our detailed review of the literature shows, in the last decade, the awareness on the usefulness of these structures is, however, dynamically growing. A broad variety of benefits of using EVs secreted by probiotics have already been shown, including regulation of intestinal homeostasis on both microbiota and host metabolism levels, anti-depressive activity, and immunostimulation, leading to a better control of microbial and carcinogenic disorders. We hope that the coming years will bring even more groundbreaking discoveries on these topics.

Supplementary Materials: The following supporting information can be downloaded at: https://www.mdpi.com/article/10.3390/pharmaceutics15020522/s1, Table S1: Detailed data on physicochemical properties of extracellular vesicles produced by probiotics.

Author Contributions: Conceptualization, P.K. and R.G.; methodology, P.K.; formal analysis, P.K., B.M., I.V.; writing—original draft preparation, P.K., B.M. and I.V.; writing—review and editing, P.K., B.M., I.V. and R.G.; visualization, P.K.; supervision, P.K. and R.G.; funding acquisition, P.K. All authors have read and agreed to the published version of the manuscript.

Funding: The study was supported by the Wroclaw Medical University grant No: SUBZ.A130.23.070. The funders had no role in the study design, data collection, and analysis, decision to publish, or preparation of the manuscript.

Conflicts of Interest: The authors declare no conflict of interest.

References

1. You, S.; Ma, Y.; Yan, B.; Pei, W.; Wu, Q.; Ding, C.; Huang, C. The Promotion Mechanism of Prebiotics for Probiotics: A Review. *Front. Nutr.* **2022**, *9*, 1000517. [CrossRef]
2. Ogunrinola, G.A.; Oyewale, J.O.; Oshamika, O.O.; Olasehinde, G.I. The Human Microbiome and Its Impacts on Health. *Int. J. Microbiol.* **2020**, *2020*, 8045646. [CrossRef]
3. Hou, K.; Wu, Z.X.; Chen, X.Y.; Wang, J.Q.; Zhang, D.; Xiao, C.; Zhu, D.; Koya, J.B.; Wei, L.; Li, J.; et al. Microbiota in Health and Diseases. *Signal Transduct. Target. Ther.* **2022**, *7*, 135. [CrossRef]
4. Depoorter, L.; Vandenplas, Y. Probiotics in Pediatrics. A Review and Practical Guide. *Nutrients* **2021**, *13*, 2176. [CrossRef]
5. Varela-Trinidad, G.U.; Domínguez-Díaz, C.; Solórzano-Castanedo, K.; Íñiguez-Gutiérrez, L.; Hernández-Flores, T.D.J.; Fafutis-Morris, M. Probiotics: Protecting Our Health from the Gut. *Microorganisms* **2022**, *10*, 1428. [CrossRef]
6. Ranjha, M.M.A.N.; Shafique, B.; Batool, M.; Kowalczewski, P.Ł.; Shehzad, Q.; Usman, M.; Manzoor, M.F.; Zahra, S.M.; Yaqub, S.; Aadil, R.M. Nutritional and Health Potential of Probiotics: A Review. *Appl. Sci.* **2021**, *11*, 11204. [CrossRef]
7. Wang, G.; Chen, Y.; Xia, Y.; Song, X.; Ai, L. Characteristics of Probiotic Preparations and Their Applications. *Foods* **2022**, *11*, 2472. [CrossRef]
8. Thorakkattu, P.; Khanashyam, A.C.; Shah, K.; Babu, K.S.; Mundanat, A.S.; Deliephan, A.; Deokar, G.S.; Santivarangkna, C.; Nirmal, N.P. Postbiotics: Current Trends in Food and Pharmaceutical Industry. *Foods* **2022**, *11*, 3094. [CrossRef]
9. Maccelli, A.; Carradori, S.; Puca, V.; Sisto, F.; Lanuti, P.; Crestoni, M.E.; Lasalvia, A.; Muraro, R.; Bysell, H.; Sotto, A.D.; et al. Correlation between the Antimicrobial Activity and Metabolic Profiles of Cell Free Supernatants and Membrane Vesicles Produced by *Lactobacillus reuteri* DSM 17938. *Microorganisms* **2020**, *8*, 1653. [CrossRef]
10. Sabahi, S.; Homayouni Rad, A.; Aghebati-Maleki, L.; Sangtarash, N.; Ozma, M.A.; Karimi, A.; Hosseini, H.; Abbasi, A. Postbiotics as the New Frontier in Food and Pharmaceutical Research. *Crit. Rev. Food Sci. Nutr.* **2022**, 1–28. [CrossRef]
11. Srivastava, P.; Kim, K. Membrane Vesicles Derived from Gut Microbiota and Probiotics: Cutting-Edge Therapeutic Approaches for Multidrug-Resistant Superbugs Linked to Neurological Anomalies. *Pharmaceutics* **2022**, *14*, 2370. [CrossRef] [PubMed]
12. Aggarwal, S.; Sabharwal, V.; Kaushik, P.; Joshi, A.; Aayushi, A.; Suri, M. Postbiotics: From Emerging Concept to Application. *Front. Sustain. Food Syst.* **2022**, *6*, 887642. [CrossRef]
13. Viswanathan, K.; Muthusamy, S. Review on the Current Trends and Future Perspectives of Postbiotics for Developing Healtheir Foods. *eFood* **2022**, *3*, e47. [CrossRef]
14. Salminen, S.; Collado, M.C.; Endo, A.; Hill, C.; Lebeer, S.; Quigley, E.M.M.; Sanders, M.E.; Shamir, R.; Swann, J.R.; Szajewska, H.; et al. The International Scientific Association of Probiotics and Prebiotics (ISAPP) Consensus Statement on the Definition and Scope of Postbiotics. *Nat. Rev. Gastroenterol. Hepatol.* **2021**, *18*, 649–667. [CrossRef]
15. Zou, C.; Zhang, Y.; Liu, H.; Wu, Y.; Zhou, X. Extracellular Vesicles: Recent Insights Into the Interaction Between Host and Pathogenic Bacteria. *Front. Immunol.* **2022**, *13*, 840550. [CrossRef]
16. Combo, S.; Mendes, S.; Nielsen, K.M.; da Silva, G.J.; Domingues, S. The Discovery of the Role of Outer Membrane Vesicles against Bacteria. *Biomedicines* **2022**, *10*, 2399. [CrossRef]
17. Srivatsav, A.T.; Kapoor, S. The Emerging World of Membrane Vesicles: Functional Relevance, Theranostic Avenues and Tools for Investigating Membrane Function. *Front. Mol. Biosci.* **2021**, *8*, 59. [CrossRef]
18. Théry, C.; Witwer, K.W.; Aikawa, E.; Alcaraz, M.J.; Anderson, J.D.; Andriantsitohaina, R.; Antoniou, A.; Arab, T.; Archer, F.; Atkin-Smith, G.K.; et al. Minimal Information for Studies of Extracellular Vesicles 2018 (MISEV2018): A Position Statement of the International Society for Extracellular Vesicles and Update of the MISEV2014 Guidelines. *J. Extracell. Vesicles* **2018**, *7*, 1535750. [CrossRef]
19. Liu, H.; Zhang, Q.; Wang, S.; Weng, W.; Jing, Y.; Su, J. Bacterial Extracellular Vesicles as Bioactive Nanocarriers for Drug Delivery: Advances and Perspectives. *Bioact. Mater.* **2022**, *14*, 169–181. [CrossRef]
20. Huang, Y.; Nieh, M.P.; Chen, W.; Lei, Y. Outer Membrane Vesicles (OMVs) Enabled Bio-applications: A Critical Review. *Biotechnol. Bioeng.* **2022**, *119*, 34–47. [CrossRef]
21. Macion, A.; Wyszyńska, A.; Godlewska, R. Delivery of Toxins and Effectors by Bacterial Membrane Vesicles. *Toxins* **2021**, *13*, 845. [CrossRef]
22. Wang, W.; Chanda, W.; Zhong, M. The Relationship between Biofilm and Outer Membrane Vesicles: A Novel Therapy Overview. *FEMS Microbiol. Lett.* **2015**, *362*, fnv117. [CrossRef]
23. Reid, G.; Gadir, A.A.; Dhir, R. Probiotics: Reiterating What They Are and What They Are Not. *Front. Microbiol.* **2019**, *10*, 424. [CrossRef] [PubMed]
24. Quinto, E.J.; Jiménez, P.; Caro, I.; Tejero, J.; Mateo, J.; Girbés, T.; Quinto, E.J.; Jiménez, P.; Caro, I.; Tejero, J.; et al. Probiotic Lactic Acid Bacteria: A Review. *Food Nutr. Sci.* **2014**, *5*, 1765–1775. [CrossRef]
25. Wang, Y.; Wu, J.; Lv, M.; Shao, Z.; Hungwe, M.; Wang, J.; Bai, X.; Xie, J.; Wang, Y.; Geng, W. Metabolism Characteristics of Lactic Acid Bacteria and the Expanding Applications in Food Industry. *Front. Bioeng. Biotechnol.* **2021**, *9*, 612285. [CrossRef] [PubMed]
26. Nataraj, B.H.; Shivanna, S.K.; Rao, P.; Nagpal, R.; Behare, P.V. Evolutionary Concepts in the Functional Biotics Arena: A Mini-review. *Food Sci. Biotechnol.* **2021**, *30*, 487–496. [CrossRef]
27. Derrien, M.; Vaughan, E.E.; Plugge, C.M.; de Vos, W.M. *Akkermansia muciniphila* gen. nov., sp. nov., a Human Intestinal Mucin-Degrading Bacterium. *Int. J. Syst. Evol. Microbiol.* **2004**, *54*, 1469–1476. [CrossRef]

28. Si, J.; Kang, H.; You, H.J.; Ko, G.P. Revisiting the Role of *Akkermansia muciniphila* as a Therapeutic Bacterium. *Gut Microbes* **2022**, *14*, 2078619. [CrossRef] [PubMed]
29. Hu, R.; Lin, H.; Li, J.; Zhao, Y.; Wang, M.; Sun, X.; Min, Y.; Gao, Y.; Yang, M. Probiotic *Escherichia coli* Nissle 1917-Derived Outer Membrane Vesicles Enhance Immunomodulation and Antimicrobial Activity in RAW264.7 Macrophages. *BMC Microbiol.* **2020**, *20*, 268. [CrossRef]
30. Liu, H.; Zhao, F.; Zhang, K.; Zhao, J.; Wang, Y. Investigating the Growth Performance, Meat Quality, Immune Function and Proteomic Profiles of Plasmal Exosomes in *Lactobacillus plantarum*-Treated Broilers with Immunological Stress. *Food Funct.* **2021**, *12*, 11790–11807. [CrossRef]
31. Müller, L.; Kuhn, T.; Koch, M.; Fuhrmann, G. Stimulation of Probiotic Bacteria Induces Release of Membrane Vesicles with Augmented Anti-inflammatory Activity. *ACS Appl. Bio Mater.* **2021**, *4*, 3739–3748. [CrossRef] [PubMed]
32. Li, M.; Lee, K.; Hsu, M.; Nau, G.; Mylonakis, E.; Ramratnam, B. *Lactobacillus*-Derived Extracellular Vesicles Enhance Host Immune Responses against Vancomycin-Resistant Enterococci. *BMC Microbiol.* **2017**, *17*, 66. [CrossRef]
33. Harrison, N.A.; Gardner, C.L.; da Silva, D.R.; Gonzalez, C.F.; Lorca, G.L. Identification of Biomarkers for Systemic Distribution of Nanovesicles from *Lactobacillus johnsonii* N6.2. *Front. Immunol.* **2021**, *12*, 3491. [CrossRef] [PubMed]
34. Hu, R.; Lin, H.; Wang, M.; Zhao, Y.; Liu, H.; Min, Y.; Yang, X.; Gao, Y.; Yang, M. *Lactobacillus reuteri*-Derived Extracellular Vesicles Maintain Intestinal Immune Homeostasis against Lipopolysaccharide-Induced Inflammatory Responses in Broilers. *J. Anim. Sci. Biotechnol.* **2021**, *12*, 25. [CrossRef] [PubMed]
35. Bäuerl, C.; Coll-Marqués, J.M.; Tarazona-González, C.; Pérez-Martínez, G. *Lactobacillus casei* Extracellular Vesicles Stimulate EGFR Pathway Likely Due to the Presence of Proteins P40 and P75 Bound to Their Surface. *Sci. Rep.* **2020**, *10*, 19237. [CrossRef] [PubMed]
36. Rubio, A.P.D.; Martínez, J.H.; Casillas, D.C.M.; Leskow, F.C.; Piuri, M.; Pérez, O.E. *Lactobacillus casei* BL23 Produces Microvesicles Carrying Proteins That Have Been Associated with Its Probiotic Effect. *Front. Microbiol.* **2017**, *8*, 1783. [CrossRef]
37. Vargoorani, M.E.; Modarressi, M.H.; Vaziri, F.; Motevaseli, E.; Siadat, S.D. Stimulatory Effects of *Lactobacillus casei* Derived Extracellular Vesicles on Toll-Like Receptor 9 Gene Expression and Cytokine Profile in Human Intestinal Epithelial Cells. *J. Diabetes Metab. Disord.* **2020**, *19*, 223–231. [CrossRef]
38. Dean, S.N.; Leary, D.H.; Sullivan, C.J.; Oh, E.; Walper, S.A. Isolation and Characterization of *Lactobacillus*-Derived Membrane Vesicles. *Sci. Rep.* **2019**, *9*, 877. [CrossRef]
39. Grande, R.; Celia, C.; Mincione, G.; Stringaro, A.; Di Marzio, L.; Colone, M.; Di Marcantonio, M.C.; Savino, L.; Puca, V.; Santoliquido, R.; et al. Detection and Physicochemical Characterization of Membrane Vesicles (MVs) of *Lactobacillus reuteri* DSM 17938. *Front. Microbiol.* **2017**, *8*, 1040. [CrossRef]
40. Shao, H.; Im, H.; Castro, C.M.; Breakefield, X.; Weissleder, R.; Lee, H. New Technologies for Analysis of Extracellular Vesicles. *Chem. Rev.* **2018**, *118*, 1917–1950. [CrossRef]
41. Hilton, S.H.; White, I.M. Advances in the Analysis of Single Extracellular Vesicles: A Critical Review. *Sens. Actuators Rep.* **2021**, *3*, 100052. [CrossRef]
42. Alpdundar Bulut, E.; Bayyurt Kocabas, B.; Yazar, V.; Aykut, G.; Guler, U.; Salih, B.; Surucu Yilmaz, N.; Ayanoglu, I.C.; Polat, M.M.; Akcali, K.C.; et al. Human Gut Commensal Membrane Vesicles Modulate Inflammation by Generating M2-like Macrophages and Myeloid-Derived Suppressor Cells. *J. Immunol.* **2020**, *205*, 2707–2718. [CrossRef] [PubMed]
43. Campoccia, D.; Montanaro, L.; Arciola, C.R. Extracellular DNA (eDNA). A Major Ubiquitous Element of the Bacterial Biofilm Architecture. *Int. J. Mol. Sci.* **2021**, *22*, 9100. [CrossRef] [PubMed]
44. Okshevsky, M.; Meyer, R.L. The Role of Extracellular DNA in the Establishment, Maintenance and Perpetuation of Bacterial Biofilms. *Crit. Rev. Microbiol.* **2015**, *41*, 341–352. [CrossRef] [PubMed]
45. Puca, V.; Ercolino, E.; Celia, C.; Bologna, G.; Di Marzio, L.; Mincione, G.; Marchisio, M.; Miscia, S.; Muraro, R.; Lanuti, P.; et al. Detection and Quantification of eDNA-Associated Bacterial Membrane Vesicles by Flow Cytometry. *Int. J. Mol. Sci.* **2019**, *20*, 5307. [CrossRef]
46. Zingl, F.G.; Leitner, D.R.; Thapa, H.B.; Schild, S. Outer Membrane Vesicles as Versatile Tools for Therapeutic Approaches. *microLife* **2021**, *2*, uqab006. [CrossRef]
47. Caruana, J.C.; Walper, S.A. Bacterial Membrane Vesicles as Mediators of Microbe—Microbe and Microbe—Host Community Interactions. *Front. Microbiol.* **2020**, *11*, 432. [CrossRef]
48. Díaz-Garrido, N.; Badia, J.; Baldomà, L. Microbiota-Derived Extracellular Vesicles in Interkingdom Communication in the Gut. *J. Extracell. Vesicles* **2021**, *10*, e12161. [CrossRef]
49. Kim, H.; Kim, M.; Myoung, K.; Kim, W.; Ko, J.; Kim, K.P.; Cho, E.G. Comparative Lipidomic Analysis of Extracellular Vesicles Derived from *Lactobacillus plantarum* APsulloc 331261 Living in Green Tea Leaves Using Liquid Chromatography-Mass Spectrometry. *Int. J. Mol. Sci.* **2020**, *21*, 8076. [CrossRef]
50. Kim, W.; Lee, E.J.; Bae, I.H.; Myoung, K.; Kim, S.T.; Park, P.J.; Lee, K.H.; Pham, A.V.Q.; Ko, J.; Oh, S.H.; et al. *Lactobacillus plantarum*-Derived Extracellular Vesicles Induce Anti-Inflammatory M2 Macrophage Polarization *In Vitro*. *J. Extracell. Vesicles* **2020**, *9*, 1793514. [CrossRef]
51. Pérez-Cruz, C.; Cañas, M.A.; Giménez, R.; Badia, J.; Mercade, E.; Baldomà, L.; Aguilera, L. Membrane Vesicles Released by a Hypervesiculating *Escherichia coli* Nissle 1917 *tolR* Mutant Are Highly Heterogeneous and Show Reduced Capacity for Epithelial Cell Interaction and Entry. *PLoS ONE* **2016**, *11*, e0169186. [CrossRef]

52. Aguilera, L.; Toloza, L.; Giménez, R.; Odena, A.; Oliveira, E.; Aguilar, J.; Badia, J.; Baldomà, L. Proteomic Analysis of Outer Membrane Vesicles from the Probiotic Strain *Escherichia coli* Nissle 1917. *Proteomics* **2014**, *14*, 222–229. [CrossRef]
53. Ghaderi, F.; Sotoodehnejadnematalahi, F.; Hajebrahimi, Z.; Fateh, A.; Siadat, S.D. Effects of Active, Inactive, and Derivatives of *Akkermansia muciniphila* on The Expression of The Endocannabinoid System and PPARs Genes. *Sci. Rep.* **2022**, *12*, 10031. [CrossRef]
54. Bajic, S.S.; Cañas, M.A.; Tolinacki, M.; Badia, J.; Sánchez, B.; Golic, N.; Margolles, A.; Baldomá, L.; Ruas-Madiedo, P. Proteomic Profile of Extracellular Vesicles Released by *Lactiplantibacillus plantarum* BGAN8 and Their Internalization by Non-Polarized HT29 Cell Line. *Sci. Rep.* **2020**, *10*, 21829. [CrossRef]
55. Kim, M.H.; Choi, S.J.; Choi, H., II; Choi, J.P.; Park, H.K.; Kim, E.K.; Kim, M.J.; Moon, B.S.; Min, T.K.; Rho, M.; et al. *Lactobacillus plantarum*-Derived Extracellular Vesicles Protect Atopic Dermatitis Induced by *Staphylococcus aureus*-Derived Extracellular Vesicles. *Allergy. Asthma Immunol. Res.* **2018**, *10*, 516–532. [CrossRef]
56. Behzadi, E.; Mahmoodzadeh Hosseini, H.; Imani Fooladi, A.A. The Inhibitory Impacts of *Lactobacillus rhamnosus* GG-Derived Extracellular Vesicles on the Growth of Hepatic Cancer Cells. *Microb. Pathog.* **2017**, *110*, 1–6. [CrossRef]
57. Keyhani, G.; Hosseini, H.M.; Salimi, A. Effect of Extracellular Vesicles of *Lactobacillus rhamnosus* GG on The Expression of CEA Gene and Protein Released by Colorectal Cancer Cells. *Iran. J. Microbiol.* **2022**, *14*, 90–96. [CrossRef]
58. Choi, J.H.; Moon, C.M.; Shin, T.S.; Kim, E.K.; McDowell, A.; Jo, M.K.; Joo, Y.H.; Kim, S.E.; Jung, H.K.; Shim, K.N.; et al. *Lactobacillus paracasei*-Derived Extracellular Vesicles Attenuate the Intestinal Inflammatory Response by Augmenting the Endoplasmic Reticulum Stress Pathway. *Exp. Mol. Med.* **2020**, *52*, 423–437. [CrossRef]
59. Shiraishi, T.; Yokota, S.; Sato, Y.; Ito, T.; Fukiya, S.; Yamamoto, S.; Sato, T.; Yokota, A. Lipoteichoic Acids are Embedded in Cell Walls during Logarithmic Phase, but Exposed on Membrane Vesicles in *Lactobacillus gasseri* JCM 1131 T. *Benef. Microbes* **2018**, *9*, 653–662. [CrossRef]
60. Seo, M.K.; Park, E.J.; Ko, S.Y.; Choi, E.W.; Kim, S. Therapeutic Effects of Kefir Grain *Lactobacillus*-Derived Extracellular Vesicles in Mice with 2,4,6-Trinitrobenzene Sulfonic Acid-Induced Inflammatory Bowel Disease. *J. Dairy Sci.* **2018**, *101*, 8662–8671. [CrossRef]
61. Yamasaki-Yashiki, S.; Miyoshi, Y.; Nakayama, T.; Kunisawa, J.; Katakura, Y. IgA-Enhancing Effects of Membrane Vesicles Derived from *Lactobacillus sakei* subsp. *sakei NBRC15893. Biosci. Microbiota, Food Health* **2019**, *38*, 29.
62. Liu, Y.; Tempelaars, M.H.; Boeren, S.; Alexeeva, S.; Smid, E.J.; Abee, T. Extracellular Vesicle Formation in *Lactococcus lactis* is Stimulated by Prophage-Encoded Holin–Lysin System. *Microb. Biotechnol.* **2022**, *15*, 1281–1295. [CrossRef] [PubMed]
63. Fábrega, M.J.; Aguilera, L.; Giménez, R.; Varela, E.; Cañas, M.A.; Antolín, M.; Badía, J.; Baldomà, L. Activation of Immune and Defense Responses in the Intestinal Mucosa by Outer Membrane Vesicles of Commensal and Probiotic *Escherichia coli* Strains. *Front. Microbiol.* **2016**, *7*, 705. [CrossRef]
64. Nishiyama, K.; Takaki, T.; Sugiyama, M.; Fukuda, I.; Aiso, M.; Mukai, T.; Odamaki, T.; Xiao, J.Z.; Osawa, R.; Okada, N. Extracellular Vesicles Produced by *Bifidobacterium longum* Export Mucin-Binding Proteins. *Appl. Environ. Microbiol.* **2020**, *86*, e01464-20. [CrossRef] [PubMed]
65. Fábrega, M.J.; Rodríguez-Nogales, A.; Garrido-Mesa, J.; Algieri, F.; Badía, J.; Giménez, R.; Gálvez, J.; Baldomà, L. Intestinal Anti-inflammatory Effects of Outer Membrane Vesicles from *Escherichia coli* Nissle 1917 in DSS-Experimental Colitis in Mice. *Front. Microbiol.* **2017**, *8*, 1274. [CrossRef] [PubMed]
66. Hirayama, S.; Nakao, R. Glycine Significantly Enhances Bacterial Membrane Vesicle Production: A Powerful Approach for Isolation of LPS-Reduced Membrane Vesicles of Probiotic *Escherichia coli*. *Microb. Biotechnol.* **2020**, *13*, 1162–1178. [CrossRef]
67. Ashrafian, F.; Shahriary, A.; Behrouzi, A.; Moradi, H.R.; Keshavarz Azizi Raftar, S.; Lari, A.; Hadifar, S.; Yaghoubfar, R.; Ahmadi Badi, S.; Khatami, S.; et al. *Akkermansia muciniphila*-Derived Extracellular Vesicles as a Mucosal Delivery Vector for Amelioration of Obesity in Mice. *Front. Microbiol.* **2019**, *10*, 2155. [CrossRef]
68. Ashrafian, F.; Behrouzi, A.; Shahriary, A.; Badi, S.A.; Davari, M.; Khatami, S.; Jamnani, F.R.; Fateh, A.; Vaziri, F.; Siadat, S.D. Comparative Study of Effect of *Akkermansia muciniphila* and Its Extracellular Vesicles on Toll-Like Receptors and Tight Junction. *Gastroenterol. Hepatol. Bed Bench* **2019**, *12*, 168.
69. Ashrafian, F.; Keshavarz Azizi Raftar, S.; Lari, A.; Shahryari, A.; Abdollahiyan, S.; Moradi, H.R.; Masoumi, M.; Davari, M.; khatami, S.; Omrani, M.D.; et al. Extracellular Vesicles and Pasteurized Cells Derived from *Akkermansia muciniphila* Protect against High-Fat Induced Obesity in Mice. *Microb. Cell Fact.* **2021**, *20*, 219. [CrossRef]
70. Keshavarz Azizi Raftar, S.; Ashrafian, F.; Yadegar, A.; Lari, A.; Moradi, H.R.; Shahriary, A.; Azimirad, M.; Alavifard, H.; Mohsenifar, Z.; Davari, M.; et al. The Protective Effects of Live and Pasteurized *Akkermansia muciniphila* and Its Extracellular Vesicles against HFD/CCl4-Induced Liver Injury. *Microbiol. Spectr.* **2021**, *9*, e0048421. [CrossRef]
71. Yaghoubfar, R.; Behrouzi, A.; Zare Banadkoki, E.; Ashrafian, F.; Lari, A.; Vaziri, F.; Nojoumi, S.A.; Fateh, A.; Khatami, S.; Siadat, S.D. Effect of *Akkermansia muciniphila, Faecalibacterium prausnitzii*, and Their Extracellular Vesicles on the Serotonin System in Intestinal Epithelial Cells. *Probiotics Antimicrob. Proteins* **2021**, *13*, 1546–1556. [CrossRef] [PubMed]
72. Hong, J.; Dauros-Singorenko, P.; Whitcombe, A.; Payne, L.; Blenkiron, C.; Phillips, A.; Swift, S. Analysis of the *Escherichia coli* Extracellular Vesicle Proteome Identifies Markers of Purity and Culture Conditions. *J. Extracell. Vesicles* **2019**, *8*, 1632099. [CrossRef] [PubMed]
73. Lee, B.H.; Wu, S.C.; Shen, T.L.; Hsu, Y.Y.; Chen, C.H.; Hsu, W.H. The Applications of *Lactobacillus plantarum*-Derived Extracellular Vesicles as a Novel Natural Antibacterial Agent for Improving Quality and Safety in Tuna Fish. *Food Chem.* **2021**, *340*, 128104. [CrossRef]

74. Ñahui Palomino, R.A.; Vanpouille, C.; Laghi, L.; Parolin, C.; Melikov, K.; Backlund, P.; Vitali, B.; Margolis, L. Extracellular Vesicles from Symbiotic Vaginal Lactobacilli Inhibit HIV-1 Infection of Human Tissues. *Nat. Commun.* **2019**, *10*, 5656. [CrossRef] [PubMed]
75. West, C.L.; Stanisz, A.M.; Mao, Y.K.; Champagne-Jorgensen, K.; Bienenstock, J.; Kunze, W.A. Microvesicles from *Lactobacillus reuteri* (DSM-17938) Completely Reproduce Modulation of Gut Motility by Bacteria in Mice. *PLoS ONE* **2020**, *15*, e0225481. [CrossRef]
76. Chen, C.Y.; Rao, S.S.; Yue, T.; Tan, Y.J.; Yin, H.; Chen, L.J.; Luo, M.J.; Wang, Z.; Wang, Y.Y.; Hong, C.G.; et al. Glucocorticoid-Induced Loss of Beneficial Gut Bacterial Extracellular Vesicles Is Associated with The Pathogenesis of Osteonecrosis. *Sci. Adv.* **2022**, *8*, eabg8335. [CrossRef]
77. Yoon, Y.C.; Ahn, B.H.; Min, J.W.; Lee, K.R.; Park, S.H.; Kang, H.C. Stimulatory Effects of Extracellular Vesicles Derived from *Leuconostoc holzapfelii* That Exists in Human Scalp on Hair Growth in Human Follicle Dermal Papilla Cells. *Curr. Issues Mol. Biol.* **2022**, *44*, 845–866. [CrossRef]
78. de Rodovalho, V.R.; da Luz, B.S.R.; Rabah, H.; do Carmo, F.L.R.; Folador, E.L.; Nicolas, A.; Jardin, J.; Briard-Bion, V.; Blottière, H.; Lapaque, N.; et al. Extracellular Vesicles Produced by the Probiotic *Propionibacterium freudenreichii* CIRM-BIA 129 Mitigate Inflammation by Modulating the NF-κB Pathway. *Front. Microbiol.* **2020**, *11*, 1544. [CrossRef]
79. de Rezende Rodovalho, V.; da Luz, B.S.R.; Nicolas, A.; do Carmo, F.L.R.; Jardin, J.; Briard-Bion, V.; Jan, G.; Loir, Y.L.; de Carvalho Azevedo, V.A.; Guédon, E. Environmental Conditions Modulate the Protein Content and Immunomodulatory Activity of Extracellular Vesicles Produced by the Probiotic *Propionibacterium freudenreichii*. *Appl. Environ. Microbiol.* **2020**, *87*, e02263-20.
80. Rubio, A.P.D.; Martínez, J.; Palavecino, M.; Fuentes, F.; López, C.M.S.; Marcilla, A.; Pérez, O.E.; Piuri, M. Transcytosis of *Bacillus subtilis* Extracellular Vesicles through an *In Vitro* Intestinal Epithelial Cell Model. *Sci. Rep.* **2020**, *10*, 3120. [CrossRef]
81. Ma, L.; Shen, Q.; Lyu, W.; Lv, L.; Wang, W.; Yu, M.; Yang, H.; Tao, S.; Xiao, Y. *Clostridium butyricum* and Its Derived Extracellular Vesicles Modulate Gut Homeostasis and Ameliorate Acute Experimental Colitis. *Microbiol. Spectr.* **2022**, *10*, e0136822. [CrossRef] [PubMed]
82. Liang, L.; Yang, C.; Liu, L.; Mai, G.; Li, H.; Wu, L.; Jin, M.; Chen, Y. Commensal Bacteria-Derived Extracellular Vesicles Suppress Ulcerative Colitis through Regulating The Macrophages Polarization and Remodeling The Gut Microbiota. *Microb. Cell Fact.* **2022**, *21*, 88. [CrossRef] [PubMed]
83. Kuhn, T.; Koch, M.; Fuhrmann, G.; Kuhn, T.; Fuhrmann, G.; Koch, M. Probiomimetics—Novel *Lactobacillus*-Mimicking Microparticles Show Anti-Inflammatory and Barrier-Protecting Effects in Gastrointestinal Models. *Small* **2020**, *16*, 2003158. [CrossRef] [PubMed]
84. Morishita, M.; Sagayama, R.; Yamawaki, Y.; Yamaguchi, M.; Katsumi, H.; Yamamoto, A. Activation of Host Immune Cells by Probiotic-Derived Extracellular Vesicles via TLR2-Mediated Signaling Pathways. *Biol. Pharm. Bull.* **2022**, *45*, 354–359. [CrossRef]
85. Morishita, M.; Horita, M.; Higuchi, A.; Marui, M.; Katsumi, H.; Yamamoto, A. Characterizing Different Probiotic-Derived Extracellular Vesicles as a Novel Adjuvant for Immunotherapy. *Mol. Pharm.* **2021**, *18*, 1080–1092. [CrossRef]
86. Yang, Z.; Gao, Z.; Yang, Z.; Zhang, Y.; Chen, H.; Yang, X.; Fang, X.; Zhu, Y.; Zhang, J.; Ouyang, F.; et al. *Lactobacillus plantarum*-Derived Extracellular Vesicles Protect against Ischemic Brain Injury via The MicroRNA-101a-3p/c-Fos/TGF-β Axis. *Pharmacol. Res.* **2022**, *182*, 106332. [CrossRef]
87. Jo, C.S.; Myung, C.H.; Yoon, Y.C.; Ahn, B.H.; Min, J.W.; Seo, W.S.; Lee, D.H.; Kang, H.C.; Heo, Y.H.; Choi, H.; et al. The Effect of *Lactobacillus plantarum* Extracellular Vesicles from Korean Women in Their 20s on Skin Aging. *Curr. Issues Mol. Biol.* **2022**, *44*, 526–540. [CrossRef]
88. Champagne-Jorgensen, K.; Mian, M.F.; McVey Neufeld, K.A.; Stanisz, A.M.; Bienenstock, J. Membrane Vesicles of *Lacticaseibacillus rhamnosus* JB-1 Contain Immunomodulatory Lipoteichoic Acid and Are Endocytosed by Intestinal Epithelial Cells. *Sci. Rep.* **2021**, *11*, 13756. [CrossRef]
89. Champagne-Jorgensen, K.; Jose, T.A.; Stanisz, A.M.; Mian, M.F.; Hynes, A.P.; Bienenstock, J. Bacterial Membrane Vesicles and Phages in Blood After Consumption of *Lacticaseibacillus rhamnosus* JB-1. *Gut Microbes* **2021**, *13*, e1993583. [CrossRef]
90. Shi, Y.; Meng, L.; Zhang, C.; Zhang, F.; Fang, Y. Extracellular Vesicles of *Lacticaseibacillus paracasei* PC-H1 Induce Colorectal Cancer Cells Apoptosis via PDK1/AKT/Bcl-2 Signaling Pathway. *Microbiol. Res.* **2021**, *255*, 126921. [CrossRef]
91. Chelakkot, C.; Choi, Y.; Kim, D.K.; Park, H.T.; Ghim, J.; Kwon, Y.; Jeon, J.; Kim, M.S.; Jee, Y.K.; Gho, Y.S.; et al. *Akkermansia muciniphila*-Derived Extracellular Vesicles Influence Gut Permeability through the Regulation of Tight Junctions. *Exp. Mol. Med.* **2018**, *50*, e450. [CrossRef] [PubMed]
92. Luo, Z.W.; Xia, K.; Liu, Y.W.; Liu, J.H.; Rao, S.S.; Hu, X.K.; Chen, C.Y.; Xu, R.; Wang, Z.X.; Xie, H. Extracellular Vesicles from *Akkermansia muciniphila* Elicit Antitumor Immunity Against Prostate Cancer via Modulation of CD8 + T Cells and Macrophages. *Int. J. Nanomed.* **2021**, *16*, 2949–2963. [CrossRef] [PubMed]
93. Hao, H.; Zhang, X.; Tong, L.; Liu, Q.; Liang, X.; Bu, Y.; Gong, P.; Liu, T.; Zhang, L.; Xia, Y.; et al. Effect of Extracellular Vesicles Derived From *Lactobacillus plantarum* Q7 on Gut Microbiota and Ulcerative Colitis in Mice. *Front. Immunol.* **2021**, *12*, 5167. [CrossRef]
94. Tong, L.; Zhang, X.; Hao, H.; Liu, Q.; Zhou, Z.; Liang, X.; Liu, T.; Gong, P.; Zhang, L.; Zhai, Z.; et al. *Lactobacillus rhamnosus* GG Derived Extracellular Vesicles Modulate Gut Microbiota and Attenuate Inflammatory in DSS-Induced Colitis Mice. *Nutrients* **2021**, *13*, 3319. [CrossRef]

95. Lee, D.H.; Park, H.K.; Lee, H.R.; Sohn, H.; Sim, S.; Park, H.J.; Shin, Y.S.; Kim, Y.K.; Choi, Y.; Park, H.S. Immunoregulatory Effects of *Lactococcus lactis*-Derived Extracellular Vesicles in Allergic Asthma. *Clin. Transl. Allergy* **2022**, *12*, e12138. [CrossRef] [PubMed]
96. Nagakubo, T.; Nomura, N.; Toyofuku, M. Cracking Open Bacterial Membrane Vesicles. *Front. Microbiol.* **2020**, *10*, 3026. [CrossRef]
97. Lee, J.; Kim, O.Y.; Gho, Y.S. Proteomic Profiling of Gram-negative Bacterial Outer Membrane Vesicles: Current Perspectives. *PROTEOMICS—Clin. Appl.* **2016**, *10*, 897–909. [CrossRef]
98. Pedersen, S.K.; Harry, J.L.; Sebastian, L.; Baker, J.; Traini, M.D.; McCarthy, J.T.; Manoharan, A.; Wilkins, M.R.; Gooley, A.A.; Righetti, P.G.; et al. Unseen Proteome: Mining Below the Tip of the Iceberg To Find Low Abundance and Membrane Proteins. *J. Proteome Res.* **2003**, *2*, 303–311. [CrossRef]
99. Ahmed, N.; Rice, G.E. Strategies for Revealing Lower Abundance Proteins in Two-Dimensional Protein Maps. *J. Chromatogr. B. Analyt. Technol. Biomed. Life Sci.* **2005**, *815*, 39–50. [CrossRef]
100. Klimentová, J.; Stulík, J. Methods of Isolation and Purification of Outer Membrane Vesicles from Gram-Negative Bacteria. *Microbiol. Res.* **2015**, *170*, 1–9. [CrossRef]
101. Graf, A.C.; Leonard, A.; Schäuble, M.; Rieckmann, L.M.; Hoyer, J.; Maass, S.; Lalk, M.; Becher, D.; Pané-Farré, J.; Riedel, K. Virulence Factors Produced by *Staphylococcus aureus* Biofilms Have a Moonlighting Function Contributing to Biofilm Integrity. *Mol. Cell. Proteomics* **2019**, *18*, 1053. [CrossRef] [PubMed]
102. Kesavan, D.; Vasudevan, A.; Wu, L.; Chen, J.; Su, Z.; Wang, S.; Xu, H. Integrative Analysis of Outer Membrane Vesicles Proteomics and Whole-Cell Transcriptome Analysis of Eravacycline Induced *Acinetobacter baumannii* Strains. *BMC Microbiol.* **2020**, *20*, 31. [CrossRef]
103. Sung, K.; Chon, J.; Kweon, O.; Nho, S.; Kim, S.; Park, M.; Paredes, A.; Lim, J.H.; Khan, S.A.; Phillips, K.S.; et al. Dynamic Adaptive Response of *Pseudomonas aeruginosa* to Clindamycin/Rifampicin-Impregnated Catheters. *Antibiotics* **2021**, *10*, 752. [CrossRef]
104. Rolhion, N.; Barnich, N.; Bringer, M.A.; Glasser, A.L.; Ranc, J.; Hébuterne, X.; Hofman, P.; Darfeuille-Michaud, A. Abnormally Expressed ER Stress Response Chaperone Gp96 in CD Favours Adherent-Invasive *Escherichia coli* Invasion. *Gut* **2010**, *59*, 1355–1362. [CrossRef]
105. Taheri, N.; Mahmud, A.K.M.F.; Sandblad, L.; Fällman, M.; Wai, S.N.; Fahlgren, A. *Campylobacter jejuni* Bile Exposure Influences Outer Membrane Vesicles Protein Content and Bacterial Interaction with Epithelial Cells. *Sci. Rep.* **2018**, *8*, 16996. [CrossRef] [PubMed]
106. Kim, S.I.; Kim, S.; Kim, E.; Hwang, S.Y.; Yoon, H. Secretion of *Salmonella* Pathogenicity Island 1-Encoded Type III Secretion System Effectors by Outer Membrane Vesicles in *Salmonella enterica* Serovar Typhimurium. *Front. Microbiol.* **2018**, *9*, 2810. [CrossRef]
107. Avila-Calderón, E.D.; del Ruiz-Palma, M.S.; Aguilera-Arreola, M.G.; Velázquez-Guadarrama, N.; Ruiz, E.A.; Gomez-Lunar, Z.; Witonsky, S.; Contreras-Rodríguez, A. Outer Membrane Vesicles of Gram-Negative Bacteria: An Outlook on Biogenesis. *Front. Microbiol.* **2021**, *12*, 345. [CrossRef]
108. Clarke, A.J. The "Hole" Story of Predatory Outer-Membrane Vesicles. *Can. J. Microbiol.* **2018**, *64*, 589–599. [CrossRef] [PubMed]
109. Peng, X.-P.; Nie, C.; Guan, W.-Y.; Qiao, L.-D.; Lu, L.; Cao, S.-J. Regulation of Probiotics on Metabolism of Dietary Protein in Intestine. *Curr. Protein Pept. Sci.* **2019**, *21*, 766–771. [CrossRef]
110. Díez-Sainz, E.; Lorente-Cebrián, S.; Aranaz, P.; Riezu-Boj, J.I.; Martínez, J.A.; Milagro, F.I. Potential Mechanisms Linking Food-Derived MicroRNAs, Gut Microbiota and Intestinal Barrier Functions in the Context of Nutrition and Human Health. *Front. Nutr.* **2021**, *8*, 85. [CrossRef]
111. Villard, A.; Boursier, J.; Andriantsitohaina, R. Microbiota-Derived Extracellular Vesicles and Metabolic Syndrome. *Acta Physiol.* **2021**, *231*, e13600. [CrossRef]
112. McMillan, H.M.; Kuehn, M.J. The Extracellular Vesicle Generation Paradox: A Bacterial Point of View. *EMBO J.* **2021**, *40*, e108174. [CrossRef]
113. Bitto, N.J.; Zavan, L.; Johnston, E.L.; Stinear, T.P.; Hill, A.F.; Kaparakis-Liaskos, M. Considerations for the Analysis of Bacterial Membrane Vesicles: Methods of Vesicle Production and Quantification Can Influence Biological and Experimental Outcomes. *Microbiol. Spectr.* **2021**, *9*, e01273-21. [CrossRef]
114. Papadimitriou, K.; Zoumpopoulou, G.; Foligné, B.; Alexandraki, V.; Kazou, M.; Pot, B.; Tsakalidou, E. Discovering Probiotic Microorganisms: *In Vitro, In Vivo*, Genetic And Omics Approaches. *Front. Microbiol.* **2015**, *6*, 58. [CrossRef] [PubMed]
115. Sagheddu, V.; Guidesi, E.; Galletti, S.; Elli, M. Selection and Characterization Criteria of Probiotics Intended for Human Use from the Past to the Future. *Food Sci. Nutr. Stud.* **2019**, *3*, p73. [CrossRef]
116. Suzuki, T. Regulation of Intestinal Epithelial Permeability By Tight Junctions. *Cell. Mol. Life Sci.* **2013**, *70*, 631–659. [CrossRef] [PubMed]
117. Turner, J.R. Intestinal Mucosal Barrier Function in Health and Disease. *Nat. Rev. Immunol.* **2009**, *9*, 799–809. [CrossRef]
118. Kang, E.A.; Choi, H.I.; Hong, S.W.; Kang, S.; Jegal, H.Y.; Choi, E.W.; Park, B.S.; Kim, J.S. Extracellular Vesicles Derived from Kefir Grain *Lactobacillus* Ameliorate Intestinal Inflammation via Regulation of Proinflammatory Pathway and Tight Junction Integrity. *Biomedicines* **2020**, *8*, 522. [CrossRef]
119. Xu, X.; Lin, S.; Yang, Y.; Gong, X.; Tong, J.; Li, K.; Li, Y. Histological and Ultrastructural Changes of the Colon in Dextran Sodium Sulfate-Induced Mouse Colitis. *Exp. Ther. Med.* **2020**, *20*, 1987. [CrossRef]
120. Hu, Y.; Ye, Z.; Wu, M.; She, Y.; Li, L.; Xu, Y.; Qin, K.; Hu, Z.; Yang, M.; Lu, F.; et al. The Communication Between Intestinal Microbiota and Ulcerative Colitis: An Exploration of Pathogenesis, Animal Models, and Potential Therapeutic Strategies. *Front. Med.* **2021**, *8*, 766126. [CrossRef]

121. Petersson, J.; Schreiber, O.; Hansson, G.C.; Gendler, S.J.; Velcich, A.; Lundberg, J.O.; Roos, S.; Holm, L.; Phillipson, M. Importance and Regulation of the Colonic Mucus Barrier In A Mouse Model of Colitis. *Am. J. Physiol.* **2011**, *300*, G327. [CrossRef] [PubMed]
122. Tomasi, M.; Caproni, E.; Benedet, M.; Zanella, I.; Giorgetta, S.; Dalsass, M.; König, E.; Gagliardi, A.; Fantappiè, L.; Berti, A.; et al. Outer Membrane Vesicles From The Gut Microbiome Contribute to Tumor Immunity by Eliciting Cross-Reactive T Cells. *Front. Oncol.* **2022**, *12*, 912639. [CrossRef]
123. Hiam-Galvez, K.J.; Allen, B.M.; Spitzer, M.H. Systemic Immunity in Cancer. *Nat. Rev. Cancer* **2021**, *21*, 345–359. [CrossRef] [PubMed]
124. Fessler, J.; Matson, V.; Gajewski, T.F. Exploring the Emerging Role of the Microbiome in Cancer Immunotherapy. *J. Immunother. Cancer* **2019**, *7*, 108. [CrossRef] [PubMed]
125. Miyoshi, Y.; Saika, A.; Nagatake, T.; Matsunaga, A.; Kunisawa, J.; Katakura, Y.; Yamasaki-Yashiki, S. Mechanisms Underlying Enhanced IgA Production in Peyer's Patch Cells by Membrane Vesicles Derived from *Lactobacillus sakei*. *Biosci. Biotechnol. Biochem.* **2021**, *85*, 1536–1545. [CrossRef] [PubMed]
126. Geuking, M.B.; Köller, Y.; Rupp, S.; McCoy, K.D. The Interplay Between the Gut Microbiota and the Immune System. *Gut Microbes* **2014**, *5*, 411. [CrossRef]
127. Kamada, N.; Seo, S.U.; Chen, G.Y.; Núñez, G. Role of The Gut Microbiota in Immunity and Inflammatory Disease. *Nat. Rev. Immunol.* **2013**, *13*, 321–335. [CrossRef]
128. Wang, X.; Zhang, P.; Zhang, X. Probiotics Regulate Gut Microbiota: An Effective Method to Improve Immunity. *Molecules* **2021**, *26*, 6076. [CrossRef]
129. Choi, J.; Kim, Y.K.; Han, P.L. Extracellular Vesicles Derived from *Lactobacillus plantarum* Increase BDNF Expression in Cultured Hippocampal Neurons and Produce Antidepressant-Like Effects in Mice. *Exp. Neurobiol.* **2019**, *28*, 158–171. [CrossRef]
130. Choi, J.; Kwon, H.; Kim, Y.K.; Han, P.L. Extracellular Vesicles from Gram-positive and Gram-negative Probiotics Remediate Stress-Induced Depressive Behavior in Mice. *Mol. Neurobiol.* **2022**, *59*, 2715–2728. [CrossRef]
131. Alvarez, C.S.; Giménez, R.; Cañas, M.A.; Vera, R.; Díaz-Garrido, N.; Badia, J.; Baldomà, L. Extracellular Vesicles and Soluble Factors Secreted by *Escherichia coli* Nissle 1917 and ECOR63 Protect against Enteropathogenic *E. coli*-Induced Intestinal Epithelial Barrier Dysfunction. *BMC Microbiol.* **2019**, *19*, 166. [CrossRef]
132. Cañas, M.A.; Fábrega, M.J.; Giménez, R.; Badia, J.; Baldomà, L. Outer Membrane Vesicles From Probiotic and Commensal *Escherichia coli* Activate NOD1-Mediated Immune Responses in Intestinal Epithelial Cells. *Front. Microbiol.* **2018**, *9*, 498. [CrossRef] [PubMed]
133. Díaz-Garrido, N.; Bonnin, S.; Riera, M.; Gíménez, R.; Badia, J.; Baldomà, L. Transcriptomic microRNA Profiling of Dendritic Cells in Response to Gut Microbiota-Secreted Vesicles. *Cells* **2020**, *9*, 1534. [CrossRef]
134. Raftar, S.K.A.; Ashrafian, F.; Abdollahiyan, S.; Yadegar, A.; Moradi, H.R.; Masoumi, M.; Vaziri, F.; Moshiri, A.; Siadat, S.D.; Zali, M.R. The Anti-Inflammatory Effects of *Akkermansia muciniphila* and Its Derivates in HFD/CCL4-Induced Murine Model of Liver Injury. *Sci. Rep.* **2022**, *12*, 2453. [CrossRef] [PubMed]
135. Mata Forsberg, M.; Björkander, S.; Pang, Y.; Lundqvist, L.; Ndi, M.; Ott, M.; Escribá, I.B.; Jaeger, M.C.; Roos, S.; Sverremark-Ekström, E. Extracellular Membrane Vesicles from Lactobacilli Dampen IFN-γ Responses in a Monocyte-Dependent Manner. *Sci. Rep.* **2019**, *9*, 17109. [CrossRef] [PubMed]
136. Teixeira, L.D.; Harrison, N.A.; da Silva, D.R.; Mathews, C.E.; Gonzalez, C.F.; Lorca, G.L. Nanovesicles From *Lactobacillus johnsonii* N6.2 Reduce Apoptosis in Human Beta Cells by Promoting AHR Translocation and IL10 Secretion. *Front. Immunol.* **2022**, *13*, 899413. [CrossRef]
137. Kim, J.H.; Jeun, E.J.; Hong, C.P.; Kim, S.H.; Jang, M.S.; Lee, E.J.; Moon, S.J.; Yun, C.H.; Im, S.H.; Jeong, S.G.; et al. Extracellular Vesicle-Derived Protein from *Bifidobacterium longum* Alleviates Food Allergy through Mast Cell Suppression. *J. Allergy Clin. Immunol.* **2016**, *137*, 507–516.e8. [CrossRef]
138. López, P.; González-Rodríguez, I.; Sánchez, B.; Gueimonde, M.; Margolles, A.; Suárez, A. Treg-Inducing Membrane Vesicles from *Bifidobacterium bifidum* LMG13195 as Potential Adjuvants in Immunotherapy. *Vaccine* **2012**, *30*, 825–829. [CrossRef] [PubMed]
139. Kim, S.; Han, S.-Y.; Lee, J.; Kim, N.-R.; Lee, B.R.; Kim, H.; Kwon, M.; Ahn, K.; Noh, Y.; Kim, S.J.; et al. *Bifidobacterium longum* and Galactooligosaccharide Improve Skin Barrier Dysfunction and Atopic Dermatitis-Like Skin. *Allergy. Asthma Immunol. Res.* **2022**, *14*, 564. [CrossRef]
140. An, J.J.; Ha, E.M. Extracellular Vesicles Derived from *Lactobacillus plantarum* Restore Chemosensitivity through the PDK2-Mediated Glucose Metabolic Pathway in 5-FU-Resistant Colorectal Cancer Cells. *J. Microbiol.* **2022**, *60*, 735–745. [CrossRef]
141. Pang, Y.; Ermann Lundberg, L.; Mata Forsberg, M.; Ahl, D.; Bysell, H.; Pallin, A.; Sverremark-Ekström, E.; Karlsson, R.; Jonsson, H.; Roos, S. Extracellular Membrane Vesicles from *Limosilactobacillus reuteri* Strengthen the Intestinal Epithelial Integrity, Modulate Cytokine Responses and Antagonize Activation of TRPV1. *Front. Microbiol.* **2022**, *13*, 1032202. [CrossRef]
142. Kurata, A.; Kiyohara, S.; Imai, T.; Yamasaki-Yashiki, S.; Zaima, N.; Moriyama, T.; Kishimoto, N.; Uegaki, K. Characterization of Extracellular Vesicles from *Lactiplantibacillus plantarum*. *Sci. Rep.* **2022**, *12*, 13330. [CrossRef] [PubMed]
143. Nakao, R.; Kobayashi, H.; Iwabuchi, Y.; Kawahara, K.; Hirayama, S.; Ramstedt, M.; Sasaki, Y.; Kataoka, M.; Akeda, Y.; Ohnishi, M. A Highly Immunogenic Vaccine Platform against Encapsulated Pathogens Using Chimeric Probiotic *Escherichia coli* Membrane Vesicles. *NPJ Vaccines* **2022**, *7*, 153. [CrossRef] [PubMed]

144. da Silva Barreira, D.; Lapaquette, P.; Novion Ducassou, J.; Couté, Y.; Guzzo, J.; Rieu, A. Spontaneous Prophage Induction Contributes to the Production of Membrane Vesicles by the Gram-positive Bacterium *Lacticaseibacillus casei* BL23. *MBio* **2022**, *13*, e0237522. [CrossRef]
145. Díez-Sainz, E.; Milagro, F.I.; Riezu-Boj, J.I.; Lorente-Cebrián, S. Effects of Gut Microbiota-Derived Extracellular Vesicles on Obesity and Diabetes and Their Potential Modulation through Diet. *J. Physiol. Biochem.* **2022**, *78*, 485–499. [CrossRef] [PubMed]
146. Jahromi, L.P.; Fuhrmann, G. Bacterial Extracellular Vesicles: Understanding Biology Promotes Applications as Nanopharmaceuticals. *Adv. Drug Deliv. Rev.* **2021**, *173*, 125–140. [CrossRef] [PubMed]
147. Domínguez Rubio, A.P.; D'Antoni, C.L.; Piuri, M.; Pérez, O.E. Probiotics, Their Extracellular Vesicles and Infectious Diseases. *Front. Microbiol.* **2022**, *13*, 864720. [CrossRef]
148. González-Lozano, E.; García-García, J.; Gálvez, J.; Hidalgo-García, L.; Rodríguez-Nogales, A.; Rodríguez-Cabezas, M.E.; Sánchez, M. Novel Horizons in Postbiotics: Lactobacillaceae Extracellular Vesicles and Their Applications in Health and Disease. *Nutrients* **2022**, *14*, 5296. [CrossRef]
149. Yuan, Y.; Sun, J.; You, T.; Shen, W.; Xu, W.; Dong, Q.; Cui, M. Extracellular Vesicle-Based Therapeutics in Neurological Disorders. *Pharmaceutics* **2022**, *14*, 2652. [CrossRef]
150. Sun, K.; Zheng, X.; Jin, H.; Yu, F.; Zhao, W. Exosomes as CNS Drug Delivery Tools and Their Applications. *Pharmaceutics* **2022**, *14*, 2252. [CrossRef]
151. Abid, R.; Waseem, H.; Ali, J.; Ghazanfar, S.; Ali, G.M.; Elasbali, A.M.; Alharethi, S.H. Probiotic Yeast *Saccharomyces*: Back to Nature to Improve Human Health. *J. Fungi* **2022**, *8*, 444. [CrossRef] [PubMed]
152. Saarela, M.H. Safety Aspects of Next Generation Probiotics. *Curr. Opin. Food Sci.* **2019**, *30*, 8–13. [CrossRef]
153. Cunningham, M.; Azcarate-Peril, M.A.; Barnard, A.; Benoit, V.; Grimaldi, R.; Guyonnet, D.; Holscher, H.D.; Hunter, K.; Manurung, S.; Obis, D.; et al. Shaping the Future of Probiotics and Prebiotics. *Trends Microbiol.* **2021**, *29*, 667–685. [CrossRef] [PubMed]
154. Cieślik, M.; Nazimek, K.; Bryniarski, K. Extracellular Vesicles-Oral Therapeutics of the Future. *Int. J. Mol. Sci.* **2022**, *23*, 7554. [CrossRef]
155. Chang, X.; Wang, S.L.; Zhao, S.B.; Shi, Y.H.; Pan, P.; Gu, L.; Yao, J.; Li, Z.S.; Bai, Y. Extracellular Vesicles with Possible Roles in Gut Intestinal Tract Homeostasis and IBD. *Mediators Inflamm.* **2020**, *2020*, 1945832. [CrossRef]
156. Hendrix, A.; De Wever, O. Systemically Circulating Bacterial Extracellular Vesicles: Origin, Fate, and Function. *Trends Microbiol.* **2022**, *30*, 213–216. [CrossRef]

pharmaceutics

MDPI

Review

Production and Utility of Extracellular Vesicles with 3D Culture Methods

Mar Casajuana Ester and Richard M. Day *

Applied Biomedical Engineering Group, Centre for Precision Healthcare, UCL Division of Medicine, University College London, London WC1E 6JF, UK
* Correspondence: r.m.day@ucl.ac.uk; Tel.: +44-203-108-2183

Abstract: In recent years, extracellular vesicles (EVs) have emerged as promising biomarkers, cell-free therapeutic agents, and drug delivery carriers. Despite their great clinical potential, poor yield and unscalable production of EVs remain significant challenges. When using 3D culture methods, such as scaffolds and bioreactors, large numbers of cells can be expanded and the cell environment can be manipulated to control the cell phenotype. This has been employed to successfully increase the production of EVs as well as to enhance their therapeutic effects. The physiological relevance of 3D cultures, such as spheroids, has also provided a strategy for understanding the role of EVs in the pathogenesis of several diseases and to evaluate their role as tools to deliver drugs. Additionally, 3D culture methods can encapsulate EVs to achieve more sustained therapeutic effects as well as prevent premature clearance of EVs to enable more localised delivery and concentrated exosome dosage. This review highlights the opportunities and drawbacks of different 3D culture methods and their use in EV research.

Keywords: extracellular vesicles; 3D culture; scaffolds; bioreactors; spheroids

Citation: Casajuana Ester, M.; Day, R.M. Production and Utility of Extracellular Vesicles with 3D Culture Methods. *Pharmaceutics* **2023**, *15*, 663. https://doi.org/10.3390/pharmaceutics15020663

Academic Editor: Tania Limongi

Received: 7 December 2022
Revised: 13 February 2023
Accepted: 13 February 2023
Published: 16 February 2023

1. Introduction

Extracellular vesicles (EVs) are lipid-bound vesicles which are important mediators in intercellular communication and which are secreted by most eukaryotic and prokaryotic cells, including animal cells and bacteria [1,2]. The presence of EVs in the extracellular space was identified in 1980 [3]. However, the secretion of EVs was initially seen as a form of secreting unwanted proteins or cellular waste resulting from either cellular damage or homeostasis [4,5]. In the mid-1990s, EVs were shown to induce vital immune responses, and in the last decade, with the advance of research methods and techniques, numerous studies have identified EVs as significant mediators in cell–cell communication [6]. EVs therefore play a fundamental biological role in cellular interactions in health and disease [1]. EVs are heterogenous vesicles and are classified based upon their biogenesis, contents, and sizes. Exosomes are lipid-bilayer-enclosed small EVs that originate from the endosomal plasma membrane [6–8]. Given their roles as vesicles in intracellular communication, EVs are involved in many physiological processes. This characteristic, together with their molecular composition, which reflects the status of the secreting cell, gives EVs the capacity to provide great clinical potential. There is a large number of ongoing pre-clinical and clinical studies evaluating the safety and efficacy of EVs for use as drug delivery agents, therapeutics, and novel tools for diagnostics [9–11]. EVs have uniquely high targeting capabilities and many studies have demonstrated both their autocrine and paracrine effects. Cancer cells, for example, can interact with each other through EV-supported cell–cell communication, promoting metastasis. Further concerning their naïve targeting capabilities, it is also possible to engineer EVs (e.g., with a particular type of antibody) to alter their targeting behaviour [12]. EVs also have lower immunogenicity than the cells they are derived from, offering a great opportunity for the improvement of current therapeutic systems [11]. An example of this is the use of EVs in cardiovascular diseases. Given their capability to transport cell–cell transferring proteins and messenger RNAs (mRNAs) amongst others, they have been proven to have pro-angiogenetic, pro-coagulant and anti-inflammatory effects as well as the ability to modulate cardiomyocytes and endothelial cells, inducing blood vessel formation and restoring oxygen supply to hypoxic regions [8].

EVs play a key role during cancer and tumour growth. EVs released from cancerous cells have been shown to promote tumour growth by promoting cell proliferation, angiogenesis, increasing the migratory and invasive capacity of cancerous cells that contribute to metastatic lesions, and increasing resistance to certain drugs [13,14]. They may therefore provide disease biomarkers suitable for non-invasive, detailed disease prognosis and diagnostic tools [15]. Several studies have shown that certain mRNAs and proteins are upregulated in EVs derived from cancer cells and could therefore be used as biomarkers for a range of malignancies including ovarian, breast, cervical, gastric, pancreatic, and lung cancers. EVs can be found in a variety of body fluids, such as plasma, saliva, and urine, and can therefore be used as disease biomarkers [16]. Furthermore, EVs are highly attractive as drug delivery agents due to their low toxicity, low immunogenicity, and ability to penetrate tight boundaries, such as the blood–brain barrier (BBB) [17]. The unique capacity to cross the BBB makes EVs very attractive carriers for carrying therapeutic drugs and genes to treat neurologic and psychiatric disorders [18].

The methods used for the isolation and purification of EVs must be standardised to ensure EV production is consistent and reproducible. Common isolation techniques, which are discussed later in the review, are often challenging for scaling up production. However, in recent years, new technologies—such as microfluidics, which are also discussed later in the review—have emerged as promising tools for EV research, offering higher EV yields and purities [19]. This review focuses on research studies performed on all EV subtypes, with a particular emphasis on exosomes, which are the most widely studied EV subtype in clinical and pharmacological fields. Where reviewed articles refer to research conducted specifically on exosomes, this has been stated. Where the articles refer to EVs, this may include exosomes or other types of EVs, such as microvesicles (MVs).

Studies are also focusing on enhancing the therapeutic potential of EVs as well as on strategies to achieve their sustained release. Three-dimensional (3D) culture systems are increasingly recognised as tools in bioprocessing and biomedical research. Three-dimensional cell culture consists of creating an in vitro environment that mimics the native tissue. This approach may consist of culturing a single cell type or co-culturing multiple cell types [20]. Culturing cells in 3D enables cells the formation of cell–cell and cell–extracellular matrix (ECM) interactions not achievable with two-dimensional (2D) culture systems. This is suggested to improve control of cell physiology, such as cell morphology, proliferation and differentiation, response to stimuli, drug metabolism, and protein synthesis [21,22]. Three-dimensional cell culture can be achieved by either encouraging cell–cell contact so that cells form only cell–cell interactions (e.g., with spheroids) or by providing an exogenous matrix material that cells can attach to (e.g., scaffolds) [23]. Several studies have used 3D culture models to study EVs as drug carriers. Nooshabadi et al., for example, loaded exosomes obtained from endometrial cells with atorvastatin and assessed their activity in the growth of glioblastoma spheroids [24]. Three-dimensional cell culture systems have also been used to investigate EVs as novel biomarkers. EVs secreted from 3D systems differed in molecular signalling and protein profiles compared to EVs secreted from 2D cultures [23,25]. Three-dimensional culture models have also been used to study the therapeutic effect of EVs, and several studies have shown that EVs secreted from 3D cultures have enhanced therapeutic effects, such as superior anti-inflammatory and pro-angiogenic effects [26–28]. Finally, 3D culture methods enable the growth of larger quantities of cells via more space- and cost-efficient methods, translating to a larger EV production, which is necessary to clinically translate EV-based therapies [20].

2. Subtypes of Extracellular Vesicles

EVs are heterogenous populations of lipid-bound vesicles and are naturally secreted by cells into the extracellular space. They can broadly be divided into four main subtypes—exomeres, exosomes, MVs, and apoptotic bodies—characterised based upon their biogenesis, release pathways, sizes, contents, and functions (Table 1) [29].

Table 1. The different types of extracellular vesicles and their defining characteristics.: miRNA, microRNA; MVs, microvesicles.

Vesicle	Size	Origin	Contents	Markers	References
Exomeres	≤50 nm	Unknown	DNA, RNA, miRNAs and lipids	Unclear—More studies are required	[7,30]
Exosomes	30–200 nm *	Intra-luminal budding into MVBs and release by MVB fusion with cell membrane	Membrane proteins, different RNA species, lipids and DNA	Tetraspanins, heat-shock proteins, integrins, TSG101, flotillin, MFGE8 and ESCRT components. They include cell-type-specific proteins	[1,3,31,32]
MVs	10–1000 nm	Outward budding or blebbing of cell plasma membrane	Membrane proteins, different RNA species, lipids, and DNA	Annexin A1 (on MVs that shed directly from the plasma membrane), integrins, selectins, and CD40 ligand, phosphatidylserine	[3,29,31–33]
Apoptotic bodies	1–5 µm	Outward blebbing of apoptotic cell plasma membrane	Nuclear fractions, cell organelles and degraded proteins	Annexin V and high amounts of phosphatidylserine	[3,31,32]

* The size range of exosomes reported in published literature differs. For example, Sun et al. reported a size of range of 30–120 nm [34], Jeppesen et al. reported 40–150 nm [33], and diameters of up to ~200 nm have been measured using cryogenic transmission electron microscopy (cryo-TEM) [35]. Inconsistency in methodology used for the collection, isolation, and analysis of exosomes, as well as size variation between exosomes from different cell types, is likely to have contributed to these differences.

3. Exosomes as a Subset of Extracellular Vesicles—Their Origin and Characteristics

The biogenesis of exosomes starts with endocytosis, a process which consists in the inward budding of the cell membrane to form endosomes, also known as intraluminal vessels (ILV). As part of this, nucleic acids, proteins, and lipids are wrapped into ILV [3,31]. These early endosomes mature into late endosomes as a result of their membrane undergoing a series of inward invaginations that subsequently close [3]. Late endosomes are also known as multivesicular bodies (MVB), and these contain multiple vesicles, each enclosing a small part of the cytosol, including various proteins and nucleic acids [4]. MVB can then fuse with lysosomes, which cause them to degrade, or alternatively with the plasma membrane, releasing exosomes into the extracellular space (Figure 1) [3,4,31].

The processes by which ILV are loaded with a particular cargo and by which MVB release their content are not yet fully understood [29]. To date, researchers have found several pathways involved in the biogenesis of exosomes [31]. The endosomal sorting complexes required for transport (ESCRT) pathways play a prominent role in the biogenesis and secretion of exosomes [3,36]. Additionally, SNARE proteins and their effectors, such as RAB GTPases, have also been shown to have a major impact on exosome secretion [29]. By delivering these cargos to neighbouring cells, they can reprogram them, and therefore, exosomes play a role in vital cellular processes, such as immune responses, signal transduction, and antigen presentation [3].

Exosomes are enclosed in a lipid bilayer, and their characteristics are dependent on the cells that secrete them. The conditions of the cells secreting them (such as cellular health status and the microenvironment the cells are grown in) [1] are reflected in the exosomal cargo, comprising proteins and lipids as well as nucleic acids [37]. Proteins, such as receptors, transcription factors, and enzymes, can reflect the physiological status of a cell and are involved in regulating essential cellular processes. An example of this is exosomal protein transfer between cells, which can contribute to the spread of aggressive-phenotype cancer cells within heterogenous tumours [38].

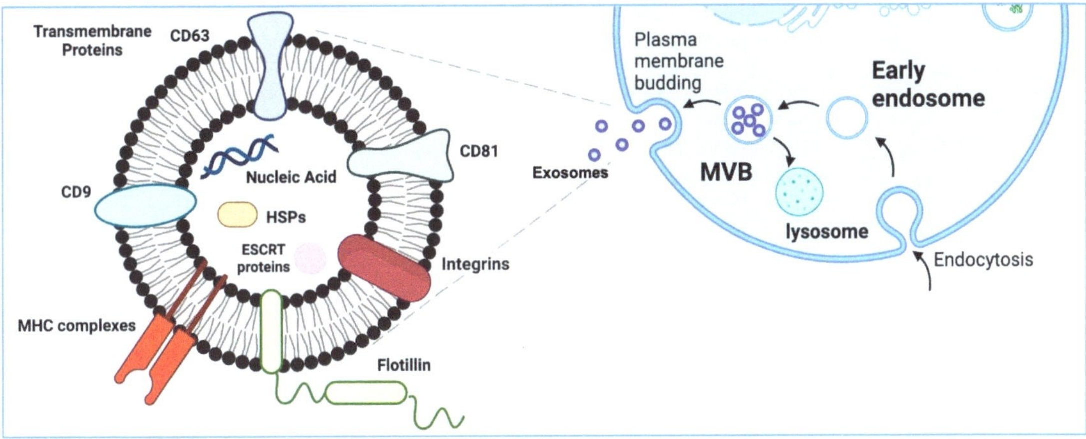

Figure 1. Biogenesis and main components of exosomes.

Exosomes contain annexins; tetraspanin proteins (CD9, CD63, and CD81), which act as exosomal markers; ESCRT proteins; actins; and integrins (Alix and TSG101), important for cell communication. They also contain heat shock proteins (Hsp60, Hsp70, and Hsp90), which are involved in the folding and unfolding of proteins and in the protection of infectious diseases [39], as well as flotillins, which are involved in endocytosis, intracellular transport, and signalling [40]. Proteins such as heat shock proteins, CD63, and ESCRT are found in all exosomes, however, some of the proteins found in exosomal membranes reflect the cells they are derived from. For example, CD80 and CD86 are expressed on dendritic-cell-derived exosomes, and CD19 is expressed on B-cell-derived exosomes and as such, they can be used as disease biomarkers [36,41]. Additionally, antigen-presenting cells secrete EVs, expressing major histocompatibility peptide complexes (MHC) that induce specific T cell responses [42]. As such, exosomes carrying MHC-peptide complexes could promote adaptive immune responses by partially or fully activating helper and cytolytic T cells to kill tumour cells [43].

Exosomes also have a lipid composition, leading to characteristics which are specific to their cellular source. Exosomal lipid components include cholesterols, sphingolipids, phosphoglycerides, and ceramide (sometimes used to differentiate exosomes from lysosomes). The outer surface of exosomes is rich in saccharide chains, such as mannose, polylactosamine, alpha-2,6 sialic acid, and N-linked glycans [44]. These lipids have an effect in the exosomal sorting of cargo, their secretion, their structure, and signalling between exosomes and cells [45]. Exosomes, similarly to liposomes, have a membranous lipid bilayer which protects the exosomal cargo [29]. Additionally, exosomes contain a complex of nucleic acids. MicroRNAs (miRNAs) are the most abundant RNA species in exosomes [3]. They play a role in several biological processes such as exocytosis, haematopoiesis, and angiogenesis and are known to regulate cell–cell communication. Other exosomal RNA species include ribosomal RNA (rRNA), which differs from cellular RNA in that it makes up over 95% of the human transcriptome [46].

Internalisation of exosomes by target cells makes them attractive for use in disease diagnosis, drug delivery, and as therapeutic modulators.

3.1. EVs in Diagnostics

As mentioned previously, exosomal cargo reflects the cellular origin and physiological state of the donor. EVs derived from tumour, stromal, and immune cells contribute to the multiple stages of tumour growth, signalling, and progression as well as to resistance to therapy [43]. Hence, EVs have the potential to be used as disease biomarkers [47]. EVs have been found and isolated from a variety of body fluids, including blood, saliva, and amniotic fluids and therefore offer a non-invasive method of diagnosing patients and of monitoring their response to cancer immunotherapy [48].

The use of EVs could allow for earlier detection of several cancers [49]. Composition and concentration of exosomal miRNAs vary between diseased and healthy individuals [16]. For example, exosomal miR-21 has been reported to correspond with tumour progression and aggressiveness, making it possible to distinguish between patients with oesophageal squamous cell cancer from patients who have benign diseases without systemic inflammation [50]. Munagala et al. isolated and characterised exosomes from conditioned media of lung cancer and normal bronchial epithelial cells and found that 77 miRNAs were significantly modulated in lung cancer cells compared to healthy epithelial cells. miR-21 and miR-155 were found to be significantly upregulated in recurrent tumours compared to primary tumours [51]. Machida et al. studied the salivary exosomes from patients with pancreatic cancer and demonstrated that the levels of certain miRNAs were higher than those in healthy control patients [52]. Exosomal miRNAs have also been studied as potential markers to predict patients' therapeutic responses to cancer treatments. Yuwen et al. demonstrated that increased levels of exosomal miR-146a-5p correlated with a better response to cisplatin, a common chemotherapy drug used to treat a variety of cancers [53,54].

EV proteins are also being studied as potential biomarkers for cancers. Exosomes containing CD24, EDIL3 and fibronectin proteins can be used to detect early breast cancer [55]. Additionally, exosomes containing CD24 Ala/Val single nucleotide polymorphisms (SNPs) genotype are associated with fast progressing autoimmune diseases and can therefore be used to detect this [56]. Additionally, exosomal PD-L1 expression levels are significantly correlated with tumour PDL-1 levels and can therefore be used as tool to evaluate the clinical efficacy of lung cancer immunotherapy [53,54,57]. Hoshino et al. demonstrated that exosomal integrins $\alpha6\beta4$ and $\alpha6\beta1$ were associated with lung metastasis and that exosomal integrin $\alpha v\beta5$ correlates to liver metastasis [58]. The same research group investigated the proteomic profiles of EVs and particles (EVPs) in human samples from tissue explants, plasma, and other bodily fluids and found that EV-specific proteins, such as VCAN, TNC, and THBS2, could distinguish tumours from normal tissues and could be used to determine the cancer's origin [59].

Furthermore, EVs can be found in cerebrospinal fluid (CSF) and have been found to cross the BBB, emerging as novel biomarker sources to study neurodegenerative diseases [60,61]. For example, exosomes found in amyloid beta ($A\beta$) plaques, characteristic of Alzheimer's disease, have been found to contain specific proteins, suggesting that they could serve as indicators of such [49]. Additionally, Ebrahimkhani et al. demonstrated that miRNAs associated with exosomes found in CSF can be used to diagnose multiple sclerosis (MS) [62].

Another condition for which EV research could be beneficial is diabetes. It was recently revealed that plasma-derived exosomes from patients with type 1 diabetes express a distinct miRNA signature [63]. Additionally, EVs have been associated in the pathogenesis of type 2 diabetes and could therefore be used as biomarkers for such [64]. EVs can be taken up by hepatocytes, muscle cells and other insulin target cell types and can cause an alteration in insulin signalling activation leading to disrupted normal metabolic responses of recipient sites to insulin causing insulin resistance [65]. An example of this is shown by hepatic EVs which contain miR-130a-3p, which attenuates glucose and lipid intolerance in adipose tissues by supressing the PHLPP2 gene [66]. Another example of this is miR-26a found in pancreatic β-cell-derived EVs, which decreases in obese animals, causing an increase to insulin resistance [67]. EVs can be used to detect multiple cardiovascular diseases such as atherosclerosis, myocardial ischaemia, cardiac fibrosis and ischaemia-reperfusion injury [68,69]. For example, Zampetaki et al. demonstrated that in patients with subsequent myocardial infarction, the expression of miR-126 in exosomes increased and could therefore be used as a biomarker for vascular injury [70].

The use of EVs as diagnostic markers is challenging in part because there are few unique cell-specific proteins and because EVs are able to circulate around the body, making it difficult to determine their tissue of origin [49]. There is a large number of non-EV particles, such as lipoproteins and protein complexes, in clinical samples. This could mean that biological effects and biomarkers assigned to EVs in some studies could be caused by contaminant constituents, which may interfere with EV-based biomarker discovery [71].

3.2. Therapeutic Application of EVs

Cells isolated from adult tissues, such as mesenchymal stem cells (MSC) have the ability to inhibit cell apoptosis, promote angiogenesis, and trigger cells that have survived in damaged tissues to proliferate [72]. Similar effects have been observed with the delivery of EVs secreted by MSC. One of the advantages of using EVs over their cells of origin is that cells can be subject to apoptosis and abnormal differentiation caused by stress during cell transplantation. Additionally, transplanted cells are at risk of immune rejection and do not possess the ease of targeting capabilities of EVs that enables them to target specific tissue areas [73]. As such, the therapeutic benefit of EVs is currently being explored in cancers, neurodegenerative diseases, immune-mediated conditions, and a variety of other fields [74,75].

Currently, a large number of stem cell research focuses on MSC due to their ability to replicate, differentiate into several cell lineages, and to participate in immunomodulation [76]. Research has explored the use of the paracrine signalling properties of MSC-derived EVs to treat and ameliorate a multitude of conditions. Yin et al. demonstrated that adipose-derived MSC (AD-MSC)-secreted exosomes led to a marked increase in H9C2 cell viability under hypoxic conditions in vitro and protected ischaemic myocardium from myocardial ischaemia reperfusion injury in vivo [77]. Another example of the therapeutic potential of MSC-derived EVs was demonstrated by Wang et al. Their studies demonstrated that exosomes secreted by bone marrow-derived MSC (BM-MSC) and AD-MSC cause superior cardioprotection compared to the cells they are derived from [78]. Another investigation demonstrated that BM-MSC-derived EVs promoted functional recovery of injured sciatic peripheral nerves using a rat model by improving nerve regeneration and increasing the expression of GAP-43, a marker for axon regeneration. [79]

In 2022, there were 33 registered exosome therapy clinical trials, of which 20 made use of MSC-derived exosomes [80]. Furthermore, biotechnology companies are developing MSC-derived exosomes to treat Alzheimer's disease (Celltex Therapeutics, Houston, TX, USA), neural-stem-cell-derived exosomes for penetrating the blood–brain barrier (Aruna Bio, Athens, GA, USA), and an exosome-based vaccine platform to prevent infectious diseases (Codiak BioSciences, Cambridge, MA, USA) [81].

3.3. EVs as Drug Carriers

Compared to synthetic drug carriers, EVs isolated from a patient's own cells offer higher biocompatibility and lower toxicity. EVs can penetrate tissues and cross tight boundaries, such as the BBB, making them attractive drug delivery vehicles. Additionally, it is possible to chemically modify the surface proteins found on EVs, increasing tissue specificity [17,82]. As a result, the first clinical trials in which EVs were used as drug delivery systems have already been reported [72]. The first clinical trial started in 2011 and investigated the ability of plant exosomes to more effectively deliver curcumin—a natural hydrophobic phenol extracted from turmeric—which has anti-inflammatory, anti-neoplastic, and anti-cancer properties to normal colon tissues and colon tumours [83].

Several research studies have also demonstrated the benefits of using EVs as drug carriers. For example, Kim et al. used exosomes to encapsulate the anti-cancer drug agent doxorubicin (Dox). Prolonged exposure to Dox caused significant cytotoxicity, limiting its prolonged use. Dox-loaded exosomes, on the other hand, were easily taken up by cells compared to unencapsulated Dox and Dox encapsulated by liposomes, reducing cytotoxicity [84]. Martins-Marques et al. demonstrated that the presence of the gap junction protein connexin43 (Cx43) in Dox-loaded EVs reduced the toxicity of the drug [85].

Additionally, several researchers have evaluated the exosomal delivery of paclitaxel (PTX), another commonly used anti-cancer agent. Kim et al., for example, showed that exosomes secreted by macrophages loaded with PTX showed higher anticancer efficacy in a mouse model of pulmonary metastases. They also demonstrated that it is possible to engineer these exosomes, leading to superior structures and higher therapeutic indices [86]. In another study, exosomes derived from human BM-MSC (hBM-MSC) were loaded with PTX, and their effect on triple negative breast cancer (TNBC) cells was investigated. Both in vitro and in vivo results showed significant tumour growth inhibition [87].

Li et al. demonstrated that exosomes can be used to deliver gemcitabine, the first-line chemotherapeutic drug for pancreatic cancer treatment. Results showed that exosomes loaded with gemcitabine supressed tumour growth with prolonged survival and caused minimal damage to normal tissues [88]. Another study showed that dopamine-loaded exosomes show a much better therapeutic effect in a Parkinson's disease (PD) mouse model and a lower systemic toxicity when compared to free dopamine, which cannot cross the BBB, following intravenous administration [89].

There are, however, a few limitations to this field and challenges that still must be overcome. A major limitation is the lack of standardised techniques for the isolation and purification of EVs, which leads to impure and low EV yields as well as variation between different groups when studying the drug delivery potential of EVs [49,90]. Additionally, due to variation between EVs derived from the same cell type, the drug delivery potential remains unknown [49]. The different exosome isolation techniques are described later in this review. Briefly, these include common isolation techniques, such as differential centrifugation (dUC), density gradient centrifugation, ultrafiltration (UF), precipitation, size exclusion chromatography (SEC), and immunoaffinity capture, and emerging technologies, such as microfluidics. They each comprise a unique set of advantages and disadvantages [19,68,91]. One of the main challenges involving EV isolation is the presence of abundant protein mixtures which can be co-isolated with EVs. Additionally, these can coat EV membranes, influencing their recovery yield and biological activity [92]. In order to clinically translate EV research, the isolation method should be robust, easy-to use, economical, reproducible, time-saving, and high-throughput [93]. Common isolation methods do not meet these criteria, and significant efforts, including the development of microfluidics for EV isolation and membrane-based separation in which exosomes are isolated by binding their phosphate groups to some metal oxides, are being combined to achieve large-scale EV GMP production [19].

Another challenge involving drug-based EV delivery involves efficiently loading drugs and therapeutic cargoes into EVs. Loading methods can be mainly divided into two categories. The first category, passive loading, involves incubating the EVs with drugs; the drugs diffuse into the EVs along a concentration gradient, the cells they are derived from are treated with a drug so that they secrete EVs which are loaded with the drug. These methods tend to have low loading efficiencies and make it difficult to control the amount of drug being loaded into the EVs [94,95]. Additionally, the drug may be cytotoxic to the treated cells and may influence the EVs secreted. Pascucci et al. treated SR4987 MSCs with PTX. The isolated PTX-loaded EVs demonstrated strong anti-proliferative activity against CFPAC-1 human pancreatic cells in vitro. However, when loading PTX onto SR4987 MSC, ~15% of them underwent apoptosis due to PTX cytotoxicity [96]. The second category involves active cargo loading methods. These include sonication, electroporation, extrusion, freeze/thaw cycles, saponin pretreatment, and incubation with membrane permeabilisers amongst others [93]. Each of these have different loading capacities which will vary depending on the hydrophilicity/hydrophobicity of the drug being loaded as well on its molecular weight [95,97]. Haney et al. compared some of these loading methods for the loading of catalase, a potent antioxidant, and reported that sonication, extrusion, and saponin treatment provided the highest loading efficiencies when compared to freeze/thaw cycles and passive incubation. It is important to note though that these resulted in an increase in EV size [98]. Additionally, other studies have found that these loading methods compromise the structure and integrity of EV membranes, therefore influencing the therapeutic and immunogenic properties of the drug-loaded EVs [93,97,99].

As mentioned earlier, drug size is also a challenge when loading drugs onto EVs. Large enzymes have been passively loaded onto EVs using saponin-assisted loaded treatment [9,98,99]. Encapsulation of large-scale functional mRNA has also been achieved using cellular nanoporation. Yang et al. transfected various cell sources with plasmid DNAs and stimulated these with electrical stimuli. This enhanced EV production and exosomal mRNA transcripts. However, this requires additional steps during transfection and electrical stimulation, making its industrial translation difficult [9,100].

4. Extracellular Vesicle Production and Isolation Methods and Strategies to Enhance Cellular Production of Extracellular Vesicles

When culturing cells in 2D flasks, the surface area of the culture vessel is proportional to cell growth and the quantity of EVs cells produced [101]. Various approaches are currently being explored to increase the yield and quality of exosome secretion, as well as their therapeutic and drug carrier properties, including 3D culture methods, stress inducing factors, genetically manipulating cells, exposing cells to physical stimulation, and chemically treating cells with drugs and other molecules. Additionally, it is also possible to engineer artificial EVs—EV-mimetic nanovesicles—which mimic natural EVs in morphology, size, and function (Figure 2) [102,103].

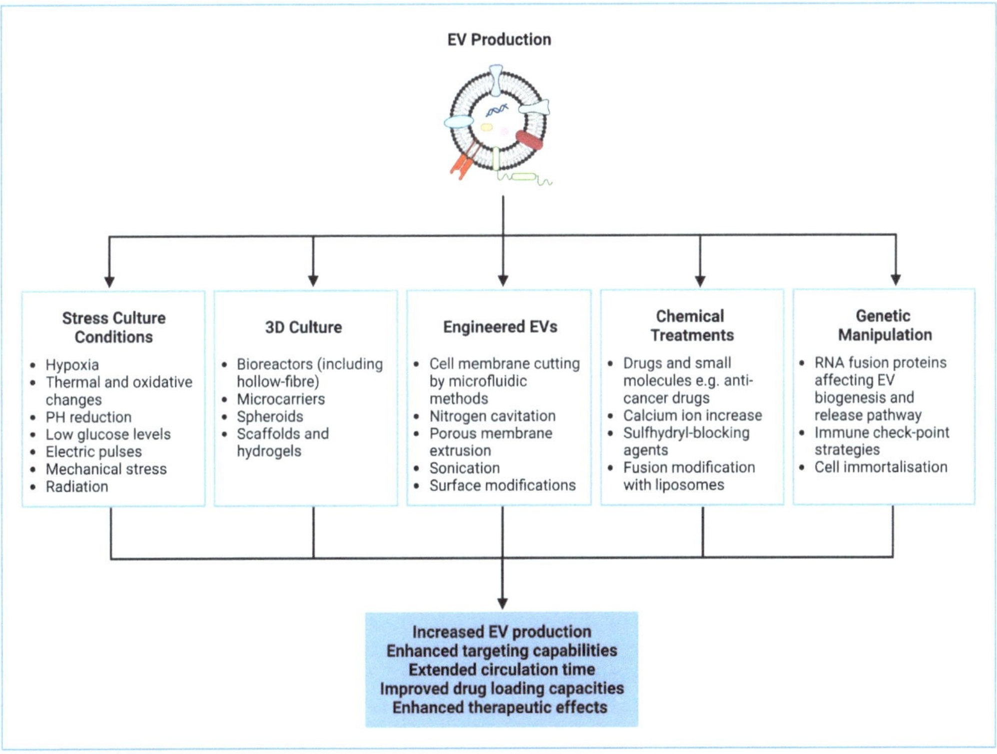

Figure 2. Strategies for enhancing extracellular vesicle production.

Although all of the methods suggested above can increase the production of EVs, as well as enhance their properties, the majority of these either induce cellular stress or change the content of the cells secreting them, which will have an impact on the EVs secreted. To overcome this, 3D culture systems have been used for the production of EVs [101].

It is important to mention that despite the effort to enhance EV production, the yields and purities of the isolated EVs will also be dependent on different isolation methods. Different techniques make use of particular EV traits, such as their densities, shapes, sizes, and surface proteins, to achieve isolation. Each of these techniques have different advantages and disadvantages; the most notable are summarised in Table 2.

Table 2. Different methods of isolating EVs and their associated advantages and disadvantages.

Method	Principles & Materials	Advantages	Disadvantages	References
Differential Ultracentrifugation (dUC)	Physical—Components with imparity of size and density possess various sediment speeds	Gold standard Low cost Pure samples Suitable for large sample volumes	Time-consuming Low yield Repeated and high-speed steps might damage EVs	[19,41,44,91]
Density Gradient Centrifugation	Physical—Components with imparity of size and density possess various sediment speeds	Higher purity than dUC Maintains EVs intact	Time-consuming Low yield	[19,68]
Ultrafiltration (UF)	Physical—Filters particles with various sizes and molecular weights	Quick and simple High yield	Low purity EV deformation	[19,41,68,81,91]
Precipitation	Physical/Chemical—High hydrophilic polymers influence the solubility of EVs	High yield Easy Low cost Concentrates diluted samples	Low purity Potential contaminants (co-purifying protein aggregates)	[19,41,44,81,88]
Size Exclusion Chromatography (SEC)	Physical/Chemical—Columns packed with pore beads separate particles of various sizes and molecular weights	High yield Pure samples Maintains EVs intact	Potential contaminants (co-purifying protein aggregates) Samples can be diluted	[19,41,44,68,91]
Immunoaffinity Capture	Chemical—Uses antibodies to interact with specific membrane proteins	Quick High yield Pure samples	Expensive Lack of standardisation	[19,41,44,68,81, 91]
Microfluidics	Physical/Chemical—Based on several principles including immunoaffinity, size and density	High yield Very pure samples	Expensive	[19,44,91]

There are discrepancies between papers on whether UC and dUC are perceived as expensive or not and on whether the isolation produces pure samples. Lai et al., for example, state that UC leads to low-purity samples caused—for example—by protein aggregates [81].

As highlighted in Table 2, microfluidic platforms make it possible to isolate EVs at high purities and yields. Compared to UC, microfluidic chips show higher yields. Zhao et al. developed a microfluidic chip that isolated ~80% of small EVs (below 150 nm) compared to UC, which isolated ~61% [104]. Another advantage of microfluidics over other EV isolation platforms is that it allows for the combined isolation and characterisation of EVs. An example of a useful application of this is liquid biopsies, which offer minimally invasive and real-time molecular profiling of patients [105]. Different isolation methods can be employed within microfluidic platforms, which can be used alone or in combination. These include immunoaffinity, membrane-based filtration, EV trapping on nanowires, acoustic nanofiltration, and deterministic lateral displacement. Detection of EVs can then also be performed using a variety of methods, such as fluorescence and colorimetry detection of EV markers or via assays such as ELISA [106]. In some cases, checking for common exosomal surface markers (CD9, CD63, and CD81), can serve as a disease biomarker diagnosis. For example, the number of exosomes found in human plasma from patients suffering from NSCLC and ovarian cancer was higher than that in healthy patients [107].

In 2014, Kanwar et al. developed the first microfluidic device used for exosome isolation and characterisation. This consisted of a PDMS chip functionalised with antibodies which were able to capture the CD63 exosomal marker. Kanwar et al. used this chip to detect the number of exosomes in serum from healthy and pancreatic cancer patients and showed that there was an increase in the number of exosomes found in pancreatic cancer patient serum [108]. Since then, multiple studies have demonstrated the use of microfluidic platforms to quantify not only EVs generally but also disease-specific EVs by using EV markers specific to each disease. Additionally, it is also possible to use microfluidic platforms to analyse EV miRNAs [109–111]. Lim et al., for example, developed a vacuum-driven power-free hydrogel microfluidic chip which was able to detect ERBB2 (a breast cancer marker gene) and a reference gene by amplifying a fluorescent signal via an enzyme-free catalytic hairpin assembly reaction at room temperature. It was tested both in vivo and in vitro and was shown to be effective for the use of liquid biopsies to detect breast cancer [109].

Microfluidics therefore offer a customisable, automatable, scalable, fast, and reliable diagnosis based on EV contents and characteristics. There is still, however, a long process before these can be used in a clinical setting. There is still no "golden standard" for EV isolation methods, and several concepts relating EV biogenesis and roles in cell–cell communication and disease still must be fully understood. In addition, microfluidics can be used to engineer EVs as drug delivery vehicles by encapsulating small molecules, nucleic acids, and proteins into EVs using mainly sonication and electroporation [112].

5. An Overview of Different 3D Culture Methods

Traditionally, cells are attached to a flat surface made of glass or plastic, in 2D, as a monolayer. This has become widely used due to its simplicity and convenience and has been an invaluable method of providing insight into a variety of diseases [102]. However, cells cultured in vitro in conventional 2D monolayers have reduced cell–cell and cell–ECM interactions. As such, cells can lose their characteristic morphology and the level of cellular responsiveness is limited. To grow cells in a more natural state, 3D culture methods have been widely used to provide an environment with adequate multidirectional cell–cell and cell–ECM interactions [113]. Additionally, cells cultured in 2D monolayers can lose their phenotype during passaging [114,115]. Since the biogenesis of EVs is not yet fully understood, these changes in cellular organisation could influence our understanding of the characteristics and functions of EVs [41,116].

A wide variety of techniques currently exists to culture cells in 3D. These can be grouped into two main categories: scaffold-based methods and scaffold-free methods (Figure 3). Scaffold-free methods involve mostly spheroids, which are formed without attachment to a scaffold; therefore, cell–cell adhesion is required for their formation [113]. Scaffold-based methods, on the other hand, use exogenous materials to provide a substitute for the tissue's native ECM. Modification of the chemical and physical properties of these allows mimicry of the microenvironment found in specific tissues and provide greater structural integrity for larger tissue engineered constructs [117]. Scaffold-based methods include hydrogels, fibrous and porous scaffolds, and microcarriers amongst others. The wide range of techniques available make it possible to choose from a range of biocompatible materials which give rise to different structures and architectures and mechanical and degradation properties, which can be tailored for different applications [118].

6. Spheroids

Spheroid culture consists of cell aggregates (usually ranging in diameter from 50–1000 μm) caused by the self-assembly of cells when cultured in suspension [117]. Spheroid 3D culture methods allow for cell–cell communication, better mimicking of in vivo environments, and retention of the intrinsic phenotypic properties of cells [119]. Due to their simplicity, low cost, and reproducibility, spheroid cultures allow for automated production of hundreds to thousands of spheroids within 24 h, which is advantageous for high-throughput drug toxicity screening and other applications [117].

For spheroids in the size range of hundreds of micrometres, it becomes difficult to transport oxygen and nutrients to the core and to dispose of metabolic waste products via simple diffusion [114]. This causes concentration gradients in which the inner cells have less access to nutrients and suffer accumulation of toxic waste products, causing necrosis in the centre of spheroids, which leads to self-disassembly. The sizes of spheroids for which this occurs are dependent on the cell type [119]. Necrosis is characteristic of tumour environments and therefore makes spheroids attractive for studying cancer-associated pathways and the effects of anticancer drugs [120].

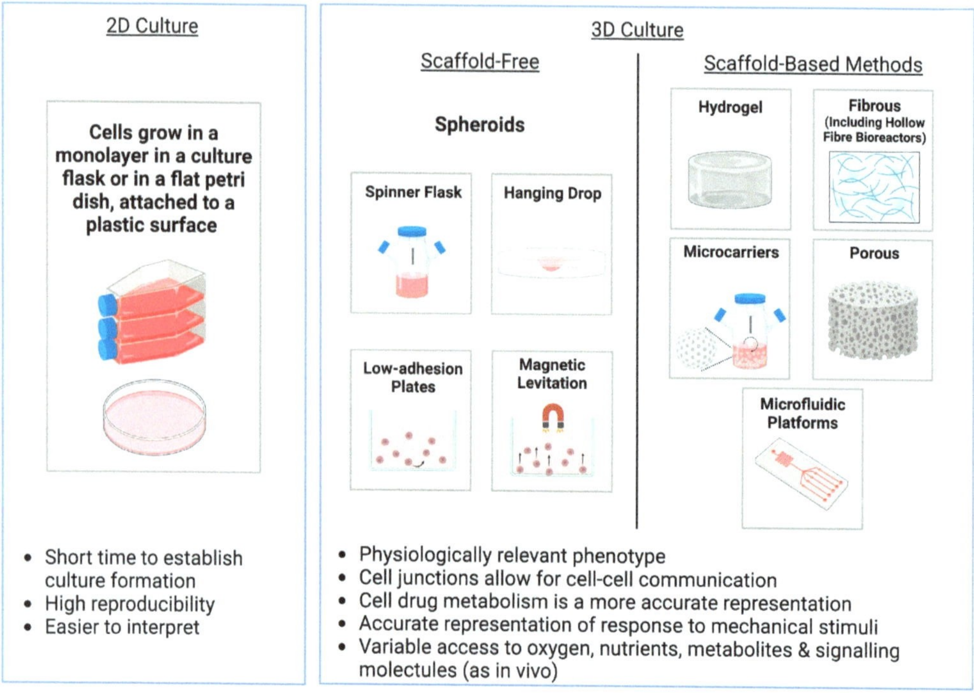

Figure 3. Advantages of 2D and 3D culture methods and the different types of 3D culture approaches.

Although spheroid 3D cultured cells are not provided with an external ECM, spheroid cells are able to secrete ECM proteins. ECM protein secretion in spheroid culture is dependent on the size of the spheroid and cell type [117]. For example, when staining human glioma and human thyroid cancer cell lines grown in spheroid culture for fibronectin, laminin, and collagen (ECM proteins), it was found that both spheroid types presented ECM proteins [121]. In contrast, spheroid culture of fibroblasts leads to nemosis, caused by cell–cell contact inhibition and the need for a sufficiently rigid mechanical environment, which eventually causes cell death. The major signalling pathway associated with this is the Hippo signalling pathway, which leads to an inhibition of the transcriptional effectors YAP and TAZ, which have essential roles in cell proliferation, migration, and survival [122,123].

Over the past decade, a variety of methods have been developed in order to achieve spheroid culturing techniques. The most commonly used methods of obtaining spheroid culture are the hanging drop method, using low-adhesion plates, stirring cells in a spinner flask, and magnetic levitation. The hanging drop method consists of placing culture medium on petri dish lids. Cells then accumulate at the tip of a drop and aggregate spontaneously, leading to the formation of spheroids. However, this method does not allow for change in culture medium, limiting the duration of cell culture, making scaling-up processes not feasible [124]. Alternatively, cells can be placed in a low-adhesion plate so that the cells cannot attach to the substrate and instead aggregate with each other, forming spheroids [125]. Another method of forming spheroids is placing cells in a spinner flask. This will agitate the cells to form spheroids, allowing for larger scale production [126]. Magnetic levitation involves labelling cells with magnetic nanoparticles and subsequently applying an external magnetic field, encouraging cells to self-assemble into multicellular spheroids. This technique overcomes the limitation of core spheroid necrosis and includes other advantages, such as the ability to image and track the cells [127].

Spheroid culture has been used successfully to culture cells and isolate EVs. Faruqu et al., for example, isolated exosomes from umbilical-cord-derived MSC (UC-MSC) spheroids. These exosomes caused increased migration and proliferation of murine fibroblasts in vitro, therefore having the potential of accelerating wound healing [128]. Many studies have also shown that MSC cultured in 3D spheroid conditions produced more EVs compared to when being cultured in 2D methods. This was shown by Kim et al., who demonstrated that when seeding MSC at the same density, a higher number of exosomes was produced from spheroid culture vs. traditional culture methods [129]. Xie et al. isolated MVs from MSC cultured in 2D and in spheroid conditions and found that, compared to 2D-MSC-MVs, 3D-MSC-MVs significantly decreased the chemotactic index of CD14+ cells and experienced an increased capability to induce signal factors as well as to improve immunomodulating activities, suggesting that these might be a better regenerative therapy for retinal degenerative diseases [130]. Miceli et al. compared the immunosuppressive and angiogenic properties of MSC-derived exosomes between 2D and 3D spheroid culture and found that there was no significant difference between 2D- and 3D-spheroid-culture-derived exosomes inducing capillary-like formation and endothelial cell migration. However, there was an increased capillary maturation and inhibition of peripheral blood mononuclear cells (PBMC) in the presence of 3D-spheroid-culture-derived condition medium (CM) compared to 2D-culture-derived CM and 2D-culture-derived exosomes [131].

Similar results have also been obtained with different cell types. A study by Hu et al. showed that exosomes secreted by spheroid culture of dermal papilla (DP) cells had a more profound therapeutic effect. Their group investigated the effect of these in hair growth and showed that miR-218-5p was notably up-regulated in exosomes from DP cells grown in spheroid culture when compared to 2D methods. This enhanced the expression of β-catenin and down-regulated secreted frizzled-related protein (SFRP2), which positively regulated hair follicle growth and maintained the anagen phase of the hair cycle [132].

The same research group (Hu et al.) also compared the effects of human dermal fibroblasts (HDF)-derived 2D and 3D spheroid exosomes on skin photoaging. They demonstrated that 3D spheroid-culture-derived exosomes caused increased procollagen type I expression and a significant decrease in matrix metalloproteinases 1 (MMP-1) expression as well as a higher levels of dermal collagen deposition. This indicated that exosomes derived from HDF spheroid 3D culture have anti-skin-aging properties and the potential to prevent and treat cutaneous ageing [133].

Tu et al., used exosomes to demonstrate that cancer cell spheroids are more physiologically relevant to native tumour tissue than 2D cultured cells. Exosomes were isolated from a pancreatic cancer cell line (PANC-1) grown in 3D spheroids and in 2D culture flasks. Spheroid 3D culture methods yielded a higher number of exosomes which contained miRNA and *Glypican-1* (GPC-1), more closely resembling the progression of pancreatic cancer [134]. Naseri et al., cultured cancer stem cells (CSC) in spheroid form and tested the exosomes secreted by these and their impact on dendritic cells (DC) maturation in order to better understand the therapeutic impact of DC against CSC. DC spheroid exosomes increased the ratio of interleukin-12 (IL-12) to interleukin-10 (IL-10) supernatants of mature DC, favouring immunostimulation and promoting T cell proliferation. T cells treated with these exosomes disrupted spheroid structure presenting an alternative immunotherapy strategy to reduce cancer spread [135]. Liu et al. also analysed the effect of exosomes from CSC and found that breast CSC spheroid exosomes had a significant impact in breast cancer cell glycolysis by miR-1252-5p/PFKB2 [136].

In 2020, a series of studies were conducted by Dinh et al. in which lung spheroid-cell-derived secretome (LSC-Sec), lung spheroid-cell-derived exosomes (LSC-exo), and MSC-derived secretome and exosomes were used to treat different models of lung injury and fibrosis. This study revealed that all secretome- and exosome-treated groups had a therapeutic benefit: decreased fibrosis and reduced lung apoptosis. However, only LSC-Sec and LSC-exo showed a more notable effect and decreased collagen deposition [137].

Additionally, spheroids have also been used to mimic a more representative form of the in vivo microenvironment to test the effect of exosomes. Choi et al., compared the effects of exosomes isolated from the CM of head and neck squamous cell carcinoma (HNSCC) and primary-cancer-associated fibroblasts (CAF) coculture from 2D conditions and 3D spheroids on angiogenesis in HSNCC. Their results showed that exosomes derived from 3D spheroid culture upregulated angiogenesis-related genes in HNSCC 3D spheroid culture when compared to 2D. Their results also showed that vasculature was significantly increased in mouse tumour xenograft models derived from 3D spheroids of HNSCC cells with primary CAF when compared to tumours derived from cells cultured in monolayers. This makes the tumour model derived from spheroids a more reliable model for studying the function of exosomes and for obtaining chemotherapy drug screening results [138].

Verdera et al. performed a set of experiments to characterise the cellular mechanisms involved in EV uptake. In their work, they showed that the uptake of EVs in 3D spheroids was restricted to the outer few cell layers in contrast to the 2D monolayer, where all cells had taken up EVs within 4 h. The 3D spheroid model mimics more closely in vivo cellular organisation, suggesting that spheroids might be best to test EV internalisation and therefore EV therapeutics and drug delivery [139].

Organoid systems also take advantage of the self-organising capabilities of cells to recreate in vitro miniaturised and simplified model systems of organs. Organoids have also been used for the research of EVs. The current review does not cover the production of EVs from scaffold-free multicellular organoids, which has been reviewed elsewhere [140].

7. Hydrogels

Hydrogels are 3D hydrophilic polymers that have attracted attention due to their low cost, ease of use and range of materials they comprise of [141]. Hydrogels can be made of either natural polymers (e.g., gelatin, fibrin, alginate, agarose) or synthetic polymers (e.g., polyethylene glycol (PEG), poly(acrylic acid) (PAA), polyethylene oxide (PEO), polyvinyl alcohol (PVA)). When cross-linked through either covalent or non-covalent bonds, hydrophilic polymers absorb water (up to ~95% of hydrogel content) [142] and swell without dissolving. Higher cross-linking results in lower swelling [143]. In the swollen state, they are often soft and elastic, making them ideal for mimicking soft tissue. Additionally, hydrogels allow free diffusion of soluble factors such as cytokines and growth factors needed for cell growth [119]. Control of hydrogels' swelling can be used to tailor their mechanical properties, such as rigidity, making it possible to match different tissue stiffness [144]. Their rate of degradation can also be tailored, allowing sustained release of encapsulated materials [114,141,145].

Porosity can also be introduced into hydrogels either through cross-linking or phase separation during synthesis. The pore size, distribution, and interconnections all have an impact on the mechanical properties of the hydrogel. However, in hydrogels, it can be difficult to obtain homogenous pore distributions and sizes, which may have an impact on the surface area for cell growth [146]. Pore sizes are important in enabling adequate tissue growth and are dependent on the specific type of cell. For example, hydrogels with pore sizes of 25–500 μm are required for cartilage growth, ~166 μm for vascular network formation, and 50–200 μm for the growth of smooth muscle cells [147,148].

The relatively low mechanical strength of hydrogels limits their application in tissue engineering to mainly soft tissues, such as skin [146,149,150]. Nonetheless, hydrogels have been proven to be useful in EV research. Using stiffness tuneable ECM hydrogel scaffolds, Patwardhan et al. reported that stiff ECMs promote exosome secretion in a YAP/TAZ-pathway-dependent manner. To do this, MCF-7 and MDA-MB-231 cells (epithelial human breast cancer cell lines) were grown in polyacrylamide gels (PA), which were coated with different amounts of collagen to obtain hydrogels with different stiffness. This study showed that hydrogels can be used to increase exosome production as well as to provide a better method of understanding breast cancer [151].

Other studies have used hydrogels to grow cells and isolate the EVs secreted. Thippabhotla et al. used peptide hydrogels to grow HeLa cells and compared the EVs secreted by these to those secreted by HeLa cells grown in 2D monolayers. Their study showed that hydrogel 3D-culture-derived EV small RNAs were different from their originator cells' RNA profile, possibly indicating a specific sorting process. Additionally, they showed that hydrogel-derived 3D EV small RNAs exhibited a much higher similarity to in-vivo-circulating EVs derived from cervical cancer patient plasma. However, DNA sequencing analysis revealed that there was no difference in the genomic information carried by EVs based on the cell growth conditions. Their work shows that EVs could be used as molecular indicators in models used to study the effect of drugs or treatments and that hydrogel scaffolds are a more physiologically representative models to grow cells compared to 2D monolayers [25].

Han et al. used gelatin methacryloyl (GelMA) hydrogels to grow MSC and then compared the exosomes secreted by these with exosomes secreted by MSC cultured in 2D monolayers. They found that exosomes derived from hydrogel 3D cultures showed better neuroprotective effects compared to exosomes derived from 2D cultures. Additionally, exosomes derived from hydrogel 3D cultures contained a higher component of neuroprotective-related proteins and miRNAs that regulate the transcription of cellular immune responses genes. Furthermore, exosomes derived from hydrogel 3D cultures contained a higher amount of anti-inflammatory and anti-apoptotic factors which could be beneficial for the treatment of spinal cord injury (SCI). The same hydrogel was investigated for the delivery of exosomes derived from hydrogel 3D cultures to a SCI lesion site. This significantly improved their retention at the site and achieved a more sustained release when compared to repeated local injection of exosomes [152].

Other research groups have similarly used hydrogels for sustained delivery of EVs. These hydrogels tend to have low viscosity fluid with shear-thinning properties, improving retention at the site of injection [153]. There are three common approaches by which EV encapsulation into hydrogels is achieved. The first involves combining exosomes with polymers followed by the addition of crosslinkers inducing gelation. The second approach is commonly known as the "breathing technique" and involves soaking the swollen hydrogel in a solution containing exosomes, which will enter the porous hydrogel network. The third approach involves mixing the exosomes with both the polymer in solution and the crosslinkers simultaneously, causing in situ gelation [141,154]. Chen et al., for example, used an injectable hyaluronic acid (HA) hydrogel to deliver endothelial progenitor cell (EPC)-derived EVs into the ischaemic myocardium. This study showed increased therapeutic efficiency and efficacy towards cardiomyocyte recovery [155]. The most commonly used methods for EV delivery using hydrogel-based systems are summarised in Table 3.

Table 3. Commonly used hydrogel-based systems for the delivery of EVs.

Materials Used	Type of Cells/EVs	Applications	References
Hyaluronic Acid	MSC secretome	Asherman's syndrome (injured endometrium)	[156]
Alginate	PPR exosomes/AD-MSC exosomes	Skin regeneration	[157,158]
Chitosan-based hydrogel with silk fibroin	hUC-MSC treated with miR-675-exosomes/gingival MSC exosomes	Aging-induced vascular disfunction/skin wound healing	[159,160]
Methylcellulose-chitosan	Placental MSC exosomes	Wound healing	[161]
Chitosan/chitosan-hyaluronic acid composite hydrogels	miR-126-3p overexpressing MSC exosomes/MSC exosomes/ BM-MSC exosomes	Wound healing Ischaemia Skin regeneration	[162–165]
Hydroxyapatite embedded hyaluronic acid	UC-MSC exosomes	Bone regeneration	[166]
Polypetide-based FHE hydrogel	AD-MSC exosomes	Wound healing	[167]

Table 3. *Cont.*

Materials Used	Type of Cells/EVs	Applications	References
RGD peptide/peptide-modified adhesive hydrogel	MSC exosomes	AKI repair/SCI treatment	[168,169]
Polyethylene glycol (PEG) hydrogel	MSC EVs	Chronic liver regeneration	[170]
Crosslinked hyaluronic acid/PEG hydrogel	MSC EVs	Osteoarthritis	[171]

Abbreviations: PPR, platelet rich plasma; hUC-MSC, human UC-MSC; FHE, pluronic F127, oxidative hyaluronic acid, and Poly-ε-L-lysine composite; AKI, acute kidney injury.

8. Hard Porous and Fibrous Scaffolds

Hard scaffolds consisting of 3D structures with interconnected pores or fibres are also widely used to provide a physical support for cell growth and attachment. Compared to hydrogel scaffolds, they have higher mechanical strength, stiffness, and wear resistance [172]. As with hydrogels, hard scaffolds can be made of natural or synthetic polymers. Natural polymers often have inherent bioactivity and may be more biocompatible. Synthetic polymers, on the other hand, are more versatile, have increased reproducibility, and are easier to process, allowing for more control over structural features [173]. Pore and fibre structures, such as their interconnection and arrangement (orientated or random), determine the scaffold's surface area and mechanical properties, which may influence cell phenotype, vascularisation, and ECM deposition [141]. These will also influence cellular penetration and migration to the scaffold's interior and access to nutrients and oxygen [114].

Currently, the most common applications of hard scaffolds are to recreate the physical and structural environment of tissues, such as bone, cartilage, vascular, ligament, and skeletal muscle, as well as applications in preclinical in vitro testing of spheroids, tumoroids, and organoids [174]. It is often important that the scaffold's mechanical properties mirror those of the target tissue and enable stress transfer and load bearing. The degradation profile should also be chosen carefully so that the scaffold provides the necessary support during tissue formation [115].

Traditional techniques for scaffold fabrication include solvent casting and particulate leaching, gas foaming, thermally induced phase separation (TIPS), and freeze-drying. These techniques have poor reproducibility and poor control over defined pore and fibre structures [118]. Advanced scaffold fabrication techniques have been developed in order to achieve better control over the aforementioned parameters. These include fused deposition modelling, stereolithography, 3D printing, the integration of computer aided design (CAD) software, electrospinning, and rapid prototyping [175].

Electrospinning has the capability of controlling the diameter of the nanoscale thin fibres, obtaining a homogenous fibrous scaffold. Electrospun scaffolds have been used for cell culture and EV collection. Kadir et al. generated electrospun fibre sheet scaffolds to grow MSC. Their results compared the CM generated from MSC grown on the fibres to the CM of MSC grown in traditional culture plates. CM from scaffold 3D culture showed enhanced migration and proliferation of MSC and chondrocytes as well as reduced inflammation. They also investigated different fibre alignments and found that these also had an effect on the properties of the CM [176].

Hu et al. showed similar results. Sericin-deprived spun silk from comber (a waste material derived from cotton manufacturing) was bonded via mechanical hydroentanglement in order to achieve web formation. Adult HDF were then cultured on the silk fibroin woven scaffolds. Compared to the exosomes from HDF grown in standard 2D flasks, 3D exosomes carried higher amounts of angiogenic growth factors, and they also induced human dermal microvascular endothelial cells (hDMVEC) to form a higher number of tubes in vitro [177].

Three-dimensional printing can also influence scaffold pore configuration, and therefore, scaffolds can be tailored to increase EV production and/or enhance their clinical potential. Gao et al. cultured BM-MSC on 3D-printed hydroxyapatite scaffolds and investigated the effect of the isolated exosomes on cell proliferation, migration, tube formation, and angiogenesis in vivo. These exhibited stronger effects than exosomes isolated from the same cell line cultured using traditional culture methods [178]. Man et al. also showed that culturing cells in 3D-printed scaffolds enhanced the therapeutic potential of the isolated EVs. In their study, osteoblasts were cultured on 3D-printed titanium scaffolds coated with hydroxyapatite with different pore sizes and shapes, and the effect this had on EV secretion yield and on the EV capacity to induce osteogenic differentiation was studied. Triangular pore geometry and coating increased bone mineralisation and EV production (2.2-fold and 4.5-fold), demonstrating that it is possible to harness bone-mimetic culture platforms, enhancing the production of pro-regenerative EVs [179]. Liu et al. used 3D printing for exosome delivery. They pretreated a 3D printed collagen/silk fibroin scaffold with hypoxia-pretreated human UC-MSC (hUC-MSC)-derived exosomes and implanted this into a traumatic brain injury (TBI) beagle model. Their study revealed that the implanted exosome scaffold inhibited nerve cell apoptosis and inflammation, enhancing the motor functional recovery of TBI [180]. Chen et al. used coaxial 3D printing to print a meter-long hollow hydrogel microfibre, which allowed for the expansion of MSC. Their platform enriched particles ~1009-fold when compared to 2D culture, and EVs secreted from scaffold 3D cultures conserved their pro-angiogenic properties [181].

It is also possible to incorporate EVs into 3D-printable bio-ink. Born et al. incorporated MSC-derived EVs into GelMA hydrogel bio-ink and demonstrated that increasing the concentration of a crosslinker during gelation can improve the sustained release of the pro-angiogenic EVs [182]. Chen et al., used a bio-ink composed of MSC-derived exosomes, decellularized cartilage ECM, and GelMA hydrogel to 3D print a biocompatible scaffold which was implanted on a rabbit model with an osteochondral defect. Their results showed that the ECM/GelMA/exosome scaffold was able to facilitate cartilage regeneration in vivo [183].

Pavia et al. used TIPS to prepare poly-L-lactic acid (PLLA) scaffolds and changed the processing parameters to compare two different morphologies. Their results showed that astrocytes were able to secrete exosomes when cultured on both scaffold morphologies [184]. Another example of this was shown by Zhang et al., who demonstrated that culturing hBM-MSC in 3D collagen scaffolds had a stronger outcome in enhancing spatial learning compared to exosomes obtained from hBM-MSC cultured in 2D platforms when injected in a TBI rat model [185]. Scaffolds and grafts have been used widely in bone regeneration by fabrication of hybrid biomaterials with multipotential cells and their released factors [139]. Table 4 summarises exosome-integrated bone engineering scaffolds strategies used to date.

Scaffolds have also been used for the sustained delivery of EVs as drug delivery vehicles. Zhang et al. encapsulated paclitaxel (PTX) onto MSC-derived exosomes and seeded these onto a collagen scaffold. This allowed for the controlled release of exosome encapsulated PTX and showed superior performance for motor functional recovery when implanted on SCI rat models. [186]

Table 4. Scaffold–exosome approaches for bone regeneration.

Type of Scaffold	Cell Type	Applications	References
Type I collagen and fibronectin matrix proteins	MSC	Augment performance of lineage specific differentiation of naïve MSCs in bone transplantation	[187]
Porous β-tricalcium phosphate	iPSC and MSC	Increased angiogenesis and osteogenesis	[188–190]
PCL	MSC and chondrogenic ATDC5 cells	Enhanced osteogenic differentiation	[191–193]
Mineral-doped PLA porous	hAD-MSC	Enhanced osteogenic MSC differentiation	[194]
Biodegradable PLGA	hAD-MSC	Enhanced osteogenic differentiation and enhanced mineralisation by endogenous cell recruitment	[195,196]
Tannic-acid-modified sulfonated SPEEK	BM-MSC	Enhanced osteoimmunomodulation by promotion of macrophage polarisation	[197]
3D-printed porous Ti alloy (Ti6Al4V)	SC	Improved efficacy of Ti alloy scaffolds in bone repair	[198]
Calcium sulphate hydroxyapatite nanocement	MSC	Enhanced bone mineralisation	[199]

Abbreviations: iPSC, induced pluripotent stem cells; PCL, polycaprolactone; hAD-MSC, human AD-MSC; PLA, poly(L-lactide) acid; PLGA, poly(lactic-co-glycolic acid); SPEEK, polyetheretherketone; Ti, titanium; SC, Schwann cells.

9. Microcarriers

The use of microcarriers to culture cells in suspension has been applied for the production of vaccines and pharmaceuticals, as a delivery method, and to expand cell populations. Microcarriers were successfully introduced in 1967, and there is now a large number of commercially available microcarriers comprising different sizes, materials and surface topographies [111]. Microcarriers are spherical beads with sizes typically in the range of 100–300 μm. They provide a substrate that enables attachment of adherent cells in bioreactors that can be maintained in suspension using agitation [200]. Several studies have demonstrated that the process of agitation may mechanically stimulate the cultured cells resulting in a higher EV yield [97]. Patel et al., for example, demonstrated that applying a low shear rate on human dermal microvascular endothelial cells (HDMEC) cultured on a perfusion bioreactor system increased EV secretion 100-fold [201]. Additionally, agitation creates a homogenous environment that allows cells to obtain uniform exposure to oxygen and nutrients [202]. However, agitation must be carefully controlled to avoid cell damage and cellular shedding of the microcarriers. To grow cells in a bioreactor, two strategies are typically implemented. The first consists of spheroid formation, as described in Section 6, and the second one consists of using suspension culture systems such as microcarriers, to which adherent cells can attach and grow [203].

Many mammalian cells are anchorage-dependent, and therefore, cell attachment to the microcarriers' surface is a crucial parameter influencing metabolic activity, growth, and culture productivity [204,205]. The process of cell attachment results from interaction between the cell's transmembrane surface receptors, such as integrins, and proteins expressed on the surface of the microcarrier. Under normal culture conditions, attachment proteins such as vitronectin and fibronectin found in the serum added to culture medium coat the surface of the microcarrier [204,206]. However, certain cells, such as fibroblasts, secrete high amounts of fibronectin and therefore do not require exogenous proteins for attachment [207]. Additionally, all vertebrate cells possess unevenly distributed negative charge on their surface and will therefore attach to positively charged microcarriers. Non-charged and negatively charged microcarriers are also available; these tend to be coated with ECM proteins to facilitate cell attachment [208]. Microcarriers can be hydrophilic or hydrophobic. Hydrophilic surfaces allow for better protein absorption and therefore lead to a higher cell attachment [204].

Microcarriers can be divided into three main categories: non-porous, micro-porous, and macro-porous microcarriers (Figure 4). In solid and micro-porous microcarriers (pores are ≤10 μm), cells grow as monolayers on their surfaces. However, in macro-porous microcarriers (pores are 10–50 μm), cells can potentially migrate and proliferate within the porous matrix as well as on the microcarrier's surface, providing a larger surface area for growth. Furthermore, cells found within the pores of the microcarriers are protected from exposure to mechanical damage that may occur during agitation [209,210]. Macro-porous microcarriers are also suitable for immobilising non-adherent cell types. The microcarrier's shape (such as spherical, disc, or cylindrical) also influences cell attachment. For example, Schmidt et al. demonstrated that MSC have a lower proliferative index with more curved microcarrier surfaces due to increased cell exposure to high shear stresses in bioreactors [211].

The material a microcarrier is made of is very important since it can affect the stiffness, hydrophobic/hydrophilic properties, permeability (important for the transport of oxygen and nutrients), and topography of the microcarrier [208]. The materials used to produce microcarriers can be divided into two categories: synthetic and natural polymers. Synthetic polymers are often biocompatible and biodegradable, including poly(lactic-co-glycolic acid) (PLGA), polylactic acid (PLA), poly(ε-caprolactone) (PCL), polystyrene, and dextran. Natural polymers include cellulose, gelatine, collagen, alginate, and chitosan [111,198,200]. Additionally, multiple culture parameters, such as the cell and microcarrier seeding density, can also impact cell attachment and growth [208].

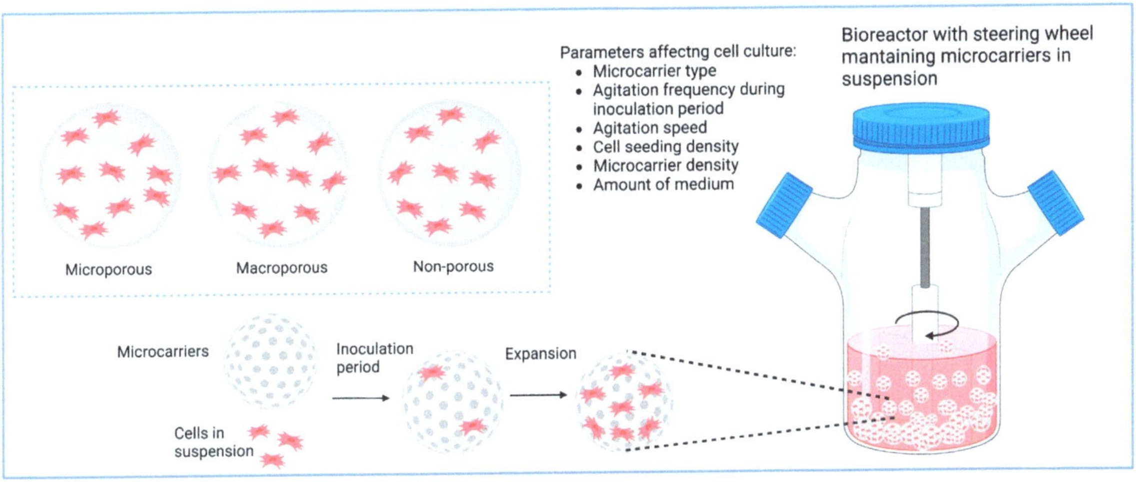

Figure 4. Schematic of cell attachment onto microcarriers and the different parameters affecting their culture.

Multiple research groups have successfully obtained EVs from cells attached to microcarriers (Table 5). In 2018, Čebatariūnienė et al. grew periodontal ligament stem cells (PLSC) on gelatin-coated alginate microcarriers using a bioreactor. NFkB reporter assays demonstrated that the EVs secreted by these stem cells suppressed basal and lipopolysaccharide (LPS) induced activity of NFκB activity, suggesting that these could potentially be used for targeting chronic inflammation during periodontitis [212].

Table 5. Microcarrier culture methods used to increase the yield or enhance the properties of EVs.

Cellular Origin	Fold Increase	Characteristic Alteration	Reference
MSC (BM-, AD- and hUC-)	5.7-fold increase	Increased purity	[202]
hUC-MSC	18.38-fold increase	Increased inhibition of silica-induced PF	[213]
hUC-MSC	20-fold increase	More potent siRNA transfer to neurons	[214]
BM-MSC	24-fold increase	Increased neurite length in TG neurons	[215]
hSF-MSC	1.6-fold increase	NA	[216]
SHED	NA	Induce apoptosis in dopaminergic neurons	[217]

Abbreviations: SHED, human exfoliated deciduous teeth.

Additionally, multiple papers have focused on looking at the implication of using microcarriers to culture cells to produce higher yields of EVs (Table 5). Fuzeta et al. used a serum-free/xeno-free microcarrier-based culture system implemented in a vertical wheel bioreactor in order to achieve the scalable production of exosomes derived from MSC obtained from different tissue sources. This allowed production of exosomes at a higher concentrations, productivities and purities [202].

Xu et al. demonstrated that the exosomes derived from microcarrier-based 3D-cultured hUC-MSC had the potential to inhibit silica-induced pulmonary fibrosis in vivo and improved lung function as a result. These results were confirmed in vitro, where it was shown that the exosomes reduced collagen deposition in NIH-3T3 cells [213].

Haraszti et al. cultivated hUC-MSC on spherical support matrix beads (Star-Plus Microcarriers) stirred in a spinner flask using serum-free medium and compared the exosomes secreted by these cells to those secreted by hUC-MSC grown in 2D culture flasks. They also compared two different exosome isolation methods: UC and tangential flow filtration (TFF). This research group showed that microcarrier-based 3D culture yielded up to 20-fold more exosomes compared to 2D culture. Additionally, their findings also reported that microcarrier 3D-TFF exosomes were seven times more potent in small interfering RNA (siRNA) transfer to neurons when compared to 2D exosomes [214].

Additionally, Jalilian et al. also successfully demonstrated that EVs derived from cells isolated in microcarriers have a more potent clinical potential. Jalilian et al. cultured BM-MSC in 2D monolayer and in a vertical wheel bioreactor using Corning's Low Concentration Synthemax II microcarriers and isolated the secreted EVs in order to investigate the potential differences in neuroregenerative properties of the EVs generated in 2D and micro-carrier-based 3D culture conditions. NTA showed that there was a 24-fold increase in EV concentration for microcarrier-based 3D culture. Additionally, a notable shift toward a more heterogenous phenotype was observed in microcarrier-based 3D-culture-derived EVs when compared to 2D-culture-derived EVs. Both 2D and microcarrier-based 3D-culture-derived EVs induced neurite growth, but microcarrier-based 3D-culture-derived EVs showed a significant increase in neurite length in trigeminal ganglia (TG) neurons when compared to 2D EVs in vitro [215].

In 2022, Cytodex microcarriers were used in order to grow human synovial fluid MSC (hSF-MSC) in a perfusion bioreactor. Compared to 2D culture, hSF-MSC prolifer-ated more quickly from 6 days onwards. After 14 days, exosomes were isolated using UC, and the samples were subsequently analysed. Both nanoparticle tracking analysis (NTA) and western blots revealed a higher exosomal concentration for microcarrier-based 3D culture samples. Exosomes derived from the microcarrier-based 3D culture system also delivered miRNAs into cells, suggesting that culturing MSC is a microcarrier-based culture system does not interfere with exosome function. Microbial and endotoxin detection results suggested that the protocol can produce exosomes which are biologically safe and promising for osteoarthritis therapy [216].

In 2015, a study revealed that exosomes derived from the microcarrier-based 3D culture of stem cells derived from dental pulp of human exfoliated deciduous teeth (SHED) supressed 6-hydroxy-dopamine (6-OHDAe), which induced apoptosis in dopaminergic neurons. This was not observed from exosomes derived from SHED grown in standard 2D culture flasks and could be a hallmark discovery for the treatment of treatment of Parkinson's disease [217].

Additionally, microcarriers have also been used to encapsulate EVs as diagnostics tools. Hou et al. used hydrogel microcarriers to identify tumour-derived exosomes by immobilising microcarriers with HER2 aptamers, which are transmembrane proteins expressed in HepG2 exosomes [218].

10. Hollow Fibre Bioreactor

A hollow fibre bioreactor is a type of bioreactor used for culturing cells in 3D that can also be used to obtain high concentrations of EVs [219]. The device consists of many small, semi-permeable hollow fibres bundled together in a tubular shell. In this way, cells can be seeded on the outside of the hollow fibres and media can be delivered through the fibre lumen. The system comprises a large surface area, which allows for a high seeding density and cell growth under a homogenous controlled culture environment. Using this system over microcarriers has the advantage of fibres protecting cells from shear stresses and allows for culture medium to circulate through the fibres where the cells are attached, while serum-free media can be applied in the extra capillary space (where EVs are secreted for isolation), preventing cross-contamination from other protein aggregates (Figure 5) [220–222].

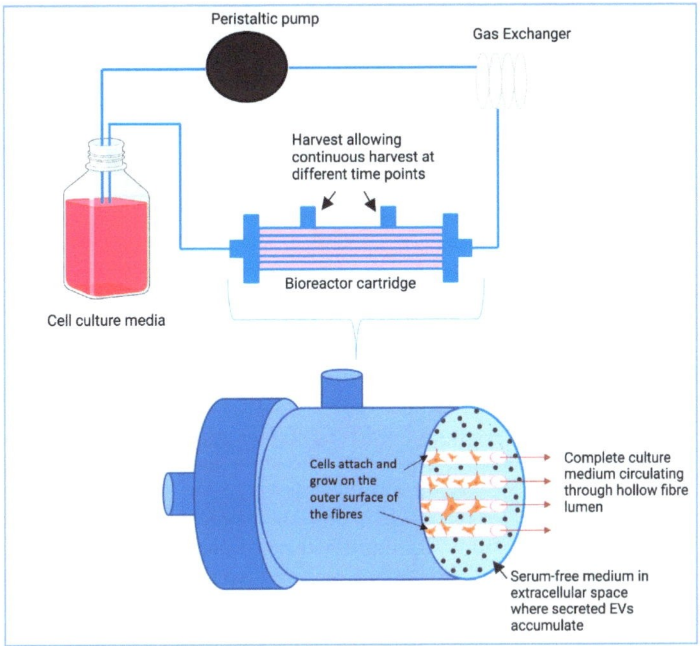

Figure 5. Schematic diagram of a hollow fibre bioreactor. Adapted with permission from I. K. Yan, N. Shukla, D. A. Borrelli and T. Patel, Methods in Molecular Biology; published by Springer Nature, 2018 [222].

In 2020, a study by Cao et al., evaluated the effect of culturing hUC-MSC in a hollow fibre bioreactor on the secreted exosomes. This culturing method yielded up to a 19.4-fold increase (as shown by protein assays) in exosome concentration when compared to traditional 2D culture. Tubular epithelial cells (TEC) were used to compare the therapeutic effect of exosomes derived from 2D cultures with exosomes derived from hollow fibre bioreactor 3D cultures. The results showed that exosomes derived from 3D cultures were more easily taken up by TEC and had a higher ability to reduce cisplatin-induced inflammation and to improve the viability of TEC. Furthermore, after injecting AKI mice models with exosomes derived from 2D and hollow fibre bioreactor 3D cultures, it was found that exosomes derived from hollow fibre bioreactor 3D cultures were more effective at alleviating AKI, which was shown by improved renal function, attenuated pathological changes of renal tubules, reduced inflammatory factors, and repressed T cell and macrophage infiltration [28].

Yan et al. investigated the use of hollow fibre bioreactors in producing exosomes for cartilage repair. UC-MSC were grown in a hollow fibre bioreactor, and these were found to yield 5.7 times more exosomes than 2D culture methods when compared using NTA. Additionally, results indicated that exosomes derived from 2D and hollow fibre bioreactor 3D cultures stimulated chondrocyte proliferation, migration, and matrix synthesis and also inhibited apoptosis, with exosomes derived from hollow fibre 3D cultures exerting a stronger effect. The exosomal therapeutic effects were then assessed by injecting exosomes derived from 2D and 3D cultures in cartilage defect areas. Exosomes derived from hollow fibre bioreactor 3D cultures showed a superior therapeutic effect [223].

Waston et al., also used a hollow fibre bioreactor for the efficient production of EVs. In their work, HEK293 cells expressing hetIL-15 were grown on a hollow fibre culture system and compared to those grown in conventional culture methods. They showed that this method yielded ~40-fold more EVs per mL while retaining their surface properties. Additionally, biophysical, and comparative proteomics suggested a more diverse population of EVs in the bioreactor preparations, while serum protein contaminants were detectable only in conventional culture EV preparations [224].

11. Conclusions

In recent years, there has been an increasing number of preclinical and clinical studies that have confirmed the therapeutic impact, drug delivery capacity and diagnostic potential of EVs. EV yield is a major limitation to the clinical translation of EV technology and as a result a wide range of studies have focused on different strategies to increase EV production.

Currently, to obtain EVs, cells are grown in 2D flaks, for which the surface area of the culture vessel is a limitation to the amount of EVs that can be obtained. Growing cells in monolayers results in reduced cell–cell interactions, influencing EV components and functions, which can hinder EV research for medical applications. The use of 3D culture methods has been shown to allow the expansion of a large number of cells, reducing cost and time required for culture. Additionally, 3D-cultured cells retain their phenotype and several studies have shown that 3D-culture-derived EVs have more enhanced clinical use. Furthermore, 3D culture methods have also been used for the delivery of EVs, allowing for a more sustained release and greater retention at the target site.

Different 3D culture methods present unique sets of advantages and disadvantages and have been used for different applications in EV research. Spheroid culture is cost efficient and reproducible; however, the transport of oxygen and nutrients to the inner cells in large spheroids is difficult, leading to cell death and therefore reducing the amount of EVs that can be obtained from spheroid 3D cell culture. Spheroid culture has been used successfully to culture cells and isolate in-vivo-like EVs. Additionally, the 3D spheroid model mimics more closely in vivo cellular organisation and therefore has been used to test EV therapeutics and drug delivery. Hydrogels offer low cost and ease of use and are comprised of a range of materials that are readily available. However, it is difficult to control pore size and distributions. This and hydrogels' low stiffness limit their application to mainly soft tissues. Hydrogels have, as spheroids, been used to grow cells and isolate EVs with stronger therapeutic effects both in vivo and for the sustained delivery of EVs. Hard and porous scaffolds have also been used to isolate EVs from cells grown in a microenvironment more closely resembling in vivo and for the delivery of EV's to certain tissue, achieving an enhanced therapeutic effect. Compared to hydrogel scaffolds, they have higher mechanical strength, stiffness, and wear resistance. They also have increased reproducibility and are easier to process, allowing for more control over structural features. However, producing scaffolds with controlled structures is expensive. Microcarriers, on the other hand, are widely commercially available, making them more affordable and offering a range of different sizes, materials, and surface topographies. When growing cells using microcarriers, these are steered in a bioreactor, and shear stress could potentially damage these cells. Multiple research groups have successfully used microcarriers to grow cells to obtain EVs with enhanced therapeutic effects and to increase EV production yield. Hollow fibre bioreactors offer a larger surface area and have an advantage over microcarriers, as the fibres protect cells from shear stress. They also allow for the growth of cells in a different space from where EVs are secreted, preventing cross-contamination from other EVs found in the cell culture medium.

Three-dimensional delivery and cell growth platforms can be tailored depending on the application and scale required. This review article summarises the different methods used for EV production and delivery. Careful consideration should be taken by the user before choosing the 3D methods for EV studies to obtain the desired clinical application.

Author Contributions: Conceptualization, M.C.E. and R.M.D.; writing—original draft preparation, M.C.E.; writing—review and editing, M.C.E. and R.M.D., visualization, M.C.E. and R.M.D.; funding acquisition, R.M.D. All authors have read and agreed to the published version of the manuscript.

Funding: M.C.E. is a doctoral student on the London Interdisciplinary Biosciences Consortium (BBSRC Grant No.: BB/M009513/1).

Institutional Review Board Statement: Not applicable.

Informed Consent Statement: Not applicable.

Data Availability Statement: Data sharing not applicable.

Acknowledgments: All figures were created with BioRender.com (accessed on 25 September 2022).

Conflicts of Interest: The authors declare no conflict of interest. The funders had no role in the design of the study, in the writing of the manuscript, or in the decision to publish the study.

References

1. Kalluri, R.; LeBleu, V.S. The biology, function, and biomedical applications of exosomes. *Science* **2020**, *367*, eaau6977. [CrossRef] [PubMed]
2. Gill, S.; Catchpole, R.; Forterre, P. Extracellular membrane vesicles in the three domains of life and beyond. *FEMS Microbiol. Rev.* **2018**, *43*, 273–303. [CrossRef] [PubMed]
3. Zhang, Y.; Liu, Y.; Liu, H.; Tang, W.H. Exosomes: Biogenesis, biologic function and clinical potential. *Cell Biosci.* **2019**, *9*, 19. [CrossRef] [PubMed]
4. Whiteside, T.L. Tumor-Derived Exosomes and Their Role in Cancer Progression. *Adv. Clin. Chem.* **2016**, *74*, 103–141. [CrossRef] [PubMed]
5. Feng, Z.-Y.; Zhang, Q.-Y.; Tan, J.; Xie, H.-Q. Techniques for increasing the yield of stem cell-derived exosomes: What factors may be involved? *Sci. China Life Sci.* **2021**, *65*, 1325–1341. [CrossRef] [PubMed]
6. Rashed, M.H.; Bayraktar, E.; Helal, G.K.; Abd-Ellah, M.F.; Amero, P.; Chavez-Reyes, A.; Rodriguez-Aguayo, C. Exosomes: From Garbage Bins to Promising Therapeutic Targets. *Int. J. Mol. Sci.* **2017**, *18*, 538. [CrossRef]
7. Zhang, Q.; Jeppesen, D.K.; Higginbotham, J.N.; Graves-Deal, R.; Trinh, V.Q.; Ramirez, M.A.; Sohn, Y.; Neininger, A.C.; Taneja, N.; McKinley, E.T.; et al. Supermeres are functional extracellular nanoparticles replete with disease biomarkers and therapeutic targets. *Nature* **2021**, *23*, 1240–1254. [CrossRef] [PubMed]
8. Fu, S.; Zhang, Y.; Li, Y.; Luo, L.; Zhao, Y.; Yao, Y. Extracellular vesicles in cardiovascular diseases. *Cell Death Discov.* **2020**, *6*, 68. [CrossRef]
9. Herrmann, I.K.; Wood, M.J.A.; Fuhrmann, G. Extracellular vesicles as a next-generation drug delivery platform. *Nat. Nanotechnol.* **2021**, *16*, 748–759. [CrossRef]
10. Ciferri, M.; Quarto, R.; Tasso, R. Extracellular Vesicles as Biomarkers and Therapeutic Tools: From Pre-Clinical to Clinical Applications. *Biology* **2021**, *10*, 359. [CrossRef]
11. Luo, R.; Liu, M.; Tan, T.; Yang, Q.; Wang, Y.; Men, L.; Zhao, L.; Zhang, H.; Wang, S.; Xie, T.; et al. Emerging Significance and Therapeutic Potential of Extracellular vesicles. *Int. J. Biol. Sci.* **2021**, *17*, 2476–2486. [CrossRef]
12. Limongi, T.; Susa, F.; Dumontel, B.; Racca, L.; Perrone Donnorso, M.; Debellis, D.; Cauda, V. Extracellular vesicles tropism: A comparative study between passive innate tropism and the active engineered targeting capability of lymphocyte-derived evs. *Membranes* **2021**, *11*, 886. [CrossRef] [PubMed]
13. Tai, Y.-L.; Chen, K.-C.; Hsieh, J.-T.; Shen, T.-L. Exosomes in cancer development and clinical applications. *Cancer Sci.* **2018**, *109*, 2364–2374. [CrossRef]
14. Osaki, M.; Okada, F. Exosomes and Their Role in Cancer Progression. *Yonago Acta Medica* **2019**, *62*, 182–190. [CrossRef] [PubMed]
15. Logozzi, M.; Mizzoni, D.; Di Raimo, R.; Fais, S. Exosomes: A Source for New and Old Biomarkers in Cancer. *Cancers* **2020**, *12*, 2566. [CrossRef] [PubMed]
16. Sumrin, A.; Moazzam, S.; Khan, A.A.; Ramzan, I.; Batool, Z.; Kaleem, S.; Ali, M.; Bashir, H.; Bilal, M. Exosomes as Biomarker of Cancer. *Braz. Arch. Biol. Technol.* **2018**, *61*, e18160730. [CrossRef]
17. Liang, Y.; Duan, L.; Lu, J.; Xia, J. Engineering exosomes for targeted drug delivery. *Theranostics* **2021**, *11*, 3183–3195. [CrossRef]
18. Soliman, H.M.; Ghonaim, G.A.; Gharib, S.M.; Chopra, H.; Farag, A.K.; Hassanin, M.H.; Nagah, A.; Emad-Eldin, M.; Hashem, N.E.; Yahya, G.; et al. Exosomes in Alzheimer's Disease: From Being Pathological Players to Potential Diagnostics and Therapeutics. *Int. J. Mol. Sci.* **2021**, *22*, 10794. [CrossRef]
19. Chen, J.; Li, P.; Zhang, T.; Xu, Z.; Huang, X.; Wang, R.; Du, L. Review on Strategies and Technologies for Exosome Isolation and Purification. *Front. Bioeng. Biotechnol.* **2022**, *9*, 811971. [CrossRef]
20. Bordanaba-Florit, G.; Madarieta, I.; Olalde, B.; Falcón-Pérez, J.; Royo, F. 3D Cell Cultures as Prospective Models to Study Extracellular Vesicles in Cancer. *Cancers* **2021**, *13*, 307. [CrossRef]
21. Wu, X.; Su, J.; Wei, J.; Jiang, N.; Ge, X. Recent Advances in Three-Dimensional Stem Cell Culture Systems and Applications. *Stem Cells Int.* **2021**, *2021*, 9477332. [CrossRef] [PubMed]
22. Jensen, C.; Teng, Y. Is It Time to Start Transitioning From 2D to 3D Cell Culture? *Front. Mol. Biosci.* **2020**, *7*, 33. [CrossRef] [PubMed]
23. Edmondson, R.; Broglie, J.; Adcock, A.; Yang, L. Three-dimensional cell culture systems and their applications in drug discovery and cell-based biosensors. *Assay Drug Dev. Technol.* **2014**, *12*, 207–218. [CrossRef]
24. Nooshabadi, V.T.; Khanmohammadi, M.; Shafei, S.; Banafshe, H.R.; Malekshahi, Z.V.; Ebrahimi-Barough, S.; Ai, J. Impact of atorvastatin loaded exosome as an anti-glioblastoma carrier to induce apoptosis of U87 cancer cells in 3D culture model. *Biochem. Biophys. Rep.* **2020**, *23*, 100792. [CrossRef] [PubMed]
25. Thippabhotla, S.; Zhong, C.; He, M. 3D cell culture stimulates the secretion of in vivo like extracellular vesicles. *Sci. Rep.* **2019**, *9*, 13012. [CrossRef]

26. Zhang, Y.; Chen, J.; Fu, H.; Kuang, S.; He, F.; Zhang, M.; Shen, Z.; Qin, W.; Lin, Z.; Huang, S. Exosomes derived from 3D-cultured MSCs improve therapeutic effects in periodontitis and experimental colitis and restore the Th17 cell/Treg balance in inflamed periodontium. *Int. J. Oral Sci.* **2021**, *13*, 43. [CrossRef]
27. Yu, W.; Li, S.; Guan, X.; Zhang, N.; Xie, X.; Zhang, K.; Bai, Y. Higher yield and enhanced therapeutic effects of exosomes derived from MSCs in hydrogel-assisted 3D culture system for bone regeneration. *Biomater. Adv.* **2022**, *133*, 112646. [CrossRef]
28. Cao, J.; Wang, B.; Tang, T.; Lv, L.; Ding, Z.; Li, Z.; Hu, R.; Wei, Q.; Shen, A.; Fu, Y.; et al. Three-dimensional culture of MSCs produces exosomes with improved yield and enhanced therapeutic efficacy for cisplatin-induced acute kidney injury. *Stem Cell Res. Ther.* **2020**, *11*, 206. [CrossRef]
29. Doyle, L.; Wang, M. Overview of Extracellular Vesicles, Their Origin, Composition, Purpose, and Methods for Exosome Isolation and Analysis. *Cells* **2019**, *8*, 727. [CrossRef]
30. Anand, S.; Samuel, M.; Mathivanan, S. Exomeres: A New Member of Extracellular Vesicles Family. *New Front. Extracell. Vesicles* **2021**, *97*, 89–97. [CrossRef]
31. Gurung, S.; Perocheau, D.; Touramanidou, L.; Baruteau, J. The exosome journey: From biogenesis to uptake and intracellular signalling. *Cell Commun. Signal.* **2021**, *19*, 47. [CrossRef] [PubMed]
32. De Palma, G.; Sallustio, F.; Schena, F.P. Clinical Application of Human Urinary Extracellular Vesicles in Kidney and Urologic Diseases. *Int. J. Mol. Sci.* **2016**, *17*, 1043. [CrossRef] [PubMed]
33. Jeppesen, D.K.; Fenix, A.M.; Franklin, J.L.; Higginbotham, J.N.; Zhang, Q.; Zimmerman, L.J.; Liebler, D.C.; Ping, J.; Liu, Q.; Evans, R.; et al. Reassessment of Exosome Composition. *Cell* **2019**, *177*, 428–445.e18. [CrossRef] [PubMed]
34. Sun, Z.; Hao, T.; Tian, J. Identification of exosomes and its signature miRNAs of male and female Cynoglossus semilaevis. *Sci. Rep.* **2017**, *7*, 860. [CrossRef]
35. Paulaitis, M.; Agarwal, K.; Nana-Sinkam, P. Dynamic Scaling of Exosome Sizes. *Langmuir* **2018**, *34*, 9387–9393. [CrossRef]
36. Schmidt, O.; Teis, D. The ESCRT machinery. *Curr. Biol.* **2012**, *22*, R116–R120. [CrossRef]
37. Alcayaga-Miranda, F.; Varas-Godoy, M.; Khoury, M. Harnessing the Angiogenic Potential of Stem Cell-Derived Exosomes for Vascular Regeneration. *Stem Cells Int.* **2016**, *2016*, 3409169. [CrossRef]
38. Zaborowski, M.P.; Balaj, L.; Breakefield, X.O.; Lai, C.P. Extracellular Vesicles: Composition, Biological Relevance, and Methods of Study. *Bioscience* **2015**, *65*, 783–797. [CrossRef]
39. Zügel, U.; Kaufmann, S.H.E. Role of heat shock proteins in protection from and pathogenesis of infectious diseases. *Clin. Microbiol. Rev.* **1999**, *12*, 19–39. [CrossRef]
40. Phuyal, S.; Hessvik, N.P.; Skotland, T.; Sandvig, K.; Llorente, A. Regulation of exosome release by glycosphingolipids and flotillins. *FEBS J.* **2014**, *281*, 2214–2227. [CrossRef]
41. Joo, H.S.; Suh, J.H.; Lee, H.J.; Bang, E.S.; Lee, J.M. Current knowledge and future perspectives on mesenchymal stem cell-derived exosomes as a new therapeutic agent. *Int. J. Mol. Sci.* **2020**, *21*, 727. [CrossRef] [PubMed]
42. Raposo, G.; Nijman, H.W.; Stoorvogel, W.; Liejendekker, R.; Harding, C.V.; Melief, C.J.; Geuze, H.J. B lymphocytes secrete antigen-presenting vesicles. *J. Exp. Med.* **1996**, *183*, 1161–1172. [CrossRef] [PubMed]
43. Wang, X.; Tian, L.; Lu, J.; Ng, I.O.-L. Exosomes and cancer—Diagnostic and prognostic biomarkers and therapeutic vehicle. *Oncogenesis* **2022**, *11*, 54. [CrossRef] [PubMed]
44. Li, P.; Kaslan, M.; Lee, S.H.; Yao, J.; Gao, Z. Progress in Exosome Isolation Techniques. *Theranostics* **2017**, *7*, 789–804. [CrossRef] [PubMed]
45. Skotland, T.; Hessvik, N.P.; Sandvig, K.; Llorente, A. Exosomal lipid composition and the role of ether lipids and phosphoinositides in exosome biology. *J. Lipid Res.* **2019**, *60*, 9–18. [CrossRef]
46. Li, I.; Nabet, B.Y. Exosomes in the tumor microenvironment as mediators of cancer therapy resistance. *Mol. Cancer* **2019**, *18*, 32. [CrossRef]
47. Lin, J.; Li, J.; Huang, B.; Liu, J.; Chen, X.; Chen, X.-M.; Xu, Y.-M.; Huang, L.-F.; Wang, X.-Z. Exosomes: Novel Biomarkers for Clinical Diagnosis. *Sci. World J.* **2015**, *2015*, 657086. [CrossRef]
48. Mathew, M.; Zade, M.; Mezghani, N.; Patel, R.; Wang, Y.; Momen-Heravi, F. Extracellular Vesicles as Biomarkers in Cancer Immunotherapy. *Cancers* **2020**, *12*, 2825. [CrossRef]
49. Li, X.; Corbett, A.L.; Taatizadeh, E.; Tasnim, N.; Little, J.P.; Garnis, C.; Daugaard, M.; Guns, E.; Hoorfar, M.; Li, I.T.S. Challenges and opportunities in exosome research—Perspectives from biology, engineering, and cancer therapy. *APL Bioeng.* **2019**, *3*, 011503. [CrossRef]
50. Tanaka, Y.; Kamohara, H.; Kinoshita, K.; Kurashige, J.; Ishimoto, T.; Iwatsuki, M.; Watanabe, M.; Baba, H. Clinical impact of serum exosomal microRNA-21 as a clinical biomarker in human esophageal squamous cell carcinoma. *Cancer* **2012**, *119*, 1159–1167. [CrossRef]
51. Munagala, R.; Aqil, F.; Gupta, R.C. Exosomal miRNAs as biomarkers of recurrent lung cancer. *Tumor Biol.* **2016**, *37*, 10703–10714. [CrossRef] [PubMed]
52. Machida, T.; Tomofuji, T.; Maruyama, T.; Yoneda, T.; Ekuni, D.; Azuma, T.; Miyai, H.; Mizuno, H.; Kato, H.; Tsutsumi, K.; et al. miR-1246 and miR-4644 in salivary exosome as potential biomarkers for pancreatobiliary tract cancer. *Oncol. Rep.* **2016**, *36*, 2375–2381. [CrossRef] [PubMed]
53. Yuwen, D.-L.; Sheng, B.-B.; Liu, J.; Wenyu, W.; Shu, Y.-Q. MiR-146a-5p level in serum exosomes predicts therapeutic effect of cisplatin in non-small cell lung cancer. *Eur. Rev. Med. Pharmacol. Sci.* **2017**, *21*, 2650–2658. [PubMed]

54. Wang, Y.; Niu, X.; Cheng, Y.; Zhang, Y.; Xia, L.; Xia, W.; Lu, S. Exosomal PD-L1 predicts response with immunotherapy in NSCLC patients. *Clin. Exp. Immunol.* **2022**, *208*, 316–322. [CrossRef]
55. Soung, Y.H.; Ford, S.; Zhang, V.; Chung, J. Exosomes in Cancer Diagnostics. *Cancers* **2017**, *9*, 8. [CrossRef]
56. Keller, S.; Ridinger, J.; Rupp, A.-K.; Janssen, J.W.G.; Altevogt, P. Body fluid derived exosomes as a novel template for clinical diagnostics. *J. Transl. Med.* **2011**, *9*, 86. [CrossRef]
57. Chen, G.; Huang, A.C.; Zhang, W.; Zhang, G.; Wu, M.; Xu, W.; Yu, Z.; Yang, J.; Wang, B.; Sun, H.; et al. Exosomal PD-L1 contributes to immunosuppression and is associated with anti-PD-1 response. *Nature* **2018**, *560*, 382–386. [CrossRef]
58. Hoshino, A.; Costa-Silva, B.; Shen, T.-L.; Rodrigues, G.; Hashimoto, A.; Mark, M.T.; Molina, H.; Kohsaka, S.; Di Giannatale, A.; Ceder, S.; et al. Tumour exosome integrins determine organotropic metastasis. *Nature* **2015**, *527*, 329–335. [CrossRef]
59. Hoshino, A.; Kim, H.S.; Bojmar, L.; Gyan, K.E.; Cioffi, M.; Hernandez, J.; Zambirinis, C.P.; Rodrigues, G.; Molina, H.; Heissel, S.; et al. Extracellular vesicle and particle biomarkers define multiple human cancers. *Cell* **2020**, *182*, 1044–1061.e18. [CrossRef]
60. D'Anca, M.; Fenoglio, C.; Serpente, M.; Arosio, B.; Cesari, M.; Scarpini, E.A.; Galimberti, D. Exosome Determinants of Physiological Aging and Age-Related Neurodegenerative Diseases. *Front. Aging Neurosci.* **2019**, *11*, 232. [CrossRef]
61. Dardet, J.P.; Serrano, N.; András, I.E.; Toborek, M. Overcoming Blood-Brain Barrier Resistance: Implications for Extracellular Vesicle-Mediated Drug Brain Delivery. *Front. Drug Deliv.* **2022**, *2*, 5. [CrossRef]
62. Ebrahimkhani, S.; Vafaee, F.; Young, P.E.; Hur, S.S.J.; Hawke, S.; Devenney, E.; Beadnall, H.; Barnett, M.H.; Suter, C.M.; Buckland, M.E. Exosomal microRNA signatures in multiple sclerosis reflect disease status. *Sci. Rep.* **2017**, *7*, 14293. [CrossRef] [PubMed]
63. Garcia-Contreras, M.; Shah, S.H.; Tamayo, A.; Robbins, P.D.; Golberg, R.B.; Mendez, A.J.; Ricordi, C. Plasma-derived exosome characterization reveals a distinct microRNA signature in long duration Type 1 diabetes. *Sci. Rep.* **2017**, *7*, 5998. [CrossRef] [PubMed]
64. Sun, Y.; Tao, Q.; Wu, X.; Zhang, L.; Liu, Q.; Wang, L. The Utility of Exosomes in Diagnosis and Therapy of Diabetes Mellitus and Associated Complications. *Front. Endocrinol.* **2021**, *12*, 1360. [CrossRef]
65. Liu, J.; Sun, X.; Zhang, F.-L.; Jin, H.; Yan, X.-L.; Huang, S.; Guo, Z.-N.; Yang, Y. Clinical Potential of Extracellular Vesicles in Type 2 Diabetes. *Front. Endocrinol.* **2021**, *11*, 1058. [CrossRef] [PubMed]
66. Wu, J.; Dong, T.; Chen, T.; Sun, J.; Luo, J.; He, J.; Wei, L.; Zeng, B.; Zhang, H.; Li, W.; et al. Hepatic exosome-derived miR-130a-3p attenuates glucose intolerance via suppressing PHLPP2 gene in adipocyte. *Metabolism* **2019**, *103*, 154006. [CrossRef] [PubMed]
67. Xu, H.; Du, X.; Xu, J.; Zhang, Y.; Tian, Y.; Liu, G.; Wang, X.; Ma, M.; Du, W.; Liu, Y.; et al. Pancreatic β cell microRNA-26a alleviates type 2 diabetes by improving peripheral insulin sensitivity and preserving β cell function. *PLoS Biol.* **2020**, *18*, e3000603. [CrossRef]
68. Liu, Q.; Piao, H.; Wang, Y.; Zheng, D.; Wang, W. Circulating exosomes in cardiovascular disease: Novel carriers of biological information. *Biomed. Pharmacother.* **2021**, *135*, 111148. [CrossRef]
69. Chong, S.Y.; Lee, C.K.; Huang, C.; Ou, Y.H.; Charles, C.J.; Richards, A.M.; Neupane, Y.R.; Pavon, M.V.; Zharkova, O.; Pastorin, G.; et al. Extracellular Vesicles in Cardiovascular Diseases: Alternative Biomarker Sources, Therapeutic Agents, and Drug Delivery Carriers. *Int. J. Mol. Sci.* **2019**, *20*, 3272. [CrossRef]
70. Zampetaki, A.; Willeit, P.; Tilling, L.; Drozdov, I.; Prokopi, M.; Renard, J.-M.; Mayr, A.; Weger, S.; Schett, G.; Shah, A.; et al. Prospective study on circulating microRNAs and risk of myocardial infarction. *J. Am. Coll. Cardiol.* **2012**, *60*, 290–299. [CrossRef]
71. Zhang, X.; Borg, E.G.F.; Liaci, A.M.; Vos, H.R.; Stoorvogel, W. A novel three step protocol to isolate extracellular vesicles from plasma or cell culture medium with both high yield and purity. *J. Extracell. Vesicles* **2020**, *9*, 1791450. [CrossRef] [PubMed]
72. Ratajczak, M.Z.; Ratajczak, J. Extracellular microvesicles/exosomes: Discovery, disbelief, acceptance, and the future? *Leukemia* **2020**, *34*, 3126–3135. [CrossRef] [PubMed]
73. Wei, W.; Ao, Q.; Wang, X.; Cao, Y.; Liu, Y.; Zheng, S.G.; Tian, X. Mesenchymal Stem Cell–Derived Exosomes: A Promising Biological Tool in Nanomedicine. *Front. Pharmacol.* **2021**, *11*, 1954. [CrossRef] [PubMed]
74. Muthu, S.; Bapat, A.; Jain, R.; Jeyaraman, N.; Jeyaraman, M. Exosomal therapy—A new frontier in regenerative medicine. *Stem Cell Investig.* **2021**, *8*, 7. [CrossRef]
75. Fuloria, S.; Subramaniyan, V.; Dahiya, R.; Dahiya, S.; Sudhakar, K.; Kumari, U.; Sathasivam, K.; Meenakshi, D.; Wu, Y.; Sekar, M.; et al. Mesenchymal Stem Cell-Derived Extracellular Vesicles: Regenerative Potential and Challenges. *Biology* **2021**, *10*, 172. [CrossRef]
76. Musiał-Wysocka, A.; Kot, M.; Majka, M. The Pros and Cons of Mesenchymal Stem Cell-Based Therapies. *Cell Transplant.* **2019**, *28*, 801–812. [CrossRef]
77. Yin, K.; Wang, S.; Zhao, R.C. Exosomes from mesenchymal stem/stromal cells: A new therapeutic paradigm. *Biomark. Res.* **2019**, *7*, 8. [CrossRef]
78. Wang, K.; Jiang, Z.; Webster, K.A.; Chen, J.; Hu, H.; Zhou, Y.; Zhao, J.; Wang, L.; Wang, Y.; Zhong, Z.; et al. Enhanced Cardioprotection by Human Endometrium Mesenchymal Stem Cells Driven by Exosomal MicroRNA-21. *Stem Cells Transl. Med.* **2016**, *6*, 209–222. [CrossRef]
79. Ma, Y.; Ge, S.; Zhang, J.; Zhou, D.; Li, L.; Wang, X.; Su, J. Mesenchymal stem cell-derived extracellular vesicles promote nerve regeneration after sciatic nerve crush injury in rats. *Int. J. Clin. Exp. Pathol.* **2017**, *10*, 10032–10039.
80. Rezaie, J.; Feghhi, M.; Etemadi, T. A review on exosomes application in clinical trials: Perspective, questions, and challenges. *Cell Commun. Signal.* **2022**, *20*, 1–13. [CrossRef]

81. Lai, J.J.; Chau, Z.L.; Chen, S.; Hill, J.J.; Korpany, K.V.; Liang, N.; Lin, L.; Lin, Y.; Liu, J.K.; Liu, Y.; et al. Exosome Processing and Characterization Approaches for Research and Technology Development. *Adv. Sci.* **2022**, *9*, 2103222. [CrossRef] [PubMed]
82. N'Diaye, E.-R.; Orefice, N.S.; Ghezzi, C.; Boumendjel, A. Chemically Modified Extracellular Vesicles and Applications in Radiolabeling and Drug Delivery. *Pharmaceutics* **2022**, *14*, 653. [CrossRef] [PubMed]
83. Dryden, G.W. Study Investigating the Ability of Plant Exosomes to Deliver Curcumin to Normal and Colon Cancer Tissue—Full Text View—ClinicalTrials.gov Identifier NCT01294072. Available online: https://clinicaltrials.gov/ct2/show/NCT01294072 (accessed on 6 January 2023).
84. Kim, M.S.; Haney, M.J.; Zhao, Y.; Mahajan, V.; Deygen, I.; Klyachko, N.L.; Inskoe, E.; Piroyan, A.; Sokolsky, M.; Okolie, O.; et al. Development of exosome-encapsulated paclitaxel to overcome mdr in cancer cells. *Nanomed. Nanotechnol. Biol. Med.* **2016**, *12*, 655–664. [CrossRef] [PubMed]
85. Martins-Marques, T.; Pinho, M.J.; Zuzarte, M.; Oliveira, C.; Pereira, P.; Sluijter, J.P.G.; Gomes, C.; Girao, H. Presence of Cx43 in extracellular vesicles reduces the cardiotoxicity of the anti-tumour therapeutic approach with doxorubicin. *J. Extracell. Vesicles* **2016**, *5*, 32538. [CrossRef]
86. Kim, M.S.; Haney, M.J.; Zhao, Y.; Yuan, D.; Deygen, I.; Klyachko, N.L.; Kabanov, A.V.; Batrakova, E.V. Engineering macrophage-derived exosomes for targeted paclitaxel delivery to pulmonary metastases: In vitro and in vivo evaluations. *Nanomedicine* **2018**, *14*, 195–204. [CrossRef]
87. Kalimuthu, S.; Gangadaran, P.; Rajendran, R.L.; Zhu, L.; Oh, J.M.; Lee, H.W.; Gopal, A.; Baek, S.H.; Jeong, S.Y.; Lee, S.-W.; et al. A New Approach for Loading Anticancer Drugs Into Mesenchymal Stem Cell-Derived Exosome Mimetics for Cancer Therapy. *Front. Pharmacol.* **2018**, *9*, 1116. [CrossRef]
88. Li, Y.-J.; Wu, J.-Y.; Wang, J.-M.; Hu, X.-B.; Cai, J.-X.; Xiang, D.-X. Gemcitabine loaded autologous exosomes for effective and safe chemotherapy of pancreatic cancer. *Acta Biomater.* **2019**, *101*, 519–530. [CrossRef]
89. Qu, M.; Lin, Q.; Huang, L.; Fu, Y.; Wang, L.; He, S.; Fu, Y.; Yang, S.; Zhang, Z.; Zhang, L.; et al. Dopamine-loaded blood exosomes targeted to brain for better treatment of Parkinson's disease. *J. Control. Release* **2018**, *287*, 156–166. [CrossRef]
90. De Jong, O.G.; Kooijmans, S.A.A.; Murphy, D.E.; Jiang, L.; Evers, M.J.W.; Sluijter, J.P.G.; Vader, P.; Schiffelers, R.M. Drug Delivery with Extracellular Vesicles: From Imagination to Innovation. *Acc. Chem. Res.* **2019**, *52*, 1761–1770. [CrossRef]
91. Sidhom, K.; Obi, P.; Saleem, A. A Review of Exosomal Isolation Methods: Is Size Exclusion Chromatography the Best Option? *Int. J. Mol. Sci.* **2020**, *21*, 6466. [CrossRef]
92. Villa, F.; Quarto, R.; Tasso, R. Extracellular Vesicles as Natural, Safe and Efficient Drug Delivery Systems. *Pharmaceutics* **2019**, *11*, 557. [CrossRef] [PubMed]
93. Meng, W.; He, C.; Hao, Y.; Wang, L.; Li, L.; Zhu, G. Prospects and challenges of extracellular vesicle-based drug delivery system: Considering cell source. *Drug Deliv.* **2020**, *27*, 585–598. [CrossRef] [PubMed]
94. Zhang, F.; Guo, J.; Zhang, Z.; Duan, M.; Wang, G.; Qian, Y.; Zhao, H.; Yang, Z.; Jiang, X. Application of engineered extracellular vesicles for targeted tumor therapy. *J. Biomed. Sci.* **2022**, *29*, 14. [CrossRef] [PubMed]
95. Luan, X.; Sansanaphongpricha, K.; Myers, I.; Chen, H.; Yuan, H.; Sun, D. Engineering exosomes as refined biological nanoplatforms for drug delivery. *Acta Pharmacol. Sin.* **2017**, *38*, 754–763. [CrossRef]
96. Pascucci, L.; Coccè, V.; Bonomi, A.; Ami, D.; Ceccarelli, P.; Ciusani, E.; Viganò, L.; Locatelli, A.; Sisto, F.; Doglia, S.M.; et al. Paclitaxel is incorporated by mesenchymal stromal cells and released in exosomes that inhibit in vitro tumor growth: A new approach for drug delivery. *J. Control. Release* **2014**, *192*, 262–270. [CrossRef]
97. Vader, P.; Mol, E.A.; Pasterkamp, G.; Schiffelers, R.M. Extracellular vesicles for drug delivery. *Adv. Drug Deliv. Rev.* **2016**, *106*, 148–156. [CrossRef]
98. Haney, M.J.; Klyachko, N.L.; Zhao, Y.; Gupta, R.; Plotnikova, E.G.; He, Z.; Patel, T.; Piroyan, A.; Sokolsky, M.; Kabanov, A.V.; et al. Exosomes as drug delivery vehicles for Parkinson's disease therapy. *J. Control. Release* **2015**, *207*, 18–30. [CrossRef]
99. Fuhrmann, G.; Chandrawati, R.; Parmar, P.A.; Keane, T.J.; Maynard, S.A.; Bertazzo, S.; Stevens, M.M. Engineering Extracellular Vesicles with the Tools of Enzyme Prodrug Therapy. *Adv. Mater.* **2018**, *30*, e1706616. [CrossRef]
100. Yang, Z.; Shi, J.; Xie, J.; Wang, Y.; Sun, J.; Liu, T.; Zhao, Y.; Zhao, X.; Wang, X.; Ma, Y.; et al. Large-scale generation of functional mRNA-encapsulating exosomes via cellular nanoporation. *Nat. Biomed. Eng.* **2020**, *4*, 69–83. [CrossRef]
101. Hahm, J.; Kim, J.; Park, J. Strategies to Enhance Extracellular Vesicle Production. *Tissue Eng. Regen. Med.* **2021**, *18*, 513–524. [CrossRef]
102. Syromiatnikova, V.; Prokopeva, A.; Gomzikova, M. Methods of the Large-Scale Production of Extracellular Vesicles. *Int. J. Mol. Sci.* **2022**, *23*, 10522. [CrossRef] [PubMed]
103. Du, C.R.; Wang, L. Zhu, Y. Yang. Extracellular Vesicles as Delivery Vehicles for Therapeutic Nucleic Acids in Cancer Gene Therapy: Progress and Challenges. *Pharmaceutics* **2022**, *14*, 2236. [CrossRef] [PubMed]
104. Zhao, Z.; Yang, Y.; Zeng, Y.; He, M. A microfluidic ExoSearch chip for multiplexed exosome detection towards blood-based ovarian cancer diagnosis. *Lab. Chip* **2016**, *16*, 489–496. [CrossRef] [PubMed]
105. Lin, B.; Lei, Y.; Wang, J.; Zhu, L.; Wu, Y.; Zhang, H.; Wu, L.; Zhang, P.; Yang, C. Microfluidic-Based Exosome Analysis for Liquid Biopsy. *Small Methods* **2021**, *5*, 2001131. [CrossRef]
106. Contreras-Naranjo, J.C.; Wu, H.-J.; Ugaz, V.M. Microfluidics for exosome isolation and analysis: Enabling liquid biopsy for personalized medicine. *Lab Chip* **2017**, *17*, 3558–3577. [CrossRef]

107. He, M.; Crow, J.; Roth, M.; Zeng, Y.; Godwin, A. From chip-in-a-lab to lab-on-a-chip: Towards a single handheld electronic system for multiple application-specific lab-on-a-chip (ASLOC). *Lab Chip* **2014**, *19*, 3773. [CrossRef]
108. Kanwar, S.S.; Dunlay, C.J.; Simeone, D.M.; Nagrath, S. Microfluidic device (ExoChip) for on-chip isolation, quantification and characterization of circulating exosomes. *Lab Chip* **2014**, *14*, 1891–1900. [CrossRef]
109. Lim, J.; Kang, B.; Son, H.Y.; Mun, B.; Huh, Y.-M.; Rho, H.W.; Kang, T.; Moon, J.; Lee, J.-J.; Seo, S.B.; et al. Microfluidic device for one-step detection of breast cancer-derived exosomal mRNA in blood using signal-amplifiable 3D nanostructure. *Biosens. Bioelectron.* **2022**, *197*, 113753. [CrossRef]
110. Ko, J.; Bhagwat, N.; Yee, S.S.; Ortiz, N.; Sahmoud, A.; Black, T.; Aiello, N.M.; McKenzie, L.; O'Hara, M.; Redlinger, C.; et al. Combining Machine Learning and Nanofluidic Technology To Diagnose Pancreatic Cancer Using Exosomes. *ACS Nano* **2017**, *11*, 11182–11193. [CrossRef]
111. Ibsen, S.D.; Wright, J.; Lewis, J.M.; Kim, S.; Ko, S.-Y.; Ong, J.; Manouchehri, S.; Vyas, A.; Akers, J.; Chen, C.C.; et al. Rapid Isolation and Detection of Exosomes and Associated Biomarkers from Plasma. *ACS Nano* **2017**, *11*, 6641–6651. [CrossRef]
112. Tian, F.; Liu, C.; Deng, J.; Sun, J. Microfluidic Separation, Detection, and Engineering of Extracellular Vesicles for Cancer Diagnostics and Drug Delivery. *Acc. Mater. Res.* **2022**, *3*, 498–510. [CrossRef]
113. Białkowska, K.; Komorowski, P.; Bryszewska, M.; Miłowska, K. Spheroids as a Type of Three-Dimensional Cell Cultures—Examples of Methods of Preparation and the Most Important Application. *Int. J. Mol. Sci.* **2020**, *21*, 6225. [CrossRef] [PubMed]
114. Huang, L.; Abdalla, A.M.; Xiao, L.; Yang, G. Biopolymer-Based Microcarriers for Three-Dimensional Cell Culture and Engineered Tissue Formation. *Int. J. Mol. Sci.* **2020**, *21*, 1895. [CrossRef] [PubMed]
115. Li, B.; Wang, X.; Wang, Y.; Gou, W.; Yuan, X.; Peng, J.; Guo, Q.; Lu, S. Past, present, and future of microcarrier-based tissue engineering. *J. Orthop. Transl.* **2015**, *3*, 51–57. [CrossRef] [PubMed]
116. Xie, S.; Zhang, Q.; Jiang, L. Current Knowledge on Exosome Biogenesis, Cargo-Sorting Mechanism and Therapeutic Implications. *Membranes* **2022**, *12*, 498. [CrossRef]
117. Valdoz, J.C.; Johnson, B.C.; Jacobs, D.J.; Franks, N.A.; Dodson, E.L.; Sanders, C.; Cribbs, C.G.; Van Ry, P.M. The ECM: To Scaffold, or Not to Scaffold, That Is the Question. *Int. J. Mol. Sci.* **2021**, *22*, 12690. [CrossRef]
118. Carletti, E.; Motta, A.; Migliaresi, C. Scaffolds for tissue engineering and 3D cell culture. *Methods Mol. Biol.* **2010**, *695*, 17–39.
119. Habanjar, O.; Diab-Assaf, M.; Caldefie-Chezet, F.; Delort, L. 3D Cell Culture Systems: Tumor Application, Advantages, and Disadvantages. *Int. J. Mol. Sci.* **2021**, *22*, 12200. [CrossRef]
120. Minchinton, A.I.; Tannock, I.F. Drug penetration in solid tumours. *Nat. Rev. Cancer* **2006**, *6*, 583–592. [CrossRef]
121. Nederman, T.; Norling, B.; Glimelius, B.; Carlsson, J.; Brunk, U. Demonstration of an extracellular matrix in multicellular tumor spheroids. *Cancer Res.* **1984**, *44*, 3090–3097.
122. Jorgenson, A.; Choi, K.; Sicard, D.; Smith, K.; Hiemer, S.; Varelas, X.; Tschumperlin, D. TAZ activation drives fibroblast spheroid growth, expression of profibrotic paracrine signals, and context-dependent ECM gene expression. *Am. J. Physiol. Cell Physiol.* **2017**, *312*, C277–C285. [CrossRef] [PubMed]
123. Salmenperä, P.; Kankuri, E.; Bizik, J.; Sirén, V.; Virtanen, I.; Takahashi, S.; Leiss, M.; Fässler, R.; Vaheri, A. Formation and activation of fibroblast spheroids depend on fibronectin–integrin interaction. *Exp. Cell Res.* **2008**, *314*, 3444–3452. [CrossRef] [PubMed]
124. Huang, S.-W.; Tzeng, S.-C.; Chen, J.-K.; Sun, J.-S.; Lin, F.-H. A Dynamic Hanging-Drop System for Mesenchymal Stem Cell Culture. *Int. J. Mol. Sci.* **2020**, *21*, 4298. [CrossRef] [PubMed]
125. Liu, D.; Chen, S.; Naing, M.W. A review of manufacturing capabilities of cell spheroid generation technologies and future development. *Biotechnol. Bioeng.* **2020**, *118*, 542–554. [CrossRef]
126. Lee, S.Y.; Lee, J.W. 3D Spheroid Cultures of Stem Cells and Exosome Applications for Cartilage Repair. *Life* **2022**, *12*, 939. [CrossRef]
127. Lewis, N.S.; EL Lewis, E.; Mullin, M.; Wheadon, H.; Dalby, M.J.; Berry, C.C. Magnetically levitated mesenchymal stem cell spheroids cultured with a collagen gel maintain phenotype and quiescence. *J. Tissue Eng.* **2017**, *8*, 2041731417704428. [CrossRef]
128. Faruqu, F.N.; Liam-Or, R.; Zhou, S.; Nip, R.; Al-Jamal, K.T. Defined serum-free three-dimensional culture of umbilical cord-derived mesenchymal stem cells yields exosomes that promote fibroblast proliferation and migration in vitro. *FASEB J.* **2020**, *35*, e21206. [CrossRef]
129. Kim, M.; Yun, H.-W.; Park, D.Y.; Choi, B.H.; Min, B.-H. Three-Dimensional Spheroid Culture Increases Exosome Secretion from Mesenchymal Stem Cells. *Tissue Eng. Regen. Med.* **2018**, *15*, 427–436. [CrossRef]
130. Xie, L.; Mao, M.; Zhou, L.; Zhang, L.; Jiang, B. Signal Factors Secreted by 2D and Spheroid Mesenchymal Stem Cells and by Cocultures of Mesenchymal Stem Cells Derived Microvesicles and Retinal Photoreceptor Neurons. *Stem Cells Int.* **2017**, *2017*, 2730472. [CrossRef]
131. Miceli, V.; Pampalone, M.; Vella, S.; Carreca, A.P.; Amico, G.; Conaldi, P.G. Comparison of Immunosuppressive and Angiogenic Properties of Human Amnion-Derived Mesenchymal Stem Cells between 2D and 3D Culture Systems. *Stem Cells Int.* **2019**, *2019*, 7486279. [CrossRef]
132. Hu, S.; Li, Z.; Lutz, H.; Huang, K.; Su, T.; Cores, J.; Dinh, P.-U.C.; Cheng, K. Dermal exosomes containing miR-218-5p promote hair regeneration by regulating β-catenin signaling. *Sci. Adv.* **2020**, *6*, eaba1685. [CrossRef]
133. Hu, S.; Li, Z.; Cores, J.; Huang, K.; Su, T.; Dinh, P.-U.; Cheng, K. Needle-Free Injection of Exosomes Derived from Human Dermal Fibroblast Spheroids Ameliorates Skin Photoaging. *ACS Nano* **2019**, *13*, 11273–11282. [CrossRef] [PubMed]

134. Tu, J.; Luo, X.; Liu, H.; Zhang, J.; He, M. Cancer spheroids derived exosomes reveal more molecular features relevant to progressed cancer. *Biochem. Biophys. Rep.* **2021**, *26*, 101026. [CrossRef] [PubMed]
135. Naseri, M.; Zöller, M.; Hadjati, J.; Ghods, R.; Pirmardan, E.R.; Kiani, J.; Eini, L.; Bozorgmehr, M.; Madjd, Z. Dendritic cells loaded with exosomes derived from cancer stem cell-enriched spheroids as a potential immunotherapeutic option. *J. Cell. Mol. Med.* **2021**, *25*, 3312–3326. [CrossRef] [PubMed]
136. Liu, Y.; Ma, L.; Hua, F.; Min, Z.; Zhan, Y.; Zhang, W.; Yao, J. Exosomal circCARM1 from spheroids reprograms cell metabolism by regulating PFKFB2 in breast cancer. *Oncogene* **2022**, *41*, 2012–2025. [CrossRef] [PubMed]
137. Dinh, P.-U.C.; Paudel, D.; Brochu, H.; Popowski, K.D.; Gracieux, M.C.; Cores, J.; Huang, K.; Hensley, M.T.; Harrell, E.; Vandergriff, A.C.; et al. Inhalation of lung spheroid cell secretome and exosomes promotes lung repair in pulmonary fibrosis. *Nat. Commun.* **2020**, *11*, 1064. [CrossRef]
138. Choi, S.-Y.; Kang, S.; Oh, S.; Lee, K.; Lee, H.-J.; Gum, S.; Kwon, T.-G.; Kim, J.-W.; Lee, S.-T.; Hong, Y.; et al. Differential Angiogenic Potential of 3-Dimension Spheroid of HNSCC Cells in Mouse Xenograft. *Int. J. Mol. Sci.* **2021**, *22*, 8245. [CrossRef]
139. Verdera, H.C.; Gitz-Francois, J.J.; Schiffelers, R.M.; Vader, P. Cellular uptake of extracellular vesicles is mediated by clathrin-independent endocytosis and macropinocytosis. *J. Control. Release* **2017**, *266*, 100–108. [CrossRef]
140. Abdollahi, S. Extracellular vesicles from organoids and 3D culture systems. *Biotechnol. Bioeng.* **2020**, *118*, 1029–1049. [CrossRef]
141. Khayambashi, P.; Iyer, J.; Pillai, S.; Upadhyay, A.; Zhang, Y.; Tran, S. Hydrogel Encapsulation of Mesenchymal Stem Cells and Their Derived Exosomes for Tissue Engineering. *Int. J. Mol. Sci.* **2021**, *22*, 684. [CrossRef]
142. Langhans, S.A. Three-Dimensional in Vitro Cell Culture Models in Drug Discovery and Drug Repositioning. *Front. Pharmacol.* **2018**, *9*, 6. [CrossRef] [PubMed]
143. Nikolova, M.P.; Chavali, M.S. Recent advances in biomaterials for 3D scaffolds: A review. *Bioact. Mater.* **2019**, *4*, 271–292. [CrossRef] [PubMed]
144. Schmidt, J.J.; Jeong, J.H.; Chan, V.; Cha, C.; Baek, K.; Lai, M.-H.; Bashir, R.; Kong, H. Tailoring the Dependency between Rigidity and Water Uptake of a Microfabricated Hydrogel with the Conformational Rigidity of a Polymer Cross-Linker. *Biomacromolecules* **2013**, *14*, 1361–1369. [CrossRef] [PubMed]
145. Tibbitt, M.W.; Anseth, K.S. Hydrogels as extracellular matrix mimics for 3D cell culture. *Biotechnol. Bioeng.* **2009**, *103*, 655–663. [CrossRef] [PubMed]
146. Hoffman, A.S. Hydrogels for biomedical applications. *Adv. Drug Deliv. Rev.* **2012**, *64*, 18–23. [CrossRef]
147. Martinez-Garcia, F.D.; Fischer, T.; Hayn, A.; Mierke, C.T.; Burgess, J.K.; Harmsen, M.C. A Beginner's Guide to the Characterization of Hydrogel Microarchitecture for Cellular Applications. *Gels* **2022**, *8*, 535. [CrossRef] [PubMed]
148. Akther, F.; Little, P.; Li, Z.; Nguyen, N.-T.; Ta, H.T. Hydrogels as artificial matrices for cell seeding in microfluidic devices. *RSC Adv.* **2020**, *10*, 43682–43703. [CrossRef]
149. Radulescu, D.-M.; Neacsu, I.A.; Grumezescu, A.-M.; Andronescu, E. New Insights of Scaffolds Based on Hydrogels in Tissue Engineering. *Polymers* **2022**, *14*, 799. [CrossRef]
150. Lin, X.; Zhao, X.; Xu, C.; Wang, L.; Xia, Y. Progress in the mechanical enhancement of hydrogels: Fabrication strategies and underlying mechanisms. *J. Polym. Sci.* **2022**, *60*, 2525–2542. [CrossRef]
151. Patwardhan, S.; Mahadik, P.; Shetty, O.; Sen, S. ECM stiffness-tuned exosomes drive breast cancer motility through thrombospondin-1. *Biomaterials* **2021**, *279*, 121185. [CrossRef]
152. Han, M.; Yang, H.; Lu, X.; Li, Y.; Liu, Z.; Li, F.; Shang, Z.; Wang, X.; Li, X.; Li, J.; et al. Three-Dimensional-Cultured MSC-Derived Exosome-Hydrogel Hybrid Microneedle Array Patch for Spinal Cord Repair. *Nano Lett.* **2022**, *22*, 6391–6401. [CrossRef]
153. Safari, B.; Aghazadeh, M.; Davaran, S.; Roshangar, L. Exosome-loaded hydrogels: A new cell-free therapeutic approach for skin regeneration. *Eur. J. Pharm. Biopharm.* **2021**, *171*, 50–59. [CrossRef] [PubMed]
154. Ju, Y.; Hu, Y.; Yang, P.; Xie, X.; Fang, B. Extracellular vesicle-loaded hydrogels for tissue repair and regeneration. *Mater. Today Bio* **2023**, *18*, 100522. [CrossRef]
155. Chen, C.W.; Wang, L.L.; Zaman, S.; Gordon, J.; Arisi, M.F.; Venkataraman, C.M.; Chung, J.J.; Hung, G.; Gaffey, A.C.; Spruce, L.A.; et al. Sustained release of endothelial progenitor cell-derived extracellular vesicles from shear-thinning hydrogels improves angiogenesis and promotes function after myocardial infarction. *Cardiovasc. Res.* **2018**, *114*, 1029–1040. [CrossRef] [PubMed]
156. Liu, F.; Hu, S.; Yang, H.; Li, Z.; Huang, K.; Su, T.; Wang, S.; Cheng, K. Hyaluronic Acid Hydrogel Integrated with Mesenchymal Stem Cell-Secretome to Treat Endometrial Injury in a Rat Model of Asherman's Syndrome. *Adv. Health Mater.* **2019**, *8*, e1900411. [CrossRef] [PubMed]
157. Guo, S.-C.; Tao, S.-C.; Yin, W.-J.; Qi, X.; Yuan, T.; Zhang, C.-Q. Exosomes derived from platelet-rich plasma promote the re-epithelization of chronic cutaneous wounds via activation of YAP in a diabetic rat model. *Theranostics* **2017**, *7*, 81–96. [CrossRef] [PubMed]
158. Shafei, S.; Khanmohammadi, M.; Heidari, R.; Ghanbari, H.; Taghdiri Nooshabadi, V.; Farzamfar, S.; Akbariqomi, M.; Sanikhani, N.S.; Absalan, M.; Tavoosidana, G. Exosome loaded alginate hydrogel promotes tissue regeneration in full-thickness skin wounds: An in vivo study. *J. Biomed. Mater. Res. Part A* **2020**, *108*, 545–556. [CrossRef] [PubMed]
159. Han, C.; Zhou, J.; Liu, B.; Liang, C.; Pan, X.; Zhang, Y.; Zhang, Y.; Wang, Y.; Shao, L.; Zhu, B.; et al. Delivery of miR-675 by stem cell-derived exosomes encapsulated in silk fibroin hydrogel prevents aging-induced vascular dysfunction in mouse hindlimb. *Mater. Sci. Eng. C* **2019**, *99*, 322–332. [CrossRef] [PubMed]

160. Shi, Q.; Qian, Z.; Liu, D.; Sun, J.; Wang, X.; Liu, H.; Xu, J.; Guo, X. GMSC-Derived Exosomes Combined with a Chitosan/Silk Hydrogel Sponge Accelerates Wound Healing in a Diabetic Rat Skin Defect Model. *Front. Physiol.* **2017**, *8*, 904. [CrossRef]
161. Wang, C.; Liang, C.; Wang, R.; Yao, X.; Guo, P.; Yuan, W.; Liu, Y.; Song, Y.; Li, Z.; Xie, X. The fabrication of a highly efficient self-healing hydrogel from natural biopolymers loaded with exosomes for the synergistic promotion of severe wound healing. *Biomater. Sci.* **2020**, *8*, 313–324. [CrossRef]
162. Li, M.; Ke, Q.-F.; Tao, S.-C.; Guo, S.-C.; Rui, B.-Y.; Guo, Y.-P. Fabrication of hydroxyapatite/chitosan composite hydrogels loaded with exosomes derived from miR-126-3p overexpressed synovial mesenchymal stem cells for diabetic chronic wound healing. *J. Mater. Chem. B* **2016**, *4*, 6830–6841. [CrossRef] [PubMed]
163. Zhang, K.; Zhao, X.; Chen, X.; Wei, Y.; Du, W.; Wang, Y.; Liu, L.; Zhao, W.; Han, Z.; Kong, D.; et al. Enhanced Therapeutic Effects of Mesenchymal Stem Cell-Derived Exosomes with an Injectable Hydrogel for Hindlimb Ischemia Treatment. *ACS Appl. Mater Interfaces* **2018**, *10*, 30081–30091. [CrossRef] [PubMed]
164. Zhao, X.; Liu, Y.; Jia, P.; Cheng, H.; Wang, C.; Chen, S.; Huang, H.; Han, Z.; Han, Z.-C.; Marycz, K.; et al. Chitosan hydrogel-loaded MSC-derived extracellular vesicles promote skin rejuvenation by ameliorating the senescence of dermal fibroblasts. *Stem Cell Res. Ther.* **2021**, *12*, 196. [CrossRef] [PubMed]
165. Tao, S.-C.; Guo, S.-C.; Li, M.; Ke, Q.-F.; Guo, Y.-P.; Zhang, C.-Q. Chitosan Wound Dressings Incorporating Exosomes Derived from MicroRNA-126-Overexpressing Synovium Mesenchymal Stem Cells Provide Sustained Release of Exosomes and Heal Full-Thickness Skin Defects in a Diabetic Rat Model. *STEM CELLS Transl. Med.* **2016**, *6*, 736–747. [CrossRef] [PubMed]
166. Yang, S.; Zhu, B.; Yin, P.; Zhao, L.; Wang, Y.; Fu, Z.; Dang, R.; Xu, J.; Zhang, J.; Wen, N. Integration of Human Umbilical Cord Mesenchymal Stem Cells-Derived Exosomes with Hydroxyapatite-Embedded Hyaluronic Acid-Alginate Hydrogel for Bone Regeneration. *ACS Biomater. Sci. Eng.* **2020**, *6*, 1590–1602. [CrossRef] [PubMed]
167. Wang, C.; Wang, M.; Xu, T.; Zhang, X.; Lin, C.; Gao, W.; Xu, H.; Lei, B.; Mao, C. Engineering Bioactive Self-Healing Antibacterial Exosomes Hydrogel for Promoting Chronic Diabetic Wound Healing and Complete Skin Regeneration. *Theranostics* **2019**, *9*, 65–76. [CrossRef] [PubMed]
168. Zhang, C.; Shang, Y.; Chen, X.; Midgley, A.C.; Wang, Z.; Zhu, D.; Wu, J.; Chen, P.; Wu, L.; Wang, X.; et al. Supramolecular Nanofibers Containing Arginine-Glycine-Aspartate (RGD) Peptides Boost Therapeutic Efficacy of Extracellular Vesicles in Kidney Repair. *ACS Nano* **2020**, *14*, 12133–12147. [CrossRef] [PubMed]
169. Li, L.; Zhang, Y.; Mu, J.; Chen, J.; Zhang, C.; Cao, H.; Gao, J.; Gao, J. Transplantation of Human Mesenchymal Stem-Cell-Derived Exosomes Immobilized in an Adhesive Hydrogel for Effective Treatment of Spinal Cord Injury. *Nano Lett.* **2020**, *20*, 4298–4305. [CrossRef]
170. Mardpour, S.; Ghanian, M.H.; Sadeghi-Abandansari, H.; Mardpour, S.; Nazari, A.; Shekari, F.; Baharvand, H. Hydrogel-Mediated Sustained Systemic Delivery of Mesenchymal Stem Cell-Derived Extracellular Vesicles Improves Hepatic Regeneration in Chronic Liver Failure. *ACS Appl. Mater. Interfaces* **2019**, *11*, 37421–37433. [CrossRef]
171. Yang, Y.; Zhu, Z.; Gao, R.; Yuan, J.; Zhang, J.; Li, H.; Xie, Z.; Wang, Y. Controlled release of MSC-derived small extracellular vesicles by an injectable Diels-Alder crosslinked hyaluronic acid/PEG hydrogel for osteoarthritis improvement. *Acta Biomater.* **2021**, *128*, 163–174. [CrossRef]
172. DiCerbo, M.; Benmassaoud, M.M.; Vega, S.L. Porous Scaffold-Hydrogel Composites Spatially Regulate 3D Cellular Mechanosensing. *Front. Med. Technol.* **2022**, *4*, 22. [CrossRef] [PubMed]
173. Liu, X.; Holzwarth, J.M.; Ma, P.X. Functionalized Synthetic Biodegradable Polymer Scaffolds for Tissue Engineering. *Macromol. Biosci.* **2012**, *12*, 911–919. [CrossRef] [PubMed]
174. Rider, P.; Kačarević, P.; Alkildani, S.; Retnasingh, S.; Barbeck, M. Bioprinting of tissue engineering scaffolds. *J. Tissue Eng.* **2018**, *9*, 2041731418802090. [CrossRef] [PubMed]
175. Lv, D.; Hu, Z.; Lu, L.; Lu, H.; Xu, X. Three-dimensional cell culture: A powerful tool in tumor research and drug discovery (Review). *Oncol. Lett.* **2017**, *14*, 6999–7010. [CrossRef]
176. Kadir, N.D.; Yang, Z.; Hassan, A.; Denslin, V.; Lee, E.H. Electrospun fibers enhanced the paracrine signaling of mesenchymal stem cells for cartilage regeneration. *Stem Cell Res. Ther.* **2021**, *12*, 3. [CrossRef] [PubMed]
177. Hu, P.; Chiarini, A.; Wu, J.; Freddi, G.; Nie, K.; Armato, U.; Dal Prà, I. Exosomes of adult human fibroblasts cultured on 3D silk fibroin nonwovens intensely stimulate neoangiogenesis. *Burns Trauma* **2021**, *9*, tkab003. [CrossRef] [PubMed]
178. Gao, W.; Liang, T.; He, R.; Ren, J.; Yao, H.; Wang, K.; Zhu, L.; Xu, Y. Exosomes from 3D culture of marrow stem cells enhances endothelial cell proliferation, migration, and angiogenesis via activation of the HMGB1/AKT pathway. *Stem Cell Res.* **2020**, *50*, 102122. [CrossRef] [PubMed]
179. Man, K.; Brunet, M.Y.; Louth, S.; Robinson, T.E.; Fernandez-Rhodes, M.; Williams, S.; Federici, A.S.; Davies, O.G.; Hoey, D.A.; Cox, S.C. Development of a Bone-Mimetic 3D Printed Ti6Al4V Scaffold to Enhance Osteoblast-Derived Extracellular Vesicles' Therapeutic Efficacy for Bone Regeneration. *Front. Bioeng. Biotechnol.* **2021**, *9*, 1003. [CrossRef]
180. Liu, X.; Wang, J.; Wang, P.; Zhong, L.; Wang, S.; Feng, Q.; Wei, X.; Zhou, L. Hypoxia-pretreated mesenchymal stem cell-derived exosomes-loaded low-temperature extrusion 3D-printed implants for neural regeneration after traumatic brain injury in canines. *Front. Bioeng. Biotechnol.* **2022**, *10*, 1828. [CrossRef]
181. Chen, J.; Zhou, D.; Nie, Z.; Lu, L.; Lin, Z.; Zhou, D.; Zhang, Y.; Long, X.; Fan, S.; Xu, T. A scalable coaxial bioprinting technology for mesenchymal stem cell microfiber fabrication and high extracellular vesicle yield. *Biofabrication* **2022**, *14*, 015012. [CrossRef]

182. Born, L.J.; McLoughlin, S.T.; Dutta, D.; Mahadik, B.; Jia, X.; Fisher, J.P.; Jay, S.M. Sustained released of bioactive mesenchymal stromal cell-derived extracellular vesicles from 3D-printed gelatin methacrylate hydrogels. *J. Biomed. Mater. Res. Part A* **2022**, *110*, 1190–1198. [CrossRef] [PubMed]
183. Chen, P.; Zheng, L.; Wang, Y.; Tao, M.; Xie, Z.; Xia, C.; Gu, C.; Chen, J.; Qiu, P.; Mei, S.; et al. Desktop-stereolithography 3D printing of a radially oriented extracellular matrix/mesenchymal stem cell exosome bioink for osteochondral defect regeneration. *Theranostics* **2019**, *9*, 2439–2459. [CrossRef] [PubMed]
184. Di Bella, M.A.; Brucato, V.; Blanda, V.; Zummo, F.; Vitrano, I.; Di Liegro, C.M.; Ghersi, G.; Di Liegro, I.; Schiera, G. A 3D-scaffold of PLLA induces the morphological differentiation and migration of primary astrocytes and promotes the production of extracellular vesicles. *Mol. Med. Rep.* **2019**, *20*, 1288–1296. [CrossRef]
185. Zhang, Y.; Chopp, M.; Zhang, Z.G.; Katakowski, M.; Xin, H.; Qu, C.; Ali, M.; Mahmood, A.; Xiong, Y. Systemic administration of cell-free exosomes generated by human bone marrow derived mesenchymal stem cells cultured under 2D and 3D conditions improves functional recovery in rats after traumatic brain injury. *Neurochem. Int.* **2017**, *111*, 69–81. [CrossRef]
186. Zhang, L.; Fan, C.; Hao, W.; Zhuang, Y.; Liu, X.; Zhao, Y.; Chen, B.; Xiao, Z.; Chen, Y.; Dai, J. NSCs Migration Promoted and Drug Delivered Exosomes-Collagen Scaffold via a Bio-Specific Peptide for One-Step Spinal Cord Injury Repair. *Adv. Health Mater.* **2021**, *10*, e2001896. [CrossRef]
187. Narayanan, R.; Huang, C.-C.; Ravindran, S. Hijacking the Cellular Mail: Exosome Mediated Differentiation of Mesenchymal Stem Cells. *Stem Cells Int.* **2016**, *2016*, 3808674. [CrossRef]
188. Qi, X.; Zhang, J.; Yuan, H.; Xu, Z.; Li, Q.; Niu, X.; Hu, B.; Wang, Y.; Li, X. Exosomes Secreted by Human-Induced Pluripotent Stem Cell-Derived Mesenchymal Stem Cells Repair Critical-Sized Bone Defects through Enhanced Angiogenesis and Osteogenesis in Osteoporotic Rats. *Int. J. Biol. Sci.* **2016**, *12*, 836–849. [CrossRef]
189. Zhang, J.; Liu, X.; Li, H.; Chen, C.; Bin Hu, B.; Niu, X.; Li, Q.; Zhao, B.; Xie, Z.; Wang, Y. Exosomes/tricalcium phosphate combination scaffolds can enhance bone regeneration by activating the PI3K/Akt signaling pathway. *Stem Cell Res. Ther.* **2016**, *7*, 136. [CrossRef]
190. Ying, C.; Wang, R.; Wang, Z.; Tao, J.; Yin, W.; Zhang, J.; Yi, C.; Qi, X.; Han, D. BMSC-Exosomes Carry Mutant HIF-1α for Improving Angiogenesis and Osteogenesis in Critical-Sized Calvarial Defects. *Front. Bioeng. Biotechnol.* **2020**, *8*, 565561. [CrossRef]
191. Sanchez, M.A.; Felice, B.; Sappia, L.D.; Moura, S.L.; Martí, M.; Pividori, M.I. Osteoblastic exosomes. A non-destructive quantitative approach of alkaline phosphatase to assess osteoconductive nanomaterials. *Mater. Sci. Eng. C* **2020**, *115*, 110931. [CrossRef]
192. Wang, X.; Ao, J.; Lu, H.; Zhao, Q.; Ma, Y.; Zhang, J.; Ren, H.; Zhang, Y. Osteoimmune Modulation and Guided Osteogenesis Promoted by Barrier Membranes Incorporated with S-Nitrosoglutathione (GSNO) and Mesenchymal Stem Cell-Derived Exosomes. *Int. J. Nanomed.* **2020**, *15*, 3483–3496. [CrossRef] [PubMed]
193. Zha, Y.; Li, Y.; Lin, T.; Chen, J.; Zhang, S.; Wang, J. Progenitor cell-derived exosomes endowed with VEGF plasmids enhance osteogenic induction and vascular remodeling in large segmental bone defects. *Theranostics* **2021**, *11*, 397–409. [CrossRef] [PubMed]
194. Gandolfi, M.G.; Gardin, C.; Zamparini, F.; Ferroni, L.; Degli Esposti, M.; Parchi, G.; Ercan, B.; Manzoli, L.; Fava, F.; Fabbri, P.; et al. Mineral-Doped Poly(L-lactide) Acid Scaffolds Enriched with Exosomes Improve Osteogenic Commitment of Human Adipose-Derived Mesenchymal Stem Cells. *Nanomaterials* **2020**, *10*, 432. [CrossRef] [PubMed]
195. Li, W.; Liu, Y.; Zhang, P.; Tang, Y.; Zhou, M.; Jiang, W.; Zhang, X.; Wu, G.; Zhou, Y. Tissue-Engineered Bone Immobilized with Human Adipose Stem Cells-Derived Exosomes Promotes Bone Regeneration. *ACS Appl. Mater. Interfaces* **2018**, *10*, 5240–5254. [CrossRef] [PubMed]
196. Swanson, W.B.; Zhang, Z.; Xiu, K.; Gong, T.; Eberle, M.; Wang, Z.; Ma, P.X. Scaffolds with controlled release of pro-mineralization exosomes to promote craniofacial bone healing without cell transplantation. *Acta Biomater.* **2020**, *118*, 215–232. [CrossRef] [PubMed]
197. Fan, L.; Guan, P.; Xiao, C.; Wen, H.; Wang, Q.; Liu, C.; Luo, Y.; Ma, L.; Tan, G.; Yu, P.; et al. Exosome-functionalized polyetheretherketone-based implant with immunomodulatory property for enhancing osseointegration. *Bioact. Mater.* **2021**, *6*, 2754–2766. [CrossRef]
198. Wu, Z.; Pu, P.; Su, Z.; Zhang, X.; Nie, L.; Chang, Y. Schwann Cell-derived exosomes promote bone regeneration and repair by enhancing the biological activity of porous Ti6Al4V scaffolds. *Biochem. Biophys. Res. Commun.* **2020**, *531*, 559–565. [CrossRef]
199. Teotia, A.K.; Qayoom, I.; Singh, P.; Mishra, A.; Jaiman, D.; Seppälä, J.; Lidgren, L.; Kumar, A. Exosome-Functionalized Ceramic Bone Substitute Promotes Critical-Sized Bone Defect Repair in Rats. *ACS Appl. Bio Mater.* **2021**, *4*, 3716–3726. [CrossRef]
200. Koh, B.; Sulaiman, N.; Fauzi, M.B.; Law, J.X.; Ng, M.H.; Idrus, R.B.H.; Yazid, M.D. Three dimensional microcarrier system in mesenchymal stem cell culture: A systematic review. *Cell Biosci.* **2020**, *10*, 75. [CrossRef]
201. Patel, D.B.; Luthers, C.R.; Lerman, M.J.; Fisher, J.P.; Jay, S.M. Enhanced extracellular vesicle production and ethanol-mediated vascularization bioactivity via a 3D-printed scaffold-perfusion bioreactor system. *Acta Biomater.* **2018**, *95*, 236–244. [CrossRef]
202. Fuzeta, M.D.A.; Bernardes, N.; Oliveira, F.D.; Costa, A.C.; Fernandes-Platzgummer, A.; Farinha, J.P.; Rodrigues, C.A.V.; Jung, S.; Tseng, R.-J.; Milligan, W.; et al. Scalable Production of Human Mesenchymal Stromal Cell-Derived Extracellular Vesicles Under Serum-/Xeno-Free Conditions in a Microcarrier-Based Bioreactor Culture System. *Front. Cell Dev. Biol.* **2020**, *8*, 553444. [CrossRef] [PubMed]
203. Bellani, C.F.; Ajeian, J.; Duffy, L.; Miotto, M.; Groenewegen, L.; Connon, C.J. Scale-Up Technologies for the Manufacture of Adherent Cells. *Front. Nutr.* **2020**, *7*, 575146. [CrossRef] [PubMed]
204. Bodiou, V.; Moutsatsou, P.; Post, M.J. Microcarriers for Upscaling Cultured Meat Production. *Front. Nutr.* **2020**, *7*, 10. [CrossRef]

205. Nam, J.H.; Ermonval, M.; Sharfstein, S.T. Cell Attachment to Microcarriers Affects Growth, Metabolic Activity, and Culture Productivity in Bioreactor Culture. *Biotechnol. Prog.* **2008**, *23*, 652–660. [CrossRef] [PubMed]
206. Derakhti, S.; Safiabadi-Tali, S.H.; Amoabediny, G.; Sheikhpour, M. Attachment and detachment strategies in microcarrier-based cell culture technology: A comprehensive review. *Mater. Sci. Eng. C* **2019**, *103*, 109782. [CrossRef]
207. Grinneli, F.; Feld, M.K. Spreading of human fibroblasts in serum-free medium: Inhibition by dithiothreitol and the effect of cold insoluble globulin (plasma fibronectin). *J. Cell. Physiol.* **1980**, *104*, 321–334. [CrossRef] [PubMed]
208. Healthcare, G.E.; Biosciences, A. *Microcarrier Cell Culture: Principles and Methods*; General Electric Company: Fairfield, CT, USA, 2005.
209. Berthiaume, F.; Yarmush, M. Tissue Engineering, Encyclopedia of Physical Science and Technology. *Tissue Eng.* **2003**, *3*, 817–842. [CrossRef]
210. Badenes, S.; Fernandes-Platzgummer, A.; Rodrigues, C.; Diogo, M.; da Silva, C.; Cabral, J. Microcarrier Culture Systems for Stem Cell Manufacturing. In *Stem Cell Manufacturing*; Elsevier: Amsterdam, the Netherlands, 2016; pp. 77–104. [CrossRef]
211. Schmidt, J.J.; Jeong, J.; Kong, H. The Interplay Between Cell Adhesion Cues and Curvature of Cell Adherent Alginate Microgels in Multipotent Stem Cell Culture. *Tissue Eng. Part A* **2011**, *17*, 2687–2694. [CrossRef]
212. Čebatariūnienė, A.; Kriaučiūnaitė, K.; Prunskaitė, J.; Tunaitis, V.; Pivoriūnas, A. Extracellular Vesicles Suppress Basal and Lipopolysaccharide-Induced NFκB Activity in Human Periodontal Ligament Stem Cells. *Stem Cells Dev.* **2019**, *28*, 1037–1049. [CrossRef]
213. Xu, C.; Zhao, J.; Li, Q.; Hou, L.; Wang, Y.; Li, S.; Jiang, F.; Zhu, Z.; Tian, L. Exosomes derived from three-dimensional cultured human umbilical cord mesenchymal stem cells ameliorate pulmonary fibrosis in a mouse silicosis model. *Stem Cell Res. Ther.* **2020**, *11*, 503. [CrossRef]
214. Haraszti, R.A.; Miller, R.; Stoppato, M.; Sere, Y.Y.; Coles, A.; Didiot, M.-C.; Wollacott, R.; Sapp, E.; Dubuke, M.L.; Li, X.; et al. Exosomes Produced from 3D Cultures of MSCs by Tangential Flow Filtration Show Higher Yield and Improved Activity. *Mol. Ther.* **2018**, *26*, 2838–2847. [CrossRef] [PubMed]
215. Jalilian, E.; Massoumi, H.; Bigit, B.; Amin, S.; Katz, E.A.; Guaiquil, V.H.; Anwar, K.N.; Hematti, P.; Rosenblatt, M.I.; Djalilian, A.R. Bone marrow mesenchymal stromal cells in a 3D system produce higher concentration of extracellular vesicles (EVs) with increased complexity and enhanced neuronal growth properties. *Stem Cell Res. Ther.* **2022**, *13*, 425. [CrossRef] [PubMed]
216. Duan, L.; Li, X.; Xu, X.; Xu, L.; Wang, D.; Ouyang, K.; Liang, Y. Large-Scale Preparation of Synovial Fluid Mesenchymal Stem Cell-Derived Exosomes by 3D Bioreactor Culture. *J. Vis. Exp.* **2022**, *185*, e62221. [CrossRef]
217. Jarmalavičiūtė, A.; Tunaitis, V.; Pivoraitė, U.; Venalis, A.; Pivoriūnas, A. Exosomes from dental pulp stem cells rescue human dopaminergic neurons from 6-hydroxy-dopamine–induced apoptosis. *Cytotherapy* **2015**, *17*, 932–939. [CrossRef] [PubMed]
218. Hou, M.; Shi, L.; Zhou, Y.; Wang, J.; Jiang, J.; Jiang, J.; He, J. Expanding the codes: The development of density-encoded hydrogel microcarriers for suspension arrays. *Biosens. Bioelectron.* **2021**, *181*, 113133. [CrossRef] [PubMed]
219. Phan, J.; Kumar, P.; Hao, D.; Gao, K.; Farmer, D.; Wang, A. Engineering mesenchymal stem cells to improve their exosome efficacy and yield for cell-free therapy. *J. Extracell. Vesicles* **2018**, *7*, 1522236. [CrossRef] [PubMed]
220. Storm, M.P.; Sorrell, I.; Shipley, R.; Regan, S.; Luetchford, K.A.; Sathish, J.; Webb, S.; Ellis, M.J. Hollow Fiber Bioreactors for In Vivo-like Mammalian Tissue Culture. *J. Vis. Exp.* **2016**, *111*, e53431. [CrossRef]
221. Gobin, J.; Muradia, G.; Mehic, J.; Westwood, C.; Couvrette, L.; Stalker, A.; Bigelow, S.; Luebbert, C.C.; Bissonnette, F.S.-D.; Johnston, M.J.W.; et al. Hollow-fiber bioreactor production of extracellular vesicles from human bone marrow mesenchymal stromal cells yields nanovesicles that mirrors the immuno-modulatory antigenic signature of the producer cell. *Stem Cell Res. Ther.* **2021**, *12*, 127. [CrossRef]
222. Yan, I.K.; Shukla, N.; Borrelli, D.A.; Patel, T. Use of a Hollow Fiber Bioreactor to Collect Extracellular Vesicles from Cells in Culture. *Extracell. RNA Methods Protoc.* **2018**, 35–41. [CrossRef]
223. Yan, L.; Wu, X. Exosomes produced from 3D cultures of umbilical cord mesenchymal stem cells in a hollow-fiber bioreactor show improved osteochondral regeneration activity. *Cell Biol. Toxicol.* **2019**, *36*, 165–178. [CrossRef]
224. Watson, D.C.; Bayik, D.; Srivatsan, A.; Bergamaschi, C.; Valentin, A.; Niu, G.; Bear, J.; Monninger, M.; Sun, M.; Morales-Kastresana, A.; et al. Efficient production and enhanced tumor delivery of engineered extracellular vesicles. *Biomaterials* **2016**, *105*, 195–205. [CrossRef] [PubMed]

pharmaceutics

Review

Engineered Exosomes for Tumor-Targeted Drug Delivery: A Focus on Genetic and Chemical Functionalization

Ali Akbari [1], Fereshteh Nazari-Khanamiri [2], Mahdi Ahmadi [3], Maryam Shoaran [4] and Jafar Rezaie [1,2,*]

1 Solid Tumor Research Center, Cellular and Molecular Medicine Research Institute, Urmia University of Medical Sciences, Urmia 5714783734, Iran
2 Hematology, Immune Cell Therapy, and Stem Cells Transplantation Research Center, Clinical Research Institute, Urmia University of Medical Sciences, Urmia 5714783734, Iran
3 Drug Applied Research Center, Tabriz University of Medical Sciences, Tabriz 5665665811, Iran
4 Pediatric Health Research Center, Tabriz University of Medical Sciences, Tabriz 5665665811, Iran
* Correspondence: rezaie.j@umsu.ac.ir; Tel.: +98-914-854-8503; Fax: +98-443-222-2010

Abstract: Cancer is the main cause of death worldwide. The limitations in traditional cancer therapies provoked the advance and use of several nanotechnologies for more effective and nontoxic cancer treatment. Along with synthetic nanocarriers, extracellular vesicles (EVs)-mediated drug delivery systems have aroused substantial interest. The term EVs refers to cell-derived nanovesicles, such as exosomes, with phospholipid-bound structures, participating in cell-to-cell communication. Exosomes are 30–150 nm vesicles that can transfer many biological molecules between cells. From a drug delivery standpoint, exosomes can be loaded with various therapeutic cargo, with the several advantages of low immunogenicity, high biocompatibility, transformative, and effective tumor targeting aptitude. The exosomal surface can be functionalized to improve tumor targeting ability of them. Researchers have genetically expressed or chemically linked various molecules on the surface of exosomes. Despite extensive investigation, clinical translation of exosome-based drug delivery remains challenging. In this review, we discuss various methods used to loading exosomes with therapeutic cargo. We describe examples of functionalized exosomes surface using genetic and chemical modification methods. Finally, this review attempts to provide future outlooks for exosome-based targeted drug delivery.

Keywords: exosomes; extracellular vesicles; drug delivery; nanocarriers

Citation: Akbari, A.; Nazari-Khanamiri, F.; Ahmadi, M.; Shoaran, M.; Rezaie, J. Engineered Exosomes for Tumor-Targeted Drug Delivery: A Focus on Genetic and Chemical Functionalization. *Pharmaceutics* **2023**, *15*, 66. https://doi.org/10.3390/pharmaceutics15010066

Academic Editor: Haibing Zhou

Received: 28 November 2022
Revised: 19 December 2022
Accepted: 22 December 2022
Published: 26 December 2022

1. Introduction

Cancer is one of the most terrible illnesses worldwide. In 2022, there will be an estimated 1.9 million new cancer cases diagnosed and 609,360 cancer deaths in the United States [1]. In recent years, cancer management including detection and therapy application has been postponed because of the COVID-19 pandemic [2]. Various methods such as chemotherapy, radiation, and surgery are commonly used for malignancy treatment [3,4]. In addition, other approaches such as immunotherapy, magnetic resonance imaging, computed tomography, imaging techniques with X-ray, endoscopy, and cells/tissues morphological studies such as cytology and histopathology can assist the diagnosis and treatment of cancers [5–7]. However, important challenges are still ongoing in cancer therapy, which include resistance to therapies, immune escape, and metastasis. In the field of nanotechnology, nanotherapy, nanoparticles or nanocarriers at the nanoscale collection are being used to combat several diseases, which show amended drug solubility and stability, drug effectiveness, and with low side effects. In addition, the use of nanoparticles for cancer therapy is an attainment interest of researchers due to its gene silencing and tumor targeting abilities [8]. Over the decades, researchers have designed various nanocarriers for use in drug delivery systems comprising polymeric nanoparticles, micelles, liposomes, and dendrimers for increasing therapeutic efficiency. However, immunogenicity, acute hypersensitivity reaction, and biocompatibility problems are associated with these particles [9,10]. Recently, nanotechnology has progressed considerably to advance smart carriers [11]. Particularly, lipid-based nanocarriers exhibit a useful policy for drug loading that has directed to the clinical translation of some inventions [11]. With the advance of new synthetic carriers, cell derivatives particles, extracellular vesicles (EVs) have emerged as novel tools for drug delivery system [12,13]. EVs are phospholipid-bound vesicles heterogeneously deriving from cells that regulate many biological processes [14]. They carry many types of biomolecules including non-coding RNAs, proteins, signaling molecules, lipids, and DNA strands between cells, therefore trafficking to several tissues and organs and contributing to cell communication [14,15]. Various types of EVs have been characterized based on generation way and size distribution know apoptotic bodies (1000–6000 nm), microvesicles (100–1000 nm), and exosomes (30–150 nm) [16,17]. Exosomes are formed within the late endosomal compartment named multivesicular bodies, which can fuse with the plasma membrane and secrete exosomes into the extracellular matrix [18] (Figure 1). Exosomes generation and intracellular trafficking comprise many signaling processes and machinery such as tetraspanins, The endosomal sorting complexes required for transport (ESCRT) machinery, lipid rafts, Rab proteins, and SNARs [17,19,20]. Microvesicles are generated from the outward budding of the cell membrane through cytoskeleton rearrangement, the reorganization of phospholipids in the cell membrane [21,22]. Apoptotic bodies are formed by apoptotic cells through membrane blebbing, and nuclear and cytoplasmic fragmentation [23]. An increasing number of studies have shown that exosomes can carry exogenous therapeutic cargo to cells [24]. In this regard, exosomes are equivalent to liposomes because both have phospholipid membranes. However, exosomes contain a complex structure of several lipids and lumen and surface proteins; some of these surface proteins help tissue targeting [24]. The lipid bilayer of exosomes can shield their cargo from degradation. Previous studies have shown that various cargo can be loaded into exosomes with different methods. Exosomes offer several advantages because of their exceptional physicochemical characterizations [25] such as natural origin, low immunogenicity, high biocompatibility, increased stability in vivo and blood circulation time, and low toxicity [25–27]. Moreover, exosomes can interact with target cells through several mechanisms, allowing exosome-mediated drug delivery to a cell or tissue [28]. Exosomes surface inherits receptors from parent cells, giving confident inherent targeting capabilities. This feature is favorable to increasing the accumulation of therapeutic cargo at the target site after systemic administration, thus decreasing drug dosage for exosomal loading with low toxic side effects [29,30]. Exosome-based drug delivery can avoid the P-glycoprotein drug efflux system, which can lessen the drug resistance response in tumor cells [31]. Most importantly, exosomes are flexible regarding surface modification and engineering [32,33]. Functionalization of exosomes surface is a greatly interesting approach to increase exosomes efficacy for delivering cargo into targeted site especially in tumor studies [34]. Exosomes modification may be useful for cancer detection and imaging studies [35]. In this review, we discuss the exosome-loading methods with special focus on methods used to improve the tumor-targeting potential of exosomes.

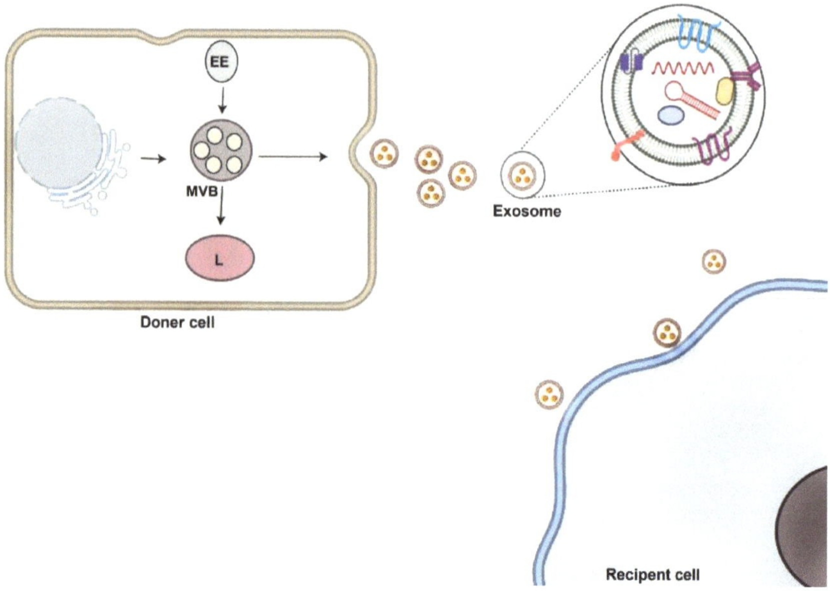

Figure 1. Biogenesis and secretion of exosomes. Many cells produce exosomes within multivesicular bodies (MVBs) via a complex mechanism. MVBs (a type of late endosomes) can fuse with the plasma membrane and secrete exosomes into the extracellular matrix. Now, exosomes can reach recipient cells located nearby or far from, inducing alteration in cell signaling. EE: early endosomes, L: lysosome.

2. Cargo Loading Methods

Exosomes from various cells are used for drug delivery systems (Figure 2). Overall, two main methods are used for cargo loading into exosomes or other EVs, known: indirect or pre-loading method and the direct or post-loading method [36] (Figure 3). In this review, we use the terms pre-loading and post-loading methods. In preloading methods, parent cells are modified and loaded with genes/cargo to produce optional exosomes. In post-loading methods, exosomes/EVs isolated from cells are directly loaded with cargo by active or passive methods. In addition, a survey on clinical trials shows that exosomes are being used for the delivery of therapeutic drugs (https://clinicaltrials.gov/ct2/home, accessed on 1 December 2022). We found that there are 6 clinical trials registered. Three clinical trials (NCT03608631, NCT03384433, and NCT05043181) were aimed at genetically modifying MSCs for producing overexpressing exosomes. Two clinical trials aimed to load curcumin into plant-derived EVs for the treatment of colon cancer Irritable Bowel Disease (NCT01294072 and NCT04879810). None of these studies is completed and results are not currently accessible. In this section, we describe loading methods used for producing exosomes.

2.1. Pre-Loading Method

Pre-loading methods allow continuous and easy production of cargo-loaded exosomes without conceding membrane integrity. In this method, cells were co-incubated with cargo or genetically transfected with target genes to produce cargo-loading exosomes. Therefore, co-incubation and genetic modification are two common approaches to the pre-loading method (Figure 3).

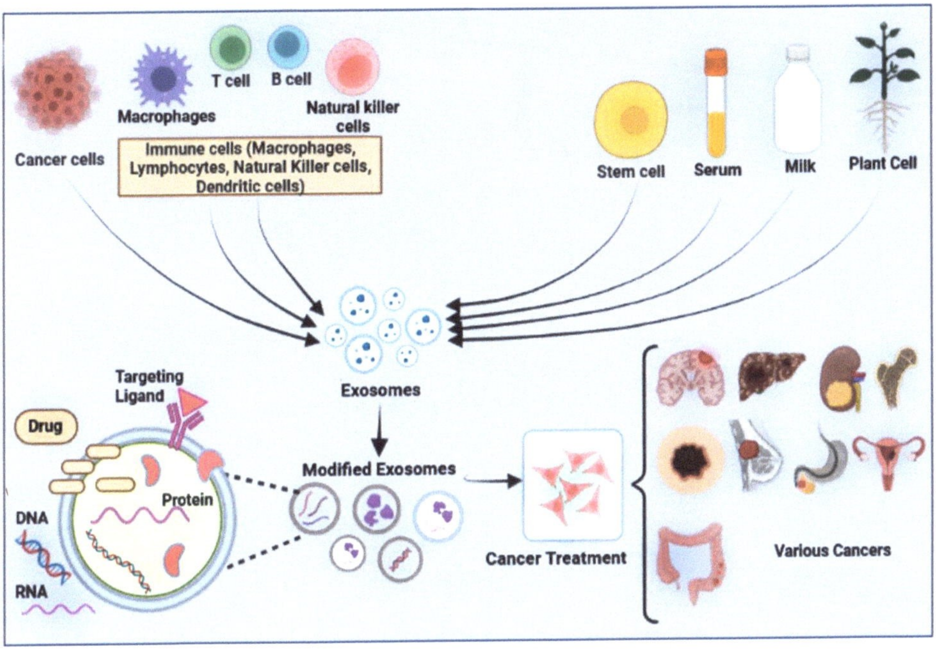

Figure 2. Various exosomes from different cells or body fluids are used for drug delivery system.

2.1.1. Co-Incubation

Co-incubation is used to load different chemotherapeutic drugs, particularly hydrophobic drugs such as paclitaxel and doxorubicin [37–39]. In this approach, chemotherapeutic drugs are co-cultured with parental cells, then they can pass through the cell membrane and enter into MVBs where exosomes are formed and loaded. After secretion, exosomes loaded with drugs can be isolated for downstream experiments. This method is easy and straightforward on its own; however, its loading efficiency is generally low and is dependent on drug dose gradient, drug characteristics, and type of parent cell [40]. For example, doxorubicin enters into different cells with different concentrations. In other words, its loading efficacy depends on cell types [41]. To overcome this challenge, there is evidence that the pre-conditioning of cells can significantly increase loading efficacy. In this regard, low current electricity and UV irradiation may encourage the loading rate of drugs or nanoparticles into exosomes [42,43].

2.1.2. Genetic Modification

In this method, therapeutic molecules including RNAs, proteins, ligands, and receptors are overexpressed in parent cells through transfection and genetic modification. Therefore, these molecules appear in the exosomes lumen or surface. Different cells such as tumor cells and stem cells were genetically modified to produce exosomes [44,45]. We focused on this method in the section below.

2.2. Post-loading

Through the post-loading approach, cargo are directly encapsulated cargo into isolated exosomes (Figure 3). The headmost step is selecting a safe and confident parental cell to produce mass exosomes. The second step is selecting a suitable and efficient method for inserting cargo, as loading methods may affect exosomes kinetics and structure. Active loading and passive loading are the two main methods of post-loading.

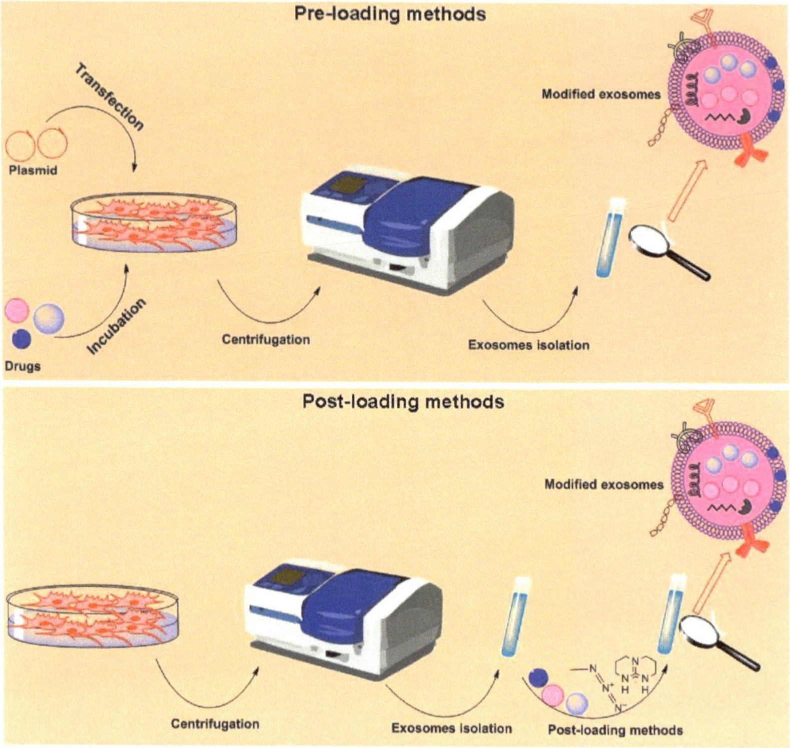

Figure 3. Exosomes loading methods. In general, two methods are used to load therapeutic cargo into exosomes including the pre-loading method and the post-loading method.

2.2.1. Active Loading

Some therapeutic cargo cannot cross exosomal membranes, therefore researchers use different methods to insert cargo into exosomes by temporary induction of the permeability of exosomes membranes. As shown by Table 1, active loading methods can be mainly divided into two methods, namely physical induction and chemical induction. In physical induction methods, exosomes membrane was rapidly disrupted by external forces, including sonication, electroporation, freeze-thaw cycle, and extrusion. We summarized active loading methods in Table 1 with advantages and limitations.

Table 1. Advantages and limitations of exosomes loading methods.

Active Methods	Examples	Advantages	Limitations	Ref.
physical induction	electroporation	High efficacy and is more efficient than chemical transfection	Depends on cargo types May affect the Zeta potential and colloid stability of exosomes Induce aggregation of siRNAs	[46,47]
	sonication	Compared with co-incubation and electroporation, sonication produces the highest loading efficiency	Damage the EVs structure Must be performed in an ice bath	[48,49]
	freeze-thaw cycle	Rapid and easy loading	Low loading efficiency, increase the size of EVs, induces aggregation	[50,51]
	extrusion	Compared with co-incubation, extrusion can produce homogeneous EVs	change the Zeta potential and membrane proteins in EVs	[52–54]

Table 1. *Cont.*

Active Methods	Examples	Advantages	Limitations	Ref.
Chemical induction				
	saponins	High loading efficiency	Potential toxicity; cause hemolysis Need extra purification phase	[55,56]
	liposomes	High loading efficiency, quickly and easily load	Potential toxicity	[57,58]
	calcium chloride	High loading efficiency simple and stable	Potential toxicity	[59]

2.2.2. Passive Loading

In this method, isolated exosomes/EVs are co-cultured with high concentrations of drugs where drugs can diffuse into the exosomes' lumen passively. This method is simple and easy to operate and preserves membrane integrity. A growing body of evidence indicates that passive loading is widely used for cancer studies [60–62]. Nonetheless, this method has limitations such as low loading efficiency and dependent on the nature of drugs (hydrophobic compounds). For example, the loading efficacy of paclitaxel and curcumin is different upon co-incubation at the same condition [63,64].

3. Improve Tumor-Targeting Potential of Exosomes

Native exosomes/EVs have shown many advantages against synthetic nanocarriers; however, they cannot effectively accumulate in the target organs after systemic administration, particularly in targets sheltered by physiological barriers [40,65]. In recent years, scientists have been motivated to increase the targeting ability of exosomes in delivering therapeutic agents to target cells. Previous evidence shows that two main methods, genetic modification and chemical modification, are being used by researchers (Figure 4). In general, in the genetic modification strategy, exosome-producing cells are genetically modified to express biomolecules on the exosomes lumen or surface [66,67]. In the chemical modification, isolated exosomes are functionalized by chemical reactions such as click chemistry and non-covalent reactions to link therapeutic molecules to exosomes' surface for increasing their targeting ability and for other applications such as imaging and tracking [68,69]. Exosomes produced by these ways are sometimes known as engineered exosomes, which we discuss here as the functionalization of exosomes. In the next sections, we describe and give examples of studies done in this field.

3.1. Genetic Modification

Genetic modification of exosomes is a useful method for the functionalization of exosomes with new properties [70,71]. In this context, exosome surface is functionalized by ligands or peptides to improve their targeting ability of them (Figure 4). In this method, as mentioned above, source cells are transfected with optional plasmids to produce exosomes containing the target protein [72]. We summarized studies that used genetic modification for drug delivery systems. Different molecules are present on exosome surfaces that can be harnessed for connecting target molecules on them. Lysosomal-associated membrane protein 2B (LAMP-2B) is present on exosomes surface, which is commonly used to fuse optional biomolecules on it. Indeed, a large N-terminal extramembrane domain of LAMP-2B is presented on the exosomes surface, providing an opportunity for researchers to connect therapeutic agents and biomolecules [73]. For example, Bellavia et al. genetically fused interleukin-3 (IL-3) to the N-terminal of LAMP-2B to improve the targeting potential of exosomes for the treatment of chronic myeloid leukemia (CML). Interleukin-3 receptor α (IL-3Rα), a receptor for IL-3, is highly expressed in CML cells. Then, they loaded these exosomes with the breakpoint cluster region (BCR)-ABL siRNA and imatinib and showed a profound anticancer effect. In vivo experiments showed that these exosomes were successfully accumulated in tumor site and suppressed cancer cells with an increase in the survival rate of xenografted mice [74]. In a similar vein, Liang and co-workers fused Her2 to the N-terminus of LAMP-2 to target colon cancer cells efficiently. The Her2-LAMP2 fusion protein was revealed to be expressed on the surface of the exosomes, which expedited the targeted cellular uptake via EGFR receptor-mediated endocytosis in tumor cells. Then, they incorporated 5-FU and miRNA-21i into these exosomes (target-Her2-LAMP2-GFP) by electroporation and incubation methods, respectively. Results showed that these exosomes accumulated in colon cancer cells and profoundly suppressed them both in vitro and xenografts BALB/c nude mice model [75]. In a study, the HEK293T cells were transduced by a lentiviral vector bearing-LAMP2b-DARPin G3 chimeric gene to produce exosomes containing DARPin G3 and then loaded them with siRNA for delivery to tumor cells, SKBR3 cells. These exosomes could specifically target SKBR3 cells and deliver siRNA molecules, inhibiting the gene expression [46]. Dendritic cells were used to express $\alpha\gamma$ integrin-specific iRGD peptide (CRGDKGPDC) on exosomes surface. The tumor-targeting ability of exosomes was improved by engineering Lamp2b fused to CRGDKGPDC. These exosomes are loaded with doxorubicin via electroporation. Doxorubicin-loaded iRGD exosomes displayed highly effective targeting ability and transfer to αv integrin-positive breast cancer cells in vitro. Intravenous injection of exosomes showed that these exosomes delivered doxorubicin specifically to tumor site, causing inhibition in tumor growth [76]. In addition, HEK293T cells were reprogrammed to concurrently express Lamp2b and KRAS siRNA in fusion with the CRGDKGPDC, iRGD peptide. Intravenous administration of iRGD-exosomes precisely could target tumor mass in vivo. The therapeutic effects were shown by the profound suppression of tumor growth in a mouse model [77]. Bai et al. prepared tLyp-1-lamp2b plasmids and transfect those into HEK293T cells. Next, the synthesized siRNA was sorted into tLyp-1 exosomes by electroporation method. In vitro experiments showed that the tLyp-1-siRNAs- exosomes had a high delivery efficacy into lung cancer and cancer stem cells [78]. Even though the efficiency of the genetic technique, the targeting peptide may be degraded in some conditions. To improve the firmness of peptides presented on the surface of the exosomes, a glycosylation motif may be linked to the N-terminus of peptide-LAMP-2B fusions [79]. Other exosomal surface proteins are the tetraspanin proteins such as CD63, CD81, and CD9, highly expressed in exosomes, which can be used to fuse with targeting molecules. For example, in mdx mice, Ran et al. fused myostatin propeptide with the second extracellular loop of CD63, which meaningfully increased its delivery efficacy and serum stability. Administration of myostatin propeptide-loaded exosomes helped muscle renovation and proliferation, causing prominent inhibition in muscle degradation and pathology [80]. ApoA-1, the key functional protein of high-density lipoprotein (HDL), is present in exosomes surface and binds to scavenger receptor class B type 1 (SR-B1) abundantly located on hepatocellular carcinoma cells. In a study, researchers genetically inserted ApoA-1 into the small extracellular loop of CD63 in 293T cells and subsequently on the surface of exosomes. Exosomes purified from ApoA-1-overexpressing donor cells were loaded with miR-26a by electroporation method. These exosomes were revealed to bind to HepG2 cells selectively via SR-B1 and at that time, captured by receptor-mediated endocytosis. The successful release of miRNA-26a in HepG2 cells reduced cell migration and proliferation [81]. Transfection with plasmid DNA encoding an OVA Ag fused to CD63 (pCD63-OVA) resulted in producing OVA-carrying exosomes. Vaccinating mice with these exosomes increased strong Ag-specific T cell responses, principally those from $CD8^+$ T cells [82]. These exosomes delivered DNA vaccination meaningfully repressed tumor growth. In addition, the fluorescent protein pHluorin was fused into the small extracellular loop of CD63 to visualize the exosome secretion and uptake [83]. The transmembrane protein platelet-derived growth factor receptor (PDGFR) is also used for the functionalizing exosomes surface. Chen et al. genetically presented two types of antibodies (αCD3 UCHT1 and scFv fragments of αEGFR cetuximab) on exosome surface. In both in vitro and in vivo experiments, these exosomes were shown to encourage cross-linking of T cells and EGFR-expressing breast cancer cells and increase effective antitumor immunity [84]. Furthermore, the 37-residue glycosylphosphatidylinositol (GPI) signal peptide DAF on exosomes surface can be used to link the C-terminus of different proteins, such as a reporter protein, an antibody, or a nanobody. For example, GPI-anchored EGFR-specific nanobodies were used to target EGFR-positive human epidermoid squamous carcinoma cells [67]. In addition, exosome targeting is realized by linking the antigen to the C1C2 domain of the lactadherin protein. Treatment of mice with these exosomes results in a prominent rise in the immune response and a decrease in tumor growth [31]. In other studies, streptavidin-lactadherin and Gaussia luciferase-lactadherin were fused with lactadherin for exosome display and tracking in biological systems [85,86].

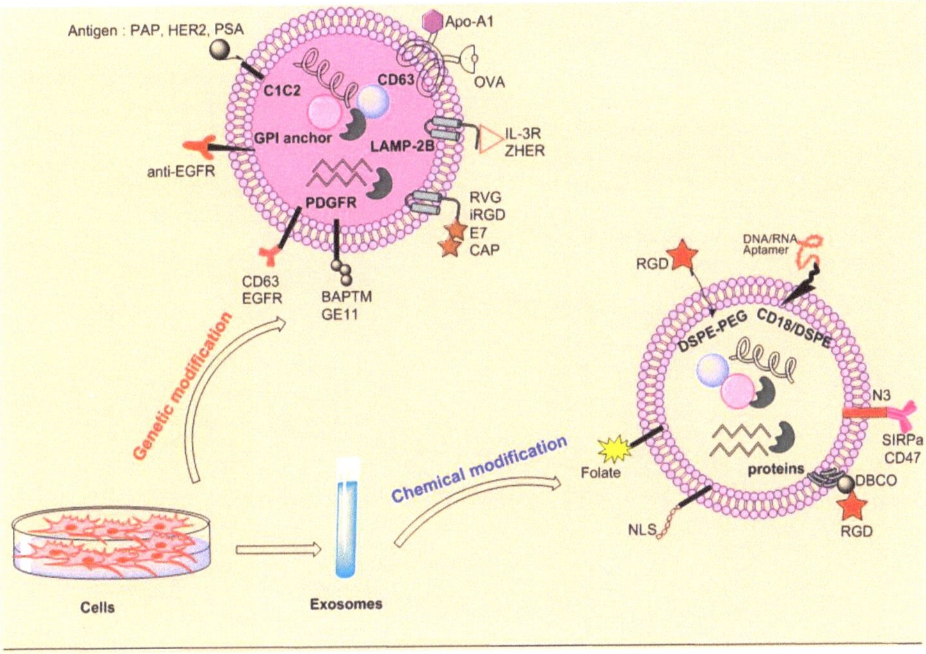

Figure 4. Schematic figure of the functionalization of exosomes surface. Exosomal surfaces can be functionalized by genetic modification and chemical modification. These approaches improve tumor targeting ability of exosomes.

3.2. Chemical Modification

Exosomes have some interesting properties such as biocompatibility, homing ability, non-immunogenicity, blood distribution, cell specific targeting, and so on, which made them a versatile tool for drug delivery. Moreover, the chemical modifications of EVs/exosomes could not only increase their stability but also maximize their efficacy of targeting and delivery [87,88] (Figure 4). In this regard, covalent and non-covalent binding approaches have been used as two efficient chemical strategies. Non-covalent binding methods are used to load cargo on the surface of EVs/exosomes. For example, Pi et al. modified exosomes surface with cholesterol-connected RNA aptamers or folate by noncovalent binding reaction [89]. These exosomes transferred miRNA and siRNA to the tumor region with greater antitumor efficacy. Researchers used diacyllipid-aptamer as the targeting ligand to progress an aptamer-functionalized exosomes (Apt-Exos) nanoplatforms for cell type-specific delivery of molecular therapeutics. These exosomes could efficiently transfer therapeutic drugs/fluorophores to target tumor cells [88]. A membrane-targeted chimeric peptide (ChiP) was established to link a nuclear localization signal (NLS) peptide to the exosome membrane [90]. ChiP exosomes expedited the nuclear delivery of photosensitizers and improved photodynamic tumor therapy both in vitro and in vivo [90]. In case of non-covalent binding, electrostatic interactions between surface peptides and EVs played a critical role for improving exosome's cellular uptake and cytosolic release. In one report, cationic lipid known as lipofectamine (LTX) with positive charge interacted electrostatically with the negatively charged surface membrane of a CD63-green fluorescent protein (GFP)-tagged exosome [91]. Cellular uptake investigation of prepared complex was evaluated towards HeLa and CHO-K1 cells. Results showed an increasing the cellular uptake of synthesized complex 15 and 175-fold by HeLa and CHO-K1 cells, respectively. These modifications can simultaneously improve the targeted ability of exosomes and the targeted delivery of drug-loaded exosomes. Click chemistry as an important covalent binding reaction has been widely employed to functionalize EVs. The term "click chemistry", which was first used in its entirety by Sharpless in 2001, refers to a set of distinct and controllable reactions that must satisfy several requirements, including high yield, high specificity, simplicity, only non-toxic byproducts, and high atom economy [92]. Under physiological conditions, click chemistry reactions can take place, and the resulting chemical bonds are irreversible. As a result, click chemistry is frequently used to modify biomolecules such as proteins, lipids, and nucleic acids with different compounds. The copper (I)-catalyzed azide-alkyne 1,3-dipolar cycloaddition (CuAAC) reaction is an example of the click chemistry processes (Figure 5) that has been applied as a bioorthogonal process in the study of health sciences [93,94].

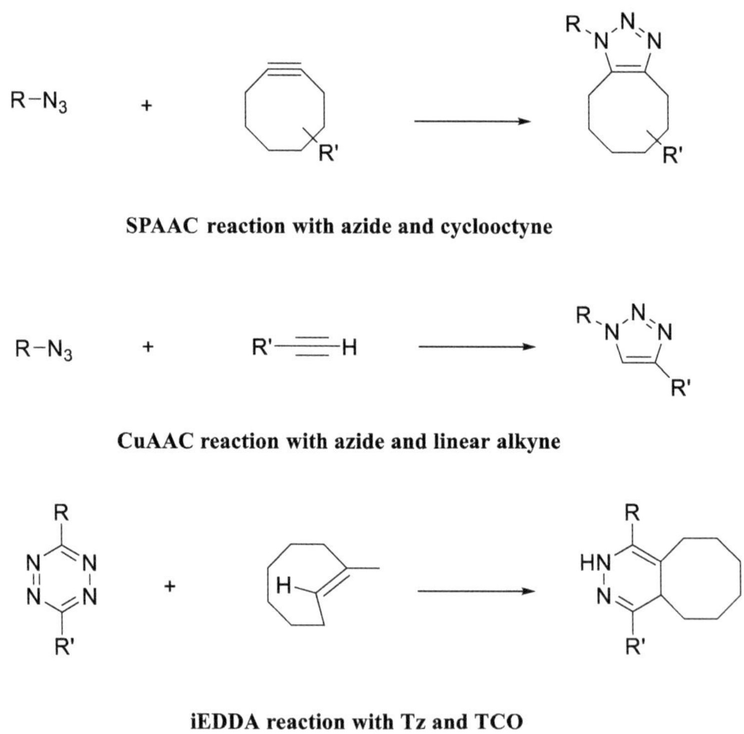

Figure 5. Schematics of various click chemistry reactions used to modify exosomes.

By presenting an azido moiety on the surface of the exosome through metabolic glycan synthesis and then conjugating a fluorescent dye with a strain-promoted dye, Lee and coworkers introduced a simple and efficient exosome labeling strategy. To better understand the biology and distribution of exosomes and develop exosome-based therapeutic approaches, their metabolic exosome labeling strategy may prove to be a useful tool [95]. Incorporating radioactive technetium (^{99m}Tc) on the surface of the exosomes membrane is one of the alternatives to the click chemistry method. In a different fascinating study, Hwang created a straightforward technique for radiolabeling macrophage-derived exosome-mimetic nanovesicles (ENVs) with ^{99m}TcHMPAO under physiological conditions, and then tracked the in vivo distribution of 99mTc-HMPAO-ENVs using SPECT/CT in living mice. Their noninvasive imaging of radiolabeled-ENVs promises a better understanding of exosome behavior in vivo for future biomedical applications [96]. The other technique uses PEG-conjugated exosomes that have been radiolabeled. It is well known that PEGylation of exosomes enhances their pharmacokinetics, permits greater tumor accumulation, and reduces their premature hepatic sequestration and clearance [96]. Recent research has shown that click chemistry can effectively be used to alter exosome-producing cells or purified exosomes to produce "tailored" vesicles.

This field is novel and several studies have been done on cancer treatment. Chemical functionalization of exosomes by click chemistry depends on the transformation of exosomal amine groups to alkynes. For example, Tian et al. by using click chemistry conjugated the peptide c(RGDyK) (Arg-Gly-Asp-D-Tyr-Lys) to the exosome surface. Then, c(RGDyK) exosomes were loaded with curcumin and injected to a transient middle cerebral artery occlusion mouse model. Results showed that these exosomes efficiently infiltrate the BBB and reduce apoptosis and inflammatory responses [97]. Similarly, in a study using click chemistry, the glioma-targeting RGE peptide (RGERPPR) was linked to exosomes by a cycloaddition reaction with sulfonyl azide. Intravenous injection of RGE exosomes caused an accumulation of exosomes in tumor regions. These glioma-targeting exosomes could be loaded with curcumin, which successfully delivered curcumin-SPION to tumor cells and induced a potent antitumor effect in mice cancer model [98]. SPION cargo of exosomes expedited magnetic flow hyperthermia therapy. By click chemistry, copper-catalyzed azide alkyne cycloaddition was used to conjugate both macromolecules and small molecules to the surface of the exosomes. This reaction showed that exosomes cross-linked with alkyne groups using carbodiimide chemistry were conjugated to a model azide, azide-fluor-545 [68]. Therefore, the exosomal amine groups can be simply functionalized with alkyne groups. Modification of exosomes surface was used to enhance immune responses against tumor cells. In this regard, Koh et al. used click chemistry to link dibenzocyclooctyne-derivatized SIRPα antibodies to Azide-modified exosomes. Tumor cells express CD47 on their surface, which can interact with SIRPα on phagocytes, resulting in phagocytosis activity of macrophages. Therefore, decorating exosomes surface with dibenzocyclooctyne-derivatized SIRPα antibodies can suppress tumor cells [99]. Therefore, these exosomes can block the CD47-SIRPα checkpoint on the surface of cancer cells. Click chemistry was used to insert amphipathic molecules into the lipid bilayer of exosomes. For instance, Kim et al. constructed and improved a formulation of paclitaxel-loaded exosomes with chemically inserted aminoethylanisamide-polyethylene glycol (AA-PEG) vector moiety to target the sigma receptor that overexpressed by lung tumor cells. The AA-PEG-vectorized exosomes enriched with paclitaxel (AA-PEG-exoPTX) displayed a high loading ability, intense capability to amass in tumor cells upon intravenous injection, and improved therapeutic effects [100]. Zhou and co-workers prepared cancer-targeting exosomes from MSCs to regulate tumor microenvironment in pancreatic ductal adenocarcinoma (PDAC) [101]. They loaded MSCs-derived exosomes with galectin-9 siRNA using an electroporation technique, and then superficially changed with oxaliplatin (OXA) as immunogenic cell death (ICD)-inducer, iEXO-OXA platform. These exosomes significantly improved tumor targeting ability and delivered the drug in the tumor region. Although click chemistry is a simple and rapid reaction method, some challenges remain. For example, this method commonly does not work specifically on a distinct exosomal amine group. In addition, non-site-specific chemical modification may guard some protein–protein interactions and change the pharmaceutics and biochemistry of the exosomes.

4. Future Outlooks

Exosomes may be utilized as carrier particles for several drug delivery applications. As mentioned, compared with conventional and synthetic delivery approaches, exosomes have been revealed to deliver therapeutic cargo with a low immune clearance level when injected systemically in vivo. Exosomes are flexible regarding the modification of their content and surface via different methods as well as production by various cells. For clinical translation of exosomes, there are still some problems that remain to be answered. In Box 1, we prepared the facts and gaps in exosomes biology and application. The main question is "which cells are suitable for the production of exosomes?" Several researchers used various cells for drug delivery systems. For example, animal cells (from tumor cells to stem cells), plant cells, bacteria, and body fluids are employed to load cargo. Another issue is that mass and reproducible production methods are needed to obtain continual exosomes. Although several procedures are used to obtain massive exosomes, there is no standard for this purpose and methods are relatively scattered [102,103]. In addition, exosomes isolation and characterization need technological progress to achieve pure and homogenous exosomes with a high yield efficiency [104]. Even though the therapeutic cargo can be loaded into exosomes [105], technological and reproducible handy and standard methods are required to load exosomes with the favorite drugs at a high level. The productivity of pre-loading methods is rather low, and most post-loading methods could harm the stability and integrity of exosomes [48,106]. Functionalization of exosomes is still in the beginning and it is of utmost importance that it be tested before clinical application. For improving the efficiency of the targeting ability of exosomes, further multidisciplinary research is needed to introduce a gold-standard method. Genetic modification may harm the safe nature of exosomes and chemical modification may harm exosomes' integrity and disrupt functional molecules on the exosome surface. Progress in cancer molecular science, materials science, nanoscience, and pharmacology may overcome these problems and increase the efficacy of exosome-based cancer treatment.

Box 1. Facts and gaps of exosomes biology and application

Facts

- Exosomes are nanovesicles with a diameter size between 30 and 150 nm, originating from inside cells with different biological cargo.
- Exosomes are present in most body fluids and therefore can travel to different organs throughout the body.
- Exosome entity from different cells is highly variable regarding their function and cargo.
- Exosomes can encapsulate various exogenous therapeutic cargo and deliver them to target cells.
- The exosomal surface can be engineered for imaging, targeting, and therapy objects.

Gaps

- What are/is the common way/s for isolation and purification of exosomes? Exosomes are heterogeneous both in size and function, and different methods are used to isolate and purify exosomes from various sources such as cell culture medium or body fluids. Therefore, a gold-standard method is needed.
- Which source cells are suitable for the massive production of exosomes? The most important issue is large-scale good manufacturing practice (GMP)—exosome production under GMP-compliant procedures to safeguard quality, safety, and reliability. Therefore, safe and confident parental cells must be selected for exosomes yield.
- What are/is the standard/s method/s for loading exosomes with exogenous cargo?
- Which surface modification approach/es is/are most common for the improving exosomes targeting abilities? Mainly two methods, namely genetic and chemical modification approaches, are used to functionalize the surface of exosomes for increasing the tumor-targeting ability of exosomes. Exosomal surfaces are decorated with various biomolecules with a certain function. This may make it difficult for selecting a suitable and safe target residual on the surface of the exosomes.
- Do surface modification methods damage exosome structure and function? Surface modification (functionalization), especially chemical ones, may blind or harm available residuals on exosome surface. Therefore, this may affect exosomes' pharmacokinetics and biodistribution in the body.

5. Conclusions

Several approaches have been used for therapeutic cargo-loading into exosomes such as pre-loading and post-loading methods. These approaches are associated with advantages and disadvantages. The inconsistency in some studies may relate to divergences in the source cells, exosomes isolation methods, and cargo properties. Large-scale production of exosomes needs GMP-compliant procedures to safeguard quality, safety, and reliability of exosomes. Therefore, for clinical application, a gold standard and universal loading method remains a challenge. In recent years, researchers have focused on the surface functionalization of exosomes for increasing their tumor-targeting ability. In this regard, isolated exosomes are genetically and/or chemically modified to link some agents such as ligands, peptides, aptamers, and antibodies. It seems that click chemistry has quickly appeared as a widespread and main method for the functionalization of exosomes chemically. For exosome modification, it is essential to fully comprehend the structure and cargo of the exosomes membrane at the target site, and choose the suitable targeting ligands. In addition, for the effective progress of clinically appropriate exosome-based therapy for cancer, forming approaches for the precise measurement of therapeutic cargo/drugs in exosomes would be required to discover a therapeutically operative concentration of exosomes. Thus, approaches for the measureable and qualitative observing of exosomes and exosome-loaded drugs to the tumor microenvironment should be advanced. Despite a robust attempt at explaining different aspects of exosomes—such as the biogenesis pathway, interactions with target cells, loading methods, and exosomal surface modification—there is still much scrutinizing to be done around incorporating the multidimensional abilities of exosomes into the drug delivery system.

Funding: This research received no external funding.

Institutional Review Board Statement: Not applicable.

Informed Consent Statement: Not applicable.

Data Availability Statement: Not applicable.

Conflicts of Interest: The authors have declared that no competing interest exists.

References

1. Siegel, R.L.; Miller, K.D.; Fuchs, H.E.; Jemal, A. Cancer statistics, 2022. *CA A Cancer J. Clin.* **2022**, *72*, 7–33. [CrossRef]
2. Cantini, L.; Mentrasti, G.; Russo, G.L.; Signorelli, D.; Pasello, G.; Rijavec, E.; Russano, M.; Antonuzzo, L.; Rocco, D.; Giusti, R.; et al. Evaluation of COVID-19 impact on DELAYing diagnostic-therapeutic pathways of lung cancer patients in Italy (COVID-DELAY study): Fewer cases and higher stages from a real-world scenario. *ESMO Open* **2022**, *7*, 100406. [CrossRef] [PubMed]
3. Liu, Y.P.; Zheng, C.C.; Huang, Y.N.; He, M.L.; Xu, W.W.; Li, B. Molecular mechanisms of chemo-and radiotherapy resistance and the potential implications for cancer treatment. *Med. Comm.* **2021**, *2*, 315–340. [CrossRef] [PubMed]
4. Bao, Y.; Liu, S.; Zhou, Q.; Cai, P.; Anfossi, S.; Li, Q.; Hu, Y.; Liu, M.; Fu, J.; Rong, T. Three-dimensional conformal radiotherapy with concurrent chemotherapy for postoperative recurrence of esophageal squamous cell carcinoma: Clinical efficacy and failure pattern. *Radiat. Oncol.* **2013**, *8*, 1–8. [CrossRef] [PubMed]
5. Yagawa, Y.; Tanigawa, K.; Kobayashi, Y.; Yamamoto, M. Cancer immunity and therapy using hyperthermia with immunotherapy, radiotherapy, chemotherapy, and surgery. *J. Cancer Metastasis Treat.* **2017**, *3*, 218–230. [CrossRef]
6. Bach, P.B.; Jett, J.R.; Pastorino, U.; Tockman, M.S.; Swensen, S.J.; Begg, C.B. Computed tomography screening and lung cancer outcomes. *JAMA* **2007**, *297*, 953–961. [CrossRef]
7. Zusman, I.; Zimber, A.; Nyska, A. Role of morphological methods in the analysis of chemically induced colon cancer in rats. *Cells Tissues Organs* **1991**, *142*, 351–356. [CrossRef]
8. Gomes-da-Silva, L.C.; Fonseca, N.A.; Moura, V.; Pedroso de Lima, M.C.; Simões, S.; Moreira, J.N. Lipid-based nanoparticles for siRNA delivery in cancer therapy: Paradigms and challenges. *Acc. Chem. Res.* **2012**, *45*, 1163–1171. [CrossRef]
9. Edis, Z.; Wang, J.; Waqas, M.K.; Ijaz, M.; Ijaz, M. Nanocarriers-mediated drug delivery systems for anticancer agents: An overview and perspectives. *Int. J. Nanomed.* **2021**, *16*, 1313. [CrossRef]
10. Ramanathan, S.; Gopinath, S.C.B.; Arshad, M.K.M.; Poopalan, P.; Perumal, V. 2-Nanoparticle Synthetic Methods: Strength and Limitations. In *Nanoparticles in Analytical and Medical Devices*; Gopinath, S.C.B., Gang, F., Eds.; Elsevier: Amsterdam, The Netherlands, 2021; pp. 31–43. [CrossRef]
11. van der Meel, R.; Sulheim, E.; Shi, Y.; Kiessling, F.; Mulder, W.J.; Lammers, T. Smart cancer nanomedicine. *Nat. Nanotechnol.* **2019**, *14*, 1007–1017. [CrossRef]

12. Elsharkasy, O.M.; Nordin, J.Z.; Hagey, D.W.; de Jong, O.G.; Schiffelers, R.M.; Andaloussi, S.E.; Vader, P. Extracellular vesicles as drug delivery systems: Why and how? *Adv. Drug Deliv. Rev.* **2020**, *159*, 332–343. [CrossRef] [PubMed]
13. Rahbarghazi, R.; Jabbari, N.; Sani, N.A.; Asghari, R.; Salimi, L.; Kalashani, S.A.; Feghhi, M.; Etemadi, T.; Akbariazar, E.; Mahmoudi, M.; et al. Tumor-derived extracellular vesicles: Reliable tools for Cancer diagnosis and clinical applications. *Cell Commun. Signal.* **2019**, *17*, 73. [CrossRef] [PubMed]
14. Rezaie, J.; Ahmadi, M.; Ravanbakhsh, R.; Mojarad, B.; Mahbubfam, S.; Shaban, S.A.; Shadi, K.; Berenjabad, N.J.; Etemadi, T. Tumor-derived extracellular vesicles: The metastatic organotropism drivers. *Life Sci.* **2021**, 120216. [CrossRef]
15. Shaban, S.A.; Rezaie, J.; Nejati, V. Exosomes Derived from Senescent Endothelial Cells Contain Distinct Pro-angiogenic miRNAs and Proteins. *Cardiovasc. Toxicol.* **2022**, *22*, 592–601. [CrossRef] [PubMed]
16. Brennan, K.; Martin, K.; FitzGerald, S.P.; O'Sullivan, J.; Wu, Y.; Blanco, A.; Richardson, C.; Mc Gee, M.M. A comparison of methods for the isolation and separation of extracellular vesicles from protein and lipid particles in human serum. *Sci. Rep.* **2020**, *10*, 1039. [CrossRef] [PubMed]
17. Doyle, L.M.; Wang, M.Z. Overview of extracellular vesicles, their origin, composition, purpose, and methods for exosome isolation and analysis. *Cells* **2019**, *8*, 727. [CrossRef] [PubMed]
18. Hassanpour, M.; Rezaie, J.; Darabi, M.; Hiradfar, A.; Rahbarghazi, R.; Nouri, M. Autophagy modulation altered differentiation capacity of CD146+ cells toward endothelial cells, pericytes, and cardiomyocytes. *Stem Cell Res. Ther.* **2020**, *11*, 1–14. [CrossRef]
19. Feghhi, M.; Rezaie, J.; Akbari, A.; Jabbari, N.; Jafari, H.; Seidi, F.; Szafert, S. Effect of multi-functional polyhydroxylated polyhedral oligomeric silsesquioxane (POSS) nanoparticles on the angiogenesis and exosome biogenesis in human umbilical vein endothelial cells (HUVECs). *Mater. Des.* **2021**, *197*, 109227. [CrossRef]
20. Soraya, H.; Sani, N.A.; Jabbari, N.; Rezaie, J. Metformin increases exosome biogenesis and secretion in U87 MG human glioblastoma cells: A possible mechanism of therapeutic resistance. *Arch. Med. Res.* **2021**, *52*, 151–162. [CrossRef]
21. Kou, X.; Xu, X.; Chen, C.; Sanmillan, M.L.; Cai, T.; Zhou, Y.; Giraudo, C.; Le, A.; Shi, S. The Fas/Fap-1/Cav-1 complex regulates IL-1RA secretion in mesenchymal stem cells to accelerate wound healing. *Sci. Transl. Med.* **2018**, *10*, eaai8524. [CrossRef]
22. Tricarico, C.; Clancy, J.; D'Souza-Schorey, C. Biology and biogenesis of shed microvesicles. *Small GTPases* **2017**, *8*, 220–232. [CrossRef] [PubMed]
23. Elmore, S. Apoptosis: A review of programmed cell death. *Toxicol. Pathol.* **2007**, *35*, 495–516. [CrossRef] [PubMed]
24. Patil, S.M.; Sawant, S.S.; Kunda, N.K. Exosomes as drug delivery systems: A brief overview and progress update. *Eur. J. Pharm. Biopharm.* **2020**, *154*, 259–269. [CrossRef] [PubMed]
25. Kreimer, S.; Belov, A.M.; Ghiran, I.; Murthy, S.K.; Frank, D.A.; Ivanov, A.R. Mass-spectrometry-based molecular characterization of extracellular vesicles: Lipidomics and proteomics. *J. Proteome Res.* **2015**, *14*, 2367–2384. [CrossRef] [PubMed]
26. Van Deun, J.; Mestdagh, P.; Agostinis, P.; Akay, Ö.; Anand, S.; Anckaert, J.; Martinez, Z.A.; Baetens, T.; Beghein, E.; Bertier, L. EV-TRACK: Transparent reporting and centralizing knowledge in extracellular vesicle research. *Nat. Methods* **2017**, *14*, 228–232.
27. Jafari, H.; Hassanpour, M.; Akbari, A.; Rezaie, J.; Gohari, G.; Mahdavinia, G.R.; Jabbari, E. Characterization of pH-sensitive chitosan/hydroxypropyl methylcellulose composite nanoparticles for delivery of melatonin in cancer therapy. *Mater. Lett.* **2021**, *282*, 128818. [CrossRef]
28. Mulcahy, L.A.; Pink, R.C.; Carter, D.R.F. Routes and mechanisms of extracellular vesicle uptake. *J. Extracell. Vesicles* **2014**, *3*, 24641. [CrossRef]
29. Valadi, H.; Ekström, K.; Bossios, A.; Sjöstrand, M.; Lee, J.J.; Lötvall, J.O. Exosome-mediated transfer of mRNAs and microRNAs is a novel mechanism of genetic exchange between cells. *Nat. Cell Biol.* **2007**, *9*, 654–659. [CrossRef]
30. Welsh, J.A.; van der Pol, E.; Bettin, B.A.; Carter, D.R.; Hendrix, A.; Lenassi, M.; Langlois, M.-A.; Llorente, A.; van de Nes, A.S.; Nieuwland, R. Towards defining reference materials for measuring extracellular vesicle refractive index, epitope abundance, size and concentration. *J. Extracell. Vesicles* **2020**, *9*, 1816641. [CrossRef]
31. Rountree, R.B.; Mandl, S.J.; Nachtwey, J.M.; Dalpozzo, K.; Do, L.; Lombardo, J.R.; Schoonmaker, P.L.; Brinkmann, K.; Dirmeier, U.; Laus, R. Exosome Targeting of Tumor Antigens Expressed by Cancer Vaccines Can Improve Antigen Immunogenicity and Therapeutic EfficacyExosome Targeting of Tumor Antigens Improves Efficacy. *Cancer Res.* **2011**, *71*, 5235–5244. [CrossRef]
32. Alvarez-Erviti, L.; Seow, Y.; Yin, H.; Betts, C.; Lakhal, S.; Wood, M.J. Delivery of siRNA to the mouse brain by systemic injection of targeted exosomes. *Nat. Biotechnol.* **2011**, *29*, 341–345. [CrossRef] [PubMed]
33. Liang, Y.; Duan, L.; Lu, J.; Xia, J. Engineering exosomes for targeted drug delivery. *Theranostics* **2021**, *11*, 3183. [CrossRef] [PubMed]
34. Zhang, Z.; Dombroski, J.A.; King, M.R. Engineering of exosomes to target cancer metastasis. *Cell. Mol. Bioeng.* **2020**, *13*, 1–16. [CrossRef] [PubMed]
35. Gomari, H.; Moghadam, M.F.; Soleimani, M. Targeted cancer therapy using engineered exosome as a natural drug delivery vehicle. *OncoTargets Ther.* **2018**, *11*, 5753. [CrossRef]
36. Rodrigues, P.; Melim, C.; Veiga, F.; Figueiras, A. An Overview of Exosomes in Cancer Therapy: A Small Solution to a Big Problem. *Processes* **2020**, *8*, 1561. [CrossRef]
37. Pascucci, L.; Coccè, V.; Bonomi, A.; Ami, D.; Ceccarelli, P.; Ciusani, E.; Viganò, L.; Locatelli, A.; Sisto, F.; Doglia, S.M. Paclitaxel is incorporated by mesenchymal stromal cells and released in exosomes that inhibit in vitro tumor growth: A new approach for drug delivery. *J. Control. Release* **2014**, *192*, 262–270. [CrossRef]

38. Bonomi, A.; Sordi, V.; Dugnani, E.; Ceserani, V.; Dossena, M.; Coccè, V.; Cavicchini, L.; Ciusani, E.; Bondiolotti, G.; Piovani, G. Gemcitabine-releasing mesenchymal stromal cells inhibit in vitro proliferation of human pancreatic carcinoma cells. *Cytotherapy* **2015**, *17*, 1687–1695. [CrossRef]
39. Toffoli, G.; Hadla, M.; Corona, G.; Caligiuri, I.; Palazzolo, S.; Semeraro, S.; Gamini, A.; Canzonieri, V.; Rizzolio, F. Exosomal doxorubicin reduces the cardiac toxicity of doxorubicin. *Nanomedicine* **2015**, *10*, 2963–2971. [CrossRef]
40. Smyth, T.; Kullberg, M.; Malik, N.; Smith-Jones, P.; Graner, M.W.; Anchordoquy, T.J. Biodistribution and delivery efficiency of unmodified tumor-derived exosomes. *J. Control. Release* **2015**, *199*, 145–155. [CrossRef]
41. Kanchanapally, R.; Deshmukh, S.K.; Chavva, S.R.; Tyagi, N.; Srivastava, S.K.; Patel, G.K.; Singh, A.P.; Singh, S. Drug-loaded exosomal preparations from different cell types exhibit distinctive loading capability, yield, and antitumor efficacies: A comparative analysis. *Int. J. Nanomed.* **2019**, *14*, 531. [CrossRef]
42. Ye, Z.; Zhang, T.; He, W.; Jin, H.; Liu, C.; Yang, Z.; Ren, J. Methotrexate-loaded extracellular vesicles functionalized with therapeutic and targeted peptides for the treatment of glioblastoma multiforme. *ACS Appl. Mater. Interfaces* **2018**, *10*, 12341–12350. [CrossRef] [PubMed]
43. Fukuta, T.; Nishikawa, A.; Kogure, K. Low level electricity increases the secretion of extracellular vesicles from cultured cells. *Biochem. Biophys. Rep.* **2020**, *21*, 100713. [CrossRef] [PubMed]
44. Mendt, M.; Kamerkar, S.; Sugimoto, H.; McAndrews, K.M.; Wu, C.-C.; Gagea, M.; Yang, S.; Blanko, E.V.R.; Peng, Q.; Ma, X. Generation and testing of clinical-grade exosomes for pancreatic cancer. *JCI Insight* **2018**, *3*, e99263. [CrossRef] [PubMed]
45. Lin, Y.; Wu, J.; Gu, W.; Huang, Y.; Tong, Z.; Huang, L.; Tan, J. Exosome–liposome hybrid nanoparticles deliver CRISPR/Cas9 system in MSCs. *Adv. Sci.* **2018**, *5*, 1700611. [CrossRef] [PubMed]
46. Limoni, S.K.; Moghadam, M.F.; Moazzeni, S.M.; Gomari, H.; Salimi, F. Engineered exosomes for targeted transfer of siRNA to HER2 positive breast cancer cells. *Appl. Biochem. Biotechnol.* **2019**, *187*, 352–364. [CrossRef]
47. Kamerkar, S.; LeBleu, V.S.; Sugimoto, H.; Yang, S.; Ruivo, C.F.; Melo, S.A.; Lee, J.J.; Kalluri, R. Exosomes facilitate therapeutic targeting of oncogenic KRAS in pancreatic cancer. *Nature* **2017**, *546*, 498–503. [CrossRef]
48. Haney, M.J.; Klyachko, N.L.; Zhao, Y.; Gupta, R.; Plotnikova, E.G.; He, Z.; Patel, T.; Piroyan, A.; Sokolsky, M.; Kabanov, A.V. Exosomes as drug delivery vehicles for Parkinson's disease therapy. *J. Control. Release* **2015**, *207*, 18–30. [CrossRef]
49. Lamichhane, T.N.; Jeyaram, A.; Patel, D.B.; Parajuli, B.; Livingston, N.K.; Arumugasaamy, N.; Schardt, J.S.; Jay, S.M. Oncogene knockdown via active loading of small RNAs into extracellular vesicles by sonication. *Cell. Mol. Bioeng.* **2016**, *9*, 315–324. [CrossRef]
50. Sato, Y.T.; Umezaki, K.; Sawada, S.; Mukai, S.-A.; Sasaki, Y.; Harada, N.; Shiku, H.; Akiyoshi, K. Engineering hybrid exosomes by membrane fusion with liposomes. *Sci. Rep.* **2016**, *6*, 1–11. [CrossRef]
51. Goh, W.J.; Lee, C.K.; Zou, S.; Woon, E.C.; Czarny, B.; Pastorin, G. Doxorubicin-loaded cell-derived nanovesicles: An alternative targeted approach for anti-tumor therapy. *Int. J. Nanomed.* **2017**, *12*, 2759. [CrossRef]
52. Fuhrmann, G.; Serio, A.; Mazo, M.; Nair, R.; Stevens, M.M. Active loading into extracellular vesicles significantly improves the cellular uptake and photodynamic effect of porphyrins. *J. Control. Release* **2015**, *205*, 35–44. [CrossRef]
53. Wang, Q.; Zhuang, X.; Mu, J.; Deng, Z.-B.; Jiang, H.; Zhang, L.; Xiang, X.; Wang, B.; Yan, J.; Miller, D. Delivery of therapeutic agents by nanoparticles made of grapefruit-derived lipids. *Nat. Commun.* **2013**, *4*, 1–13. [CrossRef]
54. Zhang, M.; Xiao, B.; Wang, H.; Han, M.K.; Zhang, Z.; Viennois, E.; Xu, C.; Merlin, D. Edible ginger-derived nano-lipids loaded with doxorubicin as a novel drug-delivery approach for colon cancer therapy. *Mol. Ther.* **2016**, *24*, 1783–1796. [CrossRef] [PubMed]
55. Sancho-Albero, M.; del Mar Encabo-Berzosa, M.; Beltran-Visiedo, M.; Fernandez-Messina, L.; Sebastian, V.; Sanchez-Madrid, F.; Arruebo, M.; Santamaria, J.; Martin-Duque, P. Efficient encapsulation of theranostic nanoparticles in cell-derived exosomes: Leveraging the exosomal biogenesis pathway to obtain hollow gold nanoparticle-hybrids. *Nanoscale* **2019**, *11*, 18825–18836. [CrossRef] [PubMed]
56. Podolak, I.; Galanty, A.; Sobolewska, D. Saponins as cytotoxic agents: A review. *Phytochem. Rev.* **2010**, *9*, 425–474. [CrossRef]
57. Yang, T.; Fogarty, B.; LaForge, B.; Aziz, S.; Pham, T.; Lai, L.; Bai, S. Delivery of small interfering RNA to inhibit vascular endothelial growth factor in zebrafish using natural brain endothelia cell-secreted exosome nanovesicles for the treatment of brain cancer. *AAPS J.* **2017**, *19*, 475–486. [CrossRef]
58. Zheng, Z.; Li, Z.; Xu, C.; Guo, B.; Guo, P. Folate-displaying exosome mediated cytosolic delivery of siRNA avoiding endosome trapping. *J. Control. Release* **2019**, *311*, 43–49. [CrossRef]
59. Zhang, D.; Lee, H.; Zhu, Z.; Minhas, J.K.; Jin, Y. Enrichment of selective miRNAs in exosomes and delivery of exosomal miRNAs in vitro and in vivo. *Am. J. Physiol. Lung Cell. Mol. Physiol.* **2017**, *312*, L110–L121. [CrossRef]
60. Munagala, R.; Aqil, F.; Jeyabalan, J.; Gupta, R.C. Bovine milk-derived exosomes for drug delivery. *Cancer Lett.* **2016**, *371*, 48–61. [CrossRef]
61. Agrawal, A.K.; Aqil, F.; Jeyabalan, J.; Spencer, W.A.; Beck, J.; Gachuki, B.W.; Alhakeem, S.S.; Oben, K.; Munagala, R.; Bondada, S. Milk-derived exosomes for oral delivery of paclitaxel. *Nanomed. Nanotechnol. Biol. Med.* **2017**, *13*, 1627–1636. [CrossRef]
62. Li, Y.; Gao, Y.; Gong, C.; Wang, Z.; Xia, Q.; Gu, F.; Hu, C.; Zhang, L.; Guo, H.; Gao, S. A33 antibody-functionalized exosomes for targeted delivery of doxorubicin against colorectal cancer. *Nanomed. Nanotechnol. Biol. Med.* **2018**, *14*, 1973–1985. [CrossRef] [PubMed]
63. Wei, H.; Chen, J.; Wang, S.; Fu, F.; Zhu, X.; Wu, C.; Liu, Z.; Zhong, G.; Lin, J. A nanodrug consisting of doxorubicin and exosome derived from mesenchymal stem cells for osteosarcoma treatment in vitro. *Int. J. Nanomed.* **2019**, *14*, 8603. [CrossRef] [PubMed]

64. Sun, D.; Zhuang, X.; Xiang, X.; Liu, Y.; Zhang, S.; Liu, C.; Barnes, S.; Grizzle, W.; Miller, D.; Zhang, H.-G. A novel nanoparticle drug delivery system: The anti-inflammatory activity of curcumin is enhanced when encapsulated in exosomes. *Mol. Ther.* **2010**, *18*, 1606–1614. [CrossRef]
65. Gourlay, J.; Morokoff, A.; Luwor, R.; Zhu, H.-J.; Kaye, A.; Stylli, S. The emergent role of exosomes in glioma. *J. Clin. Neurosci.* **2017**, *35*, 13–23. [CrossRef] [PubMed]
66. Ohno, S.-I.; Takanashi, M.; Sudo, K.; Ueda, S.; Ishikawa, A.; Matsuyama, N.; Fujita, K.; Mizutani, T.; Ohgi, T.; Ochiya, T.; et al. Systemically Injected Exosomes Targeted to EGFR Deliver Antitumor MicroRNA to Breast Cancer Cells. *Mol. Ther.* **2013**, *21*, 185–191. [CrossRef]
67. Kooijmans, S.A.A.; Aleza, C.G.; Roffler, S.R.; van Solinge, W.W.; Vader, P.; Schiffelers, R.M. Display of GPI-anchored anti-EGFR nanobodies on extracellular vesicles promotes tumour cell targeting. *J. Extracell. Vesicles* **2016**, *5*, 31053. [CrossRef]
68. Smyth, T.; Petrova, K.; Payton, N.M.; Persaud, I.; Redzic, J.S.; Graner, M.W.; Smith-Jones, P.; Anchordoquy, T.J. Surface Functionalization of Exosomes Using Click Chemistry. *Bioconjugate Chem.* **2014**, *25*, 1777–1784. [CrossRef]
69. Zhu, Q.; Ling, X.; Yang, Y.; Zhang, J.; Li, Q.; Niu, X.; Hu, G.; Chen, B.; Li, H.; Wang, Y.; et al. Embryonic Stem Cells-Derived Exosomes Endowed with Targeting Properties as Chemotherapeutics Delivery Vehicles for Glioblastoma Therapy. *Adv. Sci.* **2019**, *6*, 1801899. [CrossRef]
70. Liang, Y.; Xu, X.; Li, X.; Xiong, J.; Li, B.; Duan, L.; Wang, D.; Xia, J. Chondrocyte-targeted microRNA delivery by engineered exosomes toward a cell-free osteoarthritis therapy. *ACS Appl. Mater. Interfaces* **2020**, *12*, 36938–36947. [CrossRef]
71. Yang, J.; Zhang, X.; Chen, X.; Wang, L.; Yang, G. Exosome mediated delivery of miR-124 promotes neurogenesis after ischemia. *Mol. Ther. Nucleic Acids* **2017**, *7*, 278–287. [CrossRef]
72. Wang, X.; Chen, Y.; Zhao, Z.; Meng, Q.; Yu, Y.; Sun, J.; Yang, Z.; Chen, Y.; Li, J.; Ma, T. Engineered exosomes with ischemic myocardium-targeting peptide for targeted therapy in myocardial infarction. *J. Am. Heart Assoc.* **2018**, *7*, e008737. [CrossRef]
73. Terasawa, K.; Tomabechi, Y.; Ikeda, M.; Ehara, H.; Kukimoto-Niino, M.; Wakiyama, M.; Podyma-Inoue, K.A.; Rajapakshe, A.R.; Watabe, T.; Shirouzu, M. Lysosome-associated membrane proteins-1 and-2 (LAMP-1 and LAMP-2) assemble via distinct modes. *Biochem. Biophys. Res. Commun.* **2016**, *479*, 489–495. [CrossRef] [PubMed]
74. Bellavia, D.; Raimondo, S.; Calabrese, G.; Forte, S.; Cristaldi, M.; Patinella, A.; Memeo, L.; Manno, M.; Raccosta, S.; Diana, P. Interleukin 3-receptor targeted exosomes inhibit in vitro and in vivo Chronic Myelogenous Leukemia cell growth. *Theranostics* **2017**, *7*, 1333. [CrossRef] [PubMed]
75. Liang, G.; Zhu, Y.; Ali, D.J.; Tian, T.; Xu, H.; Si, K.; Sun, B.; Chen, B.; Xiao, Z. Engineered exosomes for targeted co-delivery of miR-21 inhibitor and chemotherapeutics to reverse drug resistance in colon cancer. *J. Nanobiotechnology* **2020**, *18*, 1–15. [CrossRef] [PubMed]
76. Tian, Y.; Li, S.; Song, J.; Ji, T.; Zhu, M.; Anderson, G.J.; Wei, J.; Nie, G. A doxorubicin delivery platform using engineered natural membrane vesicle exosomes for targeted tumor therapy. *Biomaterials* **2014**, *35*, 2383–2390. [CrossRef]
77. Zhou, Y.; Yuan, Y.; Liu, M.; Hu, X.; Quan, Y.; Chen, X. Tumor-specific delivery of KRAS siRNA with iRGD-exosomes efficiently inhibits tumor growth. *ExRNA* **2019**, *1*, 1–7. [CrossRef]
78. Bai, J.; Duan, J.; Liu, R.; Du, Y.; Luo, Q.; Cui, Y.; Su, Z.; Xu, J.; Xie, Y.; Lu, W. Engineered targeting tLyp-1 exosomes as gene therapy vectors for efficient delivery of siRNA into lung cancer cells. *Asian J. Pharm. Sci.* **2020**, *15*, 461–471. [CrossRef]
79. Hung, M.E.; Leonard, J.N. Stabilization of exosome-targeting peptides via engineered glycosylation. *J. Biol. Chem.* **2015**, *290*, 8166–8172. [CrossRef]
80. Ran, N.; Gao, X.; Dong, X.; Li, J.; Lin, C.; Geng, M.; Yin, H. Effects of exosome-mediated delivery of myostatin propeptide on functional recovery of mdx mice. *Biomaterials* **2020**, *236*, 119826. [CrossRef]
81. Liang, G.; Kan, S.; Zhu, Y.; Feng, S.; Feng, W.; Gao, S. Engineered exosome-mediated delivery of functionally active miR-26a and its enhanced suppression effect in HepG2 cells. *Int. J. Nanomed.* **2018**, *13*, 585. [CrossRef]
82. Kanuma, T.; Yamamoto, T.; Kobiyama, K.; Moriishi, E.; Masuta, Y.; Kusakabe, T.; Ozasa, K.; Kuroda, E.; Jounai, N.; Ishii, K.J. CD63-mediated antigen delivery into extracellular vesicles via DNA vaccination results in robust CD8+ T cell responses. *J. Immunol.* **2017**, *198*, 4707–4715. [CrossRef] [PubMed]
83. Sung, B.H.; von Lersner, A.; Guerrero, J.; Krystofiak, E.S.; Inman, D.; Pelletier, R.; Zijlstra, A.; Ponik, S.M.; Weaver, A.M. A live cell reporter of exosome secretion and uptake reveals pathfinding behavior of migrating cells. *Nat. Commun.* **2020**, *11*, 1–15. [CrossRef] [PubMed]
84. Cheng, Q.; Shi, X.; Han, M.; Smbatyan, G.; Lenz, H.-J.; Zhang, Y. Reprogramming exosomes as nanoscale controllers of cellular immunity. *J. Am. Chem. Soc.* **2018**, *140*, 16413–16417. [CrossRef] [PubMed]
85. Takahashi, Y.; Nishikawa, M.; Shinotsuka, H.; Matsui, Y.; Ohara, S.; Imai, T.; Takakura, Y. Visualization and in vivo tracking of the exosomes of murine melanoma B16–BL6 cells in mice after intravenous injection. *J. Biotechnol.* **2013**, *165*, 77–84. [CrossRef]
86. Morishita, M.; Takahashi, Y.; Nishikawa, M.; Sano, K.; Kato, K.; Yamashita, T.; Imai, T.; Saji, H.; Takakura, Y. Quantitative analysis of tissue distribution of the B16–BL6-derived exosomes using a streptavidin-lactadherin fusion protein and iodine-125-labeled biotin derivative after intravenous injection in mice. *J. Pharm. Sci.* **2015**, *104*, 705–713. [CrossRef]
87. Cui, G.-H.; Guo, H.-D.; Li, H.; Zhai, Y.; Gong, Z.-B.; Wu, J.; Liu, J.-S.; Dong, Y.-R.; Hou, S.-X.; Liu, J.-R. RVG-modified exosomes derived from mesenchymal stem cells rescue memory deficits by regulating inflammatory responses in a mouse model of Alzheimer's disease. *Immun. Ageing* **2019**, *16*, 10. [CrossRef]

88. Zou, J.; Shi, M.; Liu, X.; Jin, C.; Xing, X.; Qiu, L.; Tan, W. Aptamer-Functionalized Exosomes: Elucidating the Cellular Uptake Mechanism and the Potential for Cancer-Targeted Chemotherapy. *Anal. Chem.* **2019**, *91*, 2425–2430. [CrossRef]
89. Pi, F.; Binzel, D.W.; Lee, T.J.; Li, Z.; Sun, M.; Rychahou, P.; Li, H.; Haque, F.; Wang, S.; Croce, C.M.; et al. Nanoparticle orientation to control RNA loading and ligand display on extracellular vesicles for cancer regression. *Nat. Nanotechnol.* **2018**, *13*, 82–89. [CrossRef]
90. Cheng, H.; Fan, J.-H.; Zhao, L.-P.; Fan, G.-L.; Zheng, R.-R.; Qiu, X.-Z.; Yu, X.-Y.; Li, S.-Y.; Zhang, X.-Z. Chimeric peptide engineered exosomes for dual-stage light guided plasma membrane and nucleus targeted photodynamic therapy. *Biomaterials* **2019**, *211*, 14–24. [CrossRef]
91. Nakase, I.; Futaki, S. Combined treatment with a pH-sensitive fusogenic peptide and cationic lipids achieves enhanced cytosolic delivery of exosomes. *Sci. Rep.* **2015**, *5*, 1–13. [CrossRef]
92. Takayama, Y.; Kusamori, K.; Nishikawa, M. Click chemistry as a tool for cell engineering and drug delivery. *Molecules* **2019**, *24*, 172. [CrossRef] [PubMed]
93. Yang, M.; Li, J.; Chen, P.R. Transition metal-mediated bioorthogonal protein chemistry in living cells. *Chem. Soc. Rev.* **2014**, *43*, 6511–6526. [CrossRef] [PubMed]
94. Li, L.; Zhang, Z. Development and applications of the copper-catalyzed azide-alkyne cycloaddition (CuAAC) as a bioorthogonal reaction. *Molecules* **2016**, *21*, 1393. [CrossRef] [PubMed]
95. Lee, T.S.; Kim, Y.; Zhang, W.; Song, I.H.; Tung, C.-H. Facile metabolic glycan labeling strategy for exosome tracking. *Biochim. Et Biophys. Acta BBA-Gen. Subj.* **2018**, *1862*, 1091–1100. [CrossRef] [PubMed]
96. Hwang, D.W.; Choi, H.; Jang, S.C.; Yoo, M.Y.; Park, J.Y.; Choi, N.E.; Oh, H.J.; Ha, S.; Lee, Y.-S.; Jeong, J.M. Noninvasive imaging of radiolabeled exosome-mimetic nanovesicle using 99mTc-HMPAO. *Sci. Rep.* **2015**, *5*, 1–10. [CrossRef]
97. Tian, T.; Zhang, H.-X.; He, C.-P.; Fan, S.; Zhu, Y.-L.; Qi, C.; Huang, N.-P.; Xiao, Z.-D.; Lu, Z.-H.; Tannous, B.A.; et al. Surface functionalized exosomes as targeted drug delivery vehicles for cerebral ischemia therapy. *Biomaterials* **2018**, *150*, 137–149. [CrossRef]
98. Jia, G.; Han, Y.; An, Y.; Ding, Y.; He, C.; Wang, X.; Tang, Q. NRP-1 targeted and cargo-loaded exosomes facilitate simultaneous imaging and therapy of glioma in vitro and in vivo. *Biomaterials* **2018**, *178*, 302–316. [CrossRef]
99. Koh, E.; Lee, E.J.; Nam, G.-H.; Hong, Y.; Cho, E.; Yang, Y.; Kim, I.-S. Exosome-SIRPα, a CD47 blockade increases cancer cell phagocytosis. *Biomaterials* **2017**, *121*, 121–129. [CrossRef]
100. Kim, M.S.; Haney, M.J.; Zhao, Y.; Yuan, D.; Deygen, I.; Klyachko, N.L.; Kabanov, A.V.; Batrakova, E.V. Engineering macrophage-derived exosomes for targeted paclitaxel delivery to pulmonary metastases: In vitro and in vivo evaluations. *Nanomed. Nanotechnol. Biol. Med.* **2018**, *14*, 195–204. [CrossRef]
101. Zhou, W.; Zhou, Y.; Chen, X.; Ning, T.; Chen, H.; Guo, Q.; Zhang, Y.; Liu, P.; Zhang, Y.; Li, C.; et al. Pancreatic cancer-targeting exosomes for enhancing immunotherapy and reprogramming tumor microenvironment. *Biomaterials* **2021**, *268*, 120546. [CrossRef]
102. Jong, A.Y.; Wu, C.-H.; Li, J.; Sun, J.; Fabbri, M.; Wayne, A.S.; Seeger, R.C. Large-scale isolation and cytotoxicity of extracellular vesicles derived from activated human natural killer cells. *J. Extracell. Vesicles* **2017**, *6*, 1294368. [CrossRef] [PubMed]
103. Watson, D.C.; Bayik, D.; Srivatsan, A.; Bergamaschi, C.; Valentin, A.; Niu, G.; Bear, J.; Monninger, M.; Sun, M.; Morales-Kastresana, A.; et al. Efficient production and enhanced tumor delivery of engineered extracellular vesicles. *Biomaterials* **2016**, *105*, 195–205. [CrossRef] [PubMed]
104. Taylor, D.D.; Shah, S. Methods of isolating extracellular vesicles impact down-stream analyses of their cargoes. *Methods* **2015**, *87*, 3–10. [CrossRef] [PubMed]
105. Jang, S.C.; Kim, O.Y.; Yoon, C.M.; Choi, D.-S.; Roh, T.-Y.; Park, J.; Nilsson, J.; Lötvall, J.; Kim, Y.-K.; Gho, Y.S. Bioinspired Exosome-Mimetic Nanovesicles for Targeted Delivery of Chemotherapeutics to Malignant Tumors. *ACS Nano* **2013**, *7*, 7698–7710. [CrossRef] [PubMed]
106. Hood, J.L.; Scott, M.J.; Wickline, S.A. Maximizing exosome colloidal stability following electroporation. *Anal. Biochem.* **2014**, *448*, 41–49. [CrossRef] [PubMed]

pharmaceutics

MDPI

Article

Genetically Engineered Extracellular Vesicles Harboring Transmembrane Scaffolds Exhibit Differences in Their Size, Expression Levels of Specific Surface Markers and Cell-Uptake

Jiayi Zhang [1,†], Annie Brown [1,†], Brendan Johnson [1], David Diebold [1], Kyle Asano [1], Gerard Marriott [2,*] and Biao Lu [1,*]

1 Department of Bioengineering, School of Engineering, Santa Clara University, 500 El Camino Real, Santa Clara, CA 95053, USA
2 Department of Bioengineering, University of California at Berkeley, Berkeley, CA 94720, USA
* Correspondence: gmlab@berkeley.edu (G.M.); blu2@scu.edu (B.L.)
† These authors contributed equally to this work.

Abstract: Background: Human cell-secreted extracellular vesicles (EVs) are versatile nanomaterials suitable for disease-targeted drug delivery and therapy. Native EVs, however, usually do not interact specifically with target cells or harbor therapeutic drugs, which limits their potential for clinical applications. These functions can be introduced to EVs by genetic manipulation of membrane protein scaffolds, although the efficiency of these manipulations and the impacts they have on the properties of EVs are for the most part unknown. In this study, we quantify the effects of genetic manipulations of different membrane scaffolds on the physicochemical properties, molecular profiles, and cell uptake of the EVs. Methods: Using a combination of gene fusion, molecular imaging, and immuno-based on-chip analysis, we examined the effects of various protein scaffolds, including endogenous tetraspanins (CD9, CD63, and CD81) and exogenous vesicular stomatitis virus glycoprotein (VSVG), on the efficiency of integration in EV membranes, the physicochemical properties of EVs, and EV uptake by recipient cells. Results: Fluorescence imaging and live cell monitoring showed each scaffold type was integrated into EVs either in membranes of the endocytic compartment, the plasma membrane, or both. Analysis of vesicle size revealed that the incorporation of each scaffold increased the average diameter of vesicles compared to unmodified EVs. Molecular profiling of surface markers in engineered EVs using on-chip assays showed the CD63-GFP scaffold decreased expression of CD81 on the membrane surface compared to control EVs, whereas its expression was mostly unchanged in EVs bearing CD9-, CD81-, or VSVG-GFP. The results from cell uptake studies demonstrated that VSVG-engineered EVs were taken up by recipient cells to a greater degree than control EVs. Conclusion: We found that the incorporation of different molecular scaffolds in EVs altered their physicochemical properties, surface protein profiles, and cell-uptake functions. Scaffold-induced changes in the physical and functional properties of engineered EVs should therefore be considered in engineering EVs for the targeted delivery and uptake of therapeutics to diseased cells.

Keywords: extracellular vesicles (EVs); exosome; CD9; CD63; CD81; vesicular stomatitis virus envelope glycoprotein (VSVG); nanotechnology; targeted drug delivery

Citation: Zhang, J.; Brown, A.; Johnson, B.; Diebold, D.; Asano, K.; Marriott, G.; Lu, B. Genetically Engineered Extracellular Vesicles Harboring Transmembrane Scaffolds Exhibit Differences in Their Size, Expression Levels of Specific Surface Markers and Cell-Uptake. *Pharmaceutics* **2022**, *14*, 2564. https://doi.org/10.3390/pharmaceutics14122564

Academic Editor: Yong Chen

Received: 21 October 2022
Accepted: 19 November 2022
Published: 23 November 2022

1. Introduction

Extracellular vesicles (EVs) are cell-derived nanocarriers that are thought to mediate cell-to-cell communication in prokaryotes and eukaryotes [1,2]. In mammals, EVs are continuously synthesized and released to the extracellular environment in a constitutive and regulated manner [3,4]. Mammalian EVs can be divided into two distinct types according to their membrane origin: for example, microvesicles have a diameter of 100–1000 nm and are formed by direct budding from the plasma membrane, while exosomes (50–150 nm) are released via exocytosis of multivesicular bodies (MVBs) [5,6].

EVs can also be divided into CD9$^+$, CD63$^+$, and CD81$^+$ subtypes, each bearing specific surface markers [7–9]. After being released from host cells, EVs may be found in significant numbers in blood plasma [10], lymph [11], ammonic fluid [12], saliva [13], urine [14], breast milk [15], and seminal fluid [16]. Consequently, they may be involved in shuttling specific signaling molecules, including proteins, nucleic acids, and lipids, to target cells in remote tissues [17,18]. EVs are known to regulate tissue growth and organ development [19,20], modulate the immune response [21–23], mediate inflammation and viral infection [24–26], and promote cancer progression and metastasis [27–29]. As a new generation of nanomaterials, EVs may offer advantages over artificial nano-vehicles such as liposomes and polymers for targeted drug delivery and therapy [30,31]. First, EVs are derived from human cells, so they are biocompatible and biodegradable and may evade rapid clearance by the immune system [32]. Second, EVs are capable of penetrating tissue to reach deep-seated cells, and there are known cases where they cross the blood-brain barrier (BBB) [33]. Third, endogenously and/or exogenously produced EVs can be genetically engineered to facilitate drug loading and targeted delivery of biologics to diseased tissue [34,35].

While EVs hold great promise in nanomedicine, endogenous EVs exhibit poor targeting to diseased cells and lack therapeutic cargo [36,37]. These functions, however, can be introduced through the use of molecular and genetic engineering techniques [38]. An essential requirement here is to identify molecular scaffolds that present a tissue-targeting moiety while enabling loading with a therapeutic agent. To this end, previous studies have examined the use of membrane-associated proteins, including CD9, CD63, and CD81, to display tissue-targeting or imaging moieties on the outer surface of exosomes [39,40]. In addition, we have reported that the viral envelope glycoprotein derived from the vesicular stomatitis virus glycoprotein (VSVG) is a suitable scaffold for loading bioactive enzymes associated with lysosomal storage disorders in the lumen of the exosome [41,42]. Moreover, El-Addloussi et al. used the lysosome-associated membrane protein 2B (LAMP2B) to install neurotrophic peptides in the lumen of exosomes for targeted delivery of siRNA cargo to the brain in a mouse model [43]. Lipid-anchoring proteins/peptides may be used as an alternative membrane scaffold to present disease-targeting agents on the outer surface of EVs. For example, the C1C2 domain of lactadherin is a popular tool to project cell-targeting proteins on the outer face of the EV membranes [44]. This approach was employed to display an antibody fragment (scFV) to target cancer cells and to present the tumor antigens, OVA and HER2, as cancer vaccines [45]. Similarly, the peptide RPPGSPFR, derived from bradykinin, was used to bind to EVs and other highly curved lipid nanovesicles via lipid chain insertion [46,47]. Collectively, these studies established the usefulness of molecular scaffolds in engineering EVs for use as targeted therapeutic vehicles. Native EVs exhibit broad heterogeneity as a result of different tissue origins, specific surface modifications, and physicochemical properties, all of which may impact their suitability for further engineering of molecular functions for the targeting and delivery of therapeutic agents. EVs derived from a single cell type, however, may alleviate this problem, while genetic manipulation of the host cell may serve to introduce a defined molecular scaffold that presents specific targeting moieties on the external face of the EV and a therapeutic biologic in the lumen.

In this study, we assess the impacts of incorporating transmembrane scaffolds, including CD9, CD63, CD81, and VSVG, on specific physical, molecular, and functional properties of the engineered EVs. Although membrane protein scaffolds have been successfully used to engineer EVs, we know little about the effects of these modifications on different EV subtypes, including potential changes in their diameters, the efficiency of their integration, and altered expression of surface markers. Herein, we employed a newly developed, high-throughput on-chip assay in a comparative study of specific physicochemical properties of engineered EVs at the level of individual vesicles. Our results show that each molecular scaffold exhibits quantitative differences in the efficiencies of their integration into different subtypes of EVs, in the expression levels of specific membrane protein surface markers, and in the uptake of engineered EVs by recipient cells. These findings are important as alterations in the physicochemical and functional properties of engineered EVs may impact their potential for applications in nanomedicine.

2. Materials and Methods

2.1. Cells and Reagents

Human embryonic kidney cells (293T) were purchased from Alstem (Richmond, CA, USA). High glucose DMEM, Opti-MEM medium, and fetal bovine serum were purchased from ThermoFisher Scientific (Waltham, MA, USA). Chemically-defined and serum-free UltraCulture medium was purchased from Lonza (Portsmouth, NH, USA). The transfection reagent, polyethyleneimine (PEI), was purchased from Sigma-Aldrich (St. Louis, MO, USA). Lipofectamine2000 was purchased from Invitrogen, and FuGene6 were sourced from Promega (Madison, WI, USA). Nuclear staining solution Hoechst 33342 was purchased from ThermoFisher Scientific (Fremont, CA, USA). The EV precipitation solution (ExoQuick-TC) was obtained from System Biosciences (Palo Alto, CA, USA).

2.2. Vectors and Fusion Genes

Scaffolds, including human tetraspanins (CD9, CD63, and CD81) and viral VSVG, were fused with copepod GFP at the C-terminus of all scaffolds, as reported previously [39,41]. All expression vectors were constructed similarly. The coding sequences for the exosome-targeting scaffold and GFP fusion were placed after the cytomegalovirus promoter (CMV) but followed by the polyadenylation signal sequences (PolyA). All final constructs were verified by double-stranded DNA sequencing to ensure fidelity.

2.3. Cell Culture and Transfection

293T cells were cultured in high-glucose DMEM supplemented with 10% fetal bovine serum, 2 mM GlutMax, and 100 U/mL penicillin-streptomycin. Unless otherwise stated, all transfections were performed in six-well culture plates. Transfection conditions were optimized so that over 80% of cells will be effectively transfected, as judged by GFP-positivity. Typically, cells grown at 40~60% density were transfected by adding plasmid DNA (1~2 μg/well) mixed with transfection reagents (Lipofectamine 2000, FuGene6, or PEI), as previously reported [48].

2.4. Isolation of EVs

Surface modification and subsequent preparation of EVs from transfected cells were performed as previously reported [42]. Briefly, 293T cells grown on 15-cm plates (70~80% confluence) were transfected with PEI reagent. 24 h following transfection, cells were switched to a serum-free UltraCulture medium to produce modified EVs. After an additional 48 h of incubation, the conditioned medium was collected, centrifuged, and filtered through a 0.22 μm filter to remove larger EVs (>220 μm). The resulting filtered medium was subsequently mixed with ExoQuick-TC and incubated at 4 °C overnight. The EVs were precipitated after a second round of centrifugation at 3000× *g* for 60 min. The pelleted EVs were gently suspended in a phosphate buffer for further analysis or stored at −80 °C for future use.

2.5. Live Cell Microscopy

Cultured cells or fluorescently labeled EVs were monitored by using either an Olympus CKX53 culture microscope or a Leica TCS SP8 confocal microscope. To demonstrate the subcellular localization of GFP reporters, we recorded fluorescence and transmitted light images from the same field. Image adjustments such as brightness and contrast were applied to the entire image frame using dedicated instrument software.

2.6. On-Chip Capture and Characterization of EVs

Antibody-based capturing and analysis of single EVs were performed using the ExoView® Tetraspanin Kits (NanoView Biosciences; Brighton, MA, USA) according to the manufacturer's instructions on the ExoView® R100 platform (NanoView Biosciences), a single particle interferometric reflectance imaging sensing (SP-IRIS) platform coupled with fluorescence detection. Briefly, isolated EVs were first diluted in PBS (~100-fold dilution), and an equal volume of EVs was further diluted in PBS to a final concentration of 0.006 μg/μL. Chips coated with anti-CD9/CD63/CD81 antibodies and murine non-specific control IgG antibodies were used for EV capturing. Fluorescent CF647-anti-CD63 and CF555-anti-CD81 antibodies were used to detect CD63 and CD81 expression on the EV surface. EV sizes were measured by the SP-IRIS mode on ExoView® R100, and the EV surface protein profile (CD63 and CD81) was measured by the fluorescence mode. For all the fluorescence images, surface CD63 and CD81 detected by the fluorescent antibodies and exogenous scaffolds fused to GFP (CD9/CD63/CD81/VSVG) were pseudocolored as red, green, and blue, respectively. The fluorescence thresholds were set to 300 a.u., 300 a.u., and 600 a.u. for the red, green, and blue channels, respectively, throughout each experiment.

2.7. Fluorescein-Labeling of EVs

EVs isolated from the conditioned medium were labeled by the ExoGlowTM-RNA EV labeling kit (SBI, Palo Alto, CA, USA) according to the manufacturer's instructions for flow cytometry analysis. The kit contained reagents specific to EV mRNAs. We labeled both engineered and non-engineered control EVs using this kit and conducted subsequent cellular uptake experiments on fluorescein-labeled EVs.

2.8. Cellular Uptake Assay

EV uptake assays were performed as previously reported [48]. Briefly, recipient 293T cells were seeded and incubated in an FBS-supplemented medium overnight for attachment before being exchanged to an FBS-free UltraCulture medium containing fluorescein-labeled EVs to allow cellular uptake to occur. The uptake process of fluorescence-labeled EVs was monitored using fluorescence microscopy. At the indicated time points, we recorded fluorescence and transmitted light images of the preparations.

2.9. Flow Cytometry Analysis

Recipient 293T cells treated with increased amounts (0, 3.12, 6.26, 12.5, 25, 50, and 100 ug/mL) of EVs for 24 h were trypsinized, washed, and re-suspended in phosphate buffer. The amount of fluorescein isothiocyanate (FITC)-labeled EV endocytosed by recipient cells was quantified using flow cytometry in an Accuri C6 Plus instrument (BD Biosciences), as described previously [49]. Control cells (not treated with EVs) were also included in the study to determine the background fluorescence level. The fluorescence intensity data from these studies were analyzed using the CFlow Plus software (BD Biosciences).

2.10. Data Analysis and Statistics

Data on single EVs were acquired by the ExoScan Software connected to the ExoView® R100 platform. Fluorescence images of the chips and analysis of the integration efficiency of different scaffolds, expression levels of EV surface markers, and sizes of individual vesicles were performed using the NanoViewer software. Statistical analysis of these data was performed using Python 3.8.3. A p-value (<0.05) using a Student's t-test was considered statistically significant.

3. Results

3.1. Engineering Strategy and Experimental Design

Membrane-embedded protein scaffolds are widely used in the engineering of EVs for cell-targeting and loading therapeutic proteins/enzymes [41,50]. Membrane anchoring scaffolds are usually based on integral transmembrane proteins and include tetraspanins, viral envelope glycoproteins [41,50], and membrane-associated proteins such as those with the C1C2 domain [44]. In this study, we focus on transmembrane scaffolds as they provide flexibility in engineering the inner and outer surfaces of EVs [50] for both cell-targeting and drug-loading functions. In particular, we engineered EVs using the intrinsic exosome proteins CD9, CD63, and CD81 (tetraspanins), and the exogenous viral envelope glycoprotein, VSVG. The goal of the study was to investigate whether different molecular scaffolds impact the efficiency of incorporation in the EV membrane, and the potential alteration of physicochemical and biological properties of engineered EVs, including their diameter and molecular profiles. To achieve this goal, we used reporter constructs tagged with GFP previously described by our groups for real-time analysis of engineered secreted EVs (Figure 1A). The GFP molecule was tagged to the C-terminus of each type of protein scaffold to locate the probe on the luminal side of the EV membrane (Figure 1B). This approach was adopted to minimize potential interferences with the membrane targeting and anchoring abilities of the scaffolds. Following the isolation of engineered EVs from conditioned medium, we performed a high-throughput analysis of individual EVs using ExoView® to determine: (1) the incorporation efficiency; (2) evidence of subtypes in the population of engineered EVs; and (3) potential alteration of the size and surface markers (Figure 1C).

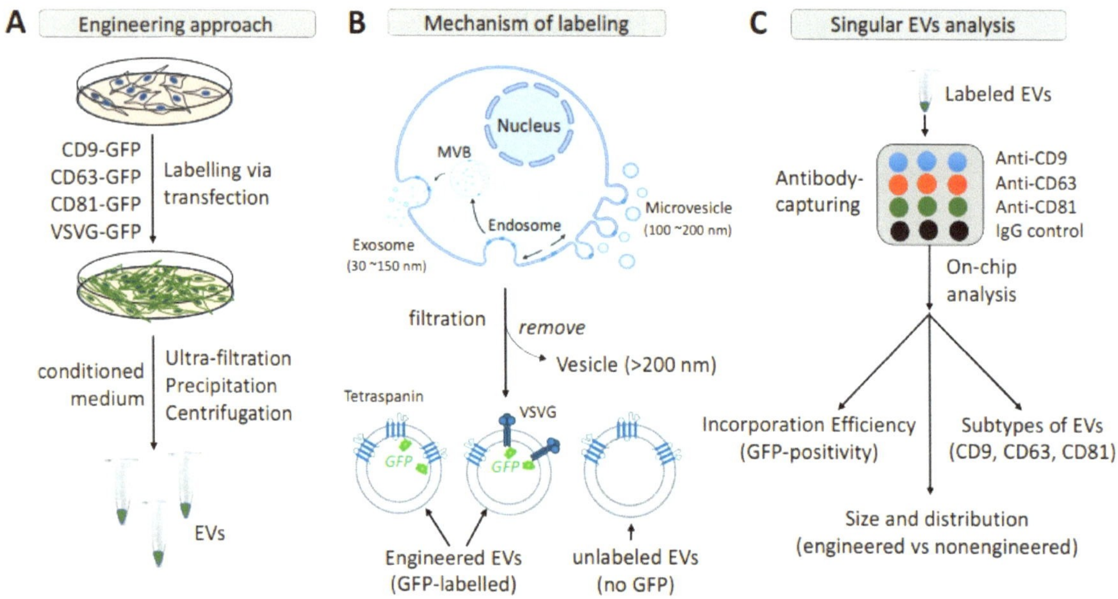

Figure 1. Strategy and molecular mechanisms underlying surface engineering of EVs via transmembrane scaffolds. (**A**) The workflow illustrates the engineering of EVs using either endogenous tetraspanins (CD9, CD63, and CD81) or exogenous vesicular stomatitis virus envelope glycoprotein (VSVG). (**B**) The molecular mechanism underlying the genetic labeling of EVs and membrane topology of the engineering scaffolds. (**C**) Methods used by on-chip analysis for characterization of scaffold-modified vs. non-modified EVs. Abbreviations: vesicular stomatitis virus envelope glycoprotein, VSVG; small extracellular vesicles, EVs; multi-vesicular bodies, MVBs.

3.2. Transmembrane Scaffolds Incorporate into Biogenic Sites of EVs in Living Human Cells

Genetic fusions of GFP with the identified transmembrane scaffolds were developed to enable real-time monitoring and imaging of their incorporation and subsequent loading into the EV membranes within live human cells. We confirmed these scaffolds were correctly targeted to EVs by first transfecting each of the GFP-fusion constructs in 293T cells and then imaging the GFP fluorescence to quantify their expression levels and integration in EV membranes. Confocal fluorescence microscopy images of GFP showed that all of the transmembrane scaffolds were able to localize to some areas of the plasma membrane (arrowheads, Figure 2(A1,A3,A7,A9)), endocytic compartments (arrows, Figure 2(A1–A12)), and sometimes the periphery of nucleus (Figure 2(A9)). Further analysis of GFP image data supports the view that all of the transmembrane scaffolds (CD9, CD63, CD81, and VSVG) were successfully targeted and incorporated in EV membranes. These findings are consistent with previous reports showing tetraspanins (CD9/CD63/CD81) and VSVG incorporate into the plasma membrane and/or endocytic compartments such as multi-vesicular bodies (MVBs) and are secreted as EVs to the extracellular environment [51–53]. While all tested GFP fusions localized to the plasma membrane and endocytic compartments, we found CD63 and VSVG were more likely to concentrate in the endocytic compartment, as seen by the larger number of GFP puncta in the cytosol (Figure 2(A4–A6,A10–A12)). In contrast, CD9 and C81 showed greater GFP fluorescence signals at the plasma membrane and less in endocytic compartments (Figure 2(A1–A3,A7–A9)). These differences in membrane distribution could suggest specific types of the transmembrane scaffold may result in the formation of different types of EVs, i.e., not just exosomes (Figure 1B). Please note that the GFP granules that appear in the cytosol are most likely MVBs rather than pre-secreted individual exosomes. Because MVBs may contain different numbers of exosomes, GFP granules tend to have different sizes (Figure 2(A4,A10)).

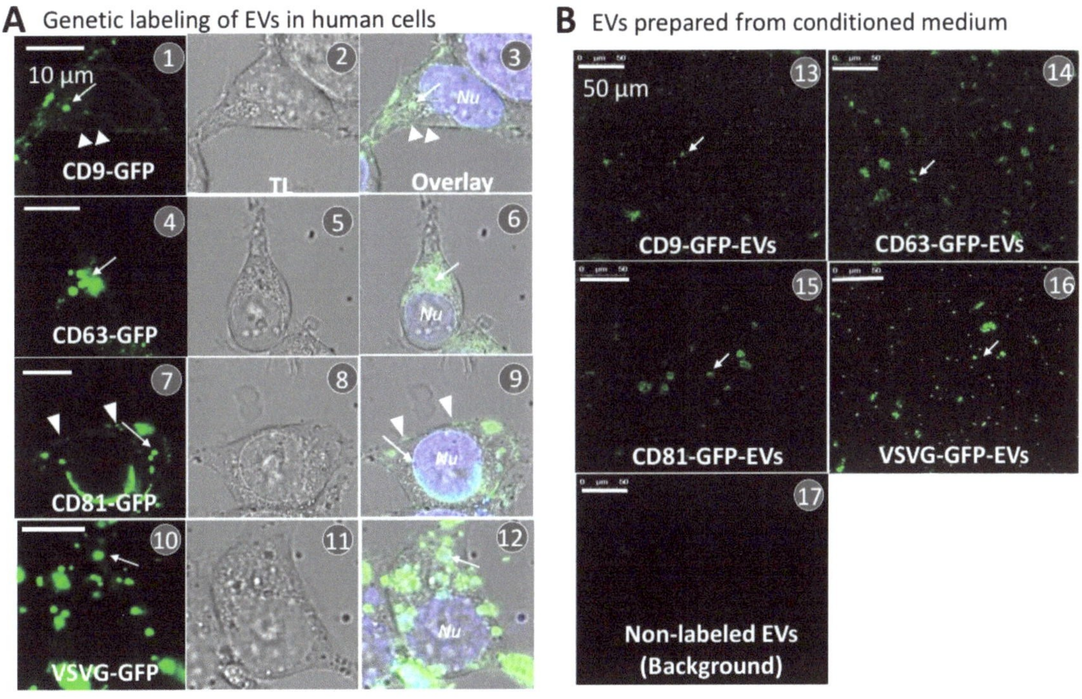

Figure 2. Transfection, expression, and isolation of genetically labeled EVs from conditioned medium of cultured 293T cells. (**A**) Cultured human 293T cells were transfected with each of the transmembrane scaffolds tagged with a GFP reporter, including CD9-GFP (**A1–A3**), CD63-GFP (**A4–A6**), CD81-GFP (**A7–A9**), and VSVG-GFP (**A10–A12**). At 48 h following the transfection, both fluorescence and transmitted light images were recorded. Arrows (→) indicate the incorporation of GFP-tagged scaffolds into the endocytic compartment of the endosome and/or MVB, while arrowheads (>) indicate focal incorporation into the plasma membrane. (**B**) EVs were prepared from the conditioned medium collected from the transfected cells, and confocal images were taken at the same dilution (0.1 µg/µL, protein of EVs) for all samples (**B13–B16**). Images were also recorded using unlabeled control samples to quantify background noise (**B17**). Arrows indicate individual/clustered EVs. Scale bar, 50 µm.

Next, we investigated whether purified EVs secreted from transfected 293T cells incorporated their respective GFP-tagged scaffolds. Briefly, EVs were purified from conditioned medium by using a combination of ultrafiltration, chemical precipitation, and centrifugation methods, as previously reported [42]. A small amount of the purified EV preparation was smeared on a microscope cover slip for subsequent fluorescence imaging and image analysis. Correct integration of each scaffold in the EV membrane was indicated by strong GFP signals (Figure 2(B13–B16)) whereas control EVs did not generate any significant fluorescence signal (Figure 2(B17)).

3.3. Each Transmembrane Scaffold Preferentially Incorporates into Different Subtypes of EVs with Various Efficiency

The ExoView system provides a powerful method to characterize individual engineered EVs (Figure 3A). Individual EVs are bonded to a layered silicon substrate chip coated with an array of capture antibodies and subsequently characterized using a combination of single-particle interferometric imaging and immunofluorescence imaging modalities. In this way, the system enables one to profile different EV subpopulations and determine the successful incorporation of each transmembrane scaffold into individual EVs. In our studies, we captured EVs at different sites on the chip using surface-attached monoclonal antibodies directed against CD9, CD63, and CD81. Bonded EVs were then fluorescently stained using the following antibody conjugates: CF647-anti-CD63 (red) and CF555-anti-CD81 (green) to profile these surface markers. The workflow used to characterize EV populations in a sample was as follows: first identify engineered EVs on the chip by imaging GFP fluorescence for each subpopulation of EV on the chip ($CD9^+$, $CD63^+$, or $CD81^+$; Figure 3B–E). For example, Figure 3(B1) shows a GFP-fluorescence image of CD9-GFP-modified EVs captured at a site with surface-attached anti-CD9 antibodies (GFP emitting is pseudotyped with blue color). High-resolution multispectral analysis of fluorescence images of immunostained EVs on the chip (Figure 3(B2–B5)) is then used to identify individual EVs with a specific surface marker profile. For example, GFP harboring EVs that emit red emissions are CD63 positive, those with green emissions are CD81 positive, and those with blue emissions are GFP positive. Overlay images of the three colors are then used to quantify the amounts of each biomarker protein on the membrane surface of the EVs. This approach was used to study the molecular profiles of EVs harboring the different molecular scaffolds, namely CD63-GFP, CD81-GFP, and VSVG-GFP, shown respectively in Figure 3(C6–C10,D11–D15,E16–E20).

Next, we characterized GFP-positive/negative EVs in terms of the molecular profile of surface markers using Venn diagrams (Figure 4(1–12)). The results show that each tetraspanin can be incorporated into its respective subgroup. More specifically, CD9-GFP preferentially modifies $CD9^+$ EVs (47.2%) as compared to $CD63^+$ (19.7%) and $CD81^+$ (32.4%) EVs. Similarly, CD63-GFP and CD81-GFP predominantly modify $CD63^+$ (58.7%) and $CD81^+$ (16.6%) EVs, respectively. In contrast, viral VSVG-GFP scaffolds have low efficacy in incorporating into all three subgroups of EVs (8.3% in $CD9^+$, 4.7% in $CD63^+$, and 8.5% in $CD81^+$ EVs) (Table 1 in Figure 4).

Table 1. Engineering efficiency with different scaffolds.

	$CD9^+$ EVs	**$CD63^+$ EVs**	**$CD81^+$ EVs**
CD9-GFP-EVs	47.2% ± 0.8%	19.7% ± 5.1%	32.4% ± 4.0%
CD63-GFP-EVs	6.7% ± 0.1%	58.7% ± 1.5%	7.3% ± 0.5%
CD81-GFP-EVs	12.3% ± 6.3%	4.9% ± 0.6%	16.6% ± 2.0%
VSVG-GFP-EVs	8.3% ± 0.2%	4.7% ± 0.8%	8.5% ± 0.1%

Note: Data is represented in mean ± standard deviation (n = 3).

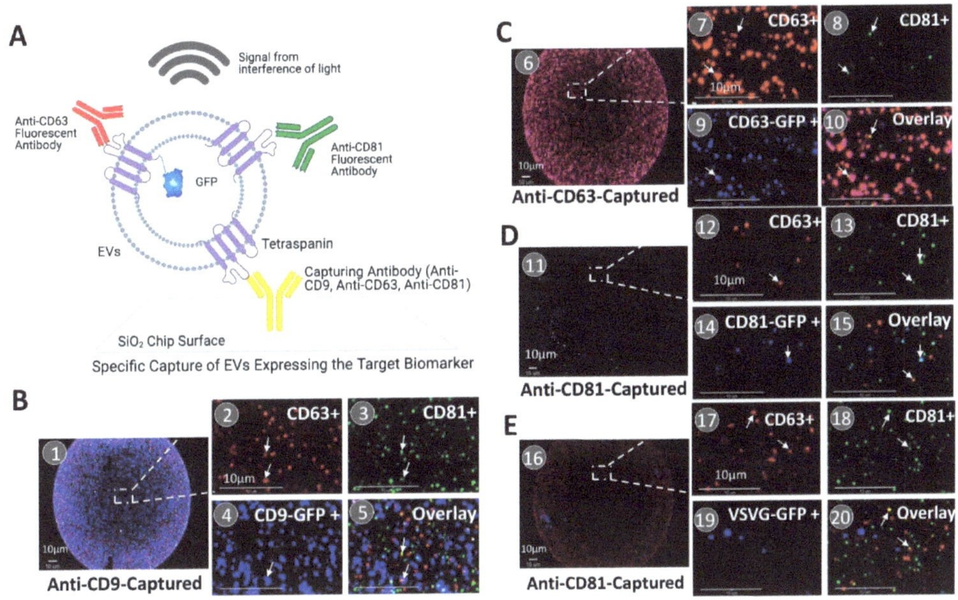

Figure 3. On-chip analysis of antibody-captured EVs. (**A**) A schematic representation of on-chip analysis of genetically labeled EVs. The size of EVs was measured and calculated using signals from the interference of light (interferometry). Surface marker profiles of EVs were specifically detected by fluorescein-labeled monoclonal antibodies. (**B–E**) Molecular profiling of various EV subtypes and subpopulations of scaffold-modified EVs. (**B1–B5**) CD9-GFP-modified EVs captured by anti-CD9 antibodies. (**C6–C10**) CD63-GFP-modified EVs captured by anti-CD63 antibodies. (**D11–D15**) CD81-GFP-modified EVs captured by anti-CD81 antibodies. (**E16–E20**) VSVG-GFP-modified EVs captured by anti-CD81 antibodies. A portion of the spots (**B1,C6,D11,E16**) was magnified to show the individual EVs and expression/co-expression of the surface markers, CD9/CD63/CD81/scaffold-GFP. Arrows indicate co-expression of surface markers on individual vesicles; Scale bar, 10 μm.

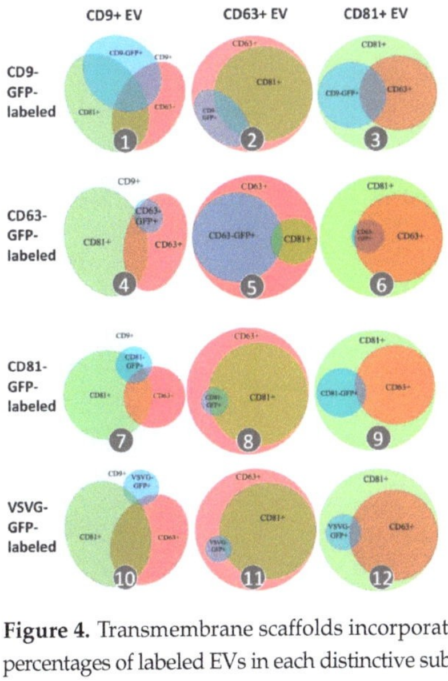

Figure 4. Transmembrane scaffolds incorporate into distinct EV subtypes. Venn diagrams summarize percentages of labeled EVs in each distinctive subpopulation of EVs. EVs captured by anti-CD9, anti-CD63,

or anti-CD81 antibodies are characterized as CD81$^+$ (green outer circle), CD63$^+$ (red outer circle), or CD9$^+$ (grey outer circle) subpopulations, respectively (columns). The percentage of EVs modified by different transmembrane scaffolds, including CD9-GFP-, CD63-GFP-, CD81-GFP, or VSVG-GFP, is represented by the blue inner circle. The surface marker profiles of CD63 and CD81 determined by fluorescein-labeled anti-CD63 and anti-CD81 antibodies were represented by the smaller red and green inner circles/ellipses, respectively. The size of all circles and ellipses was proportional to their percentages.

3.4. Surface Engineering Using Transmembrane Scaffolds Leads to an Increase in EV Size

Next, we examined the impact that different transmembrane scaffolds may have on the diameter of EVs. Taking advantage of the high-throughput power of single EV analysis via SP-IRIS (single particle interferometric reflectance image sensor), we measured the diameters of 64,861 individual EVs captured by surface-bound anti-CD9/CD63/CD81 antibodies (Supplemental Table S1). As shown in Figure 5A–D, the integration of transmembrane scaffolds in EVs led to significant increases in the diameter of all engineered EVs. The average size of unmodified EVs was 58.4 ± 8.07 nm, while the mean diameter of modified EVs was all larger than 60 nm. More specifically, CD81-GFP led to the largest increase (86.02 nm ± 34.18), followed by CD9-GFP (66.13 nm ± 16.38), VSVG-GFP (65.42 nm ± 15.62), and CD63-GFP (62.07 nm ± 14.20), respectively (Table 2). While the average percentage of unmodified EVs having a diameter ≥ 60 nm was <29%, the same measure for EVs bearing the CD81-GFP scaffold was 72.9%, 54.7% for CD9-GFP, 52.5% for VSVG-GFP, and 40.3% for CD63-GFP (Supplemental Table S2). Thus, if the diameter of the EVs was found to negatively impact their physiological function, then one would likely select EVs harboring the CD63-GFP scaffold, followed by VSVG-GFP, CD9-GFP, and CD81-GFP.

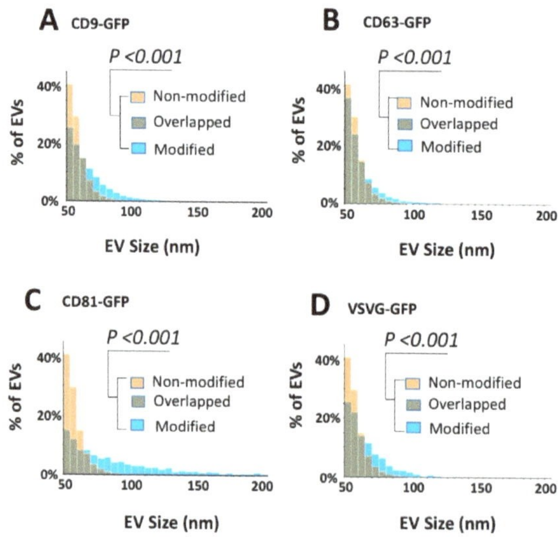

Figure 5. Transmembrane scaffolds increase the size of EVs. (**A–D**) EVs prepared from the conditioned medium were subjected to on-chip analysis. The vesicle size distributions were graphed for CD9-GFP-modified vs. non-modified EVs (**A**), CD63-GFP-modified vs. non-modified EVs (**B**), CD81-GFP-modified vs. non-modified EVs (**C**), or VSVG-GFP-modified EVs vs. non-modified EVs (**D**). Yellow and blue bars represent non-modified control and transmembrane scaffold-modified EVs, respectively, while green bars represent the overlay portion. The counts of EV numbers are normalized to the percentages of total vesicle numbers analyzed and graphed. The size differences between the modified and non-modified groups are statistically significant with a p-value < 0.001 (Student's t-test).

Table 2. Effects on the size of EVs via transmembrane scaffold.

Name of Scaffold	Unmodified EVs (nm, size)	Modified EVs (nm, size)
CD9-GFP	58.40 ± 8.07	66.13 ± 16.38
CD63-GFP		62.07 ± 14.20
CD81-GFP		86.02 ± 34.18
VSVG-GFP		65.42 ± 15.62

3.5. CD63 Scaffold Decreases the Expression Levels of CD81 Markers on Modified EVs

Next, we examined differences in the expression levels of specific tetraspanin membrane proteins such as CD63 and CD81 in EVs bearing different transmembrane scaffolds [54]. This quantitative study revealed that the CD63-GFP scaffold decreased the amount of CD81 in EVs (Figure 6B). whereas no change in the expression level of CD81 was evident when other transmembrane scaffolds such as CD9, CD81, or VSVG were used (Figure 6A,C,D). Specifically, CD81 was lowered by ~50% in EVs captured by anti-CD63 antibodies, and this decrease in the levels of CD81 was accompanied by an increase in CD63 by ~40% (indicated by stars in Figure 6B). In contrast, EVs captured by other surface marker antibodies such as CD81 and CD9 exhibited higher levels of CD81 expression than CD63. These results suggest that CD63 modification may cause a decrease in the levels of $CD81^+$ in CD63-positive EVs.

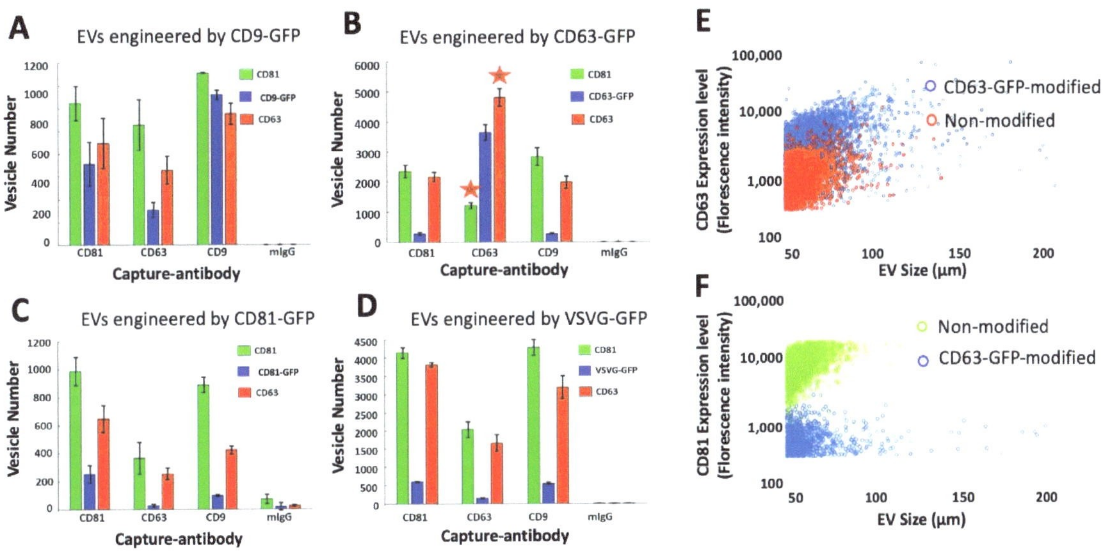

Figure 6. Effects of the engineering scaffolds on the expression of EV surface markers. (**A–D**) EVs captured on-chip by monoclonal antibodies to CD9/CD63/CD81 were further characterized for their expression of the GFP-tagged engineering scaffolds (blue) as well as CD63 and CD81, which are detected by the fluorescein CF647-labeled anti-CD63 antibody (red) and the CF555-labeled anti-CD81 antibody (green). The number of EVs that express these markers was analyzed and graphed. (**E**,**F**) Scatter plots comparing the expression levels of surface markers in CD63-GFP-modified vs. non-modified EVs. Blue dots represent CD63-GFP-EVs and red dots represent non-labeled EVs (**E**); Blue dots represent CD63-GFP-EVs and green dots represent non-labeled EVs (**F**).

Further confirmation that CD63-GFP incorporation in EVs decreases the expression of CD81 coupled with an increased CD63 expression came from an analysis of fluorescence intensity measurements of CD63 and CD81 in CD63-GFP and non-labeled control EVs. A plot of CD63 fluorescence intensity vs. average diameter reveals that individual

EVs bearing CD63-GFP have higher CD63 fluorescence compared to non-labeled EVs (Figure 6E, blue dots vs. red dots), indicating an increase in the expression of CD63. In contrast, when we plot the CD81 fluorescence intensity, the two groups show an opposite distribution pattern: the CD63-GFP-modified EVs have a lower CD81 expression level compared to the non-labeled EVs (Figure 6F, blue dots vs. green dots). This analysis confirms that engineering EVs with CD63-GFP can cause a decrease in the levels of expression of CD81 but an increase in the levels of CD63 expression.

3.6. The VSVG Scaffold Increases the Cellular Uptake of EVs

Next, we determined whether scaffold-modified EVs are capable of being endocytosed by recipient cells. Purified EVs genetically labeled with GFP-tagged scaffolds were added to the culture medium of 293T cells for either 24- or 48-h, and after washing the cells, they were imaged by confocal microscopy (Figure 7). Confocal fluorescence images showed GFP granules in cells with EVs bearing GFP fusions of CD9/CD63/CD81/VSVG-GFP (Figure 7; arrows). Consistent with previous reports [41], analysis of confocal fluorescence images seen at the 24- and 48-h time points showed EVs harboring the VSVG scaffold were taken up to a greater degree than EVs modified with tetraspanin scaffolds (Figure 7(1–18) vs. Figure 7(19–24)). Since EVs bearing each type of transmembrane scaffold were taken up by recipient cells, we conclude the integration of the scaffold protein and its GFP cargo to the EV membrane does not impact their ability to undergo internalization. Moreover, we envisage opportunities to fuse other protein cargo to the scaffold that may function as a therapeutic, for example, a functional enzyme for the treatment of a lysosomal storage disorder.

Unlike the tetraspanin-based transmembrane scaffolds, VSVG is a single-span transmembrane glycoprotein whose large ectodomain projects to the external environment of the EV. This ectodomain binds specifically to the low-density lipoprotein receptors (LDLRs) found on the surface of almost all cell types [55]. Interactions between VSVG and the receptor are known to lead to receptor-mediated endocytosis [56]. Armed with this knowledge, we propose the ectodomain of VSVG on engineered EVs is recognized by LDLRs on 293T cells, triggering their endocytosis, which may account for the increased levels of cellular uptake of EVs bearing VSVG compared to tetraspanins. To further validate that the VSVG scaffold increases the cellular uptake of modified EVs by its ectodomain, we conducted a quantitative flow cytometry analysis of cells treated with either VSVG-modified EVs, control (non-modified) EVs, or no EVs. After fluorescein labeling with the ExoGlow™ reagent, identical quantities (100 μg/mL) of VSVG-modified and non-modified control EVs were added to the culture medium of 293T cells and allowed to incubate for 24 h. Next, 293T cells were subjected to flow cytometry analysis to record the FITC intensity in individual cells. We found that the intensity of FITC fluorescence in control EVs (Figure 8A,B, blue curve + bar) was 30-times higher than the FITC intensity in cells that were not treated with EVs (Figure 8A,B, black curve + bar). In comparison, the FITC intensity in cells treated with VSVG-modified EVs was 180 times higher than the GFP-channel intensity in untreated cells and 6-fold higher than the uptake of control EVs. Thus, EVs integrating VSVG exhibit enhanced endocytosis-mediated uptake. Next, we conducted a dose-response study to determine the effective range of VSVG-modified EVs for intracellular delivery of fused molecular cargo. From the plot of the amount of VSVG-modified EVs taken up by cells versus the amount of EVs added to the medium (3.12, 6.25, 12.5, 25.0, and 50.0 μg/mL), it is evident that saturation occurs at an EV level of ~50 μg/mL (Figure 8C).

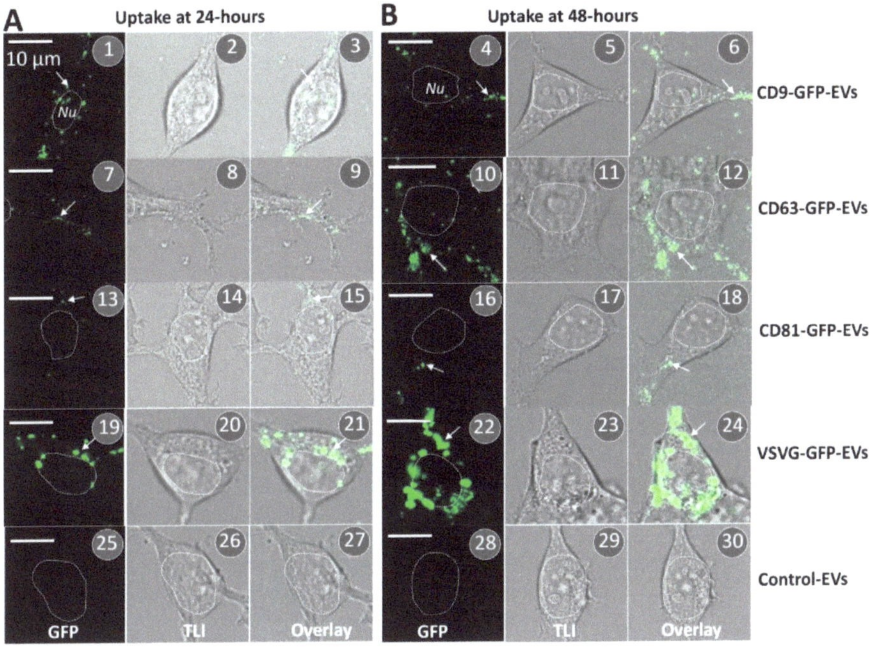

Figure 7. Cellular uptake of EVs modified by different transmembrane scaffolds. EVs prepared from the conditioned medium of transfected cells were added to the medium (30 μg EV proteins/mL) of the cultured 293T cells. Confocal images were recorded at 24 h (**A**) and 48 h (**B**) after the addition of CD9-GFP-modified EVs (**1–6**), CD63-GFP-modified EVs (**7–12**), CD81-GFP-modified EVs (**13–18**), VSVG-GFP-modified EVs (**19–24**), or non-modified controls (**25–30**). Arrows indicate internalized EVs. Scale bar, 10 μm.

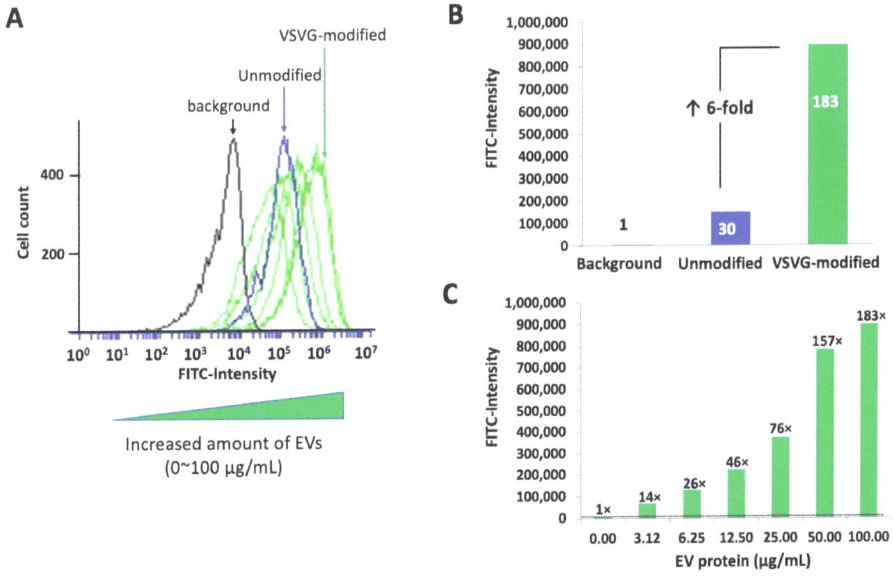

Figure 8. VSVG-GFP-modified EVs dramatically increase the cellular uptake by recipient cells. EVs prepared from the conditioned medium of either VSVG-GFP-modified cells or non-modified controls

were chemically stained by Exoflow before being added to the culture medium of human 293T cells. The cells were treated for 24 h with increased concentrations of EVs (3.12–100 EV protein/mL), then washed, collected, and subjected to flow cytometry analysis as described in Materials and Methods. The amount of EV uptake was analyzed and graphed with CFlow Plus software. (**A**) A dose-response curve of VSVG-modified EVs compared to the control. The cellular uptake of VSVG-modified EVs (green) dramatically increased (shift to the right) compared to the non-modified control (blue) at the same EV concentration (100 μg of protein/mL) and the background (black). (**B**) A bar-graph representation of the relative uptake efficiency of VSVG-GFP-modified (green) vs. non-modified control (blue) vs. the background (black). (**C**) A bar-graph representation of increasing cellular uptake of VSVG-modified EVs in a dose range of 0–100 μg EV protein/mL.

4. Discussion

The long-term goal of these studies is to optimize the design and engineering of EVs as living vehicles for the delivery of therapeutic biologics [44,57–59]. In particular, we aimed to characterize the properties of EVs harboring different molecular scaffolds that can be engineered for specific tissue targeting and uptake by recipient cells. In engineering EVs for clinical applications, it will be essential to establish how specific molecular scaffolds impact the physicochemical and biological phenotypes of modified EVs. Ultimately, this knowledge will help narrow the types of transmembrane scaffolds that are suitable for EV-based therapies [60,61]. In the present study, we employed state-of-the-art high-throughput, on-chip assays to examine how different scaffolds affect the engineering efficiency, physical properties, and biological responses of engineered EVs [39,41,60,62,63]. We found that the endogenous tetraspanin scaffolds (CD9, CD63, and CD81) were incorporated into distinct subpopulations of EVs, whereas VSVG was found equally in all EV subtypes. We also established that EVs bearing molecular scaffolds increased their average diameter compared to unmodified EVs. Although we do not know the exact mechanisms accounting for the increased size of the engineered EVs, we speculate the following three possibilities: (1) loading of GFP cargo into the lumen of engineered EVs may account for increased overall cargo loading, thus an increase in the size of engineered EVs; (2) incorporation of transmembrane scaffolds may alter the expression of endogenous surface markers; for example, the use of CD63-GFP scaffolds resulted in a decrease in the levels of CD81 (Figure 6). The change in membrane protein profile of engineered EVs may also lead to a change in EV sizes; (3) because all transmembrane scaffolds are glycoproteins, the incorporation of additional glycoproteins could increase the overall size of engineered EVs due to two mechanisms: the large and projecting ectodomain of VSVG and more sugars brought onto the outer surface by scaffold glycoproteins. We also showed EVs bearing the CD63 scaffold exhibit different expression levels of validated EV membrane biomarkers, specifically CD63 and CD81. We further demonstrated that EVs harboring VSVG were taken up by recipient cells to a greater degree (×3) compared to EVs bearing tetraspanins. Significantly, the exodomain of VSVG is known to interact with the LDL receptors on the outer membrane of most cells, where it is internalized by endocytosis. As such, this class of engineered EV may prove useful in delivering an internal cargo of functional enzymes to cells associated with LSDs [60]. In summary, our study has yielded important insights into the design and engineering of EVs with transmembrane scaffolds that may be important in the development of EVs for clinical applications.

Our study has painted a detailed picture of EV biogenesis by monitoring the subcellular localization and, finally, incorporation into different subtypes of EVs via different transmembrane scaffolds. It is well established that tetraspanins and VSVG initially enter the ER membrane after their synthesis but are quickly funneled into the plasma membrane (PM) via the route of the ER-Golgi-secretory vesicles [64,65]. After arriving at the PM, these transmembrane scaffolds may be differently sorted into distinctive microdomains, including tetraspanin-enriched microdomains or lipid rafts [66]. Existing evidence supports the hypothesis that CD9 and CD81 tend to interact with each other in certain domains that can bud off from the PM to become EVs [8,67,68]. In contrast, CD63 and VSVG may accumulate in other areas, where they undergo inward budding to form endosomes and then become intraluminal vesicles (pre-secreted exosomes) within MVBs [8]. This conjecture is supported by our image evidence that CD9 and CD81 are more enriched in the PM while CD63 and VSVG are localized mainly in endocytic compartments (Figure 2). Of note, CD9 is more often co-expressed on the same EVs as CD81 than with CD63 or VSVG, supporting the notion that CD9 and CD81 are more closely associated but divergent from CD63 and VSVG (Figure 6). Furthermore, the average size of EVs modified by CD9-GFP or CD81-GFP is slightly larger than that of those modified by CD63 or VSVG, suggesting different engineering effects on PM-derived and endosome-derived EVs (Table 2). Although molecular interactions among different tetraspanins are not mutually exclusive, overexpression of CD63-GFP appears to decrease the levels of $CD81^+$ EVs (Figure 6), supporting a stronger CD63-CD63 rather than CD63-CD81 association. Additionally, VSVG has a low co-localization rate with the tetraspanins (Table 1), indicating independent self-trimerization [69,70] rather than through interactions with tetraspanins.

The findings of our study may have important implications for the development of EV-based therapeutics using these transmembrane scaffolds. First, we find that both CD63 and VSVG preferentially modify endosome-derived EVs, which are commonly defined as exosomes. It has been established that exosomes are enriched with antigen-presenting molecules such as major histocompatibility complex I (MHC-1) and MHC-2 molecules [71,72]. Therefore, CD63 and VSVG may be more suitable for certain applications, such as the development of exosome-based nanovaccines to improve immune response [73–75]. VSVG has been used to present cancer and other antigens to elicit robust immune responses in animal models [62]. CD63 has also been proven to be a useful scaffold for the engineering of exosome-based vaccines [50,76]. On the other hand, CD9 and CD81 may be more suitable for targeted drug delivery because their modified EVs tend to become larger, allowing more drugs to be loaded into EVs [77]. Interestingly, CD9 has been successfully engineered to load cytosolic proteins or enzymes into EVs [78], while CD81 has also been mutated to gain the cancer-targeting ability for potential anticancer therapy [40].

Second, we found that individual scaffolds can only modify a small fraction of EVs, less than 50% even for the dominant subtypes of EVs (Table 1). Therefore, existing preparation protocols such as ultrafiltration, centrifugation, and even immunoaffinity capture may not be sufficient to isolate the modified EVs; hence, more robust and precise purification protocols must be individually developed. For instance, by adding a small affinity tag, such as 6xHistag, to the engineering scaffolds of CD63/VSVG, one may use nickel-coated magnetic beads to specifically capture the scaffold-modified EVs, therefore obtaining better enrichment of modified EVs. Such a specific purification method is especially important for the VSVG scaffold because VSVG-modified EVs normally lack the common surface markers (CD9, CD63, and CD81).

Third, we find that the VSVG viral scaffold may well preserve its intrinsic functions that are widely exploited, including the generation of VSVG-pseudotyped EVs for enhanced intracellular delivery via its ectodomain [41,42,56,79,80]. By the same principle, one may also use other viral glycoproteins to program EVs for tissue/cell-specific delivery. For example, spike protein from the COVID-19 coronavirus may render a tissue-specificity to epithelial/endothelial cells expressing receptor angiotensin-converting enzyme-2 receptors on their surface [81]. Lastly, we find the EVs may be vulnerable to some phenotypical alterations, including an increase in the size of modified EVs and changes in the levels of certain surface markers like CD63 and CD81 [82]. Although the biological significance of these changes remains to be determined, stringent quality control measures may be required to evaluate any changes in tissue tropics, pharmacological dynamics and kinetics, and biological activities before using them for clinical applications [83].

5. Conclusions

We have built up a set of genetic fusion reporters, which enable direct assessment of the engineering efficacy and biological impacts of various transmembrane scaffolds on modified EVs. Molecular imaging and single EV analysis reveal that these transmembrane scaffolds may have different abilities to engineer distinctive subtypes of EVs. Surface modification of EVs via various scaffolds may change physiochemical properties, such as vesicle size, surface protein marker expression, and membrane functioning via scaffold's ectodomain, of successfully modified EVs. Our findings may have important implications for the genetic engineering of EVs using transmembrane scaffolds.

Supplementary Materials: The following supporting information can be downloaded at: https://www.mdpi.com/article/10.3390/pharmaceutics14122564/s1, Table S1: Number of particles captured and measured in each subtype of EVs; Table S2: Increased sizes of EVs via various engineering scaffolds.

Author Contributions: Conceptualization, B.L.; Methodology, J.Z., A.B., D.D. and K.A.; Formal analysis, J.Z., A.B. and B.J.; Investigation, G.M.; Resources, B.L.; Data curation, J.Z., B.J. and K.A.; Writing—original draft, B.L.; Writing—review & editing, J.Z., A.B., D.D., G.M. and B.L.; Visualization, B.L.; Supervision, G.M. and B.L.; Project administration, J.Z. and B.L.; Funding acquisition, B.L. All authors have read and agreed to the published version of the manuscript.

Funding: This work was supported by funds from the School of Engineering at Santa Clara University and by the National Institute of General Medical Sciences of the National Institutes of Health under Award Number R15GM137449.

Acknowledgments: We thank Yan Jiang for kindly editing this manuscript. We also thank Clayton Deighan (NanoView Biosciences) for conducting on-chip experiments and data analysis. The content is the sole responsibility of the authors and does not necessarily represent the official views of the National Institutes of Health. Figures 1 and 3A were created with BioRender.com (accessed on 29 May 2021).

Conflicts of Interest: The authors declare no conflict of interest.

References

1. Gill, S.; Catchpole, R.; Forterre, P. Extracellular membrane vesicles in the three domains of life and beyond. *FEMS Microbiol. Rev.* **2019**, *43*, 273–303. [CrossRef] [PubMed]
2. Woith, E.; Fuhrmann, G.; Melzig, M.F. Extracellular Vesicles-Connecting Kingdoms. *Int. J. Mol. Sci.* **2019**, *20*, 5695. [CrossRef] [PubMed]
3. Yanez-Mo, M.; Siljander, P.R.; Andreu, Z.; Zavec, A.B.; Borras, F.E.; Buzas, E.I.; Buzas, K.; Casal, E.; Cappello, F.; Carvalho, J.; et al. Biological properties of extracellular vesicles and their physiological functions. *J. Extracell. Vesicles* **2015**, *4*, 27066. [CrossRef] [PubMed]
4. van Niel, G.; D'Angelo, G.; Raposo, G. Shedding light on the cell biology of extracellular vesicles. *Nat. Rev. Mol. Cell Biol.* **2018**, *19*, 213–228. [CrossRef] [PubMed]
5. Zhang, Y.; Liu, Y.; Liu, H.; Tang, W.H. Exosomes: Biogenesis, biologic function and clinical potential. *Cell Biosci.* **2019**, *9*, 19. [CrossRef]
6. Bordanaba-Florit, G.; Royo, F.; Kruglik, S.G.; Falcon-Perez, J.M. Using single-vesicle technologies to unravel the heterogeneity of extracellular vesicles. *Nat. Protoc.* **2021**, *16*, 3163–3185. [CrossRef]
7. Kowal, J.; Arras, G.; Colombo, M.; Jouve, M.; Morath, J.P.; Primdal-Bengtson, B.; Dingli, F.; Loew, D.; Tkach, M.; Thery, C. Proteomic comparison defines novel markers to characterize heterogeneous populations of extracellular vesicle subtypes. *Proc. Natl. Acad. Sci. USA* **2016**, *113*, E968–E977. [CrossRef]
8. Escola, J.M.; Kleijmeer, M.J.; Stoorvogel, W.; Griffith, J.M.; Yoshie, O.; Geuze, H.J. Selective enrichment of tetraspan proteins on the internal vesicles of multivesicular endosomes and on exosomes secreted by human B-lymphocytes. *J. Biol. Chem.* **1998**, *273*, 20121–20127. [CrossRef]
9. Simpson, R.J.; Kalra, H.; Mathivanan, S. ExoCarta as a resource for exosomal research. *J. Extracell. Vesicles* **2012**, *1*, 18374. [CrossRef]
10. Arraud, N.; Linares, R.; Tan, S.; Gounou, C.; Pasquet, J.M.; Mornet, S.; Brisson, A.R. Extracellular vesicles from blood plasma: Determination of their morphology, size, phenotype and concentration. *J. Thromb. Haemost.* **2014**, *12*, 614–627. [CrossRef]
11. Srinivasan, S.; Vannberg, F.O.; Dixon, J.B. Lymphatic transport of exosomes as a rapid route of information dissemination to the lymph node. *Sci. Rep.* **2016**, *6*, 24436. [CrossRef] [PubMed]

12. Asea, A.; Jean-Pierre, C.; Kaur, P.; Rao, P.; Linhares, I.M.; Skupski, D.; Witkin, S.S. Heat shock protein-containing exosomes in mid-trimester amniotic fluids. *J. Reprod. Immunol.* **2008**, *79*, 12–17. [CrossRef] [PubMed]
13. Zlotogorski-Hurvitz, A.; Dayan, D.; Chaushu, G.; Korvala, J.; Salo, T.; Sormunen, R.; Vered, M. Human saliva-derived exosomes: Comparing methods of isolation. *J. Histochem. Cytochem.* **2015**, *63*, 181–189. [CrossRef] [PubMed]
14. Cheruvanky, A.; Zhou, H.; Pisitkun, T.; Kopp, J.B.; Knepper, M.A.; Yuen, P.S.; Star, R.A. Rapid isolation of urinary exosomal biomarkers using a nanomembrane ultrafiltration concentrator. *Am. J. Physiol. Renal. Physiol.* **2007**, *292*, F1657–F1661. [CrossRef]
15. Adriano, B.; Cotto, N.M.; Chauhan, N.; Jaggi, M.; Chauhan, S.C.; Yallapu, M.M. Milk exosomes: Nature's abundant nanoplatform for theranostic applications. *Bioact. Mater.* **2021**, *6*, 2479–2490. [CrossRef]
16. Vojtech, L.; Woo, S.; Hughes, S.; Levy, C.; Ballweber, L.; Sauteraud, R.P.; Strobl, J.; Westerberg, K.; Gottardo, R.; Tewari, M.; et al. Exosomes in human semen carry a distinctive repertoire of small non-coding RNAs with potential regulatory functions. *Nucleic Acids Res.* **2014**, *42*, 7290–7304. [CrossRef]
17. Choi, D.S.; Kim, D.K.; Kim, Y.K.; Gho, Y.S. Proteomics, transcriptomics and lipidomics of exosomes and ectosomes. *Proteomics* **2013**, *13*, 1554–1571. [CrossRef]
18. Colombo, M.; Raposo, G.; Thery, C. Biogenesis, secretion, and intercellular interactions of exosomes and other extracellular vesicles. *Annu. Rev. Cell Dev. Biol.* **2014**, *30*, 255–289. [CrossRef]
19. Sung, B.H.; Ketova, T.; Hoshino, D.; Zijlstra, A.; Weaver, A.M. Directional cell movement through tissues is controlled by exosome secretion. *Nat. Commun.* **2015**, *6*, 7164. [CrossRef]
20. McGough, I.J.; Vincent, J.P. Exosomes in developmental signalling. *Development* **2016**, *143*, 2482–2493. [CrossRef]
21. Gutierrez-Vazquez, C.; Villarroya-Beltri, C.; Mittelbrunn, M.; Sanchez-Madrid, F. Transfer of extracellular vesicles during immune cell-cell interactions. *Immunol. Rev.* **2013**, *251*, 125–142. [CrossRef] [PubMed]
22. Raposo, G.; Nijman, H.W.; Stoorvogel, W.; Liejendekker, R.; Harding, C.V.; Melief, C.J.; Geuze, H.J. B lymphocytes secrete antigen-presenting vesicles. *J. Exp. Med.* **1996**, *183*, 1161–1172. [CrossRef] [PubMed]
23. Thery, C.; Ostrowski, M.; Segura, E. Membrane vesicles as conveyors of immune responses. *Nat. Rev. Immunol.* **2009**, *9*, 581–593. [CrossRef] [PubMed]
24. Beyer, C.; Pisetsky, D.S. The role of microparticles in the pathogenesis of rheumatic diseases. *Nat. Rev. Rheumatol.* **2010**, *6*, 21–29. [CrossRef] [PubMed]
25. Hassanpour, M.; Rezaie, J.; Nouri, M.; Panahi, Y. The role of extracellular vesicles in COVID-19 virus infection. *Infect. Genet. Evol.* **2020**, *85*, 104422. [CrossRef] [PubMed]
26. Hosseini, H.M.; Fooladi, A.A.; Nourani, M.R.; Ghanezadeh, F. The role of exosomes in infectious diseases. *Inflamm. Allergy Drug Targets* **2013**, *12*, 29–37. [CrossRef] [PubMed]
27. Melo, S.A.; Luecke, L.B.; Kahlert, C.; Fernandez, A.F.; Gammon, S.T.; Kaye, J.; LeBleu, V.S.; Mittendorf, E.A.; Weitz, J.; Rahbari, N.; et al. Glypican-1 identifies cancer exosomes and detects early pancreatic cancer. *Nature* **2015**, *523*, 177–182. [CrossRef]
28. Melo, S.A.; Sugimoto, H.; O'Connell, J.T.; Kato, N.; Villanueva, A.; Vidal, A.; Qiu, L.; Vitkin, E.; Perelman, L.T.; Melo, C.A.; et al. Cancer exosomes perform cell-independent microRNA biogenesis and promote tumorigenesis. *Cancer Cell* **2014**, *26*, 707–721. [CrossRef]
29. Peinado, H.; Aleckovic, M.; Lavotshkin, S.; Matei, I.; Costa-Silva, B.; Moreno-Bueno, G.; Hergueta-Redondo, M.; Williams, C.; Garcia-Santos, G.; Ghajar, C.; et al. Melanoma exosomes educate bone marrow progenitor cells toward a pro-metastatic phenotype through MET. *Nat. Med.* **2012**, *18*, 883–891. [CrossRef]
30. Askenase, P.W. Ancient Evolutionary Origin and Properties of Universally Produced Natural Exosomes Contribute to Their Therapeutic Superiority Compared to Artificial Nanoparticles. *Int. J. Mol. Sci.* **2021**, *22*, 1429. [CrossRef]
31. van der Pol, E.; Boing, A.N.; Harrison, P.; Sturk, A.; Nieuwland, R. Classification, functions, and clinical relevance of extracellular vesicles. *Pharmacol. Rev.* **2012**, *64*, 676–705. [CrossRef] [PubMed]
32. van der Koog, L.; Gandek, T.B.; Nagelkerke, A. Liposomes and Extracellular Vesicles as Drug Delivery Systems: A Comparison of Composition, Pharmacokinetics, and Functionalization. *Adv. Healthc. Mater.* **2022**, *11*, e2100639. [CrossRef] [PubMed]
33. Rufino-Ramos, D.; Lule, S.; Mahjoum, S.; Ughetto, S.; Cristopher Bragg, D.; Pereira de Almeida, L.; Breakefield, X.O.; Breyne, K. Using genetically modified extracellular vesicles as a non-invasive strategy to evaluate brain-specific cargo. *Biomaterials* **2022**, *281*, 121366. [CrossRef] [PubMed]
34. Cheng, L.; Hill, A.F. Therapeutically harnessing extracellular vesicles. *Nat. Rev. Drug Discov.* **2022**, *21*, 379–399. [CrossRef]
35. Vader, P.; Mol, E.A.; Pasterkamp, G.; Schiffelers, R.M. Extracellular vesicles for drug delivery. *Adv. Drug Deliv. Rev.* **2016**, *106*, 148–156. [CrossRef]
36. Burnouf, T.; Agrahari, V.; Agrahari, V. Extracellular Vesicles as Nanomedicine: Hopes And Hurdles In Clinical Translation. *Int. J. Nanomed.* **2019**, *14*, 8847–8859. [CrossRef]
37. Herrmann, I.K.; Wood, M.J.A.; Fuhrmann, G. Extracellular vesicles as a next-generation drug delivery platform. *Nat. Nanotechnol.* **2021**, *16*, 748–759. [CrossRef]
38. Garcia-Manrique, P.; Matos, M.; Gutierrez, G.; Pazos, C.; Blanco-Lopez, M.C. Therapeutic biomaterials based on extracellular vesicles: Classification of bio-engineering and mimetic preparation routes. *J. Extracell. Vesicles* **2018**, *7*, 1422676. [CrossRef]
39. Stickney, Z.; Losacco, J.; McDevitt, S.; Zhang, Z.; Lu, B. Development of exosome surface display technology in living human cells. *Biochem. Biophys. Res. Commun.* **2016**, *472*, 53–59. [CrossRef]

40. Vogt, S.; Bobbili, M.R.; Stadlmayr, G.; Stadlbauer, K.; Kjems, J.; Ruker, F.; Grillari, J.; Wozniak-Knopp, G. An engineered CD81-based combinatorial library for selecting recombinant binders to cell surface proteins: Laminin binding CD81 enhances cellular uptake of extracellular vesicles. *J. Extracell. Vesicles* **2021**, *10*, e12139. [CrossRef]
41. Meyer, C.; Losacco, J.; Stickney, Z.; Li, L.; Marriott, G.; Lu, B. Pseudotyping exosomes for enhanced protein delivery in mammalian cells. *Int. J. Nanomed.* **2017**, *12*, 3153–3170. [CrossRef] [PubMed]
42. Do, M.A.; Levy, D.; Brown, A.; Marriott, G.; Lu, B. Targeted delivery of lysosomal enzymes to the endocytic compartment in human cells using engineered extracellular vesicles. *Sci. Rep.* **2019**, *9*, 17274. [CrossRef] [PubMed]
43. El-Andaloussi, S.; Lee, Y.; Lakhal-Littleton, S.; Li, J.; Seow, Y.; Gardiner, C.; Alvarez-Erviti, L.; Sargent, I.L.; Wood, M.J. Exosome-mediated delivery of siRNA in vitro and in vivo. *Nat. Protoc.* **2012**, *7*, 2112–2126. [CrossRef] [PubMed]
44. Delcayre, A.; Estelles, A.; Sperinde, J.; Roulon, T.; Paz, P.; Aguilar, B.; Villanueva, J.; Khine, S.; Le Pecq, J.B. Exosome Display technology: Applications to the development of new diagnostics and therapeutics. *Blood Cells Mol. Dis.* **2005**, *35*, 158–168. [CrossRef] [PubMed]
45. Wang, J.H.; Forterre, A.V.; Zhao, J.; Frimannsson, D.O.; Delcayre, A.; Antes, T.J.; Efron, B.; Jeffrey, S.S.; Pegram, M.D.; Matin, A.C. Anti-HER2 scFv-Directed Extracellular Vesicle-Mediated mRNA-Based Gene Delivery Inhibits Growth of HER2-Positive Human Breast Tumor Xenografts by Prodrug Activation. *Mol. Cancer Ther.* **2018**, *17*, 1133–1142. [CrossRef]
46. Kooijmans, S.A.; Aleza, C.G.; Roffler, S.R.; van Solinge, W.W.; Vader, P.; Schiffelers, R.M. Display of GPI-anchored anti-EGFR nanobodies on extracellular vesicles promotes tumour cell targeting. *J. Extracell. Vesicles* **2016**, *5*, 31053. [CrossRef]
47. Saludes, J.P.; Morton, L.A.; Coulup, S.K.; Fiorini, Z.; Cook, B.M.; Beninson, L.; Chapman, E.R.; Fleshner, M.; Yin, H. Multivalency amplifies the selection and affinity of bradykinin-derived peptides for lipid nanovesicles. *Mol. Biosyst.* **2013**, *9*, 2005–2009. [CrossRef]
48. Levy, D.; Do, M.A.; Zhang, J.; Brown, A.; Lu, B. Orchestrating Extracellular Vesicle With Dual Reporters for Imaging and Capturing in Mammalian Cell Culture. *Front. Mol. Biosci.* **2021**, *8*, 680580. [CrossRef]
49. Levy, D.; Do, M.A.; Brown, A.; Asano, K.; Diebold, D.; Chen, H.; Zhang, J.; Lawler, B.; Lu, B. Genetic labeling of extracellular vesicles for studying biogenesis and uptake in living mammalian cells. *Methods Enzymol.* **2020**, *645*, 1–14. [CrossRef]
50. Curley, N.; Levy, D.; Do, M.A.; Brown, A.; Stickney, Z.; Marriott, G.; Lu, B. Sequential deletion of CD63 identifies topologically distinct scaffolds for surface engineering of exosomes in living human cells. *Nanoscale* **2020**, *12*, 12014–12026. [CrossRef]
51. Akers, J.C.; Gonda, D.; Kim, R.; Carter, B.S.; Chen, C.C. Biogenesis of extracellular vesicles (EV): Exosomes, microvesicles, retrovirus-like vesicles, and apoptotic bodies. *J. Neurooncol.* **2013**, *113*, 1–11. [CrossRef] [PubMed]
52. Teng, F.; Fussenegger, M. Shedding Light on Extracellular Vesicle Biogenesis and Bioengineering. *Adv. Sci.* **2020**, *8*, 2003505. [CrossRef] [PubMed]
53. Thery, C. Exosomes: Secreted vesicles and intercellular communications. *F1000 Biol. Rep.* **2021**, *3*, 15. [CrossRef] [PubMed]
54. Daaboul, G.G.; Gagni, P.; Benussi, L.; Bettotti, P.; Ciani, M.; Cretich, M.; Freedman, D.S.; Ghidoni, R.; Ozkumur, A.Y.; Piotto, C.; et al. Digital Detection of Exosomes by Interferometric Imaging. *Sci. Rep.* **2016**, *6*, 37246. [CrossRef] [PubMed]
55. Goldstein, J.L.; Brown, M.S.; Anderson, R.G.; Russell, D.W.; Schneider, W.J. Receptor-mediated endocytosis: Concepts emerging from the LDL receptor system. *Annu. Rev. Cell Biol.* **1985**, *1*, 1–39. [CrossRef] [PubMed]
56. Finkelshtein, D.; Werman, A.; Novick, D.; Barak, S.; Rubinstein, M. LDL receptor and its family members serve as the cellular receptors for vesicular stomatitis virus. *Proc. Natl. Acad. Sci. USA* **2013**, *110*, 7306–7311. [CrossRef]
57. Elsharkasy, O.M.; Nordin, J.Z.; Hagey, D.W.; de Jong, O.G.; Schiffelers, R.M.; Andaloussi, S.E.; Vader, P. Extracellular vesicles as drug delivery systems: Why and how? *Adv. Drug Deliv. Rev.* **2020**, *159*, 332–343. [CrossRef]
58. Alvarez-Erviti, L.; Seow, Y.; Yin, H.; Betts, C.; Lakhal, S.; Wood, M.J. Delivery of siRNA to the mouse brain by systemic injection of targeted exosomes. *Nat. Biotechnol.* **2011**, *29*, 341–345. [CrossRef]
59. Li, Z.; Zhou, X.; Wei, M.; Gao, X.; Zhao, L.; Shi, R.; Sun, W.; Duan, Y.; Yang, G.; Yuan, L. In Vitro and in Vivo RNA Inhibition by CD9-HuR Functionalized Exosomes Encapsulated with miRNA or CRISPR/dCas9. *Nano Lett.* **2019**, *19*, 19–28. [CrossRef]
60. Lu, B.; Ku, J.; Flojo, R.; Olson, C.; Bengford, D.; Marriott, G. Exosome- and extracellular vesicle-based approaches for the treatment of lysosomal storage disorders. *Adv. Drug Deliv. Rev.* **2022**, *188*, 114465. [CrossRef]
61. Silva, A.M.; Lazaro-Ibanez, E.; Gunnarsson, A.; Dhande, A.; Daaboul, G.; Peacock, B.; Osteikoetxea, X.; Salmond, N.; Friis, K.P.; Shatnyeva, O.; et al. Quantification of protein cargo loading into engineered extracellular vesicles at single-vesicle and single-molecule resolution. *J. Extracell. Vesicles* **2021**, *10*, e12130. [CrossRef] [PubMed]
62. Hu, K.; McKay, P.F.; Samnuan, K.; Najer, A.; Blakney, A.K.; Che, J.; O'Driscoll, G.; Cihova, M.; Stevens, M.M.; Shattock, R.J. Presentation of antigen on extracellular vesicles using transmembrane domains from viral glycoproteins for enhanced immunogenicity. *J. Extracell. Vesicles* **2022**, *11*, e12199. [CrossRef] [PubMed]
63. Segel, M.; Lash, B.; Song, J.; Ladha, A.; Liu, C.C.; Jin, X.; Mekhedov, S.L.; Macrae, R.K.; Koonin, E.V.; Zhang, F. Mammalian retrovirus-like protein PEG10 packages its own mRNA and can be pseudotyped for mRNA delivery. *Science* **2021**, *373*, 882–889. [CrossRef] [PubMed]
64. Hemler, M.E. Tetraspanin functions and associated microdomains. *Nat. Rev. Mol. Cell Biol.* **2005**, *6*, 801–811. [CrossRef]
65. Presley, J.F.; Cole, N.B.; Schroer, T.A.; Hirschberg, K.; Zaal, K.J.; Lippincott-Schwartz, J. ER-to-Golgi transport visualized in living cells. *Nature* **1997**, *389*, 81–85. [CrossRef]
66. Yanez-Mo, M.; Barreiro, O.; Gordon-Alonso, M.; Sala-Valdes, M.; Sanchez-Madrid, F. Tetraspanin-enriched microdomains: A functional unit in cell plasma membranes. *Trends Cell Biol.* **2009**, *19*, 434–446. [CrossRef]

67. Abache, T.; Le Naour, F.; Planchon, S.; Harper, F.; Boucheix, C.; Rubinstein, E. The transferrin receptor and the tetraspanin web molecules CD9, CD81, and CD9P-1 are differentially sorted into exosomes after TPA treatment of K562 cells. *J. Cell Biochem.* **2007**, *102*, 650–664. [CrossRef]
68. Fitter, S.; Sincock, P.M.; Jolliffe, C.N.; Ashman, L.K. Transmembrane 4 superfamily protein CD151 (PETA-3) associates with beta 1 and alpha IIb beta 3 integrins in haemopoietic cell lines and modulates cell-cell adhesion. *Biochem. J.* **1999**, *338 Pt 1*, 61–70. [CrossRef]
69. Nikolic, J.; Belot, L.; Raux, H.; Legrand, P.; Gaudin, Y.; Albertini, A.A. Structural basis for the recognition of LDL-receptor family members by VSV glycoprotein. *Nat. Commun.* **2018**, *9*, 1029. [CrossRef]
70. Dalton, K.P.; Rose, J.K. Vesicular stomatitis virus glycoprotein containing the entire green fluorescent protein on its cytoplasmic domain is incorporated efficiently into virus particles. *Virology* **2001**, *279*, 414–421. [CrossRef]
71. Morelli, A.E.; Larregina, A.T.; Shufesky, W.J.; Sullivan, M.L.; Stolz, D.B.; Papworth, G.D.; Zahorchak, A.F.; Logar, A.J.; Wang, Z.; Watkins, S.C.; et al. Endocytosis, intracellular sorting, and processing of exosomes by dendritic cells. *Blood* **2004**, *104*, 3257–3266. [CrossRef] [PubMed]
72. Kowal, J.; Tkach, M.; Thery, C. Biogenesis and secretion of exosomes. *Curr. Opin. Cell Biol.* **2014**, *29*, 116–125. [CrossRef] [PubMed]
73. Marsac, D.; Loirat, D.; Petit, C.; Schwartz, O.; Michel, M.L. Enhanced presentation of major histocompatibility complex class I-restricted human immunodeficiency virus type 1 (HIV-1) Gag-specific epitopes after DNA immunization with vectors coding for vesicular stomatitis virus glycoprotein-pseudotyped HIV-1 Gag particles. *J. Virol.* **2002**, *76*, 7544–7553. [CrossRef] [PubMed]
74. Temchura, V.V.; Tenbusch, M.; Nchinda, G.; Nabi, G.; Tippler, B.; Zelenyuk, M.; Wildner, O.; Uberla, K.; Kuate, S. Enhancement of immunostimulatory properties of exosomal vaccines by incorporation of fusion-competent G protein of vesicular stomatitis virus. *Vaccine* **2008**, *26*, 3662–3672. [CrossRef] [PubMed]
75. Kuate, S.; Cinatl, J.; Doerr, H.W.; Uberla, K. Exosomal vaccines containing the S protein of the SARS coronavirus induce high levels of neutralizing antibodies. *Virology* **2007**, *362*, 26–37. [CrossRef] [PubMed]
76. Kanuma, T.; Yamamoto, T.; Kobiyama, K.; Moriishi, E.; Masuta, Y.; Kusakabe, T.; Ozasa, K.; Kuroda, E.; Jounai, N.; Ishii, K.J. CD63-Mediated Antigen Delivery into Extracellular Vesicles via DNA Vaccination Results in Robust CD8(+) T Cell Responses. *J. Immunol.* **2017**, *198*, 4707–4715. [CrossRef]
77. Mathieu, M.; Nevo, N.; Jouve, M.; Valenzuela, J.I.; Maurin, M.; Verweij, F.J.; Palmulli, R.; Lankar, D.; Dingli, F.; Loew, D.; et al. Specificities of exosome versus small ectosome secretion revealed by live intracellular tracking of CD63 and CD9. *Nat. Commun.* **2021**, *12*, 4389. [CrossRef]
78. Yim, N.; Ryu, S.W.; Choi, K.; Lee, K.R.; Lee, S.; Choi, H.; Kim, J.; Shaker, M.R.; Sun, W.; Park, J.H.; et al. Exosome engineering for efficient intracellular delivery of soluble proteins using optically reversible protein-protein interaction module. *Nat. Commun.* **2016**, *7*, 12277. [CrossRef]
79. Yee, J.K.; Friedmann, T.; Burns, J.C. Generation of high-titer pseudotyped retroviral vectors with very broad host range. *Methods Cell Biol.* **1994**, *43 Pt A*, 99–112. [CrossRef]
80. Burns, J.C.; Friedmann, T.; Driever, W.; Burrascano, M.; Yee, J.K. Vesicular stomatitis virus G glycoprotein pseudotyped retroviral vectors: Concentration to very high titer and efficient gene transfer into mammalian and nonmammalian cells. *Proc. Natl. Acad. Sci. USA* **1993**, *90*, 8033–8037. [CrossRef]
81. Liu, Z.; Xiao, X.; Wei, X.; Li, J.; Yang, J.; Tan, H.; Zhu, J.; Zhang, Q.; Wu, J.; Liu, L. Composition and divergence of coronavirus spike proteins and host ACE2 receptors predict potential intermediate hosts of SARS-CoV-2. *J. Med. Virol.* **2020**, *92*, 595–601. [CrossRef] [PubMed]
82. Hemler, M.E. Targeting of tetraspanin proteins—potential benefits and strategies. *Nat. Rev. Drug Discov.* **2008**, *7*, 747–758. [CrossRef] [PubMed]
83. Hassuna, N.; Monk, P.N.; Moseley, G.W.; Partridge, L.J. Strategies for targeting tetraspanin proteins: Potential therapeutic applications in microbial infections. *BioDrugs* **2009**, *23*, 341–359. [CrossRef] [PubMed]

pharmaceutics

MDPI

Article

Doxorubicin Loading into Milk and Mesenchymal Stem Cells' Extracellular Vesicles as Drug Delivery Vehicles

Anindya Mukhopadhya [1,2], Dimitrios Tsiapalis [1,2], Niamh McNamee [1,2,3], Brian Talbot [1] and Lorraine O'Driscoll [1,2,3,*]

1 School of Pharmacy and Pharmaceutical Sciences, Panoz Institute, Trinity College Dublin, D02 PN40 Dublin, Ireland
2 Trinity Biomedical Sciences Institute, Trinity College Dublin, D02 R590 Dublin, Ireland
3 Trinity St. James's Cancer Institute, D08 W9RT Dublin, Ireland
* Correspondence: lodrisc@tcd.ie

Abstract: Extracellular vesicles (EVs) have great potential as drug delivery vehicles. While mesenchymal/stromal stem cell (MSC) conditioned medium (CM) and milk are potentially safe and scalable sources of EVs for this purpose, the suitability of MSC EVs and milk EVs as drug delivery vehicles has never been compared and so was the objective of this study. Here EVs were separated from MSCs' CM and from milk and were characterised by nanoparticle tracking analysis, transmission electron microscopy, total protein quantification, and immunoblotting. An anti-cancer chemotherapeutic drug, doxorubicin (Dox), was then loaded into the EVs by one of three methods: by passive loading or by active loading by either electroporation or sonication. Dox-loaded EVs were analysed by fluorescence spectrophotometer, high-performance liquid chromatography (HPLC), and imaging flow cytometer (IFCM). Our study showed that EVs were successfully separated from the milk and MSC CM, with significantly ($p < 0.001$) higher yields of milk EVs/mL starting material compared to MSC EVs/mL of starting material. Using a fixed amount of EVs for each comparison, electroporation achieved significantly more Dox loading when compared to passive loading ($p < 0.01$). Indeed, of 250 µg of Dox made available for loading, electroporation resulted in 90.1 ± 12 µg of Dox loading into MSC EVs and 68.0 ± 10 µg of Dox loading into milk EVs, as analysed by HPLC. Interestingly, compared to the passive loading and electroporation approach, after sonication significantly fewer CD9+ EVs/mL ($p < 0.001$) and CD63+ EVs/mL ($p < 0.001$) existed, as determined by IFCM. This observation indicates that sonication, in particular, may have detrimental effects on EVs. In conclusion, EVs can be successfully separated from both MSC CM and milk, with milk being a particularly rich source. Of the three methods tested, electroporation appears to be superior for achieving maximum drug loading while not causing damage to EV surface proteins.

Keywords: drug-loading; milk; mesenchymal/stromal stem cells; extracellular vesicles; doxorubicin; electroporation; sonication; HPLC; imaging flow cytometry

Citation: Mukhopadhya, A.; Tsiapalis, D.; McNamee, N.; Talbot, B.; O'Driscoll, L. Doxorubicin Loading into Milk and Mesenchymal Stem Cells' Extracellular Vesicles as Drug Delivery Vehicles. *Pharmaceutics* **2023**, *15*, 718. https://doi.org/10.3390/pharmaceutics15030718

Academic Editors: Yong Chen and Hugo Agostinho Machado Fernandes

Received: 10 November 2022
Revised: 13 January 2023
Accepted: 15 February 2023
Published: 21 February 2023

1. Introduction

There is a need for the development and head-to-head comparison of sources of potentially reliable, cost-effective, scalable, and easy-to-produce vehicles for the delivery of therapeutics, in addition to options such as liposomes [1,2]. The importance of this is exemplified by the fact that liposomes have been associated with adverse influences such as immunogenicity and uncontrolled toxicity, in several liposome-based drug delivery studies [3–5].

Extracellular vesicles (EVs) from various cells and biological fluids (i.e., plasma and milk) have been proposed as an ideal, nature-derived, drug-delivery vehicle [6–8]. The term EVs refers to membrane-surrounded vesicles released from cells that may be engaged in cell-to-cell communication [9]. Desirable characteristics of EVs as drug delivery carriers include their intrinsic ability to cross biological barriers including the blood-brain barrier, non-immunogenicity, and non-toxicity properties [6,10]. Moreover, EVs have been reported to demonstrate superior targeting capabilities to liposomes [8]. A proof-of-principle study from our group showed that EVs can be harnessed as anti-cancer therapeutic delivery vehicles [11]. Of course, due to the inherent other unwanted cargo in cancer cell EVs, these would not be suitable to bring forward toward clinical utility.

Two potential sources of safe EVs as vehicles for pharmaceutical agents are EVs from mesenchymal/stromal stem cells (MSCs) [12–16] and EVs from milk [17–19]. In relation to MSC EVs, a protocol was deemed suitable for separating EVs from the conditioned medium (CM) of MSC for subsequent successful administration, as therapy in the clinic in their natural (non-loaded) form has been reported [20]. For milk EVs, we recently developed an effective protocol to separate relatively pure EVs from milk, which involved the removal of caseins, which are highly abundant in milk and overlap in size with EVs [21,22].

Furthermore, both active and passive drug-loading approaches have been established to load therapeutic molecules into EVs, as reviewed by Mehryab et al. [7]. However, the is a lack of direct comparative studies of such loading approaches for EVs from different sources as delivery vehicles to help select the optimal processes to bring forward.

Hence, the overall aim of this study (Figure 1) was to collect and characterise MSC EVs and milk EVs and compare the success of their using a passive loading approach and two active loading approaches, i.e., electroporation versus sonication loading. The anti-cancer drug doxorubicin (Dox) was chosen as a cargo of interest. In this study, we focused on investigating the loading of Dox into EVs as well as evaluating the effects of loading approaches on key biological aspects of EVs.

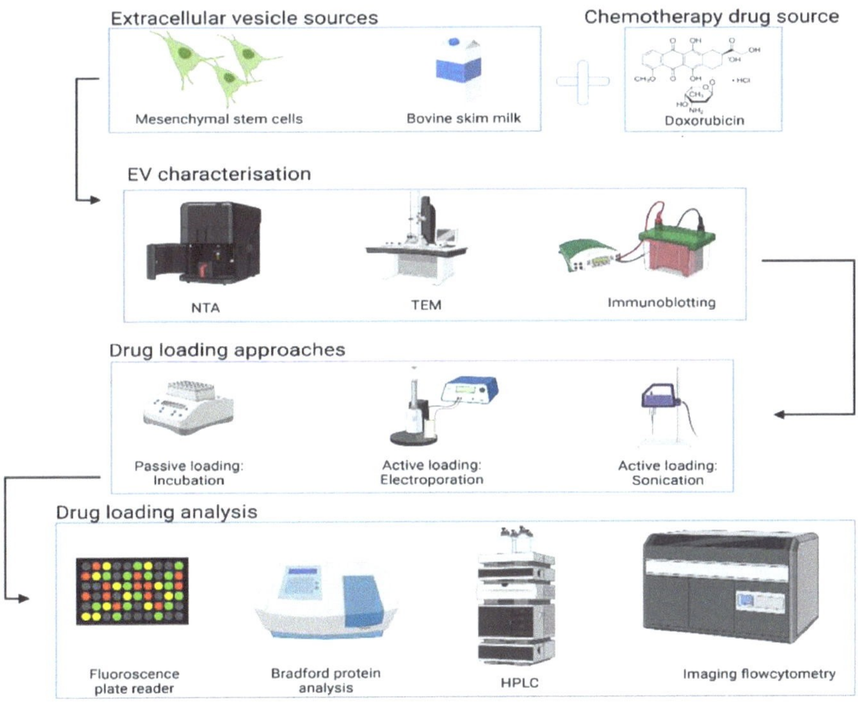

Figure 1. Illustrative summary of this comparative study. EVs were separated from MSCs and milk, characterised, and loaded with Dox by either passive loading (incubation) or active loading (electroporation or sonication). Both Dox loading successes and potential negative effects of loading on EVs (assessed for total protein as a surrogate and for established EVs surface proteins) were evaluated.

2. Materials and Methods

2.1. EVs Separation Methods

MSC EVs separation: Bone marrow MSCs (Stemcell Technologies, Cambridge, UK) were cultured in low glucose Dulbecco's modified Eagle medium (DMEM) (Sigma-Aldrich, Wicklow, Ireland) supplemented with 1% L-glutamine (Sigma-Aldrich, Wicklow, Ireland), 1% penicillin-streptomycin (Sigma-Aldrich, Wicklow, Ireland), 5 IU/mL heparin (Sigma-Aldrich, Wicklow, Ireland), and 10% human platelet lysate (hPL; Stemcell Technologies, Cambridge, UK) and maintained at 37 °C in a humidified atmosphere with 5% CO_2. The medium was changed every 3–4 days. At passage 6 and approximately 70% confluency, MSCs were washed with phosphate-buffered saline (PBS, Sigma-Aldrich, Wicklow, Ireland) and changed to a medium containing EVs-depleted FBS. After 48 h, a conditioned medium (CM) was collected. Any floating cells that remained in the medium were eliminated from the CM (100 mL) by centrifugation at 2000× *g* for 10 min. To remove cellular debris, supernatants were centrifuged at 10,000× *g* for 45 min at 4 °C in a Sorvall™ ST 8 small benchtop centrifuge using an HIGHConic™ III fixed angle rotor (Thermo Fisher Scientific, Dublin, Ireland), followed by filtration using 0.2-μm pore filters (Fisher Scientific, Dublin, Ireland). Next, EVs were separated using the polyethylene glycol 6000 (PEG) precipitation protocol, as previously described [20], with a modified centrifugation step, i.e., ultracentrifugation was performed at 100,000× *g* for 91 min using a Ti70 rotor in Optima XPN-100 Ultracentrifuge (Beckman Coulter, Brea, CA, USA) at 4 °C. MSC-EVs and preparations were resuspended in 500 μL of 10 mM Hepes/0.9% NaCl (Thermo Fisher Scientific, Dublin, Ireland). The EVs samples were stored at −80 °C until further use.

Milk EVs separation: commercially available bovine skim milk samples were used for milk EV separation using a protocol that we developed recently [21,22]. Briefly, caseins, the major EVs contaminant proteins present in milk were removed from the milk samples by isoelectric precipitation. For this, the pH was dropped to 4.6 using 6N HCl and the samples were then centrifuged at 8000× *g* at 20 °C for 30 min. Clear whey (2.33 mL) was used for density gradient ultracentrifugation following the bottom-up technique using Optiprep iodixanol solution (60%). Ultracentrifugation was performed using an SW Type 32.1 Ti rotor in Optima XPN-100 Ultracentrifuge (Beckman Coulter, Brea, CA, USA) at 186,000× *g* for 18 h at 4 °C. Pooled fractions (1.05–1.20 g/mL) were washed twice in sterile PBS, followed by 120,000× *g* for 2 h at 4 °C. The pellet was resuspended in 500 μL sterile PBS and EVs samples were stored at −80 °C until further use.

2.2. Fundamental Characterisation of EVs

For the fundamental characterisation of EVs separated from milk and MSCs, Bradford assay, nanoparticle tracking analysis (NTA), transmission electron microscopy (TEM) and immunoblotting were performed.

2.2.1. Bradford Assay for Protein Quantification

Bradford assay was performed to determine the amount of total protein in samples using Bio-Rad Protein Assay Dye Reagent Concentrate (Bio-Rad Laboratories, Watford, UK, Cat #500-0006).

2.2.2. Nanoparticle Tracking Analysis

The particle concentration and sizes were estimated using NanoSight NS300 (Malvern Instruments Ltd., Malvern, UK). Milk EVs and MSC EVs samples were automatically injected into the NTA system under constant flow conditions (flow rate = 50); videos of the particles in motion were recorded and analysed using NTA 3.1.54 software.

2.2.3. Transmission Electron Microscopy

Samples were prepared for transmission electron microscopy (TEM) analysis following the previously published protocol [23]. Specifically, 5 μL of the sample was suspended in 5 μL of 0.22 μm-filtered PBS and placed onto carbon-coated grids (Ted-Pella B 300M, Mason

Technology Ltd., Dublin, Ireland Cat. #: 01813-F) for 10 min at room temperature before fixing with 4% glutaraldehyde (Sigma-Aldrich, Wicklow, Ireland) and contrasting with 2% phosphotungstic acid (Sigma-Aldrich, Wicklow, Ireland). The grids were examined at 100 kV using a JEOL JEM-2100 TEM (JOEL, Peabody, MA, USA), as we previously described [24].

2.2.4. Immunoblotting

Immunoblotting was performed as previously described [24]. MSC EVs and milk EVs were lysed using SDS lysis buffer (250 nM Tris-HCL, pH 7.4; 2.5% SDS); cell lysates from MSCs and Hs578Ts(i)8 were used as a positive control for the proteins being analysed, respectively. A quantity of 20 µg of EVs or cell lysates was resolved on 10% SDS gels (Bio-Rad Laboratories, Watford, UK) and the protein was transferred onto PVDF membranes (Bio-Rad Laboratories, Watford, UK, Cat. #1620177). Blots were blocked with 5% (*w*/*v*) BSA in PBS containing 0.1% Tween-20 and incubated overnight at 4 °C with primary antibodies to TSG101 (1:1000; Abcam, Cambridge, UK, Cat. # ab30871), CD63 (1:500; Abcam, Cat. #: ab68418), actinin-4 (1:1000, Abcam, Cat. #: ab108198), calnexin (1:1000, Abcam, Cat. #: ab133615), syntenin-1 (1:1000, Abcam, Cat. #: ab133267), and CD9 (1:1000, Abcam, Cat. #: ab92726). Secondary antibodies used were anti-mouse (1:1000 in 5% BSA/PBS-T, Cell Signalling, Cat. #: 7076) or anti-rabbit (1:1000 in 5% BSA/PBS-T, Cell Signalling, Cat. #: 7-74). SuperSignal West Femto Chemiluminescent Substrate Kit (Fisher Scientific, Cat. # 11859290) was used for detection, imaging was performed using an automated Chemidoc exposure system (Bio-Rad Laboratories, Watford, UK).

2.3. Doxorubicin Loading into EVs

2.3.1. Passive Loading

A total of 250 µg of doxorubicin hydrochloride (Dox) (Sigma-Aldrich, Wicklow, Ireland) was added to 125 µg of MSC EVs or milk EVs, and the Dox-EVs mix was incubated on a thermo-mixer at 37 °C for 2 h.

2.3.2. Active Loading

Two different active loading approaches were performed, as described below:

(i) Electroporation: The electroporation of MSC EVs and milk EVs to load Dox was performed using a Neon™ Transfection System (Thermo Fisher Scientific, Dublin, Ireland). A total of 3 mL of Electrolytic buffer E was added to Neon™ tube and fixed to the tube stand. A total of 250 µg of Dox was mixed with 125 µg of MSC EVs or milk EVs and placed on ice. A 100 µL Neon™ Tip was attached to the Neon™ pipette and 100 µL of EV-Dox mix was pipetted up, the pipette was fixed to the Neon™ pipette station and electroporation protocol was performed using the program set on the Neon™ device at 1500 volts. The electroporated sample was collected in a fresh tube, and equal volume of Resuspension buffer R was added and incubated at 37 °C for 1 h for recovery of the EVs membrane.

(ii) Sonication: The sonication procedure was performed using a microson ultrasonic cell disruptor with a 0.25 tip (Misonix Inc., New York, NY, USA) with the following settings: 20% amplitude, and 6 cycles of 30 s on/off for 4 min with a 2 min cooling period between each cycle. The sonicated samples were incubated at 37 °C for 1 h to allow for recovery of the EVs membrane.

Following the loading step, unbound Dox was removed by washing the loaded EVs using a 300 kDa filter (Nanosep, Pall Biotech, Crosshaven, Ireland).

2.4. Fluorescence Analysis of Doxorubicin

The percentage of Dox made available that was subsequently successfully loaded in EVs was analysed by measuring the intrinsic fluorescence of doxorubicin using a fluorescence plate reader (Spectra Max Gemini System) with excitation and emission wavelengths of 485 and 535 nm, respectively. A standard curve of doxorubicin was used to interpolate unknown quantities of Dox.

2.5. High-Performance Liquid Chromatography Analysis

To evaluate Dox loading, high-performance liquid chromatography (HPLC) analysis was performed using the Waters Alliance HPLC system (Waters Corporation, Milford, MA, USA). An amount of 20 µL of lysed or non-lysed Dox-loaded milk EVs and MSC EVs samples were injected and run on a C18 column (Thermo Fisher Scientific, Dublin, Ireland) using a mobile phase of acetonitrile: water (pH 3) at a ratio of 70:30 (v/v) at a flow rate of 1 mL/min at 30 °C. Absorbance was measured at 227 nm to monitor the elution of Dox.

2.6. Imaging Flow Cytometry Analysis

The imaging flow cytometry (IFCM) analysis of Dox loaded was performed as previously described [21]. The specific antibodies used in this study were anti-CD63 conjugated with Fluorescein isothiocyanate (FITC) CD63-FITC, 1:150, Cat. #:353006, Biolegend, San Diego, CA, USA); CD9-PE (1:1500, Cat. #: 312106, Biolegend, San Diego, CA, USA); and CD81-PE-Cy7 (1:150, Cat. #: 349,512 Biolegend, San Diego, CA, USA). EVs were incubated with the antibodies for 45 min at RT in the dark and washed using a 300 kDa filter (Nanosep, Cat. #: 516-8531). Samples were resuspended in 50 µL IFCM buffer and acquired within 2 h on the ImageStream X Mk II imaging flow cytometer (Amnis/Luminex, Seattle, USA) at 60x magnification and low flow rate and EVs-free IFCM buffer, unstained EVs, single-stained controls, and fluorescence minus one (FMO) controls were run in parallel. EVs were gated as SSC-low vs. fluorescence, then as non-detectable brightfield (fluorescence vs. Raw Max Pixel Brightfield channel); gated EVs were confirmed in the IDEAS Image Gallery. Data analysis was performed using IDEAS software v6.2 (Amnis/Luminex, Seattle, WA, USA).

2.7. Data Analysis

For all experiments, data are presented as mean ± SEM. Tests for significant differences between the groups were performed using a t test or one-way ANOVA with multiple comparisons using Graph Pad Prism 9 software. A value of $p < 0.05$ was considered statistically significant.

3. Results and Discussion

3.1. MSC EVs and Milk EVs Separation and Characterisation

EVs were successfully separated from MSC CM and milk and characterised by NTA, TEM, and immunoblotting analysis. As presented in Supplementary Figure S1, the complete removal of contaminant milk protein, casein, was confirmed by comparing the same with untreated milk EV samples by polyacrylamide gel electrophoresis. The size and concentration of EVs particles obtained from MSC and milk are presented in Figure 2a. As estimated by NTA, the sizes of MSC EVs/particles (mean: 114.6 ± 2.7 nm and mode: 92.8 ± 10.8 nm) were smaller compared to milk EVs particles (mean: 169.3 ± 2.8 nm and mode: 146.8 ± 2.8 nm). The yield of EVs from MSC CM ($6.22 \times 10^8 \pm 4.46 \times 10^7$ particles/mL of starting material) was significantly lower ($p < 0.001$) than milk ($2.06 \times 10^{10} \pm 1.04 \times 10^9$ particles/mL of starting material). Generally, the use of mammalian cell cultures including MSCs to scale up EVs yield remains challenging for many reasons including specialised equipment, costs, maintaining the MSC phenotype, etc. Based on this comparison, the alternative use of milk as an EVs source would seem to be advantageous due to milk's easy accessibility, cost-effectiveness, and scalability potential. Of course, not only the source of EVs needs to be considered, but also the EVs' collection method plays a role in the yield and purity of EVs. One EVs collection method is not optimal for all biofluids, each has its own complex matrix. Therefore, although MSC CM resulted in fewer EVs/mL in this specific comparison, given that MSC EVs have some reported endogenous inflammation supressing/immune-modulatory capabilities, in instances where these additional beneficial characteristics might be considered useful then MSC seeding densities could potentially be scaled up to produce greater EVs yield/mL of CM. We would suggest, therefore, that based on yield per mL of starting material, MSC EVs should not be ruled out. Furthermore, TEM analysis of EVs samples showed that intact EVs-like structures were observed in both MSC EVs and milk EVs samples (Figure 2b), suggesting that, based on these fundamental characteristics, both MSC EVs and milk EVs were suitable to process further in their comparison as potential delivery vehicles.

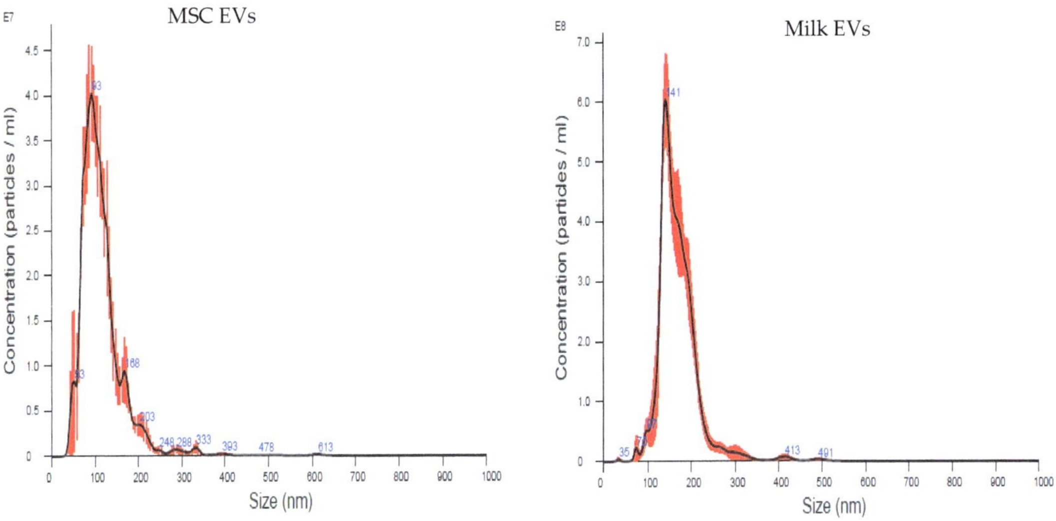

(**a**) NTA analysis

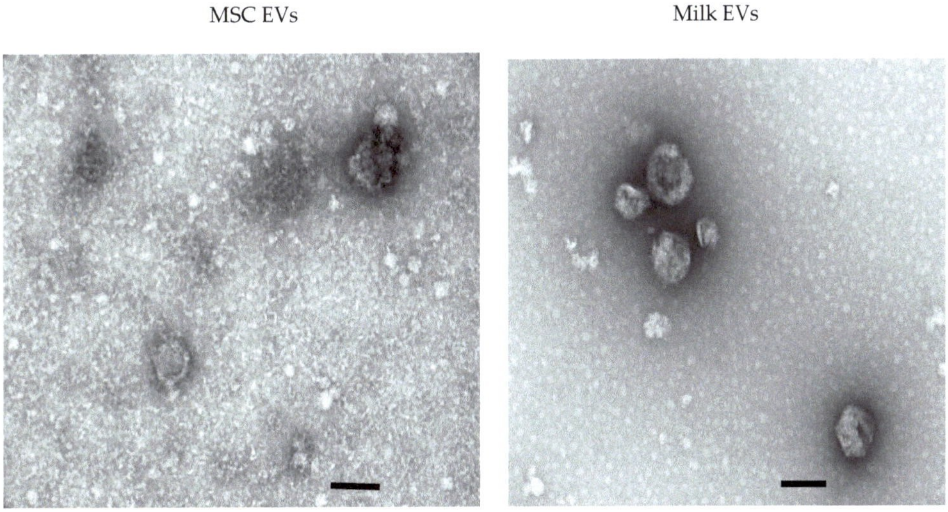

(**b**) TEM analysis

Figure 2. *Cont.*

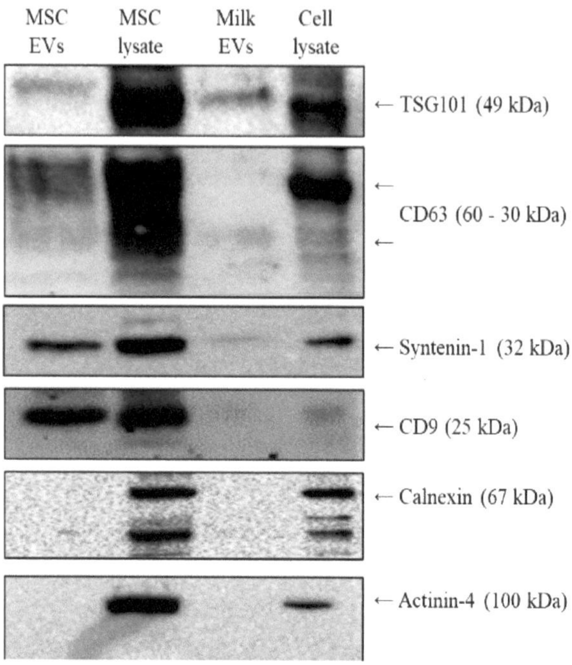

(**c**) Immunoblotting analysis

Figure 2. Fundamental characterisation of MSC EVs and milk EVs. MSC EVs and milk EVs (**a**) size distribution estimates obtained by NTA analysis and generated using NTA 3.1.54 software. (**b**) Representative TEM images (scale bar = 100 nm). (**c**) Immunoblots (using 20 μg of EVs lysates or cell lysates) for TSG101, CD63, syntenin-1, CD9, calnexin, and actinin-4.

As an additional characterisation step, in keeping with MISEV2018 guidelines, four proteins considered to be positive markers for EV populations and two proteins considered to be negative markers for EV populations were analysed by immunoblotting. Cell lysate from the Hs578Ts(i)8 human cell line was included in all gels as a positive control [21]. As presented in Figure 2c, both MSC EVs and milk EVs were positive for TSG101, CD63, syntenin-1, and CD9, whereas no signals were obtained for the negative markers actinin-4 and calnexin.

Therefore, the successful separation of intact EVs from MSC and milk was confirmed using the characterisation methodologies.

3.2. Comparison of Doxorubicin Retention and Protein Analysis Post-Drug Loading

Having successfully separated EVs from MSC CM and milk, 250 μg of the chemotherapeutic drug, Dox, was added to EVs (125 μg) from each source for loading by either passive loading or by either method of active loading (Figure 1). The apparent Dox loading achieved, i.e., the percentage of Dox that was made available with a fixed amount of EVs and that remained after removing extraneous Dox by rounds of washing is presented in Figure 3a. The electroporation approach apparently resulted in the most successful Dox loading, when compared to passive loading ($p < 0.01$) for both MSC EVs (achieving 86.4%) and milk EVs (achieving 80%). Passive loading of MSC EVs (47.2% achieved) and milk EVs (38% achieved) was also associated with significantly ($p < 0.05$) lower Dox loading capacity when compared to sonication (MSC EVs (75% achieved) and milk EVs (64% achieved) (Figure 3a). Using total protein quantities as a surrogate for the EVs post-load of those from the two sources and with each of the three methods, total protein quantities did not differ significantly from the amounts made available to the drug (Figure 3b). This indicated no substantial overall loss of EVs with any loading method.

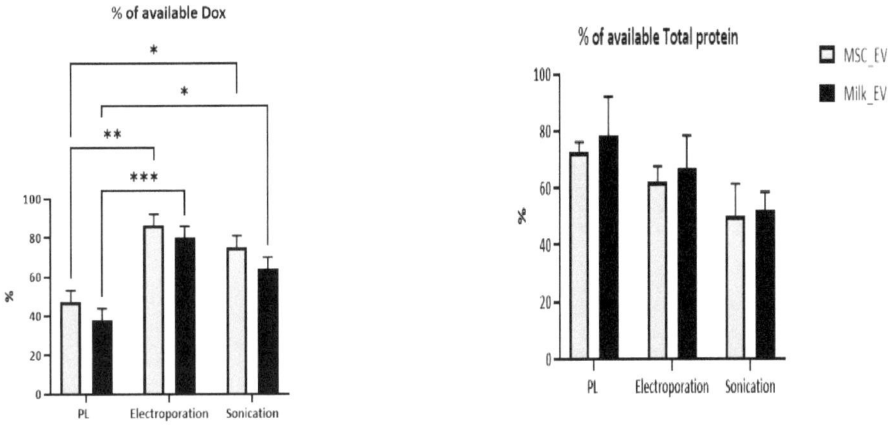

(a) (b)

Figure 3. (**a**) Percentage of Dox that was made available and that was apparently loaded into the MSC EVs or milk Evs following passive loading (PL), active loading by electroporation (ALE), or active loading by sonication (ALS). (**b**) Percentage of total protein remaining post-loading by PL, ALE, and ALS, where the total protein was used as a surrogate for Evs quantities. Results are mean from $n > 3 \pm$ SEM biological repeat experiments. A 2-way Anova analysis was performed; * represents p value < 0.05, ** $p < 0.01$, and *** $p < 0.001$.

Interestingly, in previous studies where Dox was loaded into milk EVs, 21% of encapsulation of the available drug was achieved by passive loading (Li et al. [25])and 13.4% loading via a conjugation method (Zhang et al. [26]). Crucially, neither Li et al. [25] nor Zhang et al. [26] reported the removal of the predominant milk proteins before the collection of EVs. This is particularly important as casein aggregates are abundant in the milk [27] and are of a size range overlapping with EVs [21]. Hence, their presence may lead to some Dox being caught up in these protein aggregates and so may explain the lower amount of Dox loading into EVs in those studies. In contrast, our optimised EVs separation protocol ensured maximum removal of casein aggregates [22], resulting in relatively high quantities of pure milk EVs available for loading. In the case of Dox loading to MSC EVs by electroporation, Gomari et al. [28] and Bagheri et al. [29] reported only 47% and 13% success, respectively. In contrast, using with a similar electroporation approach, we achieved 86.4% success. It has been reported that, in general, low purity and low yields of EVs are the major limitations for use of EVs in drug delivery [30,31]; therefore, our maximising purity by removing caseins seem to be a positive step in this regard.

Overall, when the results of Dox loading success achieved in the context of total protein remaining (as a surrogate of EVs quantities) are considered at this stage in the comparative study, it seemed that electroporation is the most favourable loading approach for both MSC EVs and milk EVs.

3.3. Analysis of Dox Quantity Loaded in MSC and Milk Evs by HPLC

It could be proposed that, despite the washes to remove extraneous Dox after completing the loading step, some Dox detected by fluorescence may be associated with Evs but not in the Evs as cargo. HPLC is reported to be an accurate, reproducible, and high throughput method for the quantification of small chemotherapeutic drug molecules such as Dox, paclitaxel, or curcumin [7,32]. Thus, to further investigate the amount of Dox loaded into the Evs, paired aliquots of loaded Evs, both non-lysed (so surface Dox detected) versus lysed (ruptured, so Dox cargo also detected) were analysed by HPLC. Serially diluted Dox was analysed by HPLC to prepare a standard curve (Supplementary Figure S2a). The representative Dox peaks are presented in Supplementary Figure S2b. With passive-loaded Evs, no differences were observed between non-lysed and lysed MSC Evs or milk Evs (Figure 4). This indicates that most Dox signals detected in the passive loading protocol (as presented in Figure 3a) were unlikely due to the incorporation of Dox into Evs as cargo, but rather due to a simpler association/conjugation of Dox with Evs.

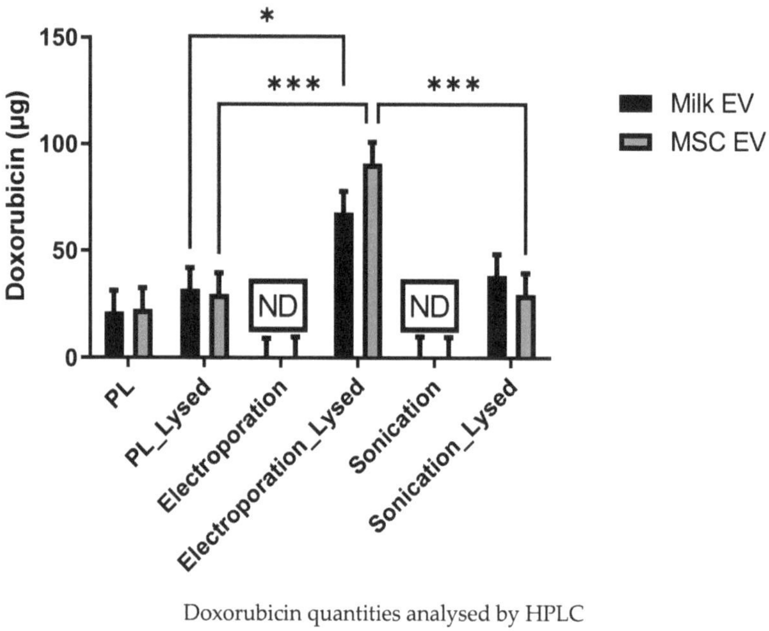

Figure 4. Dox quantities detected for non-lysed compared to lysed passive loaded (PL), electroporation loaded, and sonicated loaded MSC EVs and milk EVs. Results are mean from $n > 3 \pm$ SEM biological repeat experiments. Statistical analysis was done through 2-way Anova. * represents p value < 0.05, and *** $p < 0.001$. ND = not detected.

With respect to either the electroporation or sonication loading approaches, no peak was detected for Dox with the non-lysed samples. Rather, Dox was only detected when the Evs were lysed. This indicates that the Dox has been entrapped within the Evs as cargo. Specifically, following the electroporation method, 90.1 ± 12 µg and 68.0 ± 10 µg of Dox were detected for lysed Dox-loaded MSC Evs and milk Evs, respectively. In contrast, following the sonication method 38.3 ± 13 µg and 29.5 ± 9 µg of Dox were detected for lysed Dox-loaded MSC Evs and milk Evs, respectively. Overall, this data suggests that the electroporation process is associated with greater loading of Dox into MSC Evs and milk Evs as cargo, when compared to the passive loading and sonication approaches.

3.4. Effect of Passive and Active Loading Approaches on EVs Surface Markers

Imaging flow cytometry (IFCM) is a flow cytometry-based sophisticated method suitable for characterising EVs. This method is also useful to enumerate EVs specific surface markers and is recently reported as a robust method of EV analysis [32], even though none of the previously reported studies have analysed drug-loaded EVs with this robust technique for multi-parametric EVs analysis. Therefore, the enumeration of detectable EVs (pre- and post-loading) and amounts of three tetraspanins proteins are considered to be markers of EVs, i.e., CD9, CD63, and CD81 were analysed in order to investigate any negative effects of the various loading approaches on representative surface proteins.

The effect of loading on the number of objects/mL of MSC EVs and milk EVs are presented in Figure 5a,b, respectively. For both MSC EV and milk EV samples, there were significantly lower objects/mL detected in loaded samples compared to the non-loaded EV samples ($p < 0.00001$). Interestingly, the detected EV-like objects/mL post sonication was significantly lower compared to both passive loading ($p < 0.05$) and electroporation ($p < 0.01$) approaches, observed in both MSC EVs and milk EVs samples. There were no significant differences observed between the passive loading and electroporation approach in both MSC EVs and milk EVs samples. Hence, this observation indicates that sonication is a harsh approach that leads to the loss of intact EVs. Sonication has been known to be a harsh technique that can cause irreversible disruption to the cellular membrane [33], this may explain the lower number of detectable EVs following sonication (Figure 5a,b). Additionally, Zubair Ahmed et al. [34] reported that 'low-power sonication' altered MSC EVs membrane integrity.

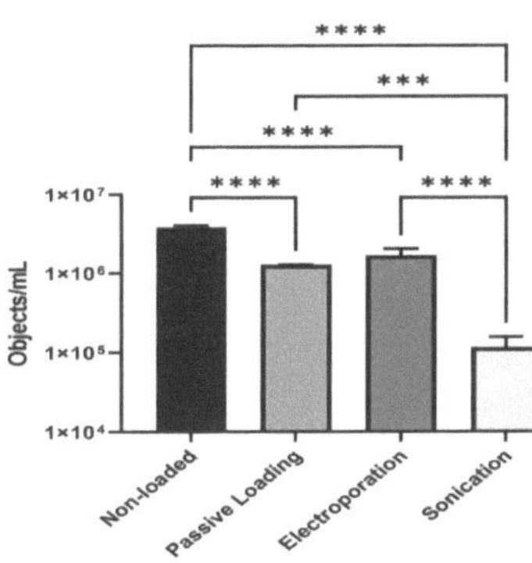

(**a**) Detectable number of MSC EVs

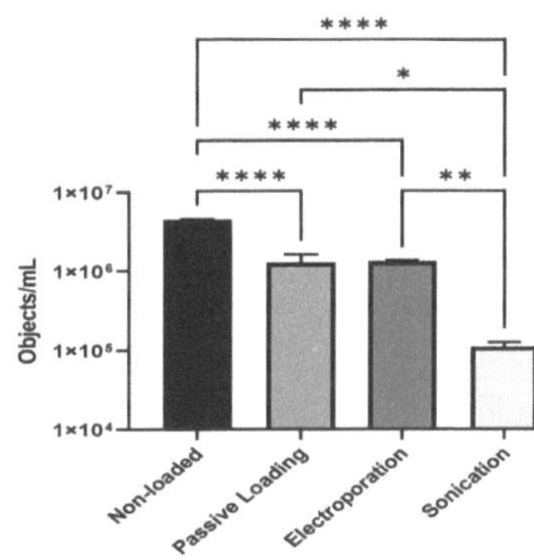

(**b**) Detectable number of milk EVs

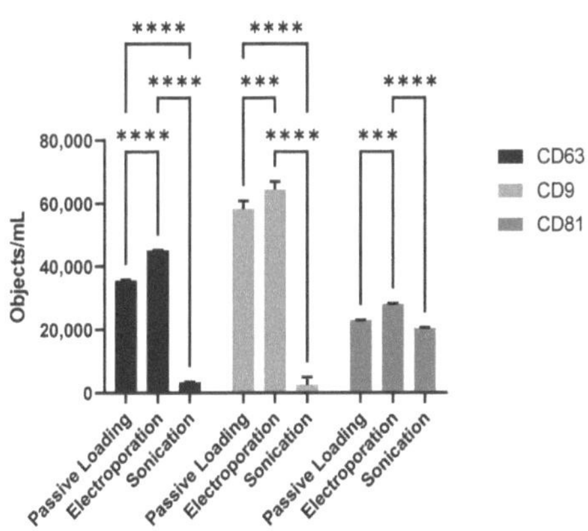

(**c**) EV marker comparison of Dox loaded MSC Evs

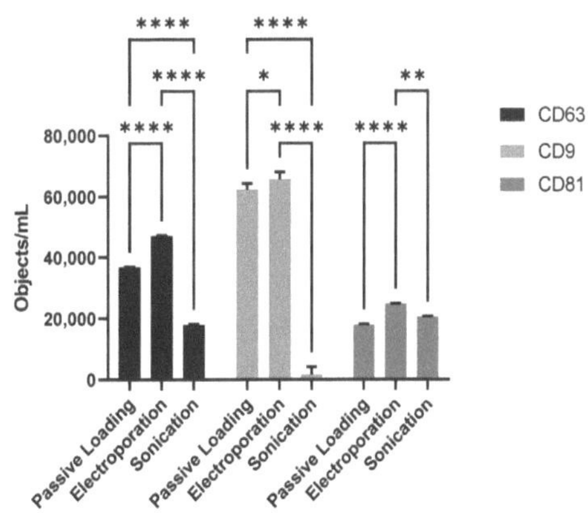

(**d**) EV marker comparison of Dox loaded milk Evs

Figure 5. MSC EVs and milk EVs loaded with Dox using passive and active loading approaches were analysed by IFCM to investigate the effect of loading on total detectable EV-like objects and representative EVs surface proteins. Total detectable number of EV-like objects/mL in non-loaded versus Dox-loaded (**a**) MSC EVs and (**b**) milk EVs are presented. Further, the results are presented as a comparison of the number of CD63+, CD9+, and CD81+ objects/EVs in samples in passive loaded and active loaded (**c**) MSC EVs and (**d**) milk EVs. Results are mean from $n > 3 \pm$ SEM biological repeat experiments. Statistical analysis was done through 2-way Anova; * represents p value < 0.05, ** $p < 0.01$, *** $p < 0.001$ and **** $p < 0.0001$.

Further analysis of representative EV surface markers was performed on the loaded MSC EVs and milk EVs.

Overall, similar quantities of surface markers, in terms of positive objects/mL, were observed in MSC EVs compared to milk EVs; CD9 was the most abundant, followed by CD63 and CD81. It is of note that when IFCM data was compared to immunoblotting data (Figure 2c), some differences were evident, especially in the abundance of CD9 and CD63. It must be considered, however, that immunoblotting is a semi-quantitative way of assessing these proteins in lysed samples of the overall pool of EVs, while IFCM is quantitative and is evaluating surface proteins on individual intact EVs.

As presented in Figure 5c, for MSC EVs sonication was associated with significantly ($p < 0.0001$) lower numbers of CD63+ and CD9+ objects/EVs, compared to passive loading and electroporation. Sonicated loaded samples also had significantly ($p < 0.05$) fewer CD81+ objects when compared to those loaded by electroporation. With milk EVs, similar observations rang through (Figure 5b) as observed with MSC EVs.

This indicates that, at least with the electroporation setting that we optimised for this study, the EVs surface protein were conserved (apparently as gentle on them as passive loading), while sonication produced detrimental effects on the EVs, i.e., lower number of EVs and proteins, particularly CD63 and CD9. This further substantiates our observation that electroporation is a preferable drug loading approach over sonication and passive loading, while no major differences were detected between milk EVs and MSC EVs in this regard.

Interestingly, a literature search indicated that a clear consensus on the 'best drug loading approach' has not been reached among EVs researchers and comparative studies focusing on loading approaches and use of different EVs sources have been lacking [8,35,36].

4. Conclusions

Our study showed that electroporation is a preferable drug loading approach, when compared to both passive loading and sonication. With electroporation, greatest success was reached in loading Dox into the EVs and minimal negative effects on surface proteins were detected, while sonication seemed to be detrimental to these proteins. When comparing MSC EVs to milk EVs, no substantial differences in Dox loading capacity were observed between electroporated MSC EVs and milk EVs, indicating that both are equally suitable. Thus, the decision to select one over the other may depend on the further future experiments that will take into consideration that MSC EVs have been shown to have some natural anti-inflammatory/immune modulating characteristics that may be of benefit to a given application in addition to its cargo/loaded therapeutic content. On the other hand, milk is cheap, easily accessible, easily scalable, and very rich source of EVs and so may be more favourable in other circumstances, e.g., for oral delivery.

Supplementary Materials: The following supporting information can be downloaded at: https://www.mdpi.com/article/10.3390/pharmaceutics15030718/s1; Figure S1. Total protein separation by polyacrylamide gel electrophoresis indicates efficient removal of casein proteins in IP treated milk samples compared to untreated milk samples; Figure S2. Serially diluted Dox samples were analysed by HPLC to obtain the standard curve and unknown concentration of Dox from loaded EV samples were calculated using the straight-line equation. Interpolation of unknown Dox was performed on GraphPad Prism 9 software.

Author Contributions: A.M. and L.O.: conceptualisation, funding acquisition; A.M.: data curation, investigation, methodology, formal analysis, writing—original draft, review & editing; D.T.: methodology, writing—review & editing; N.M.: methodology, writing—review & editing; B.T.: HPLC methodology; L.O.: conceptualisation, resources, supervision, writing—review & editing. All authors have read and agreed to the published version of the manuscript.

Funding: This research was supported by the Research Council Advanced Laureate Award EVIC to LOD [IRCLA/2019/49], Trinity College Dublin Dean's Research Award, grant number 9050610-1106-000000 to A.M., and Horizon 2020 Research and Innovation Award EVPRO to LOD [814495].

Institutional Review Board Statement: Not applicable.

Informed Consent Statement: Not applicable.

Data Availability Statement: Not applicable.

Conflicts of Interest: The authors declare no conflict of interest.

References

1. Daraee, H.; Etemadi, A.; Kouhi, M.; Alimirzalu, S.; Akbarzadeh, A. Application of liposomes in medicine and drug delivery. *Samira Alimirzalu Abolfazl Akbarzadeh* **2016**, *44*, 381–391. [CrossRef] [PubMed]
2. Busatto, S.; Pham, A.; Suh, A.; Shapiro, S.; Wolfram, J. Organotropic drug delivery: Synthetic nanoparticles and extracellular vesicles. *Biomed Microdevices* **2019**, *21*, 46. [CrossRef]
3. Desai, N. Challenges in development of nanoparticle-based therapeutics. *AAPS J.* **2012**, *14*, 282–295. [CrossRef] [PubMed]
4. Sercombe, L.; Veerati, T.; Moheimani, F.; Wu, S.Y.; Sood, A.K.; Hua, S. Advances and challenges of liposome assisted drug delivery. *Front. Pharmacol.* **2015**, *6*, 286. [CrossRef]
5. Beltrán-Gracia, E.; López-Camacho, A.; Higuera-Ciapara, I.; Velázquez-Fernández, J.B.; Vallejo-Cardona, A.A. Nanomedicine review: Clinical developments in liposomal applications. *Cancer Nanotechnol.* **2019**, *101*, 10. [CrossRef]
6. Walker, S.; Busatto, S.; Pham, A.; Tian, M.; Suh, A.; Carson, K.; Quintero, A.; Lafrence, M.; Malik, H.; Santana, M.X.; et al. Extracellular vesicle-based drug delivery systems for cancer treatment. *Theranostics* **2019**, *9*, 8001–8017. [CrossRef] [PubMed]
7. Mehryab, F.; Rabbani, S.; Shahhosseini, S.; Shekari, F.; Fatahi, Y.; Baharvand, H.; Haeri, A. Exosomes as a next-generation drug delivery system: An update on drug loading approaches, characterization, and clinical application challenges. *Acta Biomater.* **2020**, *113*, 42–62. [CrossRef]
8. Herrmann, I.K.; Wood, M.J.A.; Fuhrmann, G. Extracellular vesicles as a next-generation drug delivery platform. *Nat. Nanotechnol.* **2021**, *16*, 748–759. [CrossRef]
9. O'Driscoll, L. Expanding on exosomes and ectosomes in cancer. *N. Engl. J. Med.* **2015**, *372*, 2359–2362. [CrossRef]
10. Vader, P.; Mol, E.A.; Pasterkamp, G.; Schiffelers, R.M. Extracellular vesicles for drug delivery. *Adv. Drug. Deliv. Rev.* **2016**, *106*, 148–156. [CrossRef]
11. O'Brien, K.; Lowry, M.C.; Corcoran, C.; Martinez, V.G.; Daly, M.; Rani, S.; Gallagher, W.M.; Radomski, M.W.; MacLeod, R.A.; O'Driscoll, L. miR-134 in extracellular vesicles reduces triple-negative breast cancer aggression and increases drug sensitivity. *Oncotarget* **2015**, *6*, 32774–32789. [CrossRef]
12. Melzer, C.; Rehn, V.; Yang, Y.; Bähre, H.; von der Ohe, J.; Hass, R. Taxol-Loaded MSC-Derived Exosomes Provide a Therapeutic Vehicle to Target Metastatic Breast Cancer and Other Carcinoma Cells. *Cancers* **2019**, *11*, 798. [CrossRef] [PubMed]
13. Wei, H.; Chen, J.; Wang, S.; Fu, F.; Zhu, X.; Wu, C.; Liu, Z.; Zhong, G.; Lin, J. A Nanodrug Consisting Of Doxorubicin And Exosome Derived From Mesenchymal Stem Cells For Osteosarcoma Treatment In Vitro. *Int. J. Nanomed.* **2019**, *14*, 8603. [CrossRef] [PubMed]
14. Qiu, Y.; Sun, J.; Qiu, J.; Chen, G.; Wang, X.; Mu, Y.; Li, K.; Wang, W. Antitumor Activity of Cabazitaxel and MSC-TRAIL Derived Extracellular Vesicles in Drug-Resistant Oral Squamous Cell Carcinoma. *Cancer Manag. Res.* **2020**, *12*, 10809–10820. [CrossRef]
15. Zhou, Y.; Zhou, W.; Chen, X.; Wang, Q.; Li, C.; Chen, Q.; Zhang, Y.; Lu, Y.; Ding, X.; Jiang, C. Bone marrow mesenchymal stem cells-derived exosomes for penetrating and targeted chemotherapy of pancreatic cancer. *Acta Pharm. Sin. B* **2020**, *10*, 1563–1575. [CrossRef]
16. Liang, L.; Zhao, L.; Wang, Y.; Wang, Y. Treatment for Hepatocellular Carcinoma Is Enhanced When Norcantharidin Is Encapsulated in Exosomes Derived from Bone Marrow Mesenchymal Stem Cells. *Mol. Pharm.* **2021**, *18*, 1003–1013. [CrossRef] [PubMed]
17. Aqil, F.; Jeyabalan, J.; Agrawal, A.K.; Kyakulaga, A.-H.; Munagala, R.; Parker, L.; Gupta, R.C. Exosomal Delivery of Berry Anthocyanidins for the Management of Ovarian Cancer. 2017. Available online: https://pubs.rsc.org/en/content/articlehtml/2017/fo/c7fo00882a (accessed on 9 October 2022).
18. Munagala, R.; Aqil, F.; Jeyabalan, J. *Exosomal Formulation of Anthocyanidins Against Multiple Cancer Types*; Elsevier: Amsterdam, The Netherlands, 2017; Available online: https://www.sciencedirect.com/science/article/pii/S0304383517301040?casa_token=OsCOqVD_CQgAAAAA:1xLlN1_fsdnMHFj72F6r72_7r-XNeGTsO7LNrYrP7v_OwBPErAS8FDZnYLcmwovuBw3WCYDMsVY (accessed on 9 October 2022).
19. Vashisht, M.; Rani, P.; Onteru, S.K.; Singh, D. Curcumin Encapsulated in Milk Exosomes Resists Human Digestion and Possesses Enhanced Intestinal Permeability in Vitro. *Appl. Biochem. Biotechnol.* **2017**, *183*, 993–1007. [CrossRef]
20. Ludwig, A.-K.; De Miroschedji, K.; Doeppner, T.R.; Börger, V.; Ruesing, J.; Rebmann, V.; Durst, S.; Jansen, S.; Bremer, M.; Behrmann, E.; et al. Precipitation with polyethylene glycol followed by washing and pelleting by ultracentrifugation enriches extracellular vesicles from tissue culture supernatants in small and large scales. *J. Extracell. Vesicles* **2018**, *7*, 1528109. [CrossRef]
21. Mukhopadhya, A.; Santoro, J.; Moran, B.; Useckaite, Z.; O'Driscoll, L. Optimisation and comparison of orthogonal methods for separation and characterisation of extracellular vesicles to investigate how representative infant milk formula is of milk. *Food Chem.* **2021**, *353*, 129309. [CrossRef]
22. Mukhopadhya, A.; Santoro, J.; O'Driscoll, L. Extracellular vesicle separation from milk and infant milk formula using acid precipitation and ultracentrifugation. *STAR Protoc.* **2021**, *2*, 100821. [CrossRef]

23. Visnovitz, T.; Osteikoetxea, X.; Sódar, B.W.; Mihály, J.; Lőrincz, P.; Vukman, K.V.; Tóth, E.; Koncz, A.; Székács, I.; Horváth, R.; et al. An improved 96 well plate format lipid quantification assay for standardisation of experiments with extracellular vesicles. *J. Extracell. Vesicles* **2019**, *8*, 1565263. [CrossRef] [PubMed]
24. O'Brien, K.; Rani, S.; Corcoran, C.; Wallace, R.; Hughes, L.; Friel, A.M.; McDonnell, S.; Crown, J.; Radomski, M.W.; O'Driscoll, L. Exosomes from triple-negative breast cancer cells can transfer phenotypic traits representing their cells of origin to secondary cells. *Eur. J. Cancer* **2013**, *49*, 1845–1859. [CrossRef]
25. Li, D.; Yao, S.; Zhou, Z.; Shi, J.; Huang, Z.; Wu, Z. Hyaluronan decoration of milk exosomes directs tumor-specific delivery of doxorubicin. *Carbohydr. Res.* **2020**, *493*, 108032. [CrossRef]
26. Zhang, Q.; Xiao, Q.; Yin, H.; Xia, C.; Pu, Y.; He, Z.; Hu, Q.; Wang, J.; Wang, Y. Milk-exosome based pH/light sensitive drug system to enhance anticancer activity against oral squamous cell carcinoma. *RSC Adv.* **2020**, *10*, 28314–28323. [CrossRef]
27. O'Regan, J.; Ennis, M.P.; Mulvihill, D.M. *"Milk Proteins," in Handbook of Hydrocolloids*; Elsevier: Amsterdam, The Netherlands, 2009; pp. 298–358.
28. Gomari, H.; Moghadam, M.F.; Soleimani, M.; Ghavami, M.; Khodashenas, S. Targeted delivery of doxorubicin to HER2 positive tumor models. *Int. J. Nanomed.* **2019**, *14*, 5679–5690. [CrossRef]
29. Bagheri, E.; Abnous, K.; Farzad, S.A.; Taghdisi, S.M.; Ramezani, M.; Alibolandi, M. Targeted doxorubicin-loaded mesenchymal stem cells-derived exosomes as a versatile platform for fighting against colorectal cancer. *Life Sci.* **2020**, *261*, 118369. [CrossRef] [PubMed]
30. Hernandez-Oller, L.; Seras-Franzoso, J.; Andrade, F.; Rafael, D.; Abasolo, I.; Gener, P.; Schwartz, S., Jr. Extracellular Vesicles as Drug Delivery Systems in Cancer. *Pharmaceutics* **2020**, *12*, 1146. [CrossRef] [PubMed]
31. Stam, J.; Bartel, S.; Bischoff, R.; Wolters, J.C. Isolation of extracellular vesicles with combined enrichment methods. *J. Chromatogr. B* **2021**, *1169*, 122604. [CrossRef] [PubMed]
32. Rankin-Turner, S.; Vader, P.; O'Driscoll, L.; Giebel, B.; Heaney, L.M.; Davies, O.G. A call for the standardised reporting of factors affecting the exogenous loading of extracellular vesicles with therapeutic cargos. *Adv. Drug Deliv. Rev.* **2021**, *173*, 479–491. [CrossRef]
33. Srivastava, A.; Amreddy, N.; Pareek, V.; Chinnappan, M.; Ahmed, R.; Mehta, M.; Razaq, M.; Munshi, A.; Ramesh, R. Progress in extracellular vesicle biology and their application in cancer medicine. *Wiley Interdiscip. Rev. Nanomed. Nanobiotech.* **2020**, *12*, e1621. [CrossRef]
34. Nizamudeen, Z.A.; Xerri, R.; Parmenter, C.; Suain, K.; Markus, R.; Chakrabarti, L.; Sottile, V. Low-power sonication can alter extracellular vesicle size and properties. *Cells* **2021**, *10*, 2413. [CrossRef] [PubMed]
35. De Jong, O.G.; Kooijmans, S.A.A.; Murphy, D.E.; Jiang, L.; Evers, M.J.W.; Sluijter, J.P.G.; Vader, P.; Schiffelers, R.M. Drug Delivery with Extracellular Vesicles: From Imagination to Innovation. *Acc. Chem. Res.* **2019**, *52*, 1761–1770. [CrossRef] [PubMed]
36. Han, Y.; Jones, T.W.; Dutta, S.; Zhu, Y.; Wang, X.; Narayanan, S.P.; Fagan, S.C.; Zhang, D. Overview and update on methods for cargo loading into extracellular vesicles. *Processes* **2021**, *9*, 356. [CrossRef] [PubMed]

pharmaceutics

MDPI

Review

The CRISPR/Cas9 System Delivered by Extracellular Vesicles

Xinglong Zhu [1,†], Mengyu Gao [1,†], Yongfeng Yang [2,3], Weimin Li [2,3,4], Ji Bao [1,*] and Yi Li [2,3,*]

1 Key Laboratory of Transplant Engineering and Immunology, Institute of Clinical Pathology, West China Hospital, Sichuan University, Chengdu 610041, China
2 Institute of Respiratory Health, West China Hospital, Sichuan University, Chengdu 610041, China
3 Precision Medicine Key Laboratory, West China Hospital, Sichuan University, Chengdu 610041, China
4 Department of Respiratory and Critical Care Medicine, West China Hospital, Sichuan University, Chengdu 610041, China
* Correspondence: baoji@scu.edu.cn (J.B.); peach_adore@hotmail.com (Y.L.); Tel.: +86-28-85164030 (J.B.); +86-28-85423998 (Y.L.)
† These authors contributed equally to this work.

Abstract: Clustered regularly interspaced short palindromic repeat (CRISPR)/CRISPR-associated protein (Cas) systems can precisely manipulate DNA sequences to change the characteristics of cells and organs, which has potential in the mechanistic research on genes and the treatment of diseases. However, clinical applications are restricted by the lack of safe, targeted and effective delivery vectors. Extracellular vesicles (EVs) are an attractive delivery platform for CRISPR/Cas9. Compared with viral and other vectors, EVs present several advantages, including safety, protection, capacity, penetrating ability, targeting ability and potential for modification. Consequently, EVs are profitably used to deliver the CRISPR/Cas9 in vivo. In this review, the advantages and disadvantages of the delivery form and vectors of the CRISPR/Cas9 are concluded. The favorable traits of EVs as vectors, such as the innate characteristics, physiological and pathological functions, safety and targeting ability of EVs, are summarized. Furthermore, in terms of the delivery of the CRISPR/Cas9 by EVs, EV sources and isolation strategies, the delivery form and loading methods of the CRISPR/Cas9 and applications have been concluded and discussed. Finally, this review provides future directions of EVs as vectors of the CRISPR/Cas9 system in clinical applications, such as the safety, capacity, consistent quality, yield and targeting ability of EVs.

Keywords: CRISPR/Cas9; extracellular vesicles; delivery; biomedical applications

Citation: Zhu, X.; Gao, M.; Yang, Y.; Li, W.; Bao, J.; Li, Y. The CRISPR/Cas9 System Delivered by Extracellular Vesicles. *Pharmaceutics* **2023**, *15*, 984. https://doi.org/10.3390/pharmaceutics15030984

Academic Editor: Simon C. W. Richardson

Received: 17 February 2023
Revised: 14 March 2023
Accepted: 17 March 2023
Published: 18 March 2023

1. Introduction

In the 1970s, with the development of genetic engineering, a breakthrough dawned upon genome editing technology, which was a powerful tool for implementing fixed-point editing DNA sequences [1]. To date, genome editing tools have provided a new horizon for biomedical research, such as gene biology, biological mechanisms and treatment of disease [2]. The application of genome editing tools can be traced back to 1971, when specific DNA fragments were successfully manipulated by restriction enzymes [3]. With advances in research on endonucleases integrated with locators, a number of genome editing tools have been developed, for example, zinc finger nucleases, transcription activator-like effector nucleases and clustered regularly interspaced short palindromic repeat (CRISPR)/CRISPR-associated protein (Cas) systems [4].

For genome editing, the discovery of CRISPR/Cas systems has ushered revolutionized breakthroughs. In the study of defensive mechanisms of bacteria and archaea, CRISPR/Cas could be depicted as a defensive mechanism similar to the adaptive immune system against foreign invading nucleic acids, which was initially discovered [4,5]. When foreign invading nucleic acids enter, the acquired nucleic acid fragments are integrated and processed and finally generate CRISPR RNA (crRNA), which can complementarily pair with foreign invading nucleic acid sequences and guide the Cas protein, then form a complex with the

Cas protein and other RNA for shearing DNA [6]. Because the type II CRISPR/Cas9 system is simpler and a single Cas9 protein can cleave nucleic acid segments, the CRISPR/Cas9 system is widely used in genome editing among the numerous discovered CRISPR/Cas systems. In practical applications, a single artificial synthetic guide RNA (sgRNA), formed by the combination of crRNA and trans-activating crRNA (tracrRNA), has the ability of targeted binding and Cas9 shears DNA. The CRISPR/Cas9 system has been commonly used in basic biology, biomedicine and agriculture research [2,3,7].

To implement genome editing via CRISPR/Cas9, it is necessary to consider how to deliver it [8]. Generally, the strategies of delivering CRISPR/Cas9 are classified into two major classes (viral and nonviral vector) [9]. The delivery efficiency of CRISPR/Cas9 and gene editing efficiency can be significantly increased by viral vectors [10]. Regrettably, the intrinsic factors of viral vectors, including safety, high cost, difficult operation and limited packaging capacity, restrict their application [11,12]. Nonviral vectors are mainly based on physical methods and synthetic chemical and natural materials, such as microinjection, electroporation, liposomes, nanoparticles, and gold nanoparticles [13,14]. Although these vectors possess simple operations, cost-effectiveness and universality, their cytotoxicity, limited penetrability and imprecise targeting delivery limit their further development [8,14]. Consequently, in the process of CRISPR/Cas9 delivery, the ways in which to overcome problems of safety, efficiency, stability, targeting, penetrability and biocompatibility should be focused on. Meanwhile, novel gene delivery systems should be developed.

Extracellular vesicles (EVs), secreted by a variety of cells, possess a phospholipid bilayer-enclosed structure, which was initially described as a "cellular junk" [15,16]. Although EVs can be roughly classified into exosomes, microvesicles and apoptotic bodies by size and generation methods, it is difficult to isolate pure EVs due to their overlapping size, biomarkers and composition [16,17]. Therefore, exosomes, microvesicles and apoptotic bodies are uniformly called EVs in this review. With advances in EV research, EVs have been shown to act as indispensable messengers in intercellular communication [18]. Meanwhile, since EVs are involved in various physiological and pathological processes by regulating the immune response, tissue repair and cell growth, the potential value of EVs has been revealed in the field of diagnostic biomarkers and therapy [10,19]. EVs can effectively transport lipids, proteins and nucleic acids (for instance, mRNA, miRNA, lncRNA, circular RNA, ribosomal RNA, tRNA, and DNA fragments) [20]. In addition, recent studies have shown that EVs can be used as vectors to deliver biomolecules, especially in gene delivery systems [12].

In this review, the delivery form and vectors of the CRISPR/Cas9 system are concluded and compared; the advantages of EVs as vectors are mainly summarized; the delivery of the CRISPR/Cas9 system by EVs, including EV sources and isolation strategies, the delivery form and loading methods of the CRISPR/Cas9 system and applications in vitro and in vivo have been concluded and discussed. The CRISPR/Cas9 system delivered by EVs has potential in clinical disease treatments (Figure 1).

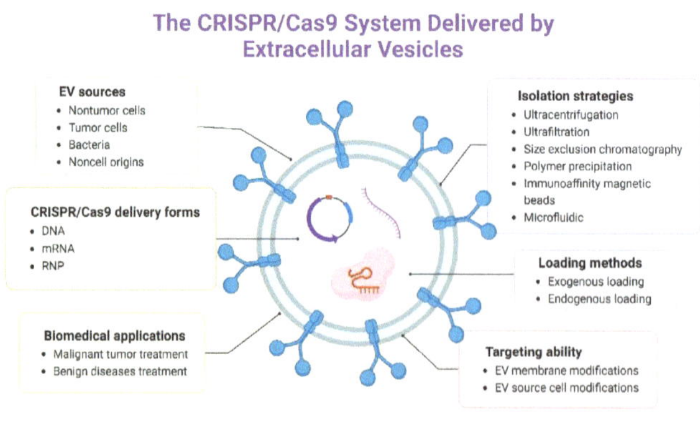

Figure 1. Key factors of extracellular vesicles (EVs) delivering the CRISPR/Cas9 system.

2. Delivery of CRISPR/Cas9

Because the molecular weight of the Cas9 protein is 160 kDa and the gRNA is negatively charged, these characteristics of the gRNA and Cas9 protein make it difficult for them to cross the cell membrane [12,21]. In the CRISPR/Cas9 gene editing system in vitro, the sgRNA and Cas9 protein should be delivered into cells to avoid degradation and move into the nucleus for gene editing [22]. Furthermore, in the more complex microenvironment in vivo, the CRISPR/Cas9 system may be degraded and neutralized by physical, chemical and biological obstacles and the immune system [10,23]. Therefore, to improve the efficiency, safety and targeting of gene editing, the delivery form of the CRISPR/Cas9 system and how to deliver the CRISPR/Cas9 system should be seriously considered.

In general, the delivery form of the CRISPR/Cas9 system can be classified as DNA, RNA or ribonucleoprotein complexes (RNPs) [12,24]. The RNP is defined as the sgRNA compounded with Cas9 protein in vitro [25]. Through plasmids carrying DNA sequences of gRNA and Cas9 protein, the CRISPR/Cas9 system is delivered into cells. This method is economical as well as convenient [12,26]. However, gRNA and Cas9 protein are further formed by transcription and translation in cells, which increases the working time and the rate of off-target effects [27]. Meanwhile, this process, which is difficult to control, could have potential risks for DNA sequences integrated into the genome [28]. Since transcription is not needed, the delivery of the RNA form of the CRISPR/Cas9 system can effectively decrease the editing efficiency [29]. Unfortunately, RNA is easily degraded, which decreases the efficiency of gene editing [30]. Gene editing immediately begins to work through the delivery of the RNP form of the CRISPR/Cas9 system in the nucleus, which leads to a higher efficiency of gene editing and a lower rate of off-target effects than DNA and RNA forms of the CRISPR/Cas9 system [31]. RNPs only temporarily exist in cells, which is beneficial for curing genetic and infectious disorders. Nevertheless, the delivery of RNPs is more costly than that of DNA and RNA [12,32].

In vitro, the efficiency of gene editing and the rate of off-target effects are mainly discussed, which is simpler than in vivo. For gene editing via CRISPR/Cas9 in vivo, several key factors should fit the following criteria: (1) safety (delivery products and strategies); (2) crossing the physiological and pathological barriers (dense characteristics of some tissue, acid and enzymes microenvironment, blood-embryo and blood–brain barrier); (3) targeting (effectively targeted tissue or organ); and (4) accurate gene editing (improving the gene editing efficiency and avoiding damage to the genome) [10,33].

For delivery of the CRISPR/Cas9 system, these strategies can be classified into viral and nonviral vectors [34]. Adeno-associated viruses (AAVs), Adenoviruses (AVs), Lentiviruses (LVs) and Baculoviruses which are some typical viral vectors, have been exploited for delivering gene editing systems [8,9]. These viral vectors can efficiently deliver the CRISPR/Cas9 system into cells crossing physiological barriers and the cell membrane and possess high transfection and gene editing efficiency [35]. However, especially in vivo, several inherent characteristics of viruses, for example, immunogenicity inducing immune responses and viral genomes randomly inserting into host genomes, have caused significant safety problems [8]. Compared with other viral vectors, AAV is safer since it cannot replicate, does not integrate into genomes and has low immunogenicity in vivo [36,37]. Nonetheless, the delivery of the CRISPR/Cas9 system may be compromised by the limited packaging capacity of AAV [38].

Electroporation and microinjection, as classical nonviral physical methods, have been used to deliver the CRISPR/Cas9 system in vitro [35]. Electroporation depends on currents, which can create numerous transient small pores in cell membranes; then, the CRISPR/Cas9 system can be delivered into cells [9]. This method is inexpensive, easy to perform and is high throughput, but the conditions of electroporation are highly variable, and cells are vulnerable [8]. Microinjection relies on microscopes and needles to inject RNPs, which are used in zygotes for the generation of small animal models. Because of the high cost of microinjection, delicate operation, low throughput and inappropriateness of in vivo editing, the applications of microinjection have been limited [39,40].

Lipid-based synthetic chemical materials have been frequently used for the delivery of the CRISPR/Cas9 system [14]. In particular, a variety of commercial liposomes have been developed. For example, liposomes can effectively deliver the DNA, RNA and RNP form of the CRISPR/Cas9 system [10,41]. With a hydrophobic tail and hydrophilic head, liposomes can spontaneously form the structure of lipid bilayers [42]. The CRISPR/Cas9 system can be encapsulated by liposomes or combined with liposomes to form complexes, and then liposome–CRISPR/Cas9 complexes fuse with cell membranes to enter cells [35]. Unlike viral vectors, liposomes are a safer method since their delivery mechanism is based on endocytosis [10]. Meanwhile, compared with electroporation, liposomes are milder to cells. Therefore, liposomes have harmonious characteristics in all aspects, including inherent structure, biocompatibility, low immunogenicity and low toxicity [9]. Gold nanoparticles can deliver the CRISPR/Cas9 system in vivo and in vitro. The advantage of gold nanoparticles is that they are biologically inert, so the immune response is hardly triggered [43,44].

In conclusion, all delivery forms of the CRISPR/Cas9 system and delivery strategies have their own benefits and drawbacks (Table 1). According to the purpose and means of research, the appropriate forms and strategies are selected.

Table 1. Comparing different delivery strategies of the CRISPR/Cas9 system, these strategies can be classified into viral and nonviral vectors. AAVs: adeno-associated viruses; AVs: adenoviruses; LVs: lentiviruses; LSCMs: lipid-based synthetic chemical materials; EVs: extracellular vesicles (EVs); RNP: ribonucleoprotein complex. + denotes low; ++ denotes medium; +++ denotes high.

Delivery Vectors	**Viral Vectors**			**Nonviral Vectors**				
	AAVs	**AVs**	**LVs**	**Electroporation**	**Microinjection**	**LSCMs**	**Gold Nanoparticles**	**EVs**
Safety	+++	++	+	+++	+++	++	++	+++
Capacity	+	++	+	−	−	++	++	+++
The form of the CRISPR/Cas9 system	DNA	DNA	DNA	DNA, RNA, RNP	DNA, RNA, RNP	DNA, RNA, RNP	RNP	DNA, RNA, RNP
Targeting ability	++	−	−	−	−	−	−	+++
Permeation	+++	+++	+++	−	−	++	++	+++
Delivery efficiency	+++	+++	+++	+++	+	++	++	+++
Applications	In vivo	In vitro and in vivo	In vitro and in vivo	In vitro	In vitro	In vitro and in vivo	In vitro and in vivo	In vitro and in vivo
Cost	+++	+++	++	+	+++	++	++	+++

3. Several Key Factors of EVs as Vectors

EVs can be generated and secreted by eukaryotes and prokaryotes and then transfer biomacromolecules (such as nucleic acids, proteins, lipids, glycoproteins, etc.) for exchange of information [18,20]. In vivo, EVs are associated with several physiological and pathophysiological processes (for instance, the immune system, viral pathogenicity, etc.) and various diseases (including liver, cardiovascular, tumor, lung and central nervous system) [16,19,45]. Consequently, EVs can reveal the biological status of biological fluids, which provides new insight for diagnosing diseases. Meanwhile, the ability of EVs to carry information indicates that EVs can deliver cargoes for therapeutics [46]. Given the loading capacity of various biomacromolecules, ability to target specific cells, immunoregulation and ease of engineering, EVs can be an ideal vector for the delivery of therapeutic agents [47]. Furthermore, these beneficial characteristics of EVs are gradually being used in CRISPR/Cas9 delivery, which has potential for gene editing in vivo [48].

3.1. Innate Characteristics of EVs

EVs are generated by several cell types. According to the EV biogenesis mechanism, EVs can be classified into exosomes, microvesicles and apoptotic bodies [16]. In general, exosomes are released by the plasma membrane fused with multivesicular bodies (MVBs), which are formed by an inward budding of the endosome, and microvesicles and apoptotic bodies are formed by an outward budding of the plasma membrane under different conditions [49]. Consequently, the EV membrane features of a phospholipid bilayer-enclosed structure containing various transmembrane and membrane-anchored proteins depend on the EV biogenesis mechanism [15,17]. These features are beneficial to the targeting and uptake of EVs.

For cargo delivery, EVs have advantages with respect to protection and capacity. With large molecules, hydrophilicity and different charges, naked nucleic acids and proteins have difficulty crossing cell membranes [10]. They were consequently encapsulated by EVs for delivery and protection. Furthermore, the EV membrane structure can effectively protect naked nucleic acids and proteins from serum endonucleases and the immune system [48]. Compared with other vectors, EVs are unique in that they can deliver different types of cargoes (saccharides, nucleic acids, proteins and lipids) [18]. A number of functional biomacromolecules, especially nucleic acids and proteins, are exogenously encapsulated and carried by EVs. In the process of EV biogenesis, several biomacromolecules related to cell communication, disease pathogenesis and therapeutic agents are innately encapsulated in EVs [16,17].

Several natural biological barriers, such as dense tissue (tumor and cartilage), acidic and enzymatic microenvironments (intestinal mucosa and gastric) and vascular endothelial cell barriers (blood-embryo barrier and blood-brain barrier (BBB)), can obstruct the delivery of cargoes in vivo [10,50]. With high biocompatibility and natural generation, EVs can cross these natural biological barriers efficiently to deliver cargoes [16,51]. The tumor microenvironment, especially high-density tumor tissue, seriously affects tumor penetration, which limits the application of nanomedicine [50]. Liposomes can permeate into the tumor tissue to deliver cargoes. However, the permeability of liposomes is mainly affected by the size, charge, type of cargo and type of tumor, which limits the applications of liposomes [52]. EVs derived from tumor cells can effectively permeate into the tumor. Sánchez et al. showed that the expression of metalloproteinases was increased, the extracellular matrix was degraded and EV penetration was improved when EV surface proteins (CD147, tetraspanin Tspan8 or CD44) and miRNAs (miRNA-494, miRNA-542-3p, and miRNA-21-5p) were overexpressed [53]. Kim et al. successfully utilized tumor-derived EVs carrying the CRISPR/Cas9 system to permeate into tumor tissue for gene editing [54]. The intestinal mucosa can hinder the uptake of several vectors that can deliver cargoes [10]. The study revealed that with small size and negative charge, these vectors performed better in permeation [55]. With their small size, negative charge and stable structure, EVs derived from milk can be easily absorbed by the intestine [56,57]. Meanwhile, EVs derived from epithelial cells also permeate across the intestine [58]. A number of biomacromolecules (curcumin and various types of RNA) could be protected by EVs from digestive juices [10]. The BBB is one of the most important natural biological barriers that can selectively allow some small molecules to cross the endothelial membrane and prevent the passage of causative agents or toxins [59]. In this way, the BBB, as a protective mechanism, also obstructs the delivery of drugs and other biomacromolecules into the brain. Nevertheless, EVs can encapsulate these drugs and biomacromolecules to cross the BBB, and their penetrable efficiency depends on the size and composition of EVs [10,60]. Morad et al. successfully showed that tumor-derived EVs could cross the BBB in vivo, which was based on the endocytosis pathway. In this process, EVs decreased the expression of Rab7 in endothelial cells to promote their transport [61].

3.2. Physiological and Pathological Functions of EVs

With extensive distribution and generation, EVs carry various biomacromolecules to orderly shuttle in vivo, which regulates numerous physiologic processes [16]. Especially in terms of immunoregulation, EVs, generated by B lymphocytes, can present antigens by histocompatibility complex (MHC) proteins located on the EV surface [62]. Recent studies have focused on the immune-regulatory functions of EVs in tumors. According to reports, tumor cell-derived EVs exhibit the ability of immunoregulation to support cancer progression or display antitumor effects [63,64]. Hoshino et al. showed that in tumor metastasis, tumor cell-derived EVs were fused with organ-specific resident cells (fibroblasts, epithelial cells, etc.) to prepare the niche through exosomal integrins, which could lead to Src phosphorylation and proinflammatory S100 expression, facilitating tumor metastasis [65]. Nevertheless, several studies have demonstrated that tumor cell-derived EVs could carry tumor antigens and then promote tumor immunity through CD8(+) and CD4(+) T cells, which could kill tumor cells and frustrate the progression of tumors [64].

Furthermore, EVs can regulate multiple intercellular communications that are related to the cell cycle (proliferation and apoptosis), tissue repair (angiogenesis and remodeling) and regeneration [16]. Since they contain a variety of coagulants, growth factors, inflammatory factors, cytokines, RNA and lipids, platelet-derived EVs regulate the clotting response, cell cycle and tissue repair and regeneration [66]. Kim et al. demonstrated that the proliferation of human umbilical vein endothelial cells (HUVECs) could be stimulated by lipids in platelet-derived EVs [67]. Meanwhile, Zhang et al. showed that in a rat model of femoral nonunion, bone marrow mesenchymal stem cell (BM-MSC)-derived EVs could effectively promote angiogenesis and bone repair. These EVs could be taken up by HUVECs, which facilitated the proliferation of HUVECs in vitro [68].

EVs are also involved in the pathological processes related to tumors and chronic and infectious diseases [16]. In the field of tumor research, EVs, which are generated from tumor, stromal, and immune cells, carry multiple DNA, RNA, protein and other metabolites to participate in tumor development, drug resistance, metastasis and immunity [63]. Tumor cell-derived EVs can affect the fate of EV-generating tumor cells and neighboring tumor and stromal cells [63]. Raimondo et al. demonstrated that chronic myeloid leukemia-derived EVs could promote the proliferation of tumor cells through the activation of antiapoptotic pathways [69]. Nedawi et al. discovered that in glioma, only a small fraction of tumor cells expressing EGFRvIII could generate EGFRvIII-carrying EVs to neighboring tumor cells, which could activate the anchorage-independent growth of neighboring tumor cells through an activation of the AKT pathway [70]. Furthermore, Antonyak et al. showed that MDA-MB-231 and U87 glioma cell-derived EVs could confer onto normal fibroblasts and epithelial cells with several characteristics of tumor cells [71].

Recent studies have also shown that EVs are involved in other chronic and infectious diseases, such as pulmonary fibrosis (PF), cardiovascular diseases and viral infection [16,19,72]. PF, as a chronic lung disease, is characterized by an increase in fibroblasts and extracellular matrix. The pathology of PF is unknown, but EVs that are associated with it have been proven [19]. Yao et al. demonstrated that with overexpression of miR-328, M2 macrophage-derived EVs promoted the proliferation of fibroblasts in vitro and the progression of PF in vivo [73]. The types of EVs, cargoes and cell types determine the effect of EVs in the process of atherothrombosis. In general, EVs play an indispensable role in every step of atherosclerosis, including lesion initiation, plaque progression, plaque rupture and thrombosis [72]. Some related RNA virus studies have shown that infected cell-derived EVs can deliver several biomacromolecules to regulate pathological processes associated with the infection process and cellular responses [16].

3.3. Safety of EVs

Compared with viral vectors (AAVs, AVs and LVs) and chemical materials (liposomes and synthetic nanoparticles), EVs have several innate characteristics (such as generation from natural sources and low immunogenicity and cytotoxicity) [17]. Kamerkar et al.

showed that compared with liposomes, the retention of EVs was improved by reducing phagocytosis by CD47-mediated protection in vivo. Furthermore, fibroblast-derived EVs carrying siRNA targeting oncogenic KRAS inhibited tumor development better than liposomes without an apparent immune response in vivo [74].

However, in the applications of EVs as therapeutic agents or cargo vectors in vivo, the safety of EVs must be thoroughly considered, such as the EV source, the cell culture conditions and the EV isolation strategies [12]. In terms of EV-generating cell sources, the type of cell determines the characteristics of the EV membrane and cargoes, which can affect the immune response, cell transformation and cell invasion [17]. MSCs are one of the most common EV-generating cell sources. A number of studies have proven the low immunogenicity of MSC-derived EVs in vivo [75]. Mendt et al. proved that when MSC-derived EVs were repeatedly administered in mice, the toxicity and immunoreaction of EVs were not obviously observed in vivo [76]. Furthermore, Zhu et al. also demonstrated that HEK293T cell-derived EVs could not elicit an immune response or toxicity in vivo [77]. However, since tumor cell-derived EVs contain multiple tumor-associated biomacromolecules that have the ability to potentially affect tumor development, the safety of these EVs is controversial [12]. Several studies have shown that in animal models of melanoma, liver tumors and colon carcinoma, tumor cell-derived EVs can inhibit tumor development through the T-cell-dependent immune response [63]. However, tumor cell-derived EVs can improve the proliferation of tumor cells, angiogenesis and metastasis and inhibit apoptosis to support tumor progression [12,78]. Consequently, an appropriate EV-generating cell source can guarantee the safety of EV applications. Moreover, the toxicity and hypoimmunogenicity of EVs should be further discussed in different application scenarios.

At present, EVs are mainly generated by transformed cell lines [12]. To fulfill the clinical demand of EV large-scale production and high quality, EV-generating cell culture conditions should comply with good manufacturing practice (GMP) to guarantee the consistent EV phenotype of different batches [79–81]. The cell culture conditions include the medium components (factors and serum), pH and cell culture type (adherent and suspension culture), which may affect the membrane structure and cargo of EVs [82]. Furthermore, EV isolation strategies also affect the quality and safety of EVs, which will be further discussed later.

3.4. Targeting Ability of EVs

In terms of in vivo delivery strategies of biomacromolecules and drugs, especially in CRISPR/Cas9 gene editing systems, the lack of tissue-specific vectors restricts their further clinical application [33]. EVs can not only encapsulate and protect cargoes but also achieve organ, tissue and cell targeting. In general, several molecules can lead to cell-specific homing, which connects with the targeting ability of EVs [48,83]. Consequently, the natural targeting ability of EVs is determined by the cell type. The glycans, proteins and lipids located in the EV membrane determine which organs, tissues and cells are targeted by EVs [17]. Hoshino et al. showed that EVs derived from lung, liver and brain tumor cells could be preferentially taken up by lung fibroblasts, Kupffer cells and brain endothelial cells, respectively. Furthermore, this study proved that the EV integrins $\alpha_6\beta_4$ and $\alpha_6\beta_1$ are associated with lung tropism, while integrin $\alpha_v\beta_5$ is associated with liver tropism [65]. Meanwhile, Kim et al. demonstrated that compared with HEK293 cell-derived EVs, SKOV3 cell-derived EVs selectively accumulated in ovarian tumors in vivo, which was likely related to cell tropism [54]. Wan et al. showed that hepatic stellate cell-derived EVs could target the liver, but there were no EVs in other organs, such as the heart, spleen, lung and kidney [33].

Specific cell types confer a certain targeting ability of EVs. However, in the applications of EVs in vivo, the poor and unstable targeting ability and off-target effects are still the principal challenges [84]. Recent studies have proposed that specific membrane modification of EVs with ligands can improve their targeting ability [17]. In general, EV modification can be classified into two broad categories: (1) direct modification of the EV membrane and (2) the generation of EVs by modifying source cells. In the former strategy, for example, Zhuang et al. showed that HEK293T cell-derived EVs were directly modified with valency-controlled tetrahedral DNA nanostructures (TDNs) conjugated with DNA aptamers, which could specifically target the liver via cholesterol anchoring [84]. In the latter strategy, Xu et al. developed EVs with a chimeric antigen receptor (CAR), which was anti-CD19, derived from anti-CD19-CAR-HEK293T cells transfected with anti-CD19CAR LVs. Consequently, these EVs could target B-cell malignancies in vivo [85].

4. Delivery of the CRISPR/Cas9 System by EVs

With precise site-specific gene editing, the CRISPR-Cas9 system has gradually become a powerful tool to cure a number of genetic disorders and tumors, especially transthyretin amyloidosis, which has entered phase 1 clinical trials [27]. As mentioned above, EVs, with good biocompatibility, low immunogenicity, capacity, protection ability, modification and targeting ability, have emerged as favorable tissue-specific vectors for delivering the CRISPR-Cas9 system and other biomacromolecules, which have been discussed. In this section, we will focus on the delivery of the CRISPR/Cas9 system by EVs, including the EV source, the isolation strategies of EVs, the delivery form of the CRISPR/Cas9 system delivered by EVs, the loading methods of the CRISPR/Cas9 system into EVs and the experimental applications of the delivery of the CRISPR/Cas9 system by EVs (Table 2).

Table 2. The CRISPR-Cas9 system delivered by EVs. UC: ultracentrifugation; SEC: size exclusion chromatography.

EV Source	Isolation Strategies	Delivery Form of CRISPR/Cas9 System	Loading Methods of CRISPR/Cas9 System	Targeting Ability	Applications	References
SKOV3 cells and HEK293 cells	UC	Plasmids	Electroporation	The tumor of SKOV3 xenograft mice	Treatment of ovarian tumor	[54]
HEK293T cells	UC	RNPs	Endogenous loading	None targeting ability	Editing cells in vitro	[86]
HEK293 cells	UC	RNPs	Endogenous loading	None targeting ability	Treatment of liver damage	[87]
Red blood cells	UC	mRNA	Electroporation	None targeting ability	Editing cells in vitro	[88]
HEK293FT cells	Polymer precipitation	Plasmids	Transfection kit	None targeting ability	Editing cells in vitro	[89]
HEK293T cells	UC	RNPs	Endogenous loading	None targeting ability	Editing cells in vitro and in vivo	[25]
HEK293T cells	UC	RNPs	Endogenous loading	None targeting ability	Editing cells in vitro	[90]
HEK293T cells	UC	RNPs	Sonication	The tumor of HepG2 xenograft mice	Treatment of liver tumor	[84]
HEK293T cells and MSCs	UC	Plasmids	Transfection kit	None targeting ability	Treatment of pancreatic tumor	[91]
Halobacterium	Centrifugation	Plasmids	Incubation	None targeting ability	Editing cells in vitro	[92]
HEK293T cells	UC	RNPs	Endogenous loading	None targeting ability	Editing cells in vitro	[93]
Expi293F cells	UC	RNPs	Endogenous loading	None targeting ability	Editing cells in vitro	[94]

Table 2. *Cont.*

EV Source	Isolation Strategies	Delivery Form of CRISPR/Cas9 System	Loading Methods of CRISPR/Cas9 System	Targeting Ability	Applications	References
LX-2 cells	UC	RNPs	Electroporation	The liver tissue	Treatment of acute liver injury, chronic liver fibrosis and hepatocellular carcinoma	[33]
A549 cells and B16-F10 cells	UC	RNPs	Endogenous loading	None targeting ability	Editing cells in vitro and in vivo	[95]
Serum	SEC	RNPs	Transfection kit	None targeting ability	Treatment of Duchenne muscular dystrophy	[96]
Anti-CD19-CAR-HEK293T cells	UC	Plasmids	Electroporation	The tumor of Raji xenograft mice	Treatment of B-cell malignancies	[85]

4.1. EV Sources

We previously discussed that the EV source determines the membrane and cargoes of EVs, which can affect the safety (toxicity and immunogenicity) and targeting ability of EVs [17]. Therefore, EV sources have been explored in the field of the delivery of the CRISPR/Cas9 system by EVs. In general, EV sources can be classified into four broad categories: (1) nontumor cells; (2) tumor cells; (3) bacteria; and (4) noncell origins. Among nontumor cells, with high EV yields, less abundant endogenous cargoes and simple culture, the human embryonic kidney cell lines HEK293 and HEK293T are widely used to generate EVs to deliver the CRISPR/Cas9 system [54,86]. Moreover, these cells are easily modified to produce engineered EVs. For example, after transfection with Cas9-sgRNA plasmids, HEK293 and HEK293T cells could produce EVs carrying RNPs to improve the efficiency of gene editing, and anti-CD19 CAR-HEK293T cells could generate anti-CD19 CAR EVs to improve tissue targeting ability [85,87]. Currently, numerous studies have proven the nontoxicity and low immunogenicity of HEK293 and HEK293T cell-derived EVs in vivo. However, the targeting ability of HEK293 and HEK293T cell-derived EVs is poor. Lainšček et al. demonstrated that after 3 h of intravenous injection into mice, HEK293 cell-derived EVs were rapidly distributed throughout the body, such as in the heart, lung, spleen, kidney and brain, and especially in the liver. With blood circulation, the EVs were still mainly distributed in the liver but were not distributed in the heart 24 h after injection [87]. Moreover, EVs can be generated by hepatic stellate cells and red blood cells to deliver the CRISPR/Cas9 system. Hepatic stellate cell-derived EVs were safe and could target the liver [33]. Usman et al. showed that with the lack of nuclear and mitochondrial DNA, the most easily available, abundant amount and safety of clinical applications, red blood cells could deliver CRISPR/Cas9 to realize gene editing [88]. MSC-derived EVs can also deliver CRISPR/Cas9 for gene editing [91].

Tumor cells, such as SKOV3, A549 and B16-F10 cells, are also used to generate EVs to deliver the CRISPR/Cas9 system [54,95]. Because of the source of tumor cells, the toxicity and immunogenicity of EVs are of serious concern. Kim et al. showed that, compared with lipopolysaccharide or CpG oligodeoxynucleotides, SKOV3 cell-derived EVs only led to human peripheral blood mononuclear cells generating a minor production of TNF-α and INF-α. Meanwhile, due to cell tropism, these EVs could target SKOV3 xenografts in vivo [54]. Furthermore, Ye et al. demonstrated that in vivo gene editing, A549 and B16-F10 cell-derived EVs could mainly accumulate in the liver. In particular, B16-F10 cell-derived EVs carried ITGβ5, which is associated with liver tropism [95].

Bacteria, such as Halobacterium, can also produce EVs that have been used to deliver the CRISPR/Cas9 system [92]. Liu et al. presented the idea that through bacteria as factories, EVs carrying RNPs and specific ligands could be produced, which is low-cost and efficient [97]. There are serum-derived EVs (noncell origin) that can deliver the CRISPR/Cas9 system. Serum-derived EVs lack immunogenicity and are easily obtained. Majeau et al. demonstrated that intravenous and intramuscular injection of serum-derived EVs did not cause adverse effects, such as inflammatory reactions, within 7 days in mice [96].

4.2. Isolation of EVs

The quality, safety, purity and yield of EVs can be controlled by isolation strategies, which is important for clinical applications in vivo. With their small size, low density and mixture with analogs (lipoprotein complexes, cell fragments and protein aggregates), the isolation of EVs is enormously challenging [80,81]. Moreover, due to the overlap of size and similar morphological characteristics, the segregation of EV subtypes, including exosomes, microvesicles and apoptotic bodies, becomes more difficult [98]. The purity, yield and integrity of EVs can be affected by the different isolation strategies [16]. Consequently, standardized and appropriate isolation strategies should be further developed. Generally, according to the principle of separation, isolation strategies can be classified into four broad categories: (1) the density of EVs (ultracentrifugation); (2) the size of EVs (ultrafiltration and size exclusion chromatography); (3) the solubility of EVs (polymer precipitation); and (4) the immunoaffinity of EVs (immunoaffinity magnetic beads).

Ultracentrifugation (UC), as the gold standard EV isolation method, is the most common strategy, accounting for almost half of EV isolation [99]. According to the density and size of EVs and their analogs, UC can remove cells, fragments and contaminants. UC possesses several advantages, for example, easy operation, low cost and largescale [98]. However, UC takes considerable time, is low throughput, cannot remove nucleic acids, lipoproteins and proteins and leads to the highly variable purity of EVs [16]. Based on the molecular size, ultrafiltration (UF) utilizes size-exclusion membranes to separate higher purity EVs than UC. However, in the process of EV isolation, the filtration membrane may be blocked by the samples, and the shear forces can destroy the membrane integrity of EVs [81]. The principle of size exclusion chromatography (SEC) is similar to that of UF [16]. Because of the porous beads, the elution speed of smaller particles is slower than that of larger particles, which can effectively protect the integrity of EVs with high purity but can lead to EVs mixed with contaminants of similar size [100]. The polymer precipitation method is used in the isolation of less soluble substances, such as EVs [98]. At present, the reagents used in the polymer precipitation method include protamine, acetate and polyethylene (PEG). With inexpensive, gentle and simple characteristics, PEG has been widely used to separate EVs, which leads to the low purity of EVs [81]. According to the immunoaffinity of EVs, immunoaffinity magnetic beads can isolate high-purity EVs. However, this method is expensive and has low yields [100]. In addition to the above methods, microfluidic approaches have also been used to isolate EVs [101]. With the development of EVs, numerous kits for EV isolation have become commercially available [81].

EV application in terms of delivering the CRISPR/Cas9 system. At present, EVs are almost completely isolated by UC. In addition, Lin et al. utilized a 500×10^{-3} M NaCl solution containing 12% PEG 6000 to separate EVs [89]. Majeau and coauthors isolated serum EVs by a size exclusion column (SEC qEV10/70 nm) and further purified them by UF [96].

4.3. The Delivery Form of the CRISPR/Cas9 System and the Loading Methods

The delivery form of the CRISPR/Cas9 system determines the efficiency of gene editing. Briefly, because they avoid the process of transcription and translation, RNPs make gene editing faster and more efficient and lower the rate of off-target effects than the DNA and RNA forms of the CRISPR/Cas9 system, but are more expensive [27]. Recent studies have demonstrated that the DNA, RNA and RNP form of the CRISPR/Cas9 system can be carried and delivered by EVs for gene editing in vitro and in vivo. For example, tumor cell-derived EVs could carry CRISPR/Cas9 plasmids to inhibit poly (ADP-ribose) polymerase-1 (PARP-1) [54]. Moreover, to improve the capacity of EVs, Lin et al. developed hybrid nanoparticles made up of EVs and liposomes [89]. Usman et al. showed that red blood cell-derived EVs could carry CRISPR/Cas9 mRNA for genome editing, and the efficiency of mRNA was higher than that of plasmids [88]. Moreover, HEK293T cell-derived EVs could also carry CRISPR/Cas9 RNPs for gene editing [86].

On the other hand, the delivery form of the CRISPR/Cas9 system can also affect the loading methods of the CRISPR/Cas9 system. Successful encapsulation of the CRISPR/Cas9 system by EVs plays a vital role in gene editing [93]. In contrast to other vectors, EVs should be intact after loading of the CRISPR/Cas9 system. The loading methods of the CRISPR/Cas9 system can be classified into two broad categories: (1) exogenous loading (directly loading the CRISPR/Cas9 system by electroporation, incubation, transfection and sonication on EVs) and (2) endogenous loading (through transforming cells to produce EVs with the loading CRISPR/Cas9 system). At present, CRISPR/Cas9 plasmids and mRNA can only be loaded by exogenous loading methods (such as electroporation and transfection kits) into EVs [54,88,89]. CRISPR/Cas9 RNPs can be loaded by exogenous loading methods (electroporation, sonication and transfection) and endogenous loading methods into EVs [33,84,86,96]. In terms of endogenous cargoes, loading cargoes of large molecular weights (such as CRISPR/Cas9 RNPs) remains challenging and under exploration [94]. Therefore, several studies have been devoted to enriching RNPs into EVs through specific interactions between modified RNPs and EVs. Wang et al. developed EVs containing arrestin domain containing protein 1 (ARRDC1), which could interact with WW-domain-containing proteins. Consequently, Cas9 was linked with WW domains to improve the enrichment of Cas9 in EVs, which did not affect the activity and functions of the Cas9 protein [86]. Yao et al. demonstrated that by utilizing the interaction between RNA aptamers and aptamer-binding proteins (ABPs), RNPs could be enriched in EVs [90]. Moreover, myristoylated Cas9 was beneficial for accumulation in EVs, which led to RNP enrichment in the EVs [93]. The RNPs could also be enriched by light-induced protein heterodimerization techniques in the EVs [94]. In addition to the above loading methods, the CRISPR/Cas9 system can potentially be loaded into EVs by the anthrax lethal toxin. Anthrax lethal toxin consists of protective antigen (PA) and lethal factor (LF). PA can form a channel to recruit and transfer LF. Based on this transporter system, foreign proteins fused with the N-terminus of LF can be delivered into cells by this system, including the Cas9 protein [102]. Meanwhile, LF is delivered not only into the cytosol but also into extracellular vesicles (EVs), which can load various cargoes into EVs, such as LFn-DTA, siRNA, ASOs and Cas9 protein [103,104].

4.4. The Application of Delivery of the CRISPR/Cas9 System by EVs

With a number of EV advantages, including safety, protection, capacity, penetrating ability, targeting ability and potential for modification, EVs are more preferably used to deliver the CRISPR/Cas9 system in vivo than in vitro [105]. At present, EVs carrying the CRISPR/Cas9 system have been used in tumor and other disease therapy.

4.4.1. Malignant Tumor Treatment

Traditional tumor treatment strategies, such as surgery, chemotherapy and radiotherapy, only effectively cure some patients and can lead to serious side effects and poor prognosis. CRISPR/Cas9 technology brings hope to tumor therapy [5,106]. Due to its connection with the DNA damage response, PARP-1 has become a promising target of tumor therapy, especially for breast and ovarian tumors [107]. Kim et al. showed that through intravenous injection of CRISPR/Cas9-loaded EVs into SKOV3 xenograft mice, PARP-1 could be effectively inhibited, reducing the tumor volume and weight [54]. Moreover, the inhibition of PARP-1 improved chemosensitivity to cisplatin. The oncogenic mutant $Kras^{G12D}$ can improve the proliferation of pancreatic tumors by Ras signaling [108]. McAndrews et al. demonstrated that MSC-derived EVs could carry and deliver the CRISPR/Cas9 plasmid to knock out the mutant $Kras^{G12D}$ oncogenic allele in KPC689 cells (derived from an autochthonous pancreatic tumor of mice), which could effectively suppress the growth of tumors in subcutaneous and orthotopic KPC689 graft mice [91]. With high overexpression in liver tumor tissue and cells, the WNT10B gene could be inhibited by siRNA to inhibit the viability and migration of HepG2 cells [109]. Zhuang et al. developed EVs modified with TDNs that could accumulate in HepG2 cells and liver tumor organoids in vitro. Meanwhile, CRISPR/Cas9 RNPs were delivered by EVs to decrease the expression of WNT10B in HepG2 xenograft mice, resulting in the inhibition of tumor growth [84]. K (lysine) acetyltransferase 5 (KAT5) plays an indispensable role in the growth of hepatocellular carcinoma. Consequently, the inhibition of KAT5 can suppress tumor growth [110]. Wan et al. showed that LX-2 cell-derived EVs could encapsulate and deliver CRISPR/Cas9 RNPs to suppress KAT5 expression in an orthotopic Huh-7 xenograft murine model, hence reducing KAT5 expression, inhibiting tumor growth and prolonging mouse survival [33]. In almost 30% of human tumors, such as Burkitt's lymphoma and other hematological malignancies, overexpression of the MYC oncogene has been detected [85]. Xu et al. developed EVs modified with anti-CD19 CAR that could accumulate in tumor tissue and deliver the CRISPR/Cas9 plasmid into subcutaneous Raji xenograft mice, leading to MYC mutation, which could induce apoptosis. Therefore, the tumor volume decreased compared with that of the control [85].

4.4.2. Benign Disease Treatment

CRISPR/Cas9 technology has gradually become a potential treatment strategy for genetic diseases and other diseases by inactivating or correcting disease-causing genes [3]. Hepatocyte growth factor (HGF) plays a crucial role in liver regeneration. Lainšček and coauthors showed that the *Hgf* gene could be improved by CRISPR/Cas9 to target the first exon in vitro. Furthermore, the alpha-naphthylisothiocyanate-induced liver damage murine model was administered EVs carrying CRISPR/Cas9 plasmids, leading to an increased HGF to induce liver regeneration and decreased ALT, bile acids, bilirubin and cholesterol [87]. The p53 upregulated modulator of apoptosis (PUMA) is associated with acetaminophen (APAP)-induced liver injury [111]. Wan and coauthors showed that, through EVs carrying CRISPR/Cas9 RNPs to inhibit the expression of PUMA protein in an APAP-induced liver injury murine model, the PUMA protein, AST and ALT levels, the number of apoptotic and necrotic cells and hyperemia could be markedly reduced, and the survival of mice was prolonged [33]. Cyclin E1 (CcnE1) can enhance the proliferation of hepatic stellate cells and is connected with liver fibrogenesis. Through the siRNA inhibition of CcnE1, the occurrence and development of fibrosis can be inhibited [112]. The CCl_4-induced chronic liver fibrosis murine model was treated with EVs carrying CRISPR/Cas9 RNPs targeting CcnE1, leading to the expression of CcnE1 and α-SMA protein being reduced. Furthermore, the initiation and development of liver fibrosis were attenuated [33]. Duchenne muscular dystrophy (DMD), caused by various mutations in the *Dmd* gene, is one of the most common genetic diseases and can reduce the expression of the dystrophin protein [113]. Majeau et al. demonstrated that with the nonsense mutation of *Dmd* gene-exon 23, *mdx* mice were injected with EVs carrying CRISPR/Cas9 RNPs to delete exons 23 and 24. Compared with the control, exons 23 and 24 were effectively deleted, and the expression of dystrophin protein was restored in muscles. Moreover, in *hDMD/mdx* mice expressing the human *Dmd* gene, the *Dmd* genes could also be modified [96].

5. Conclusions and Future Directions

The gene editing system (CRISPR/Cas9) can precisely manipulate DNA sequences to change the characteristics of cells and organs, which has potential in mechanistic research on genes and the treatment of diseases [4]. For example, in human clinical trials, genetic diseases, such as transthyretin amyloidosis (NCT04601051) and Leber congenital amaurosis (NCT03872479), are treated by CRISPR/Cas9 in vivo editing. The delivery vectors are proprietary lipid nanoparticles (LNPs) and AAVs [3,114]. Especially in terms of the treatment of clinical diseases, the CRISPR/Cas9 system should be accurately and safely delivered to the cells and organs that are needed for gene editing. Consequently, the need for appropriate vectors is urgent for clinical application [3]. At present, EVs carrying therapeutic cargoes are being evaluated for disease treatment in human clinical trials. For example, MSC-derived EVs transfected with miR-124 have been used to treat ischemic stroke (NCT03384433), and MSC-derived EVs loaded with miRNA against mutant KRAS have been used to treat pancreatic cancer (NCT03608631) [115]. However, there are no clinical trials on CRISPR/Cas9 delivered by EVs. Compared with viral and other vectors, with good biocompatibility, capacity and physiological properties, EVs are gradually regarded as the preferable "truck" with GPS carrying the CRISPR/Cas9 system for targeted delivery [48]. In this review, the delivery of the CRISPR/Cas9 system (such as vectors and the delivery form of the CRISPR/Cas9 system), the traits of EVs as vectors (including innate characteristics, physiological and pathological functions, safety and targeting ability) and the delivery of the CRISPR/Cas9 system by EVs (such as EV source and isolation strategies, the delivery form and loading methods of the CRISPR/Cas9 system and applications) have been concluded and discussed.

Ideally, with a high efficiency of gene editing and without safety problems, EVs can encapsulate CRISPR/Cas9 RNPs to target cells or tissue. At present, several studies have shown that EVs can carry and deliver the CRISPR/Cas9 system to edit genes. However, greater efforts to overcome some problems, for instance, the safety, capacity, consistent quality, yield and targeting ability of EVs, are needed. First, because of the biogenesis of EVs, a number of EV biomacromolecules have the potential to affect the physiological functions of cells. In particular, tumor-derived EVs show the ability to target tumors but contain several tumor-related molecules that have the potential to lead to tumor development and metastasis [54]. Therefore, the safety and source of EVs should be further investigated and developed. Second, the capacity of EVs and loading efficiency of CRISPR/Cas9 RNPs, which affect the efficiency of delivery and gene editing, have been mentioned. Hybrid EVs fused with other materials and enhancing the specific interaction between modified RNPs and EVs are full of prospects for improving the capacity of EVs [86]. Third, the consistent quality and yield of EVs play an indispensable role during the process of EV clinical applications, which determines the concordance and stability of EV batch to batch and the abundant supply of EVs. The stability of the EV source and isolation and further purification strategies determine the quality and yield of EVs [81]. Therefore, improving the stability of EV sources and building standard isolation and further purification strategies should be seriously considered. Fourth, the targeting ability of EVs is critical to the precise gene editing of CRISPR/Cas9 in vivo. However, the precise targeting ability of EVs, which is determined by cell tropism, is limited. At present, the targeting ability of EVs is being enhanced. There is a bright future in modifying cells to produce modified EVs with ligands and directly modifying EVs with ligands [17]. Furthermore, the advent of new CRISPR-based systems (base editors, primer editors and RNA-targeting Cas13) can remarkably improve the safety, precision and efficacy of gene editing [1]. Therefore, in the near future, with the development of EVs, genome editing can be used in clinical disease treatments.

Author Contributions: Y.L., J.B. and W.L. designed the research; X.Z., M.G. and Y.Y. contributed to the literature selection and data extraction; X.Z. and M.G. drafted the original manuscript. All authors have read and agreed to the published version of the manuscript.

Funding: The research leading to these results has received funding from the National Natural Scientific Foundations of China (No. 81900574, 82200078) and Post-Doctor Research Project, West China Hospital, Sichuan University, Grant/Award Number: 2018HXBH041.

Institutional Review Board Statement: Not applicable.

Informed Consent Statement: Not applicable.

Data Availability Statement: Not applicable.

Conflicts of Interest: The authors declare no competing interests.

References

1. Doudna, J.A. The promise and challenge of therapeutic genome editing. *Nature* **2020**, *578*, 229–236. [CrossRef] [PubMed]
2. Yang, L.; Chen, J. A Tale of Two Moieties: Rapidly Evolving CRISPR/Cas-Based Genome Editing. *Trends Biochem. Sci.* **2020**, *45*, 874–888. [CrossRef] [PubMed]
3. Pickar-Oliver, A.; Gersbach, C.A. The next generation of CRISPR-Cas technologies and applications. *Nat. Rev. Mol. Cell Biol.* **2019**, *20*, 490–507. [CrossRef]
4. Hille, F.; Richter, H.; Wong, S.P.; Bratovic, M.; Ressel, S.; Charpentier, E. The Biology of CRISPR-Cas: Backward and Forward. *Cell* **2018**, *172*, 1239–1259. [CrossRef]
5. Wang, S.W.; Gao, C.; Zheng, Y.M.; Yi, L.; Lu, J.C.; Huang, X.Y.; Cai, J.B.; Zhang, P.F.; Cui, Y.H.; Ke, A.W. Current applications and future perspective of CRISPR/Cas9 gene editing in cancer. *Mol. Cancer* **2022**, *21*, 57. [CrossRef] [PubMed]
6. Knott, G.J.; Doudna, J.A. CRISPR-Cas guides the future of genetic engineering. *Science* **2018**, *361*, 866–869. [CrossRef] [PubMed]
7. Baghini, S.S.; Gardanova, Z.R.; Abadi, S.A.H.; Zaman, B.A.; Ilhan, A.; Shomali, N.; Adili, A.; Moghaddar, R.; Yaseri, A.F. CRISPR/Cas9 application in cancer therapy: A pioneering genome editing tool. *Cell. Mol. Biol. Lett.* **2022**, *27*, 35. [CrossRef]
8. Yin, H.; Kauffman, K.J.; Anderson, D.G. Delivery technologies for genome editing. *Nat. Rev. Drug. Discov.* **2017**, *16*, 387–399. [CrossRef]
9. Yip, B.H. Recent Advances in CRISPR/Cas9 Delivery Strategies. *Biomolecules* **2020**, *10*, 839. [CrossRef]
10. Jiang, X.C.; Zhang, T.; Gao, J.Q. The in vivo fate and targeting engineering of crossover vesicle-based gene delivery system. *Adv. Drug. Deliv. Rev.* **2022**, *187*, 114324. [CrossRef]
11. Song, X.; Liu, C.; Wang, N.; Huang, H.; He, S.; Gong, C.; Wei, Y. Delivery of CRISPR/Cas systems for cancer gene therapy and immunotherapy. *Adv. Drug. Deliv. Rev.* **2021**, *168*, 158–180. [CrossRef] [PubMed]
12. Kostyushev, D.; Kostyusheva, A.; Brezgin, S.; Smirnov, V.; Volchkova, E.; Lukashev, A.; Chulanov, V. Gene Editing by Extracellular Vesicles. *Int. J. Mol. Sci.* **2020**, *21*, 7362. [CrossRef]
13. Taha, E.A.; Lee, J.; Hotta, A. Delivery of CRISPR-Cas tools for in vivo genome editing therapy: Trends and challenges. *J. Control. Release* **2022**, *342*, 345–361. [CrossRef]
14. Li, L.; Hu, S.; Chen, X. Non-viral delivery systems for CRISPR/Cas9-based genome editing: Challenges and opportunities. *Biomaterials* **2018**, *171*, 207–218. [CrossRef] [PubMed]
15. Kalluri, R.; LeBleu, V.S. The biology, function, and biomedical applications of exosomes. *Science* **2020**, *367*, eaau6977. [CrossRef] [PubMed]
16. Liu, S.; Wu, X.; Chandra, S.; Lyon, C.; Ning, B.; Jiang, L.; Fan, J.; Hu, T.Y. Extracellular vesicles: Emerging tools as therapeutic agent carriers. *Acta Pharm. Sin. B* **2022**, *12*, 3822–3842. [CrossRef]
17. Meng, W.; He, C.; Hao, Y.; Wang, L.; Li, L.; Zhu, G. Prospects and challenges of extracellular vesicle-based drug delivery system: Considering cell source. *Drug. Deliv.* **2020**, *27*, 585–598. [CrossRef]
18. Zhao, Y.; Li, X.; Zhang, W.; Yu, L.; Wang, Y.; Deng, Z.; Liu, M.; Mo, S.; Wang, R.; Zhao, J.; et al. Trends in the biological functions and medical applications of extracellular vesicles and analogues. *Acta Pharm. Sin. B* **2021**, *11*, 2114–2135. [CrossRef]
19. Yang, Y.; Huang, H.; Li, Y. Roles of exosomes and exosome-derived miRNAs in pulmonary fibrosis. *Front. Pharmacol.* **2022**, *13*, 928933. [CrossRef]
20. Massaro, C.; Sgueglia, G.; Frattolillo, V.; Baglio, S.R.; Altucci, L.; Dell'Aversana, C. Extracellular Vesicle-Based Nucleic Acid Delivery: Current Advances and Future Perspectives in Cancer Therapeutic Strategies. *Pharmaceutics* **2020**, *12*, 980. [CrossRef]
21. Jinek, M.; Jiang, F.; Taylor, D.W.; Sternberg, S.H.; Kaya, E.; Ma, E.; Anders, C.; Hauer, M.; Zhou, K.; Lin, S.; et al. Structures of Cas9 endonucleases reveal RNA-mediated conformational activation. *Science* **2014**, *343*, 1247997. [CrossRef]
22. Li, G.; Liu, Y.G.; Chen, Y. Genome-editing technologies: The gap between application and policy. *Sci. China Life Sci.* **2019**, *62*, 1534–1538. [CrossRef] [PubMed]
23. Liu, S.; Cheng, Q.; Wei, T.; Yu, X.; Johnson, L.T.; Farbiak, L.; Siegwart, D.J. Membrane-destabilizing ionizable phospholipids for organ-selective mRNA delivery and CRISPR-Cas gene editing. *Nat. Mater.* **2021**, *20*, 701–710. [CrossRef]
24. Lino, C.A.; Harper, J.C.; Carney, J.P.; Timlin, J.A. Delivering CRISPR: A review of the challenges and approaches. *Drug. Deliv.* **2018**, *25*, 1234–1257. [CrossRef]
25. Montagna, C.; Petris, G.; Casini, A.; Maule, G.; Franceschini, G.M.; Zanella, I.; Conti, L.; Arnoldi, F.; Burrone, O.R.; Zentilin, L.; et al. VSV-G-Enveloped Vesicles for Traceless Delivery of CRISPR-Cas9. *Mol. Ther. Nucleic Acids* **2018**, *12*, 453–462. [CrossRef] [PubMed]
26. Kosicki, M.; Tomberg, K.; Bradley, A. Repair of double-strand breaks induced by CRISPR-Cas9 leads to large deletions and complex rearrangements. *Nat. Biotechnol.* **2018**, *36*, 765–771. [CrossRef] [PubMed]
27. Huang, K.; Zapata, D.; Tang, Y.; Teng, Y.; Li, Y. In vivo delivery of CRISPR-Cas9 genome editing components for therapeutic applications. *Biomaterials* **2022**, *291*, 121876. [CrossRef]
28. Kim, S.; Kim, D.; Cho, S.W.; Kim, J.; Kim, J.S. Highly efficient RNA-guided genome editing in human cells via delivery of purified Cas9 ribonucleoproteins. *Genome Res.* **2014**, *24*, 1012–1019. [CrossRef]
29. Kowalski, P.S.; Rudra, A.; Miao, L.; Anderson, D.G. Delivering the Messenger: Advances in Technologies for Therapeutic mRNA Delivery. *Mol. Ther.* **2019**, *27*, 710–728. [CrossRef]
30. Mitschka, S.; Mayr, C. Context-specific regulation and function of mRNA alternative polyadenylation. *Nat. Rev. Mol. Cell Biol.* **2022**, *23*, 779–796. [CrossRef]

31. Zhang, S.; Shen, J.; Li, D.; Cheng, Y. Strategies in the delivery of Cas9 ribonucleoprotein for CRISPR/Cas9 genome editing. *Theranostics* **2021**, *11*, 614–648. [CrossRef]
32. Vakulskas, C.A.; Dever, D.P.; Rettig, G.R.; Turk, R.; Jacobi, A.M.; Collingwood, M.A.; Bode, N.M.; McNeill, M.S.; Yan, S.; Camarena, J.; et al. A high-fidelity Cas9 mutant delivered as a ribonucleoprotein complex enables efficient gene editing in human hematopoietic stem and progenitor cells. *Nat. Med.* **2018**, *24*, 1216–1224. [CrossRef] [PubMed]
33. Wan, T.; Zhong, J.; Pan, Q.; Zhou, T.; Ping, Y.; Liu, X. Exosome-mediated delivery of Cas9 ribonucleoprotein complexes for tissue-specific gene therapy of liver diseases. *Sci. Adv.* **2022**, *8*, eabp9435. [CrossRef] [PubMed]
34. Xu, X.; Liu, C.; Wang, Y.; Koivisto, O.; Zhou, J.; Shu, Y.; Zhang, H. Nanotechnology-based delivery of CRISPR/Cas9 for cancer treatment. *Adv. Drug. Deliv. Rev.* **2021**, *176*, 113891. [CrossRef] [PubMed]
35. Liu, C.; Zhang, L.; Liu, H.; Cheng, K. Delivery strategies of the CRISPR-Cas9 gene-editing system for therapeutic applications. *J. Control. Release* **2017**, *266*, 17–26. [CrossRef]
36. Wang, D.; Zhang, F.; Gao, G. CRISPR-Based Therapeutic Genome Editing: Strategies and In Vivo Delivery by AAV Vectors. *Cell* **2020**, *181*, 136–150. [CrossRef] [PubMed]
37. Verdera, H.C.; Kuranda, K.; Mingozzi, F. AAV Vector Immunogenicity in Humans: A Long Journey to Successful Gene Transfer. *Mol. Ther.* **2020**, *28*, 723–746. [CrossRef]
38. McClements, M.E.; MacLaren, R.E. Adeno-associated Virus (AAV) Dual Vector Strategies for Gene Therapy Encoding Large Transgenes. *Yale J. Biol. Med.* **2017**, *90*, 611–623.
39. Horii, T.; Arai, Y.; Yamazaki, M.; Morita, S.; Kimura, M.; Itoh, M.; Abe, Y.; Hatada, I. Validation of microinjection methods for generating knockout mice by CRISPR/Cas-mediated genome engineering. *Sci. Rep.* **2014**, *4*, 4513. [CrossRef]
40. Long, C.; McAnally, J.R.; Shelton, J.M.; Mireault, A.A.; Bassel-Duby, R.; Olson, E.N. Prevention of muscular dystrophy in mice by CRISPR/Cas9-mediated editing of germline DNA. *Science* **2014**, *345*, 1184–1188. [CrossRef]
41. Alghuthaymi, M.A.; Ahmad, A.; Khan, Z.; Khan, S.H.; Ahmed, F.K.; Faiz, S.; Nepovimova, E.; Kuca, K.; Abd-Elsalam, K.A. Exosome/Liposome-like Nanoparticles: New Carriers for CRISPR Genome Editing in Plants. *Int. J. Mol. Sci.* **2021**, *22*, 7456. [CrossRef] [PubMed]
42. Pensado, A.; Seijo, B.; Sanchez, A. Current strategies for DNA therapy based on lipid nanocarriers. *Expert Opin. Drug Deliv.* **2014**, *11*, 1721–1731. [CrossRef]
43. Lee, K.; Conboy, M.; Park, H.M.; Jiang, F.; Kim, H.J.; Dewitt, M.A.; Mackley, V.A.; Chang, K.; Rao, A.; Skinner, C.; et al. Nanoparticle delivery of Cas9 ribonucleoprotein and donor DNA in vivo induces homology-directed DNA repair. *Nat. Biomed. Eng.* **2017**, *1*, 889–901. [CrossRef] [PubMed]
44. Glass, Z.; Li, Y.; Xu, Q. Nanoparticles for CRISPR-Cas9 delivery. *Nat. Biomed. Eng.* **2017**, *1*, 854–855. [CrossRef] [PubMed]
45. Garikipati, V.N.S.; Shoja-Taheri, F.; Davis, M.E.; Kishore, R. Extracellular Vesicles and the Application of System Biology and Computational Modeling in Cardiac Repair. *Circ. Res.* **2018**, *123*, 188–204. [CrossRef]
46. Le, Q.V.; Lee, J.; Lee, H.; Shim, G.; Oh, Y.K. Cell membrane-derived vesicles for delivery of therapeutic agents. *Acta Pharm. Sin. B.* **2021**, *11*, 2096–2113. [CrossRef]
47. Du, R.; Wang, C.; Zhu, L.; Yang, Y. Extracellular Vesicles as Delivery Vehicles for Therapeutic Nucleic Acids in Cancer Gene Therapy: Progress and Challenges. *Pharmaceutics* **2022**, *14*, 2236. [CrossRef]
48. Liang, Y.; Iqbal, Z.; Wang, J.; Xu, L.; Xu, X.; Ouyang, K.; Zhang, H.; Lu, J.; Duan, L.; Xia, J. Cell-derived extracellular vesicles for CRISPR/Cas9 delivery: Engineering strategies for cargo packaging and loading. *Biomater. Sci.* **2022**, *10*, 4095–4106. [CrossRef] [PubMed]
49. He, C.; Zheng, S.; Luo, Y.; Wang, B. Exosome Theranostics: Biology and Translational Medicine. *Theranostics* **2018**, *8*, 237–255. [CrossRef]
50. Ding, J.; Chen, J.; Gao, L.; Jiang, Z.; Zhang, Y.; Li, M.; Xiao, Q.; Lee, S.S.; Chen, X. Engineered nanomedicines with enhanced tumor penetration. *Nano Today* **2019**, *29*, 100800. [CrossRef]
51. Holder, B.; Jones, T.; Shimizu, V.S.; Rice, T.F.; Donaldson, B.; Bouqueau, M.; Forbes, K.; Kampmann, B. Macrophage Exosomes Induce Placental Inflammatory Cytokines: A Novel Mode of Maternal–Placental Messaging. *Traffic* **2016**, *17*, 168–178. [CrossRef]
52. Yamamoto, S.; Kato, A.; Sakurai, Y.; Hada, T.; Harashima, H. Modality of tumor endothelial VEGFR2 silencing-mediated improvement in intratumoral distribution of lipid nanoparticles. *J. Control. Release* **2017**, *251*, 1–10. [CrossRef] [PubMed]
53. Sánchez, C.A.; Andahur, E.I.; Valenzuela, R.; Castellón, E.A.; Fullá, J.A.; Ramos, C.G.; Triviño, J.C. Exosomes from bulk and stem cells from human prostate cancer have a differential microRNA content that contributes cooperatively over local and pre-metastatic niche. *Oncotarget* **2016**, *7*, 3993–4008. [CrossRef] [PubMed]
54. Kim, S.M.; Yang, Y.; Oh, S.J.; Hong, Y.; Seo, M.; Jang, M. Cancer-derived exosomes as a delivery platform of CRISPR/Cas9 confer cancer cell tropism-dependent targeting. *J. Control. Release* **2017**, *266*, 8–16. [CrossRef]
55. Lamson, N.G.; Berger, A.; Fein, K.C.; Whitehead, K.A. Anionic nanoparticles enable the oral delivery of proteins by enhancing intestinal permeability. *Nat. Biomed. Eng.* **2020**, *4*, 84–96. [CrossRef] [PubMed]
56. Warren, M.R.; Zhang, C.; Vedadghavami, A.; Bokvist, K.; Dhal, P.K.; Bajpayee, A.G. Milk exosomes with enhanced mucus penetrability for oral delivery of siRNA. *Biomater. Sci.* **2021**, *9*, 4260–4277. [CrossRef] [PubMed]
57. Liao, Y.; Du, X.; Li, J.; Lonnerdal, B. Human milk exosomes and their microRNAs survive digestion in vitro and are taken up by human intestinal cells. *Mol. Nutr. Food Res.* **2017**, *61*, 1700082. [CrossRef]

58. Carobolante, G.; Mantaj, J.; Ferrari, E.; Vllasaliu, D. Cow Milk and Intestinal Epithelial Cell-derived Extracellular Vesicles as Systems for Enhancing Oral Drug Delivery. *Pharmaceutics* **2020**, *12*, 226. [CrossRef]
59. Sweeney, M.D.; Zhao, Z.; Montagne, A.; Nelson, A.R.; Zlokovic, B.V. Blood-Brain Barrier: From Physiology to Disease and Back. *Physiol. Rev.* **2019**, *99*, 21–78. [CrossRef]
60. Ashizawa, A.T.; Holt, J.; Faust, K.; Liu, W.; Tiwari, A.; Zhang, N.; Ashizawa, T. Intravenously Administered Novel Liposomes, DCL64, Deliver Oligonucleotides to Cerebellar Purkinje Cells. *Cerebellum* **2019**, *18*, 99–108. [CrossRef]
61. Morad, G.; Carman, C.V.; Hagedorn, E.J.; Perlin, J.R.; Zon, L.I.; Mustafaoglu, N.; Park, T.E.; Ingber, D.E.; Daisy, C.C.; Moses, M.A. Tumor-Derived Extracellular Vesicles Breach the Intact Blood-Brain Barrier via Transcytosis. *ACS Nano* **2019**, *13*, 13853–13865. [CrossRef] [PubMed]
62. Liu, J.; Jiang, F.; Jiang, Y.; Wang, Y.; Li, Z.; Shi, X.; Zhu, Y.; Wang, H.; Zhang, Z. Roles of Exosomes in Ocular Diseases. *Int. J. Nanomed.* **2020**, *15*, 10519–10538. [CrossRef] [PubMed]
63. Zhang, L.; Yu, D. Exosomes in cancer development, metastasis, and immunity. *Biochim. Biophys. Acta Rev. Cancer* **2019**, *1871*, 455–468. [CrossRef] [PubMed]
64. Kurywchak, P.; Tavormina, J.; Kalluri, R. The emerging roles of exosomes in the modulation of immune responses in cancer. *Genome Med.* **2018**, *10*, 23. [CrossRef] [PubMed]
65. Hoshino, A.; Costa-Silva, B.; Shen, T.L.; Rodrigues, G.; Hashimoto, A.; Mark, M.T.; Molina, H.; Kohsaka, S.; Di Giannatale, A.; Ceder, S.; et al. Tumour exosome integrins determine organotropic metastasis. *Nature* **2015**, *527*, 329–335. [CrossRef] [PubMed]
66. Johnson, J.; Wu, Y.W.; Blyth, C.; Lichtfuss, G.; Goubran, H.; Burnouf, T. Prospective Therapeutic Applications of Platelet Extracellular Vesicles. *Trends Biotechnol.* **2021**, *39*, 598–612. [CrossRef]
67. Kim, H.K.; Song, K.S.; Chung, J.H.; Lee, K.R.; Lee, S.N. Platelet microparticles induce angiogenesis in vitro. *Br. J. Haematol.* **2004**, *124*, 376–384. [CrossRef]
68. Zhang, L.; Jiao, G.; Ren, S.; Zhang, X.; Li, C.; Wu, W.; Wang, H.; Liu, H.; Zhou, H.; Chen, Y. Exosomes from bone marrow mesenchymal stem cells enhance fracture healing through the promotion of osteogenesis and angiogenesis in a rat model of nonunion. *Stem Cell Res. Ther.* **2020**, *11*, 38. [CrossRef]
69. Raimondo, S.; Saieva, L.; Corrado, C.; Fontana, S.; Flugy, A.; Rizzo, A.; De Leo, G.; Alessandro, R. Chronic myeloid leukemia-derived exosomes promote tumor growth through an autocrine mechanism. *Cell Commun. Signal.* **2015**, *13*, 8. [CrossRef]
70. Al-Nedawi, K.; Meehan, B.; Micallef, J.; Lhotak, V.; May, L.; Guha, A.; Rak, J. Intercellular transfer of the oncogenic receptor EGFRvIII by microvesicles derived from tumour cells. *Nat. Cell Biol.* **2008**, *10*, 619–624. [CrossRef]
71. Antonyak, M.A.; Li, B.; Boroughs, L.K.; Johnson, J.L.; Druso, J.E.; Bryant, K.L.; Holowka, D.A.; Cerione, R.A. Cancer cell-derived microvesicles induce transformation by transferring tissue transglutaminase and fibronectin to recipient cells. *Proc. Natl. Acad. Sci. USA* **2011**, *108*, 4852–4857. [CrossRef] [PubMed]
72. Giro, O.; Jimenez, A.; Pane, A.; Badimon, L.; Ortega, E.; Chiva-Blanch, G. Extracellular vesicles in atherothrombosis and cardiovascular disease: Friends and foes. *Atherosclerosis* **2021**, *330*, 61–75. [CrossRef] [PubMed]
73. Yao, M.Y.; Zhang, W.H.; Ma, W.T.; Liu, Q.H.; Xing, L.H.; Zhao, G.F. microRNA-328 in exosomes derived from M2 macrophages exerts a promotive effect on the progression of pulmonary fibrosis via FAM13A in a rat model. *Exp. Mol. Med.* **2019**, *51*, 1–16. [CrossRef]
74. Kamerkar, S.; LeBleu, V.S.; Sugimoto, H.; Yang, S.; Ruivo, C.F.; Melo, S.A.; Lee, J.J.; Kalluri, R. Exosomes facilitate therapeutic targeting of oncogenic KRAS in pancreatic cancer. *Nature* **2017**, *546*, 498–503. [CrossRef] [PubMed]
75. Wu, P.; Zhang, B.; Shi, H.; Qian, H.; Xu, W. MSC-exosome: A novel cell-free therapy for cutaneous regeneration. *Cytotherapy* **2018**, *20*, 291–301. [CrossRef]
76. Mendt, M.; Kamerkar, S.; Sugimoto, H.; McAndrews, K.M.; Wu, C.C.; Gagea, M.; Yang, S.; Blanko, E.V.R.; Peng, Q.; Ma, X.; et al. Generation and testing of clinical-grade exosomes for pancreatic cancer. *JCI Insight* **2018**, *3*, e99263. [CrossRef]
77. Zhu, X.; Badawi, M.; Pomeroy, S.; Sutaria, D.S.; Xie, Z.; Baek, A.; Jiang, J.; Elgamal, O.A.; Mo, X.; Perle, K.; et al. Comprehensive toxicity and immunogenicity studies reveal minimal effects in mice following sustained dosing of extracellular vesicles derived from HEK293T cells. *J. Extracell. Vesicles* **2017**, *6*, 1324730. [CrossRef]
78. Rahman, M.A.; Barger, J.F.; Lovat, F.; Gao, M.; Otterson, G.A.; Nana-Sinkam, P. Lung cancer exosomes as drivers of epithelial mesenchymal transition. *Oncotarget* **2016**, *7*, 54852–54866. [CrossRef]
79. Elahi, F.M.; Farwell, D.G.; Nolta, J.A.; Anderson, J.D. Preclinical translation of exosomes derived from mesenchymal stem/stromal cells. *Stem Cells* **2020**, *38*, 15–21. [CrossRef]
80. Feng, Z.Y.; Zhang, Q.Y.; Tan, J.; Xie, H.Q. Techniques for increasing the yield of stem cell-derived exosomes: What factors may be involved? *Sci. China Life Sci.* **2022**, *65*, 1325–1341. [CrossRef]
81. Chen, J.; Li, P.; Zhang, T.; Xu, Z.; Huang, X.; Wang, R.; Du, L. Review on Strategies and Technologies for Exosome Isolation and Purification. *Front. Bioeng. Biotechnol.* **2021**, *9*, 811971. [CrossRef]
82. Whitford, W.; Guterstam, P. Exosome manufacturing status. *Future Med. Chem.* **2019**, *11*, 1225–1236. [CrossRef]
83. Rana, S.; Yue, S.; Stadel, D.; Zoller, M. Toward tailored exosomes: The exosomal tetraspanin web contributes to target cell selection. *Int. J. Biochem. Cell Biol.* **2012**, *44*, 1574–1584. [CrossRef]
84. Zhuang, J.; Tan, J.; Wu, C.; Zhang, J.; Liu, T.; Fan, C.; Li, J.; Zhang, Y. Extracellular vesicles engineered with valency-controlled DNA nanostructures deliver CRISPR/Cas9 system for gene therapy. *Nucleic Acids Res.* **2020**, *48*, 8870–8882. [CrossRef]

85. Xu, Q.; Zhang, Z.; Zhao, L.; Qin, Y.; Cai, H.; Geng, Z.; Zhu, X.; Zhang, W.; Zhang, Y.; Tan, J.; et al. Tropism-facilitated delivery of CRISPR/Cas9 system with chimeric antigen receptor-extracellular vesicles against B-cell malignancies. *J. Control. Release* **2020**, *326*, 455–467. [CrossRef] [PubMed]
86. Wang, Q.; Yu, J.; Kadungure, T.; Beyene, J.; Zhang, H.; Lu, Q. ARMMs as a versatile platform for intracellular delivery of macromolecules. *Nat. Commun.* **2018**, *9*, 960. [CrossRef] [PubMed]
87. Lainscek, D.; Kadunc, L.; Keber, M.M.; Bratkovic, I.H.; Romih, R.; Jerala, R. Delivery of an Artificial Transcription Regulator dCas9-VPR by Extracellular Vesicles for Therapeutic Gene Activation. *ACS Synth. Biol.* **2018**, *7*, 2715–2725. [CrossRef] [PubMed]
88. Usman, W.M.; Pham, T.C.; Kwok, Y.Y.; Vu, L.T.; Ma, V.; Peng, B.; Chan, Y.S.; Wei, L.; Chin, S.M.; Azad, A.; et al. Efficient RNA drug delivery using red blood cell extracellular vesicles. *Nat. Commun.* **2018**, *9*, 2359. [CrossRef]
89. Lin, Y.; Wu, J.; Gu, W.; Huang, Y.; Tong, Z.; Huang, L.; Tan, J. Exosome-Liposome Hybrid Nanoparticles Deliver CRISPR/Cas9 System in MSCs. *Adv. Sci.* **2018**, *5*, 1700611. [CrossRef]
90. Yao, X.; Lyu, P.; Yoo, K.; Yadav, M.K.; Singh, R.; Atala, A.; Lu, B. Engineered extracellular vesicles as versatile ribonucleoprotein delivery vehicles for efficient and safe CRISPR genome editing. *J. Extracell. Vesicles* **2021**, *10*, e12076. [CrossRef]
91. McAndrews, K.M.; Xiao, F.; Chronopoulos, A.; LeBleu, V.S.; Kugeratski, F.G.; Kalluri, R. Exosome-mediated delivery of CRISPR/Cas9 for targeting of oncogenic Kras(G12D) in pancreatic cancer. *Life Sci. Alliance* **2021**, *4*, e202000875. [CrossRef]
92. Gao, R.; Luo, Q.; Li, Y.; Song, L.; Cai, J.S.; Xiong, Y.; Yan, F.; Liu, J. Biosynthetic Nanobubble-Mediated CRISPR/Cas9 Gene Editing of Cdh2 Inhibits Breast Cancer Metastasis. *Pharmaceutics* **2022**, *14*, 1382. [CrossRef]
93. Whitley, J.A.; Kim, S.; Lou, L.; Ye, C.; Alsaidan, O.A.; Sulejmani, E.; Cai, J.; Desrochers, E.G.; Beharry, Z.; Rickman, C.B.; et al. Encapsulating Cas9 into extracellular vesicles by protein myristoylation. *J. Extracell. Vesicles* **2022**, *11*, e12196. [CrossRef] [PubMed]
94. Osteikoetxea, X.; Silva, A.; Lazaro-Ibanez, E.; Salmond, N.; Shatnyeva, O.; Stein, J.; Schick, J.; Wren, S.; Lindgren, J.; Firth, M.; et al. Engineered Cas9 extracellular vesicles as a novel gene editing tool. *J. Extracell. Vesicles* **2022**, *11*, e12225. [CrossRef] [PubMed]
95. Ye, Y.; Shi, Q.; Yang, T.; Xie, F.; Zhang, X.; Xu, B.; Fang, J.; Chen, J.; Zhang, Y.; Li, J. In Vivo Visualized Tracking of Tumor-Derived Extracellular Vesicles Using CRISPR-Cas9 System. *Technol. Cancer Res. Treat.* **2022**, *21*, 15330338221085370. [CrossRef]
96. Majeau, N.; Fortin-Archambault, A.; Gerard, C.; Rousseau, J.; Yameogo, P.; Tremblay, J.P. Serum extracellular vesicles for delivery of CRISPR-CAS9 ribonucleoproteins to modify the dystrophin gene. *Mol. Ther.* **2022**, *30*, 2429–2442. [CrossRef]
97. Liu, Y.; Smid, E.J.; Abee, T.; Notebaart, R.A. Delivery of genome editing tools by bacterial extracellular vesicles. *Microb. Biotechnol.* **2019**, *12*, 71–73. [CrossRef] [PubMed]
98. Li, P.; Kaslan, M.; Lee, S.H.; Yao, J.; Gao, Z. Progress in Exosome Isolation Techniques. *Theranostics* **2017**, *7*, 789–804. [CrossRef]
99. Gandham, S.; Su, X.; Wood, J.; Nocera, A.L.; Alli, S.C.; Milane, L.; Zimmerman, A.; Amiji, M.; Ivanov, A.R. Technologies and Standardization in Research on Extracellular Vesicles. *Trends Biotechnol.* **2020**, *38*, 1066–1098. [CrossRef] [PubMed]
100. Zhang, Y.; Bi, J.; Huang, J.; Tang, Y.; Du, S.; Li, P. Exosome: A Review of Its Classification, Isolation Techniques, Storage, Diagnostic and Targeted Therapy Applications. *Int. J. Nanomed.* **2020**, *15*, 6917–6934. [CrossRef] [PubMed]
101. Le, M.N.; Fan, Z.H. Exosome isolation using nanostructures and microfluidic devices. *Biomed. Mater.* **2021**, *16*, 022005. [CrossRef] [PubMed]
102. Hirschenberger, M.; Stadler, N.; Fellermann, M.; Sparrer, K.M.J.; Kirchhoff, F.; Barth, H.; Papatheodorou, P. CRISPA: A Non-viral, Transient Cas9 Delivery System Based on Reengineered Anthrax Toxin. *Front. Pharmacol.* **2021**, *12*, 770283. [CrossRef] [PubMed]
103. Benedita, F.; Simon, R. Engineering protein toxins to modulate the intracellular trafficking of biologics into exosomes for third order drug targeting. *Eur. J. Extracell. Vesicles* **2022**, *2*, 1–6.
104. Simon, R.; Benedita, F. Method for Preparing Liposomes. International Patent WO2020030923A1, 13 February 2020.
105. Duan, L.; Ouyang, K.; Wang, J.; Xu, L.; Xu, X.; Wen, C.; Xie, Y.; Liang, Y.; Xia, J. Exosomes as Targeted Delivery Platform of CRISPR/Cas9 for Therapeutic Genome Editing. *ChemBioChem* **2021**, *22*, 3360–3368. [CrossRef]
106. Katti, A.; Diaz, B.J.; Caragine, C.M.; Sanjana, N.E.; Dow, L.E. CRISPR in cancer biology and therapy. *Nat. Rev. Cancer* **2022**, *22*, 259–279. [CrossRef]
107. Michels, J.; Vitale, I.; Saparbaev, M.; Castedo, M.; Kroemer, G. Predictive biomarkers for cancer therapy with PARP inhibitors. *Oncogene* **2014**, *33*, 3894–3907. [CrossRef]
108. Bryant, K.L.; Mancias, J.D.; Kimmelman, A.C.; Der, C.J. KRAS: Feeding pancreatic cancer proliferation. *Trends Biochem. Sci.* **2014**, *39*, 91–100. [CrossRef]
109. Wu, G.; Fan, X.; Sun, L. Silencing of Wnt10B reduces viability of heptocellular carcinoma HepG2 cells. *Am. J. Cancer Res.* **2015**, *5*, 1911–1920.
110. Kwan, S.Y.; Sheel, A.; Song, C.Q.; Zhang, X.O.; Jiang, T.; Dang, H.; Cao, Y.; Ozata, D.M.; Mou, H.; Yin, H.; et al. Depletion of TRRAP Induces p53-Independent Senescence in Liver Cancer by Down-Regulating Mitotic Genes. *Hepatology* **2020**, *71*, 275–290. [CrossRef]
111. Chen, D.; Ni, H.M.; Wang, L.; Ma, X.; Yu, J.; Ding, W.X.; Zhang, L. p53 Up-regulated Modulator of Apoptosis Induction Mediates Acetaminophen-Induced Necrosis and Liver Injury in Mice. *Hepatology* **2019**, *69*, 2164–2179. [CrossRef]
112. Bangen, J.M.; Hammerich, L.; Sonntag, R.; Baues, M.; Haas, U.; Lambertz, D.; Longerich, T.; Lammers, T.; Tacke, F.; Trautwein, C.; et al. Targeting CCl(4) -induced liver fibrosis by RNA interference-mediated inhibition of cyclin E1 in mice. *Hepatology* **2017**, *66*, 1242–1257. [CrossRef] [PubMed]
113. Happi Mbakam, C.; Lamothe, G.; Tremblay, G.; Tremblay, J.P. CRISPR-Cas9 Gene Therapy for Duchenne Muscular Dystrophy. *Neurotherapeutics* **2022**, *19*, 931–941. [CrossRef] [PubMed]

114. Gillmore, J.D.; Gane, E.; Taubel, J.; Kao, J.; Fontana, M.; Maitland, M.L.; Seitzer, J.; O'Connell, D.; Walsh, K.R.; Wood, K.; et al. CRISPR-Cas9 In Vivo Gene Editing for Transthyretin Amyloidosis. *N. Engl. J. Med.* **2021**, *385*, 493–502. [CrossRef] [PubMed]
115. O'Brien, K.; Breyne, K.; Ughetto, S.; Laurent, L.C.; Breakefield, X.O. RNA delivery by extracellular vesicles in mammalian cells and its applications. *Nat. Rev. Mol. Cell. Biol.* **2020**, *21*, 585–606. [CrossRef]

pharmaceutics

MDPI

Review

Oral Administration as a Potential Alternative for the Delivery of Small Extracellular Vesicles

Darío Donoso-Meneses [1,2], Aliosha I. Figueroa-Valdés [1,2], Maroun Khoury [1,2,3,4,5] and Francisca Alcayaga-Miranda [1,2,3,4,5,*]

1 Laboratory of Nano-Regenerative Medicine, Centro de Investigación e Innovación Biomédica (CiiB), Faculty of Medicine, Universidad de los Andes, Santiago 7620086, Chile
2 IMPACT, Center of Interventional Medicine for Precision and Advanced Cellular Therapy, Santiago 7620086, Chile
3 Consorcio Regenero, Chilean Consortium for Regenerative Medicine, Santiago 7550101, Chile
4 School of Medicine, Faculty of Medicine, Universidad de los Andes, Santiago 7620086, Chile
5 Cells for Cells, Santiago 7620157, Chile
* Correspondence: falcayaga@uandes.cl

Abstract: Small extracellular vesicles (sEVs) have burst into biomedicine as a natural therapeutic alternative for different diseases. Considered nanocarriers of biological origin, various studies have demonstrated the feasibility of their systemic administration, even with repeated doses. However, despite being the preferred route of physicians and patients, little is known about the clinical use of sEVs in oral administration. Different reports show that sEVs can resist the degradative conditions of the gastrointestinal tract after oral administration, accumulating regionally in the intestine, where they are absorbed for systemic biodistribution. Notably, observations demonstrate the efficacy of using sEVs as a nanocarrier system for a therapeutic payload to obtain a desired biological (therapeutic) effect. From another perspective, the information to date indicates that food-derived vesicles (FDVs) could be considered future nutraceutical agents since they contain or even overexpress different nutritional compounds of the foods from which they are derived, with potential effects on human health. In this review, we present and critically analyze the current information on the pharmacokinetics and safety profile of sEVs when administered orally. We also address the molecular and cellular mechanisms that promote intestinal absorption and that command the therapeutic effects that have been observed. Finally, we analyze the potential nutraceutical impact that FDVs would have on human health and how their oral use could be an emerging strategy to balance nutrition in people.

Keywords: small extracellular vesicles; milk-derived vesicles; food-derived vesicles; exosomes; oral delivery; oral administration; oral drug delivery; biodistribution

Citation: Donoso-Meneses, D.; Figueroa-Valdés, A.I.; Khoury, M.; Alcayaga-Miranda, F. Oral Administration as a Potential Alternative for the Delivery of Small Extracellular Vesicles. *Pharmaceutics* **2023**, *15*, 716. https://doi.org/10.3390/pharmaceutics15030716

Academic Editor: Yong Chen

Received: 25 November 2022
Revised: 11 February 2023
Accepted: 12 February 2023
Published: 21 February 2023

1. Introduction

The enteral route, including oral administration of drugs is the preferred delivery method to treat systemic diseases or local gastrointestinal (GI) pathologies due to its minimal invasiveness (pain-free), relatively low cost, and ability to self-administer [1]. However, these advantages are challenged by acidic conditions in the stomach and degrading conditions in the intestine, which affect the stability, absorption, and bioavailability of various therapeutic molecules, limiting the diversity of therapeutic compounds that can be prescribed orally [2]. Indeed, macromolecules such as proteins, peptides, or nucleic acids as free agents show only slight absorption when administered orally, as they are degraded by GI enzymes, have low stability at acidic pH and limited permeation through biological barriers [3]. Likewise, several hydrophilic and lipophilic drugs also have limitations for their oral intake since their absorption is greatly conditioned by their molecular weight, logP value, and gastrointestinal permeability, often requiring nanocarriers to generate a biological effect [4].

Nanocarriers are a colloidal transport system for drugs with a nanometric particle size (typically < 500 nm) [5]. In their oral administration, they allow the safe transport of active therapeutic molecules, improving pharmacokinetics, biodistribution, and stability, reducing toxicities, and offering a controlled release and delivery of drugs to specific sites [5]. Small extracellular vesicles (sEVs) are one of the most studied nanocarriers due to their biological origin that endows them with different and natural attributes that favor their biomedical use [6]. Defined as cell-derived nanostructures enclosed in a lipid membrane, they transport and protect an active molecular cargo composed of nucleic acids, proteins, and lipids [7–10]. In the physiologic and pathologic processes, they play a role in the regulation of intercellular communication [11,12]. As nanocarriers, they have advantageous attributes related to their proven rapid internalization, low immunogenicity even at repeated doses, high stability in physiological conditions, and the capability of modifying their internal and superficial components to generate a controlled and specific release of endogenous or loaded therapeutic molecules [13]. Compared with synthetic nanocarriers, sEVs exhibit substantial benefits in targeting, safety, and pharmacokinetics, being considered the next-generation drug delivery platform [14].

Since its introduction as a drug delivery nanosystem, research has focused on understanding the pharmacokinetics and biodistribution of intravenously (i.v.) administered sEVs [15]. The valuable information collected on this subject contrasts with the need for more knowledge about the safety, stability, pharmacokinetics, and biodistribution of orally administered sEVs, the preferred route of administration for doctors and patients. Although there are few quality studies, the data to date show that, remarkably, sEVs can withstand the harsh environment of the GI tract and reach the intestine, where they accumulate heavily. It is from the intestinal lumen where sEVs penetrate the epithelium, which is the innermost layer lining the entire GI tract and selectively regulates transport from the lumen to the underlying tissue compartment [1]. Although most of these studies are limited to a single source of sEVs, cow's milk, they remarkably demonstrate the efficacy of using sEVs as a nanocarrier system for a therapeutic payload to elicit a desired biological effect.

In this review, we first discuss the current evidence on the challenges of the ambitious concept of using sEVs as a nanocarrier system for oral prescription, focusing on the stability, bioavailability, and uptake of sEVs by intestinal cells. Second, we present a comparative analysis summarizing the biodistribution and toxicity of orally administered sEVs in murine models. Then, we investigated through the available data molecules or motifs that could explain the endogenous capacity of certain sEVs to transit the GI pathway and cause a therapeutic response, addressing the possible cellular mechanisms by which this response would be mediated. Finally, we discuss the nutraceutical perspective of the consumption of bioactive molecules within sEVs derived from food sources and their potential impact on human health.

2. Challenges of Orally Administered sEVs

sEVs are non-replicative lipid-based vesicles classified by a hydrodynamic diameter inferior to 200 nanometers (nm) [16]. They are secreted by most known cells and can be found in every biological fluid (blood, urine, saliva, breast milk, among others) [13]. Besides, their biogenesis mechanism allows the transport and protection of bioactive molecules (nucleic acids, proteins, lipids, or metabolites) from a donor towards an acceptor cell, modifying their transcriptional profile, function, or phenotype [13]. Unique properties such as high relative stability, biocompatibility, permeability, low toxicity, and low immunogenicity determine its success as a novel cell-free therapeutic agent. Their versatile properties may be modified by different bioengineering allowing the insertion of targeting motifs for specific cellular lineages in their surface, a load of therapeutic drugs or macromolecules in their membrane or lumen, or even they can be modified to increase blood circulation time (Figure 1) [17].

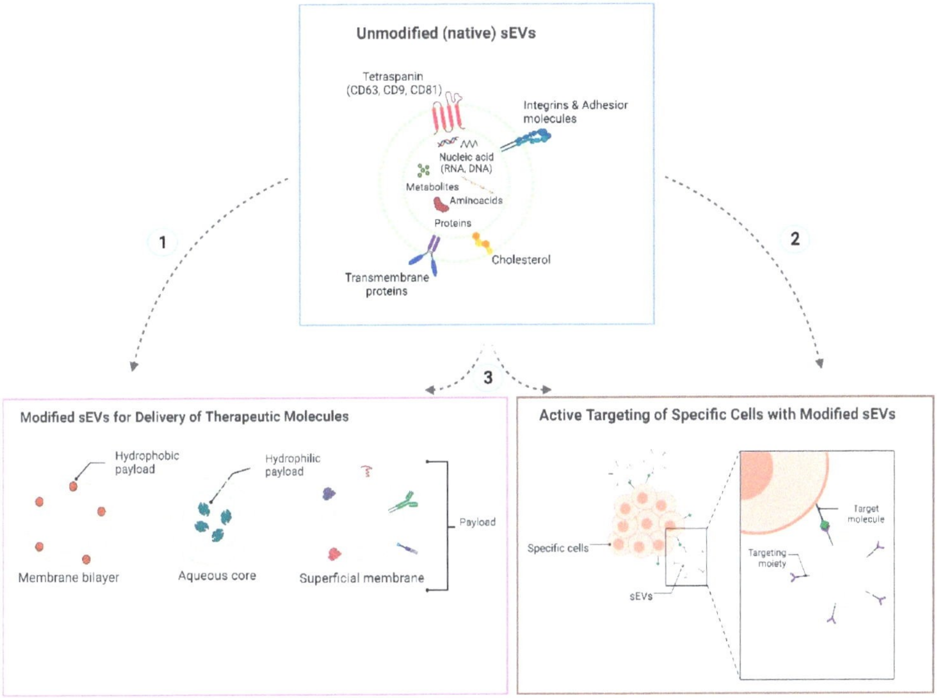

Figure 1. Diagram of the native structure of small extracellular vesicles and the functionalization strategies that can be performed on them to provide them with specific therapeutic properties. Small extracellular vesicles (sEVs) have a structure formed by a membrane composed of a lipid bilayer. Different proteins are expressed in it, which may be common to the vast majority of sEVs (such as tetraspanins for sEVs derived from eukaryotic cells) or specific proteins according to the origin of their parental cell. The core of sEVs is composed of nucleic acids, lipids, proteins, and metabolites. One of the characteristics of sEVs that make them good nanocarriers is that they can be easily modified to endow them with specific therapeutic properties. For example, to acquire a certain therapeutic efficacy, sEVs can be engineered to carry a specific therapeutic payload: drugs, proteins, or different types of nucleic acids (siRNA, miRNA, shRNA). Depending on the molecule's type and therapeutic function to be triggered, the payload can be incorporated into or anchored to the surface of the sEVs membrane. It can also be loaded into the sEVs core (1). To provide them with a better safety profile, sEVs can be functionalized to target a specific cell or tissue by incorporating a targeting moiety into their surface membrane (2). This strategy reduces off-target interactions while improving the bioavailability of the therapeutic molecule at the site of interest. Both the strategy of therapeutic loading molecules and the strategy of targeting sEVs to a specific tissue can be performed together in sEVs (3), providing the nanovesicles with better efficacy and safety profiles at the same time (created with http://www.biorender.com (accessed on 16 november 2022)).

Orally administered sEVs must survive the harsh degrading conditions of the digestive system as moisture, lubricants, mechanical forces, digestive enzymes, emulsifiers, pH neutralizers [2], commensal microbiota and their derivates [18] to successfully reach the intestine and deliver their therapeutic payload regionally or be absorbed intact for systemic distribution (Figure 2). The latter is the most challenging since once the sEVs penetrate the intestinal mucus layer, they must cross the intestinal epithelium to reach the lamina propria and cross the endothelium of blood vessels for systemic distribution [19]. When synthetic nanoparticles are orally ingested, most are degraded or eliminated, and a small fraction is effectively absorbed [20]. Nonetheless, it is currently unknown if the same proportion of orally administrated sEVs is degraded or eliminated since sEVs differs in their surface molecules, expressing receptors, peptides, saccharides, and lipids from a biological progenitor.

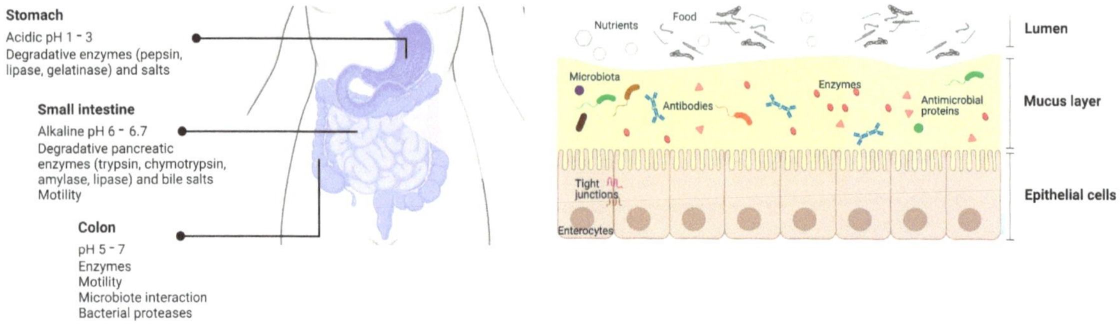

Figure 2. Scheme of the gastrointestinal tract and the physiological factors that influence the absorption of therapeutic molecules. Several physiological barriers in the gastrointestinal (GI) tract challenge drug administration by the oral route. In the GI environment, the presence of factors such as pH, degradative enzymes and salts, motility and interaction with the microbiota can alter the solubility and stability of drugs, which finally affect their permeability across the mucosal barriers. This figure is based on a schematic drawing and does not fully represent the accurate structural reality of the intestine (created with http://www.biorender.com (accessed on 21 november 2022)).

To date, it has been described that different types of nanoparticles can cross the intestinal epithelium using different mechanisms, such as paracellular transport [1]. Paracellular transport consists of the diffusion of particles between cells through tight junctions that form the intestinal epithelial barrier. However, due to limited physical dimensions between cells in physiological conditions, only particles ranging between 0.5 and 20 nm should be considered for this mechanism in a relevant proportion [21]. Conversely, a pro-inflammatory context in the intestine disrupts the epithelial barrier, allowing the passing of larger particles, as demonstrated by Tulkens et al. [22]. Thus, based on the reported results, the paracellular transport of an oral administration of sEVs (>200 nm) should only be considered in inflammatory diseases of the intestine or treatments that disrupt the epithelial barrier as side effects.

The second mechanism described by which nanoparticles cross the intestinal layers and reach systemic circulation is transcellular transport by epithelial cells (mainly enterocytes that constitute 90–95% of the cells in the GI tract) and M-cells (specialized phagocytic cells that represent 1% of the intestinal epithelium) [1]. Transcellular transport consists of the endocytosis of particles in the apical face, the intracellular transit, and posterior exocytosis in the basal face [20]. The main challenge for this route of absorption is avoiding the transport and fusion of the intracellular vesicles with lysosomes enriched in degradative enzymes. A unidirectional transport of bacterial-derived extracellular vesicles (bEVs) was demonstrated by epithelial cells in vitro, where a small proportion was "re-secreted" towards the basal face, partially supporting the proof of concept of orally ingested sEVs potential absorption and lysosome avoiding [23]. A better understanding of the molecular mechanism of uptake by these intestinal cells could contribute to an engineered increased interaction with sEVs. Macropinocytosis, caveolin, and clathrin-dependent endocytosis are the principal mechanisms described for particle uptake in enterocytes. In M-cells, the most studied are the uptake by phagocytosis and receptor-mediated endocytosis [20].

3. Biodistribution, Stability, and Safety of Oral Delivery of Native and Drug Loaded sEVs

Murine studies identifying the biodistribution pattern of orally administered sEVs are few and focus mainly on cow's milk-derived sEVs, although we have found some studies using plant-derived exosomes-like particles. These studies show that sEVs/exosomes-like particles manage to withstand the hostile environment of the gastrointestinal tract, associated with their transit through acidic conditions in the stomach and degradative conditions in the gut, in various murine models [24–26]. Cow's milk-derived sEVs cross the upper gastrointestinal tract and reach the intestine in relatively short times (1–6 h) [27,28]. The absorption of sEVs seems to occur in the gut through mechanisms that are not well understood, but that facilitates the entry of sEVs into the systemic circulation and their distribution in other organs, essentially localized in the abdominal cavity [27–31]. Unlike the "trapping" of sEVs in the organs of the mononuclear phagocytic system (liver, spleen, and lung) after systemic injection of sEVs [17], oral ingestion allows a considerable accumulation of sEVs in the intestine [27,28,30,32–34]. In the other organs of the body, the accumulation of sEVs is less but notably shows a homogeneous distribution among them. Figure 3 shows the biodistribution pattern in mice after oral and systemic administration.

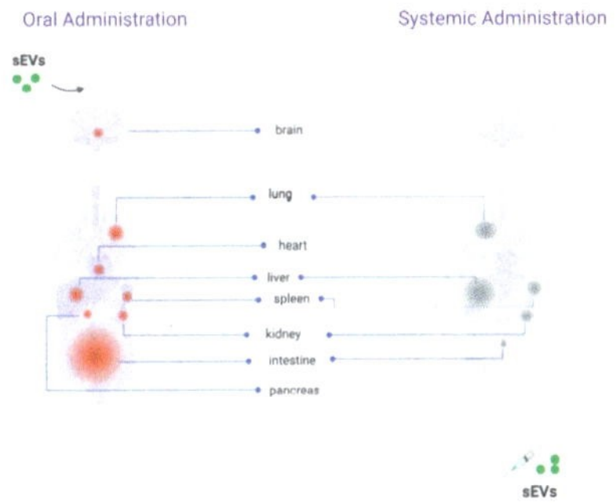

Figure 3. Comparative diagram of the biodistribution pattern of sEV administered orally and intravenously. The illustration shows the pattern of biodistribution of sEVs in different mice tissues after oral or intravenous administration. In the body on the left, the tissues and organs where the sEV would accumulate after intestinal absorption are identified in red. The considerable accumulation of sEVs in the intestine and, to a lesser extent, in the rest of the body's organs stands out. In the body on the right, the organs where sEVs would accumulate after intravenous administration are identified in gray. A considerable accumulation of sEVs is observed in the organs associated with the mononuclear phagocytic system (liver, spleen, lung), with little reach to other body organs. These data suggest that the biodistribution pattern is defined by the route of administration of the sEVs, a dependency that can be used strategically to reach a specific organ in patients (created with http://www.biorender.com (accessed on 2 february 2023)).

Interestingly, repeated oral administration of cow's milk-derived sEVs on mice seems to not alter the biodistribution pattern observed after a single oral intake of sEVs [28]. Betker et al. [29] and Samuel et al. [28] also show that orally ingested sEVs can migrate and accumulate in xenograft tumors in vivo. Other sources of sEVs studied in similar investigations are those obtained from yeast [28], beer [28], grape [34], acerola [33], ginger [32], garlic [35], tea leaves [36], and mulberry bark [37]. Yeast-, grape-, acerola-, ginger-, garlic-, tea leaves- and mulberry bark-derived sEVs showed a biodistribution pattern like that previously described for cow's milk-derived sEVs, but beer-derived sEVs in the mouse's organs could not be detected [28]. Interestingly, orally ingested ginger-derived exosomes-like particles showed a differential bio-distribution after 12 h of gavage depending on the feed condition of mice: starved mice accumulated exosomes-like particles in the stomach and small intestine, whereas non-starved mice accumulated exosomes-like particles in the colon [32]. These conditions open a new variable to consider for the pharmacokinetic profile of the oral administration of sEVs, loaded or not with drugs. Whether or not other cellular sources (of prokaryotic or eukaryotic origins) of sEVs can cross the harsh microenvironment of the gastrointestinal tract and replicate the biodistribution pattern described so far is still unknown. Table 1 summarizes the key aspects of the studies performed to determine the biodistribution pattern of sEVs/exosomes-like particles administered orally, including the type of sEVs, the cellular origin of the sEVs, doses of sEVs administered, time of detection, tissue distribution, among other variables of relevance.

Table 1. Comparative summary of the biodistribution of orally administered sEVs.

Type of sEV	Cell Source	Labeling Method	Dose	Mouse Strain	Time of Detection and Tissue Distribution	Reference
sEVs	Bovine milk	DiR	0.5 mg prot/mouse	C57BL/6 mice with DSS-induced ulcerative colitis	1 h Small intestine 6 h Colon	[27]
Exosomes	Bovine milk	DiR	1×10^{12} part/gr of mouse	Balb/c mice	24 h Intestine, lung, and liver	[30]
Exosomes	Bovine milk	DiR	40 mg prot/kg of mouse	Balb/c mice	30 min Blood 6 h Liver, spleen, kidney, heart, and lung	[29]
iRGD-Exosomes	Bovine milk	DiR	40 mg prot/kg of mouse	Tumor-bearing Balb/c mice	4 h Tumor, liver, spleen, kidney, lung, and heart	[29]
Exosomes	Bovine milk	DiR	60 mg prot/kg of mouse	Athymic nude mice	4 d Liver, lung, kidney, pancreas, spleen, ovaries, colon, and brain	[31]
sEVs	Bovine milk	DiR	25 mg prot/kg of mouse	Balb/c mice	2 and 6 h Intestine 24 h GI tract, liver, spleen, lungs, kidney, and heart	[28]
sEVs	Bovine milk	DiR	25 mg prot/kg of mouse/day × 38 days	Balb/c-Fox1nuAusb mice	24 h Tumor tissue	[28]
sEVs	Yeast	DiR	25 mg prot/kg of mouse	Not indicated	24 h GI tract, liver, spleen, kidney, lungs, and heart	[28]
sEVs	Beer	DiR	Not indicated	Not indicated	Not bioavailable in the mice	[28]
Exosomes-like	Grape	DiR, PKH26	1 mg/mouse	C57BL/6 mice	6 h Intestine	[34]
Exosomes-like	Acerola	PKH26	3×10^{9} particles/mouse	C57BL/6 mice	1 h Intestine, liver, and bladder, weak signal in brain	[33]
Exosomes-like	Ginger	DiR	0.3 mg/mouse	C57BL/6 mice	12 h Colon (in non-starved mice); 12 h Stomach and small intestine (in starved mice)	[32]
Exosomes-like	Garlic	DiR PKH26	1×10^{10} particles/mouse	C57BL/6 mice	24 h Brain, liver, small intestine, and large intestine	[35]
Exosomes-like	Tea leaves	DiR	3 mg/kg of mouse	Balb/c mice	6 h Small intestine	[36]
Exosomes-like	Mulberry bark	DiR	10×10^{10} particles/mouse	C57BL/6 mice	3 h Small intestine, colon, cecum; small fraction was observed in spleen, liver, lung, kidney, heart, and blood	[37]

Abbreviations: sEVs, small extracellular vesicles; DIR, DiIC18(7); 1,1′-dioctadecyl-3,3,3′,3′-tetramethylindotricarbocyanine iodide; part, particles; prot, protein; gr, grams; kg, kilograms; DSS, dextran sodium sulfate; min, minutes; h, hours; d, days; GI tract, gastrointestinal tract.

As mentioned, the intestine is the anatomic site where the absorption of sEVs seems to occur after oral gavage in mice, which results in their entry into the bloodstream. Transendocytosis through intestinal epithelial cells [29,38] or paracellular translocation through the epithelial barrier [22] are some proposed mechanisms for this phenomenon. Figure 4 shows the mechanisms of cellular absorption of orally administered sEVs that are expected to occur in the human intestinal epithelium. This figure was elaborated based on data obtained from preclinical studies. Recently, Wu et al. [25] determined through a series of well-established experiments that cow´s milk derived sEVs loaded with insulin exhibited efficient internalization by active multiple endocytic routes to the epithelia. Since sEVs derived from the milk (nutrient), the authors also studied the involvement of the nutrient-assimilation pathway. The data showed that the uptake of milk-derived sEVs its mediated by peptide transporter, amino acid transporters, glucose transporters, and the neonatal Fc receptor (FcRn) [25], as was first proposed by Betker et al. [29]. However, the uptake of sEVs was not affected by Niemann-Pick C1-like 1 (NPC1L1) protein, which mediates the absorption of cholesterol and phytosterols [25]. According to Sriwastva et al. [37] mulberry bark-derived exosome-like particles were predominantly taken up by gut epithelial cells, Paneth cells, and colon tissue. Furthermore, in the spleen and liver, these particles were predominantly present in F4/80+ macrophages. In this work, mice showed no adverse effects, no significant changes in body weight, skin rashes, or abnormal fecal discharge, and no abnormal effects regarding morphology of internal organs, microscopic structure of gut tissue, blood cholesterol, triglycerides, or liver enzyme alanine transaminase. Due to the complex composition and structure of sEVs, more receptors and transporters need to be investigated to elucidate the endocytic mechanisms that facilitate uptake in intestinal epithelial cells. As well as, to validate the data obtained in in vitro experimental settings in in vivo conditions.

Little information exists about other pharmacokinetic parameters of orally administered sEVs. Regarding its stability in circulation, Munagala et al. [31] observed that cow's milk-derived sEVs remained in circulation for at least 24 h after oral administration in nude mice. Results that strongly contrast with the numerous studies demonstrating the rapid clearance rate of circulating exogenous exosomes after systemic injection (~2–30 min), mainly mediated by macrophages [17]. Why sEVs absorbed from the gastrointestinal tract have a longer circulating half-life than observed in systemically administered sEVs is a question that must be answered to understand the real clinical potential of oral administration of sEVs. It is worth mentioning that the same research group subsequently tested milk-derived sEVs for oral administration of the chemotherapeutic drug paclitaxel (PAC) in a lung tumor xenograft model, demonstrating that orally administered PAC-loaded sEVs significantly inhibited tumor growth compared to the same dose of PAC administered intraperitoneally. These PAC-loaded sEVs showed remarkably lower systemic and immunologic toxicities as compared to i.v. PAC [39]. Soo Kim et al. [40] loaded murine RAW 264.7 macrophages-derived sEVs with PAC, showing a more than 50-fold increase of cytotoxicity in drug resistant $MDCK_{MDR1}$ (Pgp+) cells in vitro.

The studies that evaluated the safety profile of sEVs orally administered consistently showed that the parameters of body weight, plasma cytokine concentration, or tissue damage remain unchanged, suggesting they are well-tolerated and non-immunogenic. Although these studies were performed mainly in milk-derived sEVs, different concentrations, and even at repeated doses, toxicity data confirm preliminarily the potential clinical use of milk-derived sEVs. Table 2 details the main results that allow knowing the safety profile of oral administration of sEVs. Nonetheless, we highlight the fact that vesicles derived from food sources may not be the exclusive sEVs that possess the capacity to be absorbed after oral ingestion, emphasizing the lack of information from other sEVs sources with proven therapeutic properties such as mesenchymal stem cells [41].

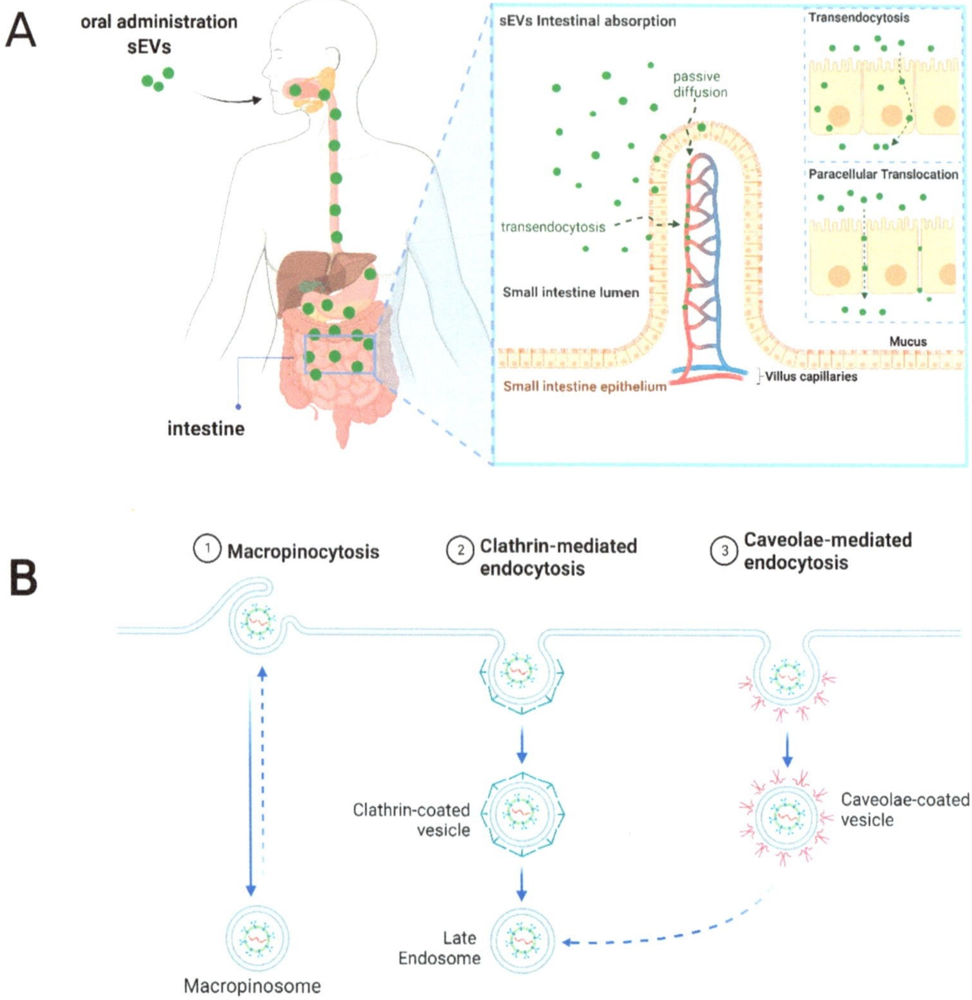

Figure 4. Scheme of the cellular mechanisms of absorption in the gastrointestinal tract of orally administered sEVs. (**A**) After oral intake, sEVs can resist the hostile degradative environment of the gastrointestinal tract and reach the intestine. At this site, the absorption of sEVs or their transport into the systemic circulation would occur, overcoming the cell permeability barrier. This figure was constructed based on preclinical in vivo/in vitro revised data and is a theorical extrapolation of what is expected in human. (**B**) In vitro studies demonstrate that multiple endocytic pathways are involved, including caveola- and clathrin-mediated pathways and macropinocytosis. Additionally, it has been described that sEVs could cross the intestinal epithelium through the intercellular spaces between epithelial cells, passively transported from the intestinal lumen to the circulation in a mechanism called paracellular translocation (created with http://www.biorender.com (accessed on 24 November 2022)).

Table 2. Summary of the main findings related to toxicity studies after oral intake of sEVs.

sEVs Type and Cell Source	Dose	Murine Strain	Time of Detection	Toxicity Profile	Reference
Cow's milk-derived exosomes	25 mg/kg (single administration) 25 mg/kg daily × 15 d	Sprague Dawley rats	6 h 15 d	No changes in clinical signs, body weight, or dietary intake in animals. Biochemical (liver and kidney function) and hematological parameters remained unchanged except for triglycerides. No changes in cytokine profile (IL-1α, IL-1β, IL-2, IL-4, IL-5, IL-6, IL-10, IL-12, IL-13, GM-CSF, IFN-γ and TNF-α), except for the anti-inflammatory cytokine GM-CSF.	[31]
Cow's milk-derived sEVs	2 mg/kg × 7 d	IRC mice	7 d	No changes in body weight in animals. Biochemical (liver function) and hematological parameters remained unchanged. Histopathology examination (H&E staining) of the heart, liver, spleen, lung, kidney, and small intestine exhibited no pathological changes.	[25]

Abbreviations: sEVs, small extracellular vesicles; mg, miligrams; kg, kilograms; h, hours; d, days.

4. sEVs Attributes for an Efficient Oral Administration

Very few studies have investigated the use of sEVs formulations for gastric drug delivery. According to Bardonnet et al. [42], nanoparticle size is essential for gastric retention because particles with a diameter < 7 mm are efficiently evacuated. Since sEVs possess a much smaller size range of 50–200 nm [13], in their native state (unmodified) is unlikely to exert any biological effect in the stomach due to weak gastric retention. However, modifying sEVs with mucoadhesion strategies using polymers or phospholipids in their surface membrane could give them time to trigger the desired biological changes [1]. Regarding intestinal drug delivery, using unmodified sEVs as nanocarriers has demonstrated promising results. Several studies have reported systemic absorption of drugs in the intestine from sEVs or a regional effect, as described in the previous section. However, a wide array of modifications has also been tested to improve sEVs stability in the GI tract, uptake by intestinal cells, and even delivery to cells independent (or far from) of the GI system. Table 3 presents a summary of these articles, where they were classified according to the source of sEVs, the attribute or modification studied, the use of sEVs as a drug nanocarrier, and the observed biological effect and the type of models utilized. As a note to mention, most articles on the oral administration of sEVs are based on the use of vesicles derived from edible compounds (fruits, vegetables, spices, milk, or its derivatives), as extensively reviewed by Ciéslik et al. [24].

Table 3. Summary of sEVs reported attributes for oral administration.

	sEV Source	sEV Attribute/ Modification/Treatment	Loaded Molecule	Biological Effect	Type of Study	References
sEVs protection in transit trough digestive tract	Bovine milk and colorectal cancer cells	Calcium chloride addition	N/A	Enhanced EV stability after acidification (pH = 2) and boiling (105 °C)	In vitro	[28]
	Human cardiosphere-derived stromal cells	Casein addition	N/A	Enhanced uptake and disease-modifying bioactivity	In vivo	[43]
sEVs uptake by gut cells	Grape juice	Phosphatidic acids, Phosphatidylethanolamines	N/A	Dextrane sulfate sodium-induced colitis protection via induction of intestinal stem cells	In vivo	[34]

Table 3. *Cont.*

	sEV Source	sEV Attribute/ Modification/Treatment	Loaded Molecule	Biological Effect	Type of Study	References
sEVs targeting beyond gut mucosa	Bovine milk	Non modified	N/A	Tumor growth reduction and accelerated metastasis, xenograft	In vivo	[28]
	Bovine milk	Folic acid functionalization	Withaferin A Anthocyanidins Curcumin Paclitaxel Docetxel	Tumor targeting, xenograft	In vivo	[31]
	Human umbilical cord	Non modified	N/A	Antioxidant and anti-apoptotic and rescue from liver failure	In vivo	[44]
	Human MSC544 cell line	Non modified	Taxol	Tumor reducing capabilities	In vivo	[45]
	Mouse suppresor T cells	Antibodies free light chains coating	miRNA-150	Immune tolerance	In vivo	[46]

Abbreviations: sEVs, small extracellular vesicles; N/A, not applicable.

Of all these sources of sEVs, notably bovine milk has reported increased stability in acidic media that emulate the conditions of the stomach lumen and structural conservation after boiling due to the presence of calcium in comparison to colorectal cancer-derived sEVs (LIM1215 cells) [28]. Besides, the addition of casein (a highly abundant protein in breast milk) has been shown to enhance the uptake of sEVs isolated from human cardiosphere-derived stromal/progenitor cells after oral ingestion [43]. The modification of sEVs with casein also presented an increased biological effect than unmodified sEVs in cardiac dysfunction [43]. This data indirectly supports the bovine milk-derived sEVs as nanocarriers for oral drug delivery since the abundant natural presence of casein in the milk should confer similar properties to those isolated vesicles. Another compound present in breast milk from various species is folic acid [47]. In a publication from Munagala et al. [31], the addition of folic acid to the surface of sEVs isolated from bovine milk and loaded with withaferin A decreased the tumor volume in a murine model of lung cancer. The modification with folic acid in the sEVs surface increased the therapeutic effect in this cancer model compared to the unmodified sEVs; however, it is not clarified if this response is attributed to enhanced stability in the GI tract or if a targeting to tumor cells after systemic circulation is reached [31].

Another approach for increasing the uptake of milk-derived sEVs was published by Warren et al. [3], where they modified the surface of the vesicles with Polyethylene glycol (PEG). Due to this modification, hydrophobic interactions with mucin (present in the lumen of the intestine) are decreased, thus enhancing the interaction, uptake by epithelial cells, and delivery of a loaded siRNA in vitro. Besides, adding PEG to the surface of the milk-derived sEVs increased the recovery after incubation in acidic conditions mimicking an infant (pH 4.5) or adult (pH 2.2) stomach acidity [3].

Another studied source of sEVs with therapeutic properties after oral delivery is grape juice. Ju et al. [34] showed that grape exosome-like nanoparticles (GELNs) isolated from grape juice possess bioactivity in intestinal stem cells, protecting from colitis in an in vivo-induced model and facilitating organoid formation in vitro. They assembled liposome-like nanoparticles with lipids from these GELNs and showed their role in in vivo targeting of intestinal stem cells through oral gavage [34]. As mentioned previously, it is currently unknown how these modifications mentioned above could modify the bioavailability of sEVs isolated from other sources different from foods or their derivatives.

5. Cellular and Molecular Mediators for sEVs Uptake after Oral Administration

Despite the incipient understanding of the cellular/molecular mechanism that regulates the biological effect of sEVs through oral administration, in the literature, it is possible to find several articles reporting therapeutic efficacy when sEVs are administered orally in models of inflammatory diseases and cancer.

In an induced cutaneous delayed-type hypersensitivity (DTH) model, Nazimek et al. [48] and Wasik et al. [49] demonstrated that T cells and B1a cells secrete a subpopulation of immunosuppressive sEVs that contain the inhibitory miRNA-150, which prevent inflammation and DTH after systemic administration in mice [48,49]. In the second of these publications [49] intravenous, intraperitoneal, intradermal, and oral administration of equivalents doses of the immunosuppressive sEVs were tested head-to-head to evaluate the anti-inflammatory response. Unexpectedly, the most potent anti-inflammatory effect was registered in the oral administration of the T cells- and B1 cells-derived sEVs. However, no further data is detailed that could explain these findings [49]. When the murine model of DTH was previously depleted of macrophages administrating clodronate liposomes, the anti-inflammatory properties of the T cells-derived sEVs were significantly lost, suggesting that the response of orally administrated T cells-derived sEVs was mediated in part by these myeloid cells [48].

This immunological effect mediated by macrophages after sEVs injection is widely described in the literature since the significant clearance of sEVs in systemic circulation occurs through these myeloid cells [17,50–52]. Peyer's patches (PPs) are subepithelial lymphoid follicles present in the intestine greatly enriched in innate and adaptive immune cells [53]. These dome-shaped clusters control antigen presentation and immunological response by several mechanisms, being the most studied the transendocytosis by specialized epithelial cells named microfold cells (M-cells) towards resident macrophages and dendritic cells [54]. The M-cells have also been previously studied for drug delivery employing synthetic nanoparticles as carrier platforms since these cells have reduced intracellular enzymatic activity and thinner mucus layer and glycocalyx in comparison to enterocytes, promoting easier access and intracellular transport [1]. In the field of drug delivery using nanoparticles, several articles study the active targeting of M-cells through surface modifications, adding peptides [55], mannose receptors ligands [56], and lectin ligands [57], but in most cases, the modification do not fully control unspecific interaction since other cellular lineages express the same receptors. In Table 4 we summarized the studies with cells present in the GI tract that potentially contribute to the uptake of sEVs after oral administration.

Table 4. Summary of cellular and molecular mediators of sEVs uptake in oral administration.

Cell Lineage	Target Cell Source	sEV Source	Findings	Type of Study	References
Microfold cells (M cells)	Several sources	N/A (Synthetic nanoparticles)	M cells possess reduced intracellular enzymatic activity, thinner mucus layer and glycocalyx, promoting easier access and intracellular transport.	In vitro In vivo	[1]
Macrophages	Ag-presenting macrophages	Ts cell-derived	Macrophage clodronate depletion abolishes anti-inflammatory effect of Ts derived sEVs observed in DTH model.	In vivo	[48]
Dendritic cells	Transgenic reporter mice	M cell-derived vesicles	M cell-derived vesicles are taken up by dendritic cells.	In vivo	[58]
Enterocytes	Rat intestinal epithelial cells (IEC-6)	Grapefruit juice	Plant EV's miRNAs are taken up by rat intestinal enterocytes.	In vitro	[59]

Table 4. *Cont.*

Cell Lineage	Target Cell Source	sEV Source	Findings	Type of Study	References
Colonocytes	Human colonocyte cell line (DLD-1) Mouse intestinal epithelial cell line (CMT-93)	Colonic luminal fluid aspirates	sEVs mRNA was present within cells, showing take up.	In vitro	[60]
Enterocytes	Porcine intestinal cells (IPEC-J2)	Porcine milk	sEVs promoted enterocytes proliferation in vitro. increased villus height, crypt depth and ratio of villus length to crypt depth of intestinal tissues was observed in vivo.	In vitro In vivo	[61]
Enterocytes	Rat intestinal epithelial cells (IEC-6) Human colon carcinoma (Caco-2)	Bovine milk	sEVs uptake decreased when incubated at low temperature (4 °C), after proteinase K treatment, using endocytosis inhibitors or carbohydrate competitors.	In vitro	[38]

Abbreviations: Ag, antigen; DTH, delayed-type hypersensitivity; Ts, suppressor T cell; N/A, not applicable.

Notably, Rubio et al. [23] demonstrated a unidirectional transport from the apical face towards the basal face of fluorescent-labeled *B. subtilis*-derived bEVs in polarized epithelial Caco-2 cells in vitro, where a fraction of those bEVs did not fuse with the cellular membranes and where secreted to the other side. From this study, three major questions arise: (1) if this described transport mechanism is conserved to all sources of sEVs (e.g., bovine milk or human derived EVs); (2) if those secreted "intact" sEVs conserve their capacity to regulate the acceptor cell function and transcriptional expression; (3) if the observed mechanism also occurs in vivo. Regarding the secretion of sEVs from epithelial cells in vivo, Sakhon et al. [58] reported in transgenic mice that M-cells constitutively release sEVs to the subepithelial space, where the highest co-localization was observed with myeloid cells (CX3CR1+/CD11b+ and CX3CR1+/CD11c+ cells). To date, diverse available data concerning the therapeutic mechanism of action of orally administered sEVs partially supports the concept of epithelial transendocytosis and uptake by the immune cells within PPs. However, this idea requires further experiments to confirm it.

The previously mentioned relationship between epithelial and immune cells from the intestine cannot fully explain the observed phenomena in inflammatory bowel disease (IBD) and cancer models. Tulkens et al. [22] demonstrated that patients with intestinal barrier dysfunction allow the paracellular translocation of bacterial bEVs (diffusion through gaps between adjacent cells), which in the end increased the production of proinflammatory cytokines. This effect was conserved for patients with different treatments (HIV infection, IBD, and chemotherapy), demonstrating that it is vinculated with intestinal barrier dysfunction rather than a particular pathology [22]. Besides, the results published by Samuel et al. [28] showed increased fluorescent signal in tumors of colorectal cancer murine models after oral gavaging of bovine milk-derived sEVs. This result, added to other articles that mention the biodistribution of orally ingested sEVs, suggests that a fraction of the vesicles enter systemic circulation, reaching other tissues and organs, as mentioned above. In a recent review, Ciéslik et al. [24] listed the therapeutic effects of orally administered sEVs from various sources assessed in different diseases. Among the cited pathologies, several articles demonstrate an effect in organs that do not belong to the GI system, suggesting that the ingested circulatory vesicles maintain therapeutic properties [24]. Nevertheless, in most articles that study the therapeutic effect of orally ingested sEVs, only the outcome is measured and characterized without a detailed explanation of a potential mechanism of action that sustains their results.

6. Food Derived Vesicles (FDVs)-Based Nutraceutical Perspectives in Infant and Elderly Health

In the last decade, structures morphologically like extracellular vesicles (EVs), called "food-derived vesicles" or FDVs, have been isolated from different foods (such as honey, pollen, milk, fruits, and vegetables, among other foods). These findings raise the question of whether FDVs contain or overexpress the nutritional compounds or nutraceutical effects of the foods from which they are derived. Several studies have shown that different FDVs have nutraceutical effects. For example, it was observed that the nanovesicles in *Apis mellifera* hypopharyngeal gland secretomal products (honey, royal jelly, and bee pollen) participate in the known antibacterial and pro-regenerative properties of bee-derived products [62]. Furthermore, Chen et al. [63] described that honey-derived nanoparticles possess anti-inflammatory properties by inhibiting the NLRP3 inflammasome, thus preventing liver damage in vivo. As the research mentioned, various other studies report the presence of FDVs and their bioactive compounds in different models of diseases such as cancer, intestinal inflammation, and autoimmune diseases [64]. In global terms, the biological effect reported for FDVs is highly associated with the source of identification. However, comparing articles is challenging since different isolation methods are employed, the doses administrated are different, and several routes of administration are tested [36,64].

Several studies have revealed the effects of sEVs derived from breast milk on the immune function of infants. The analysis of breast milk-derived sEVs showed that the molecules they contain vary depending upon the maternal allergy status [65]. Malnutrition in the elderly population is an important risk factor for sarcopenia, osteoporosis, and other age-related diseases. Protein and other components are key nutrients for the human body and affect bone and muscle mass and quality. Dairy products are rich in these nutrients, which implies that dairy products or their bioactive components, such as sEVs might be ideal for the elderly population. The use of milk sEVs as bioactive ingredients represents a novel avenue to explore in the context of human nutrition, and they might exert significant beneficial effects at multiple levels, including but not limited to intestinal health, bone and muscle metabolism, immunity, modulation of the microbiota, growth and development [66].

Due to its nutritional and immunological benefits, bovine milk-derived sEVs have become an essential fraction of proteomic research. An open online database of bovine milk proteome was established, BoMiProt (http://bomiprot.org accessed on 17 november 2022), with over 3100 proteins from whey, milk fat globule membranes (MFGM), and sEVs [67]. Interestingly, ~70% of the research on bovine milk has focused on whey proteins, followed by MFGM (20%) with a surge of sEVs in the past ten years, counting around 10%. The protein lists across milk fractions were compared to identify common and exclusive proteins among whey, MFGM, and sEVs. Interestingly, more than 1300 proteins were exclusively found in exosomes, while 801 and 294 proteins were identified in whey and MFGM, respectively. In contrast, 131 proteins were common across all the fractions [67].

To complement the content characterization, a recent lipidomic study showed eight major lipid classes found in milk sEVs, in which more than 200 fatty acid variations were identified, demonstrating the high complexity of the lipid composition of such vesicles. Also, high levels of phosphatidylcholine (PC), phosphatidylethanolamine (PE), cholesterol (Chol), and phosphatidylserine (PS) were measured. Interestingly, sEVs exhibited increased levels of phosphatidylinositol (PI) as compared to sEVs isolated from cultured cells [68]. Other cargoes, including long noncoding RNAs (lncRNAs) identified in human breast milk sEVs, are also proposed to be implicated in adult metabolism, infant metabolism, neonatal, and development [69].

Many relevant questions need to be answered to understand the value of sEVs in milk formulas since the content of sEVs, and their cargo is modest to not detectable [70]. Dietary depletion of milk sEVs elicited phenotypes such as increased purine metabolites in human and murine body fluids and tissues [71]. Dietary depletion of these sEVs also caused a variety of phenotypes in mice, including a moderate loss of grip strength, an increase in the severity of symptoms of inflammatory bowel disease, a decrease in the postnatal survival, and changes in bacterial communities in the ceca [72]. These observations raise concerns regarding infant and adult nutrition using milk formulas and the need to fortify them with sEVs supplements. However, the compatibility of adding sEVs with existing compounds is crucial for efficient absorption. A recent clinical study by Mutai et al. showed that fortification of soy formulas with milk sEVs must be done by removing lectins for a viable strategy for delivering bioavailable exosomes and their cargos. Lectins in soy formulas bind glycoprotein on the surfaces of milk sEVs, thereby preventing exosome absorption [72].

As a final reflection, this interkingdom relationship has been present throughout the entire existence of animals by dietary consumption, but little was known before the identification of the FDVs.

7. Limitation, Future Direction and Conclusions

While oral administration of sEVs presents various physiological and practical advantages over other routes, there is an existing need to investigate further the safety, stability, pharmacokinetics, and biodistribution attributes before their broad use as drug vehicles or nutritional supplements. Most biodistribution studies rely on DiR-based labeling of the sEVs, while DiR labeling does not affect sEVs morphology [73]; however, molecular dissociation between the dye and the sEVs can occur in an in vivo setting and might lead to misleading pharmacokinetic outcomes. Using foreign RNA sequences that quantitative PCR can assess could lead to more precise information devoid of possible artifacts.

The few quality studies presented in the different tables of this review display remarkable features of sEVs being able to resist the harsh acidic environment of the GI tract and reach the intestine. However, most FDVs studies are almost exclusively based on milk-derived sEVs. For this, these findings must be expanded for other FDVs of interest, membrane components, and surface markers depending on the source of isolation. Also, proper readouts must be determined to assess their capacity to elicit significant effects following oral intake.

So far, milk-derived sEVs are the most feasible option for a drug delivery application based on their published safety profile, pharmacokinetics, and endogenous stability in the GI tract. Nonetheless, this does not mean, in any case, that these properties are exclusive for this source of sEVs. As we mention in this article, studies evaluating other sources of vesicles in detail could discover an optimal sEVs-based nanocarrier for oral drug delivery.

It is interesting to mention that oral administration is getting closer to clinical-stage application. So far, we have found only one clinical trial seeking to characterize the ability of plant-derived exosomes in the delivery of curcumin to colon tissue in the context of colon cancer via oral intake (ClinicalTrials.gov Identifier: NCT01294072). This study is ongoing, and no data or results are available yet.

Several preclinical and clinical studies have failed to show a positive association between milk intake and serum miRNA levels. However, the role of miRNA cargo, the extent to which they are exported via the sEVs route, and whether they contribute to cell-cell communication are still controversial. Albanese et al. found that sEVs did not fuse detectably with cellular membranes to deliver their cargo. They engineered sEVs to be fusogenic and documented their capacity to deliver functional messenger RNAs. Engineered fusogenic sEVs, however, did not detectably alter the functionality of cells exposed to miRNA-carrying sEVs. These results suggest that sEVs-borne miRNAs do not act as effectors of cell-to-cell communication, suggesting that the delivery of different RNA species through the sEVs might be an extremely inefficient process [74].

The interaction of xeno-EVs (plant or bovine to human cells) adds another layer of complication to deciphering the fusion and cargo delivery processes, identifying the glycan features and other pathways on the EVs surface responsible for the interaction between plant/animal EVs and human cells. In conclusion, oral administration presents a reliable delivery route for EVs. The pharmacokinetics and activity of these bioactive compounds will depend on their cellular source, cargo content, and interaction with human cells.

Author Contributions: All authors contributed equally to the conceptualization, investigation, resources, writing (original draft preparation), writing (review and editing) and visualization of this article. F.A.-M. and M.K.: supervision and funding acquisition. All authors have read and agreed to the published version of the manuscript.

Funding: This work was funded by Chilean National Research and Development Agency, ANID FONDECYT Regular #1190411 grant, ANID FONDECYT Regular #1211749 grant, and ANID Basal Funding for Scientific and Technological Centers of Excellence IMPACT #FB210024 grant.

Institutional Review Board Statement: This article does not contain any studies with human or animal subjects.

Informed Consent Statement: Not applicable.

Data Availability Statement: The data that support the findings of this study are available from the corresponding author upon reasonable request.

Acknowledgments: The authors especially thank Paulina Lopez Miranda for the English revision of the manuscript.

Conflicts of Interest: Francisca Alcayaga-Miranda and Maroun Khoury received stipends from Cells for Cells. The other authors have no conflict of interest to declare.

References

1. Hua, S. Advances in Oral Drug Delivery for Regional Targeting in the Gastrointestinal Tract—Influence of Physiological, Pathophysiological and Pharmaceutical Factors. *Front. Pharmacol.* **2020**, *11*, 524. [CrossRef] [PubMed]
2. Homayun, B.; Lin, X.; Choi, H.-J. Challenges and Recent Progress in Oral Drug Delivery Systems for Biopharmaceuticals. *Pharmaceutics* **2019**, *11*, 129. [CrossRef]
3. Warren, M.R.; Zhang, C.; Vedadghavami, A.; Bokvist, K.; Dhal, P.K.; Bajpayee, A.G. Milk Exosomes with Enhanced Mucus Penetrability for Oral Delivery of SiRNA. *Biomater. Sci.* **2021**, *9*, 4260–4277. [CrossRef]
4. Siew, A.; Le, H.; Thiovolet, M.; Gellert, P.; Schatzlein, A.; Uchegbu, I. Enhanced Oral Absorption of Hydrophobic and Hydrophilic Drugs Using Quaternary Ammonium Palmitoyl Glycol Chitosan Nanoparticles. *Mol. Pharm.* **2012**, *9*, 14–28. [CrossRef] [PubMed]
5. Din, F.U.; Aman, W.; Ullah, I.; Qureshi, O.S.; Mustapha, O.; Shafique, S.; Zeb, A. Effective Use of Nanocarriers as Drug Delivery Systems for the Treatment of Selected Tumors. *Int. J. Nanomed.* **2017**, *12*, 7291–7309. [CrossRef] [PubMed]
6. Yang, B.; Chen, Y.; Shi, J. Exosome Biochemistry and Advanced Nanotechnology for Next-Generation Theranostic Platforms. *Adv. Mater.* **2019**, *31*, e1802896. [CrossRef] [PubMed]
7. Figueroa-Valdés, A.I.; de la Fuente, C.; Hidalgo, Y.; Vega-Letter, A.M.; Tapia-Limonchi, R.; Khoury, M.; Alcayaga-Miranda, F. A Chemically Defined, Xeno- and Blood-Free Culture Medium Sustains Increased Production of Small Extracellular Vesicles from Mesenchymal Stem Cells. *Front. Bioeng. Biotechnol.* **2021**, *9*, 619930. [CrossRef] [PubMed]
8. Alcayaga-Miranda, F.; Varas-Godoy, M.; Khoury, M. Harnessing the Angiogenic Potential of Stem Cell-Derived Exosomes for Vascular Regeneration. *Stem Cells Int.* **2016**, *2016*, 3409169. [CrossRef]
9. Schuh, C.M.A.P.; Cuenca, J.; Alcayaga-Miranda, F.; Khoury, M. Exosomes on the Border of Species and Kingdom Intercommunication. *Transl. Res.* **2019**, *210*, 80–98. [CrossRef]
10. Zavala, G.; Ramos, M.-P.; Figueroa-Valdés, A.I.; Cisternas, P.; Wyneken, U.; Hernández, M.; Toa, P.; Salmons, B.; Dangerfield, J.; Gunzburg, W.H.; et al. Semipermeable Cellulose Beads Allow Selective and Continuous Release of Small Extracellular Vesicles (SEV) from Encapsulated Cells. *Front. Pharmacol.* **2020**, *11*, 679. [CrossRef]
11. Rosenberger, L.; Ezquer, M.; Lillo-Vera, F.; Pedraza, P.L.; Ortúzar, M.I.; González, P.L.; Figueroa-Valdés, A.I.; Cuenca, J.; Ezquer, F.; Khoury, M.; et al. Stem Cell Exosomes Inhibit Angiogenesis and Tumor Growth of Oral Squamous Cell Carcinoma. *Sci. Rep.* **2019**, *9*, 663. [CrossRef] [PubMed]
12. Alcayaga-Miranda, F.; González, P.L.; Lopez-Verrilli, A.; Varas-Godoy, M.; Aguila-Díaz, C.; Contreras, L.; Khoury, M. Prostate Tumor-Induced Angiogenesis Is Blocked by Exosomes Derived from Menstrual Stem Cells through the Inhibition of Reactive Oxygen Species. *Oncotarget* **2016**, *7*, 44462–44477. [CrossRef] [PubMed]
13. Kalluri, R.; LeBleu, V.S. The Biology, Function, and Biomedical Applications of Exosomes. *Science* **2020**, *367*, eaau6977. [CrossRef] [PubMed]
14. Herrmann, I.K.; Wood, M.J.A.; Fuhrmann, G. Extracellular Vesicles as a Next-Generation Drug Delivery Platform. *Nat. Nanotechnol.* **2021**, *16*, 748–759. [CrossRef] [PubMed]
15. Kang, M.; Jordan, V.; Blenkiron, C.; Chamley, L.W. Biodistribution of Extracellular Vesicles Following Administration into Animals: A Systematic Review. *J. Extracell. Vesicles* **2021**, *10*, e12085. [CrossRef] [PubMed]
16. Théry, C.; Witwer, K.W.; Aikawa, E.; Alcaraz, M.J.; Anderson, J.D.; Andriantsitohaina, R.; Antoniou, A.; Arab, T.; Archer, F.; Atkin-Smith, G.K.; et al. Minimal Information for Studies of Extracellular Vesicles 2018 (MISEV2018): A Position Statement of the International Society for Extracellular Vesicles and Update of the MISEV2014 Guidelines. *J. Extracell. Vesicles* **2018**, *7*, 1535750. [CrossRef]
17. Parada, N.; Romero-Trujillo, A.; Georges, N.; Alcayaga-Miranda, F. Camouflage Strategies for Therapeutic Exosomes Evasion from Phagocytosis. *J. Adv. Res.* **2021**, *31*, 61–74. [CrossRef]

18. Azman, M.; Sabri, A.H.; Anjani, Q.K.; Mustaffa, M.F.; Hamid, K.A. Intestinal Absorption Study: Challenges and Absorption Enhancement Strategies in Improving Oral Drug Delivery. *Pharmaceuticals* **2022**, *15*, 975. [CrossRef]
19. Reinholz, J.; Landfester, K.; Mailänder, V. The Challenges of Oral Drug Delivery via Nanocarriers. *Drug Deliv.* **2018**, *25*, 1694–1705. [CrossRef]
20. Yu, M.; Yang, Y.; Zhu, C.; Guo, S.; Gan, Y. Advances in the Transepithelial Transport of Nanoparticles. *Drug Discov. Today* **2016**, *21*, 1155–1161. [CrossRef]
21. Chen, M.-C.; Mi, F.-L.; Liao, Z.-X.; Hsiao, C.-W.; Sonaje, K.; Chung, M.-F.; Hsu, L.-W.; Sung, H.-W. Recent Advances in Chitosan-Based Nanoparticles for Oral Delivery of Macromolecules. *Adv. Drug Deliv. Rev.* **2013**, *65*, 865–879. [CrossRef] [PubMed]
22. Tulkens, J.; Vergauwen, G.; Van Deun, J.; Geeurickx, E.; Dhondt, B.; Lippens, L.; De Scheerder, M.-A.; Miinalainen, I.; Rappu, P.; De Geest, B.G.; et al. Increased Levels of Systemic LPS-Positive Bacterial Extracellular Vesicles in Patients with Intestinal Barrier Dysfunction. *Gut* **2020**, *69*, 191–193. [CrossRef] [PubMed]
23. Rubio, A.P.D.; Martínez, J.; Palavecino, M.; Fuentes, F.; López, C.M.S.; Marcilla, A.; Pérez, O.E.; Piuri, M. Transcytosis of Bacillus Subtilis Extracellular Vesicles through an in Vitro Intestinal Epithelial Cell Model. *Sci. Rep.* **2020**, *10*, 3120. [CrossRef] [PubMed]
24. Cieślik, M.; Nazimek, K.; Bryniarski, K. Extracellular Vesicles—Oral Therapeutics of the Future. *Int. J. Mol. Sci.* **2022**, *23*, 7554. [CrossRef]
25. Wu, L.; Wang, L.; Liu, X.; Bai, Y.; Wu, R.; Li, X.; Mao, Y.; Zhang, L.; Zheng, Y.; Gong, T.; et al. Milk-Derived Exosomes Exhibit Versatile Effects for Improved Oral Drug Delivery. *Acta Pharm. Sin. B* **2022**, *12*, 2029–2042. [CrossRef]
26. Zhong, J.; Xia, B.; Shan, S.; Zheng, A.; Zhang, S.; Chen, J.; Liang, X.-J. High-Quality Milk Exosomes as Oral Drug Delivery System. *Biomaterials* **2021**, *277*, 121126. [CrossRef]
27. Tong, L.; Hao, H.; Zhang, Z.; Lv, Y.; Liang, X.; Liu, Q.; Liu, T.; Gong, P.; Zhang, L.; Cao, F.; et al. Milk-Derived Extracellular Vesicles Alleviate Ulcerative Colitis by Regulating the Gut Immunity and Reshaping the Gut Microbiota. *Theranostics* **2021**, *11*, 8570–8586. [CrossRef]
28. Samuel, M.; Fonseka, P.; Sanwlani, R.; Gangoda, L.; Chee, S.H.; Keerthikumar, S.; Spurling, A.; Chitti, S.V.; Zanker, D.; Ang, C.-S.; et al. Oral Administration of Bovine Milk-Derived Extracellular Vesicles Induces Senescence in the Primary Tumor but Accelerates Cancer Metastasis. *Nat. Commun.* **2021**, *12*, 3950. [CrossRef]
29. Betker, J.L.; Angle, B.M.; Graner, M.W.; Anchordoquy, T.J. The Potential of Exosomes from Cow Milk for Oral Delivery. *J. Pharm. Sci.* **2019**, *108*, 1496–1505. [CrossRef]
30. Manca, S.; Upadhyaya, B.; Mutai, E.; Desaulniers, A.T.; Cederberg, R.A.; White, B.R.; Zempleni, J. Milk Exosomes Are Bioavailable and Distinct MicroRNA Cargos Have Unique Tissue Distribution Patterns. *Sci. Rep.* **2018**, *8*, 11321. [CrossRef]
31. Munagala, R.; Aqil, F.; Jeyabalan, J.; Gupta, R.C. Bovine Milk-Derived Exosomes for Drug Delivery. *Cancer Lett.* **2016**, *371*, 48–61. [CrossRef] [PubMed]
32. Zhang, M.; Viennois, E.; Prasad, M.; Zhang, Y.; Wang, L.; Zhang, Z.; Han, M.K.; Xiao, B.; Xu, C.; Srinivasan, S.; et al. Edible Ginger-Derived Nanoparticles: A Novel Therapeutic Approach for the Prevention and Treatment of Inflammatory Bowel Disease and Colitis-Associated Cancer. *Biomaterials* **2016**, *101*, 321–340. [CrossRef] [PubMed]
33. Umezu, T.; Takanashi, M.; Murakami, Y.; Ohno, S.-I.; Kanekura, K.; Sudo, K.; Nagamine, K.; Takeuchi, S.; Ochiya, T.; Kuroda, M. Acerola Exosome-Like Nanovesicles to Systemically Deliver Nucleic acid Medicine via Oral Administration. *Mol. Ther.-Methods Clin. Dev.* **2021**, *21*, 199–208. [CrossRef] [PubMed]
34. Ju, S.; Mu, J.; Dokland, T.; Zhuang, X.; Wang, Q.; Jiang, H.; Xiang, X.; Deng, Z.-B.; Wang, B.; Zhang, L.; et al. Grape Exosome-Like Nanoparticles Induce Intestinal Stem Cells and Protect Mice from DSS-Induced Colitis. *Mol. Ther.* **2013**, *21*, 1345–1357. [CrossRef] [PubMed]
35. Sundaram, K.; Mu, J.; Kumar, A.; Behera, J.; Lei, C.; Sriwastva, M.K.; Xu, F.; Dryden, G.W.; Zhang, L.; Chen, S.Y.; et al. Garlic Exosome-Like Nanoparticles Reverse High-Fat Diet Induced Obesity via the Gut/Brain Axis. *Theranostics* **2022**, *12*, 1220–1246. [CrossRef] [PubMed]
36. Chen, Q.; Zu, M.; Gong, H.; Ma, Y.; Sun, J.; Ran, S.; Shi, X.; Zhang, J.; Xiao, B. Tea Leaf-Derived Exosome-like Nanotherapeutics Retard Breast Tumor Growth by pro-Apoptosis and Microbiota Modulation. *J. Nanobiotechnol.* **2023**, *21*, 6. [CrossRef] [PubMed]
37. Sriwastva, M.K.; Deng, Z.; Wang, B.; Teng, Y.; Kumar, A.; Sundaram, K.; Mu, J.; Lei, C.; Dryden, G.W.; Xu, F.; et al. Exosome-like Nanoparticles from Mulberry Bark Prevent DSS-Induced Colitis via the AhR/COPS8 Pathway. *EMBO Rep.* **2022**, *23*, e53365. [CrossRef]
38. Wolf, T.; Baier, S.R.; Zempleni, J. The Intestinal Transport of Bovine Milk Exosomes Is Mediated by Endocytosis in Human Colon Carcinoma Caco-2 Cells and Rat Small Intestinal IEC-6 Cells. *J. Nutr.* **2015**, *145*, 2201–2206. [CrossRef]
39. Agrawal, A.K.; Aqil, F.; Jeyabalan, J.; Spencer, W.A.; Beck, J.; Gachuki, B.W.; Alhakeem, S.S.; Oben, K.; Munagala, R.; Bondada, S.; et al. Milk-Derived Exosomes for Oral Delivery of Paclitaxel. *Nanomedicine* **2017**, *13*, 1627–1636. [CrossRef]
40. Kim, M.S.; Haney, M.J.; Zhao, Y.; Mahajan, V.; Deygen, I.; Klyachko, N.L.; Inskoe, E.; Piroyan, A.; Sokolsky, M.; Okolie, O.; et al. Development of Exosome-Encapsulated Paclitaxel to Overcome MDR in Cancer Cells. *Nanomed. Nanotechnol. Biol. Med.* **2016**, *12*, 655–664. [CrossRef]
41. Lai, P.; Weng, J.; Guo, L.; Chen, X.; Du, X. Novel Insights into MSC-EVs Therapy for Immune Diseases. *Biomark. Res.* **2019**, *7*, 6. [CrossRef] [PubMed]
42. Bardonnet, P.L.; Faivre, V.; Pugh, W.J.; Piffaretti, J.C.; Falson, F. Gastroretentive Dosage Forms: Overview and Special Case of Helicobacter Pylori. *J. Control. Release* **2006**, *111*, 1–18. [CrossRef] [PubMed]
43. Aminzadeh, M.A.; Fournier, M.; Akhmerov, A.; Jones-Ungerleider, K.C.; Valle, J.B.; Marbán, E. Casein-Enhanced Uptake and Disease-Modifying Bioactivity of Ingested Extracellular Vesicles. *J. Extracell. Vesicles* **2021**, *10*, e12045. [CrossRef] [PubMed]
44. Yan, Y.; Jiang, W.; Tan, Y.; Zou, S.; Zhang, H.; Mao, F.; Gong, A.; Qian, H.; Xu, W. HucMSC Exosome-Derived GPX1 Is Required for the Recovery of Hepatic Oxidant Injury. *Mol. Ther.* **2017**, *25*, 465–479. [CrossRef] [PubMed]

45. Melzer, C.; von der Ohe, J.; Hass, R. Anti-Tumor Effects of Exosomes Derived from Drug-Incubated Permanently Growing Human MSC. *Int. J. Mol. Sci.* **2020**, *21*, 7311. [CrossRef] [PubMed]
46. Nazimek, K.; Askenase, P.W.; Bryniarski, K. Antibody Light Chains Dictate the Specificity of Contact Hypersensitivity Effector Cell Suppression Mediated by Exosomes. *Int. J. Mol. Sci.* **2018**, *19*, 2656. [CrossRef] [PubMed]
47. Collins, R.A.; Habpeb, A.E.; Scheeibee, M.; Elvehjem, C.A. The Folio Acid and Vitamin B_{12} Content of the Milk of Various Species1. *J. Nutr.* **1951**, *43*, 313–321. [CrossRef]
48. Nazimek, K.; Bryniarski, K.; Ptak, W.; Kormelink, T.G.; Askenase, P.W. Orally Administered Exosomes Suppress Mouse Delayed-Type Hypersensitivity by Delivering Mirna-150 to Antigen-Primed Macrophage Apc Targeted by Exosome-Surface Anti-Peptide Antibody Light Chains. *Int. J. Mol. Sci.* **2020**, *21*, 5540. [CrossRef]
49. Wąsik, M.; Nazimek, K.; Nowak, B.; Askenase, P.W.; Bryniarski, K. Delayed-Type Hypersensitivity Underlying Casein Allergy Is Suppressed by Extracellular Vesicles Carrying Mirna-150. *Nutrients* **2019**, *11*, 907. [CrossRef]
50. Zhang, M.; Johnson-Stephenson, T.K.; Wang, W.; Wang, Y.; Li, J.; Li, L.; Zen, K.; Chen, X.; Zhu, D. Mesenchymal Stem Cell-Derived Exosome-Educated Macrophages Alleviate Systemic Lupus Erythematosus by Promoting Efferocytosis and Recruitment of IL-17+ Regulatory T Cell. *Stem Cell Res. Ther.* **2022**, *13*, 484. [CrossRef]
51. Imai, T.; Takahashi, Y.; Nishikawa, M.; Kato, K.; Morishita, M.; Yamashita, T.; Matsumoto, A.; Charoenviriyakul, C.; Takakura, Y. Macrophage-Dependent Clearance of Systemically Administered B16BL6-Derived Exosomes from the Blood Circulation in Mice. *J. Extracell. Vesicles* **2015**, *4*, 26238. [CrossRef] [PubMed]
52. Donoso-Meneses, D.; Figueroa-Valdés, A.I.; Georges, N.; Tobar, H.E.; Alcayaga-Miranda, F. Turning Adversity into Opportunity: Small Extracellular Vesicles as Nanocarriers for Tumor-Associated Macrophages Re-Education. *Bioeng. Transl. Med.* **2022**, *8*, e10349. [CrossRef] [PubMed]
53. Da Silva, C.; Wagner, C.; Bonnardel, J.; Gorvel, J.-P.; Lelouard, H. The Peyer's Patch Mononuclear Phagocyte System at Steady State and during Infection. *Front. Immunol.* **2017**, *8*, 1254. [CrossRef]
54. Dillon, A.; Lo, D.D. M Cells: Intelligent Engineering of Mucosal Immune Surveillance. *Front. Immunol.* **2019**, *10*, 1499. [CrossRef] [PubMed]
55. Garinot, M.; Fiévez, V.; Pourcelle, V.; Stoffelbach, F.; des Rieux, A.; Plapied, L.; Theate, I.; Freichels, H.; Jérôme, C.; Marchand-Brynaert, J.; et al. PEGylated PLGA-Based Nanoparticles Targeting M Cells for Oral Vaccination. *J. Control. Release* **2007**, *120*, 195–204. [CrossRef]
56. De Coen, R.; Vanparijs, N.; Risseeuw, M.D.P.; Lybaert, L.; Louage, B.; De Koker, S.; Kumar, V.; Grooten, J.; Taylor, L.; Ayres, N.; et al. pH-Degradable Mannosylated Nanogels for Dendritic Cell Targeting. *Biomacromolecules* **2016**, *17*, 2479–2488. [CrossRef] [PubMed]
57. Chionh, Y.-T.; Wee, J.L.K.; Every, A.L.; Ng, G.Z.; Sutton, P. M-Cell Targeting of Whole Killed Bacteria Induces Protective Immunity against Gastrointestinal Pathogens. *Infect. Immun.* **2009**, *77*, 2962–2970. [CrossRef]
58. Sakhon, O.S.; Ross, B.; Gusti, V.; Pham, A.J.; Vu, K.; Lo, D.D. M Cell-Derived Vesicles Suggest a Unique Pathway for Trans-Epithelial Antigen Delivery. *Tissue Barriers* **2015**, *3*, e1004975. [CrossRef]
59. Ito, Y.; Taniguchi, K.; Kuranaga, Y.; Eid, N.; Inomata, Y.; Lee, S.-W.; Uchiyama, K. Uptake of Micrornas from Exosome-Like Nanovesicles of Edible Plant Juice by Rat Enterocytes. *Int. J. Mol. Sci.* **2021**, *22*, 3749. [CrossRef]
60. Mitsuhashi, S.; Feldbrügge, L.; Csizmadia, E.; Mitsuhashi, M.; Robson, S.C.; Moss, A.C. Luminal Extracellular Vesicles (EVs) in Inflammatory Bowel Disease (IBD) Exhibit Proinflammatory Effects on Epithelial Cells and Macrophages. *Inflamm. Bowel Dis.* **2016**, *22*, 1587–1595. [CrossRef]
61. Chen, T.; Xie, M.-Y.; Sun, J.-J.; Ye, R.-S.; Cheng, X.; Sun, R.-P.; Wei, L.-M.; Li, M.; Lin, D.-L.; Jiang, Q.-Y.; et al. Porcine Milk-Derived Exosomes Promote Proliferation of Intestinal Epithelial Cells. *Sci. Rep.* **2016**, *6*, 33862. [CrossRef]
62. Schuh, C.M.A.P.; Aguayo, S.; Zavala, G.; Khoury, M. Exosome-Like Vesicles in *Apis mellifera* Bee Pollen, Honey and Royal Jelly Contribute to Their Antibacterial and Pro-Regenerative Activity. *J. Exp. Biol.* **2019**, *222*, jeb208702. [CrossRef] [PubMed]
63. Chen, X.; Liu, B.; Li, X.; An, T.T.; Zhou, Y.; Li, G.; Wu-Smart, J.; Alvarez, S.; Naldrett, M.J.; Eudy, J.; et al. Identification of Anti-Inflammatory Vesicle-like Nanoparticles in Honey. *J. Extracell. Vesicles* **2021**, *10*, e12069. [CrossRef] [PubMed]
64. Munir, J.; Lee, M.; Ryu, S. Exosomes in Food: Health Benefits and Clinical Relevance in Diseases. *Adv. Nutr. Int. Rev. J.* **2020**, *11*, 687–696. [CrossRef] [PubMed]
65. Paredes, P.T.; Gutzeit, C.; Johansson, S.; Admyre, C.; Stenius, F.; Alm, J.; Scheynius, A.; Gabrielsson, S. Differences in Exosome Populations in Human Breast Milk in Relation to Allergic Sensitization and Lifestyle. *Allergy Eur. J. Allergy Clin. Immunol.* **2014**, *69*, 463–471. [CrossRef] [PubMed]
66. García-Martínez, J.; Pérez-Castillo, M.; Salto, R.; López-Pedrosa, J.M.; Rueda, R.; Girón, M.D. Beneficial Effects of Bovine Milk Exosomes in Metabolic Interorgan Cross-Talk. *Nutrients* **2022**, *14*, 1442. [CrossRef] [PubMed]
67. Maity, S.; Bhat, A.H.; Giri, K.; Ambatipudi, K. BoMiProt: A Database of Bovine Milk Proteins. *J. Proteom.* **2020**, *215*, 103648. [CrossRef]
68. Grossen, P.; Portmann, M.; Koller, E.; Duschmalé, M.; Minz, T.; Sewing, S.; Pandya, N.J.; van Geijtenbeek, S.K.; Ducret, A.; Kusznir, E.-A.; et al. Evaluation of Bovine Milk Extracellular Vesicles for the Delivery of Locked Nucleic Acid Antisense Oligonucleotides. *Eur. J. Pharm. Biopharm.* **2021**, *158*, 198–210. [CrossRef]
69. Karlsson, O.; Rodosthenous, R.S.; Jara, C.; Brennan, K.J.; Wright, R.O.; Baccarelli, A.A.; Wright, R.J. Detection of Long Non-Coding RNAs in Human Breastmilk Extracellular Vesicles: Implications for Early Child Development. *Epigenetics* **2016**, *11*, 721–729. [CrossRef]
70. Leiferman, A.; Shu, J.; Upadhyaya, B.; Cui, J.; Zempleni, J. Storage of Extracellular Vesicles in Human Milk, and MicroRNA Profiles in Human Milk Exosomes and Infant Formulas. *J. Craniof. Surg.* **2019**, *69*, 235–238. [CrossRef]

71. Aguilar-Lozano, A.; Baier, S.; Grove, R.; Shu, J.; Giraud, D.; Leiferman, A.; Mercer, K.E.; Cui, J.; Badger, T.M.; Adamec, J.; et al. Concentrations of Purine Metabolites Are Elevated in Fluids from Adults and Infants and in Livers from Mice Fed Diets Depleted of Bovine Milk Exosomes and Their RNA Cargos. *J. Nutr.* **2018**, *148*, 1886–1894. [CrossRef] [PubMed]
72. Mutai, E.; Ngu, A.K.H.; Zempleni, J. Preliminary Evidence That Lectins in Infant Soy Formula Apparently BIND bovine Milk Exosomes and Prevent Their Absorption in Healthy Adults. *BMC Nutr.* **2022**, *8*, 7. [CrossRef] [PubMed]
73. Wiklander, O.P.B.; Nordin, J.Z.; O'Loughlin, A.; Gustafsson, Y.; Corso, G.; Mäger, I.; Vader, P.; Lee, Y.; Sork, H.; Seow, Y.; et al. Extracellular Vesicle in Vivo Biodistribution Is Determined by Cell Source, Route of Administration and Targeting. *J. Extracell. Vesicles* **2015**, *4*, 26316. [CrossRef] [PubMed]
74. Albanese, M.; Chen, Y.-F.A.; Hüls, C.; Gärtner, K.; Tagawa, T.; Mejias-Perez, E.; Keppler, O.T.; Göbel, C.; Zeidler, R.; Shein, M.; et al. MicroRNAs Are Minor Constituents of Extracellular Vesicles That Are Rarely Delivered to Target Cells. *PLoS Genet.* **2021**, *17*, e1009951. [CrossRef] [PubMed]

pharmaceutics

MDPI

Article

Biodistribution of Intratracheal, Intranasal, and Intravenous Injections of Human Mesenchymal Stromal Cell-Derived Extracellular Vesicles in a Mouse Model for Drug Delivery Studies

Anna Maria Tolomeo [1,2,†], Gaia Zuccolotto [3,†], Ricardo Malvicini [2,4,5], Giada De Lazzari [2,4], Alessandro Penna [6], Chiara Franco [7], Federico Caicci [8], Fabio Magarotto [4], Santina Quarta [9], Michela Pozzobon [4,10], Antonio Rosato [3,6], Maurizio Muraca [2,4,*,‡] and Federica Collino [11,12,*,‡]

1 Department of Cardiac, Thoracic and Vascular Science and Public Health, University of Padova, 35128 Padua, Italy
2 L.i.f.e.L.a.b. Program, Consorzio per la Ricerca Sanitaria (CORIS), Veneto Region, 35128 Padua, Italy
3 Istituto Oncologico Veneto IOV-Istituto di Ricovero e Cura a Carattere Scientifico IRCCS, 35128 Padua, Italy
4 Department of Women's and Children's Health, University of Padova, 35128 Padua, Italy
5 Instituto de Medicina Traslacional, Trasplante y Bioingeniería, Universidad Favaloro-Consejo Nacional de Investigaciones Científicas y Técnicas, Buenos Aires 1078, Argentina
6 Department of Surgery, Oncology and Gastroenterology, University of Padova, 35128 Padua, Italy
7 Rheumatology Unit, Department of Medicine (DIMED), University of Padova, 35128 Padua, Italy
8 Department of Biology, University of Padova, 35131 Padua, Italy
9 Department of Medicine, University of Padova, 35128 Padua, Italy
10 Fondazione Istituto di Ricerca Pediatrica Città della Speranza, 35127 Padua, Italy
11 Laboratory of Translational Research in Paediatric Nephro-Urology, Department of Clinical Sciences and Community Health, University of Milano, 20122 Milan, Italy
12 Fondazione Ca' Granda IRCCS Ospedale Maggiore Policlinico, 20122 Milan, Italy
* Correspondence: muraca@unipd.it (M.M.); federica.collino@unimi.it (F.C.); Tel.: +39-049-8213574 (M.M.); +39-02-00660360 (F.C.)
† These authors contributed equally to this work.
‡ These authors also contributed equally to this work.

Citation: Tolomeo, A.M.; Zuccolotto, G.; Malvicini, R.; De Lazzari, G.; Penna, A.; Franco, C.; Caicci, F.; Magarotto, F.; Quarta, S.; Pozzobon, M.; et al. Biodistribution of Intratracheal, Intranasal, and Intravenous Injections of Human Mesenchymal Stromal Cell-Derived Extracellular Vesicles in a Mouse Model for Drug Delivery Studies. *Pharmaceutics* **2023**, *15*, 548. https://doi.org/10.3390/pharmaceutics15020548

Academic Editor: Yong Chen

Received: 5 December 2022
Revised: 31 January 2023
Accepted: 3 February 2023
Published: 7 February 2023

Abstract: Mesenchymal stromal cell-derived extracellular vesicles (MSC-EVs) are extensively studied as therapeutic tools. Evaluation of their biodistribution is fundamental to understanding MSC-EVs' impact on target organs. In our work, MSC-EVs were initially labeled with DiR, a fluorescent lipophilic dye, and administered to BALB/c mice (2.00×10^{10} EV/mice) through the following routes: intravenous (IV), intratracheal (IT) and intranasal (IN). DiR-labeled MSC-EVs were monitored immediately after injection, and after 3 and 24 hours (h). Whole-body analysis, 3 h after IV injection, showed an accumulation of MSC-EVs in the mice abdominal region, compared to IT and IN, where EVs mainly localized at the levels of the chest and brain region, respectively. After 24 h, EV-injected mice retained a stronger positivity in the same regions identified after 3 h from injection. The analyses of isolated organs confirmed the accumulation of EVs in the spleen and liver after IV administration. Twenty-four hours after the IT injection of MSC-EVs, a stronger positivity was detected selectively in the isolated lungs, while for IN, the signal was confined to the brain. In conclusion, these results show that local administration of EVs can increase their concentration in selective organs, limiting their systemic biodistribution and possibly the extra-organ effects. Biodistribution studies can help in the selection of the most appropriate way of administration of MSC-EVs for the treatment of different diseases.

Keywords: extracellular vesicles; biodistribution; pharmacokinetics; drug delivery

1. Introduction

Extracellular vesicles (EVs) are heterogeneous small membrane structures originating from plasma membranes and containing molecules from the cells from which they are released. EVs function by transferring biological molecules to target cells that accounts for an active alteration of the cell phenotype and function [1,2], both in physiological and pathological conditions. EVs are present in almost all body fluids and can transmigrate through different tissue barriers (e.g., blood–brain barrier, BBB) reaching distant sites [3,4]. Due to these biological and functional characteristics, EVs have been proposed as a novel therapeutic platform for delivering pharmaceutical ingredients [5]. In support of their application, EVs show high biocompatibility as well as low immunogenicity in different tissues [6,7].

Mesenchymal stem cells (MSCs) play an important role in the regeneration of multiple organs [8]. It has been shown that the MSC-derived EVs (MSC-EVs) partly mediate the MSC therapeutic functions through a paracrine way. Their mechanism of action can be summarized in their capability to directly regenerate different tissues, by protecting from damage-related inflammation events and inducing pro-proliferative and angiogenic programs in different organs [9–14]. On the clinical side, MSC-EVs provide important advantages, in respect to their cells of origin, such as their reduced immunogenicity and their efficient homing and uptake by different organs [15,16]. Hence, MSC-EVs can be defined as an alternative regenerative tool to cell-based therapy. Multiple factors can affect MSC-EVs biological activity and, therefore, their translation into medical treatments. The originating cells and their surrounding microenvironment can regulate EVs function by accounting for their membrane and intravesicular composition. For instance, the injection of human-adipose-derived (AD)MSC-derived EVs, in a rat myocardial-infarction model, leads to a stronger protection of cardiomyocytes from apoptosis and to an increase in angiogenesis, compared with one prompted by the bone-marrow (BM)MSC-derived EVs [17]. By contrast, in murine acute-kidney and lung-injury models, inducible pluripotent stem cells (iPSCs) as well as BMMSC-derived EVs were shown to better induce M2 macrophage polarization, compared to that induced by ADMSC-EVs [18–20]. The routes of administration may also influence their tissue distribution and consequently their pharmacokinetic profiles, as well as the biological activity [21]. By comparing the intraarterial- and intravenous (IV)-injection strategies of umbilical cord MSC-EVs, Li et al. [22] demonstrated that the less-invasive IV approach resulted in a better clinical benefit for diabetes therapies. The same advantage was observed when MSC-EVs were administered intratracheally (IT) in an experimental model of hyperoxia-induced bronchopulmonary dysplasia (BPD) in rat pups, showing a significant therapeutic effect of the non-systemic EV injection in combination with a more feasible clinical procedure [23,24].

In this context, the development of labeling strategies able to monitor and quantify EV localization is mandatory. The approaches of the labeling developed can be categorized based on the tags used, the labeling site, and the EV modification, in two main groups: (i) membrane/surface EV labeling by the integration of the lipophilic near-infrared dyes (e.g., DiR) (ii) genetic modification-dependent labeling through the introduction of tagged fluorescent-fusion proteins in the EV-originating cells [25]. Conversely, the MSC-EVs biodistribution is challenging, due to the critical limits in imaging EV dynamics, based on their complex physical properties as well as technical labeling limitations [26].

In our work, we investigated, using fluorescence imaging strategies, the in vivo pharmacokinetic distribution patterns of DiR-labeled MSC-EVs through IV, IT and intranasal (IN) administration into healthy mice, to verify their safety and to distinguish the most efficient delivery system based on the chosen target tissue. We performed a systematic comparison of the three administration routes, evaluating the whole-body mice fluorescent signal at different times from EV administration. The ex vivo organ's fluorescent signal was also evaluated after 24 h from injection and compared to the signal from homogenized tissues. Direct tracing in vivo of DiR-labeled EVs was performed to identify the potential MSC-EVs target organs.

2. Materials and Methods

2.1. Extracellular Vesicles

Umbilical cord MSC-EVs (MSC-EVs) were kindly provided by the Cell Factory BVBA (Esperite NV, Niel, Belgium). The MSC and EV production process followed the good-manufacturing-practice (GMP) standards (ICH Q7), based on the ISO9000 quality system. For details related to source material, MSC and EV production platform and quality control, refer to Porzionato et al., 2019 [23]. Briefly, EV were isolated by concentration using tangential-flow filtration and by applying filters with a cut-off of 100 KDa. This approach was instrumental in reducing cell-culture contaminants, with a high rate of EV recovery [23].

2.2. Tunable Resistive Pulse Sensing (tRPS)

Particle concentration and size distribution were analyzed using tunable-resistive-pulse-sensing (TRPS) technology with the qNano instrument (Izon Science, Christchurch, New Zealand). NP100 or NP150 membranes were used for the analysis. The concentration of particles was standardized using a CPC100 calibration solution diluted 1:10,000 (110 nm mean carboxylate polystyrene beads; stock concentration 1.00×10^{12}) [14].

2.3. Transmission Electron Microscopy

MSC-EVs were fixed with 4% PFA for 5 min, and one drop (2.00×10^{9} particles) of EVs was placed on a 400-mesh holey-film grid for 10 min. After washing with PBS, the MSC-EVs were stained with 1% uranyl acetate for 2 min. The sample was then washed with PBS and finally observed with a Tecnai G2 (FEI; Thermo Fisher Scientific, Waltham, MA, USA) transmission electron microscope operating at 100 kV. Images were captured with a Veleta (Olympus Soft Imaging System; Münster, Germany) digital camera.

2.4. Immunophenotyping of MSC-EVs

MSC-EVs were characterized by flow cytometry using the MacsPlex Exosome Kit (Miltenyi Biotec, Bergisch Gladbach, Germany), following manufacturer's instructions. Briefly, 1.00×10^{9} particles of MSC-EVs were loaded in a 1.5 mL tube and diluted to 120 μL with MACSPlex buffer. Then, a mix of 15 μL of exosome capture beads and 15 μL of antibody were added to each tube and incubated for 1 h at RT in agitation. For blank control, only MACSPlex buffer was used. Then, 500 μL of MACSPlex buffer was added to each tube and the EVs were centrifuged at 3000× *g* for 5 min. Finally, 500 μL of the supernatant was discarded and the samples were resuspended and transferred to a flow-cytometry tube. Samples were analyzed using a Cytoflex (Beckman Coulter, Brea, CA, USA) flow cytometer.

For the Western blot analysis, MSCs and their released EVs were lysed in RIPA buffer (50 mM Tris, pH 8.0, 150 mM sodium chloride, 1.0% NP-40, 0.5% sodium deoxycholate, 0.1% SDS (sodium dodecyl sulfate)) plus a protease inhibitor cocktail (Roche, Basle, Switzerland) and incubated with Laemmli buffer with β-mercaptoethanol for 5 min at 95 °C, for complete protein denaturation. Then, 5 μg of protein were loaded and resolved in an SDS-polyacrylamide 4–12% gel at 160 V and blotted using semi-dry transfer for 7 min at 25 V to polyvinylidene difluoride membranes (PVDF) (GE Healthcare Life Science, Milan, Italy). Membranes were blocked with 5% BSA in TBS-Tween for 1 h at room temperature and then incubated with the following primary antibodies overnight: anti-TSG-101 antibody 1:1000 (ab-125011); anti-CD81 antibody 1:500 (ab-109201) anti-CD9 antibody 1:1000 (ab-92726) (all from Abcam, Cambridge, UK) and anti-calnexin 1:1000, (sc-23954; Santa Cruz biotechnology, Dallas, TX, USA), and diluted in 1% BSA in TBS-Tween. After washing, the membranes were incubated with the secondary antibodies: goat anti-rabbit HRP 1:5000 (65-6120; Thermofisher, Waltham, MA, USA) or goat anti-mouse HRP 1:5000 (sc-2005, Santa Cruz biotechnology) for 1h at room temperature. Bands were then evidenced using ECL Plus Western blotting system (32134, Thermofisher).

2.5. Labeling and Cellular Uptake of MSC-EVs

The uptake of the EVs was evaluated in the human monocyte cell line (THP-1 cells, ATCC) and human endothelial cells (HMEC cells, ATCC). The THP-1 cells were cultured in RPMI-1640 medium, supplemented with 10% FBS, while the HMEC cells were cultured in EndoGRO-LS complete culture medium (Merck Millipore, Burlington, MA, USA). MSC-EVs were labeled with DiR (2.5 µM per 1.00×10^{10} particles) and incubated for 1 h in PBS (DiR-EVs). DiR dye (2.5 µM) was diluted in PBS alone and used as control (DiR-PBS). The free, unbound dye was eliminated from the preparations, by applying 3 serial centrifugations at 4 °C at 2000× *g*, using the 100 kDa Amicon filters (Merck Millipore). The EV-DiR and PBS-DiR were then collected from the filter (around 150 µL). The same staining protocol was used for the in vivo experiments. The THP-1 and HMEC cell lines were seeded in 8-well chamber slides (2.00×10^4 cells/well and 1.00×10^4 cells/well, respectively) and incubated for 24 h. After that, DiR-PBS or DiR-EVs (1.00×10^9 particles/well) were added and incubated for 24 h. Then, cells were fixed in PFA 4% for 10 min and washed and stained with phalloidin-FITC for 20 min. After washing, Vectashield with DAPI was added. Images were taken using a Leica microscope at 40×.

2.6. In Vivo Administration

All in vivo experiments involved 6- to 8-week-old BALB/c male mice (Charles River, Wilmington, MA, USA), which were housed in our specific-pathogen-free (SPF) animal facility. Procedures involving animals and their care were in conformity with institutional guidelines that comply with national and international laws and policies (D.L. 26/2014 and subsequent implemented circulars). During in vivo experiments, animals ($n = 48$) in all experimental groups were examined for a decrease in physical activity and other signs of illness.

Intravenous administration. To evaluate the biodistribution of systemically administered DiR-labeled MSC-EVs, the mice were injected intravenously (IV) with 2.00×10^{10} DiR-labeled MSC-EVs (100 µL/mouse).

Intratracheal administration. The mice received the same dose of DiR-labeled MSC-EVs in 30 µL/mouse of PBS by intratracheal instillation under isoflurane anesthesia.

Intranasal administration. The anesthetized mice were instilled intranasally (I.N.) with 2.00×10^{10} of DiR-labeled MSC-EVs (25 µL/mouse).

2.7. IVIS Imaging of In-Vivo-Administered MSC-EVs

DiR-labeled MSC-EVs were injected in BALB/c mice of 6–8 weeks of age via intravenous (IV), intratracheal (IT) or intranasal (IN) administration and monitored over time using an IVIS® Imaging System LUMINA II (PerkinElmer, Waltham, MA, USA). Imaging was performed after injection, at 3 and 24 h after EV administration. After 24 h, the mice were sacrificed, the organs were resected, and images of the organs were captured. Ventral and dorsal images were obtained for each animal and quantified through the region of interest (ROI). We measured the fluorescence as radiance (p/s/cm^2/sr) in the live animals and excised organs, using the Living Image 3.2 software program (PerkinElmer).

2.8. Organ Biodistribution of Labeled DiR-EVs

After weighing each organ, 500 µL of homogenization buffer was added in safe seal tubes (Sarstedt, Numbrecht, Germany) and tissue homogenate was obtained (tissue lyser-Qiagen). The homogenization buffer was composed of 250 mM sucrose, 2 mM EDTA, 10 mM Hepes-Tris (pH 7.6) and protease inhibitors (Sigma Aldrich, St. Louis, MO, USA). After centrifugation at 6000× *g*, the supernatant was recovered, and 150 µL of each organ homogenate was placed in a 96-well black plate with a glass bottom (Corning) and fluorescence was quantified using the Ensight fluorimeter (PerkinElmer, excitation 745 nm and emission 770 nm). The fluorescence intensity of each organ was normalized to the respective organ weight. Furthermore, the DiR fluorescent background of the DiR-PBS of each organ (control) was subtracted from the signal intensity of the DiR-EVs-treated organs (normalized fluorescent intensity, NFI).

2.9. Immunofluorescence Staining

OCT- (Biosigma) embedded tissue slices (8 μm) were stained as follows. Tissue slices were permeabilized with Triton X-100 0.1% in PBS for 20 min and blocked with 10% horse serum for 15 min. Incubation with the primary antibody (rat anti-mouse CD31, clone RM5200-invitrogen, MA, USA) was performed overnight at 4 °C. Alexa fluor-488 secondary antibody (A11006-Life technologies, Monza, Italy) was added to the slides for 1 h at 37 °C. The slides were washed and mounted with Fluoroshield™ with DAPI (F6057-Sigma Aldrich). Pictures were taken using Zeiss LSM800 Airyscan confocal microscopy (Jena, Germany) with 63× magnification.

2.10. Statistics

All data were processed, and their statistical significance was determined using GraphPad software (version 8.0.2). Data are expressed as mean ± standard deviation (SD). Comparisons of categorical variables were carried out using one-way ANOVA followed by Bonferroni's multiple-comparison-test p values: * $p < 0.05$; ** $p < 0.01$; *** $p < 0.001$; and **** $p < 0.0001$.

3. Results

3.1. Characterization of MSC-EVs

The analysis of the GMP-grade MSC-EVs by tunable resistive pulse sensing (tRPS) demonstrated a homogeneous population with particle sizes mostly below 150 nm (Figure 1A). Transmission electron microscopy (TEM) confirmed the EV heterogeneity, with particle sizes ranging from 30 to 250 nm (Figure 1B). The tRPS and TEM analysis confirmed, therefore, that almost all the nanoparticles used in the present work can be referred to as "small EVs", according to the MISEV2018 criteria [14]. MSCs and their released EVs expressed the exosome surface markers CD9 and CD81 and the intravesicular marker TSG101, as detected by Western blot (Figure 1C). On the other hand, the MSC-EVs were negative for the endoplasmic-reticulum protein, calnexin (CNX), which was selectively expressed by MSCs (Figure 1C). The presence of different surface proteins was also analyzed by flow cytometry, using a bead-coupled assay. MSC-EVs were confirmed to be positive for the classical tetraspanin markers CD9, CD63 and CD81. Regarding the adhesion molecules, the MSC-EVs expressed relatively high levels of CD29 and the angiogenic proteoglycan MCSP, while they did not express immunological markers (Figure 1D). Finally, the vesicles' surface protein reflected those of their parental cells, as they were positive for the CD105, CD44 and SSEA4 markers, while negative for CD45 and HLA-DR. Of note, the absence of HLA-DR would suggest a low immunogenicity (Figure 1D). The MSC-EVs labeled with DiR maintained the capability of being taken up by different target cells (e.g., human endothelial cells and monocytic cells) (Supplementary Figure S1), confirming no alteration on their surface.

3.2. In Vivo Biodistribution of DiR-Labeled MSC-EVs in BALB/c Mice

To study the biodistribution of the MSC-EVs, we evaluated three different administration routes: intravenous (IV), intratracheal (IT) and intranasal (IN) administration of DiR-labeled MSC-EVs (DiR-EVs) in healthy BALB/c mice. Control mice were injected with DiR-labeled PBS (DiR-PBS). We tracked the DiR-EVs at different time points from administration in live animals (after injection, at 3 and 24 h) using the IVIS® spectrum scanner (Figure 2A). Whole-body analysis demonstrated that in IV-injected mice the accumulation of MSC-EVs was mainly in the abdominal region of the body. On the other hand, in IT-injected mice, the signal was mainly localized at the level of the chest; it was strongly visible 3 h after the EV administration and was maintained at 24 h (Figure 2A). Finally, with the IN injection, the fluorescent signal detected was mainly located in the cerebral region, at both 3 and 24 h, as observed in mice placed in posterior position (Figure 2A). Quantification of fluorescence intensity in regions of interest (ROI) was expressed as the average radiance ± standard deviation (SD) and is depicted in Figure 2B. No significant differences were observed in the intensity of the fluorescent signal among the different administration groups, or at different times after the injection.

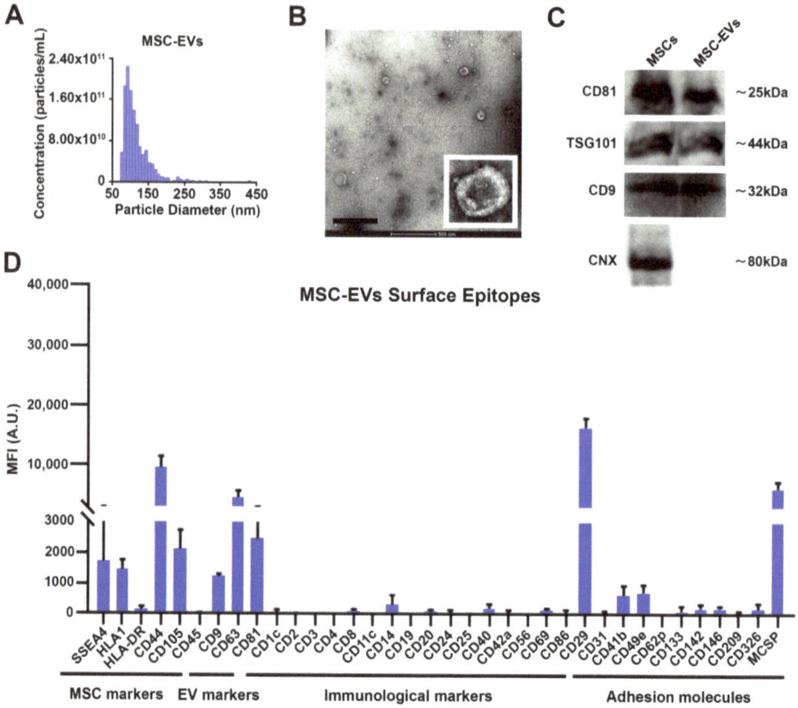

Figure 1. GMP-grade MSC-EV characterization. MSC-EV size distribution was analyzed using tRPS (**A**). MSC-EV morphology was assessed also, using TEM (**B**). Representative images of CD9, CD81, TSG101 and calnexin (CNX) markers analyzed by Western blot in MSCs and MSC-EVs (n = 3) (**C**). Finally, EV surface proteins were analyzed by flow cytometry, using a bead-coupled assay (n = 3) (**D**). Data are representative of three different independent preparations.

3.3. Ex Vivo Detection of DiR-Labeled MSC-EVs after IV, IT and IN Injection

To investigate the specific organ distribution of the injected DiR-EVs, the IVIS® spectrum scanner was used to image the harvested organs ex vivo. Images of the organs (brain, gut, heart, liver, lungs, kidneys, and spleen) harvested at 24 h after the EV administration are shown in Figure 3A. The mean radiant efficiency relative to the pixel size of the region of interest for each organ was quantified (Figure 3B). In agreement with the results from in-vivo-imaging experiments, the highest fluorescent signal after IV injection was detected in the liver, followed by the spleen and lungs. Conversely, almost no signal was detected in the kidneys, heart, and brain tissues 24 h after injection (Figure 3B). Similarly, in the IT-injected mice, after 24 h the highest signal was detected in the lungs, while the other organs did not show any significant signal (Figure 3B). Finally, after the IN injection, the signal was detected specifically in the brain, followed by a low detectable signal in the lungs, kidneys and gut (Figure 3B). Results from the DiR-EV injected groups indicated a low overall signal in the blood both 3 and 24 h after the IV, IT and IN injections, which was absent in the DiR-PBS infused mice (Supplementary Figure S2).

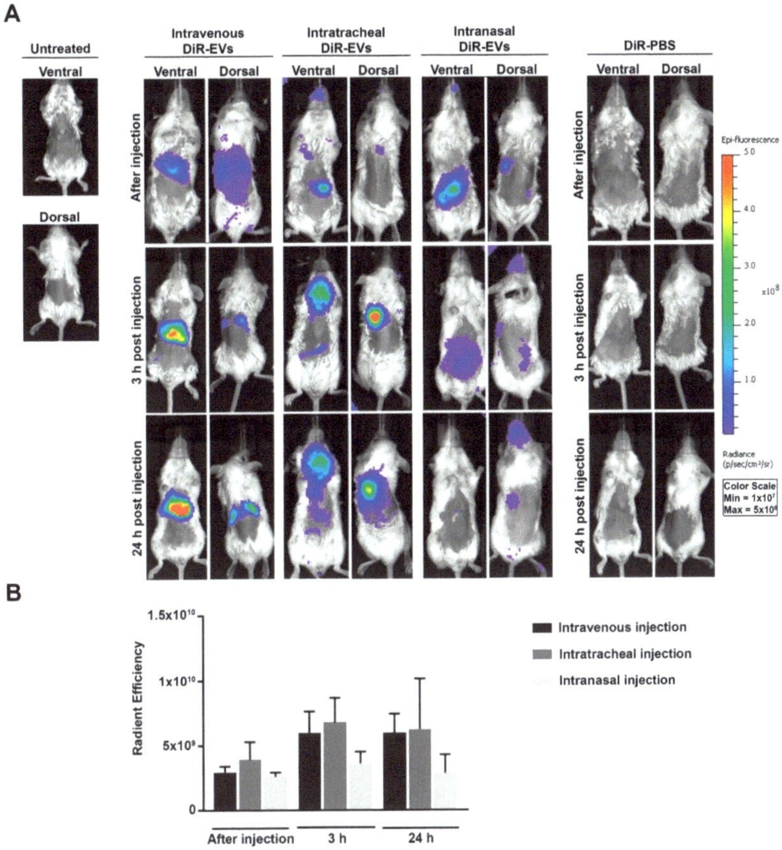

Figure 2. In-vivo DiR-labeled MSC-EV biodistribution. DiR-EVs and DiR-PBS were administered by IV, IT and IN in BALB/c mice, and fluorescence was evaluated in vivo using an IVIS® Imaging System LUMINA II. (**A**) Representative photographs of live animals are presented in supine and posterior position at different times following injection. (**B**) Quantification of fluorescence intensity through the region of interest (ROI) and measured as radiance (p/s/cm^2/sr). Data are expressed as mean ± SD; (n = 24/DiR-EVs and DiR-PBS).

To better characterize the signal derived from the DiR-EVs, the relative fluorescence was assessed also by fluorometric analysis of the homogenized tissue. After homogenization, the highest EV signal, in the IV animals, was detected in the liver and the spleen, followed by the lungs (Figure 3C). In IT-injected mice, fluorescence was mainly observed in the lung tissue, which was consistent with that observed after the IVIS® analyses (Figure 3C). Finally, the IN-injected mice exhibited a low but specific signal at the level of the brain tissue (3266.7 ± 2311.3), followed by the heart and gut (617.5 ± 437.1 and 297.7 ± 213.9, respectively), (Figure 3C). No fluorescent signal was detected in the other organs that were analyzed.

3.4. DiR-Labeled MSC-EV Tissue Detection after IV, IT and IN Administration

Data comparing the relative fluorescent signal obtained from the ex vivo analysis, for the liver, lungs, and brain, for the three administration routes, is shown in Figure 4A. In the liver, the strongest signal was detected after IV injection, compared with IT and IN injection, where the signal was significantly lower. Similarly, in the lungs the highest signal was observed after IT administration, which was significantly higher when compared to IV and IN administration. After IN injection, the highest signal was observed in the brain tissue, but significance was reached only in respect of the IT administration. Finally, immunofluorescence studies were carried out on organs targeted during the treatments, to reveal the localization of labeled EVs after IV, IT and IN injections. Specifically, DiR-EVs were directly identified in the liver, lungs, and brain after IV, IT and IN injection, respectively, as detected by confocal microscopy (Figure 4B). No fluorescent signal was found in the tissues of the DiR-PBS injected mice (Figure 4B).

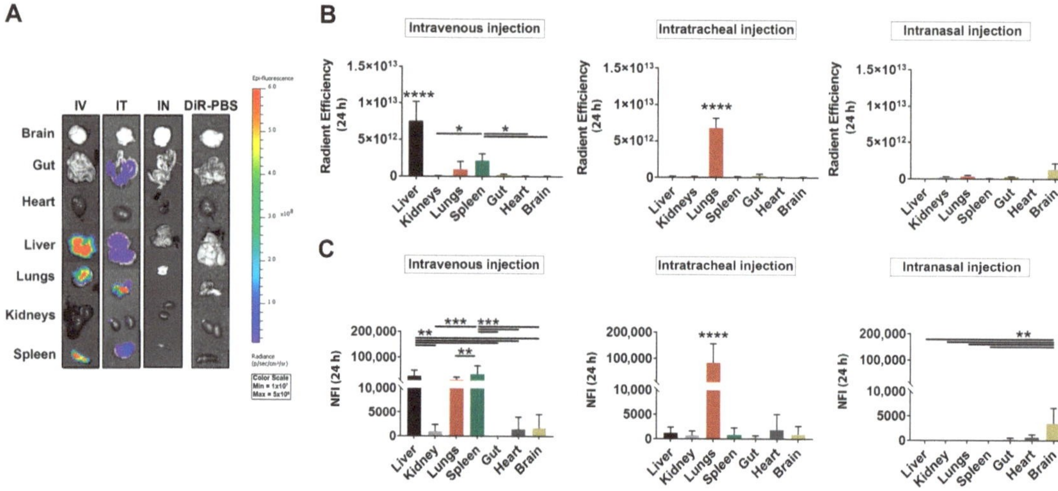

Figure 3. Ex vivo analysis of DiR-labeled MSC-EV biodistribution. Representative image of ex-vivo-organ imaging, using IVIS® (**A**). Quantification of the fluorescence as radiance (p/s/cm^2/sr) is represented in (**B**) and expressed as average radiance ± SD (n = 24/DiR-EVs and DiR-PBS). (**C**) Relative fluorescence in the different organs was assessed using fluorometric analysis after tissue homogenization, and it was calculated as AU/g of tissue. For all the data, subtraction of the DiR-PBS signal was performed (normalized fluorescent intensity, NFI). * $p < 0.05$; ** $p < 0.01$; *** $p < 0.001$ and **** $p < 0.0001$ after one-way ANOVA followed by Bonferroni's multiple comparison. For **** $p < 0.0001$ against all the other groups.

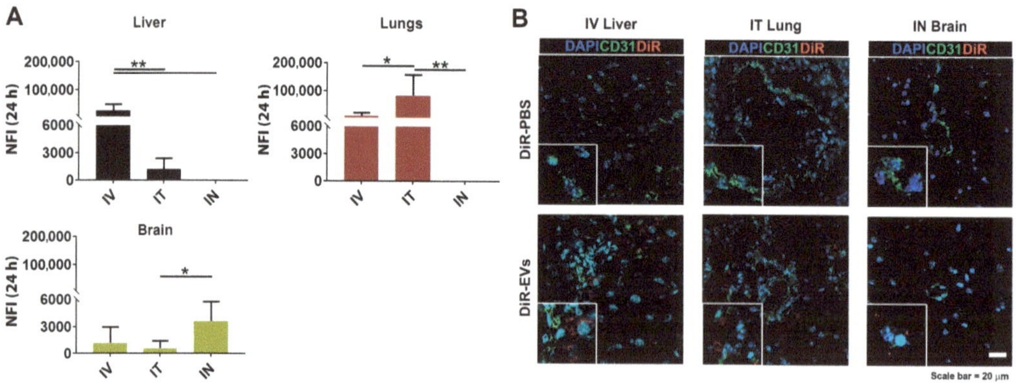

Figure 4. Fluorescent-signal detection in targeted organs. Fluorescence quantification of organ homogenates, where the signal was the highest, is depicted in (**A**); (n = 24/DiR-EVs and DiR-PBS) data are expressed as mean ± SD, among the IV, IT and IN injection route. p-values: * $p < 0.05$, ** $p < 0.01$ after one-way ANOVA followed by Bonferroni's multiple comparison. (**B**) Representative images of DiR fluorescent signal and CD31 staining detected on tissue sections of selective targeted organs.

4. Discussion

Extracellular vesicles are regarded as biological messengers, which deliver active molecules among tissues/cells in both physiological and pathological conditions. Functionally, by delivering their molecular content from donor cells into recipient cells, they modulate the recipient cells' biological responses, supporting their role as therapeutic delivery systems. Biodistribution studies are essential for understanding EVs' biology and their potential therapeutic applications. To our knowledge, this is the first time a comparative study has been performed, evaluating three different routes for the administration of GMP-grade MSC-EVs in healthy mice, in which a direct comparison between the in situ and ex vivo analysis of organs after IV, IT and IN administration is conducted.

EV biodistribution can be influenced by numerous factors, including their cells of origin and surface markers, as well as the labeling approach. We were able to potentially reduce variability in our in vivo study by controlling these critical variables. For this reason, EVs were isolated from the same GMP-grade MSC sources and administered at an equal dose into BALB/c mice by different routes. Moreover, the classical tetraspanins (e.g., CD9, CD63, CD81) and the specific adhesion molecules (e.g., Chondroitin sulfate proteoglycan-4, also called MCSP, CD44 and CD29) possibly involved in their uptake [27], were identified on the MSC-EV surface.

Focusing on the labeling protocol, numerous works were presented to evaluate the best imaging tools for in vivo and ex vivo detection, monitoring and quantification of EV localization [28]. We performed the EV labeling using a DiR lipophilic dye known for its efficient labeling properties and a deeper tissue penetration with reduced autofluorescence, together with no evidence of induction of EV chemical changes [29]. The MSC-EVs applied in this study show a heterogenous size distribution of <200 nm, which categorizes them as small EVs [30] and supports their ability to distribute homogeneously in different organs, based on their reduced size [21]. In an attempt to compare different injection routes, we chose an interval of time in which the EV signal at whole-body level was detectable, and which was previously used in other biodistribution studies [31–37]. Moreover, because we employed a labeling agent with a long half-life (5–100 days), 24 h was used as a reference point.

The EV dose that we applied was the same as the minimum amount used by [15], showing a specific signal without saturation of the liver reticuloendothelial system. Moreover, the EV concentration was ten times more than the minimum dose proposed by [38], to avoid an excess of free dye in the EV preparation before injection. Concomitantly, a purification step through PBS washing was also performed to eliminate unbound dye and enhance the labeling specificity. In our study, we applied a cross-species treatment by injecting xenotransplant MSC-EVs into BALB/c mice with no evidence of immune reactivity. Our data were supported by numerous mice preclinical studies using human-derived MSC-EVs as described in [39], which showed their capability of directly mediating biological effects without evidence of immune response [40,41]. Similarly, in a previous study, human MSC-EVs injected IV in immunocompetent mice showed the same distribution of mouse-derived EVs, supporting the absence of direct influence of the cross-species treatment in the biodistribution analysis [15].

In our model, DiR-labeled MSC-EVs intravenously administered in healthy mice were most efficiently taken up by the liver and spleen, followed by the lungs. Interestingly, Wiklander et al. [15] in the first report on MSC-EV distribution in mice, also identified the liver as the organ with the highest accumulation of bone-marrow-derived EVs. The same biodistribution was observed also for other EV sources or mice strands after IV injection, as reported by [25,31]. Moreover, the IV-distribution pattern among the examined organs was in line with previous works, evaluating the EV-biodistribution at earlier time points [21]. Interestingly, in this setting, endogenous bioluminescent-labeled cord-blood MSC-EVs, demonstrated the same pattern distribution as that of DiR-labeled EVs at the levels of the liver and lungs [42]. We also observed low levels of MSC-EV uptake by the kidneys and, to a lesser extent, by the heart, colon, and brain in IV mice. Previous biodistribution studies agree with our data, showing the increase in renal uptake of MSC-EVs only after acute kidney damage [43,44]. Furthermore, we demonstrated how the peripheral biodistribution of IV-delivered EVs was largely comparable between the two fluorescent-signal-detection methods used in our study.

After the systemic injection, the labeled EVs were retained in narrow microcapillaries without reaching uniformly the targeted organs [25]. In contrast, the uptake of labeled EVs increases when a local route of administration is chosen. Indeed, in our study, MSC-EVs administered by IT and IN were efficiently delivered to the lungs and brain, where they accumulated at more than double the concentration with respect to the IV administration, confirming the selective distribution of vesicles based on the administration route chosen. Moreover, only a minimum dispersion in other peripheral organs was observed, supporting the absence of off-target effects and EV retention by specific sites in the body when confined delivery is provided.

The different delivery routes can also generate different mechanisms of action. For instance, the IT and IV injections of bone-marrow MSC-EVs in a bleomycin-induced pulmonary-fibrosis model, were able to activate different pathways in the lung, to reduce the damage [45]. DiR-labeled MSC-EVs were efficiently taken up in vitro by endothelial and monocytic cells [46,47], confirming these cells as possible targets of EVs also in vivo, as well as the absence of any impact of the labeling procedure on the EVs' surface structure.

Another important result of our study was the detection of EV uptake in the central-nervous-system (CNS) compartments, regardless of the route of administration. EVs can enter the brain directly through the blood–brain barrier (BBB) or the choroid plexus epithelium, a more permeable counterpart of the BBB [48]. Intranasal administration of EVs has been proposed as a promising way to treat CNS diseases. When MSC-EVs were injected by IN in our mouse model, the only organ showing a significant accumulation was the brain, despite the resulting minimum signal. In accordance with this, biodistribution experiments in a non-human primate model resulted in a minimum uptake of EVs, even after intranasal delivery [49]. This may be due to the limitations for drug absorption in the nasal cavity, including low intrinsic permeability (e.g., lipophilic–hydrophilic balance), rapid mucociliary clearance, and active enzymatic degradation [50]. Interestingly, the stronger accumulation of MSC-EVs was demonstrated to occur in the brain only when neuro-inflammatory damage was present [6], suggesting that the recipient species' pathology could strongly affect EV pharmacokinetics and tissue delivery.

5. Conclusions

In the present work, we assessed the in vivo biodistribution of DiR-labeled MSC-EVs using different administration routes: intratracheal, intravenous and intranasal. Analysis of the in vivo-imaging data highlights a selective delivery and permanence of the EV cargo in specific organs, based on their route of administration, after 24 h. These results confirmed that, depending on the administration route, it is possible to deliver MSC-EVs to a target organ, limiting their systemic biodistribution and possible off-target effects.

In this context, the use of lipophilic dyes has several limitations, including their transfer between membranes and their long half-life, with possible preservation of the fluorescent signal after EV degradation [21]. Moreover, these dyes can affect the physico-chemical characteristics of EVs, resulting in altered EV distribution in favor of lipid-rich organs such as the brain [33].

Further data on EV biodistribution in multiple pathological states could better highlight the GMP-grade MSC-EVs' pharmacokinetics in disease.

Supplementary Materials: The following supporting information can be downloaded at https://www.mdpi.com/article/10.3390/pharmaceutics15020548/s1, Figure S1: In-vitro uptake experiments; Figure S2: Analysis of DiR-labeled MSC-EV organ biodistribution; Figure S3: MSC-EV biodistribution in biofluids.

Author Contributions: Conceptualization, A.M.T., M.M. and F.C. (Federica Collino); methodology, A.M.T., G.Z., R.M., G.D.L., A.P., C.F., F.C. (Federico Caicci) and F.M.; validation, A.M.T., G.Z., R.M. and G.D.L.; formal analysis, A.M.T., G.Z., R.M., G.D.L. and S.Q.; data curation, A.M.T., G.Z., R.M., G.D.L. and F.C. (Federica Collino); writing—original draft preparation, A.M.T. and F.C. (Federica Collino); writing—review and editing, A.M.T., M.P., A.R., M.M. and F.C. (Federica Collino); supervision, M.M. and F.C. (Federica Collino); funding acquisition, M.M. All authors have read and agreed to the published version of the manuscript.

Funding: This research was funded by "Consorzio per la Ricerca Sanitaria" (CORIS) of the Veneto Region, Italy (L.i.f.e.L.a.b. Program), grant number DGR1017, 17 July 2018. Part of the research was also funded by IRP Synergy grant 2019.

Institutional Review Board Statement: The animal study protocol was approved by the Institutional Review Board (or Ethics Committee) of Italian Ministry of Health, Division of Veterinary Medicine (protocol code n° 1249/2015-PR and date of approval 27 November 2015).

Informed Consent Statement: Not applicable, the study did not involve humans.

Data Availability Statement: Not applicable.

Conflicts of Interest: The authors declare no conflict of interest.

References

1. Ratajczak, J.; Miekus, K.; Kucia, M.; Zhang, J.; Reca, R.; Dvorak, P.; Ratajczak, M.Z. Embryonic Stem Cell-Derived Microvesicles Reprogram Hematopoietic Progenitors: Evidence for Horizontal Transfer of MRNA and Protein Delivery. *Leukemia* **2006**, *20*, 847–856. [CrossRef]
2. Valadi, H.; Ekström, K.; Bossios, A.; Sjöstrand, M.; Lee, J.J.; Lötvall, J.O. Exosome-Mediated Transfer of MRNAs and MicroRNAs Is a Novel Mechanism of Genetic Exchange between Cells. *Nat. Cell Biol.* **2007**, *9*, 654–659. [CrossRef] [PubMed]
3. Banks, W.A.; Sharma, P.; Bullock, K.M.; Hansen, K.M.; Ludwig, N.; Whiteside, T.L. Transport of Extracellular Vesicles across the Blood-Brain Barrier: Brain Pharmacokinetics and Effects of Inflammation. *Int. J. Mol. Sci.* **2020**, *21*, 4407. [CrossRef]
4. Matsumoto, J.; Stewart, T.; Banks, W.A.; Zhang, J. The Transport Mechanism of Extracellular Vesicles at the Blood-Brain Barrier. *Curr. Pharm. Des.* **2018**, *23*, 6206–6214. [CrossRef] [PubMed]
5. Liu, H.; Deng, S.; Han, L.; Ren, Y.; Gu, J.; He, L.; Liu, T.; Yuan, Z.X. Mesenchymal Stem Cells, Exosomes and Exosome-Mimics as Smart Drug Carriers for Targeted Cancer Therapy. *Colloids Surf. B Biointerfaces* **2022**, *209*, 112163. [CrossRef] [PubMed]
6. Perets, N.; Betzer, O.; Shapira, R.; Brenstein, S.; Angel, A.; Sadan, T.; Ashery, U.; Popovtzer, R.; Offen, D. Golden Exosomes Selectively Target Brain Pathologies in Neurodegenerative and Neurodevelopmental Disorders. *Nano Lett.* **2019**, *19*, 3422–3431. [CrossRef] [PubMed]
7. Cohen, O.; Betzer, O.; Elmaliach-Pnini, N.; Motiei, M.; Sadan, T.; Cohen-Berkman, M.; Dagan, O.; Popovtzer, A.; Yosepovich, A.; Barhom, H.; et al. 'Golden' Exosomes as Delivery Vehicles to Target Tumors and Overcome Intratumoral Barriers: In Vivo Tracking in a Model for Head and Neck Cancer. *Biomater. Sci.* **2021**, *9*, 2103–2114. [CrossRef]
8. Rohban, R.; Pieber, T.R. Mesenchymal Stem and Progenitor Cells in Regeneration: Tissue Specificity and Regenerative Potential. *Stem Cells Int.* **2017**, *2017*, 5173732. [CrossRef]
9. Psaraki, A.; Ntari, L.; Karakostas, C.; Korrou-Karava, D.; Roubelakis, M.G. Extracellular Vesicles Derived from Mesenchymal Stem/Stromal Cells: The Regenerative Impact in Liver Diseases. *Hepatology* **2022**, *75*, 1590–1603. [CrossRef]
10. Zargar, M.J.; Kaviani, S.; Vasei, M.; Soufi Zomorrod, M.; Heidari Keshel, S.; Soleimani, M. Therapeutic Role of Mesenchymal Stem Cell-Derived Exosomes in Respiratory Disease. *Stem Cell Res. Ther.* **2022**, *13*, 194. [CrossRef]
11. Vatsa, P.; Negi, R.; Ansari, U.A.; Khanna, V.K.; Pant, A.B. Insights of Extracellular Vesicles of Mesenchymal Stem Cells: A Prospective Cell-Free Regenerative Medicine for Neurodegenerative Disorders. *Mol. Neurobiol.* **2022**, *59*, 459–474. [CrossRef] [PubMed]
12. Quaglia, M.; Merlotti, G.; Colombatto, A.; Bruno, S.; Stasi, A.; Franzin, R.; Castellano, G.; Grossini, E.; Fanelli, V.; Cantaluppi, V. Stem Cell-Derived Extracellular Vesicles as Potential Therapeutic Approach for Acute Kidney Injury. *Front. Immunol.* **2022**, *13*, 849891. [CrossRef] [PubMed]
13. Magarotto, F.; Sgrò, A.; Dorigo Hochuli, A.H.; Andreetta, M.; Grassi, M.; Saggioro, M.; Nogara, L.; Tolomeo, A.M.; Francescato, R.; Collino, F.; et al. Muscle Functional Recovery Is Driven by Extracellular Vesicles Combined with Muscle Extracellular Matrix in a Volumetric Muscle Loss Murine Model. *Biomaterials* **2021**, *269*, 120653. [CrossRef] [PubMed]
14. Tolomeo, A.M.; Castagliuolo, I.; Piccoli, M.; Grassi, M.; Magarotto, F.; de Lazzari, G.; Malvicini, R.; Caicci, F.; Franzin, C.; Scarpa, M.; et al. Extracellular Vesicles Secreted by Mesenchymal Stromal Cells Exert Opposite Effects to Their Cells of Origin in Murine Sodium Dextran Sulfate-Induced Colitis. *Front. Immunol.* **2021**, *12*, 627605. [CrossRef]
15. Wiklander, O.P.B.; Nordin, J.Z.; O'Loughlin, A.; Gustafsson, Y.; Corso, G.; Mäger, I.; Vader, P.; Lee, Y.; Sork, H.; Seow, Y.; et al. Extracellular Vesicle in Vivo Biodistribution Is Determined by Cell Source, Route of Administration and Targeting. *J. Extracell. Vesicles* **2015**, *4*, 26316. [CrossRef]

16. Yoo, M.H.; Lee, A.R.; Moon, K.S. Characteristics of Extracellular Vesicles and Preclinical Testing Considerations Prior to Clinical Applications. *Biomedicines* **2022**, *10*, 869. [CrossRef] [PubMed]
17. Xu, H.; Wang, Z.; Liu, L.; Zhang, B.; Li, B. Exosomes Derived from Adipose Tissue, Bone Marrow, and Umbilical Cord Blood for Cardioprotection after Myocardial Infarction. *J. Cell Biochem.* **2020**, *121*, 2089–2102. [CrossRef]
18. Collino, F.; Lopes, J.A.; Tapparo, M.; Tortelote, G.G.; Kasai-Brunswick, T.H.; Lopes, G.M.C.; Almeida, D.B.; Skovronova, R.; Wendt, C.H.C.; Miranda, K.R.d.; et al. Extracellular Vesicles Derived from Induced Pluripotent Stem Cells Promote Renoprotection in Acute Kidney Injury Model. *Cells* **2020**, *9*, 453. [CrossRef]
19. Abreu, S.C.; Antunes, M.A.; Xisto, D.G.; Cruz, F.F.; Branco, V.C.; Bandeira, E.; Kitoko, J.Z.; de Araú Jo, A.F.; Dellatorre-Texeira, L.; Olsen, P.C.; et al. Bone Marrow, Adipose, and Lung Tissue-Derived Murine Mesenchymal Stromal Cells Release Different Mediators and Differentially Affect Airway and Lung Parenchyma in Experimental Asthma. *Stem Cells Transl. Med.* **2017**, *6*, 1557–1567. [CrossRef]
20. Liu, D.; Cheng, F.; Pan, S.; Liu, Z. Stem Cells: A Potential Treatment Option for Kidney Diseases. *Stem Cell Res. Ther.* **2020**, *11*, 249. [CrossRef]
21. Kang, M.; Jordan, V.; Blenkiron, C.; Chamley, L.W. Biodistribution of Extracellular Vesicles Following Administration into Animals: A Systematic Review. *J. Extracell. Vesicles* **2021**, *10*, e12085. [CrossRef]
22. Li, J.; Komatsu, H.; Poku, E.K.; Olafsen, T.; Huang, K.X.; Huang, L.A.; Chea, J.; Bowles, N.; Chang, B.; Rawson, J.; et al. Biodistribution of Intra-Arterial and Intravenous Delivery of Human Umbilical Cord Mesenchymal Stem Cell-Derived Extracellular Vesicles in a Rat Model to Guide Delivery Strategies for Diabetes Therapies. *Pharmaceuticals* **2022**, *15*, 595. [CrossRef] [PubMed]
23. Porzionato, A.; Zaramella, P.; Dedja, A.; Guidolin, D.; van Wemmel, K.; Macchi, V.; Jurga, M.; Perilongo, G.; de Caro, R.; Baraldi, E.; et al. Intratracheal Administration of Clinical-Grade Mesenchymal Stem Cell-Derived Extracellular Vesicles Reduces Lung Injury in a Rat Model of Bronchopulmonary Dysplasia. *Am. J. Physiol. Lung Cell. Mol. Physiol.* **2019**, *316*, L6–L19. [CrossRef]
24. Porzionato, A.; Zaramella, P.; Dedja, A.; Guidolin, D.; Bonadies, L.; Macchi, V.; Pozzobon, M.; Jurga, M.; Perilongo, G.; de Caro, R.; et al. Intratracheal Administration of Mesenchymal Stem Cell-Derived Extracellular Vesicles Reduces Lung Injuries in a Chronic Rat Model of Bronchopulmonary Dysplasia. *Am. J. Physiol. Lung Cell. Mol. Physiol.* **2021**, *320*, L688–L704. [CrossRef] [PubMed]
25. Lázaro-Ibánez, E.; Al-Jamal, K.T.; Dekker, N.; Faruqu, F.N.; Saleh, A.F.; Silva, A.M.; Wang, J.T.W.; Rak, J. Selection of Fluorescent, Bioluminescent, and Radioactive Tracers to Accurately Reflect Extracellular Vesicle Biodistribution in Vivo. *ACS Nano* **2021**, *15*, 3212–3227. [CrossRef] [PubMed]
26. Verweij, F.J.; Balaj, L.; Boulanger, C.M.; Carter, D.R.F.; Compeer, E.B.; D'Angelo, G.; el Andaloussi, S.; Goetz, J.G.; Gross, J.C.; Hyenne, V.; et al. The Power of Imaging to Understand Extracellular Vesicle Biology in Vivo. *Nat. Methods* **2021**, *18*, 1013–1026. [CrossRef] [PubMed]
27. O'Brien, K.; Ughetto, S.; Mahjoum, S.; Nair, A.V.; Breakefield, X.O. Uptake, Functionality, and Re-Release of Extracellular Vesicle-Encapsulated Cargo. *Cell Rep.* **2022**, *39*, 110651. [CrossRef]
28. Arifin, D.R.; Witwer, K.W.; Bulte, J.W.M. Non-Invasive Imaging of Extracellular Vesicles: Quo Vaditis in Vivo? *J. Extracell. Vesicles* **2022**, *11*, e12241. [CrossRef]
29. Cassidy, P.J.; Radda, G.K. Molecular Imaging Perspectives. *J. R. Soc. Interface* **2005**, *2*, 133–144. [CrossRef]
30. Théry, C.; Witwer, K.W.; Aikawa, E.; Alcaraz, M.J.; Anderson, J.D.; Andriantsitohaina, R.; Antoniou, A.; Arab, T.; Archer, F.; Atkin-Smith, G.K.; et al. Minimal Information for Studies of Extracellular Vesicles 2018 (MISEV2018): A Position Statement of the International Society for Extracellular Vesicles and Update of the MISEV2014 Guidelines. *J. Extracell. Vesicles* **2018**, *7*, 1535750. [CrossRef]
31. Grange, C.; Tapparo, M.; Bruno, S.; Chatterjee, D.; Quesenberry, P.J.; Tetta, C.; Camussi, G. Biodistribution of Mesenchymal Stem Cell-Derived Extracellular Vesicles in a Model of Acute Kidney Injury Monitored by Optical Imaging. *Int. J. Mol. Med.* **2014**, *33*, 1055–1063. [CrossRef] [PubMed]
32. Jalabert, A.; Vial, G.; Guay, C.; Wiklander, O.P.B.; Nordin, J.Z.; Aswad, H.; Forterre, A.; Meugnier, E.; Pesenti, S.; Regazzi, R.; et al. Exosome-like Vesicles Released from Lipid-Induced Insulin-Resistant Muscles Modulate Gene Expression and Proliferation of Beta Recipient Cells in Mice. *Diabetologia* **2016**, *59*, 1049–1058. [CrossRef] [PubMed]
33. Nordin, J.Z.; Lee, Y.; Vader, P.; Mäger, I.; Johansson, H.J.; Heusermann, W.; Wiklander, O.P.B.; Hällbrink, M.; Seow, Y.; Bultema, J.J.; et al. Ultrafiltration with Size-Exclusion Liquid Chromatography for High Yield Isolation of Extracellular Vesicles Preserving Intact Biophysical and Functional Properties. *Nanomedicine* **2015**, *11*, 879–883. [CrossRef] [PubMed]
34. Smyth, T.; Kullberg, M.; Malik, N.; Smith-Jones, P.; Graner, M.W.; Anchordoquy, T.J. Biodistribution and Delivery Efficiency of Unmodified Tumor-Derived Exosomes. *J. Control. Release* **2015**, *199*, 145–155. [CrossRef]
35. Wen, S.W.; Sceneay, J.; Lima, L.G.; Wong, C.S.F.; Becker, M.; Krumeich, S.; Lobb, R.J.; Castillo, V.; Wong, K.N.; Ellis, S.; et al. The Biodistribution and Immune Suppressive Effects of Breast Cancer-Derived Exosomes. *Cancer Res.* **2016**, *76*, 6816–6827. [CrossRef]
36. Zhang, P.; Dong, B.; Zeng, E.; Wang, F.; Jiang, Y.; Li, D.; Liu, D. In Vivo Tracking of Multiple Tumor Exosomes Labeled by Phospholipid-Based Bioorthogonal Conjugation. *Anal Chem.* **2018**, *90*, 11273–11279. [CrossRef]
37. Zhang, H.; Freitas, D.; Kim, H.S.; Fabijanic, K.; Li, Z.; Chen, H.; Mark, M.T.; Molina, H.; Martin, A.B.; Bojmar, L.; et al. Identification of Distinct Nanoparticles and Subsets of Extracellular Vesicles by Asymmetric Flow Field-Flow Fractionation. *Nat. Cell Biol.* **2018**, *20*, 332–343. [CrossRef]

38. Wan, L.; Xia, T.; Du, Y.; Liu, J.; Xie, Y.; Zhang, Y.; Guan, F.; Wu, J.; Wang, X.; Shi, C. Exosomes from Activated Hepatic Stellate Cells Contain GLUT1 and PKM2: A Role for Exosomes in Metabolic Switch of Liver Nonparenchymal Cells. *FASEB J.* **2019**, *33*, 8530–8542. [CrossRef]
39. Cai, J.; Wu, J.; Wang, J.; Li, Y.; Hu, X.; Luo, S.; Xiang, D. Extracellular Vesicles Derived from Different Sources of Mesenchymal Stem Cells: Therapeutic Effects and Translational Potential. *Cell Biosci.* **2020**, *10*, 69. [CrossRef]
40. Hyvärinen, K.; Holopainen, M.; Skirdenko, V.; Ruhanen, H.; Lehenkari, P.; Korhonen, M.; Käkelä, R.; Laitinen, S.; Kerkelä, E. Mesenchymal Stromal Cells and Their Extracellular Vesicles Enhance the Anti-Inflammatory Phenotype of Regulatory Macrophages by Downregulating the Production of Interleukin (IL)-23 and IL-22. *Front. Immunol.* **2018**, *9*, 771. [CrossRef]
41. Fujii, S.; Miura, Y.; Fujishiro, A.; Shindo, T.; Shimazu, Y.; Hirai, H.; Tahara, H.; Takaori-Kondo, A.; Ichinohe, T.; Maekawa, T. Graft-Versus-Host Disease Amelioration by Human Bone Marrow Mesenchymal Stromal/Stem Cell-Derived Extracellular Vesicles Is Associated with Peripheral Preservation of Naive T Cell Populations. *Stem Cells* **2018**, *36*, 434–445. [CrossRef]
42. Gupta, D.; Liang, X.; Pavlova, S.; Wiklander, O.P.B.; Corso, G.; Zhao, Y.; Saher, O.; Bost, J.; Zickler, A.M.; Piffko, A.; et al. Quantification of Extracellular Vesicles in Vitro and in Vivo Using Sensitive Bioluminescence Imaging. *J. Extracell. Vesicles* **2020**, *9*, 1800222. [CrossRef]
43. Grange, C.; Tritta, S.; Tapparo, M.; Cedrino, M.; Tetta, C.; Camussi, G.; Brizzi, M.F. Stem Cell-Derived Extracellular Vesicles Inhibit and Revert Fibrosis Progression in a Mouse Model of Diabetic Nephropathy. *Sci. Rep.* **2019**, *9*, 1–13. [CrossRef]
44. Collino, F.; Lopes, J.A.; Corrêa, S.; Abdelhay, E.; Takiya, C.M.; Wendt, C.H.C.; de Miranda, K.R.; Vieyra, A.; Lindoso, R.S. Adipose-Derived Mesenchymal Stromal Cells Under Hypoxia: Changes in Extracellular Vesicles Secretion and Improvement of Renal Recovery after Ischemic Injury. *Cell Physiol. Biochem.* **2019**, *52*, 1463–1483. [CrossRef]
45. Yang, S.; Liu, P.; Gao, T.; Song, D.; Zhao, X.; Li, Y.; Wu, J.; Wang, L.; Wang, Z.; Hao, J.; et al. Every Road Leads to Rome: Therapeutic Effect and Mechanism of the Extracellular Vesicles of Human Embryonic Stem Cell-Derived Immune and Matrix Regulatory Cells Administered to Mouse Models of Pulmonary Fibrosis through Different Routes. *Stem Cell Res. Ther.* **2022**, *13*, 163. [CrossRef]
46. Pacienza, N.; Lee, R.H.; Bae, E.H.; Kim, D.K.; Liu, Q.; Prockop, D.J.; Yannarelli, G. In Vitro Macrophage Assay Predicts the In Vivo Anti-Inflammatory Potential of Exosomes from Human Mesenchymal Stromal Cells. *Mol. Ther. Methods Clin. Dev.* **2019**, *13*, 67–76. [CrossRef]
47. Malvicini, R.; Santa-Cruz, D.; de Lazzari, G.; Tolomeo, A.M.; Sanmartin, C.; Muraca, M.; Yannarelli, G.; Pacienza, N. Macrophage Bioassay Standardization to Assess the Anti-Inflammatory Activity of Mesenchymal Stromal Cell-Derived Small Extracellular Vesicles. *Cytotherapy* **2022**, *24*, 999–1012. [CrossRef]
48. Ramos-Zaldívar, H.M.; Polakovicova, I.; Salas-Huenuleo, E.; Corvalán, A.H.; Kogan, M.J.; Yefi, C.P.; Andia, M.E. Extracellular Vesicles through the Blood–Brain Barrier: A Review. *Fluids Barriers CNS* **2022**, *19*, 60. [CrossRef]
49. Driedonks, T.; Jiang, L.; Carlson, B.; Han, Z.; Liu, G.; Queen, S.E.; Shirk, E.N.; Gololobova, O.; Liao, Z.; Nyberg, L.H.; et al. Pharmacokinetics and Biodistribution of Extracellular Vesicles Administered Intravenously and Intranasally to Macaca Nemestrina. *J. Extracell. Biol.* **2022**, *1*, e59. [CrossRef]
50. Türker, S.; Onur, E.; Ózer, Y. Nasal Route and Drug Delivery Systems. *Pharm. World Sci.* **2004**, *26*, 137–142. [CrossRef]

pharmaceutics

MDPI

Review

The Therapeutic Potential and Clinical Significance of Exosomes as Carriers of Drug Delivery System

Tianwei Li [1,†], Xiaoqing Li [2,†], Guiping Han [2,†], Ming Liang [3], Zongrui Yang [1], Congyi Zhang [1], Shizhuan Huang [1], Sheng Tai [1,*] and Shan Yu [2,*]

1 Department of Hepatic Surgery, Second Affiliated Hospital of Harbin Medical University, Harbin 150000, China
2 Department of Pathology, Second Affiliated Hospital of Harbin Medical University, Harbin 150000, China
3 Department of Infectious Diseases, Second Affiliated Hospital of Harbin Medical University, Harbin 150000, China
* Correspondence: taisheng1973@163.com (S.T.); yushan@hrbmu.edu.cn (S.Y.)
† These authors contributed equally to this work.

Abstract: Drug delivery system (DDS) realizes the drug delivery process through the drug carrier. As an important part of DDS, the selection of the drug carrier material is extremely critical, which requires the carrier material to possess excellent biocompatibility and targeting and not affect the pharmacological action of the drug. As one of the endogenous extracellular vesicles, exosomes are 30–100 nm in diameter, which are considered a new generation of a natural nanoscale delivery system. Exosomes secreted by different types of cells carry signaling molecules (such as proteins and nucleic acid) playing an important role in cell behaviors. Owing to their ability to specialize in intercellular communication, exosomes provide a distinctive method to deliver therapeutic drugs to target cells. In this concept, exosomes as the natural liposomes carry endogenous biomolecules, have excellent biocompatibility, and could be loaded with cargo both in vivo and in vitro. In addition, modifications by genetic and/or chemical engineering to part of the exosome surface or complement the desired natural effect may enhance the targeting with drug loading capability. Notably, exosomes weakly react with serum proteins prolonging cargo half-life. Overall, exosomes as natural carriers integrate the superiority of synthetic nanocarriers and cellular communication while precluding their limitations, which provides novel and reliable methods for drug delivery and treatment. Our review focuses on the therapeutic potentials and clinical values of exosomes as a carrier of drug delivery system in multiple diseases, including cancer, nervous, immune, and skeletal system diseases.

Keywords: exosome; drug delivery system; exosome carriers; tumor; CNS disease

Citation: Li, T.; Li, X.; Han, G.; Liang, M.; Yang, Z.; Zhang, C.; Huang, S.; Tai, S.; Yu, S. The Therapeutic Potential and Clinical Significance of Exosomes as Carriers of Drug Delivery System. *Pharmaceutics* **2023**, *15*, 21. https://doi.org/10.3390/pharmaceutics15010021

Academic Editor: Simon C. W. Richardson

Received: 22 November 2022
Revised: 15 December 2022
Accepted: 16 December 2022
Published: 21 December 2022

1. Introduction

Exosomes are biphospholipid bodies formed from membranes and emitted by cells [1]. In 1983, exosomes were discovered in supernatant from cultured sheep erythrocytes and were considered as secreted garbage [2]. Following in-depth investigations revealed that exosomes could be released by tumor cells, immune cells, mesenchymal stem cells, and endothelial progenitor cells and are widely detectable in blood, cerebrospinal fluid, saliva, ascites, and even urine [3]. Now, it is generally accepted that exosomes are 30–100 nm in diameter, rich in lipids (cholesterol, sphingomyelin, and ceramide), and fulfilled with active molecules including DNA, noncoding RNA, mRNA or protein (Table 1) [4]. Those unique tissue- or cell-specific proteins and genetic materials help to identify their cellular origin and the status of parental cells. Moreover, exosomes widely participate in biological activities such as cell communication, migration, angiogenesis, immunomodulation, and proliferation. During the exploiting their delivery function, exosomes from human donor cells are found to be capable of transferring chemical drugs or endogenous substances (proteins, mRNAs, miRNAs, lipids, etc.) to receiver cells for therapy. Even plant-derived exosomes have been characterized and shown to have structures similar to mammalian exosomes to mediate plant–animal intercellular communication [5]. Therefore, exosomes as naturally derived biological carriers have been refined into the concept of drug delivery. Due to the possible immune responses and lack of targeting, current studies on heterologous exosomes lack their clinical application, we mainly reviewed the role of homologous exosomes as drug delivery carriers. As an emerging drug delivery carrier, exosomes loaded with chemical or genetic drugs play a promising therapeutic role in diseases.

Table 1. Summary of the exosome compositions.

		Compositions	Reference
Protein	Cell surface protein	MHCI, MHCII, CD63, CD81, CD9, Lamp-2b, lactadherin	[6]
	Cytoplasmic proteins	Ubiquitin, ALIX, ESCRT, HSC70, HSP70, HSP60, HSP90, etc.	[7]
	Cytoskeletal protein	Actin, tubulin, Keratin 8, 10, 18 and 19, α-Actinin-4	[8]
	Enzymes	Lysosomal, AAA ATPase, kinases, fatty acid synthase	[9]
Nucleic acid		mRNA, miRNA, ncRNA, siRNA	[10]
Lipids		Ceramide, sphingomyelin, phosphatidylserine, phosphatidylcholine, steroid lipids, etc.	[11]

2. Formation and Understanding of Exosomes

2.1. Mechanism in the Secretion of Exosomes

Exosomes are mainly formed by endocytosis of cell membranes, followed by converting to multivesicular bodies (MVBs) with dynamic subcellular architecture. Parts of MVBs could be fused to lysosomes, and their contents are degraded or recycled. The remaining MVBs may merge with the membrane followed by secretion to the extracellular matrix to form new extracellular vesicles including exosomes. The biogenesis mechanism of exosomes is controlled by related proteins, including annexin and tetraspanins (CD63). The endosomal sorting complex required for transport (ESCRT) is accepted as molecular media by which exosomes have specific cargo sorting functions [12]. Studies have shown that ESCRT-0, ESCRT-I, and ESCRT-II may be regulating cargo sorting, and ESCRT-III is involved in membrane endocytosis and exocytosis. Beginning with ESCRT-0, early endosomes for cargo-specific are initiated, recruited, and assembled to eventually form MBV [13,14]. In addition, Vps4 and ALIX also participate in cargo sorting and exosome formation [15,16]. Exosome formation steps are summarized in Figure 1.

In addition, exosomes are regulated by cytokines growth factors, proteins, distinct cell types, and other physicochemical conditions at multiple stages in the production process and widely exist in cells and body fluids in vivo, making them well-tolerated and -regulated [17].

2.2. Using Exosome Carriers in Drug Delivery System for Therapeutics

The drug carrier is the key component of a successful DDS. With the progress of science and technology, artificial materials such as synthetic liposomes and polylactic acid have been exploited as carriers in the last few years. Small volume, large surface area, and high-dose drug loading are the common characteristics of these materials [18,19]. However, these materials have the following disadvantages: low transduction efficiency, lack of target specificity, rapid degradation, and toxicity. The ideal drug carrier should have the characteristics of sustained, controlled, and targeted release; be compatible with the host immune system, specifically absorbed by target cells; and maintain a sufficient circulating half-life with the loaded drug. This requires the carrier material to have appropriate biocompatibility and biodegradability without affecting drug efficacy [20]. At present, exosomes have the above conditions perfectly. As a natural liposome in the human body, exosomes are considered to have the capability of high-efficiency loading and co-transmission of therapeutic drugs [21]. Thus far, the cargo biological component is fulfilled in exosomes through incubation, sonication, freeze-thaw cycling, extrusion, and electroporation once extracted from the donor cells [22]. In vivo, an effective way to modify exosomes is by up-regulating a gene in the parental cells or culturing cell lines with a chemical drug. The gene or drug will then be gently encapsulated in vesicles according to the process of exosome biogenesis [23]. Another promising feature is that simple surface modifications by bioengineering allow exosome delivery cargo more targeted. Although exosome carriers are natural, surface modifications can be performed easily with strategies that include genetic or/and chemical engineering modification.

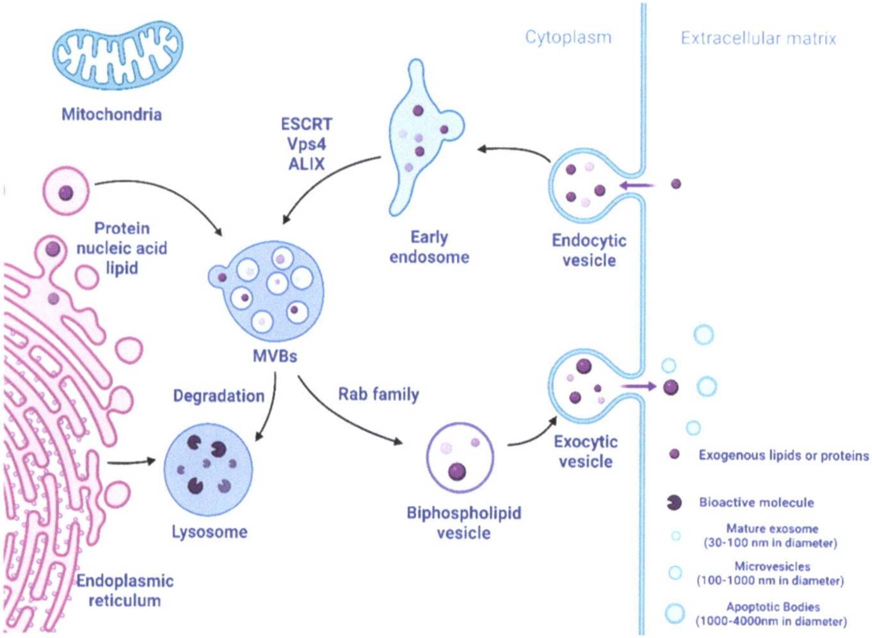

Figure 1. The illustration of exosome exchange. Bioactive components can be absorbed into the cell through endocytosis. Vesicle formation is considered to generate early endosomes, which are in turn shaped as MVBs. Part of MVBs could be degraded in lysosomes or through autophagosomes, while other parts could be returned to the plasma membrane and be secreted to the extracellular matrix, forming exosomes.

In genetic-related engineering approach, nucleic acids molecules ligands are fused to exosome surface proteins genetically and overexpressed subsequently in donor cells. The study by Zou et al. demonstrated that the constructs containing the platelet-derived growth factor receptor (PDGFR) transmembrane domain fused to single-chain variable fragments of human immunodeficiency virus (HIV)-1 Env-specific antibodies have been used to target exosomes to HIV-1-infected cells [24]. Similarly, one promising example is that Mentkowski et al. generated a highly efficient exosome delivery system that could target cardiomyocytes by modifying exosomes from cardiomyocytes (CDCs). The researchers fused cardiomyocyte targeting peptide (CMP) to the N-terminus of Lamp2b (a mouse transmembrane protein) through exosomes. After intramyocardial injection, they found that CMP-targeted CDC-derived exosomes could help in increasing cardiomyocyte uptake, decreasing apoptosis, and promoting cardiac retention. Making the groundwork supported exosomes for specific-targeting cells by drugs and gene therapy [25]. While the chemical methods rely on the bioconjugation of protein or chemical ligands to surface proteins. For example, Kim et al. used paclitaxel (PTX)-loaded exosomes with incorporated aminoethylanisamide-polyethylene glycol (AA-PEG) vector moiety to aim at binding with the sigma receptor, increasing the anticancer efficacy of PTX in lung cancer cells. Their result showed that AA-modified vesicles had a better loading capacity and therapeutic efficiency in vivo [26]. Similarly, Gao et al. used a phage-identified peptide (CP05) covalently bound to the exosome surface protein CD63. Following systemic administration of CP05-loaded exosomes, researchers found that targeting CP05-loaded exosomes increased the delivery of splice-correcting oligomers to muscle, thereby restoring muscular dystrophy [27]. It is clear that the above two major modification strategies make exosomes extremely advantageous when delivering drugs as carriers.

2.3. Advantages of Exosome Carriers for Drug Delivery

Compared with artificially synthesized carriers, the advantages of exosomes as carriers of DDS are generally known as follows: (1) A plentiful number of proteins and genetic molecules as a component in exosomes indicate that the great majority of biological substances can be loaded without unexpected interactions with the carrier. Endogenous exosomes have limited therapeutic efficacy, but exogenous exosomes can load dissimilar cargoes, including reconstituted proteins or therapeutic nucleic acids. They have superior compatibility that is critical to their function as carriers [28], which also shows a tremendous inherent capacity for receiver cells [29]. (2) Exosomes could be detected in almost any body fluids (blood, cerebrospinal fluid, saliva, etc.), indicating their transport cargo could go through membrane and be protected from degradations [30]. Furthermore, those nature-made vesicles are better tolerated in vivo. (3) The powerful targeted delivery capability and homing ability of exosomes as DDS carriers for therapeutic aims: First, exosomes can modulate targeting capabilities through loading specific binding principles of receptors and ligands, for example, dendritic cells (DC)-derived exosomes could transfer major histocompatibility complexes to antigen-presenting cell for regulating immunity [31]. Second, the targeted homing potential and cellular uptake capacity of exosomes are enhanced with the presence of vesicle surface proteins. Studies have shown that cancer-cell-derived exosomes tend to merge with their parental cells preferentially. This phenomenon created novel targeted therapies based on exosomes to deliver antitumor drugs [32]. Furthermore, integrins on exosomes determine the organotropism effect of exosomes into specific tissues. (4) Unlike synthetic liposomes, exosomes can be loaded with cargo in vivo by transfection and in vitro by electroporation and lipofection [33]. (5) Exosomes show faint nonspecific interactions with serum proteins. It was reported that serum proteins bind on the surface of synthetic nanoparticle (NP) carriers immediately after entering the bloodstream, forming so-called protein coronas [34,35]. The protein crowns can affect the properties of synthetic NP such as cell targeting, cell interactions, toxicity, etc. Furthermore, the protein corona causes an immune response and is quickly cleared from the blood (Figure 2) [36,37]. Notably, the binding of serum proteins with exosomes is weak, mainly based on exosome's endogenous nature. Therefore, exosomes have good biocompatibility as carriers, which can prolong the circulation half-time with therapeutic cargo [38].

With the above advantages, exosomes are capable to refrain from phagocytosis and cross biological barriers with therapeutic substances (proteins, mRNAs, lipids, chemical drugs) to sites that are difficult to arrive at by artificial carriers. For instance, exosomes can cross the blood–brain barrier (BBB) and transport specific drugs to the neural cell [39], significantly retaining side effects including toxicity. With the promising and highly efficient carry potentials in DDS, exosomes are showing good biocompatibility, non-immunogenicity, and biodegradability and intensively investigated in the therapeutic role for different diseases.

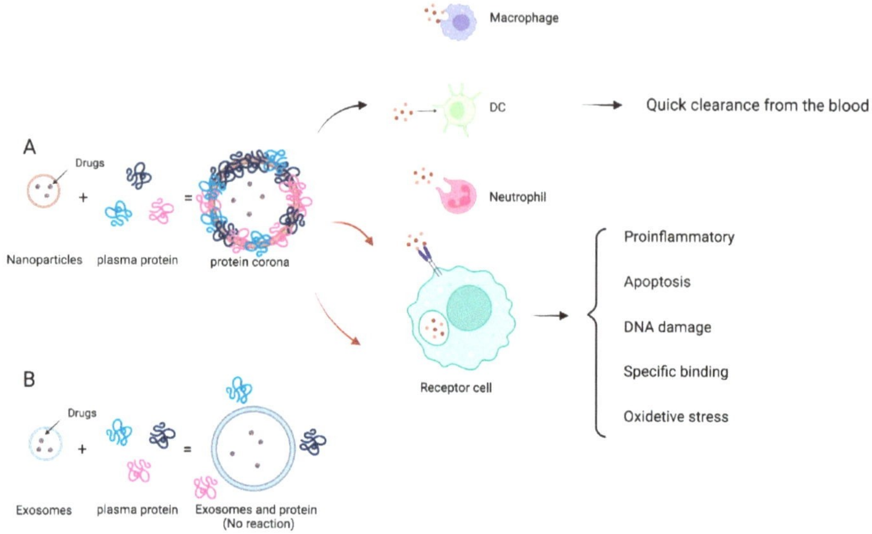

Figure 2. The schematic representation of the biological reaction of the protein crown in blood circulation. (**A**) Various plasma proteins adsorb onto NPs immediately after the synthetic NPs enter the blood, resulting in rapid clearance and cytotoxicity; (**B**) exosomes weakly bind with the serum proteins, thereby enhancing the circulation time and decreasing the cytotoxicity.

3. Tumors

Exosomes rich in genetic material, proteins, and lipids may carry effective communication information for donor cells and target cells, which may build up the tumor microenvironment (TME) [40]. Tumor-derived exosomes (TDEs) were also found to have strong associations with TME and cancer initiation. Therefore, TDEs could be devised as natural drug carriers with higher cancer cell targeting and therapeutic efficacy, low toxicity, and permeability [41].

3.1. Delivering Endogenous Biomolecules

Endogenous biomolecules contain abundant regulatory substances such as hormones, antibodies, cytokines, etc., which can also be incorporated into TDEs for therapeutic effects. Exosomes may provide a more rational way for therapeutic protein delivery to exert antitumor effects as we highlighted above [42]. In pancreatic cancer, it was shown that exosomes loaded with the survival protein-T34A protein induced apoptosis and enhanced the gemcitabine-killing effect [43]. Nie et al. synthesized exosome nano-protein bioconjugates for tumor therapy by conjugating azide-modified exosomes from M1 macrophages to dibenzocyclooctyne-modified antibodies to CD47 and SIRPα via a pH-sensitive linker. Their result showed that the nano-bioconjugates could specifically bind with cancer by recognition of CD47. Meanwhile, native M1 exosomes efficiently reprogram macrophages from pro-tumor M2 to anti-tumor M1 [44]. Furthermore, strong immunogenic proteins embedded in exosomes may provoke immune activation to inhibit cancer proliferation with the potential for developing cancer vaccines. Notably, DC-derived exosomes gain MHC-I that combines with tumor-derived peptides, and the complex could activate NK or T cells to suppress tumors [45,46]. In addition to proteins, nucleic acids (mRNA, miRNA, siRNA, piRNA, etc.) have also been reported as a potential method for cancer treatment [47,48]. In Yang et al. research, mouse embryonic fibroblast-derived exosomes were able to deliver PTEN (phosphatase and homologous tensin) mRNA to inhibit mouse glioma growth [49]. Furthermore, exosome transport solves the problem of easy degradation of miRNAs in vivo, implying a new tumor therapy [50]. Brien et al. reported that mesenchymal stem cells (MSC)-derived exosomes containing miR-379 were shown to have a therapeutic effect on breast cancer, with significantly reduced tumor growth rates in T47D breast cell line expressing miR-379 [51]. In addition, exosomes from MSCs had a higher amount of miR-1455p were displaying a strong effect on the inhibition of pancreatic cancer cells in vitro and in vivo [52]. Similarly, siRNA delivery can also be used for cancer treatment via post-transcriptional gene silencing for targeting cells. Shtam et al. showed the therapeutic potential of exosome-mediated siRNA delivery to HeLa cells (cervical cancer cell line) by targeting RAD51. These results demonstrate the cancer therapeutic capacity of using exosome carriers to deliver nucleic acids for RNAi-based gene therapy [53]. Furthermore, genetic tools can also be embedded into TDEs such as plasmids. Kim et al. used exosomes secreted from SKOV3 as a vector to express the CRISPR/Cas9 plasmid. The CRISPR/Cas9-loaded exosomes significantly down-regulated PARP-1 expression, thus causing ovarian cancer cell death [54].

3.2. Delivering Chemical Drugs

Antitumor drugs such as vincristine, curcumin, PTX, camptothecin, etc., most of which are monomer active ingredients extracted from Chinese medicine, generally have disadvantages including poor stability, low solubility, high hydrophobicity, and short half-life, etc. Therefore, their low bioavailability limited the clinical application. The efficacy of these monomeric components can be enhanced by the administration of exosome carriers [55]. For example, Saari et al. showed that tumor cell-derived exosomes could be considered a useful vehicle for paclitaxel from the parental cell, carrying the drug into recipient cells through the endocytosis pathway and increasing their cytotoxicity [56]. Similarly, Garofalo et al. showed lung tumor cell-derived exosomes can effectively carry the oncolytic virus and chemotherapeutic drugs (PTX), thus enhancing the antitumor effects in nude mice [57]. Tang et al. showed another example that exosomes pre-loaded with cisplatin could significantly decrease liver or kidney toxicities and suppress tumors in ovarian cancer mice xenograft model [58]. In general, exosome-loaded drugs display better efficacy than chemicals used alone.

3.3. Delivering Engineered Drugs

In recent years, researchers have increasingly turned to transport conjugated or modified drugs through TDEs to promote therapeutic efficacy. This procedure generally involves the reconstitution of multiple drugs through encapsulation [59]. For example, the researchers used mouse macrophage exosomes to hybridize with synthetic liposomes to obtain engineered exosomes, water-soluble doxorubicin loaded in the engineered exosomes under acidic conditions had a significantly enhanced toxicity to cancer cells. It strongly suggests that the engineered exosomes will be a promising platform for tumor-targeted drug delivery [60]. Yong et al. have innovated a biocompatible exogenous tumor-cell-exocytosed exosome-biomimetic porous silicon nanoparticles (PSiNPs) as a drug carrier for anti-tumor. After being pre-loaded with Doxorubicin, the exosome sheath enhanced tumor accumulation and vascular extravasation. In addition, this system exhibits remarkable cell absorption and cytotoxicity in tumor cells [61]. Similarly, Wu et al. synthesized sequential nano catalysts GOD-ESIONs@EVs (GE@EVs) by mixing HCC-derived exosomes as surface nanocarriers with nano-scale iron oxide particles solution (ESIONS)-arginine-glycine-aspartic acid (RGD). The RGD parts are accounting for membrane fusion to enhance cellular endocytosis and the sequential nano catalysts underwent a more effective treatment in the HCC tumor zone during a short time. In addition, Jia et al. used materials such as superparamagnetic iron oxide nanoparticles (SPION) and curcumin to coat a novel glioma-targeting exosome. Their findings demonstrated that the engineered exosome strongly improved the treatment of glioma while reducing side effects [62]. The above studies provide validations for the application of exosome carriers-loaded engineered drugs for high targeting and efficient anticancer activity.

In summary, TDEs contain tumor-associated antigens that can preferably identify tumors and targeted transmit therapeutic substances. Therefore, exosome carriers possess superior biocompatibility, causing drugs more easily uptake by the cells and avoiding drug resistance (Figure 3). Additionally, exosome carriers could hold the drug stability and half-life.

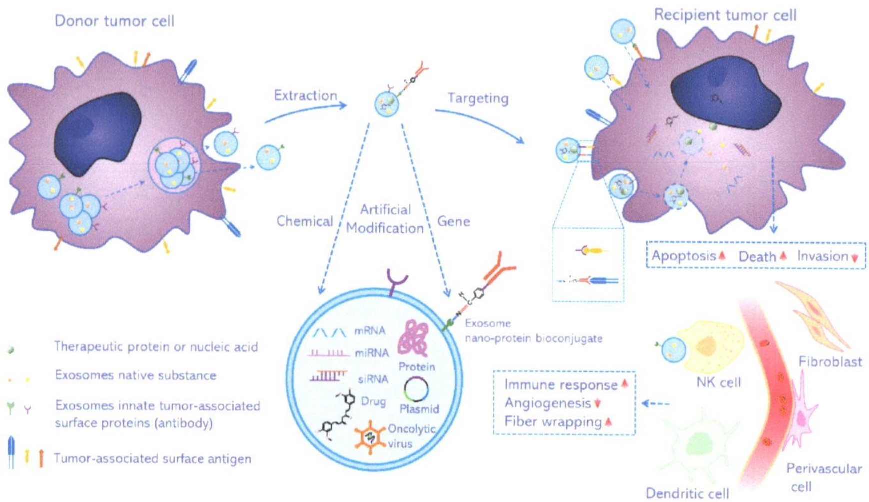

Figure 3. Schematic illustration of the tumor-derived exosomes with modification strategies for enhancing targeting. A chemical or gene modification of extracted exosomes from tumor cells may further promote the anti-tumor functions from indicated concepts.

4. Neurological Diseases

In the central nervous system (CNS), exosomes have a role in mediating intercellular communication, maintaining homeostasis, and neuroprotective (Table 2). Furthermore, exosome carriers can deliver therapeutic substances across the blood–brain barrier (BBB). Therefore, it opens up a promising possibility to deliver therapeutic substances to treat central neurological diseases, such as neurodegenerative diseases, strokes, etc. [63].

Table 2. Mechanisms of exosome neuroprotection.

Exosome Sources	The Main Molecules	Molecules or Pathways Acting in the Process	The Main Mechanism	Reference
Mesenchymal stem cells (MSC)	N/A	N/A	Increased angiogenesis after ischemia	[64]
Adipose-derived MSCs	miR-25-3p	Autophagy	Reduce neuronal autophagy	[65]
The astrocyte origin	circSHOC2	miR-7670-3p/SIRT1	Inhibition of neuronal cell apoptosis	[66]
The astrocyte origin	microRNA-34c	TLR7, NF-κB/MAPK	Reduce ischemia/reperfusion (I/R) injury	[67]

For example, traumatic brain injury (TBI) can cause severe neuronal damage, and studies have shown that exosomes from human-induced pluripotent stem cells (hiPSCs) and MSCs may heal neuronal damage [68]. Moon et al. studied the biological distribution, therapeutic effect, and action mode of MSC-derived exosomes in a rat stroke model. The results illustrated strong evidence for MSC-derived exosomes could successfully stimulate neurogenesis and angiogenesis in that model [69].

The engineered DCs-derived exosomes with Lamp2b had been generated and combined into a neuron-specific RVG peptide. After extraction of the exosome, an exogenous siRNA was loaded. Notably, exosomes specifically delivered loaded cargo to neurons in the brain, downregulating the siRNA target gene and impacted on Alzheimer's disease (AD) [70]. Others reported that exosome carriers conjugated to the surface of c (RGDyK) peptide or curcumin can target the lesion area of ischemic encephalopathy. In a mouse model, the modified exosomes provided a safe and effective delivery vehicle for ischemic stroke therapy [71]. Wang et al. studied engineered exosomes that silenced Bcl-2 and Bax with a promising result that suggested the exosomes had a therapeutic effect on apoptosis after TBI [72].

In addition, emerging engineering techniques are applied to modify the exosome to further promote its capacity to carry cargo. Ferrantelli et al. identified a negative regulatory factor mutant (Nefmut) of the HIV-encoded. The researchers loaded Nefmut into exosomes and fused a single-chain fragment variable antibody at its C-terminus to form engineered exosomes, which proposed a novel targeted strategy for endogenous engineering in the treatment of neurodegenerative diseases based on exosomes released by the cellular composition of the CNS [73]. Qu et al. established a biocompatible kit for the exosome-based delivery system across the BBB. In a mouse Parkinson's disease (PD) model, exosomes with pre-loaded dopamine exhibited better performance than free dopamine after intravenous injection [74]. Haney et al. developed engineered exosomes loaded with catalase (ExoCAT), and after intranasal administration, a major proportion of exosomes could be found in the brains of PD mice. In addition, ExoCAT showed effective neuroprotection in vivo models of PD [75]. With the development of engineered and advanced loading cargo technology, exosomes as DDS carriers will certainly have greater therapeutic potential and value for CNS diseases in the future.

5. Autoimmune Diseases

Previous studies have proved that natural or surface-modified exosomes can be used as a treatment for autoimmune diseases [76]. As conventional treatments for autoimmune diseases suffer from low bioavailability, rapid clearance, limited targeting ability, and poor therapeutic outcomes due to the unfavorable pharmacokinetic behavior of the drugs, exosomes carriers can efficiently load biologics or other inflammation inhibitors and deliver them to the target protected from enzyme-caused degradation, which provides tantalizing prospects in supporting the fight against autoimmune diseases. It was reported that miR-146a/miR-155-transduced MSC-derived exosome strongly increased Treg cell subpopulation and anti-inflammatory cytokines in collagen-induced arthritis (CIA) mice. Ultimately, this modulation may facilitate the restoration of T-cell responses in rheumatoid arthritis (RA); therefore, the use of MSC-derived exosomes to load miRNAs that can alter immune responses could serve as therapeutic targets for inflammatory diseases [77]. Riazifar et al. showed that exosome-stimulated MSCs produced by γ-interferon have been shown to have significant effects in the treatment of autoimmune encephalomyelitis (EAE) [78].

Studies have shown that glucocorticoid-loaded exosomes show therapeutic efficacy in proteolipoprotein-induced experimental autoimmune encephalomyelitis. Animals treated with glucocorticoid-loaded exosomes recovered from acute illness more rapidly than clinically used multiple sclerosis (MS) drugs, such as betafalon and copasone [79]. To suppress the side effects of methotrexate, researchers encapsulated the chemical drug in exosomes from MSCs, and it showed better retention and a 10-fold inhibition of inflammation compared to methotrexate alone [80]. Similarly, Kadry et al. found the glutathione-loaded exosomes were more able to shorten the glutathione synthesis process, increase glutathione serum levels, and meanwhile reduce rheumatoid factors. The prognostic marker malondialdehyde and C-reactive protein levels were lower than the free glutathione group [81].

Furthermore, exosomes can be modified with biological or synthetic ligands on the unique surface to enhance the targeting specific possibility to deliver cargo in different autoimmune diseases. For example, Yan et al. established biomimetic exosomes and modified them with compounds such as folic acid (FA), polyethylene glycol (PEG), and cholesterol to obtain an actively targeted drug delivery vehicle loaded with dexamethasone sodium phosphate. In vivo biodistribution experiments showed that these engineered exosomes better protected bone and cartilage in CIA mice and reduced joint inflammation without obvious liver toxicity. This approach can avoid the side effects of using corticosteroids alone [82]. Similarly, a murine microglial cell line secreted engineered exosomes loaded with IL-4 was designed by Casella. After applying the above exosomes, the experimental autoimmune encephalomyelitis score decreased sharply, significantly reducing tissue damage. The engineered exosomes can also deliver a variety of functional molecules to treat inflammatory diseases [83]. Exosomes show promising prospects for the treatment of autoimmune diseases.

6. Other Systemic Diseases

6.1. Skeletal Diseases

Traditional drug therapy for diseases of the skeletal system is mainly based on inhibiting osteoclast formation (estrogen, etc.) or inhibiting osteoclast activity (bisphosphonates, etc.). However, the prolonged use of high doses of drugs that can cause secondary adverse effects, including affecting normal osteocytes [84]. Clearly, bone drug delivery applications are not yet perfect in targeting and eliminating side effects. Due to the advent of exosome carriers, great progress in the management of drug delivery to the bone has been made [85]. Zha et al. extracted ATDC5 (chondrogenic progenitor cell line)-derived exosomes to load the vascular endothelial growth factor (VEGF) gene, which can effectively restore segmental bone defects by increasing osteogenesis and angiogenesis [86]. The result shows inspiring evidence for curing segmental bone defects. Luo et al. showed that bone marrow stromal cell (ST)-derived exosomes (STExos) could significantly enhance the osteoblast differentiation of bone mesenchymal stem cells (BMSCs) in vitro by simple surface chemical modifications. Intravenous administration of STExos could not improve osteoporotic phenotypes in mouse models. The researchers found significantly higher efficiency after conjugating the STExo surface with BMSC-specific aptamers, confirming the novel modification could help in osteoporosis and fractures [87]. Moreover, the treatment of the engineered bone scaffolds with exosomes as carriers not only provides direct bracing for bone defects but also provides a suitable status for bone regeneration. In addition, Zhang et al. found MSC-exosome/β-TCP composite scaffolds had better healing functions on rat calvarial defects [88]. Another study showed that targeting Kartogenin (KGN) to synovial fluid-derived mesenchymal stem cells (SF-MSCs) by engineered exosomes resulted in uniform dispersion of KGN in the cytoplasmic matrix, increased concentration in the target, and significantly promoted chondrogenesis of SF-MSCs. In a rat model, KGN loaded by engineered exosomes also showed better therapeutic effects than KGN alone [89]. In the future, with the further elucidation of the biological information contained in exosomes, as a natural carrier, exosomes will be able to deliver drugs more precisely and efficiently and exhibit a promising role in the treatment of bone defects, delayed healing, and other skeletal system diseases.

6.2. Cardiovascular Diseases

Cardiovascular exosomes also have a significant clinical role and therapeutic value. All cell subtypes in the cardiovascular system, including endothelial cells (ECs), cardiomyocytes, and fibroblasts, release exosomes to participate in intercellular communication and regulate cardiac function. Therefore, the superior biocompatibility of exosomes allows them potentially useful as drug carriers in cardiovascular diseases [90]. Liu et al. investigated the role of exosomes loaded with miR-19a, miR-210, and other miRNAs against oxidative stress (OS) in coronary heart disease, and the results suggest that the ability of exosomes to target loading endogenous antioxidants may make them a more effective treatment for OS than stem cell therapy [91]. In addition, exosomes with angiogenesis-related miRNAs were able to ameliorate cardiac function. For example, injecting miR-19a-3p-loaded exosomes into mouse myocardium revealed that exosomes resulted in improved angiogenesis, decreased myocardial fibrosis, and increased left ventricular ejection fraction [92]. Similarly, Chen et al. showed that bone marrow-secreted MSC exosomes carrying miRNA-125b could prevent myocardial ischemia-reperfusion injury by targeting SIRT7 [93]. A c(RGDyK) peptide-conjugated, cholesterol-modified miR-210-engineered exosomes showed up-regulated expression of integrinβ3, VEGF, and CD34 and demonstrated that miR-210 for cerebral hematogenous delivery provides angiogenic agents for alleviating ischemic diseases [94]. Wu et al. reported that molecularly engineered M2 macrophage-derived exosomes may contribute to treating atherosclerosis by suppressing inflammation via chemokine receptors and inflammation inhibitory cytokines secreted by M2 macrophages. Meanwhile, the encapsulated hexyl 5-aminolevulinate hydrochloride can diminish inflammation effectively by intrinsic biosynthesis and metabolism of heme [95]. Notably, Zhang et al. constructed novel biomimetic nanobubbles (Mel@NVs) composed of exosome-loaded melatonin (Mel) from adipose-derived stem cells (ADSCs). Further reports showed the Mel@NVs could promote the formation of microvessels and alleviate cardiac fibrosis, thereby further restoring mitochondrial dysfunction for myocardial repair. Mel@NVs proved to be a potentially promising therapy for myocardial infarction [96]. As a DDS carrier, exosome performs ideally when delivering therapeutic substances in cardiovascular diseases [97].

6.3. Urinary System Diseases

Traditionally, the signaling of cytokines and inflammatory mediators has been recognized as an important player in the pathogenesis of kidney diseases. It has been reported that exosomes can participate in renal tissue injury and regeneration by mediating inter-nephron communication [98]. Notably, exosomes are used as carriers to load therapeutic substances such as proteins and RNAs with extremely high stability, which provides an attractive method as novel therapeutic carriers for kidney disease treatment. For example, nuclear factor (NF)-kB signaling significantly participated in acute kidney injury induced by ischemia-reperfusion. Researchers used a new and optogenetically engineered exosome technology called EXPLOR to deliver exosomes with effective NF-kB inhibitors into a kidney ischemia-reperfusion mice model. Compared with the control group, the results confirmed it could improve renal injury significantly by regulating different biological components [99]. In another study, M1-Exo-GEM (pre-loading M1 macrophage-derived exosomes(M1-Exo) with Gemcitabine (GEM) by ultrasound technology) was built up for killing mouse bladder cancer MB49 cells. Compared with M1-Exo and GEM, M1-Exo-GEM had significantly up-regulated the expression of inflammatory cytokines and stronger cytotoxic effect on cancer cells [100].

6.4. Cutaneous Disease

Previous studies have revealed that exosomes could be used as a new therapeutic option for skin repair and regeneration treatment [101]. For example, exosomes derived from human umbilical vein endothelial cells (HUVECs) can promote collagen maturation and angiogenesis and regulate the keratinocytes and fibroblast growth, thereby accelerating skin wound healing [102]. Similarly, Zhang et al. found that exosomes from adipose tissue-derived stem cells can accelerate collagen synthesis and redeposition through regulating PI3K/Akt pathway. This function helps in full-thickness skin wounds, ultimately reducing healing time and scarring in mouse models [103]. In addition, exosomes can be further designed to deliver therapeutic cargos to treat skin diseases. For example, recent evidence suggests that the transport of ncRNA (including miRNA and lncRNA) target cells through the role of exosomes in the pathophysiology of psoriatic arthritis [104]. Furthermore, Shiekh et al. have shown that an antioxidant wound dressing, consisting of antioxidant polyurethane combined with ADSCs extracted exosomes, could shorten the diabetic wound healing time [105]. Similarly, Wang et al. loaded epidermal stem cell (ESC)-derived exosomes with VH298 (VH-EV), and VH-EV was shown to promote the function of HUVECs in vitro through HIF-1α signaling. This special exosome displayed great therapeutic effects on skin regeneration [106]. In addition, as carriers, exosomes provide an emerging delivery method for therapeutic miRNAs that neither penetrate the skin nor easily cross cell membranes. Xia et al. found that exosome-based miR-125b may accelerate myofibroblast differentiation and transfer to young fibroblast by targeting SIRT7. The results show a promising method for counteracting skin aging [107].

6.5. Metabolic Disease

The role of exosomes as agents for drug delivery in metabolic diseases is worth investigating [108]. However, major studies are focused on the complications of metabolic diseases, such as the diabetic skin complications discussed above [109,110]. At the same time, engineered exosomes also have broad potential in the treatment of obesity. Guo et al. designed an engineered smart exosome platform called SmartExo@Bmp7. This biological system induced local white adipose tissue browning through transporting Bmp7 mRNA to reduce obesity for C57BL/6 mice. As proof, this evidence opens a novel anti-obesity therapy [111].

7. The Conclusion and Future Breakthrough Directions of Exosome Carriers

In recent years, exosome has received special attention for its therapeutic values. A growing number of studies have proven that exosomes play a key role in the occurrence and development of diseases. Thus far, the clinical application of exosomes is mainly used for body fluid biopsy and clinical diagnosis of diseases such as cancer, nervous system diseases. and immune diseases [112]. However, the achievements are still limited by their novelty. In 2016, the world's first cancer diagnostic product based on exosome miRNAs body fluid biopsy, ExoDx Lung (ALK), was launched, which could detect EML4-ALK mutations in patients with non-small cell lung cancer in real time [113]. Similarly, Zhang et al. showed that exosome microRNAs (such as miR-193a-3p, miR-210-3p, and miR-5100) from hypoxic BMSCs were selectively taken up by lung cancer cells and could activate STAT3 signaling to induce epithelial–mesenchymal transition (EMT) to promote the invasion of lung cancer cells, which has been identified as a new biomarker for lung cancer progression [114].

Additionally, as an ideal natural cargo carrier, exosomes also have great therapeutic value in almost all types of diseases. Exosomes secreted by cells in different tissues carry different biological components, conferring unique biological roles, which enable exosomes to deliver substances such as chemical drugs, nucleic acids, and proteins, etc., to perform the therapeutic role with distinguishable advantages (Table 3). Those advantages include a higher safety profile that escapes from immune detection systems; a better-tolerated and longer-circulating half-life, which prolongs the cargo from degradation; a more easy targeting ability, by which the exosomes' surface could be artificially modified to increase biological effects as carriers and targeted transport; and easy penetration of cell membranes and biological barriers, including the BBB, due to their nanometer size and specific surface molecules.

Table 3. Exosomes derived from sources.

Exosome Sources	Function	Reference
Mesenchymal stem cells	Promote tolerant immune responses, suppress inflammatory responses	[115]
Cancer cell	Involved in tumor microenvironment and cancer development	[116]
Macrophage	Intercellular communication	[117]
Dendritic cells	Immune stimulation	[118]

Table 3. *Cont.*

Exosome Sources	Function	Reference
Mast cell	Participate in immune regulation	[119]
Other cells (such as human amniotic epithelial cells, endothelial progenitor cells, etc.)	Reflect the pathophysiological state of their cell origin and can be used to diagnose and predict disease	[120,121]
Body fluid (saliva, ascites, etc.)	Biomarker and therapeutic agent for diseases	[122]
Heterogeneity (coconut, ginger, pea, bovine or caprine milk, etc.)	Mediate plant–animal intercellular communication	[123,124]

However, most of the research on exosome carriers is still in the vitro stage. The criteria for the manufacture, purification, storage, duration of stability, loading efficiency, and dosage of exosomes also require further investigations to optimize and break through [125,126]. Moreover, existing results enhanced the interaction of exosomes with their targets by modifying exosome surface proteins, but they did not counteract the natural homing ability of exosomes, nor did they prevent off-target effects. There is currently a lack of standardized testing for drugs delivered by exosomes and also few studies investigating the ultimate fate of exosomes. Therefore, more research on the uptake mechanism of exosomes is necessary to ensure that they can deliver cargo directly to the targeted cytoplasm and exert therapeutic effects [127]. In addition, while previous studies have yielded important findings for exosome therapy, most of them only involve in vitro models, so it is unclear whether these results reflect in vivo processes. Furthermore, most of these studies simply analyzed a certain number of miRNAs or proteins. There is a lack of understanding of the exosomes with abundant biological information from distinct cell types. Although several databases of exosome contents exist, diversities between studies and techniques require extraction and purification standardization to elucidate contents and ultimately increase the diversity of cargo molecules [128]. The physical characteristics of the exosome (including size, shape, surface charge, and density) are necessary to determine its role and function. Currently, there is still a great limitation in accurately detecting these characteristics and purity [129]. Therefore, existing findings require careful analysis, and further research in this area is required to accurately measure these physicochemical properties and isolate exosomes from complex biological fluids. Commonly used isolation techniques, such as nanoparticle tracking analysis (NTA), dynamic light scattering (DLS), resistive pulse sensing (RPS), etc., cannot optimally separate exosomes and non-exosomes pollutants and still require extensive experiments studies to improve the purity of exosomes [130]. At the same time, challenges remain in reliably tracking exosomes in vivo, and this needs to be verified by extensive experiments using high-purity exosomes in vitro. The preparation of an in vitro exosome delivery cargo model may be a new method to solve this problem. In addition, the scalability or reproducibility of exosome production is also one of the challenges. Although MSCs can generate a great amount of exosomes, it requires a long time to obtain an effective therapeutic amount [131]. Similar studies are needed in the future to expand other cells or to speed up the collection of specific types of cells. Finally, the translations of exosomes into clinics are confined within existing regulatory frameworks. Therefore, these limitations are required to be fixed for the final application to the clinic.

Briefly, as we mentioned above, exosomes are involved in the occurrence and progression of various systemic diseases, which determine their intrinsic properties of high biocompatibility and low immunogenicity. As a new generation of drug delivery carriers, exosomes could deliver therapeutic drugs to target cells in a targeted manner, playing a therapeutic role in curing diseases. However, methods to regulate cargo packaging and vesicle release in vivo are still limited. Additionally, some technical, functional, and safety features of exosome-based pharmaceutical formulations have not yet been resolved. More safety validations are still required before exosome carriers could be widely performed clinically. Future research on exosomes may focus on scale-up of production and quality control and rigorous pharmacokinetic and reducing toxicology studies before eventually clinical trials. The achievement of these goals will lay the groundwork for the subsequent industrial development of exosomes as novel therapeutic interventions. In short, no difficulties could retard the emerging role of exosomes as a successful player in novel biological drug delivery systems for future clinical applications.

Author Contributions: T.L., X.L. and G.H. performed literature search and drafted the manuscript and figures; M.L., Z.Y., C.Z. and S.H. drafted parts of the manuscript and organized tables; S.Y. and S.T. designed concept of the study and revised the whole manuscript. All authors have read and agreed to the published version of the manuscript.

Funding: This study was supported by the Natural Science Foundation of China (No. 81972724).

Institutional Review Board Statement: Not applicable.

Informed Consent Statement: Not applicable.

Data Availability Statement: Not applicable.

Acknowledgments: We thank all who made contributions to the manuscript.

Conflicts of Interest: The authors declare no conflict of interest.

References

1. Boyiadzis, M.; Whiteside, T.L. Information transfer by exosomes: A new frontier in hematologic malignancies. *Blood Rev.* **2015**, *29*, 281–290. [CrossRef] [PubMed]
2. Pan, B.-T.; Johnstone, R.M. Fate of the transferrin receptor during maturation of sheep reticulocytes in vitro: Selective externalization of the receptor. *Cell* **1983**, *33*, 967–978. [CrossRef] [PubMed]
3. Lässer, C.; Alikhani, V.S.; Ekström, K.; Eldh, M.; Paredes, P.T.; Bossios, A.; Sjöstrand, M.; Gabrielsson, S.; Lötvall, J.; Valadi, H. Human saliva, plasma and breast milk exosomes contain RNA: Uptake by macrophages. *J. Transl. Med.* **2011**, *9*, 9. [CrossRef] [PubMed]
4. Kowal, J.; Tkach, M.; Théry, C. Biogenesis and secretion of exosomes. *Curr. Opin. Cell Biol.* **2014**, *29*, 116–125. [CrossRef] [PubMed]
5. Zhang, M.; Viennois, E.; Xu, C.; Merlin, D. Plant derived edible nanoparticles as a new therapeutic approach against diseases. *Tissue Barriers* **2016**, *4*, e1134415. [CrossRef] [PubMed]
6. Pathan, M.; Fonseka, P.; Chitti, S.V.; Kang, T.; Sanwlani, R.; Van Deun, J.; Hendrix, A.; Mathivanan, S. Vesiclepedia 2019: A compendium of RNA, proteins, lipids and metabolites in extracellular vesicles. *Nucleic Acids Res.* **2019**, *47*, D516–D519. [CrossRef]
7. Liang, Y.; Duan, L.; Lu, J.; Xia, J. Engineering exosomes for targeted drug delivery. *Theranostics* **2021**, *11*, 3183–3195. [CrossRef]
8. Kowal, J.; Arras, G.; Colombo, M.; Jouve, M.; Morath, J.P.; Primdal-Bengtson, B.; Dingli, F.; Loew, D.; Tkach, M.; Théry, C. Proteomic comparison defines novel markers to characterize heterogeneous populations of extracellular vesicle subtypes. *Proc. Natl. Acad. Sci. USA* **2016**, *113*, E968–E977. [CrossRef]
9. Jeppesen, D.K.; Fenix, A.M.; Franklin, J.L.; Higginbotham, J.N.; Zhang, Q.; Zimmerman, L.J.; Liebler, D.C.; Ping, J.; Liu, Q.; Evans, R.; et al. Reassessment of Exosome Composition. *Cell* **2019**, *177*, 428–445.e18. [CrossRef]
10. Ragusa, M.; Barbagallo, C.; Cirnigliaro, M.; Battaglia, R.; Brex, D.; Caponnetto, A.; Barbagallo, D.; Di Pietro, C.; Purrello, M. Asymmetric RNA Distribution among Cells and Their Secreted Exosomes: Biomedical Meaning and Considerations on Diagnostic Applications. *Front. Mol. Biosci.* **2017**, *4*, 66. [CrossRef]
11. Xu, X.; Xu, L.; Zhang, P.; Ouyang, K.; Xiao, Y.; Xiong, J.; Wang, D.; Liang, Y.; Duan, L. Effects of ATP9A on Extracellular Vesicle Release and Exosomal Lipid Composition. *Oxidative Med. Cell. Longev.* **2020**, *2020*, 8865499. [CrossRef] [PubMed]
12. Li, T.; Li, J.; Wang, H.; Zhao, J.; Yan, M.; He, H.; Yu, S. Exosomes: Potential Biomarkers and Functions in Head and Neck Squamous Cell Carcinoma. *Front. Mol. Biosci.* **2022**, *9*, 881794. [CrossRef] [PubMed]
13. Horváth, P.; Müller-Reichert, T. A Structural View on ESCRT-Mediated Abscission. *Front. Cell Dev. Biol.* **2020**, *8*, 586880. [CrossRef] [PubMed]
14. Zhen, Y.; Spangenberg, H.; Munson, M.J.; Brech, A.; Schink, K.O.; Tan, K.-W.; Sørensen, V.; Wenzel, E.M.; Radulovic, M.; Engedal, N.; et al. ESCRT-mediated phagophore sealing during mitophagy. *Autophagy* **2020**, *16*, 826–841. [CrossRef] [PubMed]
15. Jackson, C.E.; Scruggs, B.S.; Schaffer, J.E.; Hanson, P.I. Effects of Inhibiting VPS4 Support a General Role for ESCRTs in Extracellular Vesicle Biogenesis. *Biophys. J.* **2017**, *113*, 1342–1352. [CrossRef]
16. Larios, J.; Mercier, V.; Roux, A.; Gruenberg, J. ALIX- and ESCRT-III–dependent sorting of tetraspanins to exosomes. *J. Cell Biol.* **2020**, *219*. [CrossRef]
17. Meldolesi, J. Exosomes and Ectosomes in Intercellular Communication. *Curr. Biol.* **2018**, *28*, R435–R444. [CrossRef]
18. Higa, L.H.; Jerez, H.E.; de Farias, M.A.; Portugal, R.V.; Romero, E.L.; Morilla, M.J. Ultra-small solid archaeolipid nanoparticles for active targeting to macrophages of the inflamed mucosa. *Nanomedicine* **2017**, *12*, 1165–1175. [CrossRef]

19. Martínez-Carmona, M.; Lozano, D.; Colilla, M.; Vallet-Regí, M. Lectin-conjugated pH-responsive mesoporous silica nanoparticles for targeted bone cancer treatment. *Acta Biomater.* **2018**, *65*, 393–404. [CrossRef]
20. Allen, T.M.; Cullis, P.R. Drug Delivery Systems: Entering the Mainstream. *Science* **2004**, *303*, 1818–1822. [CrossRef]
21. Yang, M.; Wu, S.Y. The Advances and Challenges in Utilizing Exosomes for Delivering Cancer Therapeutics. *Front. Pharmacol.* **2018**, *9*, 735. [CrossRef] [PubMed]
22. Mehryab, F.; Rabbani, S.; Shahhosseini, S.; Shekari, F.; Fatahi, Y.; Baharvand, H.; Haeri, A. Exosomes as a next-generation drug delivery system: An update on drug loading approaches, characterization, and clinical application challenges. *Acta Biomater.* **2020**, *113*, 42–62. [CrossRef] [PubMed]
23. Familtseva, A.; Jeremic, N.; Tyagi, S.C. Exosomes: Cell-created drug delivery systems. *Mol. Cell. Biochem.* **2019**, *459*, 1–6. [CrossRef] [PubMed]
24. Zou, X.; Yuan, M.; Zhang, T.; Wei, H.; Xu, S.; Jiang, N.; Zheng, N.; Wu, Z. Extracellular vesicles expressing a single-chain variable fragment of an HIV-1 specific antibody selectively target Env+ tissues. *Theranostics* **2019**, *9*, 5657–5671. [CrossRef]
25. Mentkowski, K.; Lang, J.K. Exosomes Engineered to Express a Cardiomyocyte Binding Peptide Demonstrate Improved Cardiac Retention in Vivo. *Sci. Rep.* **2019**, *9*, 10041. [CrossRef]
26. Kim, M.S.; Haney, M.J.; Zhao, Y.; Yuan, D.; Deygen, I.; Klyachko, N.L.; Kabanov, A.V.; Batrakova, E.V. Engineering macrophage-derived exosomes for targeted paclitaxel delivery to pulmonary metastases: In vitro and in vivo evaluations. *Nanomedicine* **2018**, *14*, 195–204. [CrossRef]
27. Gao, X.; Ran, N.; Dong, X.; Zuo, B.; Yang, R.; Zhou, Q.; Moulton, H.M.; Seow, Y.; Yin, H. Anchor peptide captures, targets, and loads exosomes of diverse origins for diagnostics and therapy. *Sci. Transl. Med.* **2018**, *10*, eaat0195. [CrossRef]
28. Wei, H.; Chen, Q.; Lin, L.; Sha, C.; Li, T.; Liu, Y.; Yin, X.; Xu, Y.; Chen, L.; Gao, W.; et al. Regulation of exosome production and cargo sorting. *Int. J. Biol. Sci.* **2021**, *17*, 163–177. [CrossRef]
29. Anand, S.; Samuel, M.; Kumar, S.; Mathivanan, S. Ticket to a bubble ride: Cargo sorting into exosomes and extracellular vesicles. *Biochim. Biophys. Acta Proteins Proteom.* **2019**, *1867*, 140203. [CrossRef]
30. Lai, R.C.; Yeo, R.W.Y.; Tan, K.H.; Lim, S.K. Exosomes for drug delivery—A novel application for the mesenchymal stem cell. *Biotechnol. Adv.* **2013**, *31*, 543–551. [CrossRef]
31. Liu, Q.; Rojas-Canales, D.M.; DiVito, S.J.; Shufesky, W.J.; Stolz, D.B.; Erdos, G.; Sullivan, M.L.; Gibson, G.A.; Watkins, S.C.; Larregina, A.T.; et al. Donor dendritic cell–derived exosomes promote allograft-targeting immune response. *J. Clin. Investig.* **2016**, *126*, 2805–2820. [CrossRef] [PubMed]
32. Qiao, L.; Hu, S.; Huang, K.; Su, T.; Li, Z.; Vandergriff, A.; Cores, J.; Dinh, P.-U.; Allen, T.; Shen, D.; et al. Tumor cell-derived exosomes home to their cells of origin and can be used as Trojan horses to deliver cancer drugs. *Theranostics* **2020**, *10*, 3474–3487. [CrossRef] [PubMed]
33. Xi, X.-M.; Xia, S.-J.; Lu, R. Drug loading techniques for exosome-based drug delivery systems. *J. Pharm. Sci.* **2021**, *76*, 61–67.
34. Peng, Q.; Mu, H. The potential of protein–nanomaterial interaction for advanced drug delivery. *J. Control. Release* **2016**, *225*, 121–132. [CrossRef] [PubMed]
35. Müller, J.; Prozeller, D.; Ghazaryan, A.; Kokkinopoulou, M.; Mailänder, V.; Morsbach, S.; Landfester, K. Beyond the protein corona—Lipids matter for biological response of nanocarriers. *Acta Biomater.* **2018**, *71*, 420–431. [CrossRef]
36. Xiao, W.; Wang, Y.; Zhang, H.; Liu, Y.; Xie, R.; He, X.; Zhou, Y.; Liang, L.; Gao, H. The protein corona hampers the transcytosis of transferrin-modified nanoparticles through blood-brain barrier and attenuates their targeting ability to brain tumor. *Biomaterials* **2021**, *274*, 120888. [CrossRef]
37. Sutaria, D.S.; Badawi, M.; Phelps, M.A.; Schmittgen, T.D. Achieving the Promise of Therapeutic Extracellular Vesicles: The Devil is in Details of Therapeutic Loading. *Pharm. Res.* **2017**, *34*, 1053–1066. [CrossRef]
38. Fernandes, M.; Lopes, I.; Teixeira, J.; Botelho, C.; Gomes, A.C. Exosome-like Nanoparticles: A New Type of Nanocarrier. *Curr. Med. Chem.* **2020**, *27*, 3888–3905. [CrossRef]
39. Zhang, Y.; Chopp, M.; Meng, Y.; Katakowski, M.; Xin, H.; Mahmood, A.; Xiong, Y. Effect of exosomes derived from multipluripotent mesenchymal stromal cells on functional recovery and neurovascular plasticity in rats after traumatic brain injury. *J. Neurosurg.* **2015**, *122*, 856–867. [CrossRef]
40. Li, I.; Nabet, B.Y. Exosomes in the tumor microenvironment as mediators of cancer therapy resistance. *Mol. Cancer* **2019**, *18*, 32. [CrossRef]
41. Tarasov, V.V.; Svistunov, A.A.; Chubarev, V.N.; Dostdar, S.A.; Sokolov, A.V.; Brzecka, A.; Sukocheva, O.; Neganova, M.E.; Klochkov, S.G.; Somasundaram, S.G.; et al. Extracellular vesicles in cancer nanomedicine. Semin. *Cancer Biol.* **2021**, *69*, 212–225. [CrossRef]
42. Yim, N.; Ryu, S.W.; Choi, K.; Lee, K.R.; Lee, S.; Choi, H.; Kim, J.; Shaker, M.R.; Sun, W.; Park, J.H.; et al. Exosome engineering for efficient intracellular delivery of soluble proteins using optically reversible protein-protein interaction module. *Nat. Commun.* **2016**, *7*, 12277. [CrossRef] [PubMed]
43. Aspe, J.R.; Diaz Osterman, C.J.; Jutzy, J.M.; Deshields, S.; Whang, S.; Wall, N.R. Enhancement of Gemcitabine sensitivity in pancreatic adenocarcinoma by novel exosome-mediated delivery of the Survivin-T34A mutant. *J. Extracell. Vesicles* **2014**, *3*, 23244. [CrossRef] [PubMed]
44. Nie, W.; Wu, G.; Zhang, J.; Huang, L.; Ding, J.; Jiang, A.; Zhang, Y.; Liu, Y.; Li, J.; Pu, K.; et al. Responsive Exosome Nanobioconjugates for Synergistic Cancer Therapy. *Angew. Chem. Int. Ed.* **2019**, *59*, 2018–2022. [CrossRef] [PubMed]

45. Hartman, Z.C.; Wei, J.; Glass, O.K.; Guo, H.; Lei, G.; Yang, X.-Y.; Osada, T.; Hobeika, A.; Delcayre, A.; Le Pecq, J.-B.; et al. Increasing vaccine potency through exosome antigen targeting. *Vaccine* **2011**, *29*, 9361–9367. [CrossRef] [PubMed]
46. Romagnoli, G.G.; Zelante, B.B.; Toniolo, P.A.; Migliori, I.K.; Barbuto, J.A.M. Dendritic Cell-Derived Exosomes may be a Tool for Cancer Immunotherapy by Converting Tumor Cells into Immunogenic Targets. *Front. Immunol.* **2015**, *5*, 692.
47. Geis-Asteggiante, L.; Belew, A.T.; Clements, V.K.; Edwards, N.J.; Ostrand-Rosenberg, S.; El-Sayed, N.M.; Fenselau, C. Differential Content of Proteins, mRNAs, and miRNAs Suggests that MDSC and Their Exosomes May Mediate Distinct Immune Suppressive Functions. *J. Proteome Res.* **2018**, *17*, 486–498. [CrossRef]
48. Dvorská, D.; Braný, D.; Ňachajová, M.; Halašová, E.; Danková, Z. Breast Cancer and the Other Non-Coding RNAs. *Int. J. Mol. Sci.* **2021**, *22*, 3280. [CrossRef]
49. Yang, Z.; Shi, J.; Xie, J.; Wang, Y.; Sun, J.; Liu, T.; Zhao, Y.; Zhao, X.; Wang, X.; Ma, Y.; et al. Large-scale generation of functional mRNA-encapsulating exosomes via cellular nanoporation. *Nat. Biomed. Eng.* **2020**, *4*, 69–83. [CrossRef]
50. Ell, B.; Mercatali, L.; Ibrahim, T.; Campbell, N.; Schwarzenbach, H.; Pantel, K.; Amadori, D.; Kang, Y. Tumor-Induced Osteoclast miRNA Changes as Regulators and Biomarkers of Osteolytic Bone Metastasis. *Cancer Cell* **2013**, *24*, 542–556. [CrossRef]
51. O'Brien, K.P.; Khan, S.; Gilligan, K.; Zafar, H.; Lalor, P.; Glynn, C.; O'Flatharta, C.; Ingoldsby, H.; Dockery, P.; De Bhulbh, A.; et al. Employing mesenchymal stem cells to support tumor-targeted delivery of extracellular vesicle (EV)-encapsulated microRNA-379. *Oncogene* **2018**, *37*, 2137–2149. [CrossRef] [PubMed]
52. Ding, Y.; Cao, F.; Sun, H.; Wang, Y.; Liu, S.; Wu, Y.; Cui, Q.; Mei, W.; Li, F. Exosomes derived from human umbilical cord mesenchymal stromal cells deliver exogenous miR-145-5p to inhibit pancreatic ductal adenocarcinoma progression. *Cancer Lett.* **2019**, *442*, 351–361. [CrossRef] [PubMed]
53. Shtam, T.A.; Kovalev, R.A.; Varfolomeeva, E.Y.; Makarov, E.M.; Kil, Y.V.; Filatov, M.V. Exosomes are natural carriers of exogenous siRNA to human cells in vitro. *Cell Commun. Signal.* **2013**, *11*, 88. [CrossRef] [PubMed]
54. Kim, S.M.; Yang, Y.; Oh, S.J.; Hong, Y.; Seo, M.; Jang, M. Cancer-derived exosomes as a delivery platform of CRISPR/Cas9 confer cancer cell tropism-dependent targeting. *J. Control. Release* **2017**, *266*, 8–16. [CrossRef] [PubMed]
55. Farooqi, A.A.; Desai, N.N.; Qureshi, M.Z.; Librelotto, D.R.N.; Gasparri, M.L.; Bishayee, A.; Nabavi, S.M.; Curti, V.; Daglia, M. Exosome biogenesis, bioactivities and functions as new delivery systems of natural compounds. *Biotechnol. Adv.* **2018**, *36*, 328–334. [CrossRef] [PubMed]
56. Saari, H.; Lázaro-Ibáñez, E.; Viitala, T.; Vuorimaa-Laukkanen, E.; Siljander, P.; Yliperttula, M. Microvesicle- and exosome-mediated drug delivery enhances the cytotoxicity of Paclitaxel in autologous prostate cancer cells. *J. Control. Release* **2015**, *220*, 727–737. [CrossRef]
57. Garofalo, M.; Saari, H.; Somersalo, P.; Crescenti, D.; Kuryk, L.; Aksela, L.; Capasso, C.; Madetoja, M.; Koskinen, K.; Oksanen, T.; et al. Antitumor effect of oncolytic virus and paclitaxel encapsulated in extracellular vesicles for lung cancer treatment. *J. Control. Release* **2018**, *283*, 223–234. [CrossRef]
58. Tang, K.; Zhang, Y.; Zhang, H.; Xu, P.; Liu, J.; Ma, J.; Lv, M.; Li, D.; Katirai, F.; Shen, G.-X.; et al. Delivery of chemotherapeutic drugs in tumour cell-derived microparticles. *Nat. Commun.* **2012**, *3*, 1282. [CrossRef]
59. Palazzolo, S.; Memeo, L.; Hadla, M.; Duzagac, F.; Steffan, A.; Perin, T.; Canzonieri, V.; Tuccinardi, T.; Caligiuri, I.; Rizzolio, F. Cancer Extracellular Vesicles: Next-Generation Diagnostic and Drug Delivery Nanotools. *Cancers* **2020**, *12*, 3165. [CrossRef]
60. Rayamajhi, S.; Nguyen, T.D.T.; Marasini, R.; Aryal, S. Macrophage-derived exosome-mimetic hybrid vesicles for tumor targeted drug delivery. *Acta Biomater.* **2019**, *94*, 482–494. [CrossRef]
61. Yong, T.; Zhang, X.; Bie, N.; Zhang, H.; Zhang, X.; Li, F.; Hakeem, A.; Hu, J.; Gan, L.; Santos, H.A.; et al. Tumor exosome-based nanoparticles are efficient drug carriers for chemotherapy. *Nat. Commun.* **2019**, *10*, 3838. [CrossRef]
62. Jia, G.; Han, Y.; An, Y.; Ding, Y.; He, C.; Wang, X.; Tang, Q. NRP-1 targeted and cargo-loaded exosomes facilitate simultaneous imaging and therapy of glioma in vitro and in vivo. *Biomaterials* **2018**, *178*, 302–316. [CrossRef] [PubMed]
63. Ghosh, S.; Ghosh, S. Exosome: The "Off-the-Shelf" Cellular Nanocomponent as a Potential Pathogenic Agent, a Disease Biomarker, and Neurotherapeutics. *Front. Pharmacol.* **2022**, *13*, 878058. [CrossRef] [PubMed]
64. Doeppner, T.R.; Herz, J.; Görgens, A.; Schlechter, J.; Ludwig, A.-K.; Radtke, S.; de Miroschedji, K.; Horn, P.A.; Giebel, B.; Hermann, D.M. Extracellular Vesicles Improve Post-Stroke Neuroregeneration and Prevent Postischemic Immunosuppression. *Stem Cells Transl. Med.* **2015**, *4*, 1131–1143. [CrossRef] [PubMed]
65. Kuang, Y.; Zheng, X.; Zhang, L.; Ai, X.; Venkataramani, V.; Kilic, E.; Hermann, D.M.; Majid, A.; Bähr, M.; Doeppner, T.R. Adipose-derived mesenchymal stem cells reduce autophagy in stroke mice by extracellular vesicle transfer of miR-25. *J. Extracell. Vesicles* **2020**, *10*, e12024. [CrossRef]
66. Chen, W.; Wang, H.; Zhu, Z.; Feng, J.; Chen, L. Exosome-Shuttled circSHOC2 from IPASs Regulates Neuronal Autophagy and Ameliorates Ischemic Brain Injury via the miR-7670-3p/SIRT1 Axis. *Mol. Ther. Nucleic Acids* **2020**, *22*, 657–672. [CrossRef]
67. Wu, W.; Liu, J.; Yang, C.; Xu, Z.; Huang, J.; Lin, J. Astrocyte-derived exosome-transported microRNA-34c is neuroprotective against cerebral ischemia/reperfusion injury via TLR7 and the NF-κB/MAPK pathways. *Brain Res. Bull.* **2020**, *163*, 84–94. [CrossRef]
68. Ghosh, S.; Garg, S.; Ghosh, S. Cell-Derived Exosome Therapy: A Novel Approach to Treat Post-traumatic Brain Injury Mediated Neural Injury. *ACS Chem. Neurosci.* **2020**, *11*, 2045–2047. [CrossRef]

69. Moon, G.J.; Sung, J.H.; Kim, D.H.; Kim, E.H.; Cho, Y.H.; Son, J.P.; Cha, J.M.; Bang, O.Y. Application of Mesenchymal Stem Cell-Derived Extracellular Vesicles for Stroke: Biodistribution and MicroRNA Study. *Transl. Stroke Res.* **2019**, *10*, 509–521. [CrossRef]
70. Alvarez-Erviti, L.; Seow, Y.; Yin, H.; Betts, C.; Lakhal, S.; Wood, M.J. Delivery of siRNA to the mouse brain by systemic injection of targeted exosomes. *Nat. Biotechnol.* **2011**, *29*, 341–345. [CrossRef]
71. Tian, T.; Zhang, H.-X.; He, C.-P.; Fan, S.; Zhu, Y.-L.; Qi, C.; Huang, N.-P.; Xiao, Z.-D.; Lu, Z.-H.; Tannous, B.A.; et al. Surface functionalized exosomes as targeted drug delivery vehicles for cerebral ischemia therapy. *Biomaterials* **2018**, *150*, 137–149. [CrossRef] [PubMed]
72. Wei, H.; Chen, J.; Wang, S.; Fu, F.; Zhu, X.; Wu, C.; Liu, Z.; Zhong, G.; Lin, J. A Nanodrug Consisting of Doxorubicin And Exosome Derived From Mesenchymal Stem Cells For Osteosarcoma Treatment In Vitro. *Int. J. Nanomed.* **2019**, *14*, 8603–8610. [CrossRef] [PubMed]
73. Ferrantelli, F.; Chiozzini, C.; Leone, P.; Manfredi, F.; Federico, M. Engineered Extracellular Vesicles/Exosomes as a New Tool against Neurodegenerative Diseases. *Pharmaceutics* **2020**, *12*, 529. [CrossRef] [PubMed]
74. Qu, M.; Lin, Q.; Huang, L.; Fu, Y.; Wang, L.; He, S.; Fu, Y.; Yang, S.; Zhang, Z.; Zhang, L.; et al. Dopamine-loaded blood exosomes targeted to brain for better treatment of Parkinson's disease. *J. Control. Release* **2018**, *287*, 156–166. [CrossRef] [PubMed]
75. Haney, M.J.; Klyachko, N.L.; Zhao, Y.; Gupta, R.; Plotnikova, E.G.; He, Z.; Patel, T.; Piroyan, A.; Sokolsky, M.; Kabanov, A.V.; et al. Exosomes as drug delivery vehicles for Parkinson's disease therapy. *J. Control. Release* **2015**, *207*, 18–30. [CrossRef]
76. Zhou, X.; Xie, F.; Wang, L.; Zhang, L.; Zhang, S.; Fang, M.; Zhou, F. The function and clinical application of extracellular vesicles in innate immune regulation. *Cell. Mol. Immunol.* **2020**, *17*, 323–334. [CrossRef]
77. Tavasolian, F.; Hosseini, A.Z.; Soudi, S.; Naderi, M. miRNA-146a Improves Immunomodulatory Effects of MSC-derived Exosomes in Rheumatoid Arthritis. *Curr. Gene Ther.* **2020**, *20*, 297–312. [CrossRef]
78. Riazifar, M.; Mohammadi, M.R.; Pone, E.J.; Yeri, A.; Lässer, C.; Segaliny, A.I.; McIntyre, L.L.; Shelke, G.V.; Hutchins, E.; Hamamoto, A.; et al. Stem Cell-Derived Exosomes as Nanotherapeutics for Autoimmune and Neurodegenerative Disorders. *ACS Nano* **2019**, *13*, 6670–6688. [CrossRef]
79. Avnir, Y.; Turjeman, K.; Tulchinsky, D.; Sigal, A.; Kizelsztein, P.; Tzemach, D.; Gabizon, A.; Barenholz, Y. Fabrication Principles and Their Contribution to the Superior In Vivo Therapeutic Efficacy of Nano-Liposomes Remote Loaded with Glucocorticoids. *PLoS ONE* **2011**, *6*, e25721. [CrossRef]
80. Neupane, Y.R.; Mahtab, A.; Siddiqui, L.; Singh, A.; Gautam, N.; Rabbani, S.A.; Goel, H.; Talegaonkar, S. Biocompatible Nanovesicular Drug Delivery Systems with Targeting Potential for Autoimmune Diseases. *Curr. Pharm. Des.* **2020**, *26*, 5488–5502. [CrossRef]
81. Kadry, M.O. Liposomal glutathione as a promising candidate for immunological rheumatoid arthritis therapy. *Heliyon* **2019**, *5*, e02162. [CrossRef] [PubMed]
82. Yan, F.; Zhong, Z.; Wang, Y.; Feng, Y.; Mei, Z.; Li, H.; Chen, X.; Cai, L.; Li, C. Exosome-based biomimetic nanoparticles targeted to inflamed joints for enhanced treatment of rheumatoid arthritis. *J. Nanobiotechnol.* **2020**, *18*, 115. [CrossRef] [PubMed]
83. Casella, G.; Colombo, F.; Finardi, A.; Descamps, H.; Ill-Raga, G.; Spinelli, A.E.; Podini, P.; Bastoni, M.; Martino, G.; Muzio, L.; et al. Extracellular Vesicles Containing IL-4 Modulate Neuroinflammation in a Mouse Model of Multiple Sclerosis. *Mol. Ther.* **2018**, *26*, 2107–2118. [CrossRef]
84. Kennel, K.A.; Drake, M.T. Adverse effects of bisphosphonates: Implications for osteoporosis management. *Mayo. Clin. Proc.* **2009**, *84*, 632–637. [CrossRef]
85. Yang, X.; Chen, S.; Liu, X.; Yu, M.; Liu, X. Drug Delivery Based on Nanotechnology for Target Bone Disease. *Curr. Drug Deliv.* **2019**, *16*, 782–792. [CrossRef] [PubMed]
86. Zha, Y.; Li, Y.; Lin, T.; Chen, J.; Zhang, S.; Wang, J. Progenitor cell-derived exosomes endowed with VEGF plasmids enhance osteogenic induction and vascular remodeling in large segmental bone defects. *Theranostics* **2021**, *11*, 397–409. [CrossRef] [PubMed]
87. Luo, Z.-W.; Li, F.-X.; Liu, Y.-W.; Rao, S.-S.; Yin, H.; Huang, J.; Chen, C.-Y.; Hu, Y.; Zhang, Y.; Tan, Y.-J.; et al. Aptamer-functionalized exosomes from bone marrow stromal cells target bone to promote bone regeneration. *Nanoscale* **2019**, *11*, 20884–20892. [CrossRef] [PubMed]
88. Zhang, J.; Liu, X.; Li, H.; Chen, C.; Hu, B.; Niu, X.; Li, Q.; Zhao, B.; Xie, Z.; Wang, Y. Exosomes/tricalcium phosphate combination scaffolds can enhance bone regeneration by activating the PI3K/Akt signaling pathway. *Stem. Cell Res. Ther.* **2016**, *7*, 136. [CrossRef]
89. Xu, X.; Liang, Y.; Li, X.; Ouyang, K.; Wang, M.; Cao, T.; Li, W.; Liu, J.; Xiong, J.; Li, B.; et al. Exosome-mediated delivery of kartogenin for chondrogenesis of synovial fluid-derived mesenchymal stem cells and cartilage regeneration. *Biomaterials* **2021**, *269*, 120539. [CrossRef]
90. Liu, Q.; Piao, H.; Wang, Y.; Zheng, D.; Wang, W. Circulating exosomes in cardiovascular disease: Novel carriers of biological information. *Biomed. Pharmacother.* **2021**, *135*, 111148. [CrossRef]
91. Liu, Y.; Wang, M.; Liang, Y.; Wang, C.; Naruse, K.; Takahashi, K. Treatment of Oxidative Stress with Exosomes in Myocardial Ischemia. *Int. J. Mol. Sci.* **2021**, *22*, 1729. [CrossRef] [PubMed]

92. Gollmann-Tepeköylü, C.; Pölzl, L.; Graber, M.; Hirsch, J.; Nägele, F.; Lobenwein, D.; Hess, M.W.; Blumer, M.J.; Kirchmair, E.; Zipperle, J.; et al. miR-19a-3p containing exosomes improve function of ischaemic myocardium upon shock wave therapy. *Cardiovasc. Res.* **2010**, *116*, 1226–1236. [CrossRef]
93. Chen, Q.; Liu, Y.; Ding, X.; Li, Q.; Qiu, F.; Wang, M.; Shen, Z.; Zheng, H.; Fu, G. Bone marrow mesenchymal stem cell-secreted exosomes carrying microRNA-125b protect against myocardial ischemia reperfusion injury via targeting SIRT7. *Mol. Cell. Biochem.* **2020**, *465*, 103–114. [CrossRef] [PubMed]
94. Zhang, H.; Wu, J.; Wu, J.; Fan, Q.; Zhou, J.; Wu, J.; Liu, S.; Zang, J.; Ye, J.; Xiao, M.; et al. Exosome-mediated targeted delivery of miR-210 for angiogenic therapy after cerebral ischemia in mice. *J. Nanobiotechnol.* **2019**, *17*, 29. [CrossRef] [PubMed]
95. Wu, G.; Zhang, J.; Zhao, Q.; Zhuang, W.; Ding, J.; Zhang, C.; Gao, H.; Pang, D.-W.; Pu, K.; Xie, H.-Y. Molecularly Engineered Macrophage-Derived Exosomes with Inflammation Tropism and Intrinsic Heme Biosynthesis for Atherosclerosis Treatment. *Angew. Chem. Int. Ed.* **2020**, *59*, 4068–4074. [CrossRef] [PubMed]
96. Zhang, Y.; Yang, N.; Huang, X.; Zhu, Y.; Gao, S.; Liu, Z.; Cao, F.; Wang, Y. Melatonin Engineered Adipose-Derived Biomimetic Nanovesicles Regulate Mitochondrial Functions and Promote Myocardial Repair in Myocardial Infarction. *Front. Cardiovasc. Med.* **2022**, *9*, 789203. [CrossRef]
97. Lu, M.; Xing, H.; Xun, Z.; Yang, T.; Ding, P.; Cai, C.; Wang, D.; Zhao, X. Exosome-based small RNA delivery: Progress and prospects. *Asian J. Pharm. Sci.* **2018**, *13*, 1–11. [CrossRef]
98. Bruno, S.; Porta, S.; Bussolati, B. Extracellular vesicles in renal tissue damage and regeneration. *Eur. J. Pharmacol.* **2016**, *790*, 83–91. [CrossRef]
99. Kim, S.; A Lee, S.; Yoon, H.; Kim, M.Y.; Yoo, J.-K.; Ahn, S.-H.; Park, C.H.; Park, J.; Nam, B.Y.; Park, J.T.; et al. Exosome-based delivery of super-repressor IκBα ameliorates kidney ischemia-reperfusion injury. *Kidney Int.* **2021**, *100*, 570–584. [CrossRef]
100. Tang, Z.; Tang, C.; Sun, C.; Ying, X.; Shen, R. M1 macrophage-derived exosomes synergistically enhance the anti- bladder cancer effect of gemcitabine. *Aging* **2022**, *14*, 7364–7377. [CrossRef]
101. Wang, W.; Wu, C.; Jin, H. Exosomes in chronic inflammatory skin diseases and skin tumors. *Exp. Dermatol.* **2019**, *28*, 213–218. [CrossRef] [PubMed]
102. Zhao, D.; Yu, Z.; Li, Y.; Wang, Y.; Li, Q.; Han, D. GelMA combined with sustained release of HUVECs derived exosomes for promoting cutaneous wound healing and facilitating skin regeneration. *Histochem. J.* **2020**, *51*, 251–263. [CrossRef] [PubMed]
103. Zhang, W.; Bai, X.; Zhao, B.; Li, Y.; Zhang, Y.; Li, Z.; Wang, X.; Luo, L.; Han, F.; Zhang, J.; et al. Cell-free therapy based on adipose tissue stem cell-derived exosomes promotes wound healing via the PI3K/Akt signaling pathway. *Exp. Cell Res.* **2018**, *370*, 333–342. [CrossRef] [PubMed]
104. Yue, T.; Ji, M.; Qu, H.; Guo, M.; Bai, F.; Zhang, Z.; Wang, W.; Gong, X.; Zhang, Z. Comprehensive analyses of long non-coding RNA expression profiles by RNA sequencing and exploration of their potency as biomarkers in psoriatic arthritis patients. *BMC Immunol.* **2019**, *20*, 28. [CrossRef]
105. Shiekh, P.A.; Singh, A.; Kumar, A. Exosome laden oxygen releasing antioxidant and antibacterial cryogel wound dressing OxOBand alleviate diabetic and infectious wound healing. *Biomaterials* **2020**, *249*, 120020. [CrossRef]
106. Wang, Y.; Cao, Z.; Wei, Q.; Ma, K.; Hu, W.; Huang, Q.; Su, J.; Li, H.; Zhang, C.; Fu, X. VH298-loaded extracellular vesicles released from gelatin methacryloyl hydrogel facilitate diabetic wound healing by HIF-1α-mediated enhancement of angiogenesis. *Acta Biomater.* **2022**, *147*, 342–355. [CrossRef]
107. Xia, W.; Li, M.; Jiang, X.; Huang, X.; Gu, S.; Ye, J.; Zhu, L.; Hou, M.; Zan, T. Young fibroblast-derived exosomal microRNA-125b transfers beneficial effects on aged cutaneous wound healing. *J. Nanobiotechnol.* **2022**, *20*, 144. [CrossRef]
108. Warshauer, J.T.; Bluestone, J.A.; Anderson, M.S. New Frontiers in the Treatment of Type 1 Diabetes. *Cell Metab.* **2020**, *31*, 46–61. [CrossRef]
109. Xu, Y.-X.; Pu, S.-D.; Li, X.; Yu, Z.-W.; Zhang, Y.-T.; Tong, X.-W.; Shan, Y.-Y.; Gao, X.-Y. Exosomal ncRNAs: Novel therapeutic target and biomarker for diabetic complications. *Pharmacol. Res.* **2022**, *178*, 106135. [CrossRef]
110. He, C.; Zheng, S.; Luo, Y.; Wang, B. Exosome Theranostics: Biology and Translational Medicine. *Theranostics* **2018**, *8*, 237–255. [CrossRef]
111. Guo, Y.; Wan, Z.; Zhao, P.; Wei, M.; Liu, Y.; Bu, T.; Sun, W.; Li, Z.; Yuan, L. Ultrasound triggered topical delivery of Bmp7 mRNA for white fat browning induction via engineered smart exosomes. *J. Nanobiotechnol.* **2021**, *19*, 402. [CrossRef] [PubMed]
112. Zhou, B.; Xu, K.; Zheng, X.; Chen, T.; Wang, J.; Song, Y.; Shao, Y.; Zheng, S. Application of exosomes as liquid biopsy in clinical diagnosis. *Signal Transduct. Target. Ther.* **2020**, *5*, 144. [CrossRef] [PubMed]
113. Zhang, Y.; Bi, J.; Huang, J.; Tang, Y.; Du, S.; Li, P. Exosome: A Review of Its Classification, Isolation Techniques, Storage, Diagnostic and Targeted Therapy Applications. *Int. J. Nanomed.* **2020**, *15*, 6917–6934. [CrossRef] [PubMed]
114. Zhang, X.; Sai, B.; Wang, F.; Wang, L.; Wang, Y.; Zheng, L.; Li, G.; Tang, J.; Xiang, J. Hypoxic BMSC-derived exosomal miRNAs promote metastasis of lung cancer cells via STAT3-induced EMT. *Mol. Cancer* **2019**, *18*, 40. [CrossRef] [PubMed]
115. Xunian, Z.; Kalluri, R. Biology and therapeutic potential of mesenchymal stem cell-derived exosomes. *Cancer Sci.* **2020**, *111*, 3100–3110. [CrossRef]
116. Kok, V.C.; Yu, C.-C. Cancer-Derived Exosomes: Their Role in Cancer Biology and Biomarker Development. *Int. J. Nanomed.* **2020**, *15*, 8019–8036. [CrossRef]
117. Zheng, Y.; He, R.; Wang, P.; Shi, Y.; Zhao, L.; Liang, J. Exosomes from LPS-stimulated macrophages induce neuroprotection and functional improvement after ischemic stroke by modulating microglial polarization. *Biomater. Sci.* **2019**, *7*, 2037–2049. [CrossRef]

118. Wahlund, C.J.; Güclüler, G.; Hiltbrunner, S.; Veerman, R.E.; Näslund, T.I.; Gabrielsson, S. Exosomes from antigen-pulsed dendritic cells induce stronger antigen-specific immune responses than microvesicles in vivo. *Sci. Rep.* **2017**, *7*, 17095. [CrossRef]
119. Xie, G.; Yang, H.; Peng, X.; Lin, L.; Wang, J.; Lin, K.; Cui, Z.; Li, J.; Xiao, H.; Liang, Y.; et al. Mast cell exosomes can suppress allergic reactions by binding to IgE. *J. Allergy Clin. Immunol.* **2018**, *141*, 788–791. [CrossRef]
120. Hadley, E.E.; Sheller-Miller, S.; Saade, G.; Salomon, C.; Mesiano, S.; Taylor, R.N.; Taylor, B.D.; Menon, R. Amnion epithelial cell–derived exosomes induce inflammatory changes in uterine cells. *Am. J. Obstet. Gynecol.* **2018**, *219*, 478.e1–478.e21. [CrossRef]
121. Kong, J.; Wang, F.; Zhang, J.; Cui, Y.; Pan, L.; Zhang, W.; Wen, J.; Liu, P. Exosomes of Endothelial Progenitor Cells Inhibit Neointima Formation After Carotid Artery Injury. *J. Surg. Res.* **2018**, *232*, 398–407. [CrossRef] [PubMed]
122. Lin, J.; Li, J.; Huang, B.; Liu, J.; Chen, X.; Chen, X.-M.; Xu, Y.-M.; Huang, L.-F.; Wang, X.-Z. Exosomes: Novel Biomarkers for Clinical Diagnosis. *Sci. World J.* **2015**, *2015*, 657086. [CrossRef] [PubMed]
123. Xiao, J.; Feng, S.; Wang, X.; Long, K.; Luo, Y.; Wang, Y.; Ma, J.; Tang, Q.; Jin, L.; Li, X.; et al. Identification of exosome-like nanoparticle-derived microRNAs from 11 edible fruits and vegetables. *Peerj* **2018**, *6*, e5186. [CrossRef]
124. Yun, B.; Kim, Y.; Park, D.J.; Oh, S. Comparative analysis of dietary exosome-derived microRNAs from human, bovine and caprine colostrum and mature milk. *J. Anim. Sci. Technol.* **2021**, *63*, 593–602. [CrossRef] [PubMed]
125. Théry, C.; Witwer, K.W.; Aikawa, E.; Alcaraz, M.J.; Anderson, J.D.; Andriantsitohaina, R.; Antoniou, A.; Arab, T.; Archer, F.; Atkin-Smith, G.K.; et al. Minimal information for studies of extracellular vesicles 2018 (MISEV2018): A position statement of the International Society for Extracellular Vesicles and update of the MISEV2014 guidelines. *J. Extracell. Vesicles* **2018**, *7*, 1535750. [CrossRef] [PubMed]
126. Yáñez-Mó, M.; Siljander, P.R.-M.; Andreu, Z.; Bedina Zavec, A.; Borràs, F.E.; Buzas, E.I.; Buzas, K.; Casal, E.; Cappello, F.; Carvalho, J.; et al. Biological properties of extracellular vesicles and their physiological functions. *J. Extracell. Vesicles* **2015**, *4*, 27066. [CrossRef] [PubMed]
127. Frolova, L.; Li, I.T.S. Targeting Capabilities of Native and Bioengineered Extracellular Vesicles for Drug Delivery. *Bioengineering* **2022**, *9*, 496. [CrossRef]
128. Abels, E.R.; Breakefield, X.O. Introduction to Extracellular Vesicles: Biogenesis, RNA Cargo Selection, Content, Release, and Uptake. *Cell. Mol. Neurobiol.* **2016**, *36*, 301–312. [CrossRef]
129. Xie, S.; Zhang, Q.; Jiang, L. Current Knowledge on Exosome Biogenesis, Cargo-Sorting Mechanism and Therapeutic Implications. *Membranes* **2022**, *12*, 498. [CrossRef]
130. Tian, Y.; Gong, M.; Hu, Y.; Liu, H.; Zhang, W.; Zhang, M.; Hu, X.; Aubert, D.; Zhu, S.; Wu, L.; et al. Quality and efficiency assessment of six extracellular vesicle isolation methods by nano-flow cytometry. *J. Extracell. Vesicles* **2019**, *9*, 1697028. [CrossRef]
131. Bulut, O.; Gürsel, İ. Mesenchymal stem cell derived extracellular vesicles: Promising immunomodulators against autoimmune, autoinflammatory disorders and SARS-CoV-2 infection. *Turk. J. Biol.* **2020**, *44*, 273–282. [CrossRef]

pharmaceutics

MDPI

Review

Extracellular Non-Coding RNAs in Cardiovascular Diseases

Zeyidan Jiapaer [1,2,†], Chengyu Li [1,2,†], Xinyu Yang [3,†], Lingfei Sun [4], Emeli Chatterjee [4], Lingying Zhang [1,2], Ji Lei [5,*] and Guoping Li [4,*]

1 College of Life Science & Technology, Xinjiang University, Urumqi 830046, China
2 Xinjiang Key Laboratory of Biological Resources and Genetic Engineering, Urumqi 830046, China
3 Fangshan Hospital Beijing University of Chinese Medicine, Beijing 102400, China
4 Cardiovascular Research Center, Massachusetts General Hospital, Harvard Medical School, Boston, MA 02114, USA
5 Center for Transplantation Science, Massachusetts General Hospital, Harvard Medical School, Boston, MA 02114, USA
* Correspondence: jlei2@mgh.harvard.edu (J.L.); gli21@mgh.harvard.edu (G.L.)
† These authors contributed equally to this work.

Abstract: Cardiovascular diseases (CVDs) remain the world's leading cause of death despite the best available healthcare and therapy. Emerging as a key mediator of intercellular and inter-organ communication in CVD pathogenesis, extracellular vesicles (EVs) are a heterogeneous group of membrane-enclosed nano-sized vesicles released by virtually all cells, of which their RNA cargo, especially non-coding RNAs (ncRNA), has been increasingly recognized as a promising diagnostic and therapeutic target. Recent evidence shows that ncRNAs, such as small ncRNAs, circular RNAs, and long ncRNAs, can be selectively sorted into EVs or other non-vesicular carriers and modulate various biological processes in recipient cells. In this review, we summarize recent advances in the literature regarding the origin, extracellular carrier, and functional mechanisms of extracellular ncRNAs with a focus on small ncRNAs, circular RNAs, and long ncRNAs. The pathophysiological roles of extracellular ncRNAs in various CVDs, including atherosclerosis, ischemic heart diseases, hypertension, cardiac hypertrophy, and heart failure, are extensively discussed. We also provide an update on recent developments and challenges in using extracellular ncRNAs as biomarkers or therapeutical targets in these CVDs.

Keywords: extracellular RNAs; non-coding RNAs; cardiovascular diseases; biomarkers; therapeutical targets

Citation: Jiapaer, Z.; Li, C.; Yang, X.; Sun, L.; Chatterjee, E.; Zhang, L.; Lei, J.; Li, G. Extracellular Non-Coding RNAs in Cardiovascular Diseases. *Pharmaceutics* **2023**, *15*, 155. https://doi.org/10.3390/pharmaceutics15010155

Academic Editor: Lucio Barile

Received: 20 November 2022
Revised: 22 December 2022
Accepted: 27 December 2022
Published: 3 January 2023

1. Introduction

Cardiovascular diseases (CVDs) are widely recognized as the leading cause of death worldwide. Despite the considerable advances in both healthcare and therapies over the past decades, CVD has contributed to 17.9 million deaths in 2019 and is estimated to result in 22.2 million deaths in 2030 [1,2]. There is, therefore, an unmet medical need to develop novel diagnostics and therapeutics targeting CVDs. Emerging evidence suggests that extracellular non-coding RNAs (Ex-ncRNAs), particularly non-coding RNAs (ncRNAs) encapsulated in extracellular vesicles (EVs), function as key mediators of intercellular and inter-organ communication and play versatile roles in both homeostasis and disease [3]. EVs are continuously secreted by cells into circulation and are found in all biological fluids. The encapsulated molecular cargo inside EVs, especially RNAs, are increasingly recognized as promising biomarkers and therapeutic targets for various diseases, including CVDs [4–6].

Ex-ncRNAs are a heterogeneous group of RNAs, including small ncRNAs, long ncRNAs (lncRNAs), and circular RNAs (circRNAs), which encompass the majority of the extracellular transcriptome [7,8]. Ex-ncRNAs can be translocated into receipt cells after being secreted into the extracellular space through a variety of methods, thereby regulating various biological processes in targeted cells under both physiological and pathological conditions [9] (Figure 1). This review summarizes the recent updates of Ex-ncRNAs and discusses the diagnosis and therapeutic aspects of Ex-ncRNAs in CVDs, including atherosclerosis, ischemic heart diseases, hypertension, cardiac hypertrophy, and heart failure.

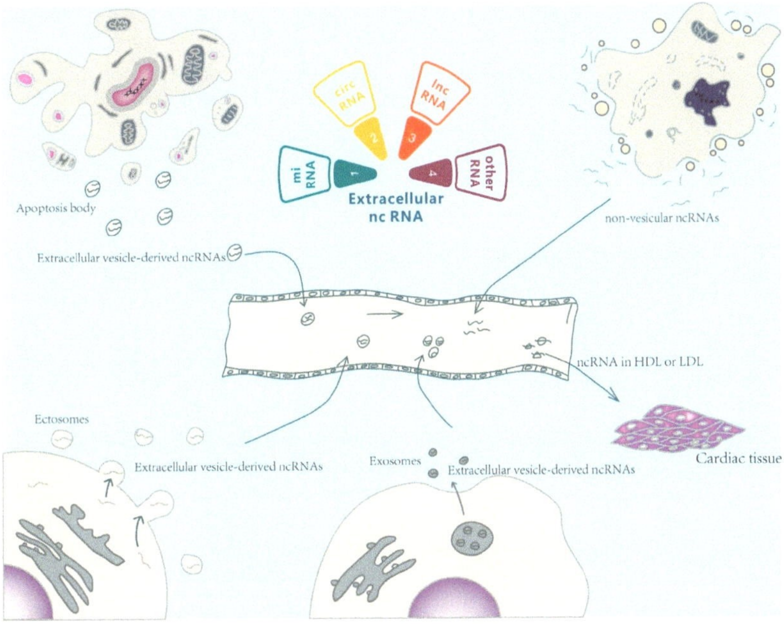

Figure 1. Extracellular non-coding RNA-mediated intercellular crosstalk. Extracellular non-coding RNAs (Ex-ncRNAs) are a heterogeneous group of RNAs and mainly include small ncRNAs, lncRNAs, and circRNAs. Ex-ncRNAs can be translocated into receipt cells and modulate the cellular functions of targeted cells (heart or other cardiovascular systems). Ex-ncRNAs can be secreted into the extracellular space through a variety of pathways, including embedded into exosomes, ectosomes, and apoptotic bodies, or partnered with ribonucleoproteins and lipoproteins.

2. Ex-ncRNAs

2.1. Extracellular Small ncRNAs

The main classes of small ncRNAs are miRNAs, small interfering RNAs (siRNAs), piwi-interacting RNAs (piRNAs), Y-RNAs, and tRNA-derived small RNAs (tDRs) [10,11]. Most small ncRNAs are capable of regulating gene expression either transcriptionally or epitranscriptionally [10,12]. Recent evidence suggests that small ncRNAs are encapsulated into EVs and modulate the transcriptome of recipient cells following release through cellular autocrine or paracrine pathways. In addition, small ncRNAs, embedded in ribonucleoproteins and lipoproteins, are found to be secreted into extracellular spaces [13]. An increasing number of studies have detected extracellular small ncRNAs in a variety of biological fluids, such as serum or plasma, and indicated that extracellular small ncRNA profiles in various body fluids could serve as novel biomarkers for different pathological conditions [14–17]. As one of the most abundant RNA species in circulation, extracellular small ncRNAs are actively involved in a variety of pathological and physiological processes. Therefore, the detection of specific circulating small ncRNAs, based on the small ncRNA profiles, could be a promising approach to diagnosing diseases.

2.2. Extracellular LncRNAs

LncRNAs are a class of transcripts with a length of more than 200 nucleotides and lack protein-coding potential [18]. There are many categories and sub-categories of lncRNAs, with major classifications including antisense, bi-directional, enhancer-associated, intergenic lncRNAs (lincRNAs), and pseudogenes [19]. They function primarily in two fashions: (1) regulating the expression of miRNA target genes by mimicking miRNA sponges via competitive endogenous RNA (ceRNA) inhibition, and (2) regulating the post-translational modification of specific proteins, thereby affecting the activity of downstream signaling pathways [20]. Recent studies have noted that EVs are the primary means through which lncRNAs are transferred outside cells [21]. Extracellular lncRNAs can affect a broad range of downstream effects. In general, lncRNAs act as heterologous RNAs that can be transferred to target cells by EVs and regulate the cellular functions of receipt cells [22]. The membrane-bound nature of EVs shields ncRNA cargos from degradation. Due to the lack of evolutionary conservation and high specificity in different cells/organs, lncRNAs continue to be investigated as potential mediators of intercellular communication, exemplifying a valuable class of therapeutic targets for disorders as well as potential biomarkers [23].

2.3. *Extracellular CircRNAs*

CircRNAs are single-stranded RNAs that are linked end-to-end by a back-splicing mechanism. According to their splicing sequence, circRNAs can be categorized into the following groups: exonic circular RNAs (ecircRNAs), circular intronic RNAs (ciRNAs), exon-intron circular RNAs (EIciRNAs), intergenic circRNAs, anti-sense circRNAs, and tRNA intronic circRNAs (tricRNAs). Until now, the functionalities of circRNAs have been mainly classified into four categories: (1) acting as ceRNAs or sponges; (2) regulation of pre-RNA cleavage; (3) regulation of gene expression; and (4) as a potential source for translation of proteins and peptides [24]. Similar to the aforementioned ncRNAs, circRNAs can also be loaded into EVs to mediate cell-cell communication [13]. CircRNAs demonstrate a notable advantage over other ncRNAs. Without a linear terminal, circRNAs have a longer half-life, allowing for accumulation in tissues with a low proliferation rate. Additionally, the lack of a linear terminal impedes RNase degradation and improves stability and integrity in the extracellular environment, thus elevating their utility as biomarkers of disease [25]. Recent evidence has identified a crucial role of several extracellular circRNAs in alleviating damage due to cardiomyocyte hypertrophy, heart failure (HF), myocardial infarction (MI), and dysfunction caused by ischemia-reperfusion (I/R) [26]. Furthermore, several studies have also reported their association with proliferation, apoptosis, and inflammatory responses, thus influencing physiological and pathological phenomena in various tissues [7,27]. Investigation of circRNAs continues to elucidate their role in the pathogenesis of CVDs and provides a potential avenue for therapeutic development.

3. Ex-ncRNAs as Biomarkers in CVDs

In recent decades, several molecular mechanisms have been identified to be associated with the induction and progression of CVDs, especially in coronary atherosclerosis and HF [28]. Although clinical management of HF is improving, incidence rates remain above 20% in the adult population, with mortality rates hovering at 50% within 5 years of diagnosis, which makes HF a leading cause of morbidity and mortality in developed countries [29]. Consequently, it is necessary to delve into the disease's underlying mechanisms and subsequent release of ncRNAs to develop more effective diagnostic and prognostic tools to reduce mortality (Table 1).

3.1. *Atherosclerosis*

Atherosclerosis is a chronic inflammatory artery disease characterized by the deposition of atherosclerotic plaque in the arteries, which leads to the hardening and narrowing of the artery lumen and subsequent obstruction of blood flow [30]. Atherosclerotic plaque results from the accumulation of circulating low-density lipoprotein (LDL) cholesterol alongside fibrous materials and inflammatory cells on the inner layers of arteries [31]. On the contrary, other cholesterol classes, namely high-density lipoproteins (HDLs), hold a significant anti-atherosclerotic role, transporting cholesterol from peripheral tissues to the liver for metabolism [32].

3.1.1. Extracellular Small ncRNAs

In 2011, a study found that circulating HDLs and LDLs can transport miRNAs, such as HDL-transported miR-223, to regulate different intercellular signaling pathways in atherosclerosis [33,34]. In addition to cholesterol-driven miRNA transport, circulating miRNAs have also been identified as potential biomarkers of atherosclerosis in hypertensive patients. By comparing the expression levels of miR-92a in plasma of different levels of carotid intima-media thickness (CIMT) and hypertensive patients, a recent study found that the increased level of miR-92a expression was positively correlated with the measured value of CIMT, ambulatory blood pressure monitoring results and carotid-femoral pulse wave velocity, all symptoms of atherosclerosis [35]. Given that lipoproteins play an important role in the progression of atherosclerosis, differential expression of HDL-miRNAs, in addition to circulating miRNAs, can help track disease progression and enable more accurate diagnosis and treatment.

3.1.2. Extracellular LncRNAs

Extracellular lncRNAs such as lncRNA Sox2 Overlapping Transcript (SOX2-OT) have also been shown to be potentially involved in the development of vascular disease [36]. Serum SOX2-OT levels were found to be significantly elevated in atherosclerotic patients. The results revealed that it could be used as a diagnostic biomarker and an excellent modality to assess patient prognosis [37].

3.1.3. Extracellular CircRNAs

Another study quantified circRNA in the plasma of patients with coronary artery disease. It was reported that the plasma level of hsa_circ_0001445 was reduced in patients with coronary artery sclerosis, and the condition remained stable in patients with reduced expression of hsa_circ_0001445. The expression level of hsa_circ_0001445 was inversely correlated with the degree of coronary atherosclerosis. Combined with coronary computed tomography, its quantification significantly improved the diagnosis of the degree of disease [38].

3.2. *Ischemic Heart Disease*

Ischemic cardiomyopathy is caused by an imbalance in the myocardial oxygen demand and available oxygen supply, most often induced by coronary artery stenosis. Based on the pathophysiology, ischemic cardiomyopathy includes coronary heart disease and myocardial infarction (MI) [39].

Although stenting is a crucial method to relieve myocardial ischemia, it may result in long-term cardiac damage when blood flow is suddenly restored, also known as ischemia-reperfusion (I/R) injury [40,41]. I/R injury after reperfusion often occurs due to cardiomyocytes undergoing anaerobic metabolism, sodium-potassium pump dysfunction, and ribosome shedding. Various intracellular ATP-dependent ion pumps become inactive, leading to ion accumulation, pH down-regulation, and up-regulation of intracellular osmolarity. Ultimately, ischemic cardiomyocytes experience cell swelling, impaired enzyme activities, and clumped nuclear chromatin. Due to the low concentration of antioxidants in ischemic cardiomyocytes, the increased reactive oxygen species after reperfusion causes oxidative stress, which further causes cellular dysfunction, DNA damage, and local inflammatory responses in cardiomyocytes. Thus, the persistence of inflammation and oxidative stress may trigger a cytokine storm that exposes cells to severe damage [42].

3.2.1. Extracellular Small ncRNAs

Currently, the primary diagnosis of MI is mainly based on the detection of MI markers like cardiac troponin [43,44]. However, there is evidence showing that elevated cardiac troponins are present outside cardiac injury and can compromise the diagnosis of MI [45]. This opens an avenue to pursue Ex-ncRNA levels as a circulating biomarker for acute myocardial infarction (AMI) [46]. A previous study observed a 1600-fold elevated expression of miR-208b in AMI compared to the control group. Further, miR-208b identified earlier detection than troponin T regarding MI progression. In addition, another study found that miR-204 was down-regulated, and lncRNA-NEAT1 and matrix metalloproteinase-9 (MMP-9) were upregulated in serum EVs from patients with acute ST-segment elevation MI [47]. Serum-derived miRNA signatures have been used to distinguish healthy volunteers from patients with coronary atherosclerosis through the expression levels of miR-370-3p and miR-409-3p, which can serve as a fingerprint for coronary heart disease [48]. By exploring the expression levels of EV-derived miRNAs in the plasma and serum of CS and AMI patients, EV miRNA landscapes facilitated disease differentiation [49].

Novel miRNAs have been found to identify the evolution of cardiac I/R injury [50]. MiRNAs with diagnostic or therapeutic potential have been identified in the context of early cardiac I/R injury with miRNA arrays conducted to screen for differential expression in a mouse model of cardiac I/R injury. A total of 1882 miRNAs were screened, among which 11 were observably down-regulated and 41 were markedly up-regulated 3 h after reperfusion. miR-3113-5P and miR-223-3p were among the most differentially expressed miRNAs and have been confirmed to be up-regulated in the early stage of cardiac tissue I/R injury [51,52]. This data confirms that cardiac miRNAs, such as miRNA-3113-5p, might be a valuable target for therapeutic purposes, and circulating miRNAs such as miRNA-3113-5p might serve as a stable marker for the early diagnosis of cardiac I/R injury.

Extracellular tDR is a newly identified small regulatory RNA species. A recent study has demonstrated that extracellular tDRs are much more dynamically regulated than intracellular tDRs and extracellular miRNAs in both cardiomyocytes and cardiac fibroblasts upon the treatments of ischemia/reperfusion-related stressors [11]. Notably, more than 3000 extracellular tDRs are significantly regulated by nutritional deprivation or ischemia, and approximately 2000 extracellular tDRs are differentially expressed upon ischemia/reoxygenation treatment mimicking ischemia/reperfusion injury in both cardiomyocytes and cardiac fibroblasts [11]. Detailedly, extracellular tDR-1:32-His-GTG-1, tDR-37:72-Val-TAC-1, tDR-1:32-Pro-AGG-1-M4, tDR-2:30-Glu-CTC-1, tDR-2:30-Glu-CTC-1-D4G, tDR-1:31-Glu-TTC-4, tDR-3:31-Gly-GCC-2-M2, and tDR-40:72-Asn-GTT-1-M2 were significantly induced by ischemia/reoxygenation from both cardiomyocytes and cardiac fibroblasts, and extracellular tDR-1:36-Glu-CTC-1, tDR-1:36-Glu-CTC-1-D5G, tDR-1:36-Asp-GTC-2-M2, and tDR-42:75-Ser-GCT-3 were downregulated considerably upon cardiac ischemia/reoxygenation [11]. Although this study is a preliminary cell culture model, the findings clearly suggest that the extracellular tDR may be a promising biomarker for diagnostic and prognostic assessments of ischemic heart diseases.

3.2.2. Extracellular LncRNAs

A previous study has shown that lncRNAs can also serve as potential biomarkers for AMI [53]. It was found that the level of circulating lncRNA ENST000005566899.1 and lncRNA ENST00000575985.1 were significantly elevated in the plasma-derived EVs of AMI patients compared to healthy individuals. Further study of these lncRNAs in combination with mature biomarkers will enhance the understanding of disease progression which is fundamental for developing lncRNA therapeutics treating MI. Owing to the similarities of disease presentation and the vast differences in management, it becomes imperative to pursue avenues that allow for identifying the types and stages of diseases using noninvasive biomarkers.

3.2.3. Extracellular CircRNAs

Previous studies have shown that the downregulation of circRNA MICRA in peripheral blood is associated with the risk of left ventricular remodeling and dysfunction after MI. Additionally, the upregulation of hsa-circ-0098964 and circRNA-284 in the serum has been found to be associated with an increased risk of hypertension and acute ischemia [54].

3.3. Hypertension

Hypertension is a significant cause of heart disease and death worldwide [55]. As the heart pumps blood, the blood applies outward pressure on the arterial wall. The maximum pressure exerted while beating is defined as systolic pressure. Conversely, blood pressure on the arterial wall during relaxation and dilatation of the heart muscles is known as diastolic pressure. Hypertension is diagnosed when systolic pressure exceeds 140 mmHg, or diastolic pressure exceeds 90 mmHg [56]. One of the leading causes of hypertension is vascular dysfunction which manifests as endothelial dysfunction, vascular inflammation, arterial remodeling, and lowered vascular elasticity [57].

Extracellular Small ncRNAs

Extracellular miR-133a, miR-21, and miR-27a have previously been reported to play an essential role in the development of hypertension [58–60]. Based on these findings, a study was conducted on a general population over five years, measuring the serum levels of miR-133a, miR-21, and miR-27a using RT-qPCR. It was found that the serum expression levels of miR-133a and miR-27a were negatively correlated with the incidence of hypertension and, as a result, could be used as diagnostic biomarkers and preventive and predictive biomarkers of hypertension [61]. Recently, a study using serum from hypertensive patients quantified miR-92a and found that its expression was significantly increased in the serum of hypertensive patients, verifying its potential as a biomarker [62]. An in vitro study further supports the potential of extracellular miR-92a as a biomarker of hypertension as it targets vascular smooth muscle cells to regulate vascular SMC phenotype, thereby causing arterial stiffness and participating in the occurrence and development of hypertension [62].

Hypertensive disorder during pregnancy is a common type of hypertension [63,64]. Commonly, severe pregnancy-induced hypertension causes irreversible damage to the mother and offspring. Previous studies have revealed that miR-200a-3p can coordinate the function of trophoblast [65]. Based on this conclusion, one study quantified miR-200a-3p in the serum of hypertensive patients during pregnancy by RT-qPCR and found that the expression level of miR-200a-3p in the serum of hypertensive patients during pregnancy was up-regulated. Moreover, its expression level was positively correlated with the development of the disease. As a result, the level of miR-200a-3p bears prognostic potential for gestational hypertension [66].

3.4. Heart Failure

HF is a clinical syndrome of structural or functional abnormalities of the heart [67]. As HF may not have symptoms at its early stage, early screening using biomarkers can significantly reduce the risk of HF. The current standard for diagnosis utilizes the N-terminal-proB-type Natriuretic Peptide (NT-proBNP) test. However, increased concentrations of BNPs are not always associated with the onset of HF and may impede accurate and earlier diagnosis of HF.

3.4.1. Extracellular Small ncRNAs

A previous study has examined the expression of Ex-ncRNAs in plasma in relation to the progression of HF [68], and found altered expression of miR-192, miR-194, and miR-134a in the plasma from patients with HF, implying the capacity of small ncRNAs to identify cardiomyocyte death and HF [68]. Similarly, another study showed that paracrine signaling via cardiomyocyte-derived EVs containing miR-30d could improve cardiac function by reducing myocardial fibrosis and cardiomyocyte apoptosis [69]. Small ncRNAs have also been assessed in the serum of acute HF patients following dilated cardiomyopathy. In this cohort, miR-92b-5p expression was up-regulated in the EVs of the patients, suggesting its use as a potential biomarker in diagnosing acute AHF caused by dilated cardiomyopathy [70].

3.4.2. Extracellular LncRNAs

Ischemic cardiomyopathy (ICM) caused by MI is a major cause of HF. In the context of circulating biomarkers, lncRNAs in ICM have been widely explored. Genome-wide transcriptome analysis has verified that a number of protein-coding genes previously reported to be associated with HF demonstrated altered expression following ICM [71,72]. Among 145 differentially expressed lncRNAs screened in ICM, 35 lncRNAs showed strong positive correlations. Expression correlation coefficient analysis of differentially expressed lncRNAs and the protein-coding genes yielded a strong correlation between lncRNAs and ECM protein-coding genes. The overexpression or knockdown of selected lncRNAs in the cardiac fibroblasts indicated that lncRNAs were significant regulators of fibrosis and ECM synthesis gene expression [73,74]. In addition, lncRNAs were found to be involved in the TGF-β pathway to regulate ECM gene expression and myofibroblast differentiation [75]. This data suggests that lncRNAs might be novel modulators of heart function and HF.

Table 1. Ex-ncRNAs as biomarkers in CVDs.

Reference	Ex-ncRNA	Carriers	Expression (↑)	(↓)	Type of CVDs
Kasey et al. [33]	miR-223	HDL	↑	-	Atherosclerosis
Huang et al. [35]	miR-92a	-	↑	-	Atherosclerosis
Tao et al. [37]	LncRNA SOX2-OT	-	↑	-	Atherosclerosis
Vilades et al. [38]	hsa_circ_0001445	-	-	↓	Atherosclerosis
Corsten et al. [46]	miR-208b	-	↑	-	Acute myocardial infarction
Li et al. [11]	tDR-1:32-His-GTG-1, tDR-37:72-Val-TAC-1, tDR-1:32-Pro-AGG-1-M4, etc.	-	↑		Cardiac ischemia/reperfusion
	tDR-1:36-Glu-CTC-1, tDR-1:36-Glu-CTC-1-D5G, tDR-1:36-Asp-GTC-2-M2, etc.	-		↓	
Chen et al. [47]	LncRNA-NEAT1, miR-204	EV	↑	↓	Acute ST-segment elevation myocardial infarction
Hildebrandt et al. [48]	miR-370-3p, miR-409-3p	EV	↑	-	Coronary heart disease
Chen et al. [50]	microRNA 3113-5P	-	↑	-	Cardiac ischemia/Reperfusion injury
Zheng et al. [53]	lncRNA ENST00000556899.1, lncRNA ENST00000575985.1	EV	↑	-	Acute myocardial infarction
Kishore et al. [54]	circRNA MICRA, circRNA-284, hsa-circ-0098964	-	↑	↓	Myocardial infarction, Ischemic heart disease, Hypertension
Suzuki et al. [61]	miR-133a, miR-27a	-	-	↓	Hypertension
Wang et al. [62]	miR-92a	-	↑	-	Hypertension
He et al. [66]	miR-200a-3p	-	↑	-	Hypertension
Janjusevic et al. [68]	lncRNA LIPCAR, miR-192, miR-134a, miR-194, miR-30d	EV	↑	↓	Heart failure
Li et al. [69]	miR-30d	EV	-	↓	Heart failure
Wu et al. [70]	miR-92b-5p	EV	↑	-	Heart failure

4. Ex-ncRNAs as Therapeutic Targets in CVDs

Over the past decade, substantial effort has been made toward better understanding the functional roles of Ex-ncRNAs in CVDs and the clinical applications of novel therapies targeting Ex-ncRNAs, based on the approaches modulating their expression or their interactions with targets. The therapeutic functions of most of the small ncRNAs can be induced by synthesized RNA oligos, known as mimics, with multiple chemical modifications that improve pharmacokinetics and pharmacodynamics [76]. With the recent success of two COVID-19 mRNA vaccines [77], long RNA mimics have been emerging as promising therapeutics to induce functional effects of lncRNAs in patients. Besides the synthetic circRNA mimics, circRNAs are usually overexpressed by gene-expressing viral or non-viral vectors [78], which can also be used to express some small and long ncRNAs. The tools exploiting the exquisite sensitivity of base-pair complementarity have been used extensively to inhibit the functions of disease-causing Ex-ncRNAs [76,78,79], which include antisense oligonucleotides (ASOs), small interfering RNAs (siRNAs), short hairpin RNAs (shRNAs), antisense, miRNA sponges, CRISPR/Cas9-based DNA editing tools, and CRISPR/Cas13-based RNA editing tools. Here, we describe recent studies that targeted Ex-ncRNAs in various CVDs (Table 2).

4.1. *Atherosclerosis*

4.1.1. Extracellular Small ncRNA

It is well-known that inflammation plays a vital role in the development of coronary atherosclerotic diseases (CAD) [80,81]. Evidence suggests that intercellular crosstalk of Ex-ncRNAs can influence the development of inflammation and subsequent CAD progression. EV-encapsulated miRNA-146a-5p treatment resulted in production of proinflammatory cytokines, injury of the coronary endothelial cell barrier, and cardiomyocyte dysfunction, by targeting inflammation-triggering Toll-like receptor 7 (TLR7) [82]. Other avenues facilitating atherosclerosis progression include Ex-ncRNAs acting as danger-associated molecular patterns (DAMPs) through stimulation of the vascular endothelial growth factor (VEGF) receptor-2 system to increase vascular permeability and inflammatory cell aggregation [83].

4.1.2. Extracellular LncRNAs

A previous study has shown that lncRNA-RNCR3 is significantly upregulated during atherosclerosis. RNCR3 acts as a ceRNA for miR-185-5p, leading to the upregulation of its target gene KLF2, a critical transcription factor for endothelial vasoprotection. Targeting RNCR3 may thereby protect from atherosclerosis-related injury [84].

4.1.3. Extracellular CircRNAs

The studies focusing on circRNAs for therapeutic application have identified a wide range of potential targets against atherosclerosis development and progression. A recent study reported the specific mechanism of hsa_circ_0001445 on endothelial injury following treatment with oxidized LDL (ox-LDL) [85]. hsa_circ_0001445 was found to directly target miR-208b-5p and lead to the upregulation of ABCG1, the direct target of miR-208b-5p [85]. The study concludes that targeting hsa_circ_0001445 promotes aortic endothelial cell proliferation and migration through the mir-208b-5p/ABCG1 axis and inhibits inflammation and extracellular matrix (ECM) to reduce the damage of ox-LDL to endothelial cells (ECs) [85].

As most Ex-ncRNAs, except circRNAs, contain linear terminals, targeting ncRNAs using RNases presents a route for therapeutic inhibition. RNases are capable of hydrolyzing Ex-ncRNAs. In linear ncRNAs, such as small and lncNRAs, RNase digestion can inhibit the development of arterial inflammation and suppress atherosclerosis [86]. Investigations on RNase-based therapies targeting Ex-ncRNAs have begun to reveal yet another critical avenue of ncRNA therapeutics [87].

4.2. *Ischemic Heart Disease*

4.2.1. Extracellular Small ncRNAs

In the immune microenvironment, EVs produced by immune cells can selectively carry Ex-ncRNAs that affect the development of MI [88]. Among the highly expressed pro-inflammatory miRNAs, miR-155 was found to inhibit angiogenesis and promote cardiac dysfunction by downregulating Rac family small GTPase 1 (RAC1), p21-activated kinase 2 (PAK2), Sirtuin 1 (Sirt1), and protein kinase AMP-activated catalytic subunit alpha 2 (AMPKα2) [89]. These proteins subsequently reduce the ability of ECs to induce angiogenesis and advance inflammation, leading to the exacerbation of MI [89]. In another vein, miR-1271-5p, carried by M2-like macrophage-derived EVs, plays a protective role in AMI [90]. It directly affects the expression of SRY-Box transcription factor 6, which prevents cardiomyocyte damage and promotes cardiac repair and cardiomyocyte viability [90]. Additionally, miR-30d, the HF biomarker mentioned above, may potentially target integrin 5 and mitogen-activated protein kinase 4 (MAPK4) in cardiac fibroblasts in response to acute cardiac damage [69].

In addition to macrophages, dendritic cells (DCs) also play an essential role in the immune microenvironment after MI. This study has found that miR-494-3p could be loaded into DC-derived EVs and promote post-MI angiogenesis by inducing VEGF expression in mice [91]. Mesenchymal stem cells (MSCs) derived Ex-ncRNAs also have been found to play a crucial role in intercellular communication. Overexpression of miR-486-5p, derived from MSCs, silences MMP19 and promotes the activity of ECs to induce angiogenesis [92]. As such, MSC EVs may be potentially used to promote angiogenesis by delivering miR-486-5p-loaded EVs. This modality may be a critical therapeutic approach in myocardial ischemic compensation [92]. MSC-derived EV transfer of miR-210 has also been found to protect cardiomyocytes from apoptotic cell death, with miR-210 downregulating the expression level of apoptosis-inducing factor mitochondria associated 3 (AIFM3) and affecting PI3K/AKT and p53 signaling pathways to reduce apoptosis in cardiomyocytes and improve cardiac function [93]. To a certain extent, MSCs under hypoxic conditions offer significant protection against I/R injury. Upregulated miR-224-5p in mouse adipose, MSC EVs were found to target thioredoxin-interacting protein (TXNIP), thereby inhibiting the degradation of GATA binding protein 4 (GATA4) and maintaining the expression of Bcl-2 [94]. TXNIP was also identified as a target for miR-150-5p [95]. Therefore, as expected, overexpression of miR-150-5p protected rat hearts during I/R by inhibiting the expression of TXNIP.

The persistence of inflammation and oxidative stress may trigger a cytokine storm that exposes cells to severe damage [42]. Bone marrow mesenchymal stem cells (BMSC) EVs exert protective effects at different levels of oxidation [96]. It is worth noting that the miR-29c was upregulated in BMCS EVs and protected against hypoxia/reoxygenation (H/R) injury by inhibiting the PTEN/Akt/mTOR axis. Additionally, two extracellular miRNAs: miR-149 and let-7c, were significantly upregulated in EVs from normal BMSCs compared to H/R BMSCs [97]. These two upregulated miRNAs downregulate the expression of the Faslg gene by promoting the miR-149/Let-7c/FASLG axis [97]. Another study using BMSC-derived EVs has shown that miR-338 is highly enriched in BMSC EVs [98]. Upregulation of miR-338 inhibits MAP3K2 gene expression by suppressing the MAP3K2/JNK axis, thus inhibiting apoptosis in cardiomyocytes. As such, it can be concluded that BMSC EVs have the potential to ameliorate cardiac conditions during MI.

Cardiac cell-derived EVs encapsulate many miRNAs like miR-146a, miR-181b, and miR-26a, and have exhibited improved cardio-protective and therapeutic effects than MSC EVs under MI conditions [99–102]. Using single RNA tracing, cardiac endothelial cells and cardiac fibroblasts have shown increased intake of cardiosphere cell-derived EVs following injury [103]. Several cardiomyocyte EC-derived miRNAs such as miR-23a-3p, miR-424, let-7f, miR-378, and miR-214 might be one of the crucial cardio protecting factors [104]. Moreover, evidence suggests that miR-19a-3p can downregulate hypoxia-inducing factor-1α (HIF-1α), leading to the inhibition of cardiomyocyte proliferation and angiogenesis. Administration of the miR-19a-3p antagomir has downregulated miR-19a-3p expression, accelerated angiogenesis, and exerted a protective effect after MI [105]. Another study has shown that the downregulated expression of miR-143 in cardiomyocyte-derived EVs leads to the induction of angiogenesis and reduces cardiac ischemic pressure through the IGF-IR/NO signaling pathway [106]. Through a small RNA sequencing study, cardiac telomeric cell-derived EVs have demonstrated the transport of miR-21-5p to ECs, where it silences Cdip1 gene expression. Silencing of Cdip1 downregulates caspase-3 protein expression and promotes angiogenesis, subsequently suppressing ischemic cardiomyopathy [107].

4.2.2. Extracellular LncRNAs

It is reported that human BMSC EVs containing lncRNA HCP5 could protect cardiomyocytes from I/R injury by inhibiting the IGF1/PI3K/AKT axis [108]. In detail, it functions as a sponge for endogenous miR-497, which targets the expression of IGF-1 [108]. Another study using human umbilical cord mesenchymal stem cell (ucMSC)-derived EVs to treat H/R cardiac microvascular ECs and I/R rats has found that human ucMSC-derived EVs containing the lncRNA UCA1 reduces the injury of cardiac microvascular ECs in vivo [109]. UCA1 sponges miR-143 and subsequently inhibits Bcl-2 via the miR-143/Bcl-2/Beclin-1 axis [109].

4.2.3. Extracellular CircRNAs

Researchers have found that circRNAs also have protective effects against MI. For example, circ-HIPK3-rich EVs were released from cardiomyocytes under hypoxic conditions and protected the heart from oxidative stress injury [110]. Circ-HIPK3 sponges miR-29a and promotes the expression of vascular endothelial growth factor A (VEGFA), accelerating the proliferation, migration, and angiogenesis of ECs. Upregulation of VEGFA thereby reduces the effects of MI and protects against MI [110]. Another study used microarray analysis to establish the circRNA expression profile of EVs derived from M2-like macrophages. This was followed by the identification, and functional characterization of M2-like macrophage-derived EVs in MI mice models [111]. From this, it was found that highly expressed circRNA-UB3A can enter cardiac fibroblasts to sponge the expression of miR-138-5p. This results in the inhibition of Rho C expression, which exacerbates myocardial fibrosis after MI [111]. In summary, Ex-ncRNAs (miRNAs, lncRNAs, and circRNAs) derived from various resources (cardiomyocytes, stem cells, immune cells) mediate crosstalk between cell-to-cell through a variety of modalities, affecting the proliferation and apoptosis of cardiomyocytes alongside promoting angiogenesis. At the same time, they can counteract the generation of ischemic injury of cardiomyocytes.

4.3. *Hypertension*

Extracellular Small ncRNAs

Endothelial dysfunction is a significant manifestation of hypertension. It was shown that miR-483 could target transforming growth factor-β (TGF-β), TGF-β receptor 2 (TGFBR2), β-catenin, connective tissue growth factor (CTGF), interleukin-1β (IL-1β), and endothelin-1 (ET-1) to obtain anti-hypertensive effects [112]. The protective mechanisms mediated by extracellular miR-483-3p derived from ECs in hypertension were also elucidated [113]. This study showed that miR-483-3p was associated with the progression of hypertension and that the expression level of miR-483-3p in serum was proportional to vascular function. Overexpression of miR-483-3p reduced the expression of TGF-β, CTGF, angiotensin-converting enzyme 1 (ACE1), and ET-1 genes both in ECs and smooth muscle cells (SMCs). Therefore, extracellular miR-483-3p may become one of the promising therapeutic targets for the treatment of various types of endothelial dysfunction represented by hypertension [113].

MiR-634, as a circulating biomarker, has been implicated in playing a role in pulmonary hypertension as well as systemic hypertension [114,115]. It was found that the expression level of miR-634 was reduced in the plasma of hypertensive patients, and miR-634 could target HASMCs through the Wnt/β-catenin signaling pathway and downregulate the expression of Wnt4, thereby inhibiting the proliferation and migration of HASMCs and influencing the course of hypertension by affecting vascular remodeling [116].

4.4. *Cardiac Hypertrophy*

Cardiac hypertrophy is mainly caused by changes in the mechanical stress of the heart. It is a compensatory mechanism of the heart to resist the increased hemodynamic pressure. The process of myocardial hypertrophy is primarily characterized by the enlargement of cardiomyocytes along with myocardial fibrosis and inflammation, resulting in myocardial dysfunction [117,118].

Extracellular Small ncRNAs

The process of myocardial hypertrophy is primarily characterized by the enlargement of cardiomyocytes along with myocardial fibrosis and inflammation, resulting in myocardial dysfunction [117,118]. It has been reported that miR-217 expression was increased in the hearts of thoracic aortic constriction (TAC) mice and CHF patients. In cases of stress overload and miR-217 overexpression in cardiac hypertrophy, fibrosis, and dysfunction, effects were reversed via miR-217-TUD-mediated miR-217 downregulation. It has been established that miR-217 directly targets PTEN, a protein involved in cell cycle regulation and proliferation. Importantly, exosomes produced from cardiomyocytes containing miR-

217 promoted fibroblast growth in vitro. Following its implications in cardiac fibrosis and hypertrophy through control of PTEN, miR-217 is undoubtedly highlighted as a potential therapeutic target for chronic HF [119].

MiR-21-3p has been identified as upregulated in cardiac fibroblast-derived EVs by miRNA profiling assay and qRT-PCR. Exploration of the crosstalk between cardiac fibroblasts and cardiomyocytes in a co-culture system further validated the paracrine function of cardiac fibroblast-derived miR-21-3p on cardiomyocytes. Co-incubation of fibroblast-derived miR-21-3p and cardiomyocytes further confirmed the capacity of miR-21-3p to mediate cardiomyocyte hypertrophy. This study further demonstrates that miR-21-3p produced by cardiac fibroblasts silenced the expression of SH3 domain-containing protein 2 (SH3P2) and the PDZ and LIM domains in cardiomyocytes, encouraging hypertrophy and fibrosis. As a result, miR-21-3p may be a crucial therapeutic target for preventing cardiac hypertrophy [120]. On the other hand, miR-21-5p is known to regulate the ERK-MAP kinase signaling pathway in cardiac fibroblasts and influence the cardiac structure and function [121–123]. Interestingly, miR-21-5p levels are selectively increased in the fibroblasts of failing hearts and have enhanced ERK-MAP kinase activity by inhibiting sprouting homolog 1 (Spry1) [121]. In a murine model of pressure overload-induced cardiac hypertrophy, silencing of miR-21-5p by miRNA inhibitors suppressed the cardiac ERK-MAP kinase activity, attenuated interstitial fibrosis, and alleviated cardiac dysfunction [121]. Therefore, miR-21 served as the disease target for myocardial fibrosis and cardiac hypertrophy and defined the therapeutic efficacy of microRNA therapeutic interventions in CVDs.

The inflammatory immune microenvironment plays an important role in the development of myocardial hypertrophy. In parallel to the micro-immune microenvironment, immune-derived exosomes have become effective regulators of inflammatory response [124]. A study confirmed that exosomes derived from angiotensin II (Ang II)-induced hypertrophic cardiomyocytes (HCs) disturbed inflammatory signaling pathways in the macrophages [125]. The incubation of mouse macrophage cell line RAW264.7 in the presence of exosomes derived from HC medium activated the secretion of inflammatory cytokines interleukin (IL)-6 and IL-8 when compared with the exosomes derived from normal cardiomyocytes (NCs). The cytokine release triggered by exosomes derived from HCs was prevented by Argonaute2 (AGO2) down-regulation, suggesting that ncRNAs were involved in the exosome-induced inflammation in the RAW 264.7 macrophages. RNA sequencing further revealed that a total of seven microRNAs were differentially expressed between NCs-derived and HCs-derived exosomes, of which miR-155 plays a crucial role in the initiation of macrophage inflammation [126]. Further analysis showed that the HC-derived exosomes abducted the phosphorylation of ERK, c-Jun N-terminal kinase (JNK), and p38 through miR-155 [126]. These findings support that exosomal microRNA has become an important inflammatory response regulator in adjusting cardiac hypertrophy.

Cardiac hypertrophy, specifically myocardial hypertrophy, is often exacerbated by valvular calcification, a progressive disease prevalent in elderly individuals. Early intervention in the development of valvular calcification is a crucial measure to prevent myocardial hypertrophy [127,128]. In the cardiac interstitium, telocytes establish a complex association between cardiac stem cells and cardiomyocytes. When valvular calcification occurs, telocytes-derived EVs modulate myocardial regeneration, reduce myocardial fibrosis, and restore some functions [129]. Extraction of T telocytes EVs and knockdown of miR-30b expression revealed that inhibition of miR-30b could reduce calcium deposition in the valve, protecting the aortic valve and mitigating cardiac hypertrophy [129].

4.5. Heart Failure

4.5.1. Extracellular Small ncRNAs

HF is a complex and progressive disease that may be caused by a variety of pathological conditions. Previous studies have indicated that Ex-ncRNAs also participate in the progression of HF. For example, a recent study demonstrated that the expression level of miR-21-5p was dysregulated in cardiac stromal cell-derived EVs from HF patients using microRNA arrays and qPCR analysis [130]. When the miR-21-5p level is downregulated, the repair effect in HF patients diminishes as it inhibits phosphatase and Tensin homologs to enhance AKT activity, thus causing the promotion of angiogenesis and protection of cardiomyocytes. This offers a promising therapeutical target for treating HF.

4.5.2. Extracellular LncRNAs

LncRNAs are significant in heart development and disease. One study verified exercise-regulated cardiac lncRNA, called lncExACT, that was evolutionarily conserved and reduced in the exercising heart but augmented in the human and experimental HF [131]. The cardiac lncExACT1 overexpression led to pathological hypertrophy and HF. LncExACT1 suppressed physiological hypertrophy and cardiomyogenesis, preventing cardiac fibrosis and dysfunction. Further, lncExACT1 regulated microRNA-222, calcineurin signaling, and Hippo/Yap1 signaling vis DCHS2 [132,133]. Overexpression of DCHS2 in the zebrafish cardiomyocytes led to pathological hypertrophy and impaired cardiac regeneration, thereby promoting scar formation after injury [134]. On the contrary, DCHS2 depletion caused physiological hypertrophy and accelerated cardiomyogenesis in mice. These data demonstrated that lncExACT1-DCHS2 was identified as a new pathway for regulating HF.

Table 2. Ex-ncRNAs as therapeutic targets in CVDs.

Reference	Donor Cells	Ex-ncRNAs	Carriers	Expression Quantity (↑) (↓)		Target/Pathway	Type of CVDs
Shimada et al. [82]	-	miR-146a-5p	EV	↑	-	TLR7	Atherosclerosis
Shan et al. [84]	Human umbilical vein endothelial cells	lncRNA-RNCR3	EV	↑	-	miR-185-5p/KLF2	Atherosclerosis
Yang et al. [85]	-	hsa_circ_0001445	-	-	↓	mir-208b-5p/ABCG1	Atherosclerosis
Liu et al. [89]	M1-like macrophage	miR-155	EV	↑	-	Sirt1/AMPKα2 and RAC1-PAK2	Acute myocardial infarction
Long et al. [90]	M2-like macrophage	miR-1271-5p	EV	↑	-	SOX6	Acute myocardial infarction
Li et al. [69]	Cardiomyocytes	miR-30d	EV	↑	-	MAP4K4 and integrin α5	Ischemic HF
Liu et al. [91]	Dendritic cell	miR-494-3p	EV	↑	-	VEGF	Myocardial infarction
Li et al. [92]	MSC	miR-486-5p	EV	↑	-	MMP 19/VEGF	Myocardial infarction
Cheng et al. [93]	MSC	miR-210	EV	↑	-	AIFM3/PI3K/AKT and p53	Myocardial infarction
Mao et al. [94]	MSC	miR-224-5p	EV	↑	-	TXNIP/GATA4/Bcl-2	Ischemia-reperfusion injury
He et al. [95]	MSC	miR-150-5p	EV	↑	-	TXNIP	Ischemia-reperfusion injury
Li et al. [96]	BMSC	miR-29c	EV	↑	-	PTEN/Akt/mTOR	Ischemia-reperfusion injury
Zou et al. [97]	-	miR-149, let-7c	EV	↑	-	miR-149/Let-7c/FASLG	Ischemia-reperfusion injury
Fu et al. [98]	BMSC	miR-338	EV	↑	-	MAP3K2/JNK axis	Myocardial infarction
Walravens et al. [99–102]	CDC	miR-26a, miR-146a, miR-181b	EV	↑	-	Adam17, TLR-NFkB, PKCδ	Myocardial infarction
Moghiman et al. [104]	MSC, Cardiomyocyte, EC	miR-23a-3p, miR-424, let-7f, miR-378, miR-214	EV	↑	-	HOXA5, GAX, p38 MAPK, Smad2/3, ATM	Myocardial infarction
Gou et al. [105]	Cardiomyocyte	miR-19a-3p	EV	↑	-	HIF-1α	Myocardial infarction
Geng et al. [106]	Cardiomyocyte	miR-143	EV	-	↓	IGF-IR/NO	Myocardial infarction
Liao et al. [107]	CT	miR-21-5p	EV	↑	-	Cdip1/caspase-3	Myocardial infarction
Li et al. [108]	BMSC	lncRNA HCP5	EV	↑	-	miR-497/IGF1/PI3K/AKT	Ischemia-reperfusion injury

Table 2. *Cont.*

Reference	Donor Cells	Ex-ncRNAs	Carriers	Expression Quantity (↑)	(↓)	Target/Pathway	Type of CVDs
Diao et al. [109]	hUCMSC	lncRNA UCA1	EV	↑	-	miR-143/Bcl-2/Beclin-1	Ischemia-reperfusion injury
Wang et al. [110]	Cardiomyocyte	circ-HIPK3	EV	↑	-	miR-29a/VEGFA	Myocardial infarction
Wang et al. [111]	M2-like macrophage	circRNA-UB3A	EV	↑	-	miR-138-5p/RhoC	Myocardial fibrosis after myocardial infarction
Zhang et al. [112]	-	miR-483	-	-	↓	TGF-β, TGFBR2, β-catenin, CTGF, IL-1β, ET-1	Hypertension
Shang et al. [113]	-	miR-483-3p	EV	↑	-	TGF-β, CTGF, ACE1, ET-1	Hypertension
Niu et al. [116]	-	miR-634	-	-	↓	Wnt/β-catenin	Hypertension
Xiang et al. [119]	Cardiomyocyte	miR-217	EV	↑	-	PTEN	Cardiac hypertrophy
Claudia et al. [120]	Cardiac fibroblast	miR-21-3p	EV	↑	-	SH3 domain-containing protein 2 and PDZ and LIM domain 5	Cardiac hypertrophy
Thum et al. [121]	-	miR-21	-	↑	-	ERK-MAPK and Spry1	Cardiac hypertrophy
Yu et al. [125]	Macrophage	miR-155	EV	↑	-	Son of Sevenless 1 and Suppressor of Cytokine Signaling 1	Cardiac hypertrophy
Yang et al. [129]	Telocyte	miR-30b	EV	↑	-	Runx2/Wnt/β-catenin	Cardiac hypertrophy
Li et al. [130]	Cardiac stromal cell	miR-21-5p	EV	↑	-	phosphatase and tensin homolog/Akt	HF
Li et al. [131–133]	-	lncExACT1	-	↑	-	DCHS2	HF

5. Clinical Developments and Applications of Ex-ncRNAs in CVDs

Recently, significant progress has been made in understanding the regulation and roles of Ex-ncRNAs in CVDs and in translating these findings into clinical applications as biomarkers or therapeutic targets [9]. Ex-ncRNAs have been identified as critical regulators in the pathogenesis of CVDs and are thus important candidates for improved diagnosis or prognosis assessment and advanced therapeutics.

5.1. Ex-ncRNAs as Biomarkers

Despite the increasing interest in searching for Ex-ncRNA as reliable biomarkers, this field still faces many significant scientific and technical hurdles, including preanalytical and analytical factors that influence data quality and reliability. These factors include sample types, Ex-ncRNA isolation, detection and processing techniques, normalization strategies, and the influence of other cofounders such as drug usage and other CVDs [9,135]. Therefore, the clinical use of Ex-ncRNAs as biomarkers for CVDs is still in its infancy, despite the promising efficacy and feasibility in animal models and a small number of patients as mentioned above. Of note, hsa-Chr8:96, a human homolog of mmu-miR-721, was identified as a novel extracellular small ncRNA for the detection of acute myocarditis in four independent cohorts of patients with myocarditis [136], which demonstrates both the unmet medical need and the enormous promise for developing Ex-ncRNAs as novel biomarkers for CVDs. Currently, more than 10 clinical trials on identifying Ex-ncRNA as novel CVD biomarkers have been initiated or are ongoing, such as ischemic heart diseases (NCT02691286, NCT01875484), atherosclerosis (NCT03279770, NCT03855891), hypertension (NCT04193046), and HF (NCT03345446). A better understanding of the biology of Ex-ncRNAs and the advances in methods for Ex-ncRNA isolation, detection, and analysis, will undoubtedly pave the way for the translation of Ex-ncRNA biomarker research to clinical routine.

5.2. Ex-ncRNAs as Therapeutics Targets

Therapeutic targeting of Ex-ncRNAs, including small ncRNAs, lncRNAs, and circRNAs either inside or outside the cells, represents an attractive strategy for treating CVDs. The RNA-targeting approaches include ASOs, siRNAs, shRNAs, antisense, miRNA sponges, CRISPR/Cas9-based DNA editing tools, and CRISPR/Cas13-based RNA editing tools. Notably, siRNAs and ASO have been approved by the United States of America Food and Drug Administration (FDA) and/or the European Medicines Agency (EMA) for clinical use. siRNA is a single- or double-stranded RNA oligo, which exploits the endogenous miRNA pathway to silence mRNAs by loading them into RNA-induced silencing complexes (RISC) for degradation [137]. The successful clinical use of siRNAs targeting proprotein convertase subtilisin/kexin type 9 (PCSK9) mRNAs for lowering circulating LDL cholesterol and then decreasing the CVD risks in human patients has proved the tremendous promise of using siRNAs targeting CVD-causing Ex-ncRNAs, in particular lncRNAs. ASO is a single-stranded DNA oligo with entire or partial complementarity to the target RNAs and may act either by inducing the degradation of target RNAs or by sequestering the interaction of target RNAs with their partner compounds [138]. ASO was first approved by FDA for silencing mRNA in 1998 and has now been widely used to target other ncRNAs, including small ncRNAs [139], lncRNAs [140], and circRNAs [78]. Over the past decades, extensive efforts have been made to clinically utilize siRNAs or ASO to target mRNAs, such as ApoA, PCSK9, Angiotensinogen, FOXO3, and SERCA2A, and only recently target ncRNAs for treating CVDs (Table 3) [141]. CDR132L, a synthetic ASO blocking the functions of miR-132, has entered the Phase II clinical trial for treating patients with reduced left ventricular ejection fraction after MI (NCT05350969). Other strategies, such as antisense, miRNA sponges, and CRISPR/Cas9-based gene editing tools, have also demonstrated promising preclinical effects and are being translated into the clinical routine.

Table 3. RNA Therapies Approved or in Clinical Trials for CVDs.

Stage	Drug	Modification and Delivery	Target Gene	Disease	Comments
Clinical trials	AZD8601	naked mRNA	VEGF-A	HF	Phase 2
	CDR132L	ASO	miR-321	HF	Phase 2
	IONIS-AGT-LRx	Antisense	Angiotensinogen	HF	Phase 2
	Olezarsen	Antisense	ApoC-III	Lipid disorders	Phase 3
	Olpasiran	siRNA	Lp(a)	Lipid disorders	Phase 2
	Pelacarsen	Antisense	Lp(a)	Lipid disorders	Phase 3
	Vupanorsen	Antisense	ANGPTL3	Lipid disorders	Phase 2
FDA/EMA approved	Inclisiran	siRNA	PCSK9	Lipid disorders	FDA approved
	Volanesorsen	ASO	APO-C3	Triglycerides	EMA approved

There are also many challenges to be overcome to further the clinical application of RNA-based therapeutics, mainly the specificity and delivery. Virtually all RNA-targeting approaches exploiting the exquisite sensitivity of base-pair complementarity have off-target effects [142]. The quality of RNA therapy is determined by both the efficacy of its on-target effects as well as the minimized off-target side effects, namely specificity. These can be achieved by the development of algorithms for improved RNAi therapeutic design and by chemical modifications. In the past 60 years, hundreds of nucleic acid chemical modifications have been characterized and synthesized, and a number of them have been successfully utilized in RNA therapeutics improving the potency and specificity [143], including the first generation of 2′-deoxy-2′-fluoro (2′-F), 2′-O-methylation (2′-OMe), and the phosphorothioates (PS) backbones, the second generation of 2′-O-(2-methoxyethylation) (2-O-MOE), and the third generation of LNA modification. Efficient and specific delivery of RNA therapeutics to organs/cells still remain the top two greatest challenges in this field [143], owing to their instability, negative charge, hydrophilic nature which prevents diffusion through cell membranes, and rapid cleaning by the liver after systematic administration. The first and second generations of chemical modifications greatly improve the stability and enhance cellular uptake [144]. Specific delivery to targeted cells/tissues can be achieved using modified lipid- and polymer-based nanoparticles, conjugation with different homing ligands, or engineering into specific EVs, among which the endosomal escape of the RNA therapeutics, also termed functional delivery, should be considered. A vast number of other strategies, such as viral vectors with cell type-specific promoters or different envelop proteins, can also be employed for specific and efficient delivery [145].

6. Conclusions and Perspectives

The poor recovery of cardiac function following heart tissue injury and the lack of effective strategies facilitating this recovery in clinical settings emphasize the importance of preventative monitoring and diagnosis [146]. Ex-ncRNAs, selectively released by different cells, play versatile roles in numerous biological processes and diseases [147]. Recently, studies elucidating the Ex-ncRNAs-mediated intercellular crosstalk in the pathogenesis of various CVDs are emerging [148], and Ex-ncRNAs are increasingly recognized as promising diagnostic biomarkers and druggable targets [149,150]. In this review, we have systematically summarized the regulation and roles of Ex-ncRNAs, including small ncRNAs, circRNAs, and lncRNAs, involved in major cardiovascular events, such as atherosclerosis, ischemic heart diseases, hypertension, cardiac hypertrophy, and HF (Figure 2). We also discussed the strategies and challenges for utilizing Ex-ncRNAs as biomarkers or therapeutical targets.

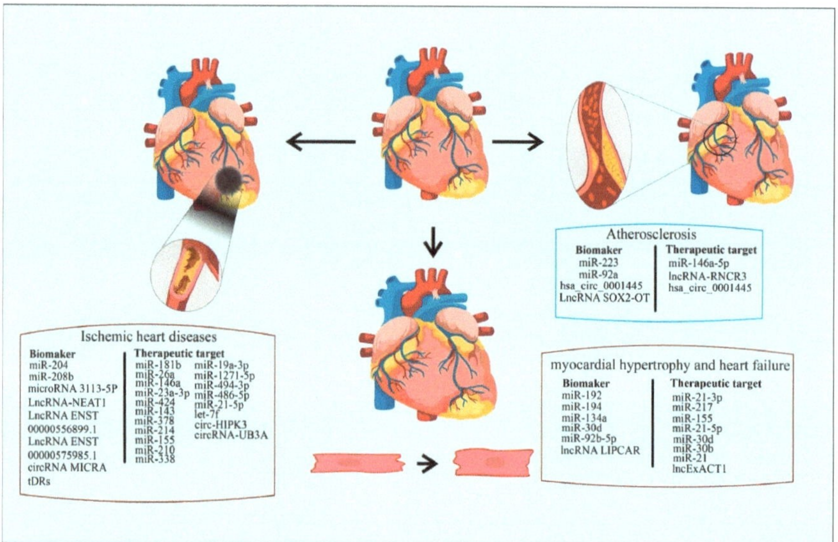

Figure 2. Extracellular non-coding RNAs as biomarkers or therapeutic targets for cardiovascular diseases. The summary of Ex-ncRNAs being identified as potential biomarkers or therapeutical targets for cardiovascular diseases.

Although increasing research interests have been attracted to the roles of Ex-ncRNAs during the onset, progression, and prognosis of CVDs [151,152], the utilization of Ex-ncRNAs as biomarkers and therapeutics is still in its infancy in its clinical routine. Due to the heterogeneity of Ex-ncRNAs in different biofluids or even in plasma samples from the same patient at different time points, a robust, reliable, and reproducible readout of specific Ex-ncRNA is indispensable for developing it as a clinical CVD biomarker, which may be achieved by a better understanding of the biology of Ex-ncRNAs and the advances in methods for Ex-ncRNA isolation, detection, and analysis. Similarly, although the specificity of RNA targeting is significantly improved, the specific delivery of RNA therapeutics to desired organs/cells still remains the leading challenge for furthering RNA therapeutics, among which EV-mediated delivery of RNA therapeutics holds the greatest potential. Further understanding of Ex-ncRNA biology and advances in related techniques will eventually establish well-defined diagnostic and therapeutic approaches using Ex-ncRNAs to alleviate the current medical burdens associated with CVDs.

Author Contributions: Conceptualization, Z.J., C.L., X.Y. and G.L.; methodology, formal analysis, investigation, resources, and data curation, Z.J., C.L., X.Y., L.S., L.Z. and G.L.; writing—original draft preparation, Z.J., C.L., X.Y., L.S., E.C. and L.Z.; writing—review and editing, X.Y., L.S., E.C., J.L. and G.L.; supervision and project administration, J.L. and G.L.; funding acquisition, Z.J., X.Y. and J.L. All authors have read and agreed to the published version of the manuscript.

Funding: This work was supported by the National Natural Science Foundation of China to Z.J (No. 81900287) and X.Y. (No. 82205088), the Tianshan Youth Foundation of Xinjiang (No. 2019Q066) to Z.J., and the Massachusetts General Hospital Institutional fund (No. 219863) to J.L.

Institutional Review Board Statement: Not applicable.

Informed Consent Statement: Not applicable.

Data Availability Statement: Not applicable.

Acknowledgments: We thank Tiffaney Hisa from the Department of Neurosurgery, Massachusetts General Hospital and Harvard Medical School, for her help with the language editing.

Conflicts of Interest: The authors declare no conflict of interest.

References

1. Campbell, N.R.C.; Ordunez, P.; Giraldo, G.; Rodriguez Morales, Y.A.; Lombardi, C.; Khan, T.; Padwal, R.; Tsuyuki, R.T.; Varghese, C. WHO HEARTS: A Global Program to Reduce Cardiovascular Disease Burden: Experience Implementing in the Americas and Opportunities in Canada. *Can. J. Cardiol.* **2021**, *37*, 744–755. [CrossRef] [PubMed]
2. Şahin, B.; İlgün, G. Risk factors of deaths related to cardiovascular diseases in World Health Organization (WHO) member countries. *Health Soc. Care Community* **2022**, *30*, 73–80. [CrossRef] [PubMed]
3. Fang, Y.; Dai, X. Emerging Roles of Extracellular Non-Coding RNAs in Vascular Diseases. *J. Cardiovasc. Transl. Res.* **2022**, *15*, 492–499. [CrossRef] [PubMed]
4. Thompson, A.G.; Gray, E.; Heman-Ackah, S.M.; Mäger, I.; Talbot, K.; Andaloussi, S.E.; Wood, M.J.; Turner, M.R. Extracellular vesicles in neurodegenerative disease—Pathogenesis to biomarkers. *Nat. Rev. Neurol.* **2016**, *12*, 346–357. [CrossRef]
5. Zijlstra, C.; Stoorvogel, W. Prostasomes as a source of diagnostic biomarkers for prostate cancer. *J. Clin. Investig.* **2016**, *126*, 1144–1151. [CrossRef]
6. Gruner, H.N.; McManus, M.T. Examining the evidence for extracellular RNA function in mammals. *Nat. Rev. Genet.* **2021**, *22*, 448–458. [CrossRef]
7. Lin, Z.; Lu, F.; Ma, X.; Xia, X.; Zou, F.; Jiang, J. Roles of circular RNAs in the pathogenesis of intervertebral disc degeneration (Review). *Exp. Ther. Med.* **2021**, *22*, 1221. [CrossRef]
8. Sato-Kuwabara, Y.; Melo, S.A.; Soares, F.A.; Calin, G.A. The fusion of two worlds: Non-coding RNAs and extracellular vesicles–diagnostic and therapeutic implications (Review). *Int. J. Oncol.* **2015**, *46*, 17–27. [CrossRef]
9. Poller, W.; Dimmeler, S.; Heymans, S.; Zeller, T.; Haas, J.; Karakas, M.; Leistner, D.M.; Jakob, P.; Nakagawa, S.; Blankenberg, S.; et al. Non-coding RNAs in cardiovascular diseases: Diagnostic and therapeutic perspectives. *Eur. Heart J.* **2018**, *39*, 2704–2716. [CrossRef]
10. Hu, Y.Y.; Cheng, X.M.; Wu, N.; Tao, Y.; Wang, X.N. Non-coding RNAs Regulate the Pathogenesis of Aortic Dissection. *Front. Cardiovasc. Med.* **2022**, *9*, 890607. [CrossRef]
11. Li, G.; Manning, A.C.; Bagi, A.; Yang, X.; Gokulnath, P.; Spanos, M.; Howard, J.; Chan, P.P.; Sweeney, T.; Kitchen, R.; et al. Distinct Stress-Dependent Signatures of Cellular and Extracellular tRNA-Derived Small RNAs. *Adv. Sci.* **2022**, *9*, e2200829. [CrossRef] [PubMed]
12. Brandão, B.B.; Guerra, B.A.; Mori, M.A. Shortcuts to a functional adipose tissue: The role of small non-coding RNAs. *Redox Biol.* **2017**, *12*, 82–102. [CrossRef] [PubMed]
13. Videira, R.F.; da Costa Martins, P.A. Non-coding RNAs in Cardiac Intercellular Communication. *Front. Physiol.* **2020**, *11*, 738. [CrossRef] [PubMed]
14. Kondkar, A.A.; Abu-Amero, K.K. Utility of circulating microRNAs as clinical biomarkers for cardiovascular diseases. *Biomed. Res. Int.* **2015**, *2015*, 821823. [CrossRef] [PubMed]
15. Peters, L.J.F.; Biessen, E.A.L.; Hohl, M.; Weber, C.; van der Vorst, E.P.C.; Santovito, D. Small Things Matter: Relevance of MicroRNAs in Cardiovascular Disease. *Front. Physiol.* **2020**, *11*, 793. [CrossRef]
16. Shang, X.; Fang, Y.; Xin, W.; You, H. The Application of Extracellular Vesicles Mediated miRNAs in Osteoarthritis: Current Knowledge and Perspective. *J. Inflamm. Res.* **2022**, *15*, 2583–2599. [CrossRef]
17. Wahid, F.; Shehzad, A.; Khan, T.; Kim, Y.Y. MicroRNAs: Synthesis, mechanism, function, and recent clinical trials. *Biochim. Biophys. Acta* **2010**, *1803*, 1231–1243. [CrossRef]
18. Xia, W.; Zhu, X.-W.; Mo, X.-B.; Wu, L.-F.; Wu, J.; Guo, Y.-F.; Zeng, K.-Q.; Wang, M.-J.; Lin, X.; Qiu, Y.-H.; et al. Integrative multi-omics analysis revealed SNP-lncRNA-mRNA (SLM) networks in human peripheral blood mononuclear cells. *Human Genet.* **2017**, *136*, 451–462. [CrossRef]

19. Robinson, E.K.; Covarrubias, S.; Carpenter, S. The how and why of lncRNA function: An innate immune perspective. *Biochim. Biophys. Acta Gene Regul. Mech.* **2020**, *1863*, 194419. [CrossRef]
20. Sun, R.; He, X.Y.; Mei, C.; Ou, C.L. Role of exosomal long non-coding RNAs in colorectal cancer. *World J. Gastrointest. Oncol.* **2021**, *13*, 867–878. [CrossRef]
21. Dragomir, M.; Chen, B.; Calin, G.A. Exosomal lncRNAs as new players in cell-to-cell communication. *Transl. Cancer Res.* **2018**, *7*, S243–S252. [CrossRef] [PubMed]
22. Xue, M.; Chen, W.; Li, X. Extracellular vesicle-transferred long noncoding RNAs in bladder cancer. *Clin. Chim. Acta* **2021**, *516*, 34–45. [CrossRef] [PubMed]
23. Ye, M.; Wang, J.; Pan, S.; Zheng, L.; Wang, Z.-W.; Zhu, X. Nucleic acids and proteins carried by exosomes of different origins as potential biomarkers for gynecologic cancers. *Mol. Ther.-Oncolytics* **2021**, *24*, 101–113. [CrossRef] [PubMed]
24. Zhang, Y.; Zhang, X.; Xu, Y.; Fang, S.; Ji, Y.; Lu, L.; Xu, W.; Qian, H.; Liang, Z.F. Circular RNA and Its Roles in the Occurrence, Development, Diagnosis of Cancer. *Front. Oncol.* **2022**, *12*, 845703. [CrossRef]
25. Tang, X.; Ren, H.; Guo, M.; Qian, J.; Yang, Y.; Gu, C. Review on circular RNAs and new insights into their roles in cancer. *Comput. Struct. Biotechnol. J.* **2021**, *19*, 910–928. [CrossRef]
26. Jiang, L.; Wang, X.; Zhan, X.; Kang, S.; Liu, H.; Luo, Y.; Lin, L. Advance in circular RNA modulation effects of heart failure. *Gene X* **2020**, *5*, 100036. [CrossRef]
27. Yan, F.; Xie, X.; Huo, Q.; Zhang, W.; Wu, T.; Daniyaer, D.; Shi, L. circ-CCND1 regulates the CCND1/P53/P21 pathway through sponging miR-138-5p in valve interstitial cells to aggravate aortic valve calcification. *J. Physiol. Biochem.* **2022**, *78*, 845–854. [CrossRef]
28. E, S.; Costa, M.C.; Kurc, S.; Drożdż, A.; Cortez-Dias, N.; Enguita, F.J. The circulating non-coding RNA landscape for biomarker research: Lessons and prospects from cardiovascular diseases. *Acta Pharmacol. Sin.* **2018**, *39*, 1085–1099. [CrossRef]
29. Shen, S.; Jiang, H.; Bei, Y.; Xiao, J.; Li, X. Long Non-Coding RNAs in Cardiac Remodeling. *Cell. Physiol. Biochem.* **2017**, *41*, 1830–1837. [CrossRef]
30. Zhang, Y.; Ying, F.; Tian, X.; Lei, Z.; Li, X.; Lo, C.-Y.; Li, J.; Jiang, L.; Yao, X. TRPM2 Promotes Atherosclerotic Progression in a Mouse Model of Atherosclerosis. *Cells* **2022**, *11*, 1423. [CrossRef]
31. Aryal, B.; Suárez, Y. Non-coding RNA regulation of endothelial and macrophage functions during atherosclerosis. *Vascul. Pharmacol.* **2019**, *114*, 64–75. [CrossRef] [PubMed]
32. Lund-Katz, S.; Phillips, M.C. High density lipoprotein structure-function and role in reverse cholesterol transport. *Subcell. Biochem.* **2010**, *51*, 183–227. [CrossRef] [PubMed]
33. Vickers, K.C.; Palmisano, B.T.; Shoucri, B.M.; Shamburek, R.D.; Remaley, A.T. MicroRNAs are transported in plasma and delivered to recipient cells by high-density lipoproteins. *Nat. Cell Biol.* **2011**, *13*, 423–433. [CrossRef] [PubMed]
34. Lu, H.; Buchan, R.J.; Cook, S.A. MicroRNA-223 regulates Glut4 expression and cardiomyocyte glucose metabolism. *Cardiovasc. Res.* **2010**, *86*, 410–420. [CrossRef]
35. Huang, Y.; Tang, S.; Ji-Yan, C.; Huang, C.; Li, J.; Cai, A.P.; Feng, Y.Q. Circulating miR-92a expression level in patients with essential hypertension: A potential marker of atherosclerosis. *J. Hum. Hypertens.* **2017**, *31*, 200–205. [CrossRef]
36. Yang, G.; Lin, C. Long Noncoding RNA SOX2-OT Exacerbates Hypoxia-Induced Cardiomyocytes Injury by Regulating miR-27a-3p/TGFβR1 Axis. *Cardiovasc. Ther.* **2020**, *2020*, 2016259. [CrossRef]
37. Tao, J.; Hu, Y. Diagnostic and prognostic significance of lncRNA SOX2-OT in patients with carotid atherosclerosis. *BMC Cardiovasc. Disord.* **2022**, *22*, 211. [CrossRef]
38. Vilades, D.; Martinez-Camblor, P.; Ferrero-Gregori, A.; Bar, C.; Lu, D.; Xiao, K.; Vea, A.; Nasarre, L.; Sanchez Vega, J.; Leta, R.; et al. Plasma circular RNA hsa_circ_0001445 and coronary artery disease: Performance as a biomarker. *FASEB J.* **2020**, *34*, 4403–4414. [CrossRef]
39. Moroni, F.; Gertz, Z.; Azzalini, L. Relief of Ischemia in Ischemic Cardiomyopathy. *Curr. Cardiol. Rep.* **2021**, *23*, 80. [CrossRef]
40. Han, D.; Kang, S.-H.; Yoon, C.-H.; Youn, T.-J.; Chae, I.-H. Attenuation of ischemia–reperfusion injury by intracoronary chelating agent administration. *Sci. Rep.* **2022**, *12*, 2050. [CrossRef]
41. Rios-Navarro, C.; Daghbouche-Rubio, N.; Gavara, J.; de Dios, E.; Perez, N.; Vila, J.M.; Chorro, F.J.; Ruiz-Sauri, A.; Bodi, V. Ischemia-reperfusion injury to coronary arteries: Comprehensive microscopic study after reperfused myocardial infarction. *Ann. Anat.* **2021**, *238*, 151785. [CrossRef] [PubMed]
42. Wu, M.Y.; Yiang, G.T.; Liao, W.T.; Tsai, A.P.; Cheng, Y.L.; Cheng, P.W.; Li, C.Y.; Li, C.J. Current Mechanistic Concepts in Ischemia and Reperfusion Injury. *Cell. Physiol. Biochem.* **2018**, *46*, 1650–1667. [CrossRef] [PubMed]
43. Kuster, D.W.; Cardenas-Ospina, A.; Miller, L.; Liebetrau, C.; Troidl, C.; Nef, H.M.; Möllmann, H.; Hamm, C.W.; Pieper, K.S.; Mahaffey, K.W.; et al. Release kinetics of circulating cardiac myosin binding protein-C following cardiac injury. *Am. J. Physiol. Heart Circ. Physiol.* **2014**, *306*, H547–H556. [CrossRef] [PubMed]
44. Okamoto, R.; Hirashiki, A.; Cheng, X.W.; Yamada, T.; Shimazu, S.; Shinoda, N.; Okumura, T.; Takeshita, K.; Bando, Y.; Kondo, T.; et al. Usefulness of serum cardiac troponins T and I to predict cardiac molecular changes and cardiac damage in patients with hypertrophic cardiomyopathy. *Int. Heart J.* **2013**, *54*, 202–206. [CrossRef] [PubMed]
45. Mannu, G.S. The non-cardiac use and significance of cardiac troponins. *Scott. Med. J.* **2014**, *59*, 172–178. [CrossRef]

46. Corsten, M.F.; Dennert, R.; Jochems, S.; Kuznetsova, T.; Devaux, Y.; Hofstra, L.; Wagner, D.R.; Staessen, J.A.; Heymans, S.; Schroen, B. Circulating MicroRNA-208b and MicroRNA-499 reflect myocardial damage in cardiovascular disease. *Circ. Cardiovasc. Genet.* **2010**, *3*, 499–506. [CrossRef]
47. Chen, Z.; Yan, Y.; Wu, J.; Qi, C.; Liu, J.; Wang, J. Expression level and diagnostic value of exosomal NEAT1/miR-204/MMP-9 in acute ST-segment elevation myocardial infarction. *IUBMB Life* **2020**, *72*, 2499–2507. [CrossRef]
48. Hildebrandt, A.; Kirchner, B.; Meidert, A.S.; Brandes, F.; Lindemann, A.; Doose, G.; Doege, A.; Weidenhagen, R.; Reithmair, M.; Schelling, G.; et al. Detection of Atherosclerosis by Small RNA-Sequencing Analysis of Extracellular Vesicle Enriched Serum Samples. *Front. Cell. Dev. Biol.* **2021**, *9*, 729061. [CrossRef]
49. Crouser, E.D.; Julian, M.W.; Bicer, S.; Ghai, V.; Kim, T.K.; Maier, L.A.; Gillespie, M.; Hamzeh, N.Y.; Wang, K. Circulating exosomal microRNA expression patterns distinguish cardiac sarcoidosis from myocardial ischemia. *PLoS ONE* **2021**, *16*, e0246083. [CrossRef]
50. Chen, Y.; Ye, X.; Yan, F. MicroRNA 3113-5p is a novel marker for early cardiac ischemia/reperfusion injury. *Diagn. Pathol.* **2019**, *14*, 121. [CrossRef]
51. Liu, X.; Xu, Y.; Deng, Y.; Li, H. MicroRNA-223 Regulates Cardiac Fibrosis After Myocardial Infarction by Targeting RASA1. *Cell. Physiol. Biochem. Int. J. Exp. Cell. Physiol. Biochem. Pharmacol.* **2018**, *46*, 1439–1454. [CrossRef] [PubMed]
52. Yang, F.; You, X.; Xu, T.; Liu, Y.; Ren, Y.; Liu, S.; Wu, F.; Xu, Z.; Zou, L.; Wang, G. Screening and Function Analysis of MicroRNAs Involved in Exercise Preconditioning-Attenuating Pathological Cardiac Hypertrophy. *Int. Heart J.* **2018**, *59*, 1069–1076. [CrossRef] [PubMed]
53. Zheng, M.L.; Liu, X.Y.; Han, R.J.; Yuan, W.; Sun, K.; Zhong, J.C.; Yang, X.C. Circulating exosomal long non-coding RNAs in patients with acute myocardial infarction. *J. Cell. Mol. Med.* **2020**, *24*, 9388–9396. [CrossRef]
54. Kishore, R.; Garikipati, V.N.S.; Gonzalez, C. Role of Circular RNAs in Cardiovascular Disease. *J. Cardiovasc. Pharmacol.* **2020**, *76*, 128–137. [CrossRef] [PubMed]
55. DeGuire, J.; Clarke, J.; Rouleau, K.; Roy, J.; Bushnik, T. Blood pressure and hypertension. *Health Rep.* **2019**, *30*, 14–21. [CrossRef] [PubMed]
56. Desai, A.N. High Blood Pressure. *JAMA* **2020**, *324*, 1254–1255. [CrossRef] [PubMed]
57. Cameron, A.C.; Lang, N.N.; Touyz, R.M. Drug Treatment of Hypertension: Focus on Vascular Health. *Drugs* **2016**, *76*, 1529–1550. [CrossRef]
58. Besler, C.; Urban, D.; Watzka, S.; Lang, D.; Rommel, K.P.; Kandolf, R.; Klingel, K.; Thiele, H.; Linke, A.; Schuler, G.; et al. Endomyocardial miR-133a levels correlate with myocardial inflammation, improved left ventricular function, and clinical outcome in patients with inflammatory cardiomyopathy. *Eur. J. Heart Fail.* **2016**, *18*, 1442–1451. [CrossRef]
59. Cengiz, M.; Yavuzer, S.; Kılıçkıran Avcı, B.; Yürüyen, M.; Yavuzer, H.; Dikici, S.A.; Karataş, Ö.F.; Özen, M.; Özen, M.; Uzun, H.; et al. Circulating miR-21 and eNOS in subclinical atherosclerosis in patients with hypertension. *Clin. Exp. Hypertens.* **2015**, *37*, 643–649. [CrossRef]
60. Zou, X.; Wang, J.; Chen, C.; Tan, X.; Huang, Y.; Jose, P.A.; Yang, J.; Zeng, C. Secreted Monocyte miR-27a, via Mesenteric Arterial Mas Receptor-eNOS Pathway, Causes Hypertension. *Am. J. Hypertens.* **2020**, *33*, 31–42. [CrossRef]
61. Suzuki, K.; Yamada, H.; Fujii, R.; Munetsuna, E.; Yamazaki, M.; Ando, Y.; Ohashi, K.; Ishikawa, H.; Mizuno, G.; Tsuboi, Y.; et al. Circulating microRNA-27a and -133a are negatively associated with incident hypertension: A five-year longitudinal population-based study. *Biomarkers* **2022**, *27*, 496–502. [CrossRef] [PubMed]
62. Wang, C.; Wu, H.; Xing, Y.; Ye, Y.; He, F.; Yin, Q.; Li, Y.; Shang, F.; Shyy, J.Y.; Yuan, Z.Y. Endothelial-derived extracellular microRNA-92a promotes arterial stiffness by regulating phenotype changes of vascular smooth muscle cells. *Sci. Rep.* **2022**, *12*, 344. [CrossRef]
63. Corsello, S.M.; Paragliola, R.M. Evaluation and Management of Endocrine Hypertension During Pregnancy. *Endocrinol. Metab. Clin. N. Am.* **2019**, *48*, 829–842. [CrossRef]
64. Shah, S.; Gupta, A. Hypertensive Disorders of Pregnancy. *Cardiol. Clin.* **2019**, *37*, 345–354. [CrossRef] [PubMed]
65. Cao, G.; Cui, R.; Liu, C.; Zhang, Z. MicroRNA regulation of transthyretin in trophoblast biofunction and preeclampsia. *Arch. Biochem. Biophys.* **2019**, *676*, 108129. [CrossRef] [PubMed]
66. He, X.; Ding, D. High miR-200a-3p expression has high diagnostic values for hypertensive disorders complicating pregnancy and predicts adverse pregnancy outcomes. *BMC Pregnancy Childbirth* **2022**, *22*, 490. [CrossRef] [PubMed]
67. Bozkurt, B.; Coats, A.J.S.; Tsutsui, H.; Abdelhamid, C.M.; Adamopoulos, S.; Albert, N.; Anker, S.D.; Atherton, J.; Böhm, M.; Butler, J.; et al. Universal definition and classification of heart failure: A report of the Heart Failure Society of America, Heart Failure Association of the European Society of Cardiology, Japanese Heart Failure Society and Writing Committee of the Universal Definition of Heart Failure. *Eur. J. Heart Fail.* **2021**, *23*, 352–380. [CrossRef]
68. Janjusevic, M.; Fluca, A.L.; Ferro, F.; Gagno, G.; D'Alessandra, Y.; Beltrami, A.P.; Sinagra, G.; Aleksova, A. Traditional and Emerging Biomarkers in Asymptomatic Left Ventricular Dysfunction-Promising Non-Coding RNAs and Exosomes as Biomarkers in Early Phases of Cardiac Damage. *Int. J. Mol. Sci.* **2021**, *22*, 4937. [CrossRef]
69. Li, J.; Salvador, A.M.; Li, G.; Valkov, N.; Ziegler, O.; Yeri, A.; Yang Xiao, C.; Meechoovet, B.; Alsop, E.; Rodosthenous, R.S.; et al. Mir-30d Regulates Cardiac Remodeling by Intracellular and Paracrine Signaling. *Circ. Res.* **2021**, *128*, e1–e23. [CrossRef]
70. Wu, T.; Chen, Y.; Du, Y.; Tao, J.; Zhou, Z.; Yang, Z. Serum Exosomal MiR-92b-5p as a Potential Biomarker for Acute Heart Failure Caused by Dilated Cardiomyopathy. *Cell. Physiol. Biochem.* **2018**, *46*, 1939–1950. [CrossRef]

71. Huang, Z.P.; Ding, Y.; Chen, J.; Wu, G.; Kataoka, M.; Hu, Y.; Yang, J.H.; Liu, J.; Drakos, S.G.; Selzman, C.H.; et al. Long non-coding RNAs link extracellular matrix gene expression to ischemic cardiomyopathy. *Cardiovasc. Res.* **2016**, *112*, 543–554. [CrossRef] [PubMed]
72. Ounzain, S.; Micheletti, R.; Beckmann, T.; Schroen, B.; Alexanian, M.; Pezzuto, I.; Crippa, S.; Nemir, M.; Sarre, A.; Johnson, R.; et al. Genome-wide profiling of the cardiac transcriptome after myocardial infarction identifies novel heart-specific long non-coding RNAs. *Eur. Heart J.* **2015**, *36*, 353–368. [CrossRef] [PubMed]
73. Kumarswamy, R.; Bauters, C.; Volkmann, I.; Maury, F.; Fetisch, J.; Holzmann, A.; Lemesle, G.; de Groote, P.; Pinet, F.; Thum, T. Circulating long noncoding RNA, LIPCAR, predicts survival in patients with heart failure. *Circ. Res.* **2014**, *114*, 1569–1575. [CrossRef]
74. Han, P.; Li, W.; Lin, C.H.; Yang, J.; Shang, C.; Nuernberg, S.T.; Jin, K.K.; Xu, W.; Lin, C.Y.; Lin, C.J.; et al. A long noncoding RNA protects the heart from pathological hypertrophy. *Nature* **2014**, *514*, 102–106. [CrossRef]
75. Piersma, B.; Bank, R.A.; Boersema, M. Signaling in Fibrosis: TGF-β, WNT, and YAP/TAZ Converge. *Front. Med.* **2015**, *2*, 59. [CrossRef]
76. Winkle, M.; El-Daly, S.M.; Fabbri, M.; Calin, G.A. Noncoding RNA therapeutics-challenges and potential solutions. *Nat. Rev. Drug Discov.* **2021**, *20*, 629–651. [CrossRef]
77. Rohner, E.; Yang, R.; Foo, K.S.; Goedel, A.; Chien, K.R. Unlocking the promise of mRNA therapeutics. *Nat. Biotechnol.* **2022**, *40*, 1586–1600. [CrossRef]
78. He, A.T.; Liu, J.; Li, F.; Yang, B.B. Targeting circular RNAs as a therapeutic approach: Current strategies and challenges. *Signal Transduct. Target. Ther.* **2021**, *6*, 185. [CrossRef]
79. Das, S.; Shah, R.; Dimmeler, S.; Freedman, J.E.; Holley, C.; Lee, J.M.; Moore, K.; Musunuru, K.; Wang, D.Z.; Xiao, J.; et al. Noncoding RNAs in Cardiovascular Disease: Current Knowledge, Tools and Technologies for Investigation, and Future Directions: A Scientific Statement from the American Heart Association. *Circ. Genom. Precis. Med.* **2020**, *13*, e000062. [CrossRef]
80. Burger, F.; Baptista, D.; Roth, A.; da Silva, R.F.; Montecucco, F.; Mach, F.; Brandt, K.J.; Miteva, K. NLRP3 Inflammasome Activation Controls Vascular Smooth Muscle Cells Phenotypic Switch in Atherosclerosis. *Int. J. Mol. Sci.* **2021**, *23*, 340. [CrossRef]
81. Cao, R.Y.; Zhang, Y.; Feng, Z.; Liu, S.; Liu, Y.; Zheng, H.; Yang, J. The Effective Role of Natural Product Berberine in Modulating Oxidative Stress and Inflammation Related Atherosclerosis: Novel Insights Into the Gut-Heart Axis Evidenced by Genetic Sequencing Analysis. *Front. Pharmacol.* **2021**, *12*, 764994. [CrossRef]
82. Shimada, B.K.; Yang, Y.; Zhu, J.; Wang, S.; Suen, A.; Kronstadt, S.M.; Jeyaram, A.; Jay, S.M.; Zou, L.; Chao, W. Extracellular miR-146a-5p Induces Cardiac Innate Immune Response and Cardiomyocyte Dysfunction. *Immunohorizons* **2020**, *4*, 561–572. [CrossRef]
83. Preissner, K.T.; Fischer, S.; Deindl, E. Extracellular RNA as a Versatile DAMP and Alarm Signal That Influences Leukocyte Recruitment in Inflammation and Infection. *Front. Cell. Dev. Biol.* **2020**, *8*, 619221. [CrossRef]
84. Shan, K.; Jiang, Q.; Wang, X.Q.; Wang, Y.N.; Yang, H.; Yao, M.D.; Liu, C.; Li, X.M.; Yao, J.; Liu, B.; et al. Role of long non-coding RNA-RNCR3 in atherosclerosis-related vascular dysfunction. *Cell Death Dis.* **2016**, *7*, e2248. [CrossRef]
85. Yang, Z.; Liang, X.; Yang, L. Circular RNA circ_0001445 alleviates the ox-LDL-induced endothelial injury in human primary aortic endothelial cells through regulating ABCG1 via acting as a sponge of miR-208b-5p. *Gen. Thorac. Cardiovasc. Surg.* **2022**, *70*, 779–792. [CrossRef]
86. Gao, X.F.; Wang, Z.M.; Chen, A.Q.; Wang, F.; Luo, S.; Gu, Y.; Kong, X.Q.; Zuo, G.F.; Jiang, X.M.; Ding, G.W.; et al. Plasma Small Extracellular Vesicle-Carried miRNA-501-5p Promotes Vascular Smooth Muscle Cell Phenotypic Modulation-Mediated In-Stent Restenosis. *Oxidative Med. Cell. Longev.* **2021**, *2021*, 6644970. [CrossRef]
87. Simsekyilmaz, S.; Cabrera-Fuentes, H.A.; Meiler, S.; Kostin, S.; Baumer, Y.; Liehn, E.A.; Weber, C.; Boisvert, W.A.; Preissner, K.T.; Zernecke, A. Role of extracellular RNA in atherosclerotic plaque formation in mice. *Circulation* **2014**, *129*, 598–606. [CrossRef]
88. Chiou, N.T.; Kageyama, R.; Ansel, K.M. Selective Export into Extracellular Vesicles and Function of tRNA Fragments during T Cell Activation. *Cell Rep.* **2018**, *25*, 3356–3370.e4. [CrossRef]
89. Liu, S.; Chen, J.; Shi, J.; Zhou, W.; Wang, L.; Fang, W.; Zhong, Y.; Chen, X.; Chen, Y.; Sabri, A.; et al. M1-like macrophage-derived exosomes suppress angiogenesis and exacerbate cardiac dysfunction in a myocardial infarction microenvironment. *Basic Res. Cardiol.* **2020**, *115*, 22. [CrossRef]
90. Long, R.; Gao, L.; Li, Y.; Li, G.; Qin, P.; Wei, Z.; Li, D.; Qian, C.; Li, J.; Yang, G. M2 macrophage-derived exosomes carry miR-1271-5p to alleviate cardiac injury in acute myocardial infarction through down-regulating SOX6. *Mol. Immunol.* **2021**, *136*, 26–35. [CrossRef]
91. Liu, H.; Zhang, Y.; Yuan, J.; Gao, W.; Zhong, X.; Yao, K.; Lin, L.; Ge, J. Dendritic cell-derived exosomal miR-494-3p promotes angiogenesis following myocardial infarction. *Int. J. Mol. Med.* **2021**, *47*, 315–325, Corrigendum in *Int. J. Mol. Med.* **2022**, *49*, 5096. [CrossRef]
92. Li, Q.; Xu, Y.; Lv, K.; Wang, Y.; Zhong, Z.; Xiao, C.; Zhu, K.; Ni, C.; Wang, K.; Kong, M.; et al. Small extracellular vesicles containing miR-486-5p promote angiogenesis after myocardial infarction in mice and nonhuman primates. *Sci. Transl. Med.* **2021**, *13*, eabb0202. [CrossRef]
93. Cheng, H.; Chang, S.; Xu, R.; Chen, L.; Song, X.; Wu, J.; Qian, J.; Zou, Y.; Ma, J. Hypoxia-challenged MSC-derived exosomes deliver miR-210 to attenuate post-infarction cardiac apoptosis. *Stem Cell Res. Ther.* **2020**, *11*, 224. [CrossRef]

94. Mao, C.; Li, D.; Zhou, E.; Gao, E.; Zhang, T.; Sun, S.; Gao, L.; Fan, Y.; Wang, C. Extracellular vesicles from anoxia preconditioned mesenchymal stem cells alleviate myocardial ischemia/reperfusion injury. *Aging* **2021**, *13*, 6156–6170. [CrossRef]
95. Ou, H.; Teng, H.; Qin, Y.; Luo, X.; Yang, P.; Zhang, W.; Chen, W.; Lv, D.; Tang, H. Extracellular vesicles derived from microRNA-150-5p-overexpressing mesenchymal stem cells protect rat hearts against ischemia/reperfusion. *Aging* **2020**, *12*, 12669–12683. [CrossRef]
96. Li, T.; Gu, J.; Yang, O.; Wang, J.; Wang, Y.; Kong, J. Bone Marrow Mesenchymal Stem Cell-Derived Exosomal miRNA-29c Decreases Cardiac Ischemia/Reperfusion Injury Through Inhibition of Excessive Autophagy via the PTEN/Akt/mTOR Signaling Pathway. *Circ. J.* **2020**, *84*, 1304–1311. [CrossRef]
97. Zou, L.; Ma, X.; Wu, B.; Chen, Y.; Xie, D.; Peng, C. Protective effect of bone marrow mesenchymal stem cell-derived exosomes on cardiomyoblast hypoxia-reperfusion injury through the miR-149/let-7c/Faslg axis. *Free Radic. Res.* **2020**, *54*, 722–731. [CrossRef]
98. Fu, D.L.; Jiang, H.; Li, C.Y.; Gao, T.; Liu, M.R.; Li, H.W. MicroRNA-338 in MSCs-derived exosomes inhibits cardiomyocyte apoptosis in myocardial infarction. *Eur. Rev. Med. Pharmacol. Sci.* **2020**, *24*, 10107–10117. [CrossRef]
99. Walravens, A.S.; Smolgovsky, S.; Li, L.; Kelly, L.; Antes, T.; Peck, K.; Quon, T.; Ibrahim, A.; Marbán, E.; Berman, B.; et al. Mechanistic and therapeutic distinctions between cardiosphere-derived cell and mesenchymal stem cell extracellular vesicle non-coding RNA. *Sci. Rep.* **2021**, *11*, 8666. [CrossRef]
100. de Couto, G.; Gallet, R.; Cambier, L.; Jaghatspanyan, E.; Makkar, N.; Dawkins, J.F.; Berman, B.P.; Marbán, E. Exosomal MicroRNA Transfer Into Macrophages Mediates Cellular Postconditioning. *Circulation* **2017**, *136*, 200–214. [CrossRef]
101. de Couto, G.; Jaghatspanyan, E.; DeBerge, M.; Liu, W.; Luther, K.; Wang, Y.; Tang, J.; Thorp, E.B.; Marbán, E. Mechanism of Enhanced MerTK-Dependent Macrophage Efferocytosis by Extracellular Vesicles. *Arterioscler. Thromb. Vasc. Biol.* **2019**, *39*, 2082–2096. [CrossRef]
102. Ibrahim, A.G.; Cheng, K.; Marbán, E. Exosomes as critical agents of cardiac regeneration triggered by cell therapy. *Stem Cell Rep.* **2014**, *2*, 606–619. [CrossRef]
103. Ciullo, A.; Li, C.; Li, L.; Ungerleider, K.C.; Peck, K.; Marbán, E.; Ibrahim, A.G.E. Biodistribution of unmodified cardiosphere-derived cell extracellular vesicles using single RNA tracing. *J. Extracell. Vesicles* **2022**, *11*, e12178. [CrossRef]
104. Moghiman, T.; Barghchi, B.; Esmaeili, S.A.; Shabestari, M.M.; Tabaee, S.S.; Momtazi-Borojeni, A.A. Therapeutic angiogenesis with exosomal microRNAs: An effectual approach for the treatment of myocardial ischemia. *Heart Fail. Rev.* **2021**, *26*, 205–213. [CrossRef]
105. Gou, L.; Xue, C.; Tang, X.; Fang, Z. Inhibition of Exo-miR-19a-3p derived from cardiomyocytes promotes angiogenesis and improves heart function in mice with myocardial infarction via targeting HIF-1α. *Aging* **2020**, *12*, 23609–23618. [CrossRef]
106. Geng, T.; Song, Z.Y.; Xing, J.X.; Wang, B.X.; Dai, S.P.; Xu, Z.S. Exosome Derived from Coronary Serum of Patients with Myocardial Infarction Promotes Angiogenesis through the miRNA-143/IGF-IR Pathway. *Int. J. Nanomed.* **2020**, *15*, 2647–2658. [CrossRef]
107. Liao, Z.; Chen, Y.; Duan, C.; Zhu, K.; Huang, R.; Zhao, H.; Hintze, M.; Pu, Q.; Yuan, Z.; Lv, L.; et al. Cardiac telocytes inhibit cardiac microvascular endothelial cell apoptosis through exosomal miRNA-21-5p-targeted cdip1 silencing to improve angiogenesis following myocardial infarction. *Theranostics* **2021**, *11*, 268–291. [CrossRef]
108. Li, K.S.; Bai, Y.; Li, J.; Li, S.L.; Pan, J.; Cheng, Y.Q.; Li, K.; Wang, Z.G.; Ji, W.J.; Zhou, Q.; et al. LncRNA HCP5 in hBMSC-derived exosomes alleviates myocardial ischemia reperfusion injury by sponging miR-497 to activate IGF1/PI3K/AKT pathway. *Int. J. Cardiol.* **2021**, *342*, 72–81. [CrossRef]
109. Diao, L.; Zhang, Q. Transfer of lncRNA UCA1 by hUCMSCs-derived exosomes protects against hypoxia/reoxygenation injury through impairing miR-143-targeted degradation of Bcl-2. *Aging* **2021**, *13*, 5967–5985. [CrossRef]
110. Wang, Y.; Zhao, R.; Shen, C.; Liu, W.; Yuan, J.; Li, C.; Deng, W.; Wang, Z.; Zhang, W.; Ge, J.; et al. Exosomal CircHIPK3 Released from Hypoxia-Induced Cardiomyocytes Regulates Cardiac Angiogenesis after Myocardial Infarction. *Oxidative Med. Cell. Longev.* **2020**, *2020*, 8418407. [CrossRef]
111. Wang, Y.; Li, C.; Zhao, R.; Qiu, Z.; Shen, C.; Wang, Z.; Liu, W.; Zhang, W.; Ge, J.; Shi, B. CircUbe3a from M2 macrophage-derived small extracellular vesicles mediates myocardial fibrosis after acute myocardial infarction. *Theranostics* **2021**, *11*, 6315–6333. [CrossRef] [PubMed]
112. Zhang, J.; He, Y.; Yan, X.; Chen, S.; He, M.; Lei, Y.; Zhang, J.; Gongol, B.; Gu, M.; Miao, Y.; et al. MicroRNA-483 amelioration of experimental pulmonary hypertension. *EMBO Mol. Med.* **2020**, *12*, e11303. [CrossRef] [PubMed]
113. Shang, F.; Guo, X.; Chen, Y.; Wang, C.; Gao, J.; Wen, E.; Lai, B.; Bai, L. Endothelial MicroRNA-483-3p Is Hypertension-Protective. *Oxidative Med. Cell. Longev.* **2022**, *2022*, 3698219. [CrossRef] [PubMed]
114. Li, S.; Zhu, J.; Zhang, W.; Chen, Y.; Zhang, K.; Popescu, L.M.; Ma, X.; Lau, W.B.; Rong, R.; Yu, X.; et al. Signature microRNA expression profile of essential hypertension and its novel link to human cytomegalovirus infection. *Circulation* **2011**, *124*, 175–184. [CrossRef] [PubMed]
115. Sarrion, I.; Milian, L.; Juan, G.; Ramon, M.; Furest, I.; Carda, C.; Cortijo Gimeno, J.; Mata Roig, M. Role of circulating miRNAs as biomarkers in idiopathic pulmonary arterial hypertension: Possible relevance of miR-23a. *Oxidative Med. Cell. Longev.* **2015**, *2015*, 792846. [CrossRef] [PubMed]
116. Niu, L.; Sun, N.; Kong, L.; Xu, Y.; Kang, Y. miR-634 inhibits human vascular smooth muscle cell proliferation and migration in hypertension through Wnt4/β-catenin pathway. *Front. Biosci. (Landmark. Ed.)* **2021**, *26*, 395–404. [CrossRef] [PubMed]
117. Shah, A.K.; Bhullar, S.K.; Elimban, V.; Dhalla, N.S. Oxidative Stress as A Mechanism for Functional Alterations in Cardiac Hypertrophy and Heart Failure. *Antioxidants* **2021**, *10*, 931. [CrossRef] [PubMed]

118. Yang, F.; Dong, A.; Mueller, P.; Caicedo, J.; Sutton, A.M.; Odetunde, J.; Barrick, C.J.; Klyachkin, Y.M.; Abdel-Latif, A.; Smyth, S.S. Coronary artery remodeling in a model of left ventricular pressure overload is influenced by platelets and inflammatory cells. *PLoS ONE* **2012**, *7*, e40196. [CrossRef]
119. Nie, X.; Fan, J.; Li, H.; Yin, Z.; Zhao, Y.; Dai, B.; Dong, N.; Chen, C.; Wang, D.W. miR-217 Promotes Cardiac Hypertrophy and Dysfunction by Targeting PTEN. *Mol. Ther. Nucleic Acids* **2018**, *12*, 254–266. [CrossRef]
120. Bang, C.; Batkai, S.; Dangwal, S.; Gupta, S.K.; Foinquinos, A.; Holzmann, A.; Just, A.; Remke, J.; Zimmer, K.; Zeug, A.; et al. Cardiac fibroblast-derived microRNA passenger strand-enriched exosomes mediate cardiomyocyte hypertrophy. *J. Clin. Investig.* **2014**, *124*, 2136–2146. [CrossRef]
121. Thum, T.; Gross, C.; Fiedler, J.; Fischer, T.; Kissler, S.; Bussen, M.; Galuppo, P.; Just, S.; Rottbauer, W.; Frantz, S.; et al. MicroRNA-21 contributes to myocardial disease by stimulating MAP kinase signalling in fibroblasts. *Nature* **2008**, *456*, 980–984. [CrossRef] [PubMed]
122. Sayed, D.; Rane, S.; Lypowy, J.; He, M.; Chen, I.Y.; Vashistha, H.; Yan, L.; Malhotra, A.; Vatner, D.; Abdellatif, M. MicroRNA-21 targets Sprouty2 and promotes cellular outgrowths. *Mol. Biol. Cell.* **2008**, *19*, 3272–3282. [CrossRef] [PubMed]
123. Tatsuguchi, M.; Seok, H.Y.; Callis, T.E.; Thomson, J.M.; Chen, J.F.; Newman, M.; Rojas, M.; Hammond, S.M.; Wang, D.Z. Expression of microRNAs is dynamically regulated during cardiomyocyte hypertrophy. *J. Mol. Cell. Cardiol.* **2007**, *42*, 1137–1141. [CrossRef] [PubMed]
124. Wu, R.; Gao, W.; Yao, K.; Ge, J. Roles of Exosomes Derived from Immune Cells in Cardiovascular Diseases. *Front. Immunol.* **2019**, *10*, 648. [CrossRef]
125. Yu, H.; Qin, L.; Peng, Y.; Bai, W.; Wang, Z. Exosomes Derived from Hypertrophic Cardiomyocytes Induce Inflammation in Macrophages via miR-155 Mediated MAPK Pathway. *Front. Immunol.* **2020**, *11*, 606045. [CrossRef]
126. Wang, C.; Zhang, C.; Liu, L.; A, X.; Chen, B.; Li, Y.; Du, J. Macrophage-Derived mir-155-Containing Exosomes Suppress Fibroblast Proliferation and Promote Fibroblast Inflammation during Cardiac Injury. *Mol. Ther. J. Am. Soc. Gene Ther.* **2017**, *25*, 192–204. [CrossRef]
127. Summerhill, V.I.; Moschetta, D.; Orekhov, A.N.; Poggio, P.; Myasoedova, V.A. Sex-Specific Features of Calcific Aortic Valve Disease. *Int. J. Mol. Sci.* **2020**, *21*, 5620. [CrossRef]
128. Duan, C.; Cao, Z.; Tang, F.; Jian, Z.; Liang, C.; Liu, H.; Xiao, Y.; Liu, L.; Ma, R. miRNA-mRNA crosstalk in myocardial ischemia induced by calcified aortic valve stenosis. *Aging* **2019**, *11*, 448–466. [CrossRef]
129. Yang, R.; Tang, Y.; Chen, X.; Yang, Y. Telocytes-derived extracellular vesicles alleviate aortic valve calcification by carrying miR-30b. *ESC Heart Fail.* **2021**, *8*, 3935–3946. [CrossRef]
130. Qiao, L.; Hu, S.; Liu, S.; Zhang, H.; Ma, H.; Huang, K.; Li, Z.; Su, T.; Vandergriff, A.; Tang, J.; et al. microRNA-21-5p dysregulation in exosomes derived from heart failure patients impairs regenerative potential. *J. Clin. Investig.* **2019**, *129*, 2237–2250. [CrossRef]
131. Li, H.; Trager, L.E.; Liu, X.; Hastings, M.H.; Xiao, C.; Guerra, J.; To, S.; Li, G.; Yeri, A.; Rodosthenous, R.; et al. lncExACT1 and DCHS2 Regulate Physiological and Pathological Cardiac Growth. *Circulation* **2022**, *145*, 1218–1233. [CrossRef] [PubMed]
132. Guo, H.; Lu, Y.W.; Lin, Z.; Huang, Z.P.; Liu, J.; Wang, Y.; Seok, H.Y.; Hu, X.; Ma, Q.; Li, K.; et al. Intercalated disc protein Xinβ is required for Hippo-YAP signaling in the heart. *Nat. Commun.* **2020**, *11*, 4666. [CrossRef] [PubMed]
133. Moya, I.M.; Halder, G. Hippo-YAP/TAZ signalling in organ regeneration and regenerative medicine. *Nat. Rev. Mol. Cell. Biol.* **2019**, *20*, 211–226. [CrossRef] [PubMed]
134. Bezzerides, V.J.; Platt, C.; Lerchenmüller, C.; Paruchuri, K.; Oh, N.L.; Xiao, C.; Cao, Y.; Mann, N.; Spiegelman, B.M.; Rosenzweig, A. CITED4 induces physiologic hypertrophy and promotes functional recovery after ischemic injury. *JCI Insight* **2016**, *1*, 5620. [CrossRef]
135. Li, K.; Rodosthenous, R.S.; Kashanchi, F.; Gingeras, T.; Gould, S.J.; Kuo, L.S.; Kurre, P.; Lee, H.; Leonard, J.N.; Liu, H.; et al. Advances, challenges, and opportunities in extracellular RNA biology: Insights from the NIH exRNA Strategic Workshop. *JCI Insight* **2018**, *3*, e98942. [CrossRef]
136. Blanco-Dominguez, R.; Sanchez-Diaz, R.; de la Fuente, H.; Jimenez-Borreguero, L.J.; Matesanz-Marin, A.; Relano, M.; Jimenez-Alejandre, R.; Linillos-Pradillo, B.; Tsilingiri, K.; Martin-Mariscal, M.L.; et al. A Novel Circulating MicroRNA for the Detection of Acute Myocarditis. *N. Engl. J. Med.* **2021**, *384*, 2014–2027. [CrossRef]
137. Elbashir, S.M.; Harborth, J.; Lendeckel, W.; Yalcin, A.; Weber, K.; Tuschl, T. Duplexes of 21-nucleotide RNAs mediate RNA interference in cultured mammalian cells. *Nature* **2001**, *411*, 494–498. [CrossRef]
138. Crooke, S.T. Molecular Mechanisms of Antisense Oligonucleotides. *Nucleic Acid Ther.* **2017**, *27*, 70–77. [CrossRef]
139. Shah, A.M.; Giacca, M. Small non-coding RNA therapeutics for cardiovascular disease. *Eur. Heart J.* **2022**, *43*, 4548–4561. [CrossRef]
140. Haemmig, S.; Feinberg, M.W. Targeting LncRNAs in Cardiovascular Disease: Options and Expeditions. *Circ. Res.* **2017**, *120*, 620–623. [CrossRef]
141. Robinson, E.L.; Port, J.D. Utilization and Potential of RNA-Based Therapies in Cardiovascular Disease. *JACC Basic Transl. Sci.* **2022**, *7*, 956–969. [CrossRef]
142. Lieberman, J. Tapping the RNA world for therapeutics. *Nat. Struct. Mol. Biol.* **2018**, *25*, 357–364. [CrossRef]
143. Egli, M.; Manoharan, M. Re-Engineering RNA Molecules into Therapeutic Agents. *Acc. Chem. Res.* **2019**, *52*, 1036–1047. [CrossRef]
144. Baumann, V.; Winkler, J. miRNA-based therapies: Strategies and delivery platforms for oligonucleotide and non-oligonucleotide agents. *Future Med. Chem.* **2014**, *6*, 1967–1984. [CrossRef]

145. Johannes, L.; Lucchino, M. Current Challenges in Delivery and Cytosolic Translocation of Therapeutic RNAs. *Nucleic Acid Ther.* **2018**, *28*, 178–193. [CrossRef]
146. Borden, A.; Kurian, J.; Nickoloff, E.; Yang, Y.; Troupes, C.D.; Ibetti, J.; Lucchese, A.M.; Gao, E.; Mohsin, S.; Koch, W.J.; et al. Transient Introduction of miR-294 in the Heart Promotes Cardiomyocyte Cell Cycle Reentry After Injury. *Circ. Res.* **2019**, *125*, 14–25. [CrossRef]
147. Žarković, M.; Hufsky, F.; Markert, U.R.; Marz, M. The Role of Non-Coding RNAs in the Human Placenta. *Cells* **2022**, *11*, 1588. [CrossRef]
148. Palazzo, C.; D'Alessio, A.; Tamagnone, L. Message in a Bottle: Endothelial Cell Regulation by Extracellular Vesicles. *Cancers* **2022**, *14*, 1969. [CrossRef]
149. Sykaras, A.G.; Christofidis, K.; Politi, E.; Theocharis, S. Exosomes on Endometrial Cancer: A Biomarkers Treasure Trove? *Cancers* **2022**, *14*, 1733. [CrossRef]
150. Samra, M.; Srivastava, K. Non-coding RNA and their potential role in cardiovascular diseases. *Gene* **2023**, *851*, 147011. [CrossRef]
151. Davidson, S.M.; Padró, T.; Bollini, S.; Vilahur, G.; Duncker, D.J.; Evans, P.C.; Guzik, T.; Hoefer, I.E.; Waltenberger, J.; Wojta, J.; et al. Progress in cardiac research: From rebooting cardiac regeneration to a complete cell atlas of the heart. *Cardiovasc. Res.* **2021**, *117*, 2161–2174. [CrossRef] [PubMed]
152. Bansal, P.; Arora, M. RNA Binding Proteins and Non-coding RNA's in Cardiovascular Diseases. *Adv. Exp. Med. Biol.* **2020**, *1229*, 105–118. [CrossRef]

pharmaceutics

MDPI

Review

Extracellular Vesicles: A New Frontier for Cardiac Repair

Benshuai You [1,2], Yang Yang [3], Zixuan Zhou [2], Yongmin Yan [1], Leilei Zhang [2], Jianhua Jin [1,*] and Hui Qian [2,*]

1 Wujin Institute of Molecular Diagnostics and Precision Cancer Medicine of Jiangsu University, Wujin Hospital Affiliated with Jiangsu University, Changzhou 213017, China
2 Jiangsu Key Laboratory of Medical Science and Laboratory Medicine, School of Medicine, Jiangsu University, Zhenjiang 212013, China
3 Clinical Laboratory Center, The Affiliated Taizhou People's Hospital of Nanjing Medical University, Taizhou 225317, China
* Correspondence: jianhuajin88@sina.com (J.J.); lstmmmlst@163.com (H.Q.)

Abstract: The ability of extracellular vesicles (EVs) to regulate a broad range of cellular processes has recently been used to treat diseases. Growing evidence indicates that EVs play a cardioprotective role in heart disease by activating beneficial signaling pathways. Multiple functional components of EVs and intracellular molecular mechanisms are involved in the process. To overcome the shortcomings of native EVs such as their heterogeneity and limited tropism, a series of engineering approaches has been developed to improve the therapeutic efficiency of EVs. In this review, we present an overview of the research and future directions for EVs-based cardiac therapies with an emphasis on EVs-mediated delivery of therapeutic agents. The advantages and limitations of various modification strategies are discussed, and possible opportunities for improvement are proposed. An in-depth understanding of the endogenous properties of EVs and EVs engineering strategies could lead to a promising cell-free therapy for cardiac repair.

Keywords: extracellular vesicles; heart disease; mesenchymal stem cells; targeted delivery

Citation: You, B.; Yang, Y.; Zhou, Z.; Yan, Y.; Zhang, L.; Jin, J.; Qian, H. Extracellular Vesicles: A New Frontier for Cardiac Repair. *Pharmaceutics* **2022**, *14*, 1848. https://doi.org/10.3390/pharmaceutics14091848

Academic Editor: Lucio Barile

Received: 9 August 2022
Accepted: 30 August 2022
Published: 1 September 2022

1. Introduction

Heart disease is a major cause of death worldwide, especially among aging populations. Approximately 17.8 million deaths globally in 2017 were caused by heart disease [1]. Thus, effective therapy for cardiac repair is required. Extracellular vesicles (EVs), nanoscale small vesicles, are secreted by many types of cells and play a key role in intercellular communication [2,3]. "EVs" is a collective term for various subtypes of membrane components released by cells, including exosomes (30–150 nm), microvesicles (200–2000 nm), and apoptotic bodies (1–10 μm) [4]. EVs contain abundant cargo such as proteins, nucleic acids, and lipids [5–7]. Compared with parental cells, EVs retain the function of the host and also have the advantages of low immunogenicity, long-term stability, easy storage, and biocompatibility [8,9]. EVs can easily diffuse to the blood, penetrate tissues through the circulatory system, and even cross the blood–brain barrier [10]. Therefore, developing novel strategies to optimize such cell-free nanoparticles could profoundly affect clinical practice.

Studies have revealed the benefits of mesenchymal stem cells (MSCs) and other cells in the treatment of cardiac disease, with the effects of paracrine playing an essential role in these benefits [11,12]. For example, conditioned medium from adipose-derived stem cells was able to attenuate ischemia-reperfusion-induced apoptosis and fibrosis through the miR-221/222/PUMA/ETS-1 pathway in a mouse model [13]. As the main paracrine component of cells, EVs exhibit regenerative properties in myocardial infarction, ischemia-reperfusion injury, and viral myocarditis [14]. Because of their acellular nature, EVs even demonstrate greater myocardial reparative capabilities than parent cells and are also safer [15]. A large body of evidence suggests that many bioactive molecules in EVs play a part in the repair processes by promoting angiogenesis, modulating immune responses and inhibiting apoptosis. The use of engineering methods can further amplify the therapeutic effects of EVs by increasing their targeting, bioactivity, retention, and yield.

In this review, we evaluate the feasibility of using natural or engineered EVs for treating myocardial injury. We present the therapeutic effects of EVs from different sources when applied to various myocardial injury models and focus on the role of multiple bioactive molecules within EVs in mediating cardioprotection. We discuss different engineering strategies and highlight the crucial challenges and opportunities in clinical translation.

2. Biosynthesis and Characteristic of EVs

Because the specific indicators of EV subtypes are still being debated, it is recommended to define EVs using operational terms on the basis of physical characteristics (e.g., size and density) or the biochemical composition or descriptions of conditions or cell of origin. For example, EVs can be divided into small EVs (sEVs, <100 nm or <200 nm) and medium/large EVs (m/lEVs, >200 nm). In previous studies, EVs have often been classified into three types: exosomes, microvesicles, and apoptotic bodies [16]. The term "exosomes" has been used frequently in previous studies, but strictly speaking, it should only be used when data demonstrating endosomal origin of an EV is provided. In this review, in order to be consistent with the original article, the names of EVs that appeared in the original article were used. Exosomes are primarily released by the fusion of multivesicular bodies (MVBs) and plasma membrane, and microvesicles and apoptotic bodies are generated through the direct budding of cell membrane [17]. The specific formation process of exosomes and microvesicles will be described below. The host cell-derived cargo carried by EVs is responsible for their diverse biological functions. Currently, research on the regeneration function of EVs mainly focuses on exosomes and microvesicles, with little attention given to apoptotic bodies. EVs deliver their contents to recipient cells through endocytosis, ligand–receptor interaction, and direct fusion with the plasma membrane (Figure 1). In recent years, some new types of EVs have been discovered, such as retractosomes [18]. However, little is known about their biogenesis and physiological function.

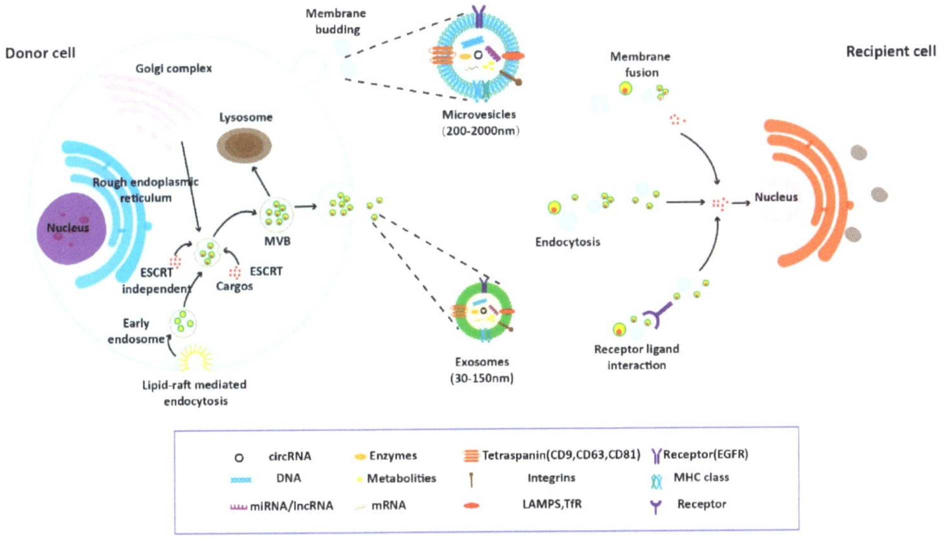

Figure 1. Classification, biogenesis, release, and uptake of EVs. Several stages–including endocytosis, endosome and MVBs formation, and exosomes release–are involved in the formation of exosomes. Microvesicles are released into the extracellular space through outward sprouting of the plasma membrane. EVs deliver their contents to recipient cells through endocytosis, ligand–receptor interaction, and direct fusion with the plasma membrane.

Several stages—including endocytosis, endosome and MVBs formation, and exosomes release—are involved in the formation of exosomes [19]. Although the exact process remains unclear, the biogenesis of exosomes has been investigated. First, the lipid raft domain of the plasma membrane forms early endosomes through the endocytosis pathway. With the assistance of the Golgi complex, these early endosomes mature into late endosomes, the bilayer membrane of which produces vesicles that accumulate in the lumen [20]. Both endosomal sorting complex required for transport (ESCRT)-dependent and ESCRT-independent pathways are involved in the process of MVBs formation [21,22]. MVBs then fuse with the plasma membrane to release exosomes or fuse with lysosomes and then degrade [23]. Once MVBs have fused with the plasma membrane, intraluminal vesicles are released into the extracellular environment.

Microvesicles are released into the extracellular space through outward sprouting of the plasma membrane [24]. The asymmetric distribution of phospholipids in the plasma membrane bilayer is involved in the formation of microvesicles. The outer membrane is dominated by phosphatidylcholine and sphingomyelin, whereas the intima is dominated by phosphatidylserine and phosphatidylethanolamine. Increased cytosolic calcium disrupts the phospholipid asymmetry by activating the phospholipid crawling enzyme and thus initiating cell budding. Ca2+-dependent proteolysis participates in the release of microvesicles through cytoskeleton degradation [25].

Given the small size of EVs and the complexity of their content, characterizing EVs accurately can be difficult and require multiple measurements. Currently, EVs are identified on the basis of their morphology, particle size, content, and surface markers [26]. EVs may collapse during fixation and dehydration, and this collapse gives them an artificial cup-shaped appearance, which can be observed using a transmission electron microscope [27]. Atomic force microscopy and cryoelectron microscopy are used to evaluate the substructural organization of EVs with high resolution [28,29]. Nanoparticle tracking analysis (NTA) is widely used to measure EVs and can provide information on their size distribution and particle concentration [30]. New detection technologies such as nanoflow cytometry are often applied in comprehensive analyses [31–33]. The development and application of specific biosensors provide a new approach for the bioanalysis of EVs [34,35]. Western blotting, mass spectrometry, and liquid chromatography are commonly adopted for protein assays [36–38]. New platform based on phage display are developed for characterization of EVs based on their different antigenic reactivities [39]. Polymerase chain reaction (PCR), high-throughput sequencing, and the newly developed droplet digital PCR are often employed for nucleic acid detection [40,41]. Moreover, chromatographic-mass spectrometry is the main method used for the lipidomic analysis of EVs [42]. A series of EVs surface proteins has been recognized as specific surface markers that can be used for EVs identification and are divided into transmembrane proteins (CD9, CD63, and CD81), heat shock proteins (Hsp70 and Hsp90), membrane fusion proteins (Alix, Annexin, and TSG101), membrane transporters (GTPases), and lipid-bound proteins [43,44]. It is also recommended to detect at least one negative protein marker such as calnexin, albumin in EVs according to the International Society for Extracellular Vesicles (ISEV) guidelines [45].

3. Natural EVs for Myocardial Injury Therapy

In the treatment of myocardial injury, stem cells are the most common donor cells selected as the source of EVs and include MSCs, embryonic stem cells (ESCs), induced pluripotent stem cells (iPSCs) and trophoblast stem cells (TSCs). Several studies have indicated that the repair that MSCs perform in myocardial injury is mainly mediated by the release of EVs [12]. MSCs-EVs were demonstrated to have a similar mechanism to MSCs in the repair of myocardial infarction. Shao et al. found that MSCs-derived exosomes had a stronger therapeutic effect than MSCs in a myocardial infarction model because of the significantly different expression of miRNAs from exosomes versus MSCs [46]. Current studies have shown that MSC-EVs aid the recovery of cardiac function mainly by inhibiting the death of cardiomyocytes, including apoptosis and ferroptosis. The EVs-mediated delivery of miRNAs (e.g., miR-23a-3p) and proteins (e.g., BMP2 and PINK1) plays a crucial role in the process [47–49]. In addition to directly inhibiting cardiomyocyte apoptosis, MSCs-EVs exert cardioprotective effects through the immunomodulation of macrophages. Zhao et al. demonstrated that MSCs-derived exosomes effectively reduced infarct size and alleviated inflammation in the heart after myocardial ischemia–reperfusion [50]. Further studies showed that exosomes-mediated miR-182 delivery to target TLR4 is essential in modifying the polarization of macrophages M1 to M2. Moreover, the miRNAs in MSCs-EVs such as miR-100-5p, miR-143-3p, miR-199a-3p, and miR-29a-3p also play functional roles in promoting the recovery of damaged myocardial tissue [51–54]. Other non-coding RNAs-such as long noncoding RNAs (lncRNA UCA1, lncRNA HCP5) and circular RNAs (circRNAs)-are involved in cardioprotective effects through the delivery of EVs [55–57].

Other stem-cell-derived EVs have also been utilized to treat heart disease. EVs derived from human-induced pluripotent stem-cell-derived cardiovascular progenitors were discovered to outperform cell injections and improve cardiac function in a myocardial infarction mouse model; this effect may have been associated with the abundant miRNAs in the tissue-repair pathways of EVs [58]. Ni et al. demonstrated that TSCs derived- exosomes were able to attenuate doxorubicin (Dox)-induced cardiac injury through anti-apoptotic and anti-inflammatory effects [59]. Further studies showed that this effect may be associated with an increase in ZEB1 expression and the inhibition of miR-200b expression in cardiomyocytes. Moreover, the research team found TSCs-derived exosomes mediated the delivery of let-7i to cardiac tissue, which inhibited myocardial apoptosis and mitigated cardiac fibrosis by downregulating YAP signaling [60]. Another study demonstrated the salutary effects of ESCs-derived exosomes on cardiac neovascularization and the reduction of apoptosis and fibrosis after myocardial infarction. ESCs-derived exosomes mediated the delivery of miR-294 to cardiac progenitor cells, thus promoting survival, cell cycle progression, and proliferation [61].

Other cells-derived EVs are also used for treating cardiovascular diseases. Under vasculogenic conditioning, subsets of proinflammatory cells in peripheral blood mononuclear cells (PBMCs) are beneficially transformed into proregenerative cells, collectively referred to as regeneration-associated cells (RAC) [62,63]. The systemic injection of RAC-EVs was superior to that of MSC-EVs for enhancing cardiac function because it delivered essential angiogenesis, antifibrosis, and anti-inflammatory miRNAs to myocardial ischemic tissue [64]. Dox and trastuzumab (Trz) are effective cancer drug treatments for HER2-positive breast cancer; the intravenous injection of cardiac-resident-mesenchymal-progenitor-cells (CPCs)-derived exosomes could attenuate Dox/Trz-induced cardiotoxicity, which includes the prevention of reactive oxygen species (ROS) production, reduction of inflammatory cell infiltration, and fibrosis [65]. Mechanism exploration revealed that miR-146a-5p that is enriched in exosomes may suppress target genes TRAF6 and MPO. In addition, CPCs-derived EVs could inhibit apoptosis in cardiomyocytes and enhance tube formation in endothelial cells by delivering miR-210 and miR-132 [66]. Many studies on EVs have been conducted in rodents; data on myocardial benefits in large animals are rare. Gallet et al. demonstrated that intramyocardial injection of exosomes secreted by cardiosphere-derived cells (CDCs) could effectively reduce scar formation, prevent adverse remodeling, and improve the left ventricular ejection fraction in acute and convalescent myocardial infarction pig models [67]. Gao et al. also demonstrated that human induced pluripotent stem-cells-derived exosomes showed benefit effects in recovery from pig myocardial infarction through improving left ventricular ejection fraction, cardiac hypertrophy, cell apoptosis, and angiogenesis [68].

The aforementioned studies focused on the role of exogenous EVs. The abundance of EVs in plasma motivated us to evaluate whether EVs play roles in mediating cardiac repair effects [69]. Studies have reported that a reduction in the infarction area through remote ischemic conditioning can be mediated by circulating EVs that accumulate in the damaged myocardium [70]. Consequently, researchers have explored the beneficial role of plasma-derived EVs in heart repair. Exosomes derived from the blood of rats and human volunteers were applied to a model of cardiac ischemia–reperfusion injury, and powerfully cardioprotective effects that were accompanied by activation of the HSP70–TLR4 communication axis were discovered [71]. To explore the intrinsic components of plasma circulating EVs, Wang and colleagues identified that miR-486 mediated the inhibition of PTEN, which then activated AKT and protected cardiomyocytes from apoptosis [72]. Additionally, the scholars used cardiac homing peptide (CHP) to link EVs and found that the infarct size in the heart was further diminished and the cardiac retention of EVs was increased in mice and dogs. Furthermore, Jin et al. observed that cotransplantation of bone marrow MSCs with plasma-derived EVs improved myocardial remodeling and promoted an increase in the myocardial capillary density by activating AKT signaling in a rat model of myocardial infarction [73].

To improve the effects of treatments, researchers have developed various methods for EVs administration. For overcoming the low efficiency of EV delivery to the heart, Yao et al. designed a minimally invasive exosome spray by using biomaterials and tested the spray's feasibility and safety in mouse and pig models of acute myocardial infarction [74]. Compared with the injected exosomes, the exosomes spray exhibited high retention in the heart, improved cardiac function, reduced fibrosis, and promoted cardiac endogenous angiomyogenesis. In addition, it is also an interesting strategy of increasing the retention of EVs in the heart to prolong the therapeutic effects. Researchers have developed a hydrogel patch by encapsulating iPSC-derived cardiomyocytes-EVs into a 7 mm diameter collagen gel-foam mesh. The hydrogel patch was found to continually release EVs into the injured heart area, significantly promote recovery of the ejection fraction, decrease the burden of arrhythmia, and reduce the extent of cardiomyocyte apoptosis after infarction [75]. The development of these new methods further enhances the efficacy and feasibility of the clinical translation of EVs (Table 1).

Table 1. Role of natural EVs from different sources for cardiac therapies.

Source	Cargo	Model	Injection	Therapeutic Effects and Mechanism	Reference
BMSCs	miRNAs	MI	Intramyocardial	Inhibit cardiac fibrosis and inflammation and improve cardiac function	[46]
UCB-MSCs	miR-23a-3p	AMI	Intramyocardial	Inhibit ferroptosis and reduce myocardial injury through suppressing DMT1 expression	[47]
UC-MSCs	PINK1	Sepsis	Intraperitoneal	Restore cardiac function and $mCa2^{+}$ efflux-induced mitochondrial calcium overload by PINK1-PKA-NCLX axis	[48]
BMSCs	BMP2	AMI	Intramyocardial	Promote angiogenesis, reduce myocardial fibrosis and inflammatory cell infiltration	[49]
BMSCs	miR-182	I/R	Intramyocardial	Reduce infarct size and alleviate inflammation through modifying the polarization of macrophages M1 to M2	[50]
BMSCs	miR-143-3p	Cellular H/R		Inhibit H/R-induced cell apoptosis and cell autophagy via CHK2-Beclin2 pathway	[51]
MSCs	miR-199a-3p	DOX-induced cardiomyopathy	Intravenous	Inhibit cardiomyocyte apoptosis by the regulation of Akt activation	[52]
BMSCs	miR-29a-3p	Severe acute pancreatitis	Intravenous	Reduce inflammatory markers and improve cardiac function	[53]
UC-MSCs	miR-100-5p	DOX-induced cardiomyopathy		Inhibit DOX-induced ROS, oxidative stress, and apoptosis through the miR-100-5p/NOX4 pathway	[54]
UC-MSCs	lncRNA UCA1	I/R	Intravenous	Inhibit cardiomyocyte apoptosis and promote angiogenesis through the miR-143/Bcl-2/Beclin-1 axis	[55]
BMSCs	LncRNA HCP5	I/R	Intramyocardial	Decrease apoptosis of cardiomyocytes via sponging miR-497 to disinhibit IGF1/PI3K/AKT signaling	[56]
UC-MSCs	circRNAs	Cellular H/R		Inhibit cardiomyocyte apoptosis through the interactions of circRNA-miRNA-PIK3CD	[57]

Table 1. *Cont.*

Source	Cargo	Model	Injection	Therapeutic Effects and Mechanism	Reference
iPSC-Pg	miRNAs	MI	Intramyocardial	Increase cell survival, proliferation, and migration through specific miRNA signature and cardioprotective pathways	[58]
TSCs		DOX-induced cardiomyopathy	Intravenous	Reduce apoptosis and inflammation with the increase of ZEB1 expression and inhibition of miR-200b	[59]
TSCs	miRNA let-7i	DOX-induced cardiomyopathy	Intramyocardial	Inhibit myocardial apoptosis and decrease inflammatory responses via the let-7i/YAP pathway	[60]
ESCs	miR-294	AMI	Intramyocardial	Promote cardiac neovascularization and reduce apoptosis and fibrosis via the delivery of miR-294 to cardiac progenitor cells	[61]
RAC	miRNAs	I/R	Intravenous	Enhance cardiac function through delivery of key angiogenesis, antifibrosis, anti-inflammatory miRNAs	[63]
CPCs	miR-146a-5p	DOX/Trz-induced cardiomyopathy	Intravenous	Prevent ROS production, reduce inflammatory cell infiltration and fibrosis by suppressing target genes Traf6 and Mpo	[65]
CPCs	miR-210/miR-132	MI	Intramyocardial	Inhibit cardiomyocytes apoptosis and enhance angiogenesis	[66]
CDCs		MI	Intramyocardial	Reduce scar formation, prevent adverse remodeling, and improve left ventricular ejection fraction	[67]
iPS		MI	Intramyocardial	Improve left ventricular ejection fraction, cardiac hypertrophy, cell apoptosis, and angiogenesis	[68]
Plasma	HSP70	I/R	Intravenous	Decrease infarct size and inhibit myocardial apoptosis through the activation of HSP70/TLR4 communication axis	[71]
Plasma	miR-486	I/R	Intracoronary	Protect cardiomyocytes from apoptosis by mediating the inhibition of PTEN, which then activates AKT	[72]
Plasma	miRNAs	MI	Intramyocardial	Promote angiogenesis and ameliorate myocardial remodeling by activating AKT signaling	[73]
MSCs		MI	Spray	Reduce fibrosis and promote cardiac angiomyogenesis	[74]
iPS	miRNAs	AMI	Hydrogel patch	Promote the recovery of ejection fraction, decrease arrhythmia burden, and reduce cardiomyocyte apoptosis	[75]

Abbreviations: BMSCs: Bone marrow MSCs; UCB-MSCs: human umbilical cord blood MSCs; UC-MSCs: umbilical cord MSCs; iPSC-Pg: human induced pluripotent stem-cell-derived cardiovascular progenitors; TSCs: human trophoblast stem cells; ESCs: embryonic stem cells; RAC: regeneration-associated cells; CPCs: cardiac-resident mesenchymal progenitor cells; CDCs: cardiosphere-derived cells; iPS: induced pluripotent stem cells.

4. Engineering EVs for Myocardial Injury Therapy

Although EVs are promising in the treatment of myocardial injury, many drawbacks exist in clinical translation such as heterogeneity and the limited tropism of EVs. Methods to increase the contents, targeting, bioactivity, kinetics, and biodistribution of EVs are necessary to overcome the shortcomings of natural EVs. Various methods have been developed to improve the treatment efficiency of EVs in heart disease. Modification of the donor cell or direct modification of the isolated EVs is often performed when bioengineering EVs (Figure 2).

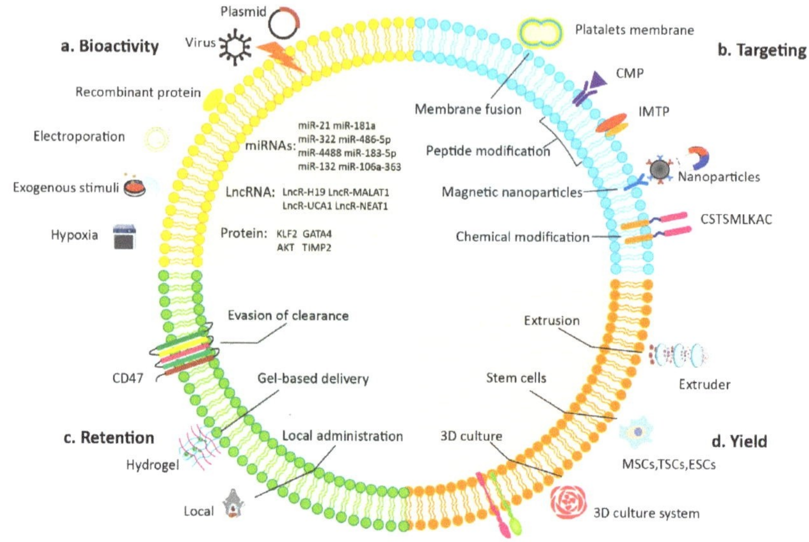

Figure 2. Modulation of EVs for cardiac therapies. Various engineered approaches have been developed to amplify the therapeutic effects of EVs by increasing the bioactivity, targeting, retention, and yield of EVs. Manipulating parental cells or direct modification of the isolated EVs is involved in bioengineering of EVs. Both genetic and nongenetic methods participate in modification strategies.

4.1. Modification of the Donor Cell

Genetic engineering using viral or plasmid vectors is a convenient means of modifying parent cells and producing engineered EVs. Various therapeutic molecules, including miRNAs and proteins, can be encapsulated into secreted EVs by transfecting cells. For example, miR-21 has been reported to inhibit apoptosis by targeting the PDCD4/AP-1 pathway in infarcted cardiomyocytes [76,77]. In a mouse model of myocardial infarction, EVs derived from HEK293T cells overexpressing miR-21 effectively delivered miR-21 to cardiomyocytes and endothelial cells, thereby inhibiting their apoptosis and promoting improvement of cardiac function [78]. Compared with liposomes and polyethylenimine, EVs significantly inhibited the degradation of miR-21. In another study, exosomes were isolated from miRNA-181a-overexpressing umbilical cord blood-derived MSCs; compared with control exosomes, these exosomes exerted stronger repairing effects on myocardium ischemia-reperfusion injury through the inhibition of c-Fos [79]. Lin et al. showed that EVs secreted by β-catenin-engineered immortal CDCs inhibited the activation of NF-κB by delivering miR-4488, which consequently reduced the level of inflammation and suppressed arrhythmogenesis in arrhythmogenic cardiomyopathy [80]. Krüppel-like factors (KLFs) are highly expressed in endothelial cells and have anti-inflammatory effects [81]. Therefore, researchers have separated EVs from KLF2-overexpressing endothelial cells and determined whether the KLF2-EVs have a protective effect on cardiac injury. Excitingly, in both myocardial ischemia-reperfusion injury and Dox-induced dilated cardiomyopathy, KLF2-EVs exerted significant anti-inflammatory effects by targeting CCR2 to prevent Ly6Chigh monocytes recruitment to the myocardium [82,83]. Additionally, in myocardial infarction models, exosomes derived from Akt-, GATA4-, and TIMP2- modified MSCs demonstrated cardiac repair capabilities by promoting angiogenesis and inhibiting apoptosis [84–86].

A common strategy to increase the targeting ability of EVs is to express cardiac-targeting proteins on the surface of EVs through gene transfection. Lamp2b, a type of EVs surface protein, is widely used for displaying targeting motifs. Bone marrow MSCs transfected with a lentivirus of Lamp2b that was fused with ischemic myocardium-targeting peptide CSTSMLKAC (IMTP) produced exosomes that accumulated greatly at myocardial ischemia sites [87]. Additionally, the IMTP-exosomes significantly restored cardiac function by reducing inflammation and fibrosis and promoting angiogenesis. In another example, the researchers constructed a plasmid that expressed Lamp2b fused to a cardiomyocyte specific peptide (CMP), WLSEAGPVVTVRALRGTGSW and transfected it into CDCs [88]. Compared with control exosomes, the CDCs-derived exosomes expressed CMP on their surface and demonstrated higher cardiac retention.

EVs elicit different effects on recipient cells depending on the cultural environment of the parent cells. Changing the culture environment of donor cells is another effective method of harvesting therapeutic EVs. When processing a culture, oxygen tension is a key factor that affects the biological behavior of cells. Hypoxia induces the expression of cytoprotective genes in stem cells and improves their differentiation potential, which alters the content of EVs [89,90]. Studies have shown that hypoxia-preconditioned stem cell-derived EVs have significantly stronger myocardial repair effects than native EVs do. Wu et al. demonstrated that EVs secreted from human pluripotent stem-cells-derived cardiovascular progenitor cells under hypoxic conditions exhibited stronger cardioprotective effects than normal EVs in myocardial infarction [91]. The enhanced effects may be attributed to targeting miR-497 due to the over-enriched lncRNA MALAT1 in EVs under hypoxic conditions. Hypoxic conditions also increased the expression of lncRNA-UCA1 in MSCs-derived exosomes [92]. The hypoxic-conditioned exosomes exerted better cardioprotective effects against myocardial injury than did normal exosomes, and these effects were exerted through the miR-873-5p–XIAP axis. To further validate the effect of hypoxia preconditioning on EVs, researchers investigated the cardiac recovery effect of hypoxia-induced EVs in a nonhuman primate model. In a cynomolgus monkey myocardial infarction, EVs from hypoxia-preconditioned MSCs were enriched in miR-486-5p and promoted cardiac angiogenesis through fibroblast MMP19-VEGFA cleavage signaling [93]. Jung et al. investigated the molecular mechanism of EVs originating from human iPSC-derived cardiomyocytes in myocardial self-repair. They discovered that hypoxic conditions resulted in significantly higher abundance of miR-106a-363 in EVs and promoted a restart of the cardiomyocyte cell cycle by inhibiting the Notch3 pathway, which consequently improved heart function [94]. These studies highlight the positive effect of altering oxygen tension on the cardiac repair potential of EVs.

Exogenous stimuli are another novel strategy used to optimize EVs through coincubation with parental cells and to deliver bioactive molecules to injured cardiomyocytes. For example, Zhuang et al. obtained exosomes from macrophage migration inhibitory factor (MIF)-pretreated MSCs (exosomeMIF) and tested the cardioprotective effects on Dox-induced cardiomyopathy [95]. The results indicated that exosomeMIF restored cardiac function and exerted anti-senescence effects through LncRNA-NEAT1 transfer, partially by inhibiting miR-221-3p and activating SIRT2. Another study reported that by promoting endothelial cell function, atorvastatin-pretreated MSCs-derived exosomes were able to significantly improve the recovery of cardiac function in rats with acute myocardial infarction. Consequently, the infarct size and cardiomyocyte apoptosis were found to decrease, which may be attributed to overexpressed lncRNA H19 in the exosomes [96]. In one report, hemin-pretreated MSCs-derived exosomes were enriched in miR-183-5p and significantly improved cardiac function and reduced fibrosis compared with blank exosomes [97]. Mechanistically, the aforementioned exosomes attenuated mitochondrial fission and the cellular senescence of cardiomyocytes by regulating the HMGB1/ERK pathway in a mouse model of myocardial infarction. However, the exact mechanisms to determine the functional cargoes enriched in EVs after exogenous stimuli remain unclear. It limits the abroad application for further discovery of unknown stimuli.

4.2. Direct Modification of Isolated EVs

Manipulating parental cells to produce engineered EVs can result in most of the biophysical properties of EVs being retained. However, parental cell manipulation may cause unforeseen consequences for the biology of EVs and ultimately interfere with EVs biogenesis and alter other biological properties. Direct modification of isolated EVs does not change the biological origin of EVs, and various methods can be used to directly impart the desired biological properties as necessary.

Many studies have shown that miRNA in EVs has a therapeutic effect by inhibiting pathological genes after myocardial injury. Therefore, electroporation of miRNA into EVs may be a promising engineering strategy to increase the therapeutic efficacy of EVs. In one study, cardiac-progenitor-cells-derived exosomes were transfected with proangiogenic miR-322 by using electroporation. The cardiac therapeutic efficacy was evaluated in a mouse model of myocardial infarction [98]. Compared with control exosomes, the bioengineered exosomes exhibited greater protection regarding the enhancement of angiogenesis in infarcted hearts. This effect may be mediated by an increase in endothelial cell migration and capillary formation through the increase in NOX2-derived ROS. Bone marrow MSCs derived exosomes were electroporated with miR-132 mimics and tested for their ability to promote angiogenesis [99]. In vivo, miR-132-loaded exosomes restored cardiac function and promoted angiogenesis better than did control exosomes following their intramyocardial injection. Kang et al. reported that peripheral blood-derived exosomes could be used for the delivery of miR21 mimic or inhibitor and change the expression of SMAD7, PTEN, and MMP2 in cardiomyocytes. In vivo, miR-21 inhibitor-loaded exosomes could also reduce cardiac fibrosis in a mouse model of myocardial infarction [100]. A distinct advantage of using this approach to deliver therapeutic cargo is the ability to precisely control the amount of drug carried by the EVs. The delivery of miRNA to EVs through electroporation is relatively efficient.

Several EVs-based heart disease therapies have exhibited good performance in experimental models. However, the high risk of off-target effects is a major barrier to the introduction of heart disease therapies in clinics. Thus, several studies have attempted to increase the cardiac targeting of EVs. Exosomes loaded with siClathrin via electroporation significantly reduced the uptake of exosomes by macrophages in vitro and in vivo and increased the exosomes' delivery to the heart [101]. Preinjection of exosomes containing siClathrin considerably improved therapeutic effects following by injection of miR-21a encapsulated exosomes in a Dox-induced mouse model. The delivery of therapeutic molecules by enhancing targeted EVs provides more possibilities for further clinical applications. The primary advantage of this strategy is that an invasive injection to the heart can be avoided if intravenous administration is employed. Liu et al. employed a nanoparticle "vesicle shuttle" for accurate capture and targeted delivery of circulating exosomes [102]. The nanoparticles consisted of a Fe3O4 core and a silica shell that conjugated through hydrazone bonds to CD63 antigens; CD63-expressing exosomes were captured and accumulated in infarcted cardiac tissue under a local magnetic field. Improvements in infarct size and angiogenesis were observed after nanoparticle injection in both rabbit and rat models. However, it is not easy to achieve targeted delivery of EVs by surface modification, and it requires strict control of the reaction conditions to avoid the destruction and aggregation of EVs due to improper temperature, pH, and osmotic pressure.

Despite less research, the EVs membrane has been chemically modified to enhance the targeting ability of engineered EVs with peptides or proteins. Although the mechanism of interaction with the myocardium is unclear, CHP has exhibited cardiac targeting [103]. Researchers have thus developed a method of conjugating exosomes and CHP through the DOPE-NHS linker and tested the repair effects on myocardial infarction in an ischemia-reperfusion rat model [104]; the engineered exosomes were discovered to increase retention in heart sections, reduce fibrosis and scar formation, and promote cellular proliferation and angiogenesis. Dibenzyl cyclooctyne groups were introduced to the surface of hypoxia-elicited MSCs-derived exosomes (Hypo-Exo) and then interacted with azide-functionalized ischemic myocardium-targeted (IMT) peptide to form stable triazide linkages [105]. The IMT-conjugated Hypo-Exo exhibited specific targeting of the ischemic myocardium due to its interaction with cTnI, which is specifically expressed in ischemic cardiomyocyte. A considerable improvement in heart function and reduced apoptosis and fibrosis were observed in a mouse model of myocardial infarction. In another study, Antes et al. designed a more general EVs membrane anchoring platform based on streptavidin by using DMPE-PEG exosome modification platform; this achieved coupling of any biotinylated molecule to modify the EVs membrane for targeted delivery [106]. CDCs-EVs were then decorated with the ischemia homing peptide (CSTSMLKAC) by using the platform. The CDCs-EVs demonstrated considerably higher localization in injured myocardium when intravenously injected. It should be noted that chemical modification of EVs by using click chemistry may result in nonspecific site reaction due to uncontrolled amino or protein modification. Therefore, there is a risk that chemical modification may shield some protein interactions on the surface of EVs.

The combination of hydrogels and EVs provides a novel approach for optimizing the therapeutic effect of functional EVs. Hydrogels are biocompatible and enable controlled release of encapsulated cargo. Bone marrow MSCs-derived EVs were incorporated into alginate hydrogel (EVs-Gel) and applied in rat models of myocardial infarction. Compared with the control group, the EVs-Gel treatment group markedly decreased cardiomyocyte apoptosis and boosted the polarization of macrophages, which improved cardiac function and infarct size [107]. Similarly, dendritic-cell-derived exosomes could activate Treg cells and promote the polarization of macrophage when they were incorporated into alginate hydrogel, thereby promoting the recovery of cardiac function after myocardial infarction [108]. Additionally, Chen et al. designed a shear-thinning gel (STG) based on the interactions between adamantane and β-cyclodextrin-modified hyaluronic acid [109]. The STG enabled the slow elution of endothelial-progenitor-cells-derived EVs in the ischemic border zone, resulting in higher proliferation of peri-infarct angiogenesis. Further research has indicated that when STG encapsulating EVs were injected on the fourth day after myocardial infarction, they improved left ventricular contractility [110]. Therefore, the therapeutic effects of STG encapsulating EVs can be optimized through strategic timing. Overall, hydrogels can increase the retention of EVs in the heart and enable their controlled release, thus improving their therapeutic effects.

4.3. Two-Step EVs Modification Strategy

In the two-step EVs delivery method, the parent cell is genetically modified, and the therapeutic cargo are then loaded into EVs. This composite modification strategy provides more possibilities for targeted delivery and enhancing the efficacy of EVs. Although in infancy, some researchers have conducted exploratory studies on this approach (Figure 3).

Kim and colleagues designed HEK-293 cells expressing cardiac-targeting peptide (CTP) fused to LAMP2b and then isolated EVs from the cell culture medium [111]. The EVs were loaded with an siRNA that targeted the receptor for advanced glycation end products (siRAGE). The modified EVs exhibited twice the siRAGE delivery efficiency of normal EVs and significantly attenuated cardiac inflammation levels in experimental autoimmune myocarditis. In another study, CD47-modified EVs were designed to solve the rapid clearance of EVs by the mononuclear phagocyte system [112]. Binding of CD47 and SIRPα results in a "do not eat me" signal, which helps cancer cells to evade phagocytosis [113]. EVs were generated from MSCs overexpressing CD47 and then loaded with miR-21a via electroporation. After being injected into an ischemia–reperfusion mouse model, the engineered EVs preferentially accumulated in the heart and significantly reduced the apoptosis and inflammation levels of injured cardiomyocyte. It is an attractive strategy to prevent immune rejection of EVs through modulating EVs' imprinting. Shao et al. isolated exosomes from β2-microglobulin (B2M)-deficient MSCs and loaded miR-24 into exosomes through electroporation [114]. The modified exosomes were able to restore cardiac function by inhibiting cardiac fibrosis in a rat model of myocardial infarction.

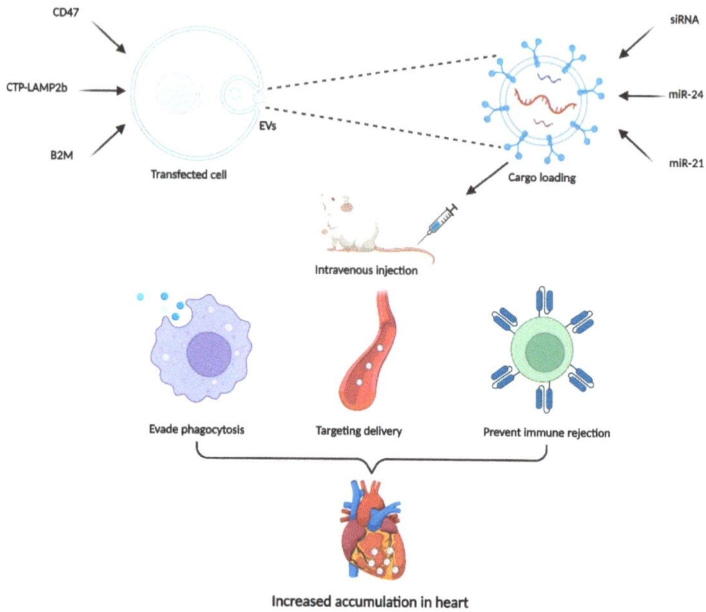

Figure 3. Two-step EVs delivery method for cardiac therapies. Two-step EVs delivery method works by genetically modifying the parent cell followed by the loading of the therapeutic cargos. CTP-Lamp2b, CD47, and B2M-modified EVs were loaded with siRAGE, miR-21, and miR-24 to impart the property of targeting delivery, evading phagocytosis and preventing immune rejection, respectively.

4.4. Biomimetic EVs for Cardiac Applications

Low yields and complicated purification processes are the main drawbacks to the clinical translation of EVs. In addition to directly or indirectly modifying EVs, scholars have applied biomimetic vesicles in cardiovascular diseases and this approach has recently garnered attention. Biomimetic EVs are synthetic particles that are engineered using the basic moieties present in natural EVs (membrane structures, proteins, lipids, and RNA) to reproduce the therapeutic effects of EVs. This approach facilitates standardization and can improve the yield of EVs because there are a wide range of sources available for the EVs production. Studies have obtained strikingly promising results with biomimetic EVs in cardiac repair processes.

Wang et al. employed a liposome extruder to generate extruded nanovesicles (NVs) from MSCs and tested the repair function of these NVs in a myocardial ischemia–reperfusion mouse model [115]. Similar to natural EVs, extruded vesicles promoted angiogenesis and cardiomyocyte proliferation in the heart after injury and reduced scarring but with the advantage that their yield is more than 20 times that of natural EVs. In a study, adipose MSCs-derived biomimetic NVs were generated by loading melatonin into MSC-extruded NVs through ultrasonic treatment [116]. The engineered NVs significantly restored cardiac function by alleviating mitochondrial dysfunction, reducing fibrosis, and promoting microvessel formation.

Another promising direction regarding biomimetic vesicles is expanding their targeting ability by using membrane-based engineering methods. In one study, mimetic extracellular NVs were extruded from iron oxide nanoparticles-incorporated MSCs [117]. Under magnetic guidance, the NVs exhibited increased retention in an infarcted heart, which consequently reduced apoptosis and fibrosis and improved angiogenesis and cardiac function recovery. Membrane fusion is a convenient method for giving EVs new properties. Li et al. designed platelet-mimetic EVs (P-EVs) by fusing the membranes of MSCs-derived EVs with platelet membranes through extrusion; their therapeutic effect was tested in a mouse model of myocardial ischemia–reperfusion [118]. The P-EVs exhibited significant myocardial targeting and favorably promoted angiogenesis. Furthermore, the P-EVs facilitated the phenotype transformation of macrophages M1 to M2, which may have been due to the release of functional miRNAs [119]. To utilize the recruitment feature of monocytes after myocardium ischemia-reperfusion, Zhang et al. modified MSCs-derived EVs with monocyte mimics through membrane fusion. The engineered EVs exhibited significantly enhanced myocardial targeting capabilities that promoted endothelial maturation for angiogenesis and modulated macrophage subpopulations [120]. These methods are noninvasive and thus clinically appealing.

Biomimetic strategies can be used to increase the retention of EVs in the blood. Avoiding the elimination of EVs by the mononuclear phagocyte system has been a focus of research. Researchers used self-assembly of MSCs membrane on the surface of miR-21-loaded mesoporous silica nanoparticle to construct an exosome-mimicking nanocomplex [121]. This nanocomplex could escape the clearance of the immunologic system and target injured myocardium. Furthermore, the nanocomplex delivered miR-21 to cardiomyocytes, which inhibited the translation of the PDCD4 and PTEN to prevent apoptosis. Platelet membrane-cloaked nanoparticles also exhibited reduced phagocytosis by the mononuclear phagocyte system [122]. Given the biological characteristics of platelet membrane, Li et al. prepared biomimetic Treg nanoparticles by camouflaging cyclosporine A and poly (5,5-dimethyl-4,6-dithio-propylene glycol azelate) within the platelet membrane through extrusion [123]. The biomimetic nanoparticles actively accumulated in the ischemic myocardium, increased the ratio of Treg and M2 type macrophages, and reduced ROS production in a mouse model of myocardial ischemia–reperfusion. The remodeling of the left ventricle and heart function were significantly improved.

5. Discussion

Various source-derived EVs have been used for myocardial repair, and each type of EVs has its own advantages. Stem-cells-derived EVs are abundant and rich in therapeutic cargo. Platelet membrane has a natural ability to target an injured vascular wall after myocardial injury. Monocyte-derived membrane is less extensively phagocytized by the mononuclear phagocyte system than are other EVs. Currently, two methods are available for administrating EVs: intramyocardial injection, which is efficient but invasive, and intravenous injection, which is noninvasive but results in low cardiac retention. Further research is necessary to develop noninvasive and efficient EV delivery for clinical applications. The delivery of therapeutic agents by bioengineered EVs leads to greater stability, a longer blood circulation time, and greater agent accumulation in the injured myocardium, all of which enhance the efficacy of the cargo and reduce the dosage required. Compared with the single-step modification strategy, the two-step EVs delivery method has garnered much attention. It works by genetically modifying the parent cell followed by the loading of the therapeutic cargos. The delivery of functional molecules can be optimized, leading to better targeting and lower dosage requirements.

EVs are rich in content, and the various molecules within them have been shown to contribute to EVs' efficacy in terms of cardiac function recovery. Among their bioactive components, miRNA is the cargo that has most widely been identified as exerting therapeutic effects. However, exogenous nucleic acid insertion, especially that of large messenger RNA, is inefficient. Therefore, an EVs-based nucleic-acid carrier platform should be developed. Additionally, other noncoding RNAs, such as lncRNAs and circRNAs, play functional roles in cardiac recovery. Studies have highlighted the role of specific single therapeutic cargo in EVs; therefore, we recommend further research on the synergistic therapeutic effects of multiple molecules in EVs, such as miRNA clusters.

A variety of mechanisms are involved in the repair process of EVs after myocardial injury. In myocardial infarction, cardiomyocyte apoptosis is the most common event. EVs have a direct inhibitory effect on cardiomyocyte apoptosis. Beyond that, the inhibition of ferroptosis, senescence, autophagy, and pyroptosis is also involved in the cardioprotective effect of EVs [124]. Moreover, regulation of mitochondrial function contributes to EVs-mediated repair. In addition to directly inhibiting apoptosis, EVs promote the recovery of cardiac function by modulating the phenotype of macrophages, a function that can be attributed to the unique miRNAs of EVs [50]. In endothelial cells, EVs promote the formation of new blood vessels. Additionally, fibroblasts can lead to antifibrosis by priming with EVs [125]. Overall, EVs-mediated repair after myocardial injury is a complex process and often combines multiple pathways (Figure 4).

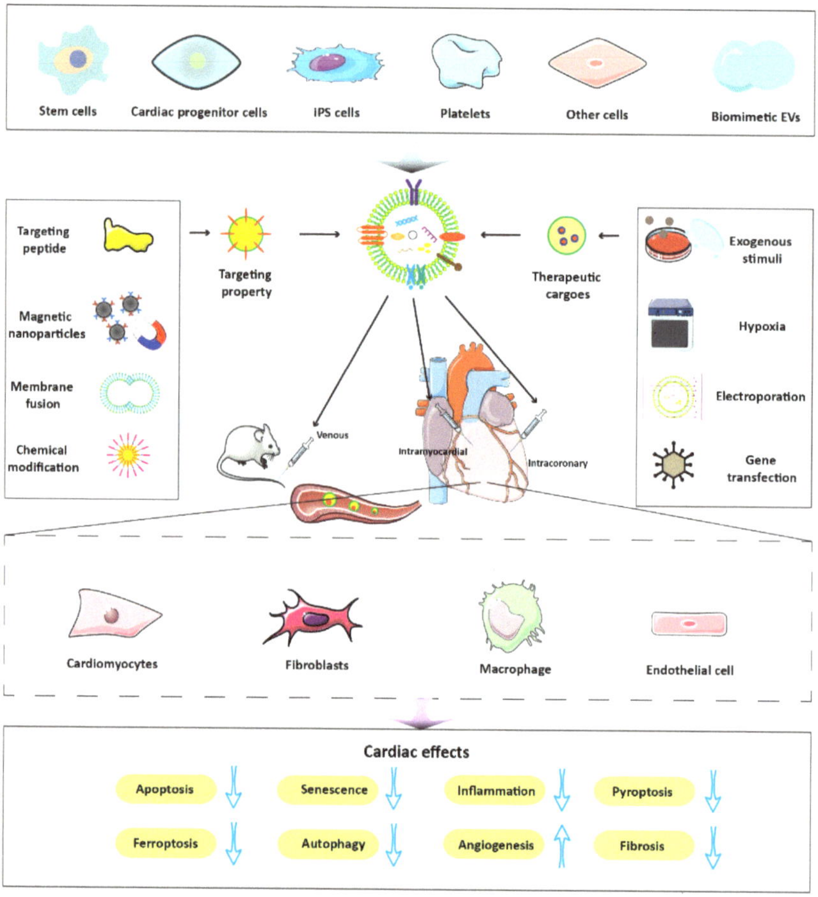

Figure 4. Examples of EVs-modulation strategies for cardiac therapies. Different sources derived-EVs can be modified to increase the therapeutic cargoes and targeting ability for cardiac repair through various injection ways. Then, EVs are able to regulate multiple effect cells including cardiomyocyte, fibroblast, macrophage, and endothelial cells for cardioprotective effects through multiple pathways.

To overcome the limitations of natural EVs, various engineering approaches have been developed. Currently, the engineering modification strategies for EVs have a few primary goals. First, several studies are performed to increase the content of therapeutic molecules in EVs through genetic or nongenetic approaches. It is a useful strategy to identify the potential key EVs miRNAs and their downstream target gene clusters via miRNA chips and computational approaches. Then, the therapeutic cargos can be loaded into EVs through modification of parent cells or isolated EVs. Second, increasing the cardiac targeting of EVs and reducing their clearance by the body's defense system can enhance the recovery function of EVs. EVs targeting is mainly increased by modifying the surface of EVs with heart-targeting homing peptides or ligands. The combination of hydrogel and EVs leads to localization of the EVs at the border of myocardial injury. Additionally, large-scale production of EVs is essential for clinical translation. A three-dimensional cell culture system is a potential candidate. A microfiber culture platform was found to enrich MSCs-derived particles 1009-fold compared with conventional two-dimensional culture but to also preserve their proangiogenic properties [126]. The biomimetic strategy-extrusion or membrane fusion-may be another means of increasing the EV yield. Notably, biomimetics may improve the standardization, scalability, automatization, cost-efficiency, biological efficacy, and safety of EVs-based cardiac therapy [127]. Overall, the application of these modification strategies can amplify the regenerative effects of EVs.

6. Conclusions

In conclusion, EVs therapy is an attractive cell-free approach for treating heart disease. The EVs-based drug delivery platform is a desired pharmacokinetics system. Attempts to modify EVs to improve their biodistribution and cardiotropic properties are still in their infancy. Further studies on EVs biogenesis, content, transfer, and interactions are necessary to develop engineering strategies for specific needs.

Funding: This work was supported by the National Natural Science Foundation of China (81871496, 82172102), Technology Development Project of Jiangsu University (20220516), the Advanced Science and Technology Foundation of the Jiangsu Province (BE2021689), Zhenjiang Key Laboratory of High Technology Research on Exosomes Foundation and Transformation Application (SS2018003), project funded by the Priority Academic Program Development of Jiangsu Higher Education Institutions (Phase III).

Institutional Review Board Statement: Not applicable.

Informed Consent Statement: Not applicable.

Data Availability Statement: Not applicable.

Conflicts of Interest: The authors declare that they have no conflict of interest.

References

1. Mensah, G.A.; Roth, G.A.; Fuster, V. The Global Burden of Cardiovascular Diseases and Risk Factors: 2020 and Beyond. *J. Am. Coll. Cardiol.* **2019**, *74*, 2529–2532. [CrossRef] [PubMed]
2. Meldolesi, J. Exosomes and Ectosomes in Intercellular Communication. *Curr. Biol.* **2018**, *28*, R435–r444. [CrossRef] [PubMed]
3. Salomon, C.; Das, S.; Erdbrügger, U.; Kalluri, R.; Lim, S.K.; Olefsky, J.M.; E Rice, G.E.; Sahoo, S.; Tao, W.A.; Vader, P.; et al. Extracellular Vesicles and Their Emerging Roles as Cellular Messengers in Endocrinology: An Endocrine Society Scientific Statement. *Endocr. Rev.* **2022**, *43*, 441–468. [CrossRef]
4. Maas, S.L.; Breakefield, X.O.; Weaver, A.M. Extracellular Vesicles: Unique Intercellular Delivery Vehicles. *Trends Cell Biol.* **2017**, *27*, 172–188. [CrossRef] [PubMed]
5. Guha, D.; Lorenz, D.R.; Misra, V.; Chettimada, S.; Morgello, S.; Gabuzda, D. Proteomic analysis of cerebrospinal fluid extracellular vesicles reveals synaptic injury, inflammation, and stress response markers in HIV patients with cognitive impairment. *J. Neuroinflamm.* **2019**, *16*, 254. [CrossRef] [PubMed]
6. Sundar, I.K.; Li, D.; Rahman, I. Small RNA-sequence analysis of plasma-derived extracellular vesicle miRNAs in smokers and patients with chronic obstructive pulmonary disease as circulating biomarkers. *J. Extracell. Vesicles* **2019**, *8*, 1684816. [CrossRef]
7. Su, H.; Rustam, Y.H.; Masters, C.L.; Makalic, E.; McLean, C.A.; Hill, A.F.; Barnham, K.J.; Reid, G.E.; Vella, L.J. Characterization of brain-derived extracellular vesicle lipids in Alzheimer's disease. *J. Extracell. Vesicles* **2021**, *10*, e12089. [CrossRef]
8. Elsharkasy, O.M.; Nordin, J.Z.; Hagey, D.W.; de Jong, O.G.; Schiffelers, R.M.; Andaloussi, S.E.; Vader, P. Extracellular vesicles as drug delivery systems: Why and how? *Adv. Drug Deliv. Rev.* **2020**, *159*, 332–343. [CrossRef]
9. Görgens, A.; Corso, G.; Hagey, D.W.; Jawad Wiklander, R.; Gustafsson, M.O.; Felldin, U.; Lee, Y.; Bostancioglu, R.B.; Sork, H.; Liang, X.; et al. Identification of storage conditions stabilizing extracellular vesicles preparations. *J. Extracell. Vesicles* **2022**, *11*, e12238. [CrossRef]
10. Muhammad, S.A. Are extracellular vesicles new hope in clinical drug delivery for neurological disorders? *Neurochem. Int.* **2021**, *144*, 104955. [CrossRef]
11. Luo, H.; Li, X.; Li, T.; Zhao, L.; He, J.; Zha, L.; Qi, Q.; Yu, Z. microRNA-423-3p exosomes derived from cardiac fibroblasts mediates the cardioprotective effects of ischaemic post-conditioning. *Cardiovasc. Res.* **2019**, *115*, 1189–1204. [CrossRef]

12. Nakamura, Y.; Kita, S.; Tanaka, Y.; Fukuda, S.; Obata, Y.; Okita, T.; Nishida, H.; Takahashi, Y.; Kawachi, Y.; Tsugawa-Shimizu, Y.; et al. Adiponectin Stimulates Exosome Release to Enhance Mesenchymal Stem-Cell-Driven Therapy of Heart Failure in Mice. *Mol. Ther.* **2020**, *28*, 2203–2219. [CrossRef]
13. Lee, T.L.; Lai, T.C.; Lin, S.R.; Lin, S.W.; Chen, Y.C.; Pu, C.M.; Lee, I.T.; Tsai, J.S.; Lee, C.W.; Chen, Y.L. Conditioned medium from adipose-derived stem cells attenuates ischemia/reperfusion-induced cardiac injury through the microRNA-221/222/PUMA/ETS-1 pathway. *Theranostics* **2021**, *11*, 3131–3149. [CrossRef]
14. De Abreu, R.C.; Fernandes, H.; da Costa Martins, P.A.; Sahoo, S.; Emanueli, C.; Ferreira, L. Native and bioengineered extracellular vesicles for cardiovascular therapeutics. *Nat. Rev. Cardiol.* **2020**, *17*, 685–697. [CrossRef]
15. Adamiak, M.; Cheng, G.; Bobis-Wozowicz, S.; Zhao, L.; Kedracka-Krok, S.; Samanta, A.; Karnas, E.; Xuan, Y.T.; Skupien-Rabian, B.; Chen, X.; et al. Induced Pluripotent Stem Cell (iPSC)-Derived Extracellular Vesicles Are Safer and More Effective for Cardiac Repair Than iPSCs. *Circ. Res.* **2018**, *122*, 296–309. [CrossRef]
16. Wu, P.; Zhang, B.; Ocansey, D.K.W.; Xu, W.; Qian, H. Extracellular vesicles: A bright star of nanomedicine. *Biomaterials* **2021**, *269*, 120467. [CrossRef]
17. Van Niel, G.; D'Angelo, G.; Raposo, G. Shedding light on the cell biology of extracellular vesicles. *Nat. Rev. Mol. Cell. Biol.* **2018**, *19*, 213–228. [CrossRef]
18. Wang, Y.; Gao, S.; Liu, Y.; Wang, D.; Liu, B.; Jiang, D.; Wong, C.C.L.; Chen, Y.; Yu, L. Retractosomes: Small extracellular vesicles generated from broken-off retraction fibers. *Cell Res.* **2022**. [CrossRef]
19. Kalluri, R.; LeBleu, V.S. The biology, function, and biomedical applications of exosomes. *Science* **2020**, *367*, eaau6977. [CrossRef]
20. Nagano, M.; Toshima, J.Y.; Siekhaus, D.E.; Toshima, J. Rab5-mediated endosome formation is regulated at the trans-Golgi network. *Commun. Biol.* **2019**, *2*, 419. [CrossRef]
21. Stuffers, S.; Wegner, C.S.; Stenmark, H.; Brech, A. Multivesicular endosome biogenesis in the absence of ESCRTs. *Traffic* **2009**, *10*, 925–937. [CrossRef]
22. Colombo, M.; Moita, C.; Van Niel, G.; Kowal, J.; Vigneron, J.; Benaroch, P.; Manel, N.; Moita, L.F.; Théry, C.; Raposo, G. Analysis of ESCRT functions in exosome biogenesis, composition and secretion highlights the heterogeneity of extracellular vesicles. *J. Cell. Sci.* **2013**, *126*, 5553–5565. [CrossRef] [PubMed]
23. Piper, R.C.; Katzmann, D.J. Biogenesis and function of multivesicular bodies. *Annu. Rev. Cell. Dev. Biol.* **2007**, *23*, 519–547. [CrossRef] [PubMed]
24. Camussi, G.; Deregibus, M.-C.; Bruno, S.; Grange, C.; Fonsato, V.; Tetta, C. Exosome/microvesicle-mediated epigenetic reprogramming of cells. *Am. J. Cancer Res.* **2011**, *1*, 98–110. [PubMed]
25. Hugel, B.; Martínez, M.C.; Kunzelmann, C.; Freyssinet, J.-M. Membrane microparticles: Two sides of the coin. *Physiology* **2005**, *20*, 22–27. [CrossRef]
26. Vinaiphat, A.; Sze, S.K. Advances in extracellular vesicles analysis. *Adv. Clin. Chem.* **2020**, *97*, 73–116. [PubMed]
27. Rikkert, L.G.; Nieuwland, R.; Terstappen, L.W.; Coumans, F.A. Quality of extracellular vesicle images by transmission electron microscopy is operator and protocol dependent. *J. Extracell. Vesicles* **2019**, *8*, 1555419. [CrossRef]
28. Sharma, S.; Rasool, H.I.; Palanisamy, V.; Mathisen, C.; Schmidt, M.; Wong, D.T.; Gimzewski, J. Structural-mechanical characterization of nanoparticle exosomes in human saliva, using correlative AFM, FESEM, and force spectroscopy. *ACS Nano* **2010**, *4*, 1921–1926. [CrossRef]
29. Milne, J.L.; Borgnia, M.J.; Bartesaghi, A.; Tran, E.E.; Earl, L.A.; Schauder, D.M.; Lengyel, J.; Pierson, J.; Patwardhan, A.; Subramaniam, S. Cryo-electron microscopy–a primer for the non-microscopist. *FEBS J.* **2013**, *280*, 28–45. [CrossRef]
30. Welsh, J.A.; van der Pol, E.; Bettin, B.A.; Carter, D.R.; Hendrix, A.; Lenassi, M.; Langlois, M.A.; Llorente, A.; van de Nes, A.S.; Nieuwland, R.; et al. Towards defining reference materials for measuring extracellular vesicle refractive index, epitope abundance, size and concentration. *J. Extracell. Vesicles* **2020**, *9*, 1816641. [CrossRef]
31. Vogel, R.; Savage, J.; Muzard, J.; Della Camera, G.; Vella, G.; Law, A.; Marchioni, M.; Mehn, D.; Geiss, O.; Peacock, B.; et al. Measuring particle concentration of multimodal synthetic reference materials and extracellular vesicles with orthogonal techniques: Who is up to the challenge? *J. Extracell. Vesicles* **2021**, *10*, e12052. [CrossRef] [PubMed]
32. Liu, H.; Tian, Y.; Xue, C.; Niu, Q.; Chen, C.; Yan, X. Analysis of extracellular vesicle DNA at the single-vesicle level by nano-flow cytometry. *J. Extracell. Vesicles* **2022**, *11*, e12206. [CrossRef]
33. Lin, B.; Lei, Y.; Wang, J.; Zhu, L.; Wu, Y.; Zhang, H.; Wu, L.; Zhang, P.; Yang, C. Microfluidic-Based Exosome Analysis for Liquid Biopsy. *Small Methods* **2021**, *5*, e2001131. [CrossRef] [PubMed]
34. Sun, Z.; Li, J.; Tong, Y.; Han, H.; Yang, Y.; Wang, C.; Li, H.; Du, L.; Jiang, Y. A ratiometric fluorescent biosensor based on self-fluorescent MOF and target-triggered rolling circle amplification for sensitive detection of exosome-derived miRNA. *Anal. Chim. Acta* **2022**, *1221*, 340136. [CrossRef]
35. Zhao, X.; Luo, C.; Mei, Q.; Zhang, H.; Zhang, W.; Su, D.; Fu, W.; Luo, Y. Aptamer-Cholesterol-Mediated Proximity Ligation Assay for Accurate Identification of Exosomes. *Anal. Chem.* **2020**, *92*, 5411–5418. [CrossRef]
36. Pocsfalvi, G.; Stanly, C.; Vilasi, A.; Fiume, I.; Capasso, G.; Turiák, L.; Buzas, E.I.; Vékey, K. Mass spectrometry of extracellular vesicles. *Mass. Spectrom. Rev.* **2016**, *35*, 3–21. [CrossRef]

37. Martínez-Greene, J.A.; Hernández-Ortega, K.; Quiroz-Baez, R.; Resendis-Antonio, O.; Pichardo-Casas, I.; Sinclair, D.A.; Budnik, B.; Hidalgo-Miranda, A.; Uribe-Querol, E.; Ramos-Godínez, M.D.P.; et al. Quantitative proteomic analysis of extracellular vesicle subgroups isolated by an optimized method combining polymer-based precipitation and size exclusion chromatography. *J. Extracell. Vesicles* **2021**, *10*, e12087. [CrossRef]
38. Nunez Lopez, Y.O.; Iliuk, A.; Petrilli, A.M.; Glass, C.; Casu, A.; Pratley, R.E. Proteomics and Phosphoproteomics of Circulating Extracellular Vesicles Provide New Insights into Diabetes Pathobiology. *Int. J. Mol. Sci.* **2022**, *23*, 5779. [CrossRef]
39. Maisano, D.; Mimmi, S.; Dattilo, V.; Marino, F.; Gentile, M.; Vecchio, E.; Fiume, G.; Nisticò, N.; Aloisio, A.; de Santo, M.P.; et al. A novel phage display based platform for exosome diversity characterization. *Nanoscale* **2022**, *14*, 2998–3003. [CrossRef]
40. Momen-Heravi, F.; Getting, S.J.; Moschos, S.A. Extracellular vesicles and their nucleic acids for biomarker discovery. *Pharmacol. Ther.* **2018**, *192*, 170–187. [CrossRef]
41. Tian, H.; Yuan, C.; Liu, Y.; Li, Z.; Xia, K.; Li, M.; Xie, F.; Chen, Q.; Chen, M.; Fu, W.; et al. A novel quantification platform for point-of-care testing of circulating MicroRNAs based on allosteric spherical nanoprobe. *J. Nanobiotechnol.* **2020**, *18*, 158. [CrossRef] [PubMed]
42. Gonçalves, D.S.; Ferreira, M.D.S.; Liedke, S.C.; Gomes, K.X.; de Oliveira, G.A.; Leão, P.E.L.; Cesar, G.V.; Seabra, S.H.; Cortines, J.R.; Casadevall, A.; et al. Extracellular vesicles and vesicle-free secretome of the protozoa Acanthamoeba castellanii under homeostasis and nutritional stress and their damaging potential to host cells. *Virulence* **2018**, *9*, 818–836. [CrossRef]
43. Andreu, Z.; Yáñez-Mó, M. Tetraspanins in extracellular vesicle formation and function. *Front. Immunol.* **2014**, *5*, 442. [CrossRef]
44. Lai, R.C.; Tan, S.S.; Yeo, R.W.; Choo, A.B.; Reiner, A.T.; Su, Y.; Shen, Y.; Fu, Z.; Alexander, L.; Sze, S.K.; et al. MSC secretes at least 3 EV types each with a unique permutation of membrane lipid, protein and RNA. *J. Extracell. Vesicles* **2016**, *5*, 29828. [CrossRef]
45. Théry, C.; Witwer, K.W.; Aikawa, E.; Alcaraz, M.J.; Anderson, J.D.; Andriantsitohaina, R.; Antoniou, A.; Arab, T.; Archer, F.; Atkin-Smith, G.K.; et al. Minimal information for studies of extracellular vesicles 2018 (MISEV2018): A position statement of the International Society for Extracellular Vesicles and update of the MISEV2014 guidelines. *J. Extracell. Vesicles* **2018**, *7*, 1535750. [CrossRef]
46. Shao, L.; Zhang, Y.; Lan, B.; Wang, J.; Zhang, Z.; Zhang, L.; Xiao, P.; Meng, Q.; Geng, Y.J.; Yu, X.Y.; et al. MiRNA-Sequence Indicates That Mesenchymal Stem Cells and Exosomes Have Similar Mechanism to Enhance Cardiac Repair. *Biomed. Res. Int.* **2017**, *2017*, 4150705. [CrossRef]
47. Song, Y.; Wang, B.; Zhu, X.; Hu, J.; Sun, J.; Xuan, J.; Ge, Z. Human umbilical cord blood-derived MSCs exosome attenuate myocardial injury by inhibiting ferroptosis in acute myocardial infarction mice. *Cell. Biol. Toxicol.* **2021**, *37*, 51–64. [CrossRef] [PubMed]
48. Zhou, Q.; Xie, M.; Zhu, J.; Yi, Q.; Tan, B.; Li, Y.; Ye, L.; Zhang, X.; Zhang, Y.; Tian, J.; et al. PINK1 contained in huMSC-derived exosomes prevents cardiomyocyte mitochondrial calcium overload in sepsis via recovery of mitochondrial Ca(2+) efflux. Stem. *Cell. Res. Ther.* **2021**, *12*, 269. [CrossRef]
49. Xuan, L.; Fu, D.; Zhen, D.; Wei, C.; Bai, D.; Yu, L.; Gong, G. Extracellular vesicles derived from human bone marrow mesenchymal stem cells protect rats against acute myocardial infarction-induced heart failure. *Cell. Tissue Res.* **2022**, *389*, 23–40. [CrossRef]
50. Zhao, J.; Li, X.; Hu, J.; Chen, F.; Qiao, S.; Sun, X.; Gao, L.; Xie, J.; Xu, B. Mesenchymal stromal cell-derived exosomes attenuate myocardial ischaemia-reperfusion injury through miR-182-regulated macrophage polarization. *Cardiovasc. Res.* **2019**, *115*, 1205–1216. [CrossRef] [PubMed]
51. Chen, G.; Wang, M.; Ruan, Z.; Zhu, L.; Tang, C. Mesenchymal stem cell-derived exosomal miR-143-3p suppresses myocardial ischemia-reperfusion injury by regulating autophagy. *Life Sci.* **2021**, *280*, 119742. [CrossRef]
52. Lee, J.Y.; Chung, J.; Byun, Y.; Kim, K.H.; An, S.H.; Kwon, K. Mesenchymal Stem Cell-Derived Small Extracellular Vesicles Protect Cardiomyocytes from Doxorubicin-Induced Cardiomyopathy by Upregulating Survivin Expression via the miR-199a-3p-Akt-Sp1/p53 Signaling Pathway. *Int. J. Mol. Sci.* **2021**, *22*, 7102. [CrossRef] [PubMed]
53. Ren, S.; Pan, L.; Yang, L.; Niu, Z.; Wang, L.; Feng, H.; Yuan, M. miR-29a-3p transferred by mesenchymal stem cells-derived extracellular vesicles protects against myocardial injury after severe acute pancreatitis. *Life Sci.* **2021**, *272*, 119189. [CrossRef]
54. Zhong, Z.; Tian, Y.; Luo, X.; Zou, J.; Wu, L.; Tian, J. Extracellular Vesicles Derived From Human Umbilical Cord Mesenchymal Stem Cells Protect Against DOX-Induced Heart Failure Through the miR-100-5p/NOX4 Pathway. *Front. Bioeng. Biotechnol.* **2021**, *9*, 703241. [CrossRef]
55. Diao, L.; Zhang, Q. Transfer of lncRNA UCA1 by hUCMSCs-derived exosomes protects against hypoxia/reoxygenation injury through impairing miR-143-targeted degradation of Bcl-2. *Aging* **2021**, *13*, 5967–5985. [CrossRef]
56. Li, K.S.; Bai, Y.; Li, J.; Li, S.L.; Pan, J.; Cheng, Y.Q.; Li, K.; Wang, Z.G.; Ji, W.J.; Zhou, Q.; et al. LncRNA HCP5 in hBMSC-derived exosomes alleviates myocardial ischemia reperfusion injury by sponging miR-497 to activate IGF1/PI3K/AKT pathway. *Int. J. Cardiol.* **2021**, *342*, 72–81. [CrossRef]
57. Zhang, C.; Wang, H.; Li, J.; Ma, L. Circular RNA Involvement in the Protective Effect of Human Umbilical Cord Mesenchymal Stromal Cell-Derived Extracellular Vesicles Against Hypoxia/Reoxygenation Injury in Cardiac Cells. *Front. Cardiovasc. Med.* **2021**, *8*, 626878. [CrossRef]
58. El Harane, N.; Kervadec, A.; Bellamy, V.; Pidial, L.; Neametalla, H.J.; Perier, M.C.; Lima Correa, B.; Thiébault, L.; Cagnard, N.; Duché, A.; et al. Acellular therapeutic approach for heart failure: In vitro production of extracellular vesicles from human cardiovascular progenitors. *Eur. Heart J.* **2018**, *39*, 1835–1847. [CrossRef] [PubMed]

59. Ni, J.; Liu, Y.; Kang, L.; Wang, L.; Han, Z.; Wang, K.; Xu, B.; Gu, R. Human trophoblast-derived exosomes attenuate doxorubicin-induced cardiac injury by regulating miR-200b and downstream Zeb1. *J. Nanobiotechnol.* **2020**, *18*, 171. [CrossRef]
60. Ni, J.; Liu, Y.; Wang, K.; Wu, M.; Kang, L.; Sha, D.; Xu, B.; Gu, R. Trophoblast Stem-Cell-Derived Exosomes Improve Doxorubicin-Induced Dilated Cardiomyopathy by Modulating the let-7i/YAP Pathway. *Mol. Ther. Nucleic Acids* **2020**, *22*, 948–956. [CrossRef]
61. Khan, M.; Nickoloff, E.; Abramova, T.; Johnson, J.; Verma, S.K.; Krishnamurthy, P.; Mackie, A.R.; Vaughan, E.; Garikipati, V.N.; Benedict, C.; et al. Embryonic stem cell-derived exosomes promote endogenous repair mechanisms and enhance cardiac function following myocardial infarction. *Circ. Res.* **2015**, *117*, 52–64. [CrossRef] [PubMed]
62. Masuda, H.; Tanaka, R.; Fujimura, S.; Ishikawa, M.; Akimaru, H.; Shizuno, T.; Sato, A.; Okada, Y.; Iida, Y.; Itoh, J.; et al. Vasculogenic conditioning of peripheral blood mononuclear cells promotes endothelial progenitor cell expansion and phenotype transition of anti-inflammatory macrophage and T lymphocyte to cells with regenerative potential. *J. Am. Heart Assoc.* **2014**, *3*, e000743. [CrossRef] [PubMed]
63. Salybekov, A.A.; Kawaguchi, A.T.; Masuda, H.; Vorateera, K.; Okada, C.; Asahara, T. Regeneration-associated cells improve recovery from myocardial infarction through enhanced vasculogenesis, anti-inflammation, and cardiomyogenesis. *PLoS ONE* **2018**, *13*, e0203244.
64. Salybekov, A.A.; Salybekova, A.; Sheng, Y.; Shinozaki, Y.; Yokoyama, K.; Kobayashi, S.; Asahara, T. Extracellular Vesicles Derived From Regeneration Associated Cells Preserve Heart Function After Ischemia-Induced Injury. *Front. Cardiovasc. Med.* **2021**, *8*, 754254. [CrossRef]
65. Milano, G.; Biemmi, V.; Lazzarini, E.; Balbi, C.; Ciullo, A.; Bolis, S.; Ameri, P.; Di Silvestre, D.; Mauri, P.; Barile, L.; et al. Intravenous administration of cardiac progenitor cell-derived exosomes protects against doxorubicin/trastuzumab-induced cardiac toxicity. *Cardiovasc. Res.* **2020**, *116*, 383–392. [CrossRef]
66. Barile, L.; Lionetti, V.; Cervio, E.; Matteucci, M.; Gherghiceanu, M.; Popescu, L.M.; Torre, T.; Siclari, F.; Moccetti, T.; Vassalli, G. Extracellular vesicles from human cardiac progenitor cells inhibit cardiomyocyte apoptosis and improve cardiac function after myocardial infarction. *Cardiovasc. Res.* **2014**, *103*, 530–541. [CrossRef]
67. Gallet, R.; Dawkins, J.; Valle, J.; Simsolo, E.; De Couto, G.; Middleton, R.; Tseliou, E.; Luthringer, D.; Kreke, M.; Smith, R.R.; et al. Exosomes secreted by cardiosphere-derived cells reduce scarring, attenuate adverse remodelling, and improve function in acute and chronic porcine myocardial infarction. *Eur. Heart J.* **2017**, *38*, 201–211. [CrossRef]
68. Gao, L.; Wang, L.; Wei, Y.; Krishnamurthy, P.; Walcott, G.P.; Menasché, P.; Zhang, J. Exosomes secreted by hiPSC-derived cardiac cells improve recovery from myocardial infarction in swine. *Sci. Transl. Med.* **2020**, *12*, eaay1318. [CrossRef]
69. Caby, M.P.; Lankar, D.; Vincendeau-Scherrer, C.; Raposo, G.; Bonnerot, C. Exosomal-like vesicles are present in human blood plasma. *Int. Immunol.* **2005**, *17*, 879–887. [CrossRef]
70. Lassen, T.R.; Just, J.; Hjortbak, M.V.; Jespersen, N.R.; Stenz, K.T.; Gu, T.; Yan, Y.; Su, J.; Hansen, J.; Bæk, R.; et al. Cardioprotection by remote ischemic conditioning is transferable by plasma and mediated by extracellular vesicles. *Basic Res. Cardiol.* **2021**, *116*, 16. [CrossRef]
71. Vicencio, J.M.; Yellon, D.M.; Sivaraman, V.; Das, D.; Boi-Doku, C.; Arjun, S.; Zheng, Y.; Riquelme, J.A.; Kearney, J.; Sharma, V.; et al. Plasma exosomes protect the myocardium from ischemia-reperfusion injury. *J. Am. Coll. Cardiol.* **2015**, *65*, 1525–1536. [CrossRef]
72. Wang, H.; Maimaitiaili, R.; Yao, J.; Xie, Y.; Qiang, S.; Hu, F.; Li, X.; Shi, C.; Jia, P.; Yang, H.; et al. Percutaneous Intracoronary Delivery of Plasma Extracellular Vesicles Protects the Myocardium Against Ischemia-Reperfusion Injury in Canis. *Hypertension* **2021**, *78*, 1541–1554. [CrossRef]
73. Jin, P.; Ding, L.; Wang, L.; Jiang, S.; Weng, J.; Gao, Y.; Fan, J.; Sun, L.-Z. Extracellular vesicles derived from myocardial infarction plasma inhibit BMSCs apoptosis and enhance cardiac function via AKT signaling pathway. *Int. Immunopharmacol.* **2021**, *96*, 107730. [CrossRef]
74. Yao, J.; Huang, K.; Zhu, D.; Chen, T.; Jiang, Y.; Zhang, J.; Mi, L.; Xuan, H.; Hu, S.; Li, J.; et al. A Minimally Invasive Exosome Spray Repairs Heart after Myocardial Infarction. *ACS Nano.* **2021**, *15*, 11099–11111. [CrossRef]
75. Liu, B.; Lee, B.W.; Nakanishi, K.; Villasante, A.; Williamson, R.; Metz, J.; Kim, J.; Kanai, M.; Bi, L.; Brown, K.; et al. Cardiac recovery via extended cell-free delivery of extracellular vesicles secreted by cardiomyocytes derived from induced pluripotent stem cells. *Nat. Biomed. Eng.* **2018**, *2*, 293–303. [CrossRef]
76. Xiao, J.; Pan, Y.; Li, X.H.; Yang, X.Y.; Feng, Y.L.; Tan, H.H.; Jiang, L.; Feng, J.; Yu, X.Y. Cardiac progenitor cell-derived exosomes prevent cardiomyocytes apoptosis through exosomal miR-21 by targeting PDCD4. *Cell Death Dis.* **2016**, *7*, e2277. [CrossRef]
77. Chen, C.H.; Hsu, S.Y.; Chiu, C.C.; Leu, S. MicroRNA-21 Mediates the Protective Effect of Cardiomyocyte-Derived Conditioned Medium on Ameliorating Myocardial Infarction in Rats. *Cells* **2019**, *8*, 935. [CrossRef]
78. Song, Y.; Zhang, C.; Zhang, J.; Jiao, Z.; Dong, N.; Wang, G.; Wang, Z.; Wang, L. Localized injection of miRNA-21-enriched extracellular vesicles effectively restores cardiac function after myocardial infarction. *Theranostics* **2019**, *9*, 2346–2360. [CrossRef]
79. Wei, Z.; Qiao, S.; Zhao, J.; Liu, Y.; Li, Q.; Wei, Z.; Dai, Q.; Kang, L.; Xu, B. miRNA-181a over-expression in mesenchymal stem cell-derived exosomes influenced inflammatory response after myocardial ischemia-reperfusion injury. *Life Sci.* **2019**, *232*, 116632. [CrossRef]
80. Lin, Y.N.; Mesquita, T.; Sanchez, L.; Chen, Y.H.; Liu, W.; Li, C.; Rogers, R.; Wang, Y.; Li, X.; Wu, D.; et al. Extracellular vesicles from immortalized cardiosphere-derived cells attenuate arrhythmogenic cardiomyopathy in desmoglein-2 mutant mice. *Eur. Heart J.* **2021**, *42*, 3558–3571. [CrossRef]

81. Chang, E.; Nayak, L.; Jain, M.K. Krüppel-like factors in endothelial cell biology. *Curr. Opin. Hematol.* **2017**, *24*, 224–229. [CrossRef] [PubMed]
82. Qiao, S.; Zhang, W.; Yin, Y.; Wei, Z.; Chen, F.; Zhao, J.; Sun, X.; Mu, D.; Xie, J.; Xu, B. Extracellular vesicles derived from Krüppel-Like Factor 2-overexpressing endothelial cells attenuate myocardial ischemia-reperfusion injury by preventing Ly6C(high) monocyte recruitment. *Theranostics* **2020**, *10*, 11562–11579. [CrossRef] [PubMed]
83. Zhang, W.; Chen, Z.; Qiao, S.; Chen, S.; Zheng, H.; Wei, X.; Li, Q.; Xu, B.; Huang, W. The effects of extracellular vesicles derived from Krüppel-Like Factor 2 overexpressing endothelial cells on the regulation of cardiac inflammation in the dilated cardiomyopathy. *J. Nanobiotechnol.* **2022**, *20*, 76. [CrossRef] [PubMed]
84. Yu, B.; Kim, H.W.; Gong, M.; Wang, J.; Millard, R.W.; Wang, Y.; Ashraf, M.; Xu, M. Exosomes secreted from GATA-4 overexpressing mesenchymal stem cells serve as a reservoir of anti-apoptotic microRNAs for cardioprotection. *Int. J. Cardiol.* **2015**, *182*, 349–360. [CrossRef] [PubMed]
85. Ma, J.; Zhao, Y.; Sun, L.; Sun, X.; Zhao, X.; Sun, X.; Qian, H.; Xu, W.; Zhu, W. Exosomes Derived from Akt-Modified Human Umbilical Cord Mesenchymal Stem Cells Improve Cardiac Regeneration and Promote Angiogenesis via Activating Platelet-Derived Growth Factor D. Stem. *Cells Transl. Med.* **2017**, *6*, 51–59. [CrossRef]
86. Ni, J.; Liu, X.; Yin, Y.; Zhang, P.; Xu, Y.-W.; Liu, Z. Exosomes Derived from TIMP2-Modified Human Umbilical Cord Mesenchymal Stem Cells Enhance the Repair Effect in Rat Model with Myocardial Infarction Possibly by the Akt/Sfrp2 Pathway. *Oxid. Med. Cell. Longev.* **2019**, *2019*, 1958941. [CrossRef]
87. Wang, X.; Chen, Y.; Zhao, Z.; Meng, Q.; Yu, Y.; Sun, J.; Yang, Z.; Chen, Y.; Li, J.; Ma, T.; et al. Engineered Exosomes With Ischemic Myocardium-Targeting Peptide for Targeted Therapy in Myocardial Infarction. *J. Am. Heart Assoc.* **2018**, *7*, e008737. [CrossRef]
88. Mentkowski, K.I.; Lang, J.K. Exosomes Engineered to Express a Cardiomyocyte Binding Peptide Demonstrate Improved Cardiac Retention in Vivo. *Sci. Rep.* **2019**, *9*, 10041. [CrossRef]
89. Gonzalez-King, H.; García, N.A.; Ontoria-Oviedo, I.; Ciria, M.; Montero, J.A.; Sepúlveda, P. Hypoxia Inducible Factor-1α Potentiates Jagged 1-Mediated Angiogenesis by Mesenchymal Stem Cell-Derived Exosomes. *Stem Cells* **2017**, *35*, 1747–1759. [CrossRef]
90. Lee, J.H.; Yoon, Y.M.; Lee, S.H. Hypoxic Preconditioning Promotes the Bioactivities of Mesenchymal Stem Cells via the HIF-1α-GRP78-Akt Axis. *Int. J. Mol. Sci.* **2017**, *18*, 1320. [CrossRef]
91. Wu, Q.; Wang, J.; Tan, W.L.W.; Jiang, Y.; Wang, S.; Li, Q.; Yu, X.; Tan, J.; Liu, S.; Zhang, P.; et al. Extracellular vesicles from human embryonic stem cell-derived cardiovascular progenitor cells promote cardiac infarct healing through reducing cardiomyocyte death and promoting angiogenesis. *Cell Death Dis.* **2020**, *11*, 354. [CrossRef]
92. Sun, L.; Zhu, W.; Zhao, P.; Wang, Q.; Fan, B.; Zhu, Y.; Lu, Y.; Chen, Q.; Zhang, J.; Zhang, F. Long noncoding RNA UCA1 from hypoxia-conditioned hMSC-derived exosomes: A novel molecular target for cardioprotection through miR-873-5p/XIAP axis. *Cell Death Dis.* **2020**, *11*, 696. [CrossRef]
93. Li, Q.; Xu, Y.; Lv, K.; Wang, Y.; Zhong, Z.; Xiao, C.; Zhu, K.; Ni, C.; Wang, K.; Kong, M.; et al. Small extracellular vesicles containing miR-486-5p promote angiogenesis after myocardial infarction in mice and nonhuman primates. *Sci. Transl. Med.* **2021**, *13*, eabb0202. [CrossRef]
94. Jung, J.H.; Ikeda, G.; Tada, Y.; von Bornstädt, D.; Santoso, M.R.; Wahlquist, C.; Rhee, S.; Jeon, Y.J.; Yu, A.C.; O'brien, C.G.; et al. miR-106a-363 cluster in extracellular vesicles promotes endogenous myocardial repair via Notch3 pathway in ischemic heart injury. *Basic Res. Cardiol.* **2021**, *116*, 19. [CrossRef]
95. Zhuang, L.; Xia, W.; Chen, D.; Ye, Y.; Hu, T.; Li, S.; Hou, M. Exosomal LncRNA-NEAT1 derived from MIF-treated mesenchymal stem cells protected against doxorubicin-induced cardiac senescence through sponging miR-221-3p. *J. Nanobiotechnol.* **2020**, *18*, 157. [CrossRef]
96. Huang, P.; Wang, L.; Li, Q.; Tian, X.; Xu, J.; Xu, J.; Xiong, Y.; Chen, G.; Qian, H.; Jin, C.; et al. Atorvastatin enhances the therapeutic efficacy of mesenchymal stem cells-derived exosomes in acute myocardial infarction via up-regulating long non-coding RNA H19. *Cardiovasc. Res.* **2020**, *116*, 353–367. [CrossRef]
97. Zheng, H.; Liang, X.; Han, Q.; Shao, Z.; Zhang, Y.; Shi, L.; Hong, Y.; Li, W.; Mai, C.; Mo, Q.; et al. Hemin enhances the cardioprotective effects of mesenchymal stem cell-derived exosomes against infarction via amelioration of cardiomyocyte senescence. *J. Nanobiotechnol.* **2021**, *19*, 332. [CrossRef] [PubMed]
98. Youn, S.W.; Li, Y.; Kim, Y.M.; Sudhahar, V.; Abdelsaid, K.; Kim, H.W.; Liu, Y.; Fulton, D.J.; Ashraf, M.; Tang, Y.; et al. Modification of Cardiac Progenitor Cell-Derived Exosomes by miR-322 Provides Protection against Myocardial Infarction through Nox2-Dependent Angiogenesis. *Antioxidants* **2019**, *8*, 18. [CrossRef]
99. Ma, T.; Chen, Y.; Chen, Y.; Meng, Q.; Sun, J.; Shao, L.; Yu, Y.; Huang, H.; Hu, Y.; Yang, Z.; et al. MicroRNA-132, Delivered by Mesenchymal Stem Cell-Derived Exosomes, Promote Angiogenesis in Myocardial Infarction. *Stem. Cells Int.* **2018**, *2018*, 3290372. [CrossRef]
100. Kang, J.Y.; Park, H.; Kim, H.; Mun, D.; Park, H.; Yun, N.; Joung, B. Human peripheral blood-derived exosomes for microRNA delivery. *Int. J. Mol. Med.* **2019**, *43*, 2319–2328. [CrossRef]
101. Wan, Z.; Zhao, L.; Lu, F.; Gao, X.; Dong, Y.; Zhao, Y.; Wei, M.; Yang, G.; Xing, C.; Liu, L. Mononuclear phagocyte system blockade improves therapeutic exosome delivery to the myocardium. *Theranostics* **2020**, *10*, 218–230. [CrossRef] [PubMed]

102. Liu, S.; Chen, X.; Bao, L.; Liu, T.; Yuan, P.; Yang, X.; Qiu, X.; Gooding, J.J.; Bai, Y.; Xiao, J.; et al. Treatment of infarcted heart tissue via the capture and local delivery of circulating exosomes through antibody-conjugated magnetic nanoparticles. *Nat. Biomed. Eng.* **2020**, *4*, 1063–1075. [CrossRef] [PubMed]
103. Kanki, S.; Jaalouk, D.E.; Lee, S.; Yu, A.Y.C.; Gannon, J.; Lee, R.T. Identification of targeting peptides for ischemic myocardium by in vivo phage display. *J. Mol. Cell. Cardiol.* **2011**, *50*, 841–848. [CrossRef] [PubMed]
104. Vandergriff, A.; Huang, K.; Shen, D.; Hu, S.; Hensley, M.T.; Caranasos, T.G.; Qian, L.; Cheng, K. Targeting regenerative exosomes to myocardial infarction using cardiac homing peptide. *Theranostics* **2018**, *8*, 1869–1878. [CrossRef]
105. Zhu, L.P.; Tian, T.; Wang, J.Y.; He, J.N.; Chen, T.; Pan, M.; Xu, L.; Zhang, H.X.; Qiu, X.T.; Li, C.C.; et al. Hypoxia-elicited mesenchymal stem cell-derived exosomes facilitates cardiac repair through miR-125b-mediated prevention of cell death in myocardial infarction. *Theranostics* **2018**, *8*, 6163–6177. [CrossRef]
106. Antes, T.J.; Middleton, R.C.; Luther, K.M.; Ijichi, T.; Peck, K.A.; Liu, W.J.; Valle, J.; Echavez, A.K.; Marbán, E. Targeting extracellular vesicles to injured tissue using membrane cloaking and surface display. *J. Nanobiotechnol.* **2018**, *16*, 61. [CrossRef]
107. Lv, K.; Li, Q.; Zhang, L.; Wang, Y.; Zhong, Z.; Zhao, J.; Lin, X.; Wang, J.; Zhu, K.; Xiao, C.; et al. Incorporation of small extracellular vesicles in sodium alginate hydrogel as a novel therapeutic strategy for myocardial infarction. *Theranostics* **2019**, *9*, 7403–7416. [CrossRef]
108. Zhang, Y.; Cai, Z.; Shen, Y.; Lu, Q.; Gao, W.; Zhong, X.; Yao, K.; Yuan, J.; Liu, H. Hydrogel-load exosomes derived from dendritic cells improve cardiac function via Treg cells and the polarization of macrophages following myocardial infarction. *J. Nanobiotechnol.* **2021**, *19*, 271. [CrossRef]
109. Chen, C.W.; Wang, L.L.; Zaman, S.; Gordon, J.; Arisi, M.F.; Venkataraman, C.M.; Chung, J.J.; Hung, G.; Gaffey, A.C.; Spruce, L.A.; et al. Sustained release of endothelial progenitor cell-derived extracellular vesicles from shear-thinning hydrogels improves angiogenesis and promotes function after myocardial infarction. *Cardiovasc. Res.* **2018**, *114*, 1029–1040. [CrossRef]
110. Chung, J.J.; Han, J.; Wang, L.L.; Arisi, M.F.; Zaman, S.; Gordon, J.; Li, E.; Kim, S.T.; Tran, Z.; Chen, C.W.; et al. Delayed delivery of endothelial progenitor cell-derived extracellular vesicles via shear thinning gel improves postinfarct hemodynamics. *J. Thorac. Cardiovasc. Surg.* **2020**, *159*, 1825–1835.e1822. [CrossRef]
111. Kim, H.; Mun, D.; Kang, J.-Y.; Lee, S.-H.; Yun, N.; Joung, B. Improved cardiac-specific delivery of RAGE siRNA within small extracellular vesicles engineered to express intense cardiac targeting peptide attenuates myocarditis. *Mol. Ther. Nucleic Acids* **2021**, *24*, 1024–1032. [CrossRef]
112. Wei, Z.; Chen, Z.; Zhao, Y.; Fan, F.; Xiong, W.; Song, S.; Yin, Y.; Hu, J.; Yang, K.; Yang, L.; et al. Mononuclear phagocyte system blockade using extracellular vesicles modified with CD47 on membrane surface for myocardial infarction reperfusion injury treatment. *Biomaterials* **2021**, *275*, 121000. [CrossRef]
113. Li, Z.; Li, Y.; Gao, J.; Fu, Y.; Hua, P.; Jing, Y.; Cai, M.; Wang, H.; Tong, T. The role of CD47-SIRPα immune checkpoint in tumor immune evasion and innate immunotherapy. *Life Sci.* **2021**, *273*, 119150. [CrossRef]
114. Shao, L.; Zhang, Y.; Pan, X.; Liu, B.; Liang, C.; Zhang, Y.; Wang, Y.; Yan, B.; Xie, W.; Sun, Y.; et al. Knockout of beta-2 microglobulin enhances cardiac repair by modulating exosome imprinting and inhibiting stem cell-induced immune rejection. *Cell. Mol. Life Sci.* **2020**, *77*, 937–952. [CrossRef]
115. Wang, X.; Hu, S.; Li, J.; Zhu, D.; Wang, Z.; Cores, J.; Cheng, K.; Liu, G.; Huang, K. Extruded Mesenchymal Stem Cell Nanovesicles Are Equally Potent to Natural Extracellular Vesicles in Cardiac Repair. *ACS Appl. Mater. Interfaces* **2021**, *13*, 55767–55779. [CrossRef]
116. Zhang, Y.; Yang, N.; Huang, X.; Zhu, Y.; Gao, S.; Liu, Z.; Cao, F.; Wang, Y. Melatonin Engineered Adipose-Derived Biomimetic Nanovesicles Regulate Mitochondrial Functions and Promote Myocardial Repair in Myocardial Infarction. *Front. Cardiovasc. Med.* **2022**, *9*, 789203. [CrossRef]
117. Lee, J.R.; Park, B.W.; Kim, J.; Choo, Y.W.; Kim, H.Y.; Yoon, J.K.; Kim, H.; Hwang, J.W.; Kang, M.; Kwon, S.P.; et al. Nanovesicles derived from iron oxide nanoparticles-incorporated mesenchymal stem cells for cardiac repair. *Sci. Adv.* **2020**, *6*, eaaz0952. [CrossRef]
118. Li, Q.; Song, Y.; Wang, Q.; Chen, J.; Gao, J.; Tan, H.; Li, S.; Wu, Y.; Yang, H.; Huang, H.; et al. Engineering extracellular vesicles with platelet membranes fusion enhanced targeted therapeutic angiogenesis in a mouse model of myocardial ischemia reperfusion. *Theranostics* **2021**, *11*, 3916–3931. [CrossRef] [PubMed]
119. Li, Q.; Huang, Z.; Wang, Q.; Gao, J.; Chen, J.; Tan, H.; Li, S.; Wang, Z.; Weng, X.; Yang, H.; et al. Targeted immunomodulation therapy for cardiac repair by platelet membrane engineering extracellular vesicles via hitching peripheral monocytes. *Biomaterials* **2022**, *284*, 121529. [CrossRef] [PubMed]
120. Zhang, N.; Song, Y.; Huang, Z.; Chen, J.; Tan, H.; Yang, H.; Fan, M.; Li, Q.; Wang, Q.; Gao, J.; et al. Monocyte mimics improve mesenchymal stem cell-derived extracellular vesicle homing in a mouse MI/RI model. *Biomaterials* **2020**, *255*, 120168. [CrossRef] [PubMed]
121. Yao, C.; Wu, W.; Tang, H.; Jia, X.; Tang, J.; Ruan, X.; Li, F.; Leong, D.T.; Luo, D.; Yang, D. Self-assembly of stem cell membrane-camouflaged nanocomplex for microRNA-mediated repair of myocardial infarction injury. *Biomaterials* **2020**, *257*, 120256. [CrossRef]
122. Hu, C.M.; Fang, R.H.; Wang, K.C.; Luk, B.T.; Thamphiwatana, S.; Dehaini, D.; Nguyen, P.; Angsantikul, P.; Wen, C.H.; Kroll, A.V.; et al. Nanoparticle biointerfacing by platelet membrane cloaking. *Nature* **2015**, *526*, 118–121. [CrossRef]

123. Li, F.; Liu, D.; Liu, M.; Ji, Q.; Zhang, B.; Mei, Q.; Cheng, Y.; Zhou, S. Tregs biomimetic nanoparticle to reprogram inflammatory and redox microenvironment in infarct tissue to treat myocardial ischemia reperfusion injury in mice. *J. Nanobiotechnol.* **2022**, *20*, 251. [CrossRef]
124. Tian, C.; Yang, Y.; Bai, B.; Wang, S.; Liu, M.; Sun, R.C.; Yu, T.; Chu, X.M. Potential of exosomes as diagnostic biomarkers and therapeutic carriers for doxorubicin-induced cardiotoxicity. *Int. J. Biol. Sci.* **2021**, *17*, 1328–1338. [CrossRef]
125. Tseliou, E.; Fouad, J.; Reich, H.; Slipczuk, L.; De Couto, G.; Aminzadeh, M.; Middleton, R.; Valle, J.; Weixin, L.; Marbán, E. Fibroblasts Rendered Antifibrotic, Antiapoptotic, and Angiogenic by Priming With Cardiosphere-Derived Extracellular Membrane Vesicles. *J. Am. Coll. Cardiol.* **2015**, *66*, 599–611. [CrossRef]
126. Chen, J.; Zhou, D.; Nie, Z.; Lu, L.; Lin, Z.; Zhou, D.; Zhang, Y.; Long, X.; Fan, S.; Xu, T. A scalable coaxial bioprinting technology for mesenchymal stem cell microfiber fabrication and high extracellular vesicle yield. *Biofabrication* **2021**, *14*, 015012. [CrossRef]
127. Villarreal-Leal, R.A.; Cooke, J.P.; Corradetti, B. Biomimetic and immunomodulatory therapeutics as an alternative to natural exosomes for vascular and cardiac applications. *Nanomedicine* **2021**, *35*, 102385. [CrossRef] [PubMed]

pharmaceutics

Article

CCR7 Mediates Dendritic-Cell-Derived Exosome Migration and Improves Cardiac Function after Myocardial Infarction

Youming Zhang [1,2], Wei Gao [3], Jie Yuan [3], Xin Zhong [3], Kang Yao [3], Rong Luo [1,*] and Haibo Liu [1,*]

1 Department of Cardiology, Qingpu Branch of Zhongshan Hospital, Fudan University, Shanghai 201700, China
2 Department of Cardiology, Shanghai East Hospital, School of Medicine, Tongji University, Shanghai 200100, China
3 Shanghai Institute of Cardiovascular Diseases, Zhongshan Hospital, Fudan University, Shanghai 200030, China
* Correspondence: luo.rong@qphospital.com (R.L.); haiboliu13@fudan.edu.cn (H.L.)

Abstract: Dendritic cells (DCs) play key roles in promoting wound healing after myocardial infarction (MI). Our previous studies have shown that exosomes derived from DCs (DEXs) could migrate to lymphoid tissue and improve cardiac function post-MI by activating CD4⁺ T cells; however, the mechanism of DEXs' migration to lymphoid tissue and the improvement of cardiac function are still unknown. In our study, we found that CCR7 expression significantly increased in MI-DEXs compared with control-DEXs; meanwhile, CCL19 and CCL21, the ligands of CCR7, significantly increased in the serum of MI-model mice. Subsequently, we overexpressed and knocked down CCR7 in MI-DEXs and found that overexpressed CCR7 enhanced the migration of MI-DEXs to the spleen; however, CCR7 knockdown attenuated MI-DEXs' migration according to near-IR fluorescence imaging. Furthermore, overexpressed CCR7 in MI-DEXs enhanced the MI-DEXs' improvement of cardiac function after MI; however, CCR7-knockdown MI-DEXs attenuated this improvement. In addition, after DEXs' migration to the spleen, MI-DEXs activated CD4⁺ T cells and induced the expression of IL-4 and IL-10, which were significantly increased in the MI-DEX group compared with the control group. In conclusion, CCR7 could mediate DEXs' migration to the spleen and improve cardiac function after MI, and we found that the mechanism was partly via activation of CD4⁺ T cells and secretion of IL-4 and IL-10. Our study presented an innovative method for improving cardiac function by enhancing the migration ability of MI-DEXs after MI, while CCR7 could be a potential candidate for MI-DEX bioengineering to enhance migration.

Keywords: CCR7; dendritic cells; exosomes; CD4⁺ T cells; myocardial infarction

Citation: Zhang, Y.; Gao, W.; Yuan, J.; Zhong, X.; Yao, K.; Luo, R.; Liu, H. CCR7 Mediates Dendritic-Cell-Derived Exosome Migration and Improves Cardiac Function after Myocardial Infarction. *Pharmaceutics* **2023**, *15*, 461. https://doi.org/10.3390/pharmaceutics15020461

Academic Editor: Dong Hyun Kim

Received: 1 November 2022
Revised: 15 January 2023
Accepted: 20 January 2023
Published: 30 January 2023

1. Introduction

Though considerable progress has been made in the diagnosis and treatment of myocardial infarction (MI), which is still the leading cause of death worldwide [1], the progression of MI often leads to adverse ventricular remodeling, eventually resulting in ventricular dysfunction and death [2–4]. The immune system plays a crucial role in the ventricular remodeling process and contributes to both the inflammatory and reparative phases [5–7]. Our previous study showed that exosomes derived from dendritic cells (DCs) could migrate to lymphoid tissue and improve cardiac function post-MI by activating CD4⁺ T cells [8]. Prolonging the retention time of DC-derived exosomes (DEXs) could result in better consequences for immunoregulation and enhance its therapeutic effects [9]. However, whether MI-DEXs' migration could affect their therapeutic effects in addition to the mechanism of DEXs' migration to lymphoid tissue is still unclear.

As the central immunoregulators in innate and adaptive immunity, DCs play crucial roles in facilitating wound healing after MI [10]. Mice depleted of DCs induced severe inflammatory reactions and worse cardiac remodeling after MI compared with the control group, which suggested that DCs have played protective roles in the pro-inflammatory response to MI [11]. In addition, infarct lysate-primed DCs activated infarct tissue-specific regulatory T cells in lymph nodes, spleen, and infarcted myocardium and facilitated wound remodeling, preserved left ventricular systolic function, and improved survival after MI [12,13]. These results suggest DCs play a protective role after MI and that their therapeutic effect is partly because of $CD4^+$ T cell activation.

Exosomes are small vesicles secreted by cells that contain proteins, DNA, and RNA and are considered messengers for cell-to-cell information exchange [14]. Exosomes from immune cells engage in intercellular communication in immune cells [15], while DEXs could also participate in antigen presentation [16] and migrate to lymphoid tissues after MI [8,9].

Chemokine receptors (CCR) and their ligands (CCL) are key factors in immune cells' migration. DCs highly express CCR7 after capturing antigens [17]. CCR7, together with its ligands, CCL19 and CCL21, promote the accurate migration of DCs to lymphocyte tissues [18]. However, whether CCR7 contributes to DEXs' migration is still unknown.

In our study, we explored the role of CCR7 and its ligands CCL19/CCL21 in DEXs' migration, including the crosstalk between DEXs' migration and its therapeutic effects on cardiac function after MI, and provided a new candidate for protecting cardiac function after MI.

2. Materials and Methods

2.1. Animals

We purchased wild-type, male C57BL/6 mice from the Shanghai Laboratory Animal Center, which we used for bone marrow-derived dendritic cell (BMDC) culture and making MI models. We raised all the mice without pathogens with a 12:12-h light–dark cycle, 22 ± 1 °C room temperature, 65–70% humidity, and free access to food and water. The Institutional Review Board of Zhongshan Hospital of Fudan University and the Shanghai Institutes of Biological Sciences-CAS (A5894-01, January 2017) approved this study, and the animal research complied with the standards of animal welfare in China.

2.2. MI Model Induction and Treatments

We used a rodent ventilator (Harvard Bioscience, Inc., Cambridge, MA, USA) for mouse ventilation and an isoflurane delivery system, and we used 2% isoflurane inhalation (RWD Life Science, Shenzhen, China) (Harvard Bioscience, Inc., Cambridge, MA, USA) for anesthetizing. Then, we opened the mouse chests and exposed the hearts. We ligated the left coronary artery (LCA) with an 8–0 silk suture. We observed the blanching of the myocardium in the infarcted area, which we determined to be myocardial infarction. We used mice receiving the same operation but without LCA ligation as the sham operation group. Finally, we evacuated the air, sutured the skin, and put the mice back in the cage before waiting for them to wake up. After 24 h of MI, we injected different DEXs or saline via the mouse tail vein.

2.3. Cell Isolation and Culture

We isolated BMDCs from the femurs of C57BL/6 mice following methods described in our previous study (8). Briefly, we sacrificed the mice and isolated the femurs; then, we washed bone marrow cells from the femurs and cultured them at 10^6 cells/mL in BD Falcon cell culture flasks (BD Biosciences, New York, NY, USA) in RPMI-1640 (Gibico, New York, NY, USA) containing 10% fetal bovine serum (FBS, Life Technologies, New York, NY, USA), 1% Penicillin/Streptomycin (Gibico, New York, NY, USA), 1 ng/mL IL-4, and 10 ng/mL granulocyte–macrophage colony-stimulating factor (both from R&D Systems, Minneapolis, MN, USA). We gently washed off non-adherent cells after 48 h and cultured the remaining loosely adherent clusters with media changes every 2 days. On day 7, we used medium without exosomes, and we collected and determined BMDCs using anti-mouse CD11c, CD40, CD80, and CD86 antibodies via flow cytometry. We collected the BMDCs' supernatants for DEX isolation.

We isolated splenic CD4$^+$ T cells from the spleens of different groups of mice using the EasySep^{TM} Mouse CD4$^+$ T Cell Isolation Kit and following the manufacturer's instructions.

2.4. Lentivirus Production and Infection

We purchased mouse CCR7 lentivirus, mouse CCR7 shRNA lentivirus, vector lentivirus, and scramble shRNA lentivirus from Genomeditech (Shanghai, China) Co., Ltd. We infected BMDCs with various plasmids using lentivirus according to the manufacturer's instructions.

2.5. Mimic MI Microenvironment

There were three methods to mimic the MI microenvironment, which were described in detail in our previous study [8]: (I) the supernatants of hypoxic primary rat cardiomyocytes; (II) the supernatants of infarcted mouse myocardium; (III) the supernatants of necrotic HL-1 cells. All three methods activate DCs in mice to a similar extent as MI. In the present study, we used the supernatants of necrotic HL-1 cells to mimic the MI microenvironment. The methods are described in detail in our previous study [8].

2.6. DEX Isolation and Characterization

We used ExoQuick-Tc^{TM} Exosome Precipitation Solution (System Biosciences Inc., Palo Alto, CA, USA) for the isolation of DEXs according to the manufacturer's instructions. We used CD63 and Alix to identify the DEX via Western blotting. We determined particle morphology via H7500 transmission electron microscopy (Hitachi, Tokyo, Japan). We determined particle size distributions via the Nanosight NS300 (Malvern, Malvern, UK).

2.7. Experimental Grouping

DEX groups: We divided DEX into four groups: (1) DEX group: DEX isolated from BMDCs treated with supernatant from normal cardiomyocytes; (2) MI-DEX group: DEX isolated from BMDCs treated with 100 μL/mL of supernatant from necrotic cardiomyocytes for 24 h; (3) CCR7^{over}-MI-DEX group: DEX from BMDCs treated with mouse CCR7 lentivirus for 72 h and then 100 μL/mL of supernatant from necrotic cardiomyocytes for 24 h; and (4) CCR7^{down}-MI-DEX group: DEX from BMDCs treated with mouse CCR7 shRNA lentivirus for 72 h and then 100 μL/mL of supernatant from necrotic cardiomyocytes for 24 h.

Animal groups: We divided the animals into six groups: (1) sham group: mice received the same surgical procedure but not ligation of the LCA; (2) MI group: mice received a saline injection after 24 h of MI; (3) DEX group: mice received a DEX injection after 24 h of MI; (4) MI-DEX group: mice received a MI-DEX injection after 24 h of MI; (5) CCR7^{over}-MI-DEX group: mice received a CCR7^{over}- MI-DEX injection after 24 h of MI; and (6) CCR7^{down}-MI-DEX group: mice received a CCR7^{down}-MI-DEX injection after 24 h of MI.

2.8. DEX Labeling and Fluorescence Imaging

We used DiR (Thermo Fisher Scientific, Waltham, MA, USA) for labeling DEX. Then, we used exosome spin columns (MW 3000; Thermo Fisher Scientific, Waltham, MA, USA) to remove the dye and purify DEX. Finally, we used the IVIS Spectrum System (PerkinElmer, Houston, TX, USA) to acquire the near-IR fluorescence images and compare the radiant efficiency of the body, spleen, and liver among different groups.

2.9. Echocardiography

On day 14, we examined the cardiac function by echocardiography (Vevo 2100, VisualSonics, Toronto, ON, Canada). We used M-mode tracings to measure LV end-systolic diameter (LVIDS) and LV end-diastolic diameter (LVIDD). We calculated percent fractional shortening (FS%) and ejection fraction (EF%) using Vevo 2100 workstation software.

2.10. Histology

On day 14, we sacrificed mice and fixed hearts with 4% paraformaldehyde for 24 h. Then, we cut the paraffin-embedded sample into 5 μm thick tissue sections, dewaxed in xylene (Sangon Biotech co., Ltd., Shanghai, China), rehydrated using ethanol, stained the sections using Masson's trichrome reagent, and finally sealed the sections using neutral gum. We calculated the wall thickness of the infarct zone and the fibrosis percentage of sections using Image J V1.53e software under an optical microscope. For each section, we took three measurements of different parts of the infarct area for thickness analysis.

2.11. Flow Cytometry Analysis

We used an Fc receptor blocker (CD16/32, BD Bioscience, New York, NY, USA) to incubate the sample to reduce non-specific antibody binding. We resuspended the freshly isolated samples and then stained them using CD45-AlexaFlour700 (Biolegend, San Diego, CA, USA), CD3-FITC (Biolegend, San Diego, CA, USA), and CD4-APC (Biolegend, San Diego, CA, USA) for 30 min at 4 °C. We performed flow cytometry using the CytoFLEX Platform (BeckmanCoulter, Brea, CA, USA) and analyzed the data with the CytExpert V2.4.0.28 software (BeckmanCoulter, Brea, CA, USA).

2.12. Quantitative Real-Time Polymerase Chain Reaction

We used a FastPure Cell/Tissue Total RNA Isolation Kit V2 (Vazyme Biotech, Nanjing, China) to extract total RNA from cells or tissue according to the manufacturer's instructions. We synthesized cDNA by reverse transcription from 500 ng of total RNA using the HiScript III RT SuperMix cDNA Synthesis Kit (Vazyme Biotech, Nanjing, China) according to the manufacturer's instructions. Then, we diluted the cDNA to 10:1 and amplified using the ChamQ Universal SYBR qPCR Master Mix Kit (Vazyme Biotech, Nanjing, China) following the manufacturer's instructions. We incubated the reaction in a 96-well plate at 95 °C for 3 min, followed by performing 40 PCR cycles at 95 °C for 5 s and 60 °C for 34 s on an Applied Biosystems 7500 Real-time PCR System (Thermo Fisher Scientific, Inc., Waltham, MA, USA). We collected and analyzed data using the $2^{\Delta\Delta Ct}$ method. First, we normalized the values of genes against GAPDH; then, we compared with the experimental controls. We synthesized primers at Tiangen Biochemical Technology Co., Ltd., and the sequences are listed below. TNF-α-F: AGAAACACAAGATGCTGGGACAGT; TNF-α-R: CCTTTGCAGAACTCAGGAATGG; IFN-γ-F: ATGAACGCTACACACTGCATC; IFN-γ-R: CCATCCTTTTGCCAGTTCCTC; IL-1β-F: GCAACTGTTCCTGAACTCAACT; IL-1β-R: ATCTTTTGGGGTCCGTCAACT; IL-6-F: TAGTCCTTCCTACCCCAATTTCC; IL-6-R: TTGGTCCTTAGCCACTCCTTC; IL-4-F: GGTCTCAACCCCCAGCTAGT; IL-4-R: GCCGATGATCTCTCTCAAGTGAT; IL-10-F: ACTGGCATGAGGATCAGCAG; IL-10-R: CTCCTTGATTTCTGGGGCCAT.

2.13. Statistical Analysis

Results are shown as mean ± SD (standard deviation). We used unpaired t-tests for the statistical analysis of the differences between two groups. We used one-way ANOVA followed by post hoc Tukey's multiple tests for the statistical analysis of the differences among three or more groups. We performed all the statistical analyses using GraphPad Prism V8.0.1. We considered $p < 0.05$ as statistically significant.

3. Results

3.1. CCR7 Was Highly Expressed in MI-DEXs as well as Its Ligand CCL19/21 in MI-Mouse Spleen

Previously, studies showed that CCR7 and its ligands, CCL19 and CCL21, promoted the accurate migration of DCs to lymphocyte tissues [18]. To investigate whether CCR7 also contributed to DEXs' migration, we generated MI-DEXs for further exploration. Figure 1A shows the ultrastructure of MI-DEXs via transmission electron microscopy (TEM). Figure 1B shows the expression of exosomal markers (CD63 and Alix). Figure 1C shows the particle size distributions of MI-DEXs determined by nanoparticle tracking analysis (NTA), and the mode diameter was 117 nm. Then, we explored CCR7 expression via Western blot. Our results showed that CCR7 was highly expressed in MI-DEXs (Figure 1D–E). Then, we also investigated its ligands, CCL19 and CCL21, in MI mouse serum and spleen (Figure 1F–J). We found that both CCL19 and CCL21 increased in MI mice, which indicated that MI-DEXs followed the same migration mechanisms as dendritic cells.

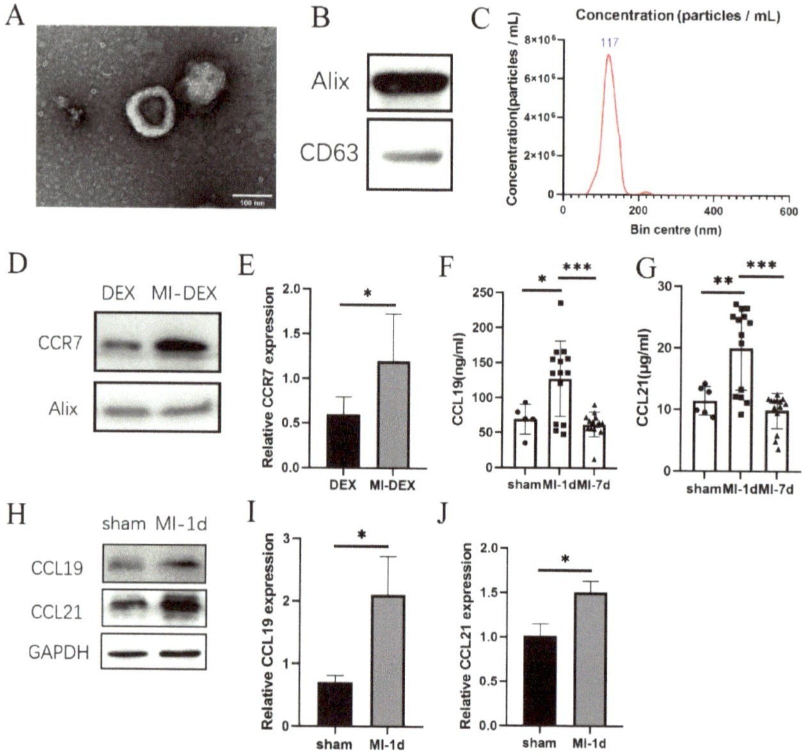

Figure 1. Characterization of MI-DEXs. Sample of MI-DEXs examined by transmission electron microscopy (TEM) image (**A**). CD63 and ALIX in MI-DEXs analyzed by Western blot analysis (**B**). The particle size distributions of MI-DEXs were analyzed by nanoparticle tracking, and the mode diameter was 117 nm (**C**). Expression of CCR7 in DEXs and MI-DEXs (**D**,**E**). $n = 3$–8. ELISA analysis of CCL19 and CCL21 in serum after MI (**F**,**G**). $n = 5$–15. Expression of CCL19 and CCL21 in the spleen after MI (**H**–**J**). $n = 3$–8, * $p < 0.05$, ** $p < 0.01$, *** $p < 0.001$.

3.2. CCR7-Mediated MI-DEX Migration to the Spleen after MI

We found CCR7 was highly expressed in MI-DEXs. To further identify CCR7's role in MI-DEXs' migration, we first compared the migration of DEXs or MI-DEXs via near-IR fluorescence imaging after MI. Figure 2A,B show that both DEXs and MI-DEXs migrated to the spleen and liver after MI; however, more MI-DEXs migrated to the spleen compared with DEXs on day 1 after injection. However, there was no significant difference between DEXs and MI-DEXs regarding migration to the liver. This indicated that CCR7 may affect the migration of MI-DEXs, mediating their movement to the spleen after MI. To further identify CCR7's role in MI-DEXs' migration, we knocked down or overexpressed CCR7 in BMDC individually, and our results showed that the overexpressed CCR7 MI-DEXs could increase MI-DEX migration to the spleen after MI, while CCR7 knockdown significantly impaired this progress. Our results indicated that CCR7 mediates MI-DEXs' migration, and CCR7 overexpression in MI-DEXs could enhance their migration to the spleen after MI.

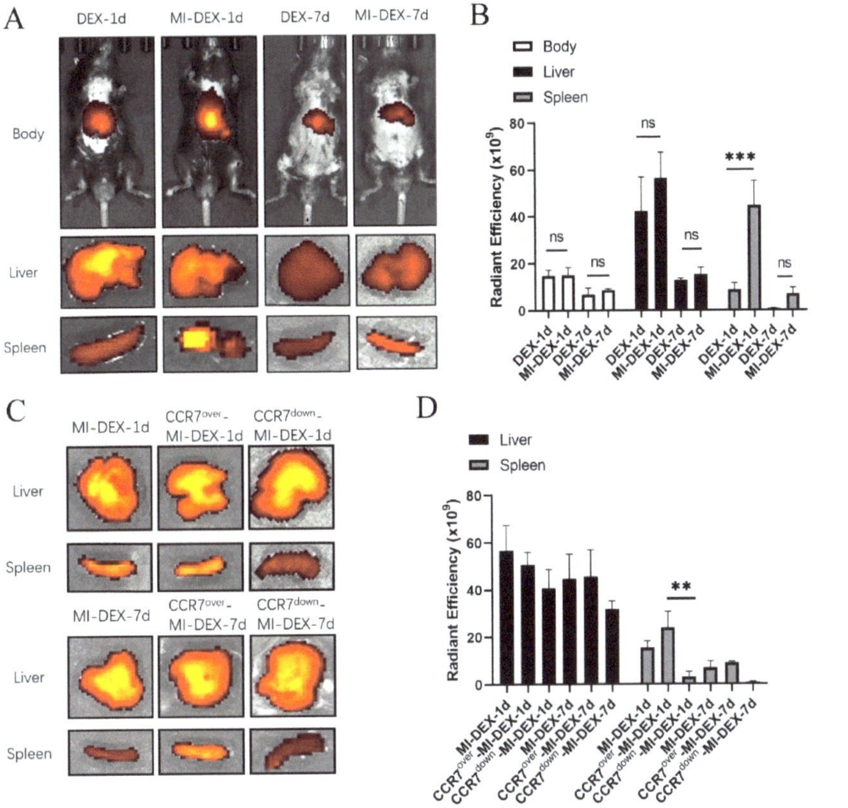

Figure 2. CCR7 mediates MI-DEXs' migration. Representative near-IR fluorescence images of the main organs and body after DEXs or MI-DEX injections (**A**). Analysis of the radiant efficiency of body, spleen, and liver (**B**). Representative near-IR fluorescence images of the liver and spleen after different MI-DEXs injections (**C**). Analysis of the radiant efficiency of the liver and spleen after different MI-DEX injections (**D**). $n = 3$, ** $p < 0.01$, *** $p < 0.001$.

3.3. *Enhancing the Migration Ability of MI-DEXs Can Improve Cardiac Function after MI*

Here, we explore the relationship between MI-DEXs' migration and cardiac function. Our previous study showed that MI-DEXs improve cardiac function post-MI by activating $CD4^+$ T cells in the spleen [8]. In addition, we found that overexpressed CCR7 could enhance the accumulation of MI-DEXs in the spleen via facilitating their migration; therefore, we needed to determine whether the accumulation of MI-DEXs would affect cardiac function post-MI. To do so, we used echocardiography and Masson staining to examine the cardiac function and remodeling on day 28 post-MI. The results showed that CCR7-overexpressed MI-DEXs received a better therapeutic effect, while CCR7 knockdown would impair the therapeutic effect (Figure 3A–E). Additionally, Masson staining results showed that MI-DEXs could retain LV-wall thickness but had no significant effect on fibrosis percentage (Figure 3F–H). In addition, though there was no significant difference among each MI-DEX group, the CCR7-knockdown group showed inferior LV-wall thickness, which may be the reason for its impaired echocardiography results.

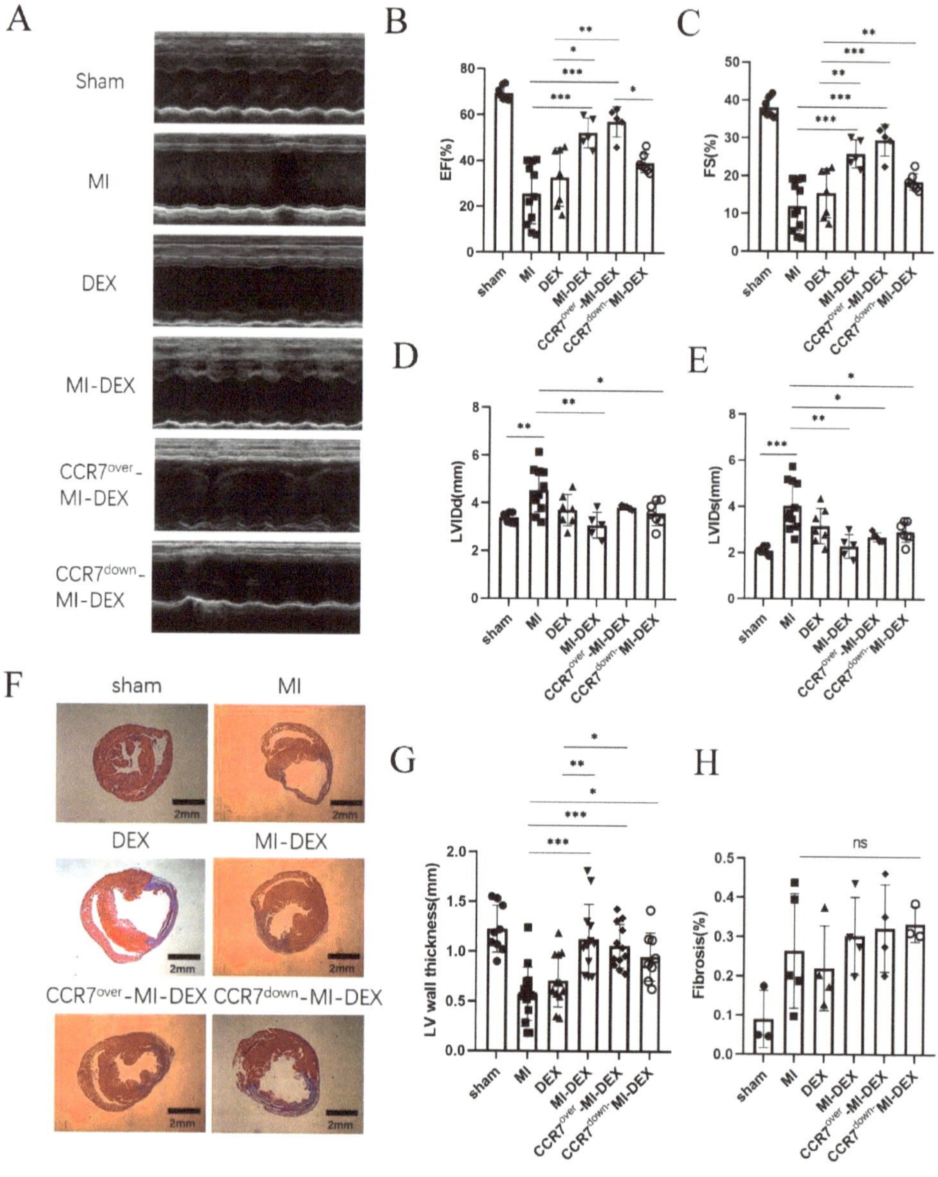

Figure 3. Enhancing MI-DEXs' migration improved cardiac function after MI. Images of MI-model mice analyzed with echocardiography in different groups (**A**). Analysis of left ventricular ejection fraction (LVEF) in different groups (**B**). Analysis of left ventricular fraction shortening (LVFS) (**C**). Analysis of left ventricular end-diastolic diameter (LVIDd) (**D**). © Analysis of left ventricular end-systolic diameter (LVID©) (**E**). $n = 5–10$. Representative images analyzed by Masson's trichrome staining in different groups (**F**). Infarct thickness (mm) in different groups (**G**). For each section, three measurements of different parts of the infarct area were taken for analysis. Analysis of fibrosis (%) in different groups (**H**). $n = 3–5$, * $p < 0.05$, ** $p < 0.01$, *** $p < 0.001$.

3.4. MI-DEXs' Activation of CD4^{+} T Cells in the Spleen

A previous study showed that the activation of CD4^{+} T cells played a key role in improving myocardial wound healing after MI [19]. To investigate the correlation between MI-DEXs and CD4^{+} T cells, we explored the CD4^{+} T cell percentage in the spleen's leukocytes via flow cytometry analysis. Our results showed that CD4^{+} T cells were slightly decreased in the spleen in the MI-model group compared with the sham group; however, they markedly increased in the MI-DEX injection group (Figure 4). These results indicated that MI-DEXs could activate CD4^{+} T cells after MI, improving cardiac function.

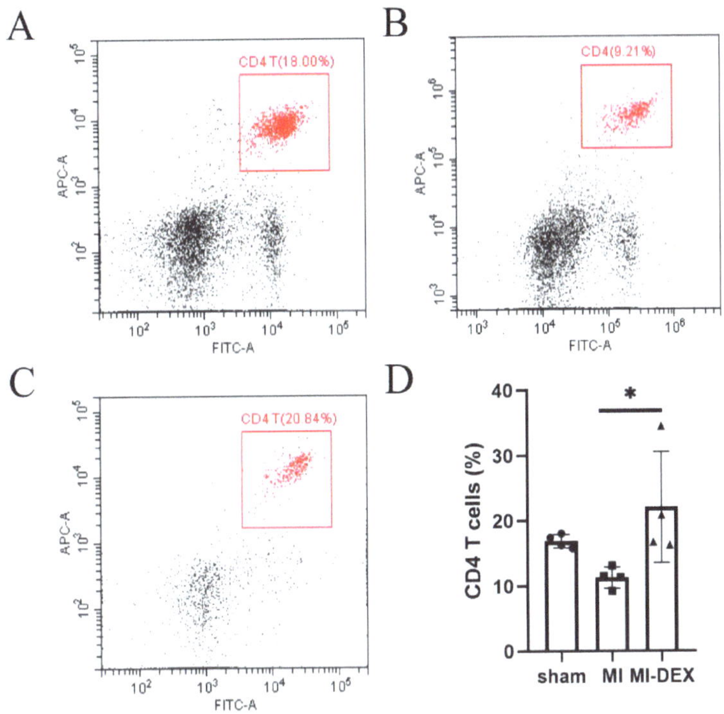

Figure 4. MI-DEXs raised the CD4^{+} T cell percentage in the spleen. Representative image of CD4^{+} T cells analyzed by flow cytometry in the sham group (**A**), MI group (**B**), and MI-DEX group (**C**); FITC-CD3; APC-CD4. Analysis of the proportions of CD45+, CD3+, and CD4+ T cells (**D**). $n = 4$, * $p < 0.05$.

3.5. MI-DEXs Induce an Anti-Inflammatory Cytokine Increase in Splenic CD4^{+} T Cells

We further explored the expression of cytokines in splenic CD4^{+} T cells in different groups and found the expression of IL-4 and IL-10 significantly increased in the MI-DEX group compared with the MI group (Figure 5). These results showed that injection of MI-DEXs could induce increases in the anti-inflammatory cytokines IL-4 and IL-10 in splenic CD4+ T cells after MI; moreover, the role of IL-4 and IL-10 as protective cytokines during cardiac remodeling after MI has been widely reported [20,21]. Thus, IL-4 and IL-10 could be functional cytokines for CD4^{+} T cells to protect cardiac function after MI. However, our results showed the expression of pro-inflammatory cytokines IFN-γ, IL-1β, and IL-6 was also significantly higher in the MI-DEX group, indicating a complex correlation between MI-DEXs and CD4^{+} T cells. Therefore, the underlying mechanism needs to be further explored.

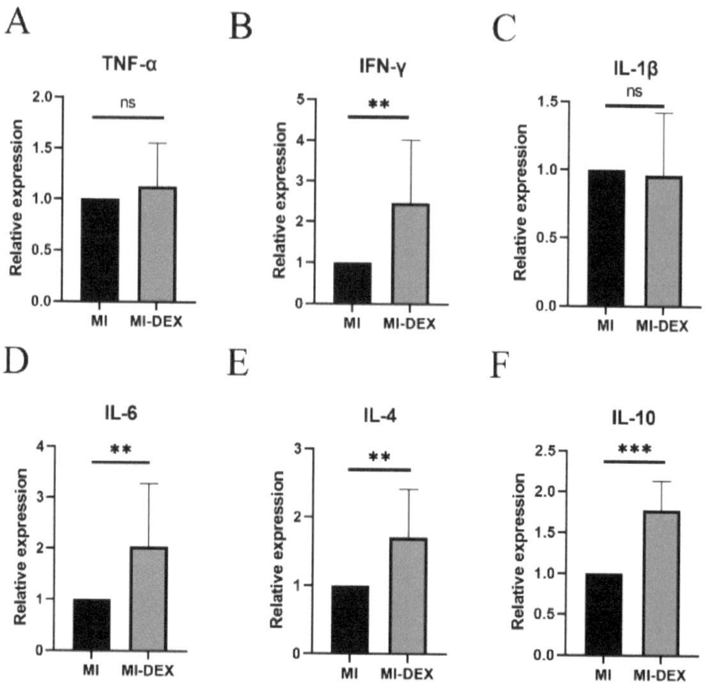

Figure 5. MI-DEXs increase anti-inflammatory cytokine expression in splenic CD4+ T cells. mRNA expression fold changes of different cytokines in different groups (**A–F**). $n = 6$–12, ** $p < 0.01$, *** $p < 0.001$; ns, no significance.

4. Discussion

Immune cells play a vital role in cardiac remodeling after MI, and our previous study showed that MI-DEXs could migrate to lymph tissues, such as the spleen and lymph nodes, improving cardiac function post-MI [8,9]. However, the mechanism of MI-DEXs' migration to lymph tissues remains unknown. A previous study showed that CCR7 interacted with its CCL19 and CCL21 ligands and guided DC trafficking toward lymph nodes via afferent lymphatics [18]. DEXs, as the exomes secreted by DCs, may have followed the same migration pattern after MI. In this study, we found CCR7 was highly expressed in MI-DEXs, as well as its ligands, CCL19/21, in the MI-mouse spleen. We also explored the role of CCR7 in MI-DEXs' migration to the spleen after MI and found that overexpressed CCR7 enhanced MI-DEXs' migration to the spleen after MI, while down-regulated CCR7 expression reduced the accumulation of MI-DEXs in the spleen. Moreover, we found that MI-DEXs' migration to the spleen could increase the infarct LV-wall thickness, decrease LV dilation, and improve cardiac function after MI. In addition, we explored the correlation between MI-DEXs and CD4+ T cells and found that MI-DEXs raised the percentage of CD4+ T cells in the spleen, as well as increasing the expression of anti-inflammatory cytokines IL-4 and IL-10 in splenic CD4+ T cells.

A previous study showed anti-inflammatory therapies could help with cardiac function recovery after MI [22], but the, inflammatory response is a double-edged sword in cardiac homeostasis and injury repair [10]. Therefore, it is important to find a proper way to mediate this process. Our previous study showed MI-DEXs could migrate to lymphoid tissue and improve cardiac function post-MI by activating CD4+ T cells [8]. Here, we focused on the mechanism of MI-DEXs' migration and found that overexpressed CCR7 in MI-DEXs enhanced MI-DEXs' migration to the spleen and improved cardiac function after MI, which indicated that modified MI-DEXs could be a useful candidate for post-MI non-cell therapy. Previous studies showed CCR7 could mediate inflammatory cells to participate in the inflammatory response [23], but our study demonstrated that CCR7 could mediate exosomes derived from DCs' migration to the spleen after MI.

We also explored the relationship between MI-DEXs and $CD4^+$ T cells. Flow cytometry analysis and qPCR results showed that MI-DEXs increased the percentage of CD4+ T cells in the spleen and increased IL-4 and IL-10 expression in splenic $CD4^+$ T cells. Previous research demonstrated the protective role of $CD4^+$ T cells in scar formation and LV dilation after MI [19]. In addition, specific cardiac antigen-triggering healing $CD4^+$ T cell activation was essential for cardiac-function recovery after MI [13]. Meanwhile, IL-4 and IL-10 were determined as protective cytokines for cardiac remodeling after MI [20,21]. Thus, our results indicated that MI-DEXs protected cardiac function via activation of $CD4^+$ T cells secreting IL-4 and IL-10 after MI. Our findings provide a new way to protect cardiac function after MI.

Exosomes act as important mediators of cell-to-cell communication and play crucial roles in regulating immune cells and immune responses post-MI [15]. A previous study showed exosomes can facilitate the reparative process of infarcted myocardium, while the exosomes' mechanism for preserving cardiac function was through the communication between lymphocytes and cardiac intrinsic cells [24]. Systemic delivery of immune-cell-derived exosomes is gradually being considered as a potent and effective new therapeutic option for healing damaged myocardium after MI [25]. In addition, because exosomes have natural material transportation properties and excellent biocompatibility characteristics, they have great potential as therapeutic drug delivery vesicles. Well-designed engineered exosomes could enhance their therapeutic effects, making them promising and inspiring tools for clinical application [26]. Our results demonstrated that CCR7 overexpression could enhance MI-DEXs' migration to the spleen and improve cardiac function after MI. Thus, CCR7 could be a potential candidate for MI-DEX bioengineering to enhance its therapeutic effects after MI.

However, there were some perplexing results in this study. We found increases in pro-inflammatory cytokine expression, such as IFN-γ, IL-1β, and IL-6, after MI-DEX injection in splenic $CD4^+$ T cells. Due to the multiple subsets of $CD4^+$ T cells existing in the spleen, including pro- and anti-inflammatory subsets, our results indicated that MI-DEXs increased anti-inflammatory cytokine expression in $CD4^+$ T cells but did not affect pro-inflammatory cytokine expression. This phenomenon showed that the correlation between MI-DEXs and $CD4^+$ T cells was complex and did not just convert $CD4^+$ T cells into an anti-inflammatory type. The underlying mechanism needs to be further explored. In addition, we also did not find significant differences among different MI-DEX groups regarding LV fibrosis; however, large variations within each group may be the primary reason.

5. Conclusions

In conclusion, DC-derived exosome migration to the spleen after MI was mediated by CCR7, and the mechanism of MI-DEX's improvement of cardiac function included the activation of $CD4^+$ T cells and secretion of IL-4 and IL-10. Our study presented an innovative way to improve cardiac function by enhancing the migration ability of MI-DEXs after MI, while CCR7 could be a potential candidate for MI-DEX bioengineering to enhance its migration and improve cardiac function after MI.

Author Contributions: Conceptualization, H.L. and Y.Z.; Animal experiments, Y.Z., W.G. and X.Z.; Cell transfection and DEX isolation and labeling: J.Y.; Cell and DEX experiments: R.L.; Data analysis and visualization: H.L. and K.Y.; Writing—original draft preparation, Y.Z. and H.L.; Writing—review and editing, H.L. All authors have read and agreed to the published version of the manuscript.

Funding: This research was supported by the National Natural Science Foundation of China (NSFC Grants 81770350; 81400263).

Institutional Review Board Statement: The Institutional Review Board of Zhongshan Hospital of Fudan University and the Shanghai Institutes of Biological Sciences-CAS (A5894-01, January 2017) approved this study, and the animal research complied with the standards of animal welfare in China.

Informed Consent Statement: Not applicable.

Data Availability Statement: The data sets used and/or analyzed during the current study can be obtained from the corresponding author if reasonably requested.

Acknowledgments: The authors thank Lu Ying for performing flow cytometry analysis and Wang Guangxue for performing small-animal echocardiography.

Conflicts of Interest: The authors declare no conflict of interest.

References

1. Bergmark, B.; Mathenge, N.; Merlini, P.; Lawrence-Wright, M.; Giugliano, R. Acute coronary syndromes. *Lancet* **2022**, *399*, 1347–1358. [CrossRef] [PubMed]
2. Murphy, S.; Ibrahim, N.; Januzzi, J., Jr. Heart Failure With Reduced Ejection Fraction: A Review. *JAMA* **2020**, *324*, 488–504. [CrossRef] [PubMed]
3. Meng, T.; Wang, P.; Ding, J.; Du, R.; Gao, J.; Li, A.; Yu, S.; Liu, J.; Lu, X.; He, Q. Global Research Trends on Ventricular Remodeling: A Bibliometric Analysis From 2012 to 2022. *Curr. Probl. Cardiol.* **2022**, *47*, 101332. [CrossRef]
4. Frantz, S.; Hundertmark, M.J.; Schulz-Menger, J.; Bengel, F.M.; Bauersachs, J. Left ventricular remodelling post-myocardial infarction: Pathophysiology, imaging, and novel therapies. *Eur. Heart J.* **2022**, *43*, 2549–2561. [CrossRef] [PubMed]
5. Andreadou, I.; Cabrera-Fuentes, H.A.; Devaux, Y.; Frangogiannis, N.G.; Frantz, S.; Guzik, T.; Liehn, E.A.; Gomes, C.P.C.; Schulz, R.; Hausenloy, D.J. Immune cells as targets for cardioprotection: New players and novel therapeutic opportunities. *Cardiovasc. Res.* **2019**, *115*, 1117–1130. [CrossRef]
6. Montrief, T.; Davis, W.; Koyfman, A.; Long, B. Mechanical, inflammatory, and embolic complications of myocardial infarction: An emergency medicine review. *Am. J. Emerg. Med.* **2019**, *37*, 1175–1183. [CrossRef]
7. Zhang, Y.; Wen, W.M.; Liu, H.M. The Role of Immune Cells in Cardiac Remodeling After Myocardial Infarction. *J. Cardiovasc. Pharmacol.* **2020**, *76*, 407–413. [CrossRef]
8. Liu, H.; Gao, W.; Yuan, J.; Wu, C.; Yao, K.; Zhang, L.; Ma, L.; Zhu, J.; Zou, Y.; Ge, J. Exosomes derived from dendritic cells improve cardiac function via activation of $CD4^+$ T lymphocytes after myocardial infarction. *J. Mol. Cell. Cardiol.* **2016**, *91*, 123–133. [CrossRef]
9. Zhang, Y.; Cai, Z.; Shen, Y.; Lu, Q.; Gao, W.; Zhong, X.; Yao, K.; Yuan, J.; Liu, H. Hydrogel-load exosomes derived from dendritic cells improve cardiac function via Treg cells and the polarization of macrophages following myocardial infarction. *J. Nanobiotechnology* **2021**, *19*, 271. [CrossRef] [PubMed]
10. Sun, K.; Li, Y.-Y.; Jin, J. A double-edged sword of immuno-microenvironment in cardiac homeostasis and injury repair. *Signal Transduct. Target. Ther.* **2021**, *6*, 1–16. [CrossRef]
11. Anzai, A.; Anzai, T.; Nagai, S.; Maekawa, Y.; Naito, K.; Kaneko, H.; Sugano, Y.; Takahashi, T.; Abe, H.; Mochizuki, S.; et al. Regulatory Role of Dendritic Cells in Postinfarction Healing and Left Ventricular Remodeling. *Circulation* **2012**, *125*, 1234–1245. [CrossRef] [PubMed]
12. Choo, E.H.; Lee, J.-H.; Park, E.-H.; Park, H.E.; Jung, N.-C.; Kim, T.-H.; Koh, Y.-S.; Kim, E.; Seung, K.-B.; Park, C.; et al. Infarcted Myocardium-Primed Dendritic Cells Improve Remodeling and Cardiac Function After Myocardial Infarction by Modulating the Regulatory T Cell and Macrophage Polarization. *Circulation* **2017**, *135*, 1444–1457. [CrossRef] [PubMed]
13. Rieckmann, M.; Delgobo, M.; Gaal, C.; Büchner, L.; Steinau, P.; Reshef, D.; Gil Cruz, C.; Ter Horst, E.N.; Kircher, M.; Reiter, T.; et al. Myocardial infarction triggers cardioprotective antigen-specific T helper cell responses. *J. Clin. Investig.* **2019**, *129*, 4922–4936. [CrossRef]
14. Yates, A.; Pink, R.; Erdbrügger, U.; Siljander, P.; Dellar, E.; Pantazi, P.; Akbar, N.; Cooke, W.; Vatish, M.; Di-as-Neto, E.; et al. In sickness and in health: The functional role of extracellular vesicles in physiology and pathology in vivo: Part I: Health and Normal Physiology: Part I: Health and Normal Physiology. *J. Extracell. Vesicles* **2022**, *11*, e12151. [PubMed]
15. Wu, R.; Gao, W.; Yao, K.; Ge, J. Roles of Exosomes Derived From Immune Cells in Cardiovascular Diseases. *Front. Immunol.* **2019**, *10*, 648. [CrossRef]
16. Hood, J.L. The association of exosomes with lymph nodes. *Semin. Cell Dev. Biol.* **2017**, *67*, 29–38. [CrossRef] [PubMed]
17. Hjortø, G.M.; Larsen, O.; Steen, A.; Daugvilaite, V.; Berg, C.; Fares, S.; Hansen, M.; Ali, S.; Rosenkilde, M.M. Differential CCR7 Targeting in Dendritic Cells by Three Naturally Occurring CC-Chemokines. *Front. Immunol.* **2016**, *7*, 568. [CrossRef]
18. Hong, W.; Yang, B.; He, Q.; Wang, J.; Weng, Q. New Insights of CCR7 Signaling in Dendritic Cell Migration and Inflammatory Diseases. *Front. Pharmacol.* **2022**, *13*, 841687. [CrossRef]
19. Hofmann, U.; Beyersdorf, N.; Weirather, J.; Podolskaya, A.; Bauersachs, J.; Ertl, G.; Kerkau, T.; Frantz, S. Activation of $CD4^+$ T Lymphocytes Improves Wound Healing and Survival After Experimental Myocardial Infarction in Mice. *Circulation* **2012**, *125*, 1652–1663. [CrossRef]
20. Shintani, Y.; Ito, T.; Fields, L.; Shiraishi, M.; Ichihara, Y.; Sato, N.; Podaru, M.; Kainuma, S.; Tanaka, H.; Suzuki, K. IL-4 as a Repurposed Biological Drug for Myocardial Infarction through Augmentation of Reparative Cardiac Macrophages: Proof-of-Concept Data in Mice. *Sci. Rep.* **2017**, *7*, 1–14. [CrossRef]

21. Shirakawa, K.; Endo, J.; Kataoka, M.; Katsumata, Y.; Yoshida, N.; Yamamoto, T.; Isobe, S.; Moriyama, H.; Goto, S.; Kitakata, H.; et al. IL (Interleukin)-10–STAT3–Galectin-3 Axis Is Essential for Osteopontin-Producing Reparative Macrophage Polarization After Myocardial Infarction. *Circulation* **2018**, *138*, 2021–2035. [CrossRef] [PubMed]
22. Huang, S.; Frangogiannis, N. Anti-inflammatory therapies in myocardial infarction: Failures, hopes and challenges. *Br. J. Pharmacol.* **2018**, *175*, 1377–1400. [CrossRef] [PubMed]
23. Van Raemdonck, K.; Umar, S.; Palasiewicz, K.; Volkov, S.; Volin, M.V.; Arami, S.; Chang, H.J.; Zanotti, B.; Sweiss, N.; Shahrara, S. CCL21/CCR7 signaling in macrophages promotes joint inflammation and Th17-mediated osteoclast formation in rheumatoid arthritis. *Cell Mol. Life Sci.* **2020**, *77*, 1387–1399. [CrossRef]
24. Barile, L.; Moccetti, T.; Marbán, E.; Vassalli, G. Roles of exosomes in cardioprotection. *Eur. Heart J.* **2016**, *38*, 1372–1379. [CrossRef] [PubMed]
25. Xiong, Y.-Y.; Gong, Z.-T.; Tang, R.-J.; Yang, Y.-J. The pivotal roles of exosomes derived from endogenous immune cells and exogenous stem cells in myocardial repair after acute myocardial infarction. *Theranostics* **2021**, *11*, 1046–1058. [CrossRef] [PubMed]
26. Liu, C.; Su, C. Design strategies and application progress of therapeutic exosomes. *Theranostics* **2019**, *9*, 1015–1028. [CrossRef]

pharmaceutics

MDPI

Review

Exosomes as CNS Drug Delivery Tools and Their Applications

Ke Sun [1], Xue Zheng [1], Hongzhen Jin [1,*], Fan Yu [2,*] and Wei Zhao [1,3]

[1] College of Pharmacy, Nankai University, Tongyan Road, Haihe Education Park, Tianjin 300350, China
[2] College of Life Sciences, Nankai University, Weijin Road, Nankai District, Tianjin 300350, China
[3] State Key Laboratory of Medicinal Chemical Biology, Nankai University, Tongyan Road, Haihe Education Park, Tianjin 300350, China
* Correspondence: jinhongzhen@nankai.edu.cn (H.J.); fanyu@nankai.edu.cn (F.Y.)

Abstract: Central nervous system (CNS) diseases threaten the health of people all over the world. However, due to the structural and functional particularities of the brain and spinal cord, CNS-targeted drug development is rather challenging. Exosomes are small cellular vesicles with lipid bilayers that can be secreted by almost all cells and play important roles in intercellular communication. The advantages of low immunogenicity, the ability to cross the blood-brain barrier, and the flexibility of drug encapsulation make them stand out among CNS drug delivery tools. Herein, we reviewed the research on exosomes in CNS drug delivery over the past decade and outlined the impact of the drug loading mode, administration route, and engineered modification on CNS targeting. Finally, we highlighted the problems and prospects of exosomes as CNS drug delivery tools.

Keywords: engineered exosomes; drug delivery system; CNS; blood-brain barrier

Citation: Sun, K.; Zheng, X.; Jin, H.; Yu, F.; Zhao, W. Exosomes as CNS Drug Delivery Tools and Their Applications. *Pharmaceutics* **2022**, *14*, 2252. https://doi.org/10.3390/pharmaceutics14102252

Academic Editor: Gert Fricker

Received: 23 September 2022
Accepted: 19 October 2022
Published: 21 October 2022

1. Introduction

The drug delivery system (DDS) can comprehensively regulate the distribution of drugs in the organism in space, time, and dose. It has multiple roles: (i) drug targeting; (ii) slow and controlled drug release; (iii) enhancing drug stability and regulating drug metabolism time; (iv) promoting drug absorption and passage through biological barriers. Modern drug delivery technology started with the advent of extended-release capsule technology in 1952, followed by oral and transdermal formulations, long-acting injectables, pegylated liposomes, drug-polymer complexes, antibody-drug conjugates, and nano-delivery systems over 70 years [1].

Delivery of drugs to the CNS has been a challenging subject to overcome. In the brain, the main biological barrier is the blood-brain barrier (BBB). Various pathways have been developed to overcome the poor penetration of the BBB [2–6]. However, so far, it remains a bottleneck in CNS drug development [7]. To overcome the BBB, lots of drug delivery systems have been developed, such as adeno-associated viral (AAV) vectors [8], erythrocyte membrane-encapsulated nanocarriers [9], cell-based delivery nanocarriers [10], extracellular vesicles (EVs) [11], injectable hydrogels [12], and immunomodulators [13]. Among them, EVs performed surprisingly well.

EVs are small membranous vesicles released into the extracellular matrix by almost all cells and are widely present in various body fluids [14]. It was initially thought that EVs were cell-secreted garbage bags as a cellular self-cleaning mechanism. Nevertheless, as research progressed, EVs were found to stably carry important signaling molecules such as proteins, mRNAs, miRNAs, and lipids, which have important roles in intercellular communication [15,16], disease diagnosis [17–19], disease development [20,21], and disease therapy [22,23]. EVs are a highly heterogeneous group of vesicles, which are broadly classified into three categories according to their biogenesis, size, and biophysical property: exosomes, microvesicles, and apoptotic bodies [14,24–26]. Among them, exosomes have received the most attention in recent decades. Exosomes are approximately 40–100 nm in diameter and float at a density of 1.13–1.19 g·mL^{-1} in sucrose density gradient solutions [27–30]. The biogenesis process of exosomes is shown in Figure 1. It is worth noting that, according to the MISEV 2018 guidelines, it is difficult to fully purify and distinguish the above EVs due to methodological difficulties in isolation, and the term "exosomes", even though widely used, is suggested to be replaced by the term "small extracellular vesicles (sEVs)" instead [31].

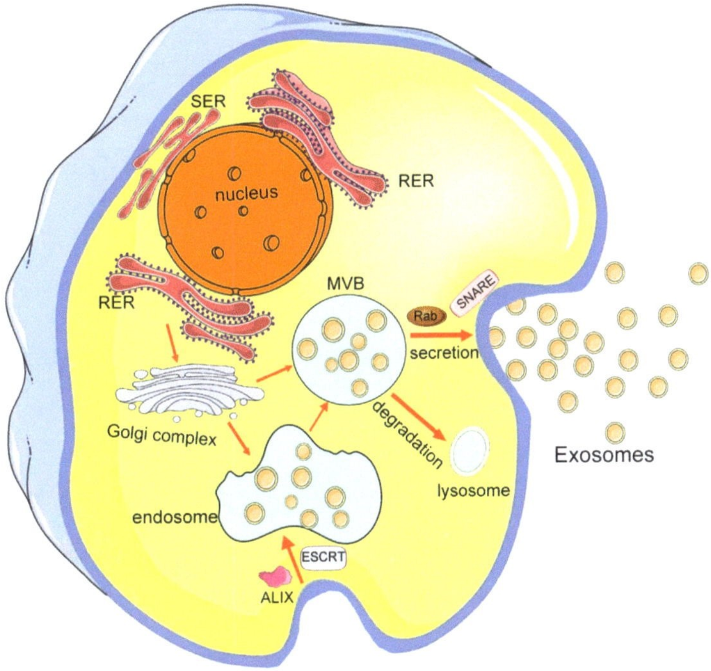

Figure 1. Biogenesis of exosomes. Cells produce small vesicles by endocytosis, which fuse to form endosomes, and are subsequently accompanied by the entry of nucleic acids, proteins, etc. into the endosomes. The endosomes gradually evolve into multivesicular bodies (MVBs), which are subsequently released extracellularly to form exosomes. RER: rough endoplasmic reticulum; SER: smooth endoplasmic reticulum; MVB: multivesicular body; ESCRT: endosomal sorting complex required for transport.

Considering the important function that exosomes contain diverse active molecules (Figure 2) and are capable of mediating cellular communications, they were vigorously developed as DDSs for the treatment of various diseases [32]. While liposomes have been used maturely in DDSs, we still cannot ignore their limitations as well as other synthetic nanoparticles, such as toxicity, immunogenicity, and short half-life due to rapid clearance by the mononuclear phagocytic system (MPS) [33]. Although PEG modification can improve the above defects to a certain extent, it may cause the acceleration of the blood clearance (ABC) phenomenon after repeated multiple dosing [34–36]. In addition, studies have shown that exposure to chemicals and cosmetics in daily life could increase PEG antibodies in the human body [37]. In contrast, when exosomes were used in DDSs, they had better biocompatibility and lower immunogenicity due to characteristics such as an endogenous biological origin [38], and longer circulation times [39]. Moreover, exosomes from different sources had different targeting capabilities and roles in crossing biological barriers [40,41].

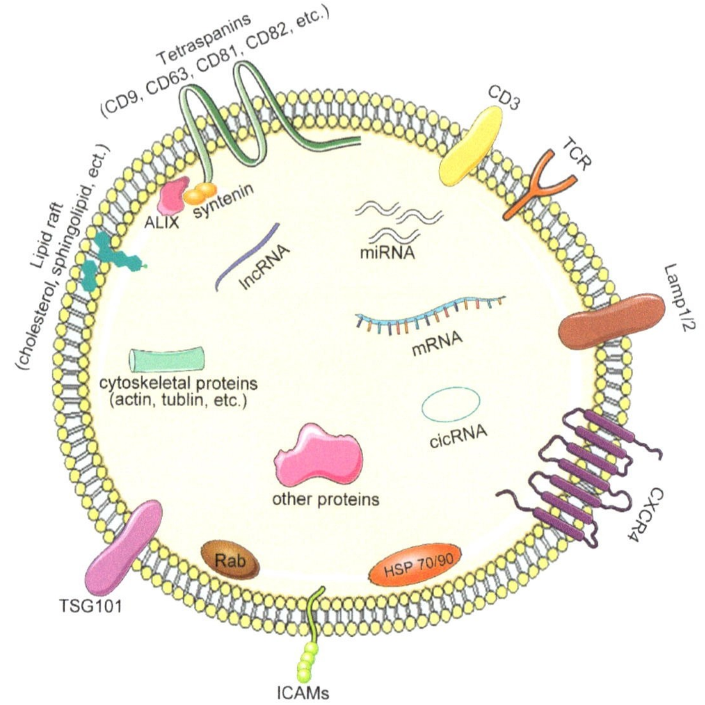

Figure 2. Rich contents and surface markers of exosomes. Exosomes are rich in cholesterol and sphingomyelin and have a lipid bilayer structure. Universally, exosomes contain tubulin, heat shock proteins, actin-binding proteins, ALIX, tetra membrane proteins, abundant nucleic acids, etc. CXCR4: CXC chemokine receptor 4; TCR: T cell receptor; HSP: heat shock proteins; ICAMs: intercellular cell adhesion molecules; TSG: tumor suppressor gene; lncRNA: Long non-coding RNA; miRNA: micro-RNA; cicRNA: circular RNA.

Since the focus of this review was the study on exosomes as CNS drug delivery tools, all authors reached a consensus on article screening. More specifically, the review was performed in PubMed and Web of Science databases using the keywords (exosomes/extracellular vesicles/CNS/brain/spinal cord/drug delivery/therapeutic molecules). At the same time, articles of potential interest should include at least three of the above keywords in their title or abstract.

2. The Roles of Exosomes in the CNS

The dense BBB protects the brain from various pathogenic microorganisms but is also the biggest obstacle to treating CNS disease. Thus, designing a safe, effective, and specific DDS to cross the BBB is the focus of current research. Numerous drug delivery technologies have been devoted to crossing the BBB [42–44], among which exosomes exhibited more unique roles and advantages.

2.1. The Blood-Brain Barrier and Its Challenges in the Treatment

The BBB consists of brain capillary endothelial cells (BCECs), the basement membrane of pericytes, and astrocyte end-feet [45–47]. In addition, the presence of enzymes and efflux pumps (e.g., P-glycoproteins and multi-drug resistance proteins (MRPs)) restricts non-specific translocation [48]. The current approaches to facilitate the passage of therapeutic compounds across the BBB can be summarized in the following three methods: (i) invasive methods; (ii) pharmacological methods; (iii) physiological methods [49]. Intracerebral or intrathecal injection directly opens the blood-brain barrier, which is highly invasive and makes it easy to cause tissue trauma or inflammation. The pharmacological approach emphasizes drug modification. However, it is not sufficient and requires the assistance of delivery tools to maximize the drug's effect. In the physiological approach, various nano-delivery systems including exosomes are used to cross the BBB.

2.2. Multiple Functions of CNS Cell-Derived Exosomes

Microglia, astrocytes, oligodendrocytes, and neurons can actively secrete exosomes [50–53] and play important roles in intercellular communications [54]. In the CNS, exosomes propagate signals not only over short distances within cells but also throughout the brain via the cerebrospinal fluid (CSF) [55]. Therefore, exosomes are involved in the maintenance of the normal physiological state of the CNS as well as in the development of pathology [56,57].

As the most fundamental structural and functional unit of the CNS, neurons play important roles in maintaining neural homeostasis. It was found that exosomes have astonishing efficacy in neurogenesis and repair [58]. Additionally, they can mediate intra-neural communication and make it better [59]. The delivery of miR-132 to vascular endothelial cells by neuronal exosomes could maintain cerebral vasculature integrity [60]. Similarly, neuronal-derived extracellular vesicles could also detect insulin/mTOR pathway changes in the brain of Down syndrome (DS) patients [61].

Microglia are important neural immune cells with active immune sensing functions [62]. Furthermore, exosomes secreted by microglia are actively involved in physiological and pathological processes in the CNS. For example, after traumatic brain injury, upregulation of miR-124-3p in microglia exosomes suppressed neuronal inflammation and promoted nerve growth via transfer to neurons [63]. Microglia could sense abnormal signals and convert from the inflammation-suppressing M2 type to the pro-inflammatory M1 type in pathologic conditions such as trauma and inflammation. Nevertheless, the involvement of exosomes may reverse this process, as exosomes from mesenchymal stem cells attenuated CNS inflammation and demyelination in EAE rats by regulating microglia polarization [64].

One important mediator of cell-to-cell communication is miRNA. For example, exosomes could transfer miR-133b from pluripotent mesenchymal stromal cells (MSC) to neuronal cells to promote nerve growth [65]. MSC-origin exosomes contained miRNAs that regulate neuroinflammation [66]. Exosomes secreted from glia and neurons mediated Alzheimer's disease (AD) development via miRNA delivery. Changes in exosomal miRNAs in the peripheral blood or cerebrospinal fluid of patients were important guides for the early diagnosis of AD. More information on the roles of exosomal miRNAs in the diagnosis and treatment of AD have been reported [67].

Astrocytes are involved in the BBB formation, which may help regulate the ionic microenvironment surrounding neurons. Nevertheless, it has been shown that increasing the release of their exosomes can mitigate β-amyloid-induced neurotoxicity [68], offering novel ideas for the treatment of AD. However, the release of astrocyte exosomes is not always beneficial, and it has been shown that the microenvironment induced by astrocyte exosomal microRNA induced PTEN loss and brain metastatic growth of tumors [69].

Neural stem cells, in contrast to the aforementioned CNS cells, have the capacity for self-renewal and can differentiate into neurons, astrocytes, oligodendrocytes, etc. Neural stem cell exosomes held great promise in the treatment of neurodegenerative diseases [70], e.g., human neural stem cell exosomes have a protective effect against Parkinson's disease [71] and could ameliorate AD [72]. Alongside this, extracellular vesicles derived from human neural stem cells have been shown to have good efficacy in the functional recovery of strokes in mice [73].

3. Strategies for Drug Loading into Exosomes

Although naked exosomes have therapeutic effects, they are limited. Drug-loaded exosomes can synergize the effects of drugs and exosomes, which have become a hotspot in DDS research.

The drug delivery system consists of two main components: one is the "outer shell", as well as the drug delivery vehicle, which in this review refers to as exosomes. The other part is the "content", which is also called the therapeutic drug. Currently, almost 20% of exosome-related topics are focused on drug loading, demonstrating its importance.

In contrast to the nano-formulations already developed, exosomes are loaded with active molecules more flexibly and diversely. Synthetic drug delivery vehicles like nanomaterials can be loaded with drugs during the synthesis. Exosomes, on the other hand, seem to be more receptive to the idea of loading active molecules before or after their secretion.

3.1. Pre-Secretory Loading

The idea of loading drugs before exosome secretion, i.e., at the biogenesis stage of exosomes, is to manipulate exosome-generating progenitor cells, which is also called cell engineering. The donor cells are capable of secreting exosomes containing the drugs.

Drugs can enter cells by transfection, e.g., transfecting HEK293T cells with circSCMH1 plasmid [74] can efficiently encapsulate them into secreted exosomes, and targeted delivery to the brain can enhance neuronal plasticity and inhibit glial reactivity, thus effectively ameliorating stroke symptoms in mice and rhesus monkeys. Ge et al. [75] transfected miR-124-3p mimics into microglia for 6 h, and exosomes containing miR-124-3p were extracted and isolated 48 h after the culture medium was changed. Intravenous injection of the above exosomes alleviated the neurodegenerative lesions in repetitive mild traumatic brain injury (rmTBI) mice.

Drugs can also be co-incubated with donor cells to gain access to the cell interior. For instance, macrophage RAW264.7 cells co-cultured with high doses of curcumin at 37 °C for 24 h were isolated by ultracentrifugation to produce exosomes containing curcumin and were effective in alleviating symptoms of middle cerebral artery occlusion (MCAO) in vivo [76].

The method of drug loading by manipulating donor cells before exosome secretion is simple to operate. However, this strategy has high requirements for the compatibility between parental cells and a drug [11], and a variety of uncontrolled factors such as cell status and culture conditions ultimately lead to unstable or low loading efficiency [77,78]. In conclusion, a lack of knowledge of the complex intracellular metabolic pathways is the main reason. A better understanding of the mechanisms by which therapeutic molecules are transported in cells and localized to exosomes may improve loading efficiency.

3.2. Post-Secretory Loading

The post-secretory approach refers to the way that naive exosomes are extracted and isolated from donor cells, and then the purified exosomes are loaded with drugs by various methods in vitro. Some common approaches include co-incubation, electroporation, sonication, repeated freeze-thawing, extrusion, and so on (Figure 3).

Exosomes have lipid bilayers, so co-incubation of exosomes with hydrophobic compounds allows passive entry of drugs into exosomes. For example, aptamer F5R1 was co-incubated with exosomes derived from the human embryonic kidney (HEK) 293T cells at 37 °C for some time [79], and an aptamer was able to efficiently enter exosomes and reduce a-synuclein aggregation, exerting a therapeutic effect on PD. It is worth mentioning that drug saturation solutions can be used to improve the efficiency of drug entry in vitro. This idea was applied by Qu et al. [80] to the experiment of dopamine loading in mouse blood exosomes. The enormous concentration difference contributed to the passive penetration of dopamine into exosomes during co-incubation. Dopamine-loaded exosomes showed a PD therapeutic effect. Co-incubation loading efficiency is related to drug hydrophobicity, molecular weight, exosome size, the lipid content of exosomes, and so on [81]. Therefore, the appropriate mixing ratio must be mastered to achieve higher loading efficiency.

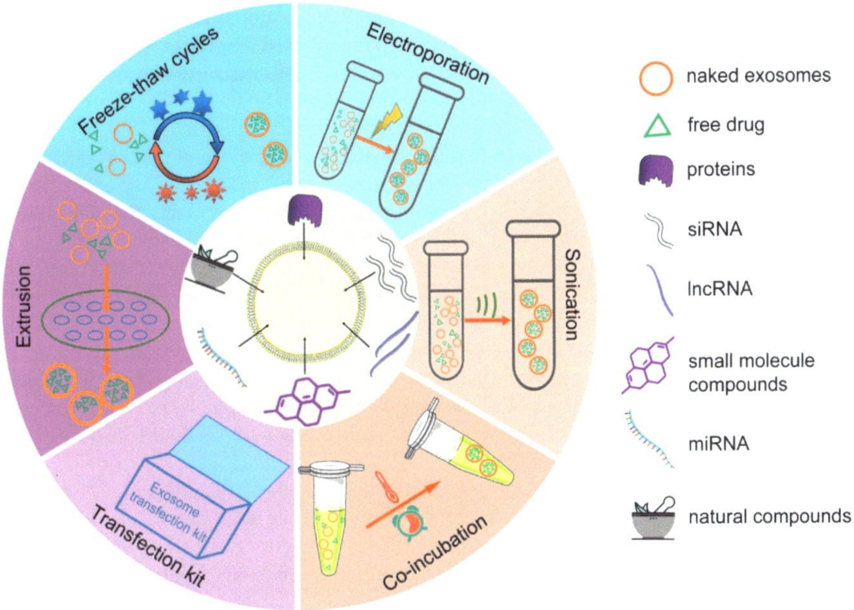

Figure 3. Post-secretory loading methods of exosomes. Drug encapsulation strategies for isolated exosomes include sonication, electroporation, co-incubation, freeze-thaw cycles, extrusion, transfection kits, etc.

Electroporation enables the membranes of exosomes to temporarily create pores in the presence of an electric current, through which the drugs enter the exosomes. For example, Zhang et al. [82] loaded ZIKV-specific siRNA into exosomes derived from HEK 293T cells at 450 V and 100 mF. They could cross the BBB and placental barrier to treat fetal microcephaly caused by ZIKV infection. Electroporation charging efficiency can be affected by voltage, electrical capacitance, discharge time, and other conditions.

Sonication is also commonly used. Luo et al. [83] isolated exosomes from fresh bovine milk and encapsulated epicatechin gallate (ECG) into exosomes using ultrasonication with a loading efficiency of 25.96%. The ultrasonically loaded exosomes were anti-apoptotic and neuroprotective against Parkinson's disease. The loading efficiency of sonication is high but may lead to the aggregation of exosomes.

Aside from the abovementioned modalities, chemical reactions have also been skillfully applied [84]. LJM-3064 potently inhibits the inflammatory response and reduces the areas of demyelinating lesions in CNS by chemically covalently binding to amine groups on exosome surfaces via EDC/NHS. There are also alternative drug loading methods using exosome transfection reagents, which can directly transfer nucleic acids including siRNAs, miRNAs, mRNAs, and even plasmid DNAs into isolated exosomes [85]. These novel ways provide new ideas that may expand the development of exosomal drug delivery.

The addition of some adjuvants like saponin will improve loading efficiency appropriately. For example, in loading catalase, the authors [86] investigated the drug loading efficiency with and without saponin separately when using co-incubation as a modality and demonstrated that the addition of saponin significantly increased the drug loading efficiency from 4.9% to 18.5%. It was worth mentioning that the study also explored comparing the differences in drug loading rates of four modalities loaded on the same drug, and it was found that the loading efficiencies of sonication and extrusion were higher, 26.1% and 22.2%, respectively. However, this may not apply to other research, and the optimal method still needs to be explored personally in the respective studies. In some cases, multiple methods may be used at the same time to improve the efficiency of drug loading. For example, to load curcumin into mouse embryonic stem cell (MESC)-derived exosomes, Anuradha et al. [87] first incubated curcumin with exosomes in a 1:4 ratio for 15 min at room temperature, followed by rapid freeze-thawing two to three times. Successfully loaded exosomes were capable of reducing vascular inflammation and promoting neurovascular recovery in mice with ischemia-reperfusion injury.

In conclusion, efficient drug loading remains one of the biggest challenges. Especially for small molecules or extremely hydrophobic molecules, although simple co-incubation is the most commonly used method, it no longer meets the requirements. Therefore, Haney et al. [88] explored the optimization of co-incubation conditions. The team found that when the pH of the co-incubation system was adjusted to 8.0, the drug loading rate increased significantly. The possible reason was that a pH close to pI reduced the molecule's charge and increased its hydrophobicity. It is reasonable to assume that optimizing other incubation conditions such as appropriate temperature increase, shaking, longer incubation time, etc. may also improve the loading rate. In addition, other suitable methods can be directly used instead of co-incubation. For example, mild sonication could significantly increase the loading rates of small molecules such as doxorubicin [88], paclitaxel [88,89], and gemcitabine [90].

Drug loading after secretion is controlled and efficient. Disadvantages, however, include destruction of exosome integrity, facile aggregation, etc. The character of the drug and the properties of exosomes may all influence the loading efficiency [91]. Therefore, the choice of drug loading mode is ultimately based on experimental needs.

4. Drug Administration Affects the Efficiency of Exosomes into the CNS

In DDS, appropriate changes in administration modes may enhance the therapeutic effect. Exosomes biodistribution was determined by cellular origin, route of administration, and targeting [92,93]. Thus, intravenous [94–96], nasal [97–100], intraperitoneal [101–103], and local [104] injections have been used extensively.

When exosomes are used as drug delivery tools, the most common administration is intravenous injection. For example, brain endothelium-derived exosomes might reach the brain after intravenous injection to deliver doxorubicin for the treatment of brain cancer in zebrafish [105]. Nevertheless, intravenously injected exosomes have restricted CNS tropism. In addition to this, the half-life of intravenous exosomes is shorter. Therefore, most of them are still surface-modified. One of the most widely used is the modification of neuron-targeting peptides (RVG) to enhance their brain-targeting capacity.

Intranasal injection allows drug delivery to the brain via intranasal deposits, olfactory bulbs, trigeminal nerves, and the respiratory epithelium [106,107]. It is therefore widely used in brain disorders [108]. For example, exosomes containing cholesterol-modified AMO181a were capable of brain delivery and exerted therapeutic effects on ischemic brain injury when administered intranasally [98]. MSC-exosomes injected intranasally could cross the BBB and migrate to the injured area of the spinal cord, achieving recovery [109].

The local administration has also attracted attention. In a recent study, Han et al. [104] explored the use of an array of patches using autonomously designed gel microneedles loaded with 3D cultured MSC-exosomes to achieve in situ repair of exosomes in spinal cord injury. MSC-exosomes could reduce the neuroinflammatory response, promote polarization of microglia to M2 phenotype, and reduce glial scar formation to facilitate the repair of neurological injury. This successful exploration will also bring more researchers to think, innovate, and achieve breakthroughs concerning the exosomes administrations.

5. Engineering Exosomes Enhance the CNS Targeting and Therapeutic Efficacy

Exosomes inherit the characteristics of donor cells [110] and have certain passive targeting abilities, also known as a homing ability [111,112]. However, this natural homing ability is weak and may be affected by various factors such as injection methods, drug doses, and individual differences [92], thereby weakening or even losing the CNS targeting capacity of exosomes. Moreover, it has been demonstrated that intravenously injected naked exosomes were easily enriched in reticuloendothelial system (RES) organs such as the liver and it was extremely difficult for them to reach the CNS [92,93].

Engineered exosomes are endowed with desired targeting capabilities because they are decorated with various functional molecules on their surfaces [113–116]. Functional molecules can utilize specific ligand/receptor binding strategies to increase brain targeting capabilities [110,117]. Strategies for surface modification of engineered exosomes include genetic engineering and chemical modification [117,118].

Genetic engineering modification of exosomes is the fusion of the gene sequence of a target functional protein or peptide with a selected exosomal membrane protein, and then donor cells transfected with the above plasmids secrete engineered exosomes with targeting ligands on their surface [119]. Lamp2b-RVG is the most widely used hybrid plasmid for genetically modified brain-targeted exosome modifications. Lamp2b is a highly abundant membrane-localized protein on exosomes. Rabies virus glycoprotein (RVG) is the more recognized brain-targeting peptide, and RVG selectively targets neurons and brain endothelial cells by binding to the nicotinic acetylcholine receptor (nAChR) [120]. For example, Alvarez-Erviti et al. [118] genetically engineered Lamp2b-RVG plasmids and transfected autologous-derived dendritic cells to make them secrete engineered exosomes. Intravenous injection of the above exosomes specifically delivered siRNA to neurons, microglia, and oligodendrocytes in the brain, leading to specific gene knockdown and offering new hope for AD treatment. Genetic engineering strategies are currently widely used, but the procedures are complex and costly.

The chemical modification enables in vitro manipulation after exosome isolation. For example, stearoyl-RVG was inserted into the phospholipid bilayer of immature DC exosomes via hydrophobic interactions. The drug-loaded exosomes were able to scavenge α-synuclein aggregates and reduce cytotoxicity in PD neurons [121]. Han et al. [122] synthesized RVG-15-PEG-DSPE and inserted it onto the surface of exosomes containing doxorubicin to achieve the treatment of glioblastoma. In addition to RVG, other types of brain-targeting small molecules can also be engineered by chemical ligations. For example, to attach RGD peptides to the surface of exosomes, Tian et al. [123] first reacted naive exosomes isolated from MSC cells with DBCO-sulfo-NHS to produce EXO-DBCO, which was chemically reacted with the exposed amino groups on the surface of exosomes using NHS. Then, EXO-DBCO was reacted with the azide-modified cRGD in a click reaction, so the azide-modified cRGD was successfully attached to EXO-DBCO. Finally, the attachment of the targeted functional peptide cRGD to the surface of the exosomes by the chemical reaction was achieved (known as the bioorthogonal reaction) [124–127]. Jia et al. [128] also modified cargo-loaded exosomes with the glioma-targeting peptide RGE by click chemistry and finally obtained engineered exosomes with therapeutic effects on glioma. The chemical modification strategy is less costly and has higher linkage efficiency, but has more influencing factors such as temperature, solvent, etc.

Although current engineered exosomes focused on increasing targeting, Kojima et al. [129] pioneered the idea of increasing exosome release. Specifically, Kojima's team constructed a triple hybrid plasmid with STEAP3 capable of participating in exosomes biogenesis, and syndecan-4 (SDC4) capable of supporting endosomal membrane outgrowth to form polycystic and L-aspartate oxidase (NadB) capable of promoting cellular metabolism by regulating the citric acid cycle. The combined expression of these genes significantly increased exosome production.

The aim of engineered exosomes is to overcome some deficiencies of naked exosomes and enable them to better serve as CNS drug delivery tools.

6. Research and Applications of Exosomal Drug Delivery Systems in CNS Diseases

As exosomes have been studied more intensively, numerous studies have been conducted on various CNS disease models to assess the efficacy of exosomal drug delivery systems and help their clinical translation.

6.1. Alzheimer's Disease

Alzheimer's disease (AD) is a progressive neurodegenerative disorder manifested by memory loss and cognitive decline [130]. There are no available therapeutic agents and the current drugs merely alleviate the associated symptoms. Neurogenic fibrillary tangles (NFT) composed of amyloid β (Aβ) plaques and abnormally phosphorylated tau protein (p-tau) are the major pathological hallmarks and AD is accompanied by neuronal death, synaptic loss, neuroinflammation, and brain injury [131–133].

Exosomes contain a wide variety of proteins, RNAs, etc., and therefore can mediate intercellular communication [134]. Because of this, exosomes have excellent performance in delivering RNA [135–137]. Small interfering RNAs (siRNAs) are among the many RNA drugs widely used, which result in gene silencing [138]. In recent years, siRNAs delivery technology has advanced rapidly, but extrahepatic and especially brain siRNA-targeted delivery has still been in the exploratory stage. Alvarez-Erviti et al. [118] made the first attempt to achieve intracerebral targeted delivery using exosomes as siRNA delivery vehicles. This study used self-derived dendritic cell exosomes to minimize immunogenicity, as well as RVG neuro-targeting peptides to modify exosomes. Suitable siRNAs were designed for the AD therapeutic target BACE1, resulting in a strong knockdown of the corresponding mRNA and proteins in mice.

6.2. Parkinson's Disease

PD is the second most common neurodegenerative disorder worldwide, the major pathological hallmark being dopaminergic (DA) neuron degenerative death [139–141].

Catalase has been shown to have a protective effect on neurons. With this in mind, Haney et al. [86] explored the use of different methods for loading catalase into RAW264.7 cell exosomes. After intranasal administration, catalase-loaded exosomes were taken up by neurons and microglia of PD mice and exhibited significant neuroprotective effects. Likewise, Kojima et al. [129] used a mixed plasmid containing peroxidase mRNA along with RVG to transfect HEK-293T cells. By subcutaneous injection of the cells, the cells produced exosomes containing peroxidase mRNA in vivo and delivered it to the brain and alleviated the neurotoxicity and neuroinflammation caused by PD.

Alpha-synuclein aggregation is closely related to Lewy body formation and dopaminergic neuron death and plays an important role in the pathogenesis of PD. Thus, the reduction of α-synuclein protofibril aggregation is an idea for PD therapy. Cooper and colleagues [142] showed a significant reduction in α-Syn mRNA and protein levels in the brains of both normal and PD mice treated with RVG exosomes loaded with anti-α-Syn siRNA. This team targeted the reduction of α-synuclein aggregation again [143] using primary dendritic cell-derived, RVG-modified exosomes encapsulating the therapeutic molecule shRNA-MCs, which were specifically delivered to the brains of PD mice by intravenous injection and attenuated α-synuclein aggregation, reducing the loss of dopaminergic neurons and thus improving PD-related symptoms. It is noteworthy that the authors considered that shRNA size could affect drug delivery efficiency during exosome electroporation and specifically designed a smaller loop shape, i.e., shRNA-MCs, to achieve better loading efficiencies and therapeutic effects. This novel approach provided insights into the exosomal drug delivery systems for the treatment of other neurodegenerative disorders. Along similar lines, RVG-exosomes loaded with aptamer F5R1 were also able to deliver to neurons in vitro and in vivo, significantly reducing the pathological aggregations induced by α-synuclein pre-formed fibers (PFFs) [79].

Dopamine is also used for PD in addition to the treatment options mentioned above, but dopamine reaching the brain is problematic. Qu et al. [80] used blood exosomes to encapsulate dopamine and successfully delivered it to the striatum and substantia nigra of the brains by intravenous injection to ameliorate symptoms of PD mice.

6.3. Huntington's Disease

Huntington's disease (HD) is a hereditary neurodegenerative disorder [144]. Disease-causing genes, also known as Huntington's genes, produce abnormal Huntington's proteins which tend to adhere and aggregate, ultimately resulting in neuronal cell death [145,146]. Thus, silencing this gene is a strategy for HD therapy. Since exosomes have been widely used for siRNA delivery [147], Didiot et al. [148] modified siRNA hydrophobically to improve loading efficiency when incubated with exosomes. After unilateral infusion of exosomes into the mice striatum, exosomes carried siRNA for diffusion to the contralateral striatum and transported it to neurons, ultimately resulting in dose-dependent silencing of Huntingtin mRNA and protein in bilateral ventricles.

6.4. Stroke

A stroke is a general term for brain tissue damage caused by sudden rupture or blockage of cerebral blood vessels, including ischemic and hemorrhagic stroke [149–151]. It is a neurological disease with a high rate of disability worldwide [152,153].

Subarachnoid hemorrhage is a major reason for hemorrhagic stroke. In one study [154], miR-193b-3p was delivered to the brains of mice by intravenous injection of exosomes, which ameliorated inflammatory response through inhibition of HDAC3. Lastly, neurobehavioral disturbances, brain edema, BBB injury, and neurodegeneration were alleviated.

Compared with hemorrhagic stroke, ischemic stroke accounts for the vast majority of the total number of strokes [155] and the main causes are occlusion and stenosis of the associated arteries. MiRNAs were involved in regulating nervous system development and function [156,157] and their therapeutic potential has been demonstrated in a variety of CNS diseases [158,159]. MSC-exosomes showed superior effects in the treatment of various neurological disorders [160–162], as evidenced by neural repair and inhibition of neuroinflammation [95,163]. Therefore, several studies [164–166] have explored the use of MSC-exosome-encapsulated miRNAs as therapeutic molecules for the treatment of ischemic strokes. For example, Zhao et al. [164] transfected MSCs with miR-223-3p to generate miRNA-loaded exosomes. After intravenous injection, the volume of cerebral infarction was greatly reduced, and neurological function was markedly improved. Its protective effect was closely associated with an increased polarization of microglia towards the M2 phenotype. MiR-124 also biased neural progenitor cells toward neuronal lineage through exosomes, greatly contributing to neurogenesis after ischemia [165]. Similarly, miR-17-92-enriched exosomes improved neurological function and promoted neurogenesis [166].

Curcumin is a natural polyphenolic compound with a potent anti-inflammatory effectivity [167,168]. RGD peptides were bound to the surface of MSC-exosomes by bioorthogonal chemistry, and curcumin entered the exosomes after co-incubation. Drug-loaded exosomes targeted microglia, neurons, and astrocytes in the brain following intravenous injection and effectively inhibited inflammatory response and apoptosis in ischemic brain injury areas [123]. Whereas the aforementioned brain targeting of exosomes was RGD mediated, He et al. [76] took advantage of the targeted migration capability of mouse macrophage RAW264.7 exosomes themselves, loading curcumin as a therapeutic agent as well. After intravenous injection, the exosomes targeted ischemic areas and exerted powerful neuroprotective effects by eliminating ROS generation and mitigating BBB destruction. Exosomes from mouse embryonic stem cells (MESC) may also bind curcumin for stroke treatment [87].

Aside from the curcumin and miRNAs mentioned above, other active molecules such as circSCMH1 [74], recombinant human NGF mRNA [169], and pigment epithelium-derived factor (PEDF) [170] could also be coated with exosomes as therapeutic molecules for strokes treatment.

6.5. Brain or Spinal Cord Injury and Neuroinflammation

Brain or spinal cord injury is a neuroinflammatory condition that endangers human health. In spinal cord injury (SCI), MSC-exosomes acquired the homing property of its progenitor cells and were able to automatically penetrate the BBB to reach the injured spinal cord region. Taking advantage of this property, Guo et al. [109] repaired SCI after intranasal injection of MSC-exosomes containing phosphatase and tensin homolog siRNA (PTEN-siRNA), which effectively reduced neuroinflammation and glial proliferation. In addition to SCI, repetitive mild TBI (rmTBI) not only triggered neuroinflammation but may also have led to long-term neurodegenerative diseases like AD [171]. Microglia, as specific resident macrophages in the CNS, play key roles in the development and regression of neuroinflammation [172,173]. One study [75] reported that intravenous administration of microglia exosomes harboring miR-124-3p could target neurons and alleviate neurodegeneration. Multiple sclerosis (MS) is a classic neuroinflammatory disorder mainly characterized by inflammatory demyelinating lesions in the white matter of the CNS [174]. The LJM-3064 aptamer, which was chemically covalently bound to the surface of MSCs exosomes, significantly ameliorated neuroinflammation by reducing areas of demyelinating lesions in the spinal cord and brain [84]. Zhuang et al. [175] verified the therapeutic effect of the exosomes' drug delivery system in three neuroinflammatory models: LPS-induced encephalitis models, experimental autoimmune encephalomyelitis (EAE) models, and brain-tumor-induced neuroinflammation. Exosomes loaded with curcumin or JSI124 (a signal transducer and activator of the transcription 3 inhibitor) could target microglia and induce microglia apoptosis to alleviate neuroinflammation after intranasal injection.

6.6. Brain Tumor

Gliomas account for 40% to 50% of brain tumors and are the most common primary intracranial tumors. Glioma has a high mortality, disability, and very poor prognosis [176]. A major reason why current drugs have difficulty in achieving the desired therapeutic effect is the difficulty in crossing the BBB to accumulate sufficient local drug concentrations at the tumor site. Exosomes, as drug delivery systems capable of crossing the blood-brain barrier, have played important roles in glioma treatment. For example, a recent study developed exosomes modified with Angiopep-2 and transcriptional peptide trans-activators and loaded doxorubicin to reach gliomas by crossing the BBB, not only improving the survival time of glioma mice by more than 2-fold but also greatly reducing the toxic effects of doxorubicin [177]. Similarly, Jia et al. [128] loaded curcumin and SPIONs (MRI contrast agents) into exosomes simultaneously by electroporation and then modified the exosomes with glioma-targeting peptides by click chemistry, ultimately showing dual antitumor effects.

In tumor therapy, overcoming drug resistance is also a major task. Glioblastoma multiforme (GBM) often exhibit chemo- and radio-resistance [178]. Yamada's group found that the main reason for the resistance of GBM to the chemotherapeutic drug temozolomide was the upregulation of miR-9 in cells, which was involved in the expression of the P-glycoprotein, a drug efflux transporter. Given this, the authors used mesenchymal stem-cell-derived exosomes carrying anti-miR-9 to eventually reverse the expression of multidrug transporter proteins and sensitize GBM cells to temozolomide [179].

Apart from gliomas, brain tumors contain astrocytoma, meningioma, neurofibroma, and so on [180]. Because of the complex and precise structures in the brain, whatever type of cytopathic brain tumor, once compressed to any part of the brain, will cause damage to different functions in the body. For the treatment of brain tumors, exosome delivery systems continue to perform well. For example, brain endothelium-derived exosomes could deliver the anticancer drug doxorubicin via the BBB for the treatment of brain cancer in zebrafish [105].

6.7. Other Brain Diseases: Viral Infection; Drug Addiction

Drug addiction is highly damaging to individuals and society, mainly because of a series of withdrawal symptoms that occur when the drug stops stimulating the CNS. Nevertheless, there are very limited treatments available [181]. Among them, opioids mediate analgesic and addictive effects through MOR receptors. Thus, Liu's team boldly attempted to use exosomes derived from RVG-modified HEK 293T cells to deliver MOR siRNA specifically to the mouse brain and downregulate MOR expression to mediate morphine addiction treatment [182].

Viruses can invade the organism and proliferate in the host cells through multiple pathways. Even some viruses invade the CNS, such as the ZIKA virus, which could cross the placenta and BBB to enter the fetal brain and cause fetal microcephaly [82]. Zhang et al. [183] designed an RVG-modified exosome derived from HEK 293T cells, which contained ZIKV-specific siRNA. Once intravenously injected, exosomes could cross the mice's placental barrier from the maternal circulatory system to the fetal mice and cross the fetal BBB to target the head, thus protecting the fetal mice from ZIKV virus infection and alleviating neuroinflammation.

In summary, exosomes have been widely used as CNS drug delivery tools. They can be loaded with a variety of therapeutic molecules, including nucleic acids, proteins, and small molecule compounds. Exosomal drug delivery systems have shown good results in treating almost all CNS diseases, from neurodegenerative diseases to neuroinflammatory diseases, from brain tumors to brain viral infections. This greatly encouraged researchers to continue to explore and utilize exosomes as drug delivery tools for the treatment of CNS diseases. Additionally, the studies on exosomal drug delivery systems for CNS diseases are summarized in Table 1.

Table 1. Preclinical studies on exosomes as DDS for CNS diseases treatment.

Disease	Donor Cell	Therapeutic Molecule	Drug Loading Method	Modification Strategy	Animal	Administration Route	Targeted Cells	Ref.
Alzheimer's disease	self-derived dendritic cells	BACE1 siRNA	electroporation	Lamp2b-RVG	Mice	intravenous	neurons, microglia, and oligodendrocytes	[118]
Parkinson's disease	HEK-293T cells	catalase mRNA	transfection	Lamp2b-RVG	Mice	subcutaneous	unknown	[129]
	primary dendritic cells	a-Syn siRNA	electroporation	Lamp2b-RVG	Mice	intravenous	unknown	[142]
	primary dendritic cells	shRNA-MCs	electroporation	Lamp2b-RVG	Mice	intravenous	unknown	[143]
	HEK-293T cells	aptamer F5R1	co-incubation	Lamp2b-RVG	Mice	intraperitoneal	microglia, neurons, and astrocytes	[79]
	mice blood	dopamine	co-incubation	None	Mice	intravenous	unknown	[80]
	RAW264.7	catalase	co-incubation, freeze-thaw, sonication, or extrusion	None	Mice	intranasal	neurons and microglia	[86]
Huntington's disease	glioblastoma U87 cells	$hsiRNA^{HTT}$	co-incubation	None	Mice	unilateral brain infusion	neurons	[148]
Stroke	mesenchymal stromal cells (MSC)	curcumin	co-incubation	c(RGDyK) peptide	Mice	intravenous	microglia, neurons, and astrocytes	[123]
	bone marrow mesenchymal stem cells (BMSC)	miR-193b-3p	electroporation	Lamp2b-RVG	Mice	intravenous	unknown	[154]
	HEK-293T cells	circ SCMH1	transfection	Lamp2b-RVG	Mice and rhesus monkeys	intravenous	microglia, neurons, and astrocytes	[74]
	mesenchymal stem cells (MSCs)	miR-223-3p	transfection	None	Rats	intravenous	unknown	[164]
	RAW264.7	curcumin	co-incubation	None	Rats	intravenous	neurons and endothelium cells	[76]
	mouse embryonic stem cells (MESCs)	curcumin	co-incubation	None	Mice	intranasal	astrocytes and neurons	[87]
	multipotent mesenchymal stromal cells (MSCs)	miR-17-92	transfection	None	Rats	intravenous	unknown	[166]
	adipose-derived stem cells (ADSCs)	PEDF	transfection	None	Rats	intravenous	unknown	[170]
	HEK-293T cells	recombinant human NGF mRNA	transfection	Lamp2b-RVG	Mice	intravenous	microglia, neurons, and astrocytes	[169]
	bone marrow mesenchymal stem cells (BMSC)	miR-124	electroporation	Lamp2b-RVG	Mice	intravenous	neurons, astrocytes, and oligodendrocytes	[165]

Table 1. *Cont.*

Disease	Donor Cell	Therapeutic Molecule	Drug Loading Method	Modification Strategy	Animal	Administration Route	Targeted Cells	Ref.
Repetitive mild traumatic brain injury (rmTBI)	microglia	miR-124-3p	transfection	None	Mice	intravenous	microglia, neurons, and astrocytes	[75]
Spinal cord injury (SCI)	mesenchymal stem cells (MSC)	PTEN-siRNA	co-incubation	None	Rats	intranasal	neurons	[109]
Multiple sclerosis	EL-4 cells	curcumin or JSI124	co-incubation	None	Mice	intranasal	microglia	[175]
	mesenchymal stem cells (MSCs)	LJM-3064 aptamer	EDC/NHS	None	Mice	intravenous	unknown	[84]
Brain tumor	brain endothelial cell (bEND.3)	doxorubicin	co-incubation	None	zebrafishes	intravenous	unknown	[105]
	RAW264.7	curcumin and SPIONs	electroporation	RGE-peptide	Mice	intravenous	glioma	[128]
ZIKV infection	HEK-293T cells	ZIKV-specific siRNA	electroporation	Lamp2b-RVG	Mice	intravenous	microglia, neurons, and astrocytes	[183]
Morphine addiction	HEK-293T cells	Mu (MOR) siRNA	transfection	Lamp2b-RVG	Mice	intravenous	neuro2A	[182]

7. Conclusions and Perspectives

According to the latest database (http://www.exocarta.org/, accessed on 23 September 2022), 9769 proteins, 3408 mRNAs, and 2838 microRNAs have been identified in exosomes. These rich contents make the role of exosomes in intercellular communication, disease development, and therapy increasingly expansive. It brings light to exosomes as CNS drug delivery tools. To date, exosome studies have involved a number of species including mice, rats, zebrafishes, and monkeys (https://evtrack.org/, accessed on 23 September 2022), which will drive the clinical translation of exosomes.

As CNS drug delivery tools, exosomes have several characteristics compared to synthetic nanoparticles: low immunogenicity, non-toxicity, high cargo carrying, protective capabilities [184–186], and the ability to cross the blood-brain barrier [187–189]. To improve the efficiency of entering the CNS, exosome surface engineering modification has been widely used. It can increase the local concentration of drugs at the lesion site and reduce toxic side effects while improving therapeutic efficacy. However, the structural and functional stability of engineered exosomes and the mechanism of improving CNS targeting efficiency have not been thoroughly studied. Therefore, more research is needed to enhance the stability, security, and standardization of these strategies.

There are various types of active molecules encapsulated in exosomes, including nucleic acids (miRNAs, siRNAs, shRNAs, mRNAs, etc.), small molecule compounds (doxorubicin, dopamine, etc.), natural products (curcumin, paclitaxel, resveratrol, etc.), and proteins (catalase, pigment epithelium-derived factor, etc.). For different types of therapeutic drugs and exosomes, various loading methods exist, both before and after the secretion of exosomes. Genetic engineering, co-incubation, electroporation, sonication, extrusion, and repeated freeze-thawing have been employed. On this basis, we need to further investigate the mechanisms of exosome internalization to better understand how they work and thus select suitable drug loading methods for different types of therapeutic molecules. There has been increasing evidence that exosomes carrying the therapeutic molecules mentioned above have made breakthroughs in various CNS diseases such as brain tumors, neurodegenerative diseases, multiple scleroses, brain or spinal cord injuries, strokes, drug addictions, and viral infections. However, progress in the isolation and purification of exosomes as well as mechanistic studies are needed to fully realize the potential of exosomes in CNS drug delivery systems.

In conclusion, engineering modifications, administration routes, type of therapeutic molecules, and encapsulation modes are all important parameters of exosomes as CNS drug delivery tools (Figure 4) and affect their clinical transformation. The majority of patients with CNS diseases will benefit if we can pay more attention to the problems already present, deepen our understanding of unexplained mechanisms, and realize their maximal clinical potential.

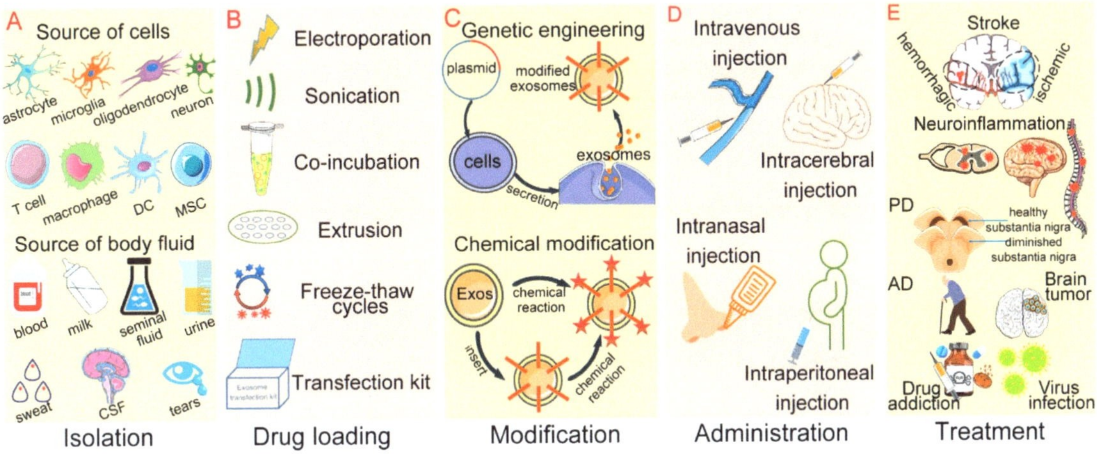

Figure 4. The research process of exosomes as CNS drug delivery tools. (**A**) Exosomes are isolated from cells or body fluids; (**B**) multiple drug loading modes of exosomes; (**C**) exosomes can be modified by genetic engineering and chemical reactions; (**D**) several administration routes of cargo-loading exosomes; (**E**) exosomes loaded with therapeutic molecules are used to treat a variety of CNS diseases. DC: dendritic cell; MSC: mesenchymal stem cell; CSF: cerebrospinal fluid; Exos: exosomes; PD: Parkinson's disease; AD: Alzheimer's disease.

Author Contributions: Writing—original draft preparation, K.S.; writing—review and editing, K.S. and X.Z.; visualization, W.Z. and F.Y.; supervision, W.Z. and H.J. All authors have read and agreed to the published version of the manuscript.

Funding: This research was funded by National Key R&D Program of China (2018YFA0507204) and the National Natural Science Foundation of China (22077068).

Institutional Review Board Statement: Not applicable.

Informed Consent Statement: Not applicable.

Data Availability Statement: Not applicable.

Conflicts of Interest: The authors declare no conflict of interest.

Abbreviations

CNS	central nervous system
RVG	rabies virus glycoprotein
DDS	drug delivery system
BBB	blood-brain barrier
AAV	adeno-associated virus
EVs	extracellular vesicles
MPS	mononuclear phagocytic system
PEG	polyethylene glycol
ABC	acceleration of blood clearance
CSF	cerebrospinal fluid

MSC	mesenchymal stem cell
SCI	spinal cord injury
TBI	traumatic brain injury
MS	multiple sclerosis
EAE	experimental allergic encephalomyelitis
RES	reticuloendothelial system
PD	Parkinson's disease
AD	Alzheimer's disease

References

1. Park, H.; Otte, A.; Park, K. Evolution of drug delivery systems: From 1950 to 2020 and beyond. *J. Control. Release* **2022**, *342*, 53–65. [CrossRef]
2. Bally, M.B.; Harvie, P.; Wong, F.M.; Kong, S.; Wasan, E.K.; Reimer, D.L. Biological barriers to cellular delivery of lipid-based DNA carriers. *Adv. Drug Deliv. Rev.* **1999**, *38*, 291–315. [CrossRef]
3. Begley, D.J. Delivery of therapeutic agents to the central nervous system: The problems and the possibilities. *Pharmacol. Ther.* **2004**, *104*, 29–45. [CrossRef]
4. Deprez, J.; Lajoinie, G.; Engelen, Y.; De Smedt, S.C.; Lentacker, I. Opening doors with ultrasound and microbubbles: Beating biological barriers to promote drug delivery. *Adv. Drug Deliv. Rev.* **2021**, *172*, 9–36. [CrossRef]
5. Henrich-Noack, P.; Nikitovic, D.; Neagu, M.; Docea, A.O.; Engin, A.B.; Gelperina, S.; Shtilman, M.; Mitsias, P.; Tzanakakis, G.; Gozes, I.; et al. The blood-brain barrier and beyond: Nano-based neuropharmacology and the role of extracellular matrix. *Nanomedicine* **2019**, *17*, 359–379. [CrossRef]
6. Yang, R.; Wei, T.; Goldberg, H.; Wang, W.; Cullion, K.; Kohane, D.S. Getting Drugs Across Biological Barriers. *Adv. Mater.* **2017**, *29*, 1606596. [CrossRef]
7. Wang, Y.I.; Abaci, H.E.; Shuler, M.L. Microfluidic blood-brain barrier model provides in vivo-like barrier properties for drug permeability screening. *Biotechnol. Bioeng.* **2017**, *114*, 184–194. [CrossRef]
8. Chen, W.; Yao, S.; Wan, J.; Tian, Y.; Huang, L.; Wang, S.; Akter, F.; Wu, Y.; Yao, Y.; Zhang, X. BBB-crossing adeno-associated virus vector: An excellent gene delivery tool for CNS disease treatment. *J. Control. Release* **2021**, *333*, 129–138. [CrossRef]
9. Castro, F.; Martins, C.; Silveira, M.J.; Moura, R.P.; Pereira, C.L.; Sarmento, B. Advances on erythrocyte-mimicking nanovehicles to overcome barriers in biological microenvironments. *Adv. Drug Deliv. Rev.* **2021**, *170*, 312–339. [CrossRef]
10. Mendanha, D.; Vieira de Castro, J.; Ferreira, H.; Neves, N.M. Biomimetic and cell-based nanocarriers—New strategies for brain tumor targeting. *J. Control. Release* **2021**, *337*, 482–493. [CrossRef]
11. Escude Martinez de Castilla, P.; Tong, L.; Huang, C.; Sofias, A.M.; Pastorin, G.; Chen, X.; Storm, G.; Schiffelers, R.M.; Wang, J.W. Extracellular vesicles as a drug delivery system: A systematic review of preclinical studies. *Adv. Drug Deliv. Rev.* **2021**, *175*, 113801. [CrossRef]
12. Akhtar, A.; Andleeb, A.; Waris, T.S.; Bazzar, M.; Moradi, A.R.; Awan, N.R.; Yar, M. Neurodegenerative diseases and effective drug delivery: A review of challenges and novel therapeutics. *J. Control. Release* **2021**, *330*, 1152–1167. [CrossRef]
13. Nash, A.; Aghlara-Fotovat, S.; Hernandez, A.; Scull, C.; Veiseh, O. Clinical translation of immunomodulatory therapeutics. *Adv. Drug Deliv. Rev.* **2021**, *176*, 113896. [CrossRef]
14. Tkach, M.; Thery, C. Communication by Extracellular Vesicles: Where We Are and Where We Need to Go. *Cell* **2016**, *164*, 1226–1232. [CrossRef]
15. Mathieu, M.; Martin-Jaular, L.; Lavieu, G.; Thery, C. Specificities of secretion and uptake of exosomes and other extracellular vesicles for cell-to-cell communication. *Nat. Cell Biol.* **2019**, *21*, 9–17. [CrossRef]
16. Valadi, H.; Ekstrom, K.; Bossios, A.; Sjostrand, M.; Lee, J.J.; Lotvall, J.O. Exosome-mediated transfer of mRNAs and microRNAs is a novel mechanism of genetic exchange between cells. *Nat. Cell Biol.* **2007**, *9*, 654–659. [CrossRef]
17. Chong, S.Y.; Lee, C.K.; Huang, C.; Ou, Y.H.; Charles, C.J.; Richards, A.M.; Neupane, Y.R.; Pavon, M.V.; Zharkova, O.; Pastorin, G.; et al. Extracellular Vesicles in Cardiovascular Diseases: Alternative Biomarker Sources, Therapeutic Agents, and Drug Delivery Carriers. *Int. J. Mol. Sci.* **2019**, *20*, 3272. [CrossRef]
18. de Jong, O.G.; Kooijmans, S.A.A.; Murphy, D.E.; Jiang, L.; Evers, M.J.W.; Sluijter, J.P.G.; Vader, P.; Schiffelers, R.M. Drug Delivery with Extracellular Vesicles: From Imagination to Innovation. *Acc. Chem. Res.* **2019**, *52*, 1761–1770. [CrossRef]
19. Pan, S.; Zhang, Y.; Natalia, A.; Lim, C.Z.J.; Ho, N.R.Y.; Chowbay, B.; Loh, T.P.; Tam, J.K.C.; Shao, H. Extracellular vesicle drug occupancy enables real-time monitoring of targeted cancer therapy. *Nat. Nanotechnol.* **2021**, *16*, 734–742. [CrossRef]
20. Fan, J.; Wei, Q.; Koay, E.J.; Liu, Y.; Ning, B.; Bernard, P.W.; Zhang, N.; Han, H.; Katz, M.H.; Zhao, Z.; et al. Chemoresistance Transmission via Exosome-Mediated EphA2 Transfer in Pancreatic Cancer. *Theranostics* **2018**, *8*, 5986–5994. [CrossRef]
21. Hutcheson, J.D.; Aikawa, E. Extracellular vesicles in cardiovascular homeostasis and disease. *Curr. Opin. Cardiol.* **2018**, *33*, 290–297. [CrossRef] [PubMed]
22. Roefs, M.T.; Sluijter, J.P.G.; Vader, P. Extracellular Vesicle-Associated Proteins in Tissue Repair. *Trends Cell Biol.* **2020**, *30*, 990–1013. [CrossRef] [PubMed]

23. Zhou, X.; Xie, F.; Wang, L.; Zhang, L.; Zhang, S.; Fang, M.; Zhou, F. The function and clinical application of extracellular vesicles in innate immune regulation. *Cell. Mol. Immunol.* **2020**, *17*, 323–334. [CrossRef] [PubMed]
24. Gyorgy, B.; Szabo, T.G.; Pasztoi, M.; Pal, Z.; Misjak, P.; Aradi, B.; Laszlo, V.; Pallinger, E.; Pap, E.; Kittel, A.; et al. Membrane vesicles, current state-of-the-art: Emerging role of extracellular vesicles. *Cell. Mol. Life Sci.* **2011**, *68*, 2667–2688. [CrossRef] [PubMed]
25. El Andaloussi, S.; Mager, I.; Breakefield, X.O.; Wood, M.J. Extracellular vesicles: Biology and emerging therapeutic opportunities. *Nat. Rev. Drug Discov.* **2013**, *12*, 347–357. [CrossRef]
26. Shao, H.; Im, H.; Castro, C.M.; Breakefield, X.; Weissleder, R.; Lee, H. New Technologies for Analysis of Extracellular Vesicles. *Chem. Rev.* **2018**, *118*, 1917–1950. [CrossRef]
27. Thery, C.; Zitvogel, L.; Amigorena, S. Exosomes: Composition, biogenesis and function. *Nat. Rev. Immunol.* **2002**, *2*, 569–579. [CrossRef]
28. Pluchino, S.; Smith, J.A. Explicating Exosomes: Reclassifying the Rising Stars of Intercellular Communication. *Cell* **2019**, *177*, 225–227. [CrossRef]
29. Willms, E.; Johansson, H.J.; Mager, I.; Lee, Y.; Blomberg, K.E.; Sadik, M.; Alaarg, A.; Smith, C.I.; Lehtio, J.; El Andaloussi, S.; et al. Cells release subpopulations of exosomes with distinct molecular and biological properties. *Sci. Rep.* **2016**, *6*, 22519. [CrossRef]
30. Farooqi, A.A.; Desai, N.N.; Qureshi, M.Z.; Librelotto, D.R.N.; Gasparri, M.L.; Bishayee, A.; Nabavi, S.M.; Curti, V.; Daglia, M. Exosome biogenesis, bioactivities and functions as new delivery systems of natural compounds. *Biotechnol. Adv.* **2018**, *36*, 328–334. [CrossRef]
31. Thery, C.; Witwer, K.W.; Aikawa, E.; Alcaraz, M.J.; Anderson, J.D.; Andriantsitohaina, R.; Antoniou, A.; Arab, T.; Archer, F.; Atkin-Smith, G.K.; et al. Minimal information for studies of extracellular vesicles 2018 (MISEV2018): A position statement of the International Society for Extracellular Vesicles and update of the MISEV2014 guidelines. *J. Extracell. Vesicles* **2018**, *7*, 1535750. [CrossRef] [PubMed]
32. Vader, P.; Mol, E.A.; Pasterkamp, G.; Schiffelers, R.M. Extracellular vesicles for drug delivery. *Adv. Drug Deliv. Rev.* **2016**, *106*, 148–156. [CrossRef] [PubMed]
33. Hua, S.; Wu, S.Y. The use of lipid-based nanocarriers for targeted pain therapies. *Front. Pharmacol.* **2013**, *4*, 143. [CrossRef] [PubMed]
34. Mima, Y.; Hashimoto, Y.; Shimizu, T.; Kiwada, H.; Ishida, T. Anti-PEG IgM Is a Major Contributor to the Accelerated Blood Clearance of Polyethylene Glycol-Conjugated Protein. *Mol. Pharm.* **2015**, *12*, 2429–2435. [CrossRef] [PubMed]
35. Ishihara, T.; Takeda, M.; Sakamoto, H.; Kimoto, A.; Kobayashi, C.; Takasaki, N.; Yuki, K.; Tanaka, K.; Takenaga, M.; Igarashi, R.; et al. Accelerated blood clearance phenomenon upon repeated injection of PEG-modified PLA-nanoparticles. *Pharm. Res.* **2009**, *26*, 2270–2279. [CrossRef] [PubMed]
36. Ishida, T.; Kashima, S.; Kiwada, H. The contribution of phagocytic activity of liver macrophages to the accelerated blood clearance (ABC) phenomenon of PEGylated liposomes in rats. *J. Control. Release* **2008**, *126*, 162–165. [CrossRef] [PubMed]
37. Armstrong, J.K.; Hempel, G.; Koling, S.; Chan, L.S.; Fisher, T.; Meiselman, H.J.; Garratty, G. Antibody against poly(ethylene glycol) adversely affects PEG-asparaginase therapy in acute lymphoblastic leukemia patients. *Cancer* **2007**, *110*, 103–111. [CrossRef]
38. van Niel, G.; D'Angelo, G.; Raposo, G. Shedding light on the cell biology of extracellular vesicles. *Nat. Rev. Mol. Cell Biol.* **2018**, *19*, 213–228. [CrossRef]
39. Batrakova, E.V.; Kim, M.S. Using exosomes, naturally-equipped nanocarriers, for drug delivery. *J. Control. Release* **2015**, *219*, 396–405. [CrossRef]
40. Ha, D.; Yang, N.; Nadithe, V. Exosomes as therapeutic drug carriers and delivery vehicles across biological membranes: Current perspectives and future challenges. *Acta Pharm. Sin. B* **2016**, *6*, 287–296. [CrossRef]
41. van der Meel, R.; Fens, M.H.; Vader, P.; van Solinge, W.W.; Eniola-Adefeso, O.; Schiffelers, R.M. Extracellular vesicles as drug delivery systems: Lessons from the liposome field. *J. Control. Release* **2014**, *195*, 72–85. [CrossRef] [PubMed]
42. de Abreu, R.C.; Fernandes, H.; da Costa Martins, P.A.; Sahoo, S.; Emanueli, C.; Ferreira, L. Native and bioengineered extracellular vesicles for cardiovascular therapeutics. *Nat. Rev. Cardiol.* **2020**, *17*, 685–697. [CrossRef] [PubMed]
43. Saeedi, M.; Eslamifar, M.; Khezri, K.; Dizaj, S.M. Applications of nanotechnology in drug delivery to the central nervous system. *Biomed. Pharmacother.* **2019**, *111*, 666–675. [CrossRef]
44. Chen, Y.; Liu, L. Modern methods for delivery of drugs across the blood-brain barrier. *Adv. Drug Deliv. Rev.* **2012**, *64*, 640–665. [CrossRef]
45. Zlokovic, B.V. The blood-brain barrier in health and chronic neurodegenerative disorders. *Neuron* **2008**, *57*, 178–201. [CrossRef]
46. Lee, J.; Kim, S.E.; Moon, D.; Doh, J. A multilayered blood vessel/tumor tissue chip to investigate T cell infiltration into solid tumor tissues. *Lab Chip* **2021**, *21*, 2142–2152. [CrossRef]
47. Deng, Z.; Sheng, Z.; Yan, F. Ultrasound-Induced Blood-Brain-Barrier Opening Enhances Anticancer Efficacy in the Treatment of Glioblastoma: Current Status and Future Prospects. *J. Oncol.* **2019**, *2019*, 2345203. [CrossRef]
48. Saint-Pol, J.; Gosselet, F.; Duban-Deweer, S.; Pottiez, G.; Karamanos, Y. Targeting and Crossing the Blood-Brain Barrier with Extracellular Vesicles. *Cells* **2020**, *9*, 851. [CrossRef]
49. Gabathuler, R. Approaches to transport therapeutic drugs across the blood-brain barrier to treat brain diseases. *Neurobiol. Dis.* **2010**, *37*, 48–57. [CrossRef]

50. Faure, J.; Lachenal, G.; Court, M.; Hirrlinger, J.; Chatellard-Causse, C.; Blot, B.; Grange, J.; Schoehn, G.; Goldberg, Y.; Boyer, V.; et al. Exosomes are released by cultured cortical neurones. *Mol. Cell. Neurosci.* **2006**, *31*, 642–648. [CrossRef]
51. Fruhbeis, C.; Frohlich, D.; Kuo, W.P.; Kramer-Albers, E.M. Extracellular vesicles as mediators of neuron-glia communication. *Front. Cell. Neurosci.* **2013**, *7*, 182. [CrossRef] [PubMed]
52. Potolicchio, I.; Carven, G.J.; Xu, X.; Stipp, C.; Riese, R.J.; Stern, L.J.; Santambrogio, L. Proteomic analysis of microglia-derived exosomes: Metabolic role of the aminopeptidase CD13 in neuropeptide catabolism. *J. Immunol.* **2005**, *175*, 2237–2243. [CrossRef] [PubMed]
53. Taylor, A.R.; Robinson, M.B.; Gifondorwa, D.J.; Tytell, M.; Milligan, C.E. Regulation of heat shock protein 70 release in astrocytes: Role of signaling kinases. *Dev. Neurobiol.* **2007**, *67*, 1815–1829. [CrossRef] [PubMed]
54. Milane, L.; Singh, A.; Mattheolabakis, G.; Suresh, M.; Amiji, M.M. Exosome mediated communication within the tumor microenvironment. *J. Control. Release* **2015**, *219*, 278–294. [CrossRef]
55. Zhang, T.; Ma, S.; Lv, J.; Wang, X.; Afewerky, H.K.; Li, H.; Lu, Y. The emerging role of exosomes in Alzheimer's disease. *Ageing Res. Rev.* **2021**, *68*, 101321. [CrossRef]
56. Ramirez, S.H.; Andrews, A.M.; Paul, D.; Pachter, J.S. Extracellular vesicles: Mediators and biomarkers of pathology along CNS barriers. *Fluids Barriers CNS* **2018**, *15*, 19. [CrossRef]
57. Basso, M.; Bonetto, V. Extracellular Vesicles and a Novel Form of Communication in the Brain. *Front. Neurosci.* **2016**, *10*, 127. [CrossRef]
58. Sharma, P.; Mesci, P.; Carromeu, C.; McClatchy, D.R.; Schiapparelli, L.; Yates, J.R., 3rd; Muotri, A.R.; Cline, H.T. Exosomes regulate neurogenesis and circuit assembly. *Proc. Natl. Acad. Sci. USA* **2019**, *116*, 16086–16094. [CrossRef]
59. Budnik, V.; Ruiz-Canada, C.; Wendler, F. Extracellular vesicles round off communication in the nervous system. *Nat. Rev. Neurosci.* **2016**, *17*, 160–172. [CrossRef]
60. Xu, B.; Zhang, Y.; Du, X.F.; Li, J.; Zi, H.X.; Bu, J.W.; Yan, Y.; Han, H.; Du, J.L. Neurons secrete miR-132-containing exosomes to regulate brain vascular integrity. *Cell Res.* **2017**, *27*, 882–897. [CrossRef]
61. Perluigi, M.; Picca, A.; Montanari, E.; Calvani, R.; Marini, F.; Matassa, R.; Tramutola, A.; Villani, A.; Familiari, G.; Domenico, F.D.; et al. Aberrant crosstalk between insulin signaling and mTOR in young Down syndrome individuals revealed by neuronal-derived extracellular vesicles. *Alzheimers Dement* **2022**, *18*, 1498–1510. [CrossRef] [PubMed]
62. Xiong, X.Y.; Liu, L.; Yang, Q.W. Functions and mechanisms of microglia/macrophages in neuroinflammation and neurogenesis after stroke. *Prog. Neurobiol.* **2016**, *142*, 23–44. [CrossRef] [PubMed]
63. Huang, S.; Ge, X.; Yu, J.; Han, Z.; Yin, Z.; Li, Y.; Chen, F.; Wang, H.; Zhang, J.; Lei, P. Increased miR-124-3p in microglial exosomes following traumatic brain injury inhibits neuronal inflammation and contributes to neurite outgrowth via their transfer into neurons. *FASEB J.* **2018**, *32*, 512–528. [CrossRef]
64. Li, Z.; Liu, F.; He, X.; Yang, X.; Shan, F.; Feng, J. Exosomes derived from mesenchymal stem cells attenuate inflammation and demyelination of the central nervous system in EAE rats by regulating the polarization of microglia. *Int. Immunopharmacol.* **2019**, *67*, 268–280. [CrossRef]
65. Xin, H.; Li, Y.; Buller, B.; Katakowski, M.; Zhang, Y.; Wang, X.; Shang, X.; Zhang, Z.G.; Chopp, M. Exosome-mediated transfer of miR-133b from multipotent mesenchymal stromal cells to neural cells contributes to neurite outgrowth. *Stem Cells* **2012**, *30*, 1556–1564. [CrossRef]
66. Giunti, D.; Marini, C.; Parodi, B.; Usai, C.; Milanese, M.; Bonanno, G.; Kerlero de Rosbo, N.; Uccelli, A. Role of miRNAs shuttled by mesenchymal stem cell-derived small extracellular vesicles in modulating neuroinflammation. *Sci. Rep.* **2021**, *11*, 1740. [CrossRef]
67. Cui, G.H.; Zhu, J.; Wang, Y.C.; Wu, J.; Liu, J.R.; Guo, H.D. Effects of exosomal miRNAs in the diagnosis and treatment of Alzheimer's disease. *Mech. Ageing Dev.* **2021**, *200*, 111593. [CrossRef]
68. Deng, Z.; Wang, J.; Xiao, Y.; Li, F.; Niu, L.; Liu, X.; Meng, L.; Zheng, H. Ultrasound-mediated augmented exosome release from astrocytes alleviates amyloid-beta-induced neurotoxicity. *Theranostics* **2021**, *11*, 4351–4362. [CrossRef]
69. Zhang, L.; Zhang, S.; Yao, J.; Lowery, F.J.; Zhang, Q.; Huang, W.C.; Li, P.; Li, M.; Wang, X.; Zhang, C.; et al. Microenvironment-induced PTEN loss by exosomal microRNA primes brain metastasis outgrowth. *Nature* **2015**, *527*, 100–104. [CrossRef]
70. Vogel, A.; Upadhya, R.; Shetty, A.K. Neural stem cell derived extracellular vesicles: Attributes and prospects for treating neurodegenerative disorders. *eBioMedicine* **2018**, *38*, 273–282. [CrossRef]
71. Lee, E.J.; Choi, Y.; Lee, H.J.; Hwang, D.W.; Lee, D.S. Human neural stem cell-derived extracellular vesicles protect against Parkinson's disease pathologies. *J. Nanobiotechnol.* **2022**, *20*, 198. [CrossRef] [PubMed]
72. Apodaca, L.A.; Baddour, A.A.D.; Garcia, C., Jr.; Alikhani, L.; Giedzinski, E.; Ru, N.; Agrawal, A.; Acharya, M.M.; Baulch, J.E. Human neural stem cell-derived extracellular vesicles mitigate hallmarks of Alzheimer's disease. *Alzheimers Res. Ther.* **2021**, *13*, 57. [CrossRef] [PubMed]
73. Webb, R.L.; Kaiser, E.E.; Scoville, S.L.; Thompson, T.A.; Fatima, S.; Pandya, C.; Sriram, K.; Swetenburg, R.L.; Vaibhav, K.; Arbab, A.S.; et al. Human Neural Stem Cell Extracellular Vesicles Improve Tissue and Functional Recovery in the Murine Thromboembolic Stroke Model. *Transl. Stroke Res.* **2018**, *9*, 530–539. [CrossRef]
74. Yang, L.; Han, B.; Zhang, Z.; Wang, S.; Bai, Y.; Zhang, Y.; Tang, Y.; Du, L.; Xu, L.; Wu, F.; et al. Extracellular Vesicle-Mediated Delivery of Circular RNA SCMH1 Promotes Functional Recovery in Rodent and Nonhuman Primate Ischemic Stroke Models. *Circulation* **2020**, *142*, 556–574. [CrossRef] [PubMed]

75. Ge, X.; Guo, M.; Hu, T.; Li, W.; Huang, S.; Yin, Z.; Li, Y.; Chen, F.; Zhu, L.; Kang, C.; et al. Increased Microglial Exosomal miR-124-3p Alleviates Neurodegeneration and Improves Cognitive Outcome after rmTBI. *Mol. Ther.* **2020**, *28*, 503–522. [CrossRef]
76. He, R.; Jiang, Y.; Shi, Y.; Liang, J.; Zhao, L. Curcumin-laden exosomes target ischemic brain tissue and alleviate cerebral ischemia-reperfusion injury by inhibiting ROS-mediated mitochondrial apoptosis. *Mater. Sci. Eng. C Mater. Biol. Appl.* **2020**, *117*, 111314. [CrossRef]
77. Sutaria, D.S.; Badawi, M.; Phelps, M.A.; Schmittgen, T.D. Achieving the Promise of Therapeutic Extracellular Vesicles: The Devil is in Details of Therapeutic Loading. *Pharm. Res.* **2017**, *34*, 1053–1066. [CrossRef]
78. Sutaria, D.S.; Jiang, J.; Elgamal, O.A.; Pomeroy, S.M.; Badawi, M.; Zhu, X.; Pavlovicz, R.; Azevedo-Pouly, A.C.P.; Chalmers, J.; Li, C.; et al. Low active loading of cargo into engineered extracellular vesicles results in inefficient miRNA mimic delivery. *J. Extracell. Vesicles* **2017**, *6*, 1333882. [CrossRef]
79. Ren, X.; Zhao, Y.; Xue, F.; Zheng, Y.; Huang, H.; Wang, W.; Chang, Y.; Yang, H.; Zhang, J. Exosomal DNA Aptamer Targeting alpha-Synuclein Aggregates Reduced Neuropathological Deficits in a Mouse Parkinson's Disease Model. *Mol. Ther. Nucleic Acids* **2019**, *17*, 726–740. [CrossRef]
80. Qu, M.; Lin, Q.; Huang, L.; Fu, Y.; Wang, L.; He, S.; Fu, Y.; Yang, S.; Zhang, Z.; Zhang, L.; et al. Dopamine-loaded blood exosomes targeted to brain for better treatment of Parkinson's disease. *J. Control. Release* **2018**, *287*, 156–166. [CrossRef]
81. Fuhrmann, G.; Serio, A.; Mazo, M.; Nair, R.; Stevens, M.M. Active loading into extracellular vesicles significantly improves the cellular uptake and photodynamic effect of porphyrins. *J. Control. Release* **2015**, *205*, 35–44. [CrossRef] [PubMed]
82. Bogoch, I.I.; Brady, O.J.; Kraemer, M.U.G.; German, M.; Creatore, M.I.; Brent, S.; Watts, A.G.; Hay, S.I.; Kulkarni, M.A.; Brownstein, J.S.; et al. Potential for Zika virus introduction and transmission in resource-limited countries in Africa and the Asia-Pacific region: A modelling study. *Lancet Infect. Dis.* **2016**, *16*, 1237–1245. [CrossRef]
83. Luo, S.; Sun, X.; Huang, M.; Ma, Q.; Du, L.; Cui, Y. Enhanced Neuroprotective Effects of Epicatechin Gallate Encapsulated by Bovine Milk-Derived Exosomes against Parkinson's Disease through Antiapoptosis and Antimitophagy. *J. Agric. Food Chem.* **2021**, *69*, 5134–5143. [CrossRef] [PubMed]
84. Hosseini Shamili, F.; Alibolandi, M.; Rafatpanah, H.; Abnous, K.; Mahmoudi, M.; Kalantari, M.; Taghdisi, S.M.; Ramezani, M. Immunomodulatory properties of MSC-derived exosomes armed with high affinity aptamer toward mylein as a platform for reducing multiple sclerosis clinical score. *J. Control. Release* **2019**, *299*, 149–164. [CrossRef] [PubMed]
85. Hu, G.; Liao, K.; Niu, F.; Yang, L.; Dallon, B.W.; Callen, S.; Tian, C.; Shu, J.; Cui, J.; Sun, Z.; et al. Astrocyte EV-Induced lincRNA-Cox2 Regulates Microglial Phagocytosis: Implications for Morphine-Mediated Neurodegeneration. *Mol. Ther. Nucleic Acids* **2018**, *13*, 450–463. [CrossRef] [PubMed]
86. Haney, M.J.; Klyachko, N.L.; Zhao, Y.; Gupta, R.; Plotnikova, E.G.; He, Z.; Patel, T.; Piroyan, A.; Sokolsky, M.; Kabanov, A.V.; et al. Exosomes as drug delivery vehicles for Parkinson's disease therapy. *J. Control. Release* **2015**, *207*, 18–30. [CrossRef] [PubMed]
87. Kalani, A.; Chaturvedi, P.; Kamat, P.K.; Maldonado, C.; Bauer, P.; Joshua, I.G.; Tyagi, S.C.; Tyagi, N. Curcumin-loaded embryonic stem cell exosomes restored neurovascular unit following ischemia-reperfusion injury. *Int. J. Biochem. Cell Biol.* **2016**, *79*, 360–369. [CrossRef]
88. Haney, M.J.; Zhao, Y.; Jin, Y.S.; Li, S.M.; Bago, J.R.; Klyachko, N.L.; Kabanov, A.V.; Batrakova, E.V. Macrophage-Derived Extracellular Vesicles as Drug Delivery Systems for Triple Negative Breast Cancer (TNBC) Therapy. *J. Neuroimmune Pharmacol.* **2020**, *15*, 487–500. [CrossRef]
89. Kim, M.S.; Haney, M.J.; Zhao, Y.; Mahajan, V.; Deygen, I.; Klyachko, N.L.; Inskoe, E.; Piroyan, A.; Sokolsky, M.; Okolie, O.; et al. Development of exosome-encapsulated paclitaxel to overcome MDR in cancer cells. *Nanomedicine* **2016**, *12*, 655–664. [CrossRef]
90. Li, Y.J.; Wu, J.Y.; Wang, J.M.; Hu, X.B.; Cai, J.X.; Xiang, D.X. Gemcitabine loaded autologous exosomes for effective and safe chemotherapy of pancreatic cancer. *Acta Biomater.* **2020**, *101*, 519–530. [CrossRef]
91. Lee, J.; Lee, H.; Goh, U.; Kim, J.; Jeong, M.; Lee, J.; Park, J.H. Cellular Engineering with Membrane Fusogenic Liposomes to Produce Functionalized Extracellular Vesicles. *ACS Appl. Mater. Interfaces* **2016**, *8*, 6790–6795. [CrossRef]
92. Wiklander, O.P.; Nordin, J.Z.; O'Loughlin, A.; Gustafsson, Y.; Corso, G.; Mager, I.; Vader, P.; Lee, Y.; Sork, H.; Seow, Y.; et al. Extracellular vesicle in vivo biodistribution is determined by cell source, route of administration and targeting. *J. Extracell. Vesicles* **2015**, *4*, 26316. [CrossRef]
93. Lai, C.P.; Mardini, O.; Ericsson, M.; Prabhakar, S.; Maguire, C.; Chen, J.W.; Tannous, B.A.; Breakefield, X.O. Dynamic biodistribution of extracellular vesicles in vivo using a multimodal imaging reporter. *ACS Nano* **2014**, *8*, 483–494. [CrossRef]
94. Nakazaki, M.; Morita, T.; Lankford, K.L.; Askenase, P.W.; Kocsis, J.D. Small extracellular vesicles released by infused mesenchymal stromal cells target M2 macrophages and promote TGF-beta upregulation, microvascular stabilization and functional recovery in a rodent model of severe spinal cord injury. *J. Extracell. Vesicles* **2021**, *10*, e12137. [CrossRef]
95. Riazifar, M.; Mohammadi, M.R.; Pone, E.J.; Yeri, A.; Lasser, C.; Segaliny, A.I.; McIntyre, L.L.; Shelke, G.V.; Hutchins, E.; Hamamoto, A.; et al. Stem Cell-Derived Exosomes as Nanotherapeutics for Autoimmune and Neurodegenerative Disorders. *ACS Nano* **2019**, *13*, 6670–6688. [CrossRef]
96. Dasgupta, D.; Nakao, Y.; Mauer, A.S.; Thompson, J.M.; Sehrawat, T.S.; Liao, C.Y.; Krishnan, A.; Lucien, F.; Guo, Q.; Liu, M.; et al. IRE1A Stimulates Hepatocyte-Derived Extracellular Vesicles That Promote Inflammation in Mice With Steatohepatitis. *Gastroenterology* **2020**, *159*, 1487–1503.e17. [CrossRef]
97. Thome, A.D.; Thonhoff, J.R.; Zhao, W.; Faridar, A.; Wang, J.; Beers, D.R.; Appel, S.H. Extracellular Vesicles Derived From Ex Vivo Expanded Regulatory T Cells Modulate In Vitro and In Vivo Inflammation. *Front. Immunol.* **2022**, *13*, 875825. [CrossRef]

98. Kim, M.; Lee, Y.; Lee, M. Hypoxia-specific anti-RAGE exosomes for nose-to-brain delivery of anti-miR-181a oligonucleotide in an ischemic stroke model. *Nanoscale* **2021**, *13*, 14166–14178. [CrossRef]
99. Moss, L.D.; Sode, D.; Patel, R.; Lui, A.; Hudson, C.; Patel, N.A.; Bickford, P.C. Intranasal delivery of exosomes from human adipose derived stem cells at forty-eight hours post injury reduces motor and cognitive impairments following traumatic brain injury. *Neurochem. Int.* **2021**, *150*, 105173. [CrossRef]
100. Thomi, G.; Joerger-Messerli, M.; Haesler, V.; Muri, L.; Surbek, D.; Schoeberlein, A. Intranasally Administered Exosomes from Umbilical Cord Stem Cells Have Preventive Neuroprotective Effects and Contribute to Functional Recovery after Perinatal Brain Injury. *Cells* **2019**, *8*, 855. [CrossRef]
101. Wang, D.; Xue, H.; Tan, J.; Liu, P.; Qiao, C.; Pang, C.; Zhang, L. Bone marrow mesenchymal stem cells-derived exosomes containing miR-539-5p inhibit pyroptosis through NLRP3/caspase-1 signalling to alleviate inflammatory bowel disease. *Inflamm. Res.* **2022**, *71*, 833–846. [CrossRef]
102. Heidari, N.; Abbasi-Kenarsari, H.; Namaki, S.; Baghaei, K.; Zali, M.R.; Ghaffari Khaligh, S.; Hashemi, S.M. Adipose-derived mesenchymal stem cell-secreted exosome alleviates dextran sulfate sodium-induced acute colitis by Treg cell induction and inflammatory cytokine reduction. *J. Cell. Physiol.* **2021**, *236*, 5906–5920. [CrossRef]
103. Tsai, S.C.; Yang, K.D.; Chang, K.H.; Lin, F.C.; Chou, R.H.; Li, M.C.; Cheng, C.C.; Kao, C.Y.; Chen, C.P.; Lin, H.C.; et al. Umbilical Cord Mesenchymal Stromal Cell-Derived Exosomes Rescue the Loss of Outer Hair Cells and Repair Cochlear Damage in Cisplatin-Injected Mice. *Int. J. Mol. Sci.* **2021**, *22*, 6664. [CrossRef]
104. Han, M.; Yang, H.; Lu, X.; Li, Y.; Liu, Z.; Li, F.; Shang, Z.; Wang, X.; Li, X.; Li, J.; et al. Three-Dimensional-Cultured MSC-Derived Exosome-Hydrogel Hybrid Microneedle Array Patch for Spinal Cord Repair. *Nano Lett.* **2022**, *22*, 6391–6401. [CrossRef]
105. Yang, T.; Martin, P.; Fogarty, B.; Brown, A.; Schurman, K.; Phipps, R.; Yin, V.P.; Lockman, P.; Bai, S. Exosome delivered anticancer drugs across the blood-brain barrier for brain cancer therapy in Danio rerio. *Pharm. Res.* **2015**, *32*, 2003–2014. [CrossRef]
106. Quintana, D.S.; Guastella, A.J.; Westlye, L.T.; Andreassen, O.A. The promise and pitfalls of intranasally administering psychopharmacological agents for the treatment of psychiatric disorders. *Mol. Psychiatry* **2016**, *21*, 29–38. [CrossRef]
107. Erdo, F.; Bors, L.A.; Farkas, D.; Bajza, A.; Gizurarson, S. Evaluation of intranasal delivery route of drug administration for brain targeting. *Brain Res. Bull.* **2018**, *143*, 155–170. [CrossRef]
108. Kou, L.; Bhutia, Y.D.; Yao, Q.; He, Z.; Sun, J.; Ganapathy, V. Transporter-Guided Delivery of Nanoparticles to Improve Drug Permeation across Cellular Barriers and Drug Exposure to Selective Cell Types. *Front. Pharmacol.* **2018**, *9*, 27. [CrossRef]
109. Guo, S.; Perets, N.; Betzer, O.; Ben-Shaul, S.; Sheinin, A.; Michaelevski, I.; Popovtzer, R.; Offen, D.; Levenberg, S. Intranasal Delivery of Mesenchymal Stem Cell Derived Exosomes Loaded with Phosphatase and Tensin Homolog siRNA Repairs Complete Spinal Cord Injury. *ACS Nano* **2019**, *13*, 10015–10028. [CrossRef]
110. Mulcahy, L.A.; Pink, R.C.; Carter, D.R. Routes and mechanisms of extracellular vesicle uptake. *J. Extracell. Vesicles* **2014**, *3*, 24641. [CrossRef]
111. Qi, Z.; Yan, Z.; Wang, Y.; Ji, N.; Yang, X.; Zhang, A.; Li, M.; Xu, F.; Zhang, J. Ginsenoside Rh2 Inhibits NLRP3 Inflammasome Activation and Improves Exosomes to Alleviate Hypoxia-Induced Myocardial Injury. *Front. Immunol.* **2022**, *13*, 883946. [CrossRef]
112. Bashyal, S.; Thapa, C.; Lee, S. Recent progresses in exosome-based systems for targeted drug delivery to the brain. *J. Control. Release* **2022**, *348*, 723–744. [CrossRef]
113. Guo, Z.; Zhang, Y.; Xu, W.; Zhang, X.; Jiang, J. Engineered exosome-mediated delivery of circDIDO1 inhibits gastric cancer progression via regulation of MiR-1307-3p/SOCS2 Axis. *J. Transl. Med.* **2022**, *20*, 326. [CrossRef]
114. Li, X.; Yu, Q.; Zhao, R.; Guo, X.; Liu, C.; Zhang, K.; Zhang, W.; Liu, J.; Yu, J.; Wang, S.; et al. Designer Exosomes for Targeted Delivery of a Novel Therapeutic Cargo to Enhance Sorafenib-Mediated Ferroptosis in Hepatocellular Carcinoma. *Front. Oncol.* **2022**, *12*, 898156. [CrossRef]
115. Huang, X.; Wu, W.; Jing, D.; Yang, L.; Guo, H.; Wang, L.; Zhang, W.; Pu, F.; Shao, Z. Engineered exosome as targeted lncRNA MEG3 delivery vehicles for osteosarcoma therapy. *J. Control. Release* **2022**, *343*, 107–117. [CrossRef]
116. Cui, Y.; Guo, Y.; Kong, L.; Shi, J.; Liu, P.; Li, R.; Geng, Y.; Gao, W.; Zhang, Z.; Fu, D. A bone-targeted engineered exosome platform delivering siRNA to treat osteoporosis. *Bioact. Mater.* **2022**, *10*, 207–221. [CrossRef]
117. Terasawa, K.; Tomabechi, Y.; Ikeda, M.; Ehara, H.; Kukimoto-Niino, M.; Wakiyama, M.; Podyma-Inoue, K.A.; Rajapakshe, A.R.; Watabe, T.; Shirouzu, M.; et al. Lysosome-associated membrane proteins-1 and -2 (LAMP-1 and LAMP-2) assemble via distinct modes. *Biochem. Biophys. Res. Commun.* **2016**, *479*, 489–495. [CrossRef]
118. Alvarez-Erviti, L.; Seow, Y.; Yin, H.; Betts, C.; Lakhal, S.; Wood, M.J. Delivery of siRNA to the mouse brain by systemic injection of targeted exosomes. *Nat. Biotechnol.* **2011**, *29*, 341–345. [CrossRef]
119. Liang, Y.; Duan, L.; Lu, J.; Xia, J. Engineering exosomes for targeted drug delivery. *Theranostics* **2021**, *11*, 3183–3195. [CrossRef]
120. Phoolcharoen, W.; Prehaud, C.; van Dolleweerd, C.J.; Both, L.; da Costa, A.; Lafon, M.; Ma, J.K. Enhanced transport of plant-produced rabies single-chain antibody-RVG peptide fusion protein across an in cellulo blood-brain barrier device. *Plant Biotechnol. J.* **2017**, *15*, 1331–1339. [CrossRef]
121. Liu, L.; Li, Y.; Peng, H.; Liu, R.; Ji, W.; Shi, Z.; Shen, J.; Ma, G.; Zhang, X. Targeted exosome coating gene-chem nanocomplex as "nanoscavenger" for clearing alpha-synuclein and immune activation of Parkinson's disease. *Sci. Adv.* **2020**, *6*, eaba3967. [CrossRef] [PubMed]

122. Han, M.; Xing, H.; Chen, L.; Cui, M.; Zhang, Y.; Qi, L.; Jin, M.; Yang, Y.; Gao, C.; Gao, Z.; et al. Efficient antiglioblastoma therapy in mice through doxorubicin-loaded nanomicelles modified using a novel brain-targeted RVG-15 peptide. *J. Drug Target.* **2021**, *29*, 1016–1028. [CrossRef] [PubMed]
123. Tian, T.; Zhang, H.X.; He, C.P.; Fan, S.; Zhu, Y.L.; Qi, C.; Huang, N.P.; Xiao, Z.D.; Lu, Z.H.; Tannous, B.A.; et al. Surface functionalized exosomes as targeted drug delivery vehicles for cerebral ischemia therapy. *Biomaterials* **2018**, *150*, 137–149. [CrossRef] [PubMed]
124. Jewett, J.C.; Bertozzi, C.R. Cu-free click cycloaddition reactions in chemical biology. *Chem. Soc. Rev.* **2010**, *39*, 1272–1279. [CrossRef]
125. Bertozzi, C.R. A decade of bioorthogonal chemistry. *Acc. Chem. Res.* **2011**, *44*, 651–653. [CrossRef]
126. Robinson, P.V.; de Almeida-Escobedo, G.; de Groot, A.E.; McKechnie, J.L.; Bertozzi, C.R. Live-Cell Labeling of Specific Protein Glycoforms by Proximity-Enhanced Bioorthogonal Ligation. *J. Am. Chem. Soc.* **2015**, *137*, 10452–10455. [CrossRef]
127. Agarwal, P.; Beahm, B.J.; Shieh, P.; Bertozzi, C.R. Systemic Fluorescence Imaging of Zebrafish Glycans with Bioorthogonal Chemistry. *Angew. Chem. Int. Ed. Engl.* **2015**, *54*, 11504–11510. [CrossRef]
128. Jia, G.; Han, Y.; An, Y.; Ding, Y.; He, C.; Wang, X.; Tang, Q. NRP-1 targeted and cargo-loaded exosomes facilitate simultaneous imaging and therapy of glioma in vitro and in vivo. *Biomaterials* **2018**, *178*, 302–316. [CrossRef]
129. Kojima, R.; Bojar, D.; Rizzi, G.; Hamri, G.C.; El-Baba, M.D.; Saxena, P.; Auslander, S.; Tan, K.R.; Fussenegger, M. Designer exosomes produced by implanted cells intracerebrally deliver therapeutic cargo for Parkinson's disease treatment. *Nat. Commun.* **2018**, *9*, 1305. [CrossRef]
130. Oboudiyat, C.; Glazer, H.; Seifan, A.; Greer, C.; Isaacson, R.S. Alzheimer's disease. *Semin. Neurol.* **2013**, *33*, 313–329. [CrossRef]
131. Karran, E.; De Strooper, B. The amyloid hypothesis in Alzheimer disease: New insights from new therapeutics. *Nat. Rev. Drug Discov.* **2022**, *21*, 306–318. [CrossRef] [PubMed]
132. Ismail, Z.; Creese, B.; Aarsland, D.; Kales, H.C.; Lyketsos, C.G.; Sweet, R.A.; Ballard, C. Psychosis in Alzheimer disease—Mechanisms, genetics and therapeutic opportunities. *Nat. Rev. Neurol.* **2022**, *18*, 131–144. [CrossRef] [PubMed]
133. Leng, F.; Edison, P. Neuroinflammation and microglial activation in Alzheimer disease: Where do we go from here? *Nat. Rev. Neurol.* **2021**, *17*, 157–172. [CrossRef] [PubMed]
134. Pitt, J.M.; Kroemer, G.; Zitvogel, L. Extracellular vesicles: Masters of intercellular communication and potential clinical interventions. *J. Clin. Investig.* **2016**, *126*, 1139–1143. [CrossRef] [PubMed]
135. Zhang, D.; Lee, H.; Wang, X.; Rai, A.; Groot, M.; Jin, Y. Exosome-Mediated Small RNA Delivery: A Novel Therapeutic Approach for Inflammatory Lung Responses. *Mol. Ther.* **2018**, *26*, 2119–2130. [CrossRef]
136. Wahlgren, J.; De, L.K.T.; Brisslert, M.; Vaziri Sani, F.; Telemo, E.; Sunnerhagen, P.; Valadi, H. Plasma exosomes can deliver exogenous short interfering RNA to monocytes and lymphocytes. *Nucleic Acids Res.* **2012**, *40*, e130. [CrossRef]
137. Shtam, T.A.; Kovalev, R.A.; Varfolomeeva, E.Y.; Makarov, E.M.; Kil, Y.V.; Filatov, M.V. Exosomes are natural carriers of exogenous siRNA to human cells in vitro. *Cell Commun. Signal.* **2013**, *11*, 88. [CrossRef]
138. Kim, B.; Park, J.H.; Sailor, M.J. Rekindling RNAi Therapy: Materials Design Requirements for In Vivo siRNA Delivery. *Adv. Mater.* **2019**, *31*, e1903637. [CrossRef]
139. Balestrino, R.; Schapira, A.H.V. Parkinson disease. *Eur. J. Neurol.* **2020**, *27*, 27–42. [CrossRef]
140. GBD 2015 Maternal Mortality Collaborators. Global, regional, and national levels of maternal mortality, 1990–2015: A systematic analysis for the Global Burden of Disease Study 2015. *Lancet* **2016**, *388*, 1775–1812. [CrossRef]
141. Olanow, C.W.; Kieburtz, K.; Katz, R. Clinical approaches to the development of a neuroprotective therapy for PD. *Exp. Neurol.* **2017**, *298*, 246–251. [CrossRef] [PubMed]
142. Cooper, J.M.; Wiklander, P.B.; Nordin, J.Z.; Al-Shawi, R.; Wood, M.J.; Vithlani, M.; Schapira, A.H.; Simons, J.P.; El-Andaloussi, S.; Alvarez-Erviti, L. Systemic exosomal siRNA delivery reduced alpha-synuclein aggregates in brains of transgenic mice. *Mov. Disord.* **2014**, *29*, 1476–1485. [CrossRef] [PubMed]
143. Izco, M.; Blesa, J.; Schleef, M.; Schmeer, M.; Porcari, R.; Al-Shawi, R.; Ellmerich, S.; de Toro, M.; Gardiner, C.; Seow, Y.; et al. Systemic Exosomal Delivery of shRNA Minicircles Prevents Parkinsonian Pathology. *Mol. Ther.* **2019**, *27*, 2111–2122. [CrossRef] [PubMed]
144. Ross, C.A.; Tabrizi, S.J. Huntington's disease: From molecular pathogenesis to clinical treatment. *Lancet Neurol.* **2011**, *10*, 83–98. [CrossRef]
145. A novel gene containing a trinucleotide repeat that is expanded and unstable on Huntington's disease chromosomes. The Huntington's Disease Collaborative Research Group. *Cell* **1993**, *72*, 971–983. [CrossRef]
146. Tabrizi, S.J.; Estevez-Fraga, C.; van Roon-Mom, W.M.C.; Flower, M.D.; Scahill, R.I.; Wild, E.J.; Munoz-Sanjuan, I.; Sampaio, C.; Rosser, A.E.; Leavitt, B.R. Potential disease-modifying therapies for Huntington's disease: Lessons learned and future opportunities. *Lancet Neurol.* **2022**, *21*, 645–658. [CrossRef]
147. Zhang, Y.; Liu, Q.; Zhang, X.; Huang, H.; Tang, S.; Chai, Y.; Xu, Z.; Li, M.; Chen, X.; Liu, J.; et al. Recent advances in exosome-mediated nucleic acid delivery for cancer therapy. *J. Nanobiotechnol.* **2022**, *20*, 279. [CrossRef]
148. Didiot, M.C.; Hall, L.M.; Coles, A.H.; Haraszti, R.A.; Godinho, B.M.; Chase, K.; Sapp, E.; Ly, S.; Alterman, J.F.; Hassler, M.R.; et al. Exosome-mediated Delivery of Hydrophobically Modified siRNA for Huntingtin mRNA Silencing. *Mol. Ther.* **2016**, *24*, 1836–1847. [CrossRef]

149. Ganguly, K.; Khanna, P.; Morecraft, R.J.; Lin, D.J. Modulation of neural co-firing to enhance network transmission and improve motor function after stroke. *Neuron* **2022**, *110*, 2363–2385. [CrossRef]
150. Debette, S.; Markus, H.S. Stroke Genetics: Discovery, Insight Into Mechanisms, and Clinical Perspectives. *Circ. Res.* **2022**, *130*, 1095–1111. [CrossRef]
151. Kelly, P.J.; Kavanagh, E.; Murphy, S. Stroke: New Developments and Their Application in Clinical Practice. *Semin. Neurol.* **2016**, *36*, 317–323. [CrossRef] [PubMed]
152. Owolabi, M.O.; Thrift, A.G.; Mahal, A.; Ishida, M.; Martins, S.; Johnson, W.D.; Pandian, J.; Abd-Allah, F.; Yaria, J.; Phan, H.T.; et al. Primary stroke prevention worldwide: Translating evidence into action. *Lancet Public Health* **2022**, *7*, e74–e85. [CrossRef]
153. Zhao, L.; Li, J.; Kalviainen, R.; Jolkkonen, J.; Zhao, C. Impact of drug treatment and drug interactions in post-stroke epilepsy. *Pharmacol. Ther.* **2022**, *233*, 108030. [CrossRef]
154. Lai, N.; Wu, D.; Liang, T.; Pan, P.; Yuan, G.; Li, X.; Li, H.; Shen, H.; Wang, Z.; Chen, G. Systemic exosomal miR-193b-3p delivery attenuates neuroinflammation in early brain injury after subarachnoid hemorrhage in mice. *J. Neuroinflamm.* **2020**, *17*, 74. [CrossRef]
155. Writing Group, M.; Mozaffarian, D.; Benjamin, E.J.; Go, A.S.; Arnett, D.K.; Blaha, M.J.; Cushman, M.; Das, S.R.; de Ferranti, S.; Despres, J.P.; et al. Heart Disease and Stroke Statistics-2016 Update: A Report From the American Heart Association. *Circulation* **2016**, *133*, e38–e360. [CrossRef]
156. Lemaire, Q.; Raffo-Romero, A.; Arab, T.; Van Camp, C.; Drago, F.; Forte, S.; Gimeno, J.P.; Begard, S.; Colin, M.; Vizioli, J.; et al. Isolation of microglia-derived extracellular vesicles: Towards miRNA signatures and neuroprotection. *J. Nanobiotechnol.* **2019**, *17*, 119. [CrossRef] [PubMed]
157. Leidinger, P.; Backes, C.; Deutscher, S.; Schmitt, K.; Mueller, S.C.; Frese, K.; Haas, J.; Ruprecht, K.; Paul, F.; Stahler, C.; et al. A blood based 12-miRNA signature of Alzheimer disease patients. *Genome Biol.* **2013**, *14*, R78. [CrossRef]
158. Hamzei Taj, S.; Kho, W.; Riou, A.; Wiedermann, D.; Hoehn, M. MiRNA-124 induces neuroprotection and functional improvement after focal cerebral ischemia. *Biomaterials* **2016**, *91*, 151–165. [CrossRef]
159. Upadhya, R.; Madhu, L.N.; Attaluri, S.; Gitai, D.L.G.; Pinson, M.R.; Kodali, M.; Shetty, G.; Zanirati, G.; Kumar, S.; Shuai, B.; et al. Extracellular vesicles from human iPSC-derived neural stem cells: miRNA and protein signatures, and anti-inflammatory and neurogenic properties. *J. Extracell. Vesicles* **2020**, *9*, 1809064. [CrossRef]
160. Mathew, B.; Ravindran, S.; Liu, X.; Torres, L.; Chennakesavalu, M.; Huang, C.C.; Feng, L.; Zelka, R.; Lopez, J.; Sharma, M.; et al. Mesenchymal stem cell-derived extracellular vesicles and retinal ischemia-reperfusion. *Biomaterials* **2019**, *197*, 146–160. [CrossRef]
161. Perets, N.; Hertz, S.; London, M.; Offen, D. Intranasal administration of exosomes derived from mesenchymal stem cells ameliorates autistic-like behaviors of BTBR mice. *Mol. Autism* **2018**, *9*, 57. [CrossRef] [PubMed]
162. Thomi, G.; Surbek, D.; Haesler, V.; Joerger-Messerli, M.; Schoeberlein, A. Exosomes derived from umbilical cord mesenchymal stem cells reduce microglia-mediated neuroinflammation in perinatal brain injury. *Stem Cell Res. Ther.* **2019**, *10*, 105. [CrossRef] [PubMed]
163. Williams, A.M.; Dennahy, I.S.; Bhatti, U.F.; Halaweish, I.; Xiong, Y.; Chang, P.; Nikolian, V.C.; Chtraklin, K.; Brown, J.; Zhang, Y.; et al. Mesenchymal Stem Cell-Derived Exosomes Provide Neuroprotection and Improve Long-Term Neurologic Outcomes in a Swine Model of Traumatic Brain Injury and Hemorrhagic Shock. *J. Neurotrauma* **2019**, *36*, 54–60. [CrossRef] [PubMed]
164. Zhao, Y.; Gan, Y.; Xu, G.; Hua, K.; Liu, D. Exosomes from MSCs overexpressing microRNA-223-3p attenuate cerebral ischemia through inhibiting microglial M1 polarization mediated inflammation. *Life Sci.* **2020**, *260*, 118403. [CrossRef]
165. Yang, J.; Zhang, X.; Chen, X.; Wang, L.; Yang, G. Exosome Mediated Delivery of miR-124 Promotes Neurogenesis after Ischemia. *Mol. Ther. Nucleic Acids* **2017**, *7*, 278–287. [CrossRef]
166. Xin, H.; Katakowski, M.; Wang, F.; Qian, J.Y.; Liu, X.S.; Ali, M.M.; Buller, B.; Zhang, Z.G.; Chopp, M. MicroRNA cluster miR-17-92 Cluster in Exosomes Enhance Neuroplasticity and Functional Recovery After Stroke in Rats. *Stroke* **2017**, *48*, 747–753. [CrossRef]
167. Lu, L.; Qi, S.; Chen, Y.; Luo, H.; Huang, S.; Yu, X.; Luo, Q.; Zhang, Z. Targeted immunomodulation of inflammatory monocytes across the blood-brain barrier by curcumin-loaded nanoparticles delays the progression of experimental autoimmune encephalomyelitis. *Biomaterials* **2020**, *245*, 119987. [CrossRef]
168. Yuan, R.; Li, Y.; Han, S.; Chen, X.; Chen, J.; He, J.; Gao, H.; Yang, Y.; Yang, S.; Yang, Y. Fe-Curcumin Nanozyme-Mediated Reactive Oxygen Species Scavenging and Anti-Inflammation for Acute Lung Injury. *ACS Cent. Sci.* **2022**, *8*, 10–21. [CrossRef]
169. Yang, J.; Wu, S.; Hou, L.; Zhu, D.; Yin, S.; Yang, G.; Wang, Y. Therapeutic Effects of Simultaneous Delivery of Nerve Growth Factor mRNA and Protein via Exosomes on Cerebral Ischemia. *Mol. Ther. Nucleic Acids* **2020**, *21*, 512–522. [CrossRef]
170. Huang, X.; Ding, J.; Li, Y.; Liu, W.; Ji, J.; Wang, H.; Wang, X. Exosomes derived from PEDF modified adipose-derived mesenchymal stem cells ameliorate cerebral ischemia-reperfusion injury by regulation of autophagy and apoptosis. *Exp. Cell Res.* **2018**, *371*, 269–277. [CrossRef]
171. Edwards, G., 3rd; Moreno-Gonzalez, I.; Soto, C. Amyloid-beta and tau pathology following repetitive mild traumatic brain injury. *Biochem. Biophys. Res. Commun.* **2017**, *483*, 1137–1142. [CrossRef] [PubMed]
172. Yim, A.; Smith, C.; Brown, A.M. Osteopontin/secreted phosphoprotein-1 harnesses glial-, immune-, and neuronal cell ligand-receptor interactions to sense and regulate acute and chronic neuroinflammation. *Immunol. Rev.* **2022**, *311*, 224–233. [CrossRef] [PubMed]
173. Spiteri, A.G.; Wishart, C.L.; Pamphlett, R.; Locatelli, G.; King, N.J.C. Microglia and monocytes in inflammatory CNS disease: Integrating phenotype and function. *Acta Neuropathol.* **2022**, *143*, 179–224. [CrossRef]

174. Kaufmann, M.; Schaupp, A.L.; Sun, R.; Coscia, F.; Dendrou, C.A.; Cortes, A.; Kaur, G.; Evans, H.G.; Mollbrink, A.; Navarro, J.F.; et al. Identification of early neurodegenerative pathways in progressive multiple sclerosis. *Nat. Neurosci.* **2022**, *25*, 944–955. [CrossRef]
175. Zhuang, X.; Xiang, X.; Grizzle, W.; Sun, D.; Zhang, S.; Axtell, R.C.; Ju, S.; Mu, J.; Zhang, L.; Steinman, L.; et al. Treatment of brain inflammatory diseases by delivering exosome encapsulated anti-inflammatory drugs from the nasal region to the brain. *Mol. Ther.* **2011**, *19*, 1769–1779. [CrossRef] [PubMed]
176. Omuro, A.; DeAngelis, L.M. Glioblastoma and other malignant gliomas: A clinical review. *JAMA* **2013**, *310*, 1842–1850. [CrossRef] [PubMed]
177. Zhu, Z.; Zhai, Y.; Hao, Y.; Wang, Q.; Han, F.; Zheng, W.; Hong, J.; Cui, L.; Jin, W.; Ma, S.; et al. Specific anti-glioma targeted-delivery strategy of engineered small extracellular vesicles dual-functionalised by Angiopep-2 and TAT peptides. *J. Extracell. Vesicles* **2022**, *11*, e12255. [CrossRef]
178. Yamada, R.; Nakano, I. Glioma stem cells: Their role in chemoresistance. *World Neurosurg.* **2012**, *77*, 237–240. [CrossRef]
179. Munoz, J.L.; Bliss, S.A.; Greco, S.J.; Ramkissoon, S.H.; Ligon, K.L.; Rameshwar, P. Delivery of Functional Anti-miR-9 by Mesenchymal Stem Cell-derived Exosomes to Glioblastoma Multiforme Cells Conferred Chemosensitivity. *Mol. Ther. Nucleic Acids* **2013**, *2*, e126. [CrossRef]
180. Shah, V.; Kochar, P. Brain Cancer: Implication to Disease, Therapeutic Strategies and Tumor Targeted Drug Delivery Approaches. *Recent Pat. Anticancer Drug Discov.* **2018**, *13*, 70–85. [CrossRef]
181. Pouletty, P. Drug addictions: Towards socially accepted and medically treatable diseases. *Nat. Rev. Drug Discov.* **2002**, *1*, 731–736. [CrossRef] [PubMed]
182. Liu, Y.; Li, D.; Liu, Z.; Zhou, Y.; Chu, D.; Li, X.; Jiang, X.; Hou, D.; Chen, X.; Chen, Y.; et al. Targeted exosome-mediated delivery of opioid receptor Mu siRNA for the treatment of morphine relapse. *Sci. Rep.* **2015**, *5*, 17543. [CrossRef] [PubMed]
183. Zhang, R.; Fu, Y.; Cheng, M.; Ma, W.; Zheng, N.; Wang, Y.; Wu, Z. sEVs(RVG) selectively delivers antiviral siRNA to fetus brain, inhibits ZIKV infection and mitigates ZIKV-induced microcephaly in mouse model. *Mol. Ther.* **2022**, *30*, 2078–2091. [CrossRef] [PubMed]
184. Bunggulawa, E.J.; Wang, W.; Yin, T.; Wang, N.; Durkan, C.; Wang, Y.; Wang, G. Recent advancements in the use of exosomes as drug delivery systems. *J. Nanobiotechnol.* **2018**, *16*, 81. [CrossRef]
185. Kooijmans, S.A.; Vader, P.; van Dommelen, S.M.; van Solinge, W.W.; Schiffelers, R.M. Exosome mimetics: A novel class of drug delivery systems. *Int. J. Nanomed.* **2012**, *7*, 1525–1541. [CrossRef]
186. Ingato, D.; Lee, J.U.; Sim, S.J.; Kwon, Y.J. Good things come in small packages: Overcoming challenges to harness extracellular vesicles for therapeutic delivery. *J. Control. Release* **2016**, *241*, 174–185. [CrossRef]
187. Aryani, A.; Denecke, B. Exosomes as a Nanodelivery System: A Key to the Future of Neuromedicine? *Mol. Neurobiol.* **2016**, *53*, 818–834. [CrossRef]
188. El Andaloussi, S.; Lakhal, S.; Mager, I.; Wood, M.J. Exosomes for targeted siRNA delivery across biological barriers. *Adv. Drug Deliv. Rev.* **2013**, *65*, 391–397. [CrossRef]
189. Grapp, M.; Wrede, A.; Schweizer, M.; Huwel, S.; Galla, H.J.; Snaidero, N.; Simons, M.; Buckers, J.; Low, P.S.; Urlaub, H.; et al. Choroid plexus transcytosis and exosome shuttling deliver folate into brain parenchyma. *Nat. Commun.* **2013**, *4*, 2123. [CrossRef]

pharmaceutics

MDPI

Review

Extracellular Vesicle-Based Therapeutics in Neurological Disorders

Yiwen Yuan [1], Jian Sun [1], Tongyao You [1], Weiwei Shen [1], Wenqing Xu [1], Qiang Dong [1,2,*] and Mei Cui [1,2,*]

1 Department of Neurology, Huashan Hospital, Fudan University, Shanghai 200031, China
2 State Key Laboratory of Medical Neurobiology and MOE Frontiers Center for Brain Science, Department of Neurology, Huashan Hospital, Fudan University, Shanghai 200031, China
* Correspondence: dong_qiang@fudan.edu.cn (Q.D.); cuimei@fudan.edu.cn (M.C.)

Abstract: Neurological diseases remain some of the major causes of death and disability in the world. Few types of drugs and insufficient delivery across the blood–brain barrier limit the treatment of neurological disorders. The past two decades have seen the rapid development of extracellular vesicle-based therapeutics in many fields. As the physiological and pathophysiological roles of extracellular vesicles are recognized in neurological diseases, they have become promising therapeutics and targets for therapeutic interventions. Moreover, advanced nanomedicine technologies have explored the potential of extracellular vesicles as drug delivery systems in neurological diseases. In this review, we discussed the preclinical strategies for extracellular vesicle-based therapeutics in neurological disorders and the struggles involved in their clinical application.

Keywords: extracellular vesicles; neurological disorders; mesenchymal stem cells; drug delivery; therapeutics; neurodegenerative diseases

Citation: Yuan, Y.; Sun, J.; You, T.; Shen, W.; Xu, W.; Dong, Q.; Cui, M. Extracellular Vesicle-Based Therapeutics in Neurological Disorders. *Pharmaceutics* **2022**, *14*, 2652. https://doi.org/10.3390/pharmaceutics14122652

Academic Editor: Maria Carafa

Received: 19 October 2022
Accepted: 26 November 2022
Published: 30 November 2022

1. Introduction

Neurological diseases such as stroke, neurodegenerative diseases, and neuromuscular diseases, are some of the leading causes of death and disability worldwide [1]. The therapeutics and drugs for treating neurological diseases are still limited. As the physiological and pathophysiological roles of extracellular vesicles (EVs) are becoming recognized, emerging evidence has demonstrated the therapeutic potential of EVs in treating neurological diseases [2,3]. EVs are heterogeneous, membrane-bound particles that are naturally released from most cells. They are generally classified into two types: endosome-origin "exosomes" and plasma-membrane-derived "ectosomes" (microvesicles) [4–6]. It is challenging to exactly distinguish exosomes and ectosomes because of their overlapping sizes and the similar markers between them [7]. Therefore, we used the generic term "EVs" to refer to both exosomes and ectosomes in this review.

EVs contain various types of cargos, including nucleic acids, proteins, and metabolites. Initial studies have focused on the regulatory and therapeutic effects of native EVs and their cargos. In the nervous system, EVs, as important mediators of intercellular communication in the brain, play a profound role in the maintenance and recovery of neural functions [8–10]. With the rapid development of nanotechnology, EVs have been modified for broader therapeutic capabilities, especially targeted drug delivery [11,12]. Some well-established synthetic nanoparticles such as liposomes, the first nano drug delivery systems, have received clinical approval and marketing authorization [13]. However, their therapeutic effects are limited because of their rapid clearance from the blood and their activation of the innate immune response [14]. Compared to synthetic drug delivery systems, EVs have emerged as a more complex and biocompatible form of liposomes with lower immunogenicity. The functional pharmacokinetic-related proteins of EVs contribute to their larger volume of biodistribution and higher retention in the circulation [15–17]. Furthermore, different molecules on the surface of EVs enable them to cross the blood–brain barrier (BBB), deliver their cargos, and evoke responses in the recipient cells [18–23]. These attributes of EVs exhibit their vast therapeutic potential in the treatments of central nervous system (CNS) disorders.

The roles of EVs in the diagnosis, progression monitoring, and treatment of neurological diseases have been gradually recognized [24,25]. Inspired by emerging studies, here, we reviewed the preclinical evidence and strategies for EV-based therapeutics in the treatment of neurological diseases (Figure 1). Finally, we discussed issues to be considered for the future clinical applications of EVs.

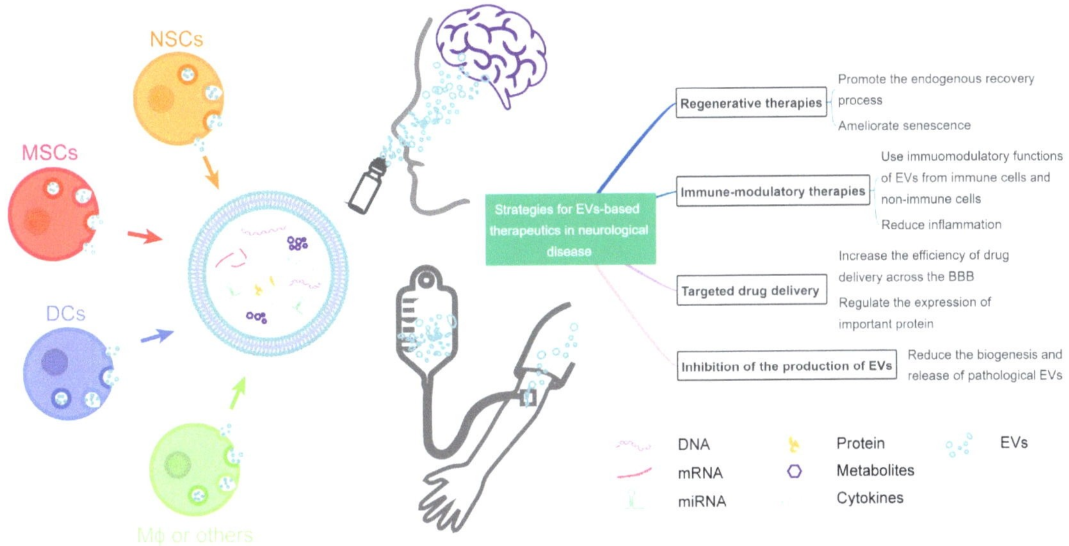

Figure 1. Strategies for EV-based therapeutics in neurological diseases. NSCs, neural stem cells; MSCs, mesenchymal stromal cells; DCs, dendritic cells; Mϕ, macrophage; BBB, blood–brain barrier; miRNA, microRNA; EVs, extracellular vesicles.

2. Strategies for EV-Based Therapeutics in Neurological Diseases

2.1. EVs in Regenerative Therapies

The pathophysiological processes underlying most neurological diseases remain to be fully defined. Despite the delicate structures and functions of the nervous system, the spontaneous recovery of neurological function is commonly found in neurological diseases. Figuring out the underlying mechanisms and promoting the endogenous recovery process are key strategies for the development of therapies. Initial attempts were cell-based therapies such as the systematic administration of mesenchymal stromal cells (MSCs) in stroke models [26,27]. The safety of intravenous stem cell therapies has been approved in many clinical trials, but there are limited therapeutic effects in patients [28–30]. After different administrations, most stem cells are trapped in capillaries or peripheral organs such as the liver, spleen, and lungs [31]. The landmark paper by Gnecchi et al. proposed that paracrine factors account for the protective effects of MSCs [32]. Subsequently, emerging evidence has suggested that EVs secreted from MSCs contribute substantially to the beneficial effects of cell-based therapies [33]. Marbán drew interesting analogies between EV production and the process whereby bees manufacture honey [34]. He proposed that compared to fragile cells (like flowers), EVs (like honey), which contain the active ingredients of their sources, are more stable, efficacious, immune tolerant, and modifiable.

Regenerative progress is particularly important in post-stroke brain recovery, and the critical process is inducing neurogenesis and angiogenesis in lesions. Many studies have proven that MSC-EVs promote these agents in vivo and enhance functional recovery in stroke patients [35–37]. Although MSC-EVs promote neuronal survival and the process of neurogenesis in peri-infarct tissue, these studies have not shown significant effects in terms of reductions in the infarct volume. The failure to reduce the infarct volume was possibly attributed to the timing, because the time taken in MSC-EV delivery is usually longer than the 3–6 h window required for tissue plasminogen activator (t-PA) therapy, the only stroke treatment. Recent studies have indicated that neural-stem-cell (NSC)-derived EVs administered both within and outside the t-PA therapeutic window result in a significant reduction in infarct volume, exhibiting better therapeutic effects in stroke compared to MSC-EVs [38]. Modified NSC-EVs loaded with triiodothyronine, a critical factor for oligodendrocyte development, successfully target the demyelinated lesion in the brain and present an effective remyelination effect in experimental autoimmune encephalomyelitis (EAE), a classical multiple sclerosis (MS) animal model [39]. In addition, an injectable hyaluronic acid hydrogel has been developed to deliver NSC-EVs into the stroke brain, enhancing EV retention and sustaining the therapeutic effects [40]. However, considering the ethical questions and problematic logistics of acquiring fetal tissues, NSC is not an optimal choice as an EV producer. Induced NSCs from somatic-cells (iNSCs)-derived EVs display comparable therapeutic effects to NSC-EVs in post-stroke functional recovery without significant adverse effects [41]. The development of iNSCs can overcome some ethical questions about NSC-derived EVs, but the mass production of iNSC-EVs for clinical use is still a problem.

The function and proliferative capacity of stem cells decline over time. In regenerative therapies, the anti-senescence effect is another tool to promote endogenous recovery. For example, embryonic-stem-cell-derived EVs reverse hippocampal NSC senescence and the corresponding reduction in neurogenesis and cognitive impairment [42,43]. In addition, cellular senescence and stem cell exhaustion are two biological hallmarks of aging, which correlate with a susceptibility to neurodegenerative diseases and other aging-related diseases [44]. Recent studies have provided evidence for the potential roles of EVs in treatments for diseases related to aging and the hallmarks of aging. For instance, circulating EVs from young mice present a pro-longevity function [45,46]; EVs from fibroblasts of young human healthy donors ameliorate senescence in old recipient fibroblasts and mice, and they especially ameliorate oxidative stress—one of the classical pathophysiology features of senescence and aging [47]. Unfortunately, these therapeutical effects of EVs have not been deeply explored in most age-related neurological diseases.

2.2. EVs in Immune-Modulatory Therapies

Immune-cell-derived EVs have been favored as promising therapeutic agents for their immune-modulatory capabilities [48–52]. Microglia, the macrophage-like immune cells of the CNS, are involved in homeostasis and in the pathophysiology of CNS diseases [53]. EVs isolated from IL-4-treated microglia could inhibit glial scar formation, reduce brain atrophy volume, and promote white matter repair and functional recovery after ischemic stroke [54–57]. Increasing studies have shown that stem-cell-derived EVs present immune-modulatory capabilities. Embryonic-stem-cell-derived EVs significantly alleviate pathology and the long-term neurological deficits after ischemic stroke in a regulatory T-cell-dependent way [58]. The intrinsic anti-inflammatory activity of NSC-EVs also contributes to an improvement in pathology and behavioral outcomes in stroke [38,59]. The inhibition of leukocytes, especially polymorphonuclear neutrophil infiltration, may be the underlying mechanism of MSC-EV-induced ischemic neuroprotection [60]. MSC-EVs conjugated with LJM-3064 aptamer, a myelin-specific DNA aptamer demonstrating remyelination induction, on their surface produce immune-modulatory properties and promote remyelination in EAE [61]. Since MS is a typical autoimmune disorder in the CNS, researchers have also proposed using the programmed cell death protein-1/programmed death ligand-1 (PD-1/PD-L1) pathway to inhibit pathological immune responses and maintain self-tolerance in MS and EAE [62]. PD-L1-expressing dendritic cells demonstrate therapeutic effects in EAE, but there is still insufficient data for the immune-modulatory functions of PD-1/PD-L1-pathway-related EVs in MS [63]. Recently developed PD-L1-overexpressed MSC-EVs significantly suppress pathogenic immune responses via the PD1/PD-L1 pathway in two different autoimmune diseases: ulcerative colitis and psoriasis [64]. The application of these PD-L1-overexpressed EVs in MS may exhibit therapeutic effects and provide insights into EV-based immune-modulatory therapies in the treatment of autoimmune neurological disorders.

Naïve macrophage (Mϕ) EVs inherit the integrin lymphocyte-function-associated antigen 1 (LFA-1) from their parental cells and interact with the intercellular adhesion molecule 1 (ICAM-1) of BBB endothelial cells. In inflammation, the upregulation of ICAM-1 promotes the uptake of Mϕ EVs to the brain parenchyma [65]. Moreover, the brain-derived neurotrophic factor (BDNF), an important neuroprotective factor, loaded in these Mϕ EVs is stable and exhibits higher brain accumulation compared to BDNF alone [65]. Considering the common inflammatory response in neurological diseases and the properties of naïve Mϕ EVs, these EVs could be simple and efficient delivery vehicles of anti-inflammatory and neuroprotective drugs to brain lesions. However, similar to the distributions of other naïve EVs in a previous study, most naïve Mϕ EVs accumulate in peripheral organs such as the liver, spleen, gastrointestinal tract, and lungs, and less than 1% of administrated EVs successfully enter the brain [66]. We still need other methods to increase the brain-targeting efficiency of EVs and their cargos. In the next part, we focused on strategies for EV-based drug delivery to the brain, including advanced techniques for the efficient delivery of anti-inflammation drugs.

2.3. EVs for Targeted Drug Delivery

Most therapeutic agents are unable to reach lesions in effective concentrations by systemic administration because of biological barriers, especially the BBB, a major hindrance to drug treatments of CNS diseases. An alternative drug administration route is intranasal administration. The intranasal delivery route help drugs bypass the BBB and delivers them directly to the brain [67,68]. It has been proven to be an effective route for the delivery of drug-loaded EVs to the brain. For example, curcumin is a natural anti-inflammatory and antioxidant nutraceutical that has been widely investigated. Tumor-derived EVs with encapsulated curcumin are taken up by microglia via intranasal administration and have shown therapeutic effects in three independent inflammation-mediated disease models [69]. The intranasal administration of embryonic stem cell EVs loaded with curcumin not only reduces inflammation but also restores the neurovascular unit in ischemia-reperfusion-injured mice [70]. However, the nasal mucosa barrier limits the efficiency of intranasal therapy, as less than 1% of administrated drugs reach the brain [71].

Remarkable advancements in nanotechnology have yielded many brain delivery technologies that have achieved a sufficient delivery of drugs for neurological diseases [72]. Although the mechanisms by which EVs traverse the BBB and target lesions are still opaque, it is becoming increasingly difficult to ignore the role of EVs as drug delivery vehicles in the treatment of CNS diseases. However, as mentioned before, most naïve EVs tend to accumulate in peripheral organs. Surface modifications of EVs have been applied to increase their brain-targeting efficiency. For instance, cyclo(Arg-Gly-Asp-D-Tyr-Lys)-peptide (c(RGDyK))-conjugated EVs exhibit a high affinity to lesions of the ischemic brain after intravenous administration [73]. Curcumin loaded in these EVs exhibits a strong suppression of the inflammatory response in the lesion region of the ischemic brain [73]. In addition, the conjugation of rabies virus glycoprotein (RVG) to EVs displays a twofold greater accumulation in the brain [66]. As shown in the seminal work by Alvarez-Erviti et al., the conjugation of RVG to the EV surface significantly increased their brain-targeting efficiency [74]. Furthermore, exogeneous short interfering (si) RNA loaded in RVG-targeted dendritic cell EVs has been successfully delivered to the brain, resulting in a specific gene knockdown [74]. This landmark study not only demonstrated that EVs can be engineered into an efficient brain delivery system but also established an siRNA RVG-EV strategy for inhibiting the production of pathological proteins in neurodegenerative diseases.

Neurodegeneration is defined as the progress of loss or dysfunction of neurons, which impairs the properties of the CNS and previously established CNS functions such as mobility, coordination, memory, and learning [75]. One of the pathological hallmarks of neurodegenerative diseases is the aggregation of characteristic proteins. Representative instances are β-amyloid (Aβ) extracellular plaques and tau neurofibrillary tangles in Alzheimer's disease (AD). Transactive response DNA-binding protein 43 (TDP-43) is a misfolded protein typical in amyotrophic lateral sclerosis (ALS) and frontotemporal dementia (FTD). Alpha-synuclein aggregates are the representative pathology in Parkinson's disease (PD), dementia with Lewy bodies (DLB), and multiple system atrophy (MSA). Disease-specific pathological proteins and rare mutations of their encoding genes raise an interlinked hypothesis that a causal association exists between these proteins and neurodegenerative diseases [76].

One of the therapeutic strategies for neurodegenerative diseases is reducing the pathological protein burden in the brain. Alvarez-Erviti and colleagues first employed RVG-EVs loaded with exogenous BACE1 siRNA to inhibit the expression of BACE1 and Aβ in the cortex by systemic injection [74]. Subsequently, systemic siRNA RVG-EV treatment successfully reduced the expression of alpha-synuclein throughout the brain of S129D transgenic mice [77]. Likewise, RVG-EVs loaded with anti-alpha-synuclein short hairpin RNA (shRNA) minicircles decreased the aggregation of alpha-synuclein, rescued dopaminergic neurons, and improved clinical symptoms in a progressive mouse model of PD [78]. Indeed, some naïve EVs exhibited a capacity for reducing the pathological protein level. EVs secreted from adipose-derived MSC effectively ameliorated neurodegeneration and rescued cognitive impairment in APP/PS1 transgenic mice, a classic AD mice model [79]. Similarly, aFGF-stimulated astrocyte-derived EVs alleviated the brain Aβ burden and cognitive deficits in the APP/PS1 mice [80]. Adipose-derived EVs also reduce the aggregation of mutant superoxide dismutase 1 (SOD1), a pathologic hallmark of familial ALS [81]. Future studies may consider a combination of these naïve EVs and pathological-protein-targeted siRNA or shRNA to increase their therapeutic effects.

Due to the complicated aeotiology and pathogenesis of neurodegenerative diseases, apart from pathological-protein-targeted therapeutics, other EV-based therapeutic strategies have been developed. To start with, neurodegenerative diseases are commonly linked to neurotoxic substances such as reactive oxygen species (ROS), and hence the delivery of antioxidant drugs to the brain can be instrumental. EVs loaded with catalase effectively protected the substantia nigra pars compacta neurons from 6-OHDA-induced oxidative stress in a typical PD mouse model [82]. In addition, compared to free dopamine, EV-based dopamine delivery in PD models displays a more than fifteen-fold increase in brain distribution and a lower systemic toxicity [83]. Additionally, in a recent review, the authors summarized a therapeutic potential of EVs and small heat-shock proteins in neurodegenerative diseases [84]. They also hypothesized that a combination of them would be an effective therapeutic in the future by targeting the autophagy and apoptosis pathways, two major pathophysiological processes in neurogenerative diseases [84].

Engineered EVs fused with RVG have also been researched to carry many other compounds such as low-molecular-weight proteins, mRNA, and miRNA. For instance, the systemic administration of RVG-EVs loaded with nerve growth factor (NGF) protein along with NGF mRNA significantly increases the expression of NGF in the infarcted cortex, reduces inflammation, and promotes cell survival in stroke [85]. Considering that some proteins need post-translational modification or act in a paracrine way, the delivery of mRNA can promote the production of intracellular bioactive proteins in the targeted region [86]. EV-mediated protein and mRNA delivery provide a stable and efficient strategy to overcome obstacles such as the rapid extracellular degradation of naked proteins and mRNA. EV-based therapeutics may promote the development of mRNA therapeutics. Similarly, modified EVs with RVG fused to the exosomal protein lysosome-associated membrane glycoprotein 2b (Lamp2b) can deliver miR-124 to the infarct site and promote neurogenesis in stroke [87]. Among the various RNA delivery systems, EVs have been proven to be more efficient than other clinically approved synthetic systems [88]. As potential therapeutic targets or drugs in neurological diseases, the role of exosomal miRNAs has been comprehensively discussed in other reviews [89].

With recent advances in therapeutic nucleic acids, EV-based delivery has demonstrated great promise in nucleic acid therapies for genetic disorders [90]. Huntington's disease (HD) and Duchenne muscular dystrophy (DMD) are two neurogenetic disorders that have been widely researched in this field.

The expansion of CAG repeats in the Huntingtin (HTT) gene leads to HD. The delivery of oligonucleotide directly targeting HTT mRNA and silencing the expression of pathological proteins is a promising strategy for HD treatment. EVs loaded with hydrophobically modified siRNAs display a significant bilateral distribution and silencing of Huntingtin mRNA in mice [91]. Recently, Zhang et al. designed an interesting genetic circuit that could reprogram hepatocytes to produce RVG-EVs loaded with mutant HTT siRNA [92]. These EVs reduced the levels of mutant HTT in the cortex and striatum and ameliorated behavioral deficits in three different mouse models of HD [92].

DMD is an X-linked recessive, progressive neuromuscular disease caused by the loss of dystrophin [93]. One of the most promising therapies for DMD is exon skipping, using antisense oligonucleotides (ASOs) to restore the function of dystrophin. Some ASOs have been tested in clinical trials, such as eteplirsen and drisapersen, based on phosphorodiamidate morpholino oligomer (PMO) and a 2′-O-methyl phosphorothioate (2OMePS), respectively [94]. Due to the unsatisfied functional benefits in large clinical trials, improving the delivery of ASOs by EVs may be an approach to promote the efficiency of exon-skipping therapy. The combination of PMO and peptide-modified EVs demonstrates an 18-fold increase in dystrophin expression in the muscle cells of mice compared to other non-exosomal components [95]. Similarly, anchoring myostatin propeptide, a natural inhibitor of myostatin, to the surface of EVs increased their stability and delivery efficiency and thus significantly promoted muscle regeneration and functional rescue in a DMD mouse model [96]. The systemic administration of EVs from different origins can rescue muscle function by stabilizing muscle membranes [97]. In addition, EVs secreted from muscle cells have been discovered for several years, and several studies have shown their effects in maintaining muscle homeostasis [98,99]. These muscle EVs may exhibit protective effects on muscle cells and slow the progress of neuromuscular diseases. However, far too little attention has been paid to these muscle EVs. Future studies are needed to explore the therapeutic effects of naïve or modified muscle EVs in treatments for neuromuscular disorders.

2.4. Inhibition of the Production of Pathological EVs

Other than their therapeutic roles, EVs are vital factors in the progression of neurological diseases [2,100,101]. For instance, EVs from B cells, rather than immunoglobulins or complement, cause apoptosis in neurons and oligodendrocytes in MS [102–104]. The contribution of EVs to the progression of neurodegenerative diseases has been well summarized [105–109]. The inhibition of EV release has emerged as a novel therapeutic strategy. There are two basic approaches currently adopted to develop pharmacological inhibitors of EVs: the inhibition of EV trafficking (e.g., calpeptin, manumycin A, and Y27632) and the inhibition of the lipid metabolism (e.g., pantethine, imipramine, and GW4869) [110]. For a comprehensive review of these inhibitors and their proposed mechanisms of action, readers may refer to the outstanding review written by Catalano and O'Driscoll [110]. In addition, some enzymes participating in EV secretion, such as peptidyl arginine deiminases, are preserved from microbes to mammals [111]. Thus, compounds that effectively inhibit the production of bacterial EVs may be potential inhibitors of EV release in mammals [111].

However, as pivotal agents of intercellular communication, some EVs transfer information and mediate physiological functions. Interference with the biogenesis of all EVs brings undesired side effects, and effective methods to inhibit specific pathological EVs are still lacking. The maturation of recombinant adeno-associated viruses (AAVs) provides cell-type-specific gene-delivery vehicles for neuroscience research [112]. Moreover, the silencing of genes such as GTPase, Rab27a, and Rab27b has been shown to significantly reduce the biogenesis and release of EVs [113]. Using cell-type-specific AAVs to silence EV genes in the parental cells of pathological EVs may increase the specificity of this therapeutic strategy.

3. Issues to Be Considered for Clinical Applications of EV-Based Therapeutics

EV-based therapeutics have attracted attention from the academic community and several pharmaceutical companies [114,115]. Clinical trials for EV-based therapeutics in humans have been approved, and the number of them is rapidly increasing [116–119]. We summarized all the registered clinical trials of EV-based therapeutics in Table 1. Among these registered trials, there are currently three registered clinical trials related to neurological problems: NCT04388982 (Alzheimer's disease), NCT03384433 (cerebrovascular disorders), and NCT05490173 (neurodevelopmental disorders). MSCs were the source of EVs in all three trials, but the tissue sources of MSCs were different. Allogenic adipose MSCs were applied in NCT04388982 (Alzheimer's disease), while allogenic bone marrow MSCs were applied in NCT03384433 (cerebrovascular disorders). Notably, NCT03384433 (cerebrovascular disorders) used allogenic MSCs transfected with miR-124, which may provide evidence for the effects of EV-based gene therapies in humans. In particular, the NCT05490173 (neurodevelopmental disorders) and NCT04388982 (Alzheimer's disease) studies adopted intranasal administration, while the intravenous administration of EVs was applied in NCT03384433 (cerebrovascular disorders). We hope these representative clinical trials will provide exciting results for EV-based therapeutics in neurological diseases in humans.

Table 1. EVs as therapeutics in registered trials.

Strategy	Study Identifier	Condition or Disease	Phase	Source of EVs	Native/Engineered	Status
Regenerative	NCT04388982	Alzheimer's disease	I/II	MSC *	Native	Unknown
	NCT05490173	Premature birth Extreme prematurity Preterm intraventricular hemorrhage Hypoxia-ischemia, cerebral Neurodevelopmental disorders	NA *	MSC	Native	Not yet recruiting
	NCT04602104	Acute respiratory distress syndrome	I/II	MSC	Native	Recruiting
	NCT05402748	Fistula perianal	I/II	MSC	Native	Recruiting
	NCT04213248	Dry eye	I/II	MSC	Native	Recruiting
	NCT03437759	Macular holes	I	MSC	Native	Active, not recruiting
	NCT05060107	Osteoarthritis, knee	I	MSC	Native	Not yet recruiting
	NCT04270006	Periodontitis	I	Adipose stem cell	Native	Unknown
	NCT05475418	Wounds and injuries	NA	Adipose tissue	Native	Not yet recruiting
Regenerative and immune-modulatory	NCT04356300	Multiple organ failure	NA	MSC	Native	Not yet recruiting
	NCT04202770	Refractory depression Anxiety disorders Neurodegenerative diseases	NA	MSC	Native	Suspended
Immune-modulatory	NCT01159288	Non-small-cell lung cancer	II	dendritic cell	Native	Completed
	NCT04389385	Coronavirus infection Pneumonia	I	COVID-19 Specific T Cell	Native	Unknown
	NCT05191381	COVID-19 Critical illness Hypercytokinemia Lung fibrosis	NA	MSC	Native	Recruiting
	NCT04276987	COVID-19	I	MSC	Native	Completed [120]
	NCT04491240	COVID-19 SARS-CoV-2 pneumonia	I/II	MSC	Native	Completed
Drug delivery	NCT03384433	Cerebrovascular disorders	I/II	MSC	Engineered (loaded with miRNA-124)	Recruiting
	NCT04879810	Irritable bowel disease	NA	Ginger	Engineered (loaded with curcumin)	Recruiting
	NCT05043181	Familial hypercholesterolemia	I	MSC	Engineered (loaded with low-density lipoprotein receptor mRNA)	Not yet recruiting
	NCT03608631	KRAS NP_004976.2:p.G12D Metastatic pancreatic adenocarcinoma Pancreatic ductal adenocarcinoma Stage IV pancreatic cancer AJCC v8	I	MSC	Engineered (loaded with KRAS G12D siRNA)	Recruiting

* MSC, mesenchymal stem cell; NA, not applicable.

As shown in Table 1, MSC-derived EVs are the most frequently used therapeutic EVs [121–125]. In the current bibliometric analysis of MSC-EV publications, 1595 articles and reviews about MSC-EV were published between 2009 and 2021; the annual publication reached as high as 555 publications in 2021 [126]. These data display a steep growth trend in MSC-EV studies in recent years. Given the rapid growth of preclinical and clinical MSC-EV publications, a systematic review has comprehensively analyzed the outcomes, methodologies, dosing, and possible mechanistic pathways of 206 animal studies using MSC-EVs as an intervention until 2020 [127]. Notably, a recent study has reported some interesting approaches that could enhance the therapeutic effects of MSC-EVs. For instance, appropriate preconditioning has been proven to enhance the therapeutic potential of MSC-EVs [128–130]. EVs of embryonic stem cells have an antisenescence activity on MSCs, which can be applied to maintain the EV production capacity of MSCs [131]. In addition, the pathology-specific homing of MSC-EVs is highly correlated with neuroinflammatory signals, suggesting that the distinct distribution pattern may be inflammatory-driven [132].

Indeed, as indicated in the explorations of MSC-EVs in laboratory and clinical studies, MSC-EV-based therapeutics have numerous problems. A major problem is their unstable therapeutic effects. For instance, studies offer contradictory findings about the effects of MSC-EVs on the angiogenesis process. MSC-EVs under hypoxic conditions promote angiogenesis, while MSC-EVs display anti-angiogenic effects in a pro-inflammatory microenvironment [133–135]. The unstable effects of native MSCs may be attributed to lots of reasons, ranging from isolation techniques, the cell source of MSCs, and distinct preconditioning. Though Gorgun and colleagues report that MSC-EVs display relatively minor changes in the microRNA landscape, they are less sensitive than soluble proteins in different microenvironments [136]. These results highlight the importance of standardized protocols in the preconditioning and elimination of soluble proteins.

The heterogeneity of EVs is another possible reason for their unstable therapeutic effects. Researchers have raised concerns about the different neuroprotective efficacy of MSC-EVs between individual preparations [60]. The latest review provides a definition of MSV-EVs and a general optimization strategy of the MSC manufacturing process for better and more homogeneous MSC-EVs [137,138]. On the other side, apart from avoiding the heterogeneity of EVs, understanding and taking advantage of the heterogeneity of EVs presents more opportunities for obtaining optimal therapeutic outcomes. For example, MSC-EVs consist of at least three types with different proteomes [139]. Recently, more exosome subpopulations have been found by asymmetric flow field-flow fractionation and high-speed ultracentrifugation [140,141]. These subpopulations within the classical subtypes of EVs mean that their therapeutic activities come from a collective effect of heterogeneous EV groups [142]. Although the biological significance and functions of these subpopulations have not been illustrated so far, some subpopulations may exhibit better therapeutic effects than other subpopulations. Thus, selecting the optimal subpopulations for treating different diseases will increase the consistency of their therapeutic effects and the accuracy of EV-based therapeutics.

Another major hindrance to clinical EV-based therapy is the production of sufficient EVs. Mendt et al. reported bioreactor-based progress in the large-scale generation of good-manufacturing-practice-grade (GMP-grade) MSC-EVs [143]. Plasma- and adipose-tissue-derived EVs have been proposed to be a cost-efficient alternative source of EVs compared to cell-culture-derived EVs [144]. Recently, a set of genetically encoded devices in EV-producer cells has been developed to enhance EV production and to specify the packaging and delivery of therapeutic mRNA in PD models [145]. In this study, the researchers designed an EV production booster, namely a tricistronic plasmid vector with a combined expression of STEAP3, syndecan-4 (SDC4), and a fragment of l-aspartate oxidase (NadB) at a fixed ratio, which produced a 15-fold to 40-fold increase in EV production in different cells. Co-transfecting the EV production booster, a potential RNA packaging device, a cytosolic delivery helper, mRNA, and RVG-Lamp2b into the EV-producer cells significantly increased the delivery of therapeutic mRNA into the target cells. Moreover, the engineered

EV-producer cells implanted in living mice constitutively produced and delivered EVs loaded with therapeutic mRNAs, attenuating 6-OHDA-induced neuroinflammation in the PD mouse model. Thus, these genetically encoded devices can serve as efficient tools to produce a great deal of designer EVs and to enable the delivery of therapeutic mRNA in situ in vivo [145]. Grangier et al. critically compared the technological advances toward the mass production of EVs and clinical production platforms in detail [146]. The upscaling, isolation, storage, production, and standardization of them have been well discussed in other outstanding reviews [12,147–151].

The difficulty in the large-scale production of EVs for clinical application prompts the development of fully synthetic EV mimetic particles by bionanotechnology. EV mimetic vesicles can be a cheaper and more scalable nanosystem for encapsulating and delivering drugs. According to García-Manrique et al., the preparation of artificial EVs consists of two types: bioengineering cells as membrane fragment precursors (top-down methodologies) and mimicking the plasma membrane with artificial bilayers (bottom-up techniques) [152]. The mass production of EV mimetics with natural immunotolerance can be obtained by the top-down methodologies, but the encapsulation of cargo is passive and lacks selectivity. On the contrary, the bottom-up techniques provide specific cargo loading and high encapsulation efficiencies, while the production of EVs is still small. Therefore, the artificial EV field is still premature. Polyethylene-glycol (PEG)-induced membrane fusion between liposomes and EVs provides another strategy for this purpose [153]. The analysis of the characterization of EVs provides insights into the targeting and efficient delivery of therapeutic cargo, while the methodologies and advanced techniques in the liposome field may help to manufacture therapeutic EVs for specific clinical uses. Given the involvement of EV-associated lipids in the pathological process of neurological diseases, the modulation of EV lipidome represents a possible therapeutic strategy [107].

Off-target activity and dilution effects block the development and progress of EV-based therapy to some extent. The precisely controlled release of drugs is another challenge in EV-based therapeutics. Intelligent EVs engineered with responsive modules can react to specific internal and/or external stimulation to release cargo. These intelligent EVs have been systematically reviewed recently [154].

4. Conclusions

Despite ongoing challenges, extracellular vesicles have emerged as promising therapeutics and drug delivery systems in recent years. Emerging EV-based therapeutics in preclinical studies of neurological diseases have set the stage for their clinical use. In addition, the combination of EV-based therapeutics and some therapeutics that are in rapid development, such as mRNA therapeutics, may provide insight into treatments for neurological diseases. However, unstable therapeutic effects, difficulties in the large-scale production of EVs, and off-target activities still limit the clinical applications of EV-based therapeutics. Although many issues remain to be addressed, as a consequence of emerging standardized protocols and guidelines for EV isolation and storage, EV-based therapeutics are not far away from clinical application in neurological diseases.

Author Contributions: Conceptualization, Y.Y., Q.D. and M.C.; writing—original draft preparation, Y.Y. and J.S.; writing—review and editing, T.Y., W.S. and W.X.; visualization, Y.Y. and J.S.; funding acquisition, Q.D. and M.C. All authors have read and agreed to the published version of the manuscript.

Funding: This study was supported by the National Natural Science Foundation of China (81971013 to M.C.; 82071197 to Q.D.).

Institutional Review Board Statement: Not applicable.

Informed Consent Statement: Not applicable.

Data Availability Statement: Not applicable.

Conflicts of Interest: The authors declare that they have no conflict of interest.

References

1. Feigin, V.L.; Nichols, E.; Alam, T.; Bannick, M.S.; Beghi, E.; Blake, N.; Culpepper, W.J.; Dorsey, E.R.; Elbaz, A.; Ellenbogen, R.G. Global, regional, and national burden of neurological disorders, 1990–2016: A systematic analysis for the Global Burden of Disease Study 2016. *Lancet Neurol.* **2019**, *18*, 459–480. [CrossRef] [PubMed]
2. Kalluri, R.; LeBleu, V.S. The biology, function, and biomedical applications of exosomes. *Science* **2020**, *367*, eaau6977. [CrossRef] [PubMed]
3. Kao, C.Y.; Papoutsakis, E.T. Extracellular vesicles: Exosomes, microparticles, their parts, and their targets to enable their biomanufacturing and clinical applications. *Curr. Opin. Biotechnol.* **2019**, *60*, 89–98. [CrossRef] [PubMed]
4. Thery, C.; Witwer, K.W.; Aikawa, E.; Alcaraz, M.J.; Anderson, J.D.; Andriantsitohaina, R.; Antoniou, A.; Arab, T.; Archer, F.; Atkin-Smith, G.K.; et al. Minimal information for studies of extracellular vesicles 2018 (MISEV2018): A position statement of the International Society for Extracellular Vesicles and update of the MISEV2014 guidelines. *J. Extracell. Vesicles* **2018**, *7*, 1535750. [CrossRef]
5. Cocucci, E.; Meldolesi, J. Ectosomes and exosomes: Shedding the confusion between extracellular vesicles. *Trends Cell Biol.* **2015**, *25*, 364–372. [CrossRef]
6. Pegtel, D.M.; Gould, S.J. Exosomes. *Annu. Rev. Biochem.* **2019**, *88*, 487–514. [CrossRef]
7. Raposo, G.; Stoorvogel, W. Extracellular vesicles: Exosomes, microvesicles, and friends. *J. Cell Biol.* **2013**, *200*, 373–383. [CrossRef]
8. Sharma, P.; Mesci, P.; Carromeu, C.; McClatchy, D.R.; Schiapparelli, L.; Yates, J.R., 3rd; Muotri, A.R.; Cline, H.T. Exosomes regulate neurogenesis and circuit assembly. *Proc. Natl. Acad. Sci. USA* **2019**, *116*, 16086–16094. [CrossRef]
9. You, Y.; Borgmann, K.; Edara, V.V.; Stacy, S.; Ghorpade, A.; Ikezu, T. Activated human astrocyte-derived extracellular vesicles modulate neuronal uptake, differentiation and firing. *J. Extracell. Vesicles* **2020**, *9*, 1706801. [CrossRef]
10. Upadhya, R.; Zingg, W.; Shetty, S.; Shetty, A.K. Astrocyte-derived extracellular vesicles: Neuroreparative properties and role in the pathogenesis of neurodegenerative disorders. *J. Control. Release* **2020**, *323*, 225–239. [CrossRef]
11. Donoso-Quezada, J.; Ayala-Mar, S.; Gonzalez-Valdez, J. State-of-the-art exosome loading and functionalization techniques for enhanced therapeutics: A review. *Crit. Rev. Biotechnol.* **2020**, *40*, 804–820. [CrossRef] [PubMed]
12. Elsharkasy, O.M.; Nordin, J.Z.; Hagey, D.W.; de Jong, O.G.; Schiffelers, R.M.; Andaloussi, S.E.; Vader, P. Extracellular vesicles as drug delivery systems: Why and how? *Adv. Drug Deliv. Rev.* **2020**, *159*, 332–343. [CrossRef] [PubMed]
13. Bulbake, U.; Doppalapudi, S.; Kommineni, N.; Khan, W. Liposomal Formulations in Clinical Use: An Updated Review. *Pharmaceutics* **2017**, *9*, 12. [CrossRef] [PubMed]
14. Sercombe, L.; Veerati, T.; Moheimani, F.; Wu, S.Y.; Sood, A.K.; Hua, S. Advances and Challenges of Liposome Assisted Drug Delivery. *Front. Pharm.* **2015**, *6*, 286. [CrossRef] [PubMed]
15. Charoenviriyakul, C.; Takahashi, Y.; Morishita, M.; Nishikawa, M.; Takakura, Y. Role of Extracellular Vesicle Surface Proteins in the Pharmacokinetics of Extracellular Vesicles. *Mol. Pharm.* **2018**, *15*, 1073–1080. [CrossRef] [PubMed]
16. Kamerkar, S.; LeBleu, V.S.; Sugimoto, H.; Yang, S.; Ruivo, C.F.; Melo, S.A.; Lee, J.J.; Kalluri, R. Exosomes facilitate therapeutic targeting of oncogenic KRAS in pancreatic cancer. *Nature* **2017**, *546*, 498–503. [CrossRef] [PubMed]
17. Clayton, A.; Harris, C.L.; Court, J.; Mason, M.D.; Morgan, B.P. Antigen-presenting cell exosomes are protected from complement-mediated lysis by expression of CD55 and CD59. *Eur. J. Immunol.* **2003**, *33*, 522–531. [CrossRef]
18. Hoshino, A.; Costa-Silva, B.; Shen, T.L.; Rodrigues, G.; Hashimoto, A.; Tesic Mark, M.; Molina, H.; Kohsaka, S.; Di Giannatale, A.; Ceder, S.; et al. Tumour exosome integrins determine organotropic metastasis. *Nature* **2015**, *527*, 329–335. [CrossRef]
19. Osawa, S.; Kurachi, M.; Yamamoto, H.; Yoshimoto, Y.; Ishizaki, Y. Fibronectin on extracellular vesicles from microvascular endothelial cells is involved in the vesicle uptake into oligodendrocyte precursor cells. *Biochem. Biophys. Res. Commun.* **2017**, *488*, 232–238. [CrossRef]
20. Wu, A.Y.T.; Sung, Y.C.; Chen, Y.J.; Chou, S.T.Y.; Guo, V.; Chien, J.C.Y.; Ko, J.J.S.; Yang, A.L.; Huang, H.C.; Chuang, J.C. Multiresolution imaging using bioluminescence resonance energy transfer identifies distinct biodistribution profiles of extracellular vesicles and exomeres with redirected tropism. *Adv. Sci.* **2020**, *7*, 2001467. [CrossRef]
21. Williams, C.; Royo, F.; Aizpurua-Olaizola, O.; Pazos, R.; Boons, G.J.; Reichardt, N.C.; Falcon-Perez, J.M. Glycosylation of extracellular vesicles: Current knowledge, tools and clinical perspectives. *J. Extracell. Vesicles* **2018**, *7*, 1442985. [CrossRef] [PubMed]
22. Murphy, D.E.; de Jong, O.G.; Brouwer, M.; Wood, M.J.; Lavieu, G.; Schiffelers, R.M.; Vader, P. Extracellular vesicle-based therapeutics: Natural versus engineered targeting and trafficking. *Exp. Mol. Med.* **2019**, *51*, 1–12. [CrossRef] [PubMed]
23. El Andaloussi, S.; Mager, I.; Breakefield, X.O.; Wood, M.J. Extracellular vesicles: Biology and emerging therapeutic opportunities. *Nat. Rev. Drug Discov.* **2013**, *12*, 347–357. [CrossRef] [PubMed]
24. Wang, R.; Wang, X.; Zhang, Y.; Zhao, H.; Cui, J.; Li, J.; Di, L. Emerging prospects of extracellular vesicles for brain disease theranostics. *J. Control. Release* **2022**, *341*, 844–868. [CrossRef]
25. Manna, I.; De Benedittis, S.; Quattrone, A.; Maisano, D.; Iaccino, E.; Quattrone, A. Exosomal miRNAs as Potential Diagnostic Biomarkers in Alzheimer's Disease. *Pharmaceuticals* **2020**, *13*, 243. [CrossRef] [PubMed]
26. Zhang, Z.G.; Chopp, M. Neurorestorative therapies for stroke: Underlying mechanisms and translation to the clinic. *Lancet Neurol.* **2009**, *8*, 491–500. [CrossRef] [PubMed]
27. Chen, J.; Li, Y.; Wang, L.; Zhang, Z.; Lu, D.; Lu, M.; Chopp, M. Therapeutic benefit of intravenous administration of bone marrow stromal cells after cerebral ischemia in rats. *Stroke* **2001**, *32*, 1005–1011. [CrossRef]

28. Hess, D.C.; Wechsler, L.R.; Clark, W.M.; Savitz, S.I.; Ford, G.A.; Chiu, D.; Yavagal, D.R.; Uchino, K.; Liebeskind, D.S.; Auchus, A.P.; et al. Safety and efficacy of multipotent adult progenitor cells in acute ischaemic stroke (MASTERS): A randomised, double-blind, placebo-controlled, phase 2 trial. *Lancet Neurol.* **2017**, *16*, 360–368. [CrossRef]
29. Chung, J.W.; Chang, W.H.; Bang, O.Y.; Moon, G.J.; Kim, S.J.; Kim, S.K.; Lee, J.S.; Sohn, S.I.; Kim, Y.H.; et al.; STARTING-2 Collaborators. Efficacy and Safety of Intravenous Mesenchymal Stem Cells for Ischemic Stroke. *Neurology* **2021**, *96*, e1012–e1023. [CrossRef]
30. Jaillard, A.; Hommel, M.; Moisan, A.; Zeffiro, T.A.; Favre-Wiki, I.M.; Barbieux-Guillot, M.; Vadot, W.; Marcel, S.; Lamalle, L.; Grand, S.; et al. Autologous Mesenchymal Stem Cells Improve Motor Recovery in Subacute Ischemic Stroke: A Randomized Clinical Trial. *Transl. Stroke Res.* **2020**, *11*, 910–923. [CrossRef]
31. Zhang, S.; Lachance, B.B.; Moiz, B.; Jia, X. Optimizing Stem Cell Therapy after Ischemic Brain Injury. *J. Stroke* **2020**, *22*, 286–305. [CrossRef] [PubMed]
32. Gnecchi, M.; He, H.; Liang, O.D.; Melo, L.G.; Morello, F.; Mu, H.; Noiseux, N.; Zhang, L.; Pratt, R.E.; Ingwall, J.S. Paracrine action accounts for marked protection of ischemic heart by Akt-modified mesenchymal stem cells. *Nat. Med.* **2005**, *11*, 367–368. [CrossRef]
33. Zhang, Z.G.; Buller, B.; Chopp, M. Exosomes—beyond stem cells for restorative therapy in stroke and neurological injury. *Nat. Rev. Neurol.* **2019**, *15*, 193–203. [CrossRef] [PubMed]
34. Marban, E. The Secret Life of Exosomes: What Bees Can Teach Us about Next-Generation Therapeutics. *J. Am. Coll. Cardiol.* **2018**, *71*, 193–200. [CrossRef] [PubMed]
35. Xin, H.; Li, Y.; Cui, Y.; Yang, J.J.; Zhang, Z.G.; Chopp, M. Systemic administration of exosomes released from mesenchymal stromal cells promote functional recovery and neurovascular plasticity after stroke in rats. *J. Cereb. Blood Flow Metab.* **2013**, *33*, 1711–1715. [CrossRef] [PubMed]
36. Xin, H.; Katakowski, M.; Wang, F.; Qian, J.Y.; Liu, X.S.; Ali, M.M.; Buller, B.; Zhang, Z.G.; Chopp, M. MicroRNA cluster miR-17–92 Cluster in Exosomes Enhance Neuroplasticity and Functional Recovery after Stroke in Rats. *Stroke* **2017**, *48*, 747–753. [CrossRef]
37. Doeppner, T.R.; Herz, J.; Gorgens, A.; Schlechter, J.; Ludwig, A.K.; Radtke, S.; de Miroschedji, K.; Horn, P.A.; Giebel, B.; Hermann, D.M. Extracellular Vesicles Improve Post-Stroke Neuroregeneration and Prevent Postischemic Immunosuppression. *Stem Cells Transl. Med.* **2015**, *4*, 1131–1143. [CrossRef]
38. Webb, R.L.; Kaiser, E.E.; Scoville, S.L.; Thompson, T.A.; Fatima, S.; Pandya, C.; Sriram, K.; Swetenburg, R.L.; Vaibhav, K.; Arbab, A.S.; et al. Human Neural Stem Cell Extracellular Vesicles Improve Tissue and Functional Recovery in the Murine Thromboembolic Stroke Model. *Transl. Stroke Res.* **2018**, *9*, 530–539. [CrossRef]
39. Xiao, Y.; Tian, J.; Wu, W.C.; Gao, Y.H.; Guo, Y.X.; Song, S.J.; Gao, R.; Wang, L.B.; Wu, X.Y.; Zhang, Y.; et al. Targeting central nervous system extracellular vesicles enhanced triiodothyronine remyelination effect on experimental autoimmune encephalomyelitis. *Bioact. Mater.* **2022**, *9*, 373–384. [CrossRef]
40. Jiang, Y.; Wang, R.; Wang, C.; Guo, Y.; Xu, T.; Zhang, Z.; Yang, G.Y.; Xu, H.; Tang, Y. Brain Microenvironment Responsive and Pro-Angiogenic Extracellular Vesicle-Hydrogel for Promoting Neurobehavioral Recovery in Type 2 Diabetic Mice after Stroke. *Adv. Healthc Mater.* **2022**, *11*, e2201150. [CrossRef]
41. Gao, G.; Li, C.; Zhu, J.; Sheng, S.; Liang, Z.; Fu, S.; Li, X.; Sun, Y.; Wang, Y.; Feng, X.; et al. Induced neural stem/progenitor cell-derived extracellular vesicles promote recovery post-stroke. *Clin. Transl. Med.* **2022**, *12*, e936. [CrossRef] [PubMed]
42. Hu, G.; Xia, Y.; Chen, B.; Zhang, J.; Gong, L.; Chen, Y.; Li, Q.; Wang, Y.; Deng, Z. ESC-sEVs Rejuvenate Aging Hippocampal NSCs by Transferring SMADs to Regulate the MYT1-Egln3-Sirt1 Axis. *Mol. Ther.* **2021**, *29*, 103–120. [CrossRef] [PubMed]
43. Saez-Atienzar, S.; Masliah, E. Cellular senescence and Alzheimer disease: The egg and the chicken scenario. *Nat. Rev. Neurosci.* **2020**, *21*, 433–444. [CrossRef] [PubMed]
44. Hou, Y.; Dan, X.; Babbar, M.; Wei, Y.; Hasselbalch, S.G.; Croteau, D.L.; Bohr, V.A. Ageing as a risk factor for neurodegenerative disease. *Nat. Rev. Neurol.* **2019**, *15*, 565–581. [CrossRef]
45. Yoshida, M.; Satoh, A.; Lin, J.B.; Mills, K.F.; Sasaki, Y.; Rensing, N.; Wong, M.; Apte, R.S.; Imai, S.I. Extracellular Vesicle-Contained eNAMPT Delays Aging and Extends Lifespan in Mice. *Cell Metab.* **2019**, *30*, 329–342.e325. [CrossRef]
46. Prattichizzo, F.; Giuliani, A.; Sabbatinelli, J.; Mensa, E.; De Nigris, V.; La Sala, L.; de Candia, P.; Olivieri, F.; Ceriello, A. Extracellular vesicles circulating in young organisms promote healthy longevity. *J. Extracell. Vesicles* **2019**, *8*, 1656044. [CrossRef]
47. Fafian-Labora, J.A.; Rodriguez-Navarro, J.A.; O'Loghlen, A. Small Extracellular Vesicles Have GST Activity and Ameliorate Senescence-Related Tissue Damage. *Cell Metab.* **2020**, *32*, 71–86.e75. [CrossRef]
48. Marar, C.; Starich, B.; Wirtz, D. Extracellular vesicles in immunomodulation and tumor progression. *Nat. Immunol.* **2021**, *22*, 560–570. [CrossRef]
49. Schneider, E.; Winzer, R.; Rissiek, A.; Ricklefs, I.; Meyer-Schwesinger, C.; Ricklefs, F.L.; Bauche, A.; Behrends, J.; Reimer, R.; Brenna, S.; et al. CD73-mediated adenosine production by CD8 T cell-derived extracellular vesicles constitutes an intrinsic mechanism of immune suppression. *Nat. Commun.* **2021**, *12*, 5911. [CrossRef]
50. Takenaka, M.; Yabuta, A.; Takahashi, Y.; Takakura, Y. Interleukin-4-carrying small extracellular vesicles with a high potential as anti-inflammatory therapeutics based on modulation of macrophage function. *Biomaterials* **2021**, *278*, 121160. [CrossRef]
51. Robbins, P.D.; Morelli, A.E. Regulation of immune responses by extracellular vesicles. *Nat. Rev. Immunol.* **2014**, *14*, 195–208. [CrossRef] [PubMed]
52. Buzas, E.I. The roles of extracellular vesicles in the immune system. *Nat. Rev. Immunol.* **2022**. [CrossRef] [PubMed]
53. Prinz, M.; Jung, S.; Priller, J. Microglia Biology: One Century of Evolving Concepts. *Cell* **2019**, *179*, 292–311. [CrossRef] [PubMed]

54. Li, Y.; Liu, Z.; Song, Y.; Pan, J.J.; Jiang, Y.; Shi, X.; Liu, C.; Ma, Y.; Luo, L.; Mamtilahun, M.; et al. M2 microglia-derived extracellular vesicles promote white matter repair and functional recovery via miR-23a-5p after cerebral ischemia in mice. *Theranostics* **2022**, *12*, 3553–3573. [CrossRef]
55. Li, Z.; Song, Y.; He, T.; Wen, R.; Li, Y.; Chen, T.; Huang, S.; Wang, Y.; Tang, Y.; Shen, F.; et al. M2 microglial small extracellular vesicles reduce glial scar formation via the miR-124/STAT3 pathway after ischemic stroke in mice. *Theranostics* **2021**, *11*, 1232–1248. [CrossRef]
56. Raffaele, S.; Gelosa, P.; Bonfanti, E.; Lombardi, M.; Castiglioni, L.; Cimino, M.; Sironi, L.; Abbracchio, M.P.; Verderio, C.; Fumagalli, M. Microglial vesicles improve post-stroke recovery by preventing immune cell senescence and favoring oligodendrogenesis. *Mol. Ther.* **2021**, *29*, 1439–1458. [CrossRef]
57. Song, Y.; Li, Z.; He, T.; Qu, M.; Jiang, L.; Li, W.; Shi, X.; Pan, J.; Zhang, L.; Wang, Y.; et al. M2 microglia-derived exosomes protect the mouse brain from ischemia-reperfusion injury via exosomal miR-124. *Theranostics* **2019**, *9*, 2910–2923. [CrossRef]
58. Xia, Y.; Hu, G.; Chen, Y.; Yuan, J.; Zhang, J.; Wang, S.; Li, Q.; Wang, Y.; Deng, Z. Embryonic Stem Cell Derived Small Extracellular Vesicles Modulate Regulatory T Cells to Protect against Ischemic Stroke. *ACS Nano* **2021**, *15*, 7370–7385. [CrossRef]
59. Tian, T.; Cao, L.; He, C.; Ye, Q.; Liang, R.; You, W.; Zhang, H.; Wu, J.; Ye, J.; Tannous, B.A.; et al. Targeted delivery of neural progenitor cell-derived extracellular vesicles for anti-inflammation after cerebral ischemia. *Theranostics* **2021**, *11*, 6507–6521. [CrossRef]
60. Wang, C.; Borger, V.; Sardari, M.; Murke, F.; Skuljec, J.; Pul, R.; Hagemann, N.; Dzyubenko, E.; Dittrich, R.; Gregorius, J.; et al. Mesenchymal Stromal Cell-Derived Small Extracellular Vesicles Induce Ischemic Neuroprotection by Modulating Leukocytes and Specifically Neutrophils. *Stroke* **2020**, *51*, 1825–1834. [CrossRef]
61. Hosseini Shamili, F.; Alibolandi, M.; Rafatpanah, H.; Abnous, K.; Mahmoudi, M.; Kalantari, M.; Taghdisi, S.M.; Ramezani, M. Immunomodulatory properties of MSC-derived exosomes armed with high affinity aptamer toward mylein as a platform for reducing multiple sclerosis clinical score. *J. Control. Release* **2019**, *299*, 149–164. [CrossRef] [PubMed]
62. Mi, Y.; Han, J.; Zhu, J.; Jin, T. Role of the PD-1/PD-L1 Signaling in Multiple Sclerosis and Experimental Autoimmune Encephalomyelitis: Recent Insights and Future Directions. *Mol. Neurobiol.* **2021**, *58*, 6249–6271. [CrossRef] [PubMed]
63. Hirata, S.; Senju, S.; Matsuyoshi, H.; Fukuma, D.; Uemura, Y.; Nishimura, Y. Prevention of experimental autoimmune encephalomyelitis by transfer of embryonic stem cell-derived dendritic cells expressing myelin oligodendrocyte glycoprotein peptide along with TRAIL or programmed death-1 ligand. *J. Immunol.* **2005**, *174*, 1888–1897. [CrossRef] [PubMed]
64. Xu, F.; Fei, Z.; Dai, H.; Xu, J.; Fan, Q.; Shen, S.; Zhang, Y.; Ma, Q.; Chu, J.; Peng, F.; et al. Mesenchymal Stem Cell-Derived Extracellular Vesicles with High PD-L1 Expression for Autoimmune Diseases Treatment. *Adv. Mater.* **2022**, *34*, e2106265. [CrossRef]
65. Yuan, D.; Zhao, Y.; Banks, W.A.; Bullock, K.M.; Haney, M.; Batrakova, E.; Kabanov, A.V. Macrophage exosomes as natural nanocarriers for protein delivery to inflamed brain. *Biomaterials* **2017**, *142*, 1–12. [CrossRef]
66. Wiklander, O.P.; Nordin, J.Z.; O'Loughlin, A.; Gustafsson, Y.; Corso, G.; Mager, I.; Vader, P.; Lee, Y.; Sork, H.; Seow, Y.; et al. Extracellular vesicle in vivo biodistribution is determined by cell source, route of administration and targeting. *J. Extracell. Vesicles* **2015**, *4*, 26316. [CrossRef]
67. Agrawal, M.; Saraf, S.; Saraf, S.; Antimisiaris, S.G.; Chougule, M.B.; Shoyele, S.A.; Alexander, A. Nose-to-brain drug delivery: An update on clinical challenges and progress towards approval of anti-Alzheimer drugs. *J. Control. Release* **2018**, *281*, 139–177. [CrossRef]
68. Sabir, F.; Ismail, R.; Csoka, I. Nose-to-brain delivery of antiglioblastoma drugs embedded into lipid nanocarrier systems: Status quo and outlook. *Drug Discov. Today* **2020**, *25*, 185–194. [CrossRef]
69. Zhuang, X.; Xiang, X.; Grizzle, W.; Sun, D.; Zhang, S.; Axtell, R.C.; Ju, S.; Mu, J.; Zhang, L.; Steinman, L.; et al. Treatment of brain inflammatory diseases by delivering exosome encapsulated anti-inflammatory drugs from the nasal region to the brain. *Mol. Ther.* **2011**, *19*, 1769–1779. [CrossRef]
70. Kalani, A.; Chaturvedi, P.; Kamat, P.K.; Maldonado, C.; Bauer, P.; Joshua, I.G.; Tyagi, S.C.; Tyagi, N. Curcumin-loaded embryonic stem cell exosomes restored neurovascular unit following ischemia-reperfusion injury. *Int. J. Biochem. Cell Biol.* **2016**, *79*, 360–369. [CrossRef]
71. Illum, L. Is nose-to-brain transport of drugs in man a reality? *J. Pharm. Pharm.* **2004**, *56*, 3–17. [CrossRef]
72. Terstappen, G.C.; Meyer, A.H.; Bell, R.D.; Zhang, W. Strategies for delivering therapeutics across the blood-brain barrier. *Nat. Rev. Drug Discov.* **2021**, *20*, 362–383. [CrossRef] [PubMed]
73. Tian, T.; Zhang, H.X.; He, C.P.; Fan, S.; Zhu, Y.L.; Qi, C.; Huang, N.P.; Xiao, Z.D.; Lu, Z.H.; Tannous, B.A.; et al. Surface functionalized exosomes as targeted drug delivery vehicles for cerebral ischemia therapy. *Biomaterials* **2018**, *150*, 137–149. [CrossRef] [PubMed]
74. Alvarez-Erviti, L.; Seow, Y.; Yin, H.; Betts, C.; Lakhal, S.; Wood, M.J. Delivery of siRNA to the mouse brain by systemic injection of targeted exosomes. *Nat. Biotechnol.* **2011**, *29*, 341–345. [CrossRef]
75. Ransohoff, R.M. How neuroinflammation contributes to neurodegeneration. *Science* **2016**, *353*, 777–783. [CrossRef]
76. Goedert, M.; Spillantini, M.G.; Serpell, L.C.; Berriman, J.; Smith, M.J.; Jakes, R.; Crowther, R.A. From genetics to pathology: Tau and alpha-synuclein assemblies in neurodegenerative diseases. *Philos. Trans. R. Soc. Lond. B Biol. Sci.* **2001**, *356*, 213–227. [CrossRef]
77. Cooper, J.M.; Wiklander, P.B.; Nordin, J.Z.; Al-Shawi, R.; Wood, M.J.; Vithlani, M.; Schapira, A.H.; Simons, J.P.; El-Andaloussi, S.; Alvarez-Erviti, L. Systemic exosomal siRNA delivery reduced alpha-synuclein aggregates in brains of transgenic mice. *Mov. Disord.* **2014**, *29*, 1476–1485. [CrossRef] [PubMed]
78. Izco, M.; Blesa, J.; Schleef, M.; Schmeer, M.; Porcari, R.; Al-Shawi, R.; Ellmerich, S.; de Toro, M.; Gardiner, C.; Seow, Y.; et al. Systemic Exosomal Delivery of shRNA Minicircles Prevents Parkinsonian Pathology. *Mol. Ther.* **2019**, *27*, 2111–2122. [CrossRef]

79. Ma, X.; Huang, M.; Zheng, M.; Dai, C.; Song, Q.; Zhang, Q.; Li, Q.; Gu, X.; Chen, H.; Jiang, G.; et al. ADSCs-derived extracellular vesicles alleviate neuronal damage, promote neurogenesis and rescue memory loss in mice with Alzheimer's disease. *J. Control. Release* **2020**, *327*, 688–702. [CrossRef]
80. Peng, D.; Wang, Y.; Xiao, Y.; Peng, M.; Mai, W.; Hu, B.; Jia, Y.; Chen, H.; Yang, Y.; Xiang, Q.; et al. Extracellular vesicles derived from astrocyte-treated with haFGF14-154 attenuate Alzheimer phenotype in AD mice. *Theranostics* **2022**, *12*, 3862–3881. [CrossRef]
81. Lee, M.; Ban, J.J.; Kim, K.Y.; Jeon, G.S.; Im, W.; Sung, J.J.; Kim, M. Adipose-derived stem cell exosomes alleviate pathology of amyotrophic lateral sclerosis in vitro. *Biochem. Biophys. Res. Commun.* **2016**, *479*, 434–439. [CrossRef] [PubMed]
82. Haney, M.J.; Klyachko, N.L.; Zhao, Y.; Gupta, R.; Plotnikova, E.G.; He, Z.; Patel, T.; Piroyan, A.; Sokolsky, M.; Kabanov, A.V.; et al. Exosomes as drug delivery vehicles for Parkinson's disease therapy. *J. Control. Release* **2015**, *207*, 18–30. [CrossRef] [PubMed]
83. Qu, M.; Lin, Q.; Huang, L.; Fu, Y.; Wang, L.; He, S.; Fu, Y.; Yang, S.; Zhang, Z.; Zhang, L.; et al. Dopamine-loaded blood exosomes targeted to brain for better treatment of Parkinson's disease. *J. Control. Release* **2018**, *287*, 156–166. [CrossRef]
84. Van den Broek, B.; Wuyts, C.; Irobi, J. Extracellular vesicle-associated small heat shock proteins as therapeutic agents in neurodegenerative diseases and beyond. *Adv. Drug Deliv. Rev.* **2021**, *179*, 114009. [CrossRef] [PubMed]
85. Yang, J.; Wu, S.; Hou, L.; Zhu, D.; Yin, S.; Yang, G.; Wang, Y. Therapeutic Effects of Simultaneous Delivery of Nerve Growth Factor mRNA and Protein via Exosomes on Cerebral Ischemia. *Mol. Ther.-Nucleic Acids* **2020**, *21*, 512–522. [CrossRef] [PubMed]
86. Rohner, E.; Yang, R.; Foo, K.S.; Goedel, A.; Chien, K.R. Unlocking the promise of mRNA therapeutics. *Nat. Biotechnol.* **2022**, *40*, 1586–1600. [CrossRef]
87. Yang, J.; Zhang, X.; Chen, X.; Wang, L.; Yang, G. Exosome mediated delivery of miR-124 promotes neurogenesis after ischemia. *Mol. Ther.-Nucleic Acids* **2017**, *7*, 278–287. [CrossRef]
88. Murphy, D.E.; de Jong, O.G.; Evers, M.J.W.; Nurazizah, M.; Schiffelers, R.M.; Vader, P. Natural or Synthetic RNA Delivery: A Stoichiometric Comparison of Extracellular Vesicles and Synthetic Nanoparticles. *Nano Lett.* **2021**, *21*, 1888–1895. [CrossRef]
89. Xia, X.; Wang, Y.; Huang, Y.; Zhang, H.; Lu, H.; Zheng, J.C. Exosomal miRNAs in central nervous system diseases: Biomarkers, pathological mediators, protective factors and therapeutic agents. *Prog. Neurobiol* **2019**, *183*, 101694. [CrossRef]
90. Ke, W.; Afonin, K.A. Exosomes as natural delivery carriers for programmable therapeutic nucleic acid nanoparticles (NANPs). *Adv. Drug Deliv. Rev.* **2021**, *176*, 113835. [CrossRef]
91. Didiot, M.C.; Hall, L.M.; Coles, A.H.; Haraszti, R.A.; Godinho, B.M.; Chase, K.; Sapp, E.; Ly, S.; Alterman, J.F.; Hassler, M.R.; et al. Exosome-mediated Delivery of Hydrophobically Modified siRNA for Huntingtin mRNA Silencing. *Mol. Ther.* **2016**, *24*, 1836–1847. [CrossRef]
92. Zhang, L.; Wu, T.; Shan, Y.; Li, G.; Ni, X.; Chen, X.; Hu, X.; Lin, L.; Li, Y.; Guan, Y.; et al. Therapeutic reversal of Huntington's disease by in vivo self-assembled siRNAs. *Brain* **2021**, *144*, 3421–3435. [CrossRef] [PubMed]
93. Duan, D.; Goemans, N.; Takeda, S.; Mercuri, E.; Aartsma-Rus, A. Duchenne muscular dystrophy. *Nat. Rev. Dis. Primers* **2021**, *7*, 13. [CrossRef]
94. Verhaart, I.E.C.; Aartsma-Rus, A. Therapeutic developments for Duchenne muscular dystrophy. *Nat. Rev. Neurol.* **2019**, *15*, 373–386. [CrossRef]
95. Gao, X.; Ran, N.; Dong, X.; Zuo, B.; Yang, R.; Zhou, Q.; Moulton, H.M.; Seow, Y.; Yin, H. Anchor peptide captures, targets, and loads exosomes of diverse origins for diagnostics and therapy. *Sci. Transl. Med.* **2018**, *10*, eaat0195. [CrossRef]
96. Ran, N.; Gao, X.; Dong, X.; Li, J.; Lin, C.; Geng, M.; Yin, H. Effects of exosome-mediated delivery of myostatin propeptide on functional recovery of mdx mice. *Biomaterials* **2020**, *236*, 119826. [CrossRef]
97. Leng, L.; Dong, X.; Gao, X.; Ran, N.; Geng, M.; Zuo, B.; Wu, Y.; Li, W.; Yan, H.; Han, G.; et al. Exosome-mediated improvement in membrane integrity and muscle function in dystrophic mice. *Mol. Ther.* **2021**, *29*, 1459–1470. [CrossRef]
98. Qin, W.; Dallas, S.L. Exosomes and Extracellular RNA in Muscle and Bone Aging and Crosstalk. *Curr. Osteoporos. Rep.* **2019**, *17*, 548–559. [CrossRef] [PubMed]
99. Isaac, R.; Reis, F.C.G.; Ying, W.; Olefsky, J.M. Exosomes as mediators of intercellular crosstalk in metabolism. *Cell Metab.* **2021**, *33*, 1744–1762. [CrossRef]
100. Gratpain, V.; Mwema, A.; Labrak, Y.; Muccioli, G.G.; van Pesch, V.; des Rieux, A. Extracellular vesicles for the treatment of central nervous system diseases. *Adv. Drug Deliv. Rev.* **2021**, *174*, 535–552. [CrossRef] [PubMed]
101. Hao, Y.; Song, H.; Zhou, Z.; Chen, X.; Li, H.; Zhang, Y.; Wang, J.; Ren, X.; Wang, X. Promotion or inhibition of extracellular vesicle release: Emerging therapeutic opportunities. *J. Control. Release* **2021**, *340*, 136–148. [CrossRef] [PubMed]
102. Benjamins, J.A.; Nedelkoska, L.; Touil, H.; Stemmer, P.M.; Carruthers, N.J.; Jena, B.P.; Naik, A.R.; Bar-Or, A.; Lisak, R.P. Exosome-enriched fractions from MS B cells induce oligodendrocyte death. *Neurol.-Neuroimmunol. Neuroinflammation* **2019**, *6*, e550. [CrossRef] [PubMed]
103. Lisak, R.P.; Nedelkoska, L.; Benjamins, J.A.; Schalk, D.; Bealmear, B.; Touil, H.; Li, R.; Muirhead, G.; Bar-Or, A. B cells from patients with multiple sclerosis induce cell death via apoptosis in neurons in vitro. *J. Neuroimmunol.* **2017**, *309*, 88–99. [CrossRef] [PubMed]
104. Lisak, R.P.; Benjamins, J.A.; Nedelkoska, L.; Barger, J.L.; Ragheb, S.; Fan, B.; Ouamara, N.; Johnson, T.A.; Rajasekharan, S.; Bar-Or, A. Secretory products of multiple sclerosis B cells are cytotoxic to oligodendroglia in vitro. *J. Neuroimmunol.* **2012**, *246*, 85–95. [CrossRef] [PubMed]
105. Delpech, J.C.; Herron, S.; Botros, M.B.; Ikezu, T. Neuroimmune Crosstalk through Extracellular Vesicles in Health and Disease. *Trends Neurosci.* **2019**, *42*, 361–372. [CrossRef] [PubMed]

106. Thompson, A.G.; Gray, E.; Heman-Ackah, S.M.; Mager, I.; Talbot, K.; Andaloussi, S.E.; Wood, M.J.; Turner, M.R. Extracellular vesicles in neurodegenerative disease—Pathogenesis to biomarkers. *Nat. Rev. Neurol.* **2016**, *12*, 346–357. [CrossRef]
107. Vanherle, S.; Haidar, M.; Irobi, J.; Bogie, J.F.J.; Hendriks, J.J.A. Extracellular vesicle-associated lipids in central nervous system disorders. *Adv. Drug Deliv. Rev.* **2020**, *159*, 322–331. [CrossRef]
108. Yu, H.; Sun, T.; An, J.; Wen, L.; Liu, F.; Bu, Z.; Cui, Y.; Feng, J. Potential Roles of Exosomes in Parkinson's Disease: From Pathogenesis, Diagnosis, and Treatment to Prognosis. *Front. Cell Dev. Biol.* **2020**, *8*, 86. [CrossRef]
109. Zhang, T.; Ma, S.; Lv, J.; Wang, X.; Afewerky, H.K.; Li, H.; Lu, Y. The emerging role of exosomes in Alzheimer's disease. *Ageing Res. Rev.* **2021**, *68*, 101321. [CrossRef]
110. Catalano, M.; O'Driscoll, L. Inhibiting extracellular vesicles formation and release: A review of EV inhibitors. *J. Extracell. Vesicles* **2020**, *9*, 1703244. [CrossRef]
111. Chen, J.; Zhang, H.; Wang, S.; Du, Y.; Wei, B.; Wu, Q.; Wang, H. Inhibitors of Bacterial Extracellular Vesicles. *Front. Microbiol.* **2022**, *13*, 835058. [CrossRef] [PubMed]
112. Challis, R.C.; Ravindra Kumar, S.; Chen, X.; Goertsen, D.; Coughlin, G.M.; Hori, A.M.; Chuapoco, M.R.; Otis, T.S.; Miles, T.F.; Gradinaru, V. Adeno-Associated Virus Toolkit to Target Diverse Brain Cells. *Annu. Rev. Neurosci.* **2022**, *45*, 447–469. [CrossRef]
113. Ostrowski, M.; Carmo, N.B.; Krumeich, S.; Fanget, I.; Raposo, G.; Savina, A.; Moita, C.F.; Schauer, K.; Hume, A.N.; Freitas, R.P.; et al. Rab27a and Rab27b control different steps of the exosome secretion pathway. *Nat. Cell Biol.* **2010**, *12*, 19–30, sup pp 11–13. [CrossRef] [PubMed]
114. Zipkin, M. Big pharma buys into exosomes for drug delivery. *Nat. Biotechnol.* **2020**, *38*, 1226–1228. [CrossRef] [PubMed]
115. Roy, S.; Hochberg, F.H.; Jones, P.S. Extracellular vesicles: The growth as diagnostics and therapeutics; a survey. *J. Extracell. Vesicles* **2018**, *7*, 1438720. [CrossRef] [PubMed]
116. Guo, M.; Wu, F.; Hu, G.; Chen, L.; Xu, J.; Xu, P.; Wang, X.; Li, Y.; Liu, S.; Zhang, S.; et al. Autologous tumor cell-derived microparticle-based targeted chemotherapy in lung cancer patients with malignant pleural effusion. *Sci. Transl. Med.* **2019**, *11*, eaat5690. [CrossRef] [PubMed]
117. Kordelas, L.; Rebmann, V.; Ludwig, A.K.; Radtke, S.; Ruesing, J.; Doeppner, T.R.; Epple, M.; Horn, P.A.; Beelen, D.W.; Giebel, B. MSC-derived exosomes: A novel tool to treat therapy-refractory graft-versus-host disease. *Leukemia* **2014**, *28*, 970–973. [CrossRef] [PubMed]
118. Zhang, X.; Liu, J.; Yu, B.; Ma, F.; Ren, X.; Li, X. Effects of mesenchymal stem cells and their exosomes on the healing of large and refractory macular holes. *Graefe's Arch. Clin. Exp. Ophthalmol.* **2018**, *256*, 2041–2052. [CrossRef] [PubMed]
119. Mendt, M.; Rezvani, K.; Shpall, E. Mesenchymal stem cell-derived exosomes for clinical use. *Bone Marrow Transplant.* **2019**, *54*, 789–792. [CrossRef]
120. Zhu, Y.G.; Shi, M.M.; Monsel, A.; Dai, C.X.; Dong, X.; Shen, H.; Li, S.K.; Chang, J.; Xu, C.L.; Li, P.; et al. Nebulized exosomes derived from allogenic adipose tissue mesenchymal stromal cells in patients with severe COVID-19: A pilot study. *Stem Cell Res. Ther.* **2022**, *13*, 220. [CrossRef]
121. Lai, R.C.; Yeo, R.W.; Tan, K.H.; Lim, S.K. Exosomes for drug delivery—A novel application for the mesenchymal stem cell. *Biotechnol. Adv.* **2013**, *31*, 543–551. [CrossRef] [PubMed]
122. Rani, S.; Ryan, A.E.; Griffin, M.D.; Ritter, T. Mesenchymal Stem Cell-derived Extracellular Vesicles: Toward Cell-free Therapeutic Applications. *Mol. Ther.* **2015**, *23*, 812–823. [CrossRef] [PubMed]
123. Yeo, R.W.; Lai, R.C.; Zhang, B.; Tan, S.S.; Yin, Y.; Teh, B.J.; Lim, S.K. Mesenchymal stem cell: An efficient mass producer of exosomes for drug delivery. *Adv. Drug Deliv. Rev.* **2013**, *65*, 336–341. [CrossRef] [PubMed]
124. Crivelli, B.; Chlapanidas, T.; Perteghella, S.; Lucarelli, E.; Pascucci, L.; Brini, A.T.; Ferrero, I.; Marazzi, M.; Pessina, A.; Torre, M.L.; et al. Mesenchymal stem/stromal cell extracellular vesicles: From active principle to next generation drug delivery system. *J. Control. Release* **2017**, *262*, 104–117. [CrossRef] [PubMed]
125. Brennan, M.A.; Layrolle, P.; Mooney, D.J. Biomaterials functionalized with MSC secreted extracellular vesicles and soluble factors for tissue regeneration. *Adv. Funct. Mater.* **2020**, *30*, 1909125. [CrossRef]
126. Zhang, X.; Lu, Y.; Wu, S.; Zhang, S.; Li, S.; Tan, J. An Overview of Current Research on Mesenchymal Stem Cell-Derived Extracellular Vesicles: A Bibliometric Analysis From 2009 to 2021. *Front. Bioeng. Biotechnol.* **2022**, *10*, 910812. [CrossRef]
127. Tieu, A.; Lalu, M.M.; Slobodian, M.; Gnyra, C.; Fergusson, D.A.; Montroy, J.; Burger, D.; Stewart, D.J.; Allan, D.S. An Analysis of Mesenchymal Stem Cell-Derived Extracellular Vesicles for Preclinical Use. *ACS Nano* **2020**, *14*, 9728–9743. [CrossRef]
128. Chen, S.; Sun, F.; Qian, H.; Xu, W.; Jiang, J. Preconditioning and Engineering Strategies for Improving the Efficacy of Mesenchymal Stem Cell-Derived Exosomes in Cell-Free Therapy. *Stem Cells Int.* **2022**, *2022*, 1779346. [CrossRef]
129. Han, M.; Yang, H.; Lu, X.; Li, Y.; Liu, Z.; Li, F.; Shang, Z.; Wang, X.; Li, X.; Li, J.; et al. Three-Dimensional-Cultured MSC-Derived Exosome-Hydrogel Hybrid Microneedle Array Patch for Spinal Cord Repair. *Nano Lett.* **2022**, *22*, 6391–6401. [CrossRef]
130. Yang, L.; Zhai, Y.; Hao, Y.; Zhu, Z.; Cheng, G. The Regulatory Functionality of Exosomes Derived from hUMSCs in 3D Culture for Alzheimer's Disease Therapy. *Small* **2020**, *16*, e1906273. [CrossRef]
131. Zhang, Y.; Xu, J.; Liu, S.; Lim, M.; Zhao, S.; Cui, K.; Zhang, K.; Wang, L.; Ji, Q.; Han, Z.; et al. Embryonic stem cell-derived extracellular vesicles enhance the therapeutic effect of mesenchymal stem cells. *Theranostics* **2019**, *9*, 6976–6990. [CrossRef] [PubMed]
132. Perets, N.; Betzer, O.; Shapira, R.; Brenstein, S.; Angel, A.; Sadan, T.; Ashery, U.; Popovtzer, R.; Offen, D. Golden Exosomes Selectively Target Brain Pathologies in Neurodegenerative and Neurodevelopmental Disorders. *Nano Lett.* **2019**, *19*, 3422–3431. [CrossRef] [PubMed]

133. Salomon, C.; Ryan, J.; Sobrevia, L.; Kobayashi, M.; Ashman, K.; Mitchell, M.; Rice, G.E. Exosomal signaling during hypoxia mediates microvascular endothelial cell migration and vasculogenesis. *PLoS ONE* **2013**, *8*, e68451. [CrossRef] [PubMed]
134. Gonzalez-King, H.; Garcia, N.A.; Ontoria-Oviedo, I.; Ciria, M.; Montero, J.A.; Sepulveda, P. Hypoxia Inducible Factor-1alpha Potentiates Jagged 1-Mediated Angiogenesis by Mesenchymal Stem Cell-Derived Exosomes. *Stem Cells* **2017**, *35*, 1747–1759. [CrossRef] [PubMed]
135. Angioni, R.; Liboni, C.; Herkenne, S.; Sanchez-Rodriguez, R.; Borile, G.; Marcuzzi, E.; Cali, B.; Muraca, M.; Viola, A. CD73(+) extracellular vesicles inhibit angiogenesis through adenosine A2B receptor signalling. *J. Extracell. Vesicles* **2020**, *9*, 1757900. [CrossRef]
136. Gorgun, C.; Ceresa, D.; Lesage, R.; Villa, F.; Reverberi, D.; Balbi, C.; Santamaria, S.; Cortese, K.; Malatesta, P.; Geris, L.; et al. Dissecting the effects of preconditioning with inflammatory cytokines and hypoxia on the angiogenic potential of mesenchymal stromal cell (MSC)-derived soluble proteins and extracellular vesicles (EVs). *Biomaterials* **2021**, *269*, 120633. [CrossRef]
137. Fernandez-Santos, M.E.; Garcia-Arranz, M.; Andreu, E.J.; Garcia-Hernandez, A.M.; Lopez-Parra, M.; Villaron, E.; Sepulveda, P.; Fernandez-Aviles, F.; Garcia-Olmo, D.; Prosper, F.; et al. Optimization of Mesenchymal Stromal Cell (MSC) Manufacturing Processes for a Better Therapeutic Outcome. *Front. Immunol.* **2022**, *13*, 918565. [CrossRef]
138. Witwer, K.W.; Van Balkom, B.W.M.; Bruno, S.; Choo, A.; Dominici, M.; Gimona, M.; Hill, A.F.; De Kleijn, D.; Koh, M.; Lai, R.C.; et al. Defining mesenchymal stromal cell (MSC)-derived small extracellular vesicles for therapeutic applications. *J. Extracell. Vesicles* **2019**, *8*, 1609206. [CrossRef]
139. Lai, R.C.; Tan, S.S.; Yeo, R.W.; Choo, A.B.; Reiner, A.T.; Su, Y.; Shen, Y.; Fu, Z.; Alexander, L.; Sze, S.K.; et al. MSC secretes at least 3 EV types each with a unique permutation of membrane lipid, protein and RNA. *J. Extracell. Vesicles* **2016**, *5*, 29828. [CrossRef]
140. Zhang, Q.; Jeppesen, D.K.; Higginbotham, J.N.; Graves-Deal, R.; Trinh, V.Q.; Ramirez, M.A.; Sohn, Y.; Neininger, A.C.; Taneja, N.; McKinley, E.T.; et al. Supermeres are functional extracellular nanoparticles replete with disease biomarkers and therapeutic targets. *Nat. Cell Biol.* **2021**, *23*, 1240–1254. [CrossRef]
141. Zhang, H.; Freitas, D.; Kim, H.S.; Fabijanic, K.; Li, Z.; Chen, H.; Mark, M.T.; Molina, H.; Martin, A.B.; Bojmar, L.; et al. Identification of distinct nanoparticles and subsets of extracellular vesicles by asymmetric flow field-flow fractionation. *Nat. Cell Biol.* **2018**, *20*, 332–343. [CrossRef] [PubMed]
142. Lasser, C.; Jang, S.C.; Lotvall, J. Subpopulations of extracellular vesicles and their therapeutic potential. *Mol. Asp. Med.* **2018**, *60*, 1–14. [CrossRef] [PubMed]
143. Mendt, M.; Kamerkar, S.; Sugimoto, H.; McAndrews, K.M.; Wu, C.C.; Gagea, M.; Yang, S.; Blanko, E.V.R.; Peng, Q.; Ma, X.; et al. Generation and testing of clinical-grade exosomes for pancreatic cancer. *JCI Insight* **2018**, *3*, e99263. [CrossRef]
144. Iannotta, D.; Yang, M.; Celia, C.; Di Marzio, L.; Wolfram, J. Extracellular vesicle therapeutics from plasma and adipose tissue. *Nano Today* **2021**, *39*, 101159. [CrossRef] [PubMed]
145. Kojima, R.; Bojar, D.; Rizzi, G.; Hamri, G.C.; El-Baba, M.D.; Saxena, P.; Auslander, S.; Tan, K.R.; Fussenegger, M. Designer exosomes produced by implanted cells intracerebrally deliver therapeutic cargo for Parkinson's disease treatment. *Nat. Commun.* **2018**, *9*, 1305. [CrossRef] [PubMed]
146. Grangier, A.; Branchu, J.; Volatron, J.; Piffoux, M.; Gazeau, F.; Wilhelm, C.; Silva, A.K.A. Technological advances towards extracellular vesicles mass production. *Adv. Drug Deliv. Rev.* **2021**, *176*, 113843. [CrossRef] [PubMed]
147. Gandham, S.; Su, X.; Wood, J.; Nocera, A.L.; Alli, S.C.; Milane, L.; Zimmerman, A.; Amiji, M.; Ivanov, A.R. Technologies and Standardization in Research on Extracellular Vesicles. *Trends Biotechnol.* **2020**, *38*, 1066–1098. [CrossRef]
148. Herrmann, I.K.; Wood, M.J.A.; Fuhrmann, G. Extracellular vesicles as a next-generation drug delivery platform. *Nat. Nanotechnol.* **2021**, *16*, 748–759. [CrossRef]
149. Kimiz-Gebologlu, I.; Oncel, S.S. Exosomes: Large-scale production, isolation, drug loading efficiency, and biodistribution and uptake. *J. Control. Release* **2022**, *347*, 533–543. [CrossRef]
150. Yang, D.; Zhang, W.; Zhang, H.; Zhang, F.; Chen, L.; Ma, L.; Larcher, L.M.; Chen, S.; Liu, N.; Zhao, Q.; et al. Progress, opportunity, and perspective on exosome isolation—Efforts for efficient exosome-based theranostics. *Theranostics* **2020**, *10*, 3684–3707. [CrossRef]
151. Colao, I.L.; Corteling, R.; Bracewell, D.; Wall, I. Manufacturing Exosomes: A Promising Therapeutic Platform. *Trends Mol. Med.* **2018**, *24*, 242–256. [CrossRef] [PubMed]
152. Garcia-Manrique, P.; Gutierrez, G.; Blanco-Lopez, M.C. Fully Artificial Exosomes: Towards New Theranostic Biomaterials. *Trends Biotechnol.* **2018**, *36*, 10–14. [CrossRef] [PubMed]
153. Piffoux, M.; Silva, A.K.A.; Wilhelm, C.; Gazeau, F.; Tareste, D. Modification of Extracellular Vesicles by Fusion with Liposomes for the Design of Personalized Biogenic Drug Delivery Systems. *ACS Nano* **2018**, *12*, 6830–6842. [CrossRef] [PubMed]
154. Fan, Z.; Jiang, C.; Wang, Y.; Wang, K.; Marsh, J.; Zhang, D.; Chen, X.; Nie, L. Engineered extracellular vesicles as intelligent nanosystems for next-generation nanomedicine. *Nanoscale Horiz* **2022**, *7*, 682–714. [CrossRef] [PubMed]

pharmaceutics

MDPI

Review

Small Extracellular Vesicles' miRNAs: Biomarkers and Therapeutics for Neurodegenerative Diseases

Wei Qing Lim [1], Kie Hoon Michelle Luk [1], Kah Yee Lee [1], Nasuha Nurul [1], Sin Jade Loh [1], Zhen Xiong Yeow [1], Qi Xuan Wong [1], Qi Hao Daniel Looi [2,*], Pan Pan Chong [3], Chee Wun How [4], Sharina Hamzah [1,5] and Jhi Biau Foo [1,5,*]

1 School of Pharmacy, Faculty of Health and Medical Sciences, Taylor's University, Subang Jaya 47500, Selangor, Malaysia; sharina.hamzah@taylors.edu.my (S.H.)
2 My CytoHealth Sdn. Bhd., Lab 6, DMC Level 2, Hive 5, Taman Teknologi MRANTI, Bukit Jalil, Kuala Lumpur 57000, Malaysia
3 National Orthopaedic Centre of Excellence for Research and Learning (NOCERAL), Department of Orthopaedic Surgery, Faculty of Medicine, Universiti Malaya, Kuala Lumpur 50603, Malaysia; panpanchong@um.edu.my
4 School of Pharmacy, Monash University Malaysia, Bandar Sunway, Subang Jaya 47500, Selangor, Malaysia; how.cheewun@monash.edu
5 Medical Advancement for Better Quality of Life Impact Lab, Taylor's University, Subang Jaya 47500, Selangor, Malaysia
* Correspondence: dr.daniellooi@cytoholdings.com (Q.H.D.L.); jhibiau.foo@taylors.edu.my (J.B.F.)

Abstract: Neurodegenerative diseases are critical in the healthcare system as patients suffer from progressive diseases despite currently available drug management. Indeed, the growing ageing population will burden the country's healthcare system and the caretakers. Thus, there is a need for new management that could stop or reverse the progression of neurodegenerative diseases. Stem cells possess a remarkable regenerative potential that has long been investigated to resolve these issues. Some breakthroughs have been achieved thus far to replace the damaged brain cells; however, the procedure's invasiveness has prompted scientists to investigate using stem-cell small extracellular vesicles (sEVs) as a non-invasive cell-free therapy to address the limitations of cell therapy. With the advancement of technology to understand the molecular changes of neurodegenerative diseases, efforts have been made to enrich stem cells' sEVs with miRNAs to increase the therapeutic efficacy of the sEVs. In this article, the pathophysiology of various neurodegenerative diseases is highlighted. The role of miRNAs from sEVs as biomarkers and treatments is also discussed. Lastly, the applications and delivery of stem cells and their miRNA-enriched sEVs for treating neurodegenerative diseases are emphasised and reviewed.

Keywords: extracellular vesicles; exosomes; miRNAs; neurodegeneration; stem cells

Citation: Lim, W.Q.; Michelle Luk, K.H.; Lee, K.Y.; Nurul, N.; Loh, S.J.; Yeow, Z.X.; Wong, Q.X.; Daniel Looi, Q.H.; Chong, P.P.; How, C.W.; et al. Small Extracellular Vesicles' miRNAs: Biomarkers and Therapeutics for Neurodegenerative Diseases. *Pharmaceutics* **2023**, *15*, 1216. https://doi.org/10.3390/pharmaceutics15041216

Academic Editor: Hugo Agostinho Machado Fernandes

Received: 20 January 2023
Revised: 10 March 2023
Accepted: 16 March 2023
Published: 11 April 2023

1. Introduction

Neurodegeneration refers to the death of neurons in the central nervous system (CNS) and peripheral nervous system (PNS). When CNS is affected, neurodegeneration causes Alzheimer's disease (AD), Parkinson's disease (PD), Huntington's disease (HD), and others [1]. Around 50 million people worldwide have dementia, which is predicted to increase rapidly to 130 million people in the next 30 years. Most of these dementia cases are caused by AD. Neurodegenerative diseases will eventually lead to disability, institutionalisation, and mortality that requires high treatment costs of up to USD 1 trillion worldwide [2].

All neurodegenerative diseases are associated with functional neuron loss—progressive and irreversible. When neuronal structures deteriorate, there will be a gradual loss of cognitive skills (dementia) and motor skills (ataxia), leading to mental impairment and debilitation [3]. Some common mechanisms involved in all neurodegenerative diseases are oxidative stress, inflammatory responses, and the aggregation of abnormal misfolded proteins in selectively vulnerable neuron populations. Neurodegenerative diseases are challenging to treat because the damaged or dead neuron cells are naturally irreplaceable [3].

Neurodegenerative diseases cannot be completely cured, and the available treatments only help to alleviate pain, control symptoms, and enhance patients' ability to move their limbs (Table 1) [4]. Various preclinical and clinical studies conducted 40 years ago revealed that cell therapy is the only rational and feasible strategy to regenerate neural tissues, mainly using stem cells. However, stem cell therapy has disadvantages as its therapeutic molecules cannot pass through the blood-brain barrier (BBB) effectively and are detrimental to patient safety [4]. Mesenchymal stem cells (MSCs) are adult multipotent progenitor cells that can renew themselves and undergo differentiation into various mesodermal cell lineages, including bone, cartilage, and adipose tissues. However, MSCs have several other disadvantages in clinical settings, which include a greater risk of transmitting infections and their potential to differentiate decreasing in long-term culture [5].

Table 1. Currently available drugs for neurodegenerative diseases.

Disease and Therapeutic Strategies	Drug Classification	Drug Example	Reference
Parkinson's Disease Maintain CNS dopamine levels or signalling	Dopamine	Levodopa, carbidopa	[6]
	Monoamine oxidase inhibitor (type B)	Selegiline, rasagiline, safinamide	
	Catechol-O-methyltransferase inhibitors	Entacapone, Tolcapone	
	Dopamine receptor agonists	Ergot: bromocriptine Non-ergot: Ropinirole, pramipexole, rotigotine, apomorphine	[7]
	Antiviral	Amantadine	[6]
	Antimuscarinic agents	Benztropine, trihexyphenidyl	
Alzheimer's Disease Improve cholinergic transmission within the CNS or prevent NMDA-glutamate receptor-mediated excitotoxicity	Acetylcholinesterase inhibitors	Donepezil, rivastigmine, galantamine	
	NMDA receptor antagonist	Memantine	
	Cognitive enhancers	Pyritinol, dihydroergotoxine, piribedil, citicholine, gingko biloba	[8]
	Amyloid beta-directed antibody	Aducanumab Lecanemab	[9]
Amyotrophic Lateral Sclerosis Improve survival time, slow progression of the disease	NMDA receptor antagonist	Riluzole	[6]
	Antioxidant	Edaravone	
Huntington's Disease Symptomatic treatment to improve motor function and quality of life and suppress chorea. Does not delay the progression of the disease	Dopamine-depleting agent	Tetrabenazine	
	Dopamine antagonist	Haloperidol Olanzapine Aripiprazole	[10]
	Benzodiazepine	Clonazepam	[7]
	NMDA antagonist	Amantadine Riluzole	[6]

Furthermore, after injecting MSCs into the body intravenously, MSCs undergo a pulmonary first-pass effect leading to the accumulation of 50% to 80% of MSCs in the lungs due to MSC's huge molecular size of 20 μm to 30 μm diameter, which is larger than circulating immune cells and lung capillaries [11]. Besides this "lung-trapping" effect, for all delivery routes such as intravenous, intratracheal, intraperitoneal, and intranasal, MSCs could only survive less than 24 h in the respiratory tract, making it difficult for

MSCs to be delivered to other organs. For instance, the effectiveness of using MSCs to treat neurodegenerative diseases is much restricted as less than 1% of MSCs are detected in the brain following administration [12].

Due to the limitations of MSC treatment, various clinical studies are being conducted based on small extracellular vesicles (sEVs) extracted from MSCs and enriched with miRNAs to treat neurodegenerative diseases more safely and effectively [13]. Studies have found that after systemic transplantation, MSCs are quickly excreted from the body but their pharmaceutical effects are usually maintained. This indicates that the molecules responsible for the therapeutic effect are secretomes of MSCs, especially sEVs. Indeed, in order to deliver therapeutic molecules to the brain more efficiently by crossing the BBB, sEVs are used as an alternative strategy to treat neurodegenerative diseases owing to their tiny molecular size of 30 nm to 100 nm [14].

Due to their ability to mediate intercellular communication, MSCs' sEVs may affect the target cells by interacting with their receptors or by delivering biologically active cargo molecules such as proteins, mRNA, and microRNAs (miRNAs). Intercellular communication occurs when the target cells receive or engulf sEVs via endocytosis or phagocytosis [15]. Non-coding RNAs with 17–21 nucleotides called miRNAs are among the most significant sEVs' cargoes. Canonically, a base pairing of nucleotides 2–7 of miRNAs (the seed) to mRNA 3′ untranslated regions (UTRs) prevents the translation of mRNAs [15]. Various studies have reported that MSCs' sEVs show a promising therapeutic potential for neurodegenerative diseases [16]. MSC-sEVs can prevent the apoptosis and inflammation caused by microglial cells and demyelination and suppress oxidative stress [17]. Hence, the functional deterioration of neurons can be prevented. Additionally, MSC-sEVs play a vital role in the regeneration of neurons via four mechanisms of action: neuroprotection, neurogenesis, neuromodulation, and angiogenesis [18]. Evidence shows that MSC-sEVs can preserve myelin sheaths and synapses [19]. In this article, the pathophysiology of various neurodegenerative diseases is reviewed. The role of miRNAs from sEVs as biomarkers and treatments is also discussed. Lastly, the applications and delivery of stem cells and their miRNA-enriched sEVs for treating neurodegenerative diseases are emphasised and reviewed.

2. Pathophysiology of Neurodegenerative Diseases

2.1. Alzheimer's Disease

Alzheimer's disease (AD) was first discovered in 1906 by the German psychiatrist Alois Alzheimer and is now hailed as one of the leading causes of dementia globally [20]. Patients with dementia experience progressive deterioration in performing mental and motor tasks. They often begin to display worrying emotional responses, which can take a toll on their caregivers in the long run. Post-mortems of patients' brains reveal an accumulation of Aβ plaques in the extracellular region and neurofibrillary tangles (NFTs) that originate due to hyperphosphorylated microtubule-associated τ intracellularly. β-secretases (BACE1) and γ-secretases cleave the amyloid precursor protein (APP) to produce insoluble Aβ fibrils [21], which then oligomerise and diffuse into synaptic clefts to disrupt synaptic signalling. Consequently, polymerisation into insoluble amyloid fibrils leads to aggregation into plaques. The polymerisation process activates protein kinases such as GSK3β and CDK5, which promote the hyperphosphorylation of the τ protein [22]. The τ proteins then oligomerise, contributing to the dissociation of microtubule subunits. The microtubules fall apart and accumulate into τ filaments, which further aggregate into insoluble NFTs [23]. This negatively affects cell-to-cell communication and signal processing, leading to neuron cell death and increased reactive oxidative stress [24].

Furthermore, this triggers the infiltration of microglia, which act as phagocytes and are vital in neuronal plasticity and synapse remodelling [25]. Aβ plaques activate receptors such as CD36, SCARA1, $\alpha_6\beta_1$ integrin, CD14, toll-like receptors, and CD47 on the microglia, leading to the activation and induction of microglia neuroinflammation through the release of pro-inflammatory cytokines and chemokines [26]. Microglia induce the endocytosis of Aβ oligomers and NFT fibrils through neprilysin and insulin-degrading enzymes through this cascade. However, AD can be exacerbated due to an excessive or insufficient inflammatory response [27]. The triggering receptor expressed on myeloid cells 2 mutation or glial cell activation prolongs the neuroinflammation process and leads to reactive oxygen species' overexpression that further damages neuronal cells. Eventually, the clearance of waste proteins is impaired [28].

2.2. Parkinson's Disease

Parkinson's disease (PD) is the second most common neurodegenerative disease globally. It is characterised by tremor, rigidity, and bradykinesia with late-stage postural instability. Although PD is not fatal, patients suffer a drastic decrease in quality of life as retardation in mobility progresses [29]. They tend to experience falls more frequently and develop aspiration pneumonia contributing to life-threatening infections. Despite being a prevalent disease, the cause of the disease is largely unknown, with some speculating that smoking, pesticide exposure, and familial history are associated risk factors [30].

Chiefly, the pathological presentation of PD begins in the substantia nigra, where declining dopaminergic neurons are observed. This is accompanied by a severe deficiency of dopamine concentration in the striatum. α-synuclein is found naturally in the brain and presents as a tertiary protein in unfolded form. It can be folded into α-helical structures at the N-terminus upon interaction with phospholipids [31]. Pathological development arises when α-synuclein is folded into a β-sheet-rich amyloid-like structure, possibly due to serine 129 phosphorylation, ubiquitination, and C-terminal truncation resulting in misfolding and aggregation [32]. Such misfolded proteins can present as unfolded monomers, soluble oligomers, protofibrils, and insoluble fibrils [33]. Among the four types, the oligomers present the largest threat due to their capability of "seeding" and accelerating α-synuclein accumulation. Researchers also note that α-synuclein interacts with the TOM20 receptor on the mitochondrial membrane, leading to the damage of complex-I, a vital component of the electron transport chain [34]. This results in mitochondrial dysfunction through impaired mitochondrial protein import machinery, reduced respiration, and excessive production of reactive oxygen species [35]. This theory is further supported by a deficiency of mitochondrial complex-I in patients' brains, skeletal muscles, and platelets. Furthermore, the exposure of individuals to neurotoxins such as MPTP, rotenone, and paraquat resulted in the inhibition of the same complex. Lastly, the PINK1 and parkin genes commonly found in hereditary PD patients have also been found to regulate the removal of dysfunctional mitochondria (Figure 1) [36].

Apart from that, dysfunctional protein clearance systems (the ubiquitin-proteasome system and autophagy-lysosome system) also play a significant role in the pathophysiology of PD. Typically, the ubiquitin-proteasome system (UPS) breaks down soluble misfolded α-synuclein through ubiquitin tagging and transportation to the proteasome for degradation. In contrast, the activity of UPS and proteasome component levels (PA700 and PA28 found in the 20S proteasome α-subunit) are reduced in the brain and peripheral blood mononuclear cells in PD patients [37]. The parkin and UCH-L1 genes in diseased patients have also been determined to regulate the ubiquitin-encoding E3 ubiquitin ligase and ubiquitin C-terminal hydrolase [38]. The autophagy-lysosome system removes abnormal proteins through macroautophagy, microautophagy, and chaperone-mediated autophagy. In PD patients, although the autophagosome marker LC3-II was found to be increased, the vital proteins of lysosomal membranes (LAMP1 and LAMP2A) and several molecular chaperones from the heat-shock protein family (hsc70 and hsp35) were decreased [39]. Again, the parkin and PINK1 genes were also found to regulate the autophagic turnover of mitochondria, confirming that altered protein clearance systems play a role in the development of the disease. Gradually, the accumulation of α-synuclein directly triggers microglial activation (similar to AD) and initiates inflammatory processes [40]. This is confirmed through post-mortem studies demonstrating evidence of microglial and complement activation, T-lymphocyte infiltration, and increased concentrations of pro-inflammatory cytokines [41].

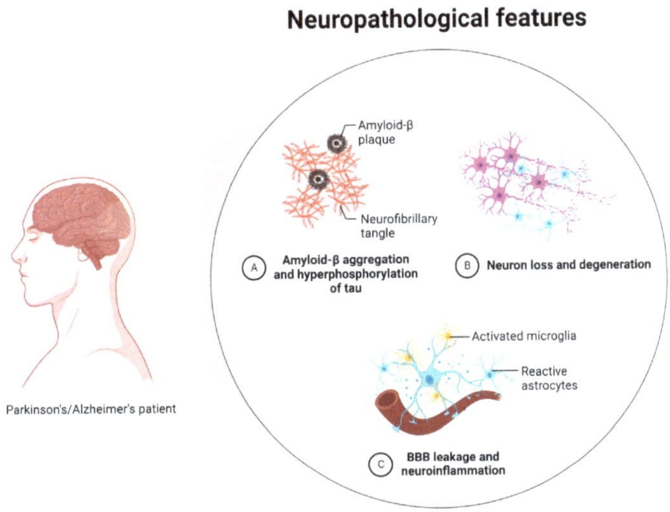

Figure 1. Pathophysiology of Alzheimer's and Parkinson's disease. Generally, the formation of amyloid-β plaques and neurofibrillary tangles results in neuron loss and degeneration. This triggers an uncontrolled immune response resulting in BBB leakage and neuroinflammation (created with BioRender.com) (accessed on 3 January 2023).

2.3. Huntington's Disease

Huntington's disease (HD) is a rare autosomal dominant condition with a prevalence of 0.4/100,000 in Asia and 5.70/100,000 in the Western population. It is characterised by progressive movement disorder and cognitive decline. Patients experience motor defects such as chorea (resulting in involuntary muscle movement) and loss of coordination. Obsessive-compulsive disorder, depression, and psychosis are also common among sufferers. The disease is currently incurable, and patients often succumb to the disease roughly 20 years after disease onset [42].

The consensus among researchers infers that the abnormal expansion of CAG repeats in the HTT gene encoding huntingtin causes HD. The protein contains a polyglutamine tract encoded by uninterrupted CAG trinucleotide repeats in the first exon of HTT. Healthy individuals possess the wild-type allele that contains up to 35 CAG repeats, while the pathogenic allele carries expansions of 36 or more repetitions [43]. Huntingtin has been revealed to be crucial in neurogenesis, synapse connectivity, and neuron cell survival by acting as a protein scaffold and transcriptional regulator. Therefore, a diseased state results in general brain shrinkage, degeneration of the striatum, and the loss of efferent medium spiny neurons [44].

As with other neurodegenerative diseases, HD is characterised by the presence of aggregates in the brain. The long CAG repeats may be cleaved by caspases and calpains to form toxic N-terminal fragments, which subsequently form β-sheets when held together by hydrogen bonds, ultimately assuming an amyloid structure. Gradually, the aggregates may sequester ubiquitin, proteasome subunits, chaperones, transcriptional factors, or wild-type alleles which induce neurotoxic effects, leading to an impairment in the ubiquitin-proteasome system. Indeed, the aggregates show abnormal axonal transport of the autophagosome-lysosome system, contributing to inefficient autophagosome-lysosome fusion and decreased degradation of the aggregates [45].

Moreover, scientists have discovered transcriptional disruption in HD patients. Mutant huntingtin has been shown to interact with regulators of transcription such as p53, cAMP response element-binding (CREB) protein, and CREB-binding protein (CBP), which are essential for cell growth and survival [46]. Furthermore, mutant huntingtin also interacts with several other molecules and affects their underlying molecular mechanisms, for instance: PGC-1α (peroxisome proliferator-activating receptor-γ coactivator-1 α), which is required for energy metabolism; Sp1 and its coactivator TAFII130, which affect the transcription of genes such as the D2 dopamine receptor; cystathionine γ-lyase, the biosynthetic enzyme for cysteine; and lastly, BDNF, a pro-survival factor that enhances the survival of striatal neurons [44]. Many also believe that huntingtin disrupts the epigenetic landscape through deregulation of histone modification by binding to histone acetyltransferase domain in CBPs to disrupt histone acetylation, induce chromatin structural modifications in downregulated genes, and change the DNA methylation of several altered genes [47]. Finally, miRNA deregulation has been shown to exacerbate HD, as cleaved CAG RNAs silence specific genes. Notably, the cleaved RNAs are potentially neurotoxic through Ago-2-mediated gene silencing of CTG-containing genes [48].

A combination of aggregates and gene silencing ultimately leads to neuronal and synaptic abnormalities. The aggregates delay axonal transport due to Huntington-associated-protein-1 disruptions, resulting in a failed delivery of GABA(A), which inhibits synaptic excitability and leads to neuronal cell death (Figure 2). The disruption in the trafficking of NMDA receptors in striatal neurons may cause an imbalance between synaptic and extrasynaptic NMDA receptors. Consequently, excitotoxicity happens either due to increased glutamate or impaired uptake and clearance [49]. Ultimately, this leads to defects in ATP production, Ca^{2+} buffering capacity, and mitochondrial apoptosis. Overexpression of the myeloid lineage-determining factors PU.1 and CCAAT/enhancer-binding proteins results in a pro-inflammatory cascade contributing to neuroinflammation. The inhibition of NF-κB signalling in the peripheral immune system also increases peripheral inflammatory responses [50].

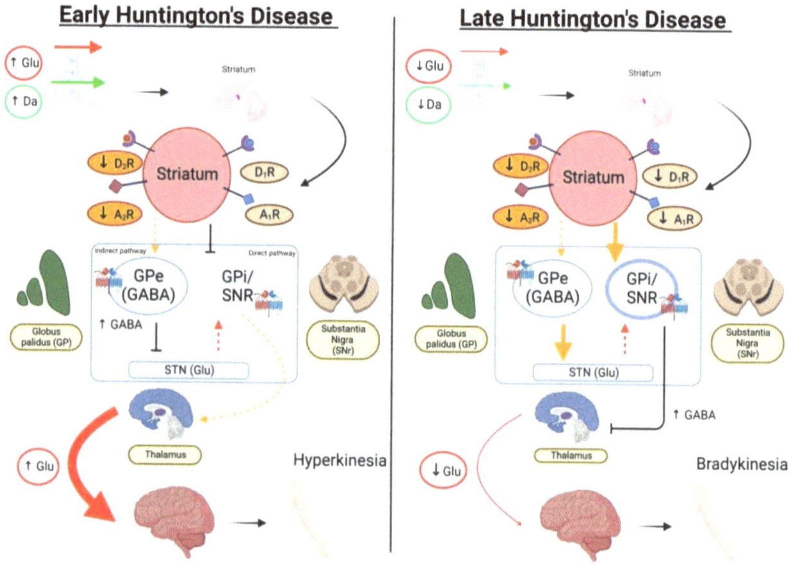

Figure 2. Pathophysiology of Huntington's disease. In the early stage, the aggregates delay axonal transport, resulting in a failed delivery of GABA(A), which inhibits the synaptic excitability of the subthalamic nucleus. As a result, the compensatory mechanism of the thalamus leads to hyperkinesia. In the late stage, the trafficking of NMDA receptors in striatal neurons is affected and may cause an imbalance between synaptic and extrasynaptic NMDA receptors. This leads to excitotoxicity either due to increased glutamate or impaired uptake and clearance. Ultimately, bradykinesia is observed (created with BioRender.com) (accessed on 5 January 2023).

2.4. Amyotrophic Lateral Sclerosis

Amyotrophic lateral sclerosis (ALS) is an agonising and rapidly progressive neurodegenerative disease characterised by motor neuron degeneration and progressive muscle weakness. Most patients receive their initial diagnosis between the ages of 40–70 and will succumb to respiratory failure within 3–5 years. Currently, researchers are unsure of the exact mechanism contributing to ALS; hence, therapeutic options remain limited. Three theories have been proposed concerning ALS pathogenesis: the dying forward hypothesis, the dying back hypothesis, and the independent hypothesis (Figure 3) [51]. In the dying forward hypothesis, it is theorised that ALS results in anterograde corticomotor neuron degeneration. Dysfunctional astrocytic excitatory amino acid transporter 2 is implicated in reduced glutamate uptake at the synaptic cleft. Ultimately, degradation of the anterior horn cells ensues due to excitotoxicity. In the dying back hypothesis, ALS begins within the neurofilaments. Mutations in the TDP-43, c9orf72, and fused in sarcoma (FUS) genes result in disruptive RNA metabolism, abnormalities of gene translation, and eventually, the formation of intracellular neuronal aggregates [52]. Aside from that, disruption of the neurofilament-L (NF-L) gene in SOD1 also increases oxidative stress and mitochondrial dysfunction, forming aberrant perikaryal and axonal aggregates of neurofilaments [53]. Neurofilament-dependent slowing of slow axonal transport mediates damage to the cargoes and deprives axons of essential nutrients. Ultimately, this leads to motor axon degeneration. The independent degeneration hypothesis argues that upper and lower motor neuron degeneration occurs independently. Separately, it is found that microglia-induced neuroinflammation is noted in ALS patients [54].

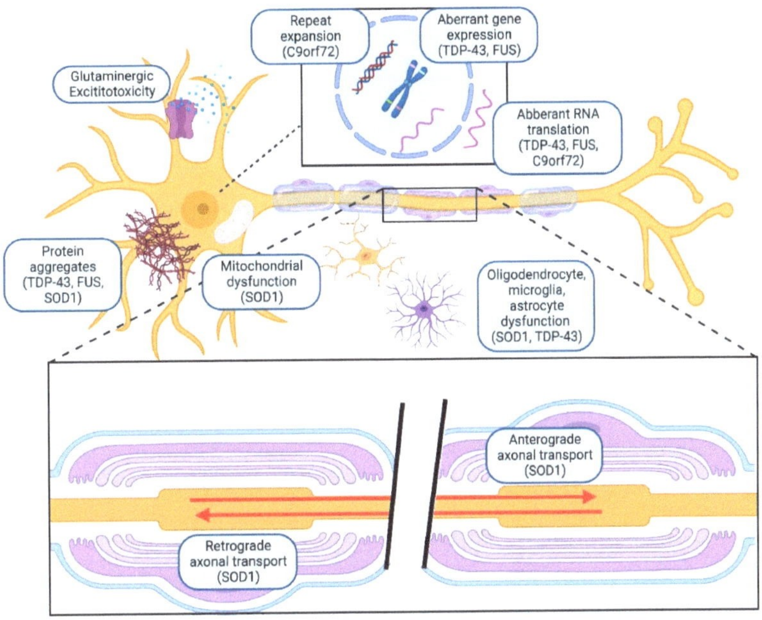

Figure 3. Pathophysiology of amyotrophic lateral sclerosis. The dying forward hypothesis states that ALS results in anterograde corticomotor neuron degeneration. In the dying back hypothesis, mutations in the TDP-43, c9orf72, and FUS genes form intracellular neuronal aggregates. The independent degeneration hypothesis argues that upper and lower motor neuron degeneration occurs independently (created with BioRender.com) (accessed on 8 January 2023).

3. Applications of Small Extracellular Vesicles' miRNAs

Numerous published papers have highlighted the cargo of sEVs, including proteins, RNA, DNA, lipids, etc. [55]. Among all these cargoes, sEVs' miRNAs have gained the spotlight in the last decade for both disease identification and treatment. It has been shown that sEVs synthesized and released by brain nerve cells can cross the BBB and present in blood and peripheral fluids [56]. Hence, temporal changes in the expression of sEVs' miRNAs during the progression of neurodegenerative diseases can be identified, which enhances their ability to act as diagnostic tools [57]. In terms of treatment, MSCs' sEVs-miRNAs have been widely reported to improve the pathophysiology of neurodegenerative diseases in preclinical studies. Although challenges are faced in the isolation of sEVs, consistent characterisation methods and techniques to increase genomic and proteomic yield are being rapidly improved to improve their usability in clinical practice [58].

3.1. Disease Biomarkers

sEVs' miRNAs are gaining traction from multiple researchers as a reliable biomarker for neurodegenerative diseases. Over 2000 types of miRNAs have been identified that influence the gene regulation of essential biological pathways such as neurogenesis and neuronal growth, cell communication, and cell death [55]. The brain is highly enriched in miR-7, miR-9, miR-23, miR-125 a-b, miR-128, miR-137, miR-132, and miR-139. There are also various brain specific miRNAs such as miR-101, miR-191, let-7 g, miR-134, miR-181a-b, miR-135, miR-107, miR-let-7c, let-7a, miR-29a, and miR-124 [59]. Due to their capacity for intercellular communication, distant cells can pick up sEVs' miRNAs that reflect the current functional status of the cell and alterations that contribute to disease pathogenesis and progression. Such alterations occur long before symptoms bud and an official diagnosis is determined, making them a valuable diagnostic tool for diseases [60]. Moreover, they can differentiate between diseases with similar symptoms, such as AD and PD, further branching into the identification of subtypes of the diseases [61]. To illustrate, a comparison of miRNA-135a, miRNA- 193b, and miRNA-384 levels in serum-derived sEVs from individuals with AD, PD, and vascular dementia can be made by observing the area under the curve from ROC curve analysis, qRT-PCR analysis, or miRNA PCR array analysis. Lastly, novel technology such as next-generation deep sequencing enables the identification of sEVs' miRNAs free of contaminant RNA from blood samples, accelerating the possibility of using sEVs' miRNAs as biomarkers. SEVs isolated from the biological fluid are protected from degradation, allowing for the easy identification of miRNAs [62].

3.2. Delivery System

As sEVs can carry diverse cargo, multiple miRNAs can be shuffled into a single preparation to treat patients with chronic medical conditions requiring multiple medications. Hence, patient compliance might be improved. Moreover, the risks associated with polypharmacy can be reduced drastically. Nowadays, scientists have successfully formulated intranasal dosage forms that allow penetration of sEVs' miRNAs across the BBB, indicating that sEVs' miRNAs could be available over the counter for patients [63]. To know more about the current status of the sEVs delivery system that can be used for neurodegenerative diseases, it is recommended to read our previous publication in which the intravenous delivery system has been critically reviewed [64]. The possible routes of administration are also critically reviewed in the later section.

3.3. Disease Treatment

miRNAs possess both pathogenetic and protective effects towards neurodegenerative diseases. Hence, sEVs' miRNAs present a possibility for use as treatments for disease. Selective modification of the sEVs' cargo or the biological production of protective sEVs' miRNAs can activate target site receptors directly. The crossover of sEVs' miRNAs through endocytosis enables them to deliver therapeutic miRNAs to intracellular components such as the cytoplasm and nucleus. Finally, modification of the sEVs with cell surface proteins allows for specific brain targeting (Figure 4) [65].

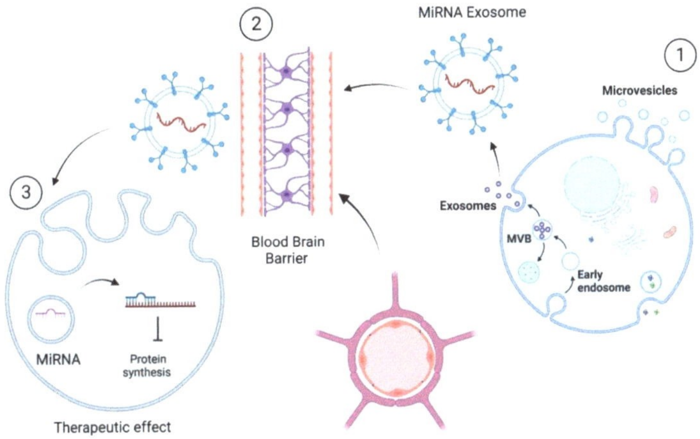

Figure 4. The ability of sEVs' miRNAs to cross the blood-brain barrier presents an opportunity to correct endogenous miRNAs' levels through miRNAs/anti-miRNAs treatment (created with BioRender.com) (accessed on 13 January 2023).

MSC-sEVs have been found to promote cell proliferation by transferring miR-17-92 clusters to the distal axons of cortical neurons. sEVs enriched with miR-124 from human CSF were able to promote neurogenesis in neural stem cells [66]. Yang et al., injected 12 μg (about 500 miRNAs per sEV) into stroke-induced mice weighing 22–25 g, in which the team observed neurogenesis [67]. Lastly, miR-132 can maintain the integrity of the BBB, postulating its significance in neurovascular communication and homeostatic functions. This is demonstrated by injecting 0.8 nmol miR-132 in 4 μL phosphate buffer solution into C57BL/6 mice weighing 20–25 g [68].

In patients experiencing a stroke, the transfer of miR-133b and miR-17-92 clusters through MSC-sEVs promoted plasticity and functional recovery. miR-133b inhibits the connective tissue growth factor and helps to encourage axonal growth by reducing microglial scarring. It also acts on the RhoA protein to promote spinal cord recovery. This effect was demonstrated by Yu et al., (2011), who injected 100 ng/μL of green fluorescent and red fluorescent protein–mRNAs solution containing 10 μM of miR-133b into adult zebrafish (approximately 2.5 cm) [69]. Furthermore, miR-17-92 inhibits PTEN gene expression in neurons, activating the PI3K/Akt/mTOR pathway. This was demonstrated by Xin et al., by injecting 100 μg/0.5 mL of phosphate buffer solution containing sEVs–miR17-92 into mice weighing 270–300 g [70]. Simultaneously, NMDA receptor activity was shown to be downregulated, while GABAA receptor activity is upregulated. This ultimately promoted axonal growth and accelerated nerve repair accompanied by reduced excitotoxicity [71].

Aside from that, Ma et al., showed that miR-181a targets Kruppel-like factor 6 and increases the permeability of the blood–tumour barrier, which allows enhanced delivery of therapeutics to treat gliomas [72]. Unsurprisingly, a downregulated level of miR-181a was observed in 80 tissue samples from glioblastoma patients [72]. Yu et al., found that sEVs–miRNA-199a inhibits glioma progression by downregulating ArfGAP with the GTPase domain, ankyrin repeat, and PH domain 2 [73]. The team also demonstrated that human MSCs transfected with miR-199a are able to inhibit tumour growth through the delivery of sEVs [73]. Interestingly, in vivo studies showed that miRNA-199a increased the chemosensitivity of glioma cells to temozolomide by inhibiting the K-RAS signalling pathway [74].

Lastly, Wang et al., transfected 10 μL of miR-146a onto dorsal root ganglia neurons of diabetic mice to prove that downregulation of miR-146a induced cell apoptosis through activation of IRAK1, TRAF6, and caspase-3 [75]. Elevations in IRAK1 and TRAF6 are known to impair wound healing and induce peripheral neuropathy in patients with type two diabetes. Therefore, the study concluded that maintenance of miR-146a levels achieves possible therapeutic effects in diabetic patients [76].

4. Small Extracellular Vesicles' miRNAs for Neurodegenerative Diseases

4.1. Small Extracellular Vesicles' miRNAs

sEVs' miRNAs, particularly those involved in neurodegenerative illnesses, are definitively being shown to play a critical role in disease progression. Three main mechanisms explain how miRNAs contribute to neurodegenerative diseases: targeting regulatory-related gene mRNA for protein translation inhibition or protein degradation, taking part in neuroinflammation by directly interacting with a toll-like receptor or controlling its mRNA expression, and producing distortion in miRNAs' formation [77]. In various neurodegenerative diseases, the expression of miRNA changes, and some of these changes have been linked to disease progression.

In addition, when the donor cells release the sEVs, miRNAs will be transmitted to the targeted cells via three distinct methods: fusion with the plasma membrane, endocytosis into the cytoplasm, and exhibiting receptor–ligand interactions for binding to target cells (Figure 5) [78]. Additionally, it has been discovered that neurons can indirectly control astrocyte protein expression by delivering miRNAs to them via sEVs. The above elaboration proposed that neurons might regulate the protein expression of astrocytes while the secretion of sEVs' miRNAs takes place [77]. On the other hand, miRNAs are also involved in the mRNA loading pathway into sEVs. Through a mechanism controlled by miR-1289, certain regions in the 3′ UTR of mRNA with around 25 nucleotides and a CTGCC motif within a stem-loop structure operate as a sorting sequence to sEVs [79,80]. With the aid of Rab5 immuno-localisation, Wnt3 protein enters the cell and carries out its role to modulate the three main Wnt signalling pathways: the β-catenin/GSK3 (glucogen synthase kinase 3) pathway, the planar cell polarity pathway, and the Wnt/Ca^{2+} pathway in the recipient cells [80].

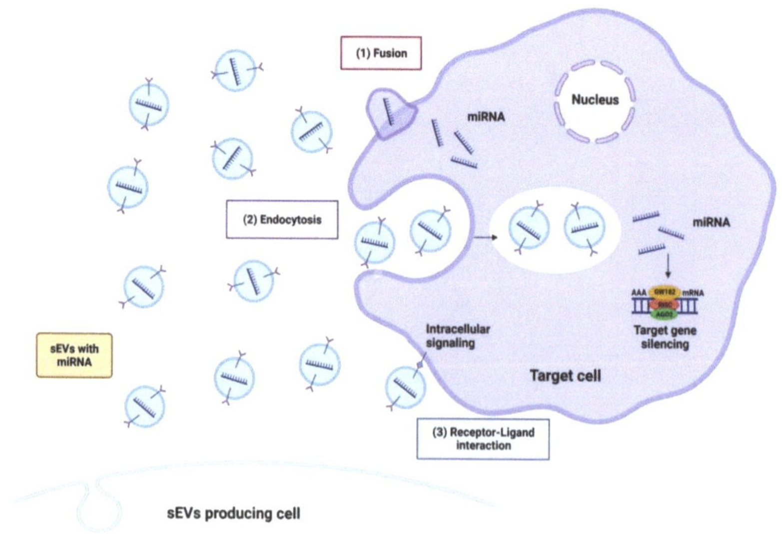

Figure 5. miRNA-enriched sEVs can be transmitted to target cells via three methods which are fusion, endocytosis, and receptor–ligand interactions (created with BioRender.com) (accessed on 13 January 2023).

4.2. Small Extracellular Vesicles' miRNAs and Alzheimer's Disease

Numerous studies have shown that sEVs reduce the signs and symptoms of AD. However, more research into precise molecular pathways is still needed [81]. sEVs made by hypoxia-pretreated MSCs showed enhanced miR-21 expression, suggesting that miR-21 can improve mice's cognitive impairments and prevent the clinical signs of AD [82]. sEVs' capacity to remove beta-amyloid was also revealed by Zhi-You Cai et al., (2018) [83]. Since sEVs–neprilysin may break down beta-amyloid, MSC-sEVs encapsulating small molecule therapies can effectively target beta-amyloid [84]. The inhibition of miR-125b-5p was found to have neuroprotective benefits against oxidative stress, as it decreased reactive oxygen species levels and mitochondrial membrane potential [85]. The result suggested that miR-125b-5p may be a new regulator of AD development and serve as a therapeutic target for AD treatment.

The hypothesis that these vesicles could be a promising source of APP cleavage was raised by the discovery of secretases (γ-, α-, and β-secretases), enzymes implicated in the proteolytic cleavage of APP, in isolated sEVs from an AD animal model. Indeed, it was discovered that APP undergoes cleavage within sEVs and is found in sEVs from human and mouse AD model brains [86]. Moreover, findings from Yuyama et al., (2014) supported the sEVs' mentioned "clearance role" through the decrease in Aβ and Aβ-mediated synaptotoxicity [87]. The neuroprotection effects of MSC-sEVs against Aβ-induced neuronal damage include decreased extracellular Aβ oligomer level, secretion of sEVs containing antioxidant enzymes such as catalase, and paracrine action via the extracellular release of anti-inflammatory cytokines and trophic factors including IL-6, IL-10, and VEGF [88]. Additionally, after being incubated with sEVs, β-amyloid oligomers (Aβo) were restricted to their surface structure by interacting with proteins, such as the prion protein (PrPC). In fact, PrPC performs a dual function: a protective one, encouraging the production of amyloidogenic fibrils and preventing the neurotoxic complications caused by Aβo or its neurotoxic action on the neuronal surface of the Aβ receptor by capturing Aβ in sEVs by superficial recognition [89]. sEVs-targeting therapeutic strategies may therefore offer promising clinical results for AD.

4.3. Small Extracellular Vesicles' miRNAs and Parkinson's Disease

Xin et al., (2012) reported that the growth of neurons was stimulated upon the transfer of miR-133b by MSC-sEVs [90]. Xin et al., (2017) discovered miR-17-92 clusters with neurogenesis activity in MSC-sEVs, stimulating oligodendrogenesis and enhancing neuronal function [70]. miR-34a was revealed to play a role in the neurotoxic pathways of PD-associated neurotoxins, namely paraquat, rotenone, and 6-hydroxydopamine (6-OHDA) [77]. The increase in miR-34a expression induced by 6-OHDA and inhibition of NRF2 in cells was reversed by the antioxidant Schisandrin B. In a 6-OHDA mouse PD model, Ba et al., (2015) discovered that lentiviral-mediated miR-34a expression could reverse the behavioural improvement affected by Schisandrin B [91]. Injected sEVs have been demonstrated to prevent gait impairments caused by 6-OHDA, in addition to improving motor function due to the normalised activity and expression of striatal tyrosine hydroxylase (TH) [92]. The release of miR-34a from astrocytes and its delivery via sEVs can augment the sensitivity of dopaminergic neurons to neurotoxins by targeting Bcl-2 in a PD model [93]. Chen et al., (2019) reported in a study that oxidative-stress-induced apoptosis can be reduced by upregulation of miR-34a [94]. Jiang et al., (2019) revealed that an increase in oxidation resistance 1 (OXR1) was observed upon upregulation of sEVs' miR-137, thus providing a neuroprotective effect against oxidative stress in PD mice [95].

Meanwhile, the Let-7 family is responsible for neurodegeneration via the activation of toll-like receptor 7 (TLR7), in addition to being discovered to downregulate the effects of leucine-rich repeat kinase (LRRK2) functional mutations, which play a role in PD pathogenesis [77]. The cleavage of extracellular α-synuclein, a crucial factor in the development of PD, by the MSC conditional media was shown in several studies to have neuroprotective effects. For instance, extracellular α-synuclein breakdown using in vitro and in vivo model tests demonstrated that matrix metalloproteinase 2 (MMP-2) in the MSC-secretome decreased insoluble-synuclein oligomers and resulted in an improvement in neuronal survival in PD diseases [96].

4.4. Small Extracellular Vesicles' miRNAs and Huntington's Disease

sEVs affect the nervous system to regulate mutant Huntington gene (mHtt) aggregation, mitochondrial dysfunction, cell death, and cell viability in HD [97]. sEVs secreted by MSCs are vital for relieving HD phenotypes, which upregulate phosphorylated CREB and PGC-1 and expedite non-apoptotic protein levels [98], in particular alleviating mHtt aggregation in R6/2 mouse neurons. Thus, sEVs-carried mHTT propagation is thought to be a novel mechanism for HD pathology, presenting a potential therapeutic target for reducing this neurodegenerative disease [99]. An increase in cyclin A2 expression is observed with the decrease in miR-124 expression, suggesting that the expression of cyclin A2 is controlled by miR-124, indicating its role in cell cycle dysregulation in HD cell models [100]. Recent research has sought to use sEVs' miR-124 to treat HD symptoms in animal models. The viability of sEVs-based miR-124 in an HD model was confirmed, even though the results did not demonstrate an improvement in the symptoms of HD animal models [101]. Given that oxidative stress might change the expression levels of miRNAs, there are not enough studies that focus explicitly on the connection between miRNAs and oxidative stress in HD. More research is required to determine whether the interaction between miR-124 and oxidative stress is significant in the pathophysiological process of HD [77,102]. Additionally, it has been reported that miR-124 expression is decreased in HD patients and can increase the expression of the neuron-restrictive silencing factor, which suppresses the expression of brain-derived neurotrophic factors. This finding raises the possibility that abnormal miR-124 expression is a major factor in the pathogenesis of HD [77].

4.5. Small Extracellular Vesicles' miRNAs and Amyotrophic Lateral Sclerosis

Rizzuti et al., (2018) established the importance of miR-34a in neurodegeneration and ALS. Sirtuin 1 (SIRT1), one of miR-34a's targets, is a factor that protects against oxidative stress-induced apoptosis [103]. In the ALS in vitro model, elevated SIRT1 is also seen, in addition to miR-34a downregulation [103]. This finding implies that inhibiting miR-34a may protect against oxidative stress-induced apoptosis in ALS via boosting SIRT1 expression. Furthermore, epigenetic modifications regulate miR-34a expression through the demethylation of the promoter region of the miR-34a gene [77]. According to Wang et al., (2017), miR-142-5p suppression can activate Nrf2, which then blocks oxidative stress and cell damage through the OGD/R pathway. Validating the involvement of miR-142 in ALS would help us to better understand the pathogenesis and progression of ALS, given the significance of inflammation and oxidative stress in the disease [77].

Recent studies suggest that remyelinating potential is demonstrated in sEVs [104]. The downregulation of IFNγ would stimulate the secretion of sEVs containing remyelinating miRNA species by dendritic cells, forming a new compact myelinating area in the lysolecithin-induced demyelinating hippocampal slice [104]. sEVs may contain miRNA clusters effective in myelin production (miR219 and miR-17-92) and anti-inflammatory effects (miR-27a-b and miR-145). miR-219 is responsible for inhibiting platelet-derived growth factor receptor alpha, promoting cell proliferation while prohibiting differentiation. miR-219 also inhibits ELOVL7, which is responsible for modulating lipid metabolism to increase myelin basic protein and actively participating in myelination, hence solidifying its significant role in the remyelination of samples of demyelinated hippocampus tissue by sEVs [105]. In a related study, administering environmental enrichment to older animals increased the miRNA-219 levels within serum-derived sEVs, which was sufficient for producing myelinating oligodendrocytes [104], reinforcing its significant role in the remyelination of samples of demyelinated hippocampus tissue by sEVs [105]. The miRNAs involved in various neurodegenerative diseases are summarised in Table 2.

Table 2. Levels of miRNAs that are upregulated or downregulated in different diseases.

Diseases	Sample	Validated Changes		References
		Upregulated	Down-Regulated	
Alzheimer's Disease	Plasma	N/A	miRNA 342-3p miRNA 342-3p, miRNA 125a-5p, miRNA 23a-3p	[106]
	Serum	miRNA 29a, miRNA 135a, miRNA 384, miRNA 15a-5p, miRNA 18b-5p	N/A	[107,108]
	CSF	N/A	miRNA 193b, miRNA 9-5p, miRNA 598	[109,110]
Parkinson's Disease	Plasma	miRNA 331-5p	N/A	[111]
	Serum	miRNA 22, miRNA 23a	N/A	[107]
	CSF	miRNA 153, miRNA 409-3p	N/A	[112]
ALS	Serum	N/A	miRNA 27a-3p	[113]
	CSF	miRNA 143-5p	miRNA 132-5p, miRNA 132-3p, ex-miR-143-3p	[114]

4.6. Roles of miRNAs and Proteins in sEVs

Among the various EV kinds described thus far, including microvesicles, microparticles, ectosomes, shedding particles, and apoptotic bodies, the sEVs are the most clearly defined. The sEVs' membrane is similar to a cell in that it is rich in signalling molecules and surface antigens. Besides that, it is also said to include both proteins and genetic material, but no organelles such as the nucleus or mitochondria exist [115]. miRNAs play essential roles in gene expression, especially in post-transcription regulation. Since the cancerous cells can release miRNA species that can be used as diagnostic indicators, extracellular miRNAs have been studied to become potential circulating biomarkers for certain cancers and diseases [116]. The recent sEVs preparations that contain miRNAs raise the possibility that these vesicles function as a form of intercellular communication and as a means of transporting miRNAs across cells. One of the intriguing theories states that >60% of all mRNAs are regulated by miRNAs. Therefore, the activity of target mRNAs can be bound and inhibited by miRNAs [117]. Epstein–Barr virus-infected cells were the first to exhibit the intercellular transfer of miRNAs via sEVs that led to functional activity in recipient cells, where viral miRNAs were transferred to uninfected recipient cells, as well as to COS-7 cells and metastatic prostate cancer cells. Numerous MSC-sEVs-mediated cellular processes, including angiogenesis and anti-angiogenesis, immunomodulation, anti-apoptosis, and anti-fibrosis, have been linked to MSC-sEVs' miRNAs. For example, sEVs' miR-146a was up-regulated and enhanced macrophage polarisation to M2 macrophages in MSCs pre-treated with interleukin-1, which in turn attenuated inflammation and improved survival in septic mice [118].

Several groups have covered the proteome of MSC-sEVs to date. Meanwhile, there are about a thousand proteins known thus far. The proteome's relationship to biological processes was mapped, and it became clear when those proteomes are known to play a significant role in crucial biological processes, including cellular communication, cellular structure, inflammation, sEVs biogenesis, development, tissue repair and regeneration, and metabolism [119]. Proteins in MSC-sEVs can affect a few biological processes involved in disease pathogenesis or tissue repair and regeneration, similar to miRNAs in MSC-sEVs. The comparison of the proteins' and MSC-sEVs–miRNAs' ability to elicit physiologically relevant activity is clear, as miRNAs are unlikely to be present in the proper structure or concentration. However, a normal sEVs dose does not include enough pre-miRNAs for a biologically meaningful reaction. According to the study by Chevillet et al., (2014), only a tiny fraction (3%) of cancer-related biomarker miRNAs were found in the recovered classical sEVs isolated using differential ultracentrifugation-based techniques. Therefore, this study suggests that these well-established biomarkers are present in plasma and serum in various physical forms, even though it does not directly address the diagnostic value of these sEVs [117]. Meanwhile, proteins in a typical therapeutic MSC-sEVs dose, as demonstrated by the example of glycolytic enzymes to create ATP, show their capacity to elicit a physiologically relevant response. Therefore, a protein-mediated mechanism of action stands out as the more likely route of the sEVs' effect. However, it should be highlighted that structural proteins might not elicit a biological reaction and the ability to evoke a physiologically meaningful response is mainly attributable to the catalytic activity of enzymes [119].

5. Administration Route of Small Extracellular Vesicles

The efficacy and efficiency of delivering neuro-specific sEVs remain significant problems. This is because the administered therapeutic sEVs may be identified by immune cells, leading to subsequent destruction by the reticuloendothelial system (RES). It is also a consensus that the BBB is a major barrier to developing CNS-targeting therapeutics [120]. The route of administration influences its distribution and its therapeutic and biological effects. The common administration routes in neurodegenerative disease treatments are intravenous (IV), stereotactic, oral, and nasal.

5.1. Intravenous Injection

Currently, sEVs are mainly administrated intravenously [120]. A recent study found that intravenously injected sEVs could travel to the brain and enhance cognitive capabilities due to reduced plasma Aβ levels and normalised cytokine levels [121]. Furthermore, in another study, parkinsonian mice were injected with catalase-containing sEVs; this intervention demonstrated a protective effect towards SNpc neurons in mice [122]. Although the IV route shows promising effects, its scalability is limited by a variable half-life ranging from minutes to hours due to macrophage clearance during circulation in blood [123].

5.2. Stereotactic Injection

The stereotactic injection is performed by dispersing or dissolving the therapeutic component in a solvent and injecting the mixture intrathecally [124]. The stereotactic injection is more advantageous compared to the IV route due to its site-specificity and superior stability. Most importantly, the side effects are reduced due to a lower dose retention time [125]. To illustrate this, PPSweInd transgenic (APP) mice were injected with biotinylated sEVs in the right hippocampus. The results show potential for AD therapy, as the sEVs successfully entrapped Aβ proteins, improving the proteins' clearance through immunological processes [87]. As with any pharmacological therapy, further improvements are required to improve therapeutic outcomes. The challenges associated with stereotactic injection are mandatory imaging guidance to locate the target position, high expertise requirement, and the potential for severe damage to the brain in cases of procedural blunders [126].

5.3. Nasal Administration

Similar to the above routes, the most significant advantage of nasal administration (IN) is its ability to bypass the BBB [127]. Moreover, there is evidence that IN might be more effective than the IV route [128]. Apart from that, IN is non-invasive. Hence, repeated administration is possible, resulting in rapid distribution to the intended active site [129]. A study on mouse models with 6-OHDA-induced brain inflammation showed that sEVs are distributed throughout the brain, specifically the cerebral frontal cortex, cerebellum central, and sulcus [122]. Furthermore, a study used intranasal delivery of gold nanoparticle (GNP)-labelled MSCs-derived sEVs and X-ray computed tomography (CT) technology, which observed that sEVs administrated intranasally were retained in the brain for up to

96 h [130]. However, the intranasal route has its limitations, as only a small dosage can be administered due to small surface areas for absorption at the olfactory epithelium and a short retention time for drug absorption [127,131].

6. Advantages of sEVs over Stem Cells

Unlike stem cell therapy, which involves classical transplantation of live stem cells from donors into patients, sEVs are extracted from the human donor's MSCs and sterilised. Hence, sEVs have several advantages over stem cells [132]. For neurodegenerative diseases, sEVs can cross the BBB more efficiently than MSCs [133]. By manipulating and optimising their lipids and membrane proteins, sEVs can recognise specific recipient cells to cross the BBB [134]. Studies have found that sEVs can be transfected and engineered to deliver miRNAs to the targeted neurons [135]. There are two possible mechanisms. Firstly, sEVs are internalised by endothelial cells, undergo transcytosis, and then are released to be internalised by the target recipient cells [136,137]. Alternatively, sEVs may enter the CNS through the intercellular junctions of endothelial cells [138].

Compared with stem cell therapy, using sEVs for treating neurodegenerative diseases is better tolerated in patients, improving safety. Life-threatening issues that may happen in stem cell therapy, such as immune rejection, pulmonary embolism and stress reactions resulting in the death of cells, and abnormal differentiation, can be prevented by using sEVs [132]. Furthermore, patients can be safe from unlimited cell growth and tumour development because sEVs are not constantly dividing cells. In the case of repeated injections for long-term treatment, MSC-sEVs also do not induce toxicity in patients [139]. sEVs do not undergo mutation nor induce metastasis [140]. Other than target tissues, sEVs do not form abnormal aggregations in the liver or lung, reducing toxicity risks [141]. As stem cell therapy poses risks for small vessel obstruction, sEVs have advantages including a lower immunogenicity without an obstructive vascular effect [135].

miRNAs are protected in sEVs from enzymatic degradation in biological fluids. Hence, sEVs can help miRNAs to maintain their integrity and functionality in the target neurons. This enhances the ability of sEVs to provide candidate biomarkers for investigating neurodegenerative diseases [142]. Modifications can be performed on sEVs to carry certain cargo for drug delivery. Hence, sEVs can be loaded with bioactive cargo such as miRNAs and transferred effectively to the target cells along short or long distances. sEVs have a slower clearance rate due to their protein contents, so they are more stable and can remain for longer in the brain or target sites [138]. With their unique lipid bilayer structure enveloping an aqueous core, sEVs have a remarkable ability to load themselves with both hydrophilic and hydrophobic materials, which helps introduce miRNAs to the target sites. This property also allows sEVs to effectively distribute themselves in blood and CSF and remain for a long time in systemic circulation [141]. Since sEVs can be engineered to target specific neuron populations, this opens more possibilities for developing different sEVs delivery methods, such as intravenous and intranasal administration. Hence, neurosurgical intervention can be avoided for the convenience of patients [143]. The preparation of sEVs can also be done without harmful preservatives such as dimethyl sulfoxide (DMSO), and the storage time is relatively long [139]. With a high surface/volume ratio, sEVs can efficiently transfer biomolecules to the target tissues by amplifying the ligand-gated signalling pathways [135].

7. Challenges and Future Perspectives

7.1. The Challenges and Opportunities in the Development of MicroRNA Therapeutics: A Multidisciplinary Viewpoint

In order to study and develop miRNA therapeutics, a few factors need to be further tested: pinpointing the significant miRNAs in a specific disease, delivering the miRNAs to the target area, target expression regulation, and minimising other unwanted nonspecific interactions. The complexity of miRNAs' biology and their physicochemical nature generates many hurdles in developing miRNA therapeutics [144] (Table 3).

Table 3. Current status in the development of miRNAs therapeutics.

miRNAs	siRNAs
Less than 20 in clinical trials	Over 60 in clinical trials
Percentage being terminated/suspended (50%)	Percentage being terminated/suspended (35%)
None in phase III trials	12% of trials in phase III

The majority of DNA or RNA-based modulators have a negative charge to interact with blood proteins. For example, phosphorothioate oligonucleotide is a negatively charged compound that only targets RNA to carry out hybridisation, leading to a suppression of protein expression and preventing pathological progression [145]. It possesses a considerably long half-life of 2–4 weeks. The combination of a long half-life with nonspecific binding causes sequence complementarity-dependent effects in the off-target cells [145]. Moreover, the negative charge of miRNAs also disrupts cellular entry due to the cell membranes being in negative charge. The complexity of the functions and off-target effects represent further challenges. One type of mRNA can be acted on by hundreds of miRNAs and, vice versa, one type of miRNA can target hundreds of mRNAs. This creates a problem where the identification and implementation of miR are exceedingly complicated [146]. Furthermore, miR modulators can act on the target gene expression in unrelated cell types and tissues, causing more unwanted adverse effects. Therefore, identifying miRNAs that possesses the optimal therapeutic outcome in each disease is one of the main challenges [144].

In addition, the stability of miRNA modulators and the escape of endosomes pose challenges in the development process. miRNAs and unmodified miRNA inhibitors are susceptible to degradation. Ribonuclease enzymes in the blood can break down miRNAs that occupy the cerebrovascular duplex by targeting the less stable 3′ terminus. To this end, chemical modifications have been developed. However, the modifications must be better implemented in the 5′ terminus [147]. This indicates the consequence of an asymmetry of molecules in the RNA interference activity. Other than that, intracellular trafficking takes place initially in early endosomes, which later combine with late endosomes and lysosomes with the assistance of an acidic environment [148]. However, they can be degraded by nuclease enzymes as well. Strategies related to photosensitive molecules and pH lipoplexes have been developed in order to enhance the escape of miRNAs [144].

Using sEVs as a miRNA delivery carrier also has its obstacles, including nonspecific distribution of sEVs into unrelated organs such as kidneys, lungs, pancreas, spleen, liver, etc., [149]. In recent years, some unmodified sEVs have been better collected in a specific tissue or organ than traditional drug carriers. For example, sEVs derived from M1 polarised macrophages were discovered to have a remarkable accumulation in tumour tissue, which promotes the stimulation of macrophages in the cancer tissues [150]. In another important piece of research, the accumulation of sEVs of pancreatic cancer cells (Panc-1 cell) at the target site was observed in male BALB/c nude mice; the pancreatic cancer cell sEVs showed an accumulation in tumour tissue 30 times greater than peg-pe micelles for 4 h after administration [75]. Moreover, further profound studies have demonstrated neural-derived sEVs′ isolation by immunoadsorption with L1CAM, the neuronal antibody [151]. These innovative discoveries can lead a whole new direction in the research of neurodegenerative diseases. However, the neural-derived sEVs require improvement in purification and more evaluations are needed regarding the specific surface proteins [151]. For instance, most neurodegenerative diseases jump-start or progress through neuroinflammation. The segregation of microglia-derived sEVs and the detection of abnormal inflammatory miRNAs will be integrated into the development of the advanced diagnosis of many neurodegenerative diseases [152].

In addition, sEVs tend to be cleared rapidly from the bloodstream when observed during in vivo tests, regardless of the sEVs having distinctive lipid and protein compositions comparable to phosphatidylcholine or cholesterol liposomes. No more than 5% of the injected dosage of sEVs remained in the blood for 3 h after administration [153]. This is primarily because of macrophage capture. Evidence suggests that IV injection of B16BL6 cell-derived sEVs results in rapid clearance from the blood by the macrophages originating from the liver and spleen [154]. Therefore, any development that can alter the sEVs to avoid detection by the reticuloendothelial system will notably enhance the action of sEVs to deliver miRNAs.

7.2. Future Perspectives

The control of miRNAs in terms of different therapy practices has progressed from bed to bench with the success of phase I and II trials. Research on miRNAs has the potential to understand the sporadic forms of AD, PD, HD, and ALS. The obstacle now is to study the position of specific miRNA and then transfer this knowledge into clinical research and development [155]. Currently, two miRNA therapeutics are being studied in vivo. miRNA-mimics and anti-miRNAs are small molecules of RNA similar to mRNA precursors and have been used to down-regulate specific target protein expression. The target can be any gene that takes part in the pathogenesis of neurodegenerative diseases or possesses a gain of function mutation. This strategy mainly relies on reducing the specific protein [148].

Moreover, vector-based, chemically modified, and "packaged" RNA oligonucleotide delivery systems have been developed in siRNAs. This knowledge can be directly translated to developing miRNA therapeutics in the future, since siRNAs and miRNAs stem from the same concept. Nevertheless, the challenge is whether these procedures will be applicable in clinical treatment due to toxicity and bioavailability. The blood-brain barrier also plays a significant part in developing drugs to act on the brain [81].

On the other hand, sEVs are part of many pathological procedures. For instance, in AD, the progression can be contributed to by sEVs through the proliferation of neurofibrillary tangles and senile plaques. sEVs are also involved in other pathogenic occurrences, such as neuroinflammation [83]. However, sEVs can bear advantageous effects regarding AD. SEVs can isolate amyloid beta and stimulate its clearance [87]. Therefore, this signifies the requirement to further study sEVs' mechanisms and exact functions in neurodegenerative diseases. Furthermore, sEVs have been revealed in the field of biomarkers in neurodegenerative diseases [55]. In recent years, three recognisable miRNAs observed in peripheral sEVs have been presented as potential biomarkers. Even though many studies still require further validation, it is indisputable that sEVs have a high potential in diagnosing and perhaps treating neurodegenerative diseases [156].

8. Conclusions

miRNA-enriched sEVs from stem cells represent a future treatment to reverse neurodegenerative disease. These could help thousands of patients live a better quality of life for the rest of their lives. Despite the many advantages of using miRNA-enriched sEVs, nevertheless, many challenges need to be addressed to make this mission possible in clinical settings (Figure 6). Particular miRNAs that could be the focus of the researchers and clinicians are the following: miR-21, miR-17-92, miR-133, miR-138, miR-124, miR-146a, etc., but the relevant miRNAs are not limited to these. If any miRNAs make a breakthrough, this will be the new chapter of cell-free therapy in neurodegenerative diseases.

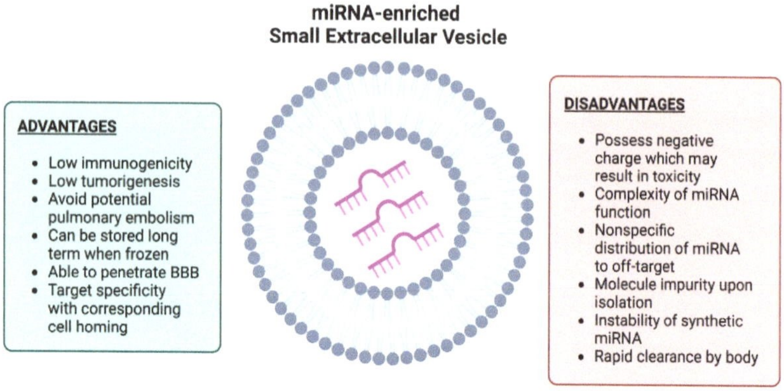

Figure 6. Advantages and disadvantages of miRNA-enriched small extracellular vesicles.

Author Contributions: Conceptualization, J.B.F., Q.H.D.L. and C.W.H.; data search and writing—original draft, W.Q.L., K.H.M.L., K.Y.L., N.N., S.J.L., Z.X.Y. and Q.X.W.; writing—review and editing, P.P.C., S.H., Q.H.D.L., C.W.H., P.P.C. and J.B.F. All authors have read and agreed to the published version of the manuscript.

Funding: This write-up did not receive any specific grant from funding agencies in the public, commercial, or not-for-profit sectors. The figures in the article were generated from a BioRender account subscribed by Taylor's University. The open access fee of this manuscript was funded by My CytoHealth Sdn. Bhd.

Institutional Review Board Statement: Not applicable.

Informed Consent Statement: Not applicable.

Data Availability Statement: Data are contained within the article.

Acknowledgments: The authors would like to thank the laboratory staffs of the Faculty of Health and Medical Sciences, Taylor University, for their resources and technical support during the present study.

Conflicts of Interest: The authors declare no conflict of interest.

References

1. Rekatsina, M.; Paladini, A.; Piroli, A.; Zis, P.; Pergolizzi, J.V.; Varrassi, G. Pathophysiology and Therapeutic Perspectives of Oxidative Stress and Neurodegenerative Diseases: A Narrative Review. *Adv. Ther.* **2020**, *37*, 113–139. [CrossRef] [PubMed]
2. Livingston, G.; Huntley, J.; Sommerlad, A.; Ames, D.; Ballard, C.; Banerjee, S.; Brayne, C.; Burns, A.; Cohen-Mansfield, J.; Cooper, C.; et al. Dementia prevention, intervention, and care: 2020 report of the Lancet Commission. *Lancet* **2020**, *396*, 413–446. [CrossRef]
3. Oladele, J.O.; Oladiji, A.T.; Oladele, O.T.; Oyeleke, O.M. Reactive Oxygen Species in Neurodegenerative Diseases: Implications in Pathogenesis and Treatment Strategies. In *Reactive Oxygen Species*; IntechOpen: London, UK, 2021; pp. 149–166.
4. Fayazi, N.; Sheykhhasan, M.; Soleimani Asl, S.; Najafi, R. Stem Cell-Derived Exosomes: A New Strategy of Neurodegenerative Disease Treatment. *Mol. Neurobiol.* **2021**, *58*, 3494–3514. [CrossRef]
5. Parambi, D.G.T.; Alharbi, K.S.; Kumar, R.; Harilal, S.; Batiha, G.E.-S.; Cruz-Martins, N.; Magdy, O.; Musa, A.; Panda, D.S.; Mathew, B. Gene Therapy Approach with an Emphasis on Growth Factors: Theoretical and Clinical Outcomes in Neurodegenerative Diseases. *Mol. Neurobiol.* **2022**, *59*, 191–233. [CrossRef]
6. Muddapu, V.; Ranjith, A.; Chakravarthy, S.; Gromiha, M. Neurodegenerative Diseases–Is Metabolic Deficiency the Root Cause? *Front. Neurosci.* **2020**, *14*, 213. [CrossRef] [PubMed]
7. Whalen, K. *Pharmacology*; Lippincott Williams & Wilkins: Philadelphia, PA, USA, 2014; pp. 181–193.
8. Ogbodo, J.O.; Agbo, C.P.; Njoku, U.O.; Ogugofor, M.O.; Egba, S.I.; Ihim, S.A.; Echezona, A.C.; Brendan, K.C.; Upaganlawar, A.B.; Upasani, C.D. Alzheimer's Disease: Pathogenesis and Therapeutic Interventions. *Curr. Aging Sci.* **2022**, *15*, 2–25. [CrossRef]
9. Shi, M.; Chu, F.; Zhu, F.; Zhu, J. Impact of Anti-amyloid-β Monoclonal Antibodies on the Pathology and Clinical Profile of Alzheimer's Disease: A Focus on Aducanumab and Lecanemab. *Front. Aging Neurosci.* **2022**, *14*, 870517. [CrossRef]

10. Kim, D.D.; Barr, A.M.; Lian, L.; Yuen, J.W.Y.; Fredrikson, D.; Honer, W.G.; Thornton, A.E.; Procyshyn, R.M. Efficacy and tolerability of aripiprazole versus D2 antagonists in the early course of schizophrenia: A systematic review and meta-analysis. *Npj Schizophr.* **2021**, *7*, 29. [CrossRef]
11. Ferrini, E.; Stellari, F.F.; Franceschi, V.; Macchi, F.; Russo, L.; Murgia, A.; Grisendi, G.; Villetti, G.; Dominici, M.; Donofrio, G. Persistency of Mesenchymal Stromal/Stem Cells in Lungs. *Front. Cell Dev. Biol.* **2021**, *9*, 1825. [CrossRef]
12. Wang, S.; Guo, L.; Ge, J.; Yu, L.; Cai, T.; Tian, R.; Jiang, Y.; Zhao, R.C.H.; Wu, Y. Excess Integrins Cause Lung Entrapment of Mesenchymal Stem Cells. *Stem Cells* **2015**, *33*, 3315–3326. [CrossRef]
13. Théry, C.; Witwer, K.W.; Aikawa, E.; Alcaraz, M.J.; Anderson, J.D.; Andriantsitohaina, R.; Antoniou, A.; Arab, T.; Archer, F.; Atkin-Smith, G.K.; et al. Minimal information for studies of extracellular vesicles 2018 (MISEV2018): A position statement of the International Society for Extracellular Vesicles and update of the MISEV2014 guidelines. *J. Extracell. Vesicles* **2018**, *7*, 1535750. [CrossRef] [PubMed]
14. Abdelaal, N.E.; Abdelhai, M.F. Differential Expression of Exosomal MicroRNAs in Neurodegenerative Diseases. In *Role of Exosomes in Biological Communication Systems*; Springer: Singapore, 2021; pp. 207–219.
15. Beatriz, M.; Vilaça, R.; Lopes, C. Exosomes: Innocent Bystanders or Critical Culprits in Neurodegenerative Diseases. *Front. Cell Dev. Biol.* **2021**, *9*, 635104. [CrossRef] [PubMed]
16. Takahashi, Y.; Takakura, Y. Extracellular vesicle-based therapeutics: Extracellular vesicles as therapeutic targets and agents. *Pharmacol. Ther.* **2023**, *242*, 108352. [CrossRef]
17. Sarvar, D.P.; Shamsasenjan, K.; Akbarzadehlaleh, P. Mesenchymal stem cell-derived exosomes: New opportunity in cell-free therapy. *Adv. Pharm. Bull.* **2016**, *6*, 293. [CrossRef] [PubMed]
18. Yang, Y.; Ye, Y.; Kong, C.; Su, X.; Zhang, X.; Bai, W.; He, X. MiR-124 Enriched Exosomes Promoted the M2 Polarization of Microglia and Enhanced Hippocampus Neurogenesis After Traumatic Brain Injury by Inhibiting TLR4 Pathway. *Neurochem. Res.* **2019**, *44*, 811–828. [CrossRef]
19. Salarpour, S.; Barani, M.; Pardakhty, A.; Khatami, M.; Pal Singh Chauhan, N. The application of exosomes and Exosome-nanoparticle in treating brain disorders. *J. Mol. Liq.* **2022**, *350*, 118549. [CrossRef]
20. Alzheimer, A. Uber einen eigenartigen schweren Erkrankungsprozess der Hirninde. *Neurol. Cent.* **1906**, *25*, 1134.
21. Genaro Gabriel, O.; Fermín, P.P.-M.; Erika, D.G.-R.; Luis, F.; Miguel, A.M.-I.; Mario Mireles, R.; Flores-Alvarado, L.J.; Angélica, S.-L.; Dhea, G.N.-P.; Irma, E.V.-B.; et al. Genetic, Biochemical and Histopathological Aspects of Familiar Alzheimer's Disease. In *Alzheimer's Disease*; Inga, Z., Ed.; IntechOpen: Rijeka, Croatia, 2015; Chapter 10; pp. 297–301.
22. Chow, H.M.; Guo, D.; Zhou, J.C.; Zhang, G.Y.; Li, H.F.; Herrup, K.; Zhang, J. CDK5 activator protein p25 preferentially binds and activates GSK3β. *Proc. Natl. Acad. Sci. USA* **2014**, *111*, E4887–E4895. [CrossRef] [PubMed]
23. Bourdenx, M.; Koulakiotis, N.S.; Sanoudou, D.; Bezard, E.; Dehay, B.; Tsarbopoulos, A. Protein aggregation and neurodegeneration in prototypical neurodegenerative diseases: Examples of amyloidopathies, tauopathies and synucleinopathies. *Prog. Neurobiol.* **2017**, *155*, 171–193. [CrossRef]
24. Singh, A.; Kukreti, R.; Saso, L.; Kukreti, S. Oxidative Stress: A Key Modulator in Neurodegenerative Diseases. *Molecules* **2019**, *24*, 1583. [CrossRef]
25. Neniskyte, U.; Gross, C.T. Errant gardeners: Glial-cell-dependent synaptic pruning and neurodevelopmental disorders. *Nat. Rev. Neurosci.* **2017**, *18*, 658–670. [CrossRef] [PubMed]
26. Suescun, J.; Chandra, S.; Schiess, M.C. Chapter 13-The Role of Neuroinflammation in Neurodegenerative Disorders. In *Translational Inflammation*; Actor, J.K., Smith, K.C., Eds.; Academic Press: Cambridge, MA, USA, 2019; pp. 241–267.
27. Zuroff, L.; Daley, D.; Black, K.L.; Koronyo-Hamaoui, M. Clearance of cerebral Aβ in Alzheimer's disease: Reassessing the role of microglia and monocytes. *Cell. Mol. Life Sci.* **2017**, *74*, 2167–2201. [CrossRef] [PubMed]
28. Wang, Y.; Cella, M.; Mallinson, K.; Ulrich, J.D.; Young, K.L.; Robinette, M.L.; Gilfillan, S.; Krishnan, G.M.; Sudhakar, S.; Zinselmeyer, B.H. TREM2 lipid sensing sustains the microglial response in an Alzheimer's disease model. *Cell* **2015**, *160*, 1061–1071. [CrossRef]
29. Khan, A.U.; Akram, M.; Daniyal, M.; Zainab, R. Awareness and current knowledge of Parkinson's disease: A neurodegenerative disorder. *Int. J. Neurosci.* **2019**, *129*, 55–93. [CrossRef] [PubMed]
30. Parashos, S.A.; Wichmann, R. *Navigating Life with Parkinson's Disease*, 2nd ed.; Oxford University Press: New York, NY, USA, 2020.
31. Bellucci, A.; Bubacco, L.; Longhena, F.; Parrella, E.; Faustini, G.; Porrini, V.; Bono, F.; Missale, C.; Pizzi, M. Nuclear Factor-κB Dysregulation and α-Synuclein Pathology: Critical Interplay in the Pathogenesis of Parkinson's Disease. *Front. Aging Neurosci.* **2020**, *12*, 68. [CrossRef]
32. Ma, L.; Yang, C.; Zhang, X.; Li, Y.; Wang, S.; Zheng, L.; Huang, K. C-terminal truncation exacerbates the aggregation and cytotoxicity of α-Synuclein: A vicious cycle in Parkinson's disease. *Biochim. Biophys. Acta (BBA) Mol. Basis Dis.* **2018**, *1864*, 3714–3725. [CrossRef]
33. Sato, H.; Arawaka, S.; Hara, S.; Fukushima, S.; Koga, K.; Koyama, S.; Kato, T. Authentically phosphorylated α-synuclein at Ser129 accelerates neurodegeneration in a rat model of familial Parkinson's disease. *J. Neurosci.* **2011**, *31*, 16884–16894. [CrossRef]
34. Park, M.J.; Cheon, S.-M.; Bae, H.-R.; Kim, S.-H.; Kim, J.W. Elevated levels of α-synuclein oligomer in the cerebrospinal fluid of drug-naïve patients with Parkinson's disease. *J. Clin. Neurol.* **2011**, *7*, 215–222. [CrossRef]

35. Di Maio, R.; Barrett, P.J.; Hoffman, E.K.; Barrett, C.W.; Zharikov, A.; Borah, A.; Hu, X.; McCoy, J.; Chu, C.T.; Burton, E.A. α-Synuclein binds to TOM20 and inhibits mitochondrial protein import in Parkinson's disease. *Sci. Transl. Med.* **2016**, *8*, 342ra78. [CrossRef]
36. Jones, R. The roles of PINK1 and Parkin in Parkinson's disease. *PLoS Biol.* **2010**, *8*, e1000299. [CrossRef]
37. Behl, T.; Kumar, S.; Althafar, Z.M.; Sehgal, A.; Singh, S.; Sharma, N.; Badavath, V.N.; Yadav, S.; Bhatia, S.; Al-Harrasi, A.; et al. Exploring the Role of Ubiquitin–Proteasome System in Parkinson's Disease. *Mol. Neurobiol.* **2022**, *59*, 4257–4273. [CrossRef] [PubMed]
38. Liu, B.; Ruan, J.; Chen, M.; Li, Z.; Manjengwa, G.; Schlüter, D.; Song, W.; Wang, X. Deubiquitinating enzymes (DUBs): Decipher underlying basis of neurodegenerative diseases. *Mol. Psychiatry* **2022**, *27*, 259–268. [CrossRef] [PubMed]
39. Zhang, J.X.; Tong, W.F.; Jiang, M.; Zhou, K.G.; Xiang, X.R.; He, Y.J.; Zhang, Z.Y.; Guan, Q.; Jin, L.J. MANF Inhibits α-Synuclein Accumulation through Activation of Autophagic Pathways. *Oxid. Med. Cell. Longev.* **2022**, *2022*, 7925686. [CrossRef]
40. Wilkaniec, A.; Lenkiewicz, A.M.; Babiec, L.; Murawska, E.; Jęśko, H.M.; Cieślik, M.; Culmsee, C.; Adamczyk, A. Exogenous Alpha-Synuclein Evoked Parkin Downregulation Promotes Mitochondrial Dysfunction in Neuronal Cells. Implications for Parkinson's Disease Pathology. *Front. Aging Neurosci.* **2021**, *13*, 591475. [CrossRef]
41. Kouli, A.; Torsney, K.M.; Kuan, W.L. Parkinson's Disease: Etiology, Neuropathology, and Pathogenesis. In *Parkinson's Disease: Pathogenesis and Clinical Aspects*; Stoker, T.B., Greenland, J.C., Eds.; Codon Publications: Brisbane, Australia, 2018.
42. Stoker, T.B.; Mason, S.L.; Greenland, J.C.; Holden, S.T.; Santini, H.; Barker, R.A. Huntington's disease: Diagnosis and management. *Pract. Neurol.* **2022**, *22*, 32. [CrossRef] [PubMed]
43. Ruff, K.M. *Determining the Molecular Mechanisms of Huntington's Disease through Multi-Scale Modeling*; ProQuest: St. Louis, MO, USA, 2017.
44. Jimenez-Sanchez, M.; Licitra, F.; Underwood, B.R.; Rubinsztein, D.C. Huntington's Disease: Mechanisms of Pathogenesis and Therapeutic Strategies. *Cold Spring Harb. Perspect. Med.* **2017**, *7*, a024240. [CrossRef]
45. Heinz, A.; Nabariya, D.K.; Krauß, S. Huntington's Disease and Neurodegeneration. In *Handbook of Neurotoxicity*; Kostrzewa, R.M., Ed.; Springer International Publishing: Cham, Switzerland, 2021; pp. 1–23.
46. Carmo, C.; Naia, L.; Lopes, C.; Rego, A.C. Mitochondrial Dysfunction in Huntington's Disease. *Adv. Exp. Med. Biol.* **2018**, *1049*, 59–83.
47. Paul, B.D.; Sbodio, J.I.; Xu, R.; Vandiver, M.S.; Cha, J.Y.; Snowman, A.M.; Snyder, S.H. Cystathionine γ-lyase deficiency mediates neurodegeneration in Huntington's disease. *Nature* **2014**, *509*, 96–100. [CrossRef]
48. Catanesi, M.; d'Angelo, M.; Tupone, M.G.; Benedetti, E.; Giordano, A.; Castelli, V.; Cimini, A. MicroRNAs Dysregulation and Mitochondrial Dysfunction in Neurodegenerative Diseases. *Int. J. Mol. Sci.* **2020**, *21*, 5986. [CrossRef]
49. Buren, C. Global Neuroprotection of Huntingtin in Culture and Alterations of Cortico-Striatal Connections in Huntington's Disease Culture and Mouse Models. Ph.D. Thesis, University of British Columbia, Vancouver, BC, Canada, 2017.
50. Raymond, L.A.; André, V.M.; Cepeda, C.; Gladding, C.M.; Milnerwood, A.J.; Levine, M.S. Pathophysiology of Huntington's disease: Time-dependent alterations in synaptic and receptor function. *Neuroscience* **2011**, *198*, 252–273. [CrossRef]
51. Watanabe, K.; Shibuya, K.; Misawa, S.; Nagashima, K.; Suzuki, Y.i.; Suichi, T.; Kojima, Y.; Nakamura, K.; Kano, H.; Prado, M. Impaired neuromuscular transmission in facial muscles of amyotrophic lateral sclerosis: A single-fiber electromyography study. *Neurol. Clin. Neurosci.* **2022**, *10*, 78–82. [CrossRef]
52. Satarker, S.; Bojja, S.L.; Gurram, P.C.; Mudgal, J.; Arora, D.; Nampoothiri, M. Astrocytic Glutamatergic Transmission and Its Implications in Neurodegenerative Disorders. *Cells* **2022**, *11*, 1139. [CrossRef] [PubMed]
53. Didonna, A.; Opal, P. The role of neurofilament aggregation in neurodegeneration: Lessons from rare inherited neurological disorders. *Mol. Neurodegener.* **2019**, *14*, 19. [CrossRef] [PubMed]
54. Van den Bos, M.A.J.; Geevasinga, N.; Higashihara, M.; Menon, P.; Vucic, S. Pathophysiology and Diagnosis of ALS: Insights from Advances in Neurophysiological Techniques. *Int. J. Mol. Sci.* **2019**, *20*, 2818. [CrossRef]
55. He, M.; Zhang, H.N.; Tang, Z.C.; Gao, S.G. Diagnostic and Therapeutic Potential of Exosomal MicroRNAs for Neurodegenerative Diseases. *Neural Plast.* **2021**, *2021*, 8884642. [CrossRef]
56. Matsumoto, J.; Stewart, T.; Sheng, L.; Li, N.; Bullock, K.; Song, N.; Shi, M.; Banks, W.A.; Zhang, J. Transmission of α-synuclein-containing erythrocyte-derived extracellular vesicles across the blood-brain barrier via adsorptive mediated transcytosis: Another mechanism for initiation and progression of Parkinson's disease? *Acta Neuropathol. Commun.* **2017**, *5*, 71. [CrossRef]
57. Manna, I.; De Benedittis, S.; Quattrone, A.; Maisano, D.; Iaccino, E.; Quattrone, A. Exosomal miRNAs as Potential Diagnostic Biomarkers in Alzheimer's Disease. *Pharmaceuticals* **2020**, *13*, 243. [CrossRef]
58. Mathew, B.; Mansuri, M.S.; Williams, K.R.; Nairn, A.C. Exosomes as Emerging Biomarker Tools in Neurodegenerative and Neuropsychiatric Disorders-A Proteomics Perspective. *Brain Sci.* **2021**, *11*, 258. [CrossRef]
59. Cheng, L.; Sharples, R.A.; Scicluna, B.J.; Hill, A.F. Exosomes provide a protective and enriched source of miRNA for biomarker profiling compared to intracellular and cell-free blood. *J. Extracell. Vesicles* **2014**, *3*, 23743. [CrossRef]
60. Fiandaca, M.S.; Kapogiannis, D.; Mapstone, M.; Boxer, A.; Eitan, E.; Schwartz, J.B.; Abner, E.L.; Petersen, R.C.; Federoff, H.J.; Miller, B.L.; et al. Identification of preclinical Alzheimer's disease by a profile of pathogenic proteins in neurally derived blood exosomes: A case-control study. *Alzheimers Dement.* **2015**, *11*, 600–607.e1. [CrossRef]
61. D'Anca, M.; Fenoglio, C.; Serpente, M.; Arosio, B.; Cesari, M.; Scarpini, E.A.; Galimberti, D. Exosome Determinants of Physiological Aging and Age-Related Neurodegenerative Diseases. *Front. Aging Neurosci.* **2019**, *11*, 232. [CrossRef] [PubMed]

62. Kumar, S.; Reddy, P.H. Are circulating microRNAs peripheral biomarkers for Alzheimer's disease? *Biochim. Biophys. Acta* **2016**, *1862*, 1617–1627. [CrossRef]
63. Thomi, G.; Surbek, D.; Haesler, V.; Joerger-Messerli, M.; Schoeberlein, A. Exosomes derived from umbilical cord mesenchymal stem cells reduce microglia-mediated neuroinflammation in perinatal brain injury. *Stem Cell Res. Ther.* **2019**, *10*, 105. [CrossRef]
64. Foo, J.B.; Looi, Q.H.; How, C.W.; Lee, S.H.; Al-Masawa, M.E.; Chong, P.P.; Law, J.X. Mesenchymal Stem Cell-Derived Exosomes and MicroRNAs in Cartilage Regeneration: Biogenesis, Efficacy, miRNA Enrichment and Delivery. *Pharmaceuticals* **2021**, *14*, 1093. [CrossRef]
65. Markoutsa, E.; Mayilsamy, K.; Gulick, D.; Mohapatra, S.S.; Mohapatra, S. Extracellular vesicles derived from inflammatory-educated stem cells reverse brain inflammation-implication of miRNAs. *Mol. Ther.* **2022**, *30*, 816–830. [CrossRef]
66. Chen, Q.Y.; Wen, T.; Wu, P.; Jia, R.; Zhang, R.; Dang, J. Exosomal Proteins and miRNAs as Mediators of Amyotrophic Lateral Sclerosis. *Front. Cell Dev. Biol.* **2021**, *9*, 718803. [CrossRef]
67. Yang, J.; Zhang, X.; Chen, X.; Wang, L.; Yang, G. Exosome Mediated Delivery of miR-124 Promotes Neurogenesis after Ischemia. *Mol. Ther. Nucleic Acids* **2017**, *7*, 278–287. [CrossRef]
68. Cheng, L.-C.; Pastrana, E.; Tavazoie, M.; Doetsch, F. MiR-124 Regulates Adult Neurogenesis in the Subventricular Zone Stem Cell Niche. *Nat. Neurosci.* **2009**, *12*, 399–408. [CrossRef]
69. Yu, Y.-M.; Gibbs, K.M.; Davila, J.; Campbell, N.; Sung, S.; Todorova, T.I.; Otsuka, S.; Sabaawy, H.E.; Hart, R.P.; Schachner, M. MicroRNA miR-133b is essential for functional recovery after spinal cord injury in adult zebrafish. *Eur. J. Neurosci.* **2011**, *33*, 1587–1597. [CrossRef]
70. Xin, H.; Katakowski, M.; Wang, F.; Qian, J.Y.; Liu, X.S.; Ali, M.M.; Buller, B.; Zhang, Z.G.; Chopp, M. MicroRNA cluster miR-17–92 Cluster in Exosomes Enhance Neuroplasticity and Functional Recovery After Stroke in Rats. *Stroke* **2017**, *48*, 747–753. [CrossRef]
71. Zuo, X.; Lu, J.; Manaenko, A.; Qi, X.; Tang, J.; Mei, Q.; Xia, Y.; Hu, Q. MicroRNA-132 attenuates cerebral injury by protecting blood-brain-barrier in MCAO mice. *Exp. Neurol.* **2019**, *316*, 12–19. [CrossRef] [PubMed]
72. Ma, J.; Yao, Y.; Wang, P.; Liu, Y.; Zhao, L.; Li, Z.; Li, h.; Xue, Y. MiR-181a Regulates Blood-Tumor Barrier Permeability by Targeting Krüppel-Like Factor 6. *J. Cereb. Blood Flow Metab.* **2014**, *34*, 1826–1836. [CrossRef]
73. Yu, L.; Gui, S.; Liu, Y.; Qiu, X.; Zhang, G.; Zhang, X.; Pan, J.; Fan, J.; Qi, S.; Qiu, B. Exosomes derived from microRNA-199a-overexpressing mesenchymal stem cells inhibit glioma progression by down-regulating AGAP2. *Aging* **2019**, *11*, 5300–5318. [CrossRef]
74. Li, W.; Wang, L.; Ji, X.B.; Wang, L.H.; Ge, X.; Liu, W.T.; Chen, L.; Zheng, Z.; Shi, Z.M.; Liu, L.Z.; et al. MiR-199a Inhibits Tumor Growth and Attenuates Chemoresistance by Targeting K-RAS via AKT and ERK Signalings. *Front. Oncol.* **2019**, *9*, 1071. [CrossRef] [PubMed]
75. Wang, J.; Chen, D.; Ho, E.A. Challenges in the development and establishment of exosome-based drug delivery systems. *J. Control. Release* **2021**, *329*, 894–906. [CrossRef]
76. Wang, L.; Chopp, M.; Szalad, A.; Zhang, Y.; Wang, X.; Zhang, R.L.; Liu, X.S.; Jia, L.; Zhang, Z.G. The role of miR-146a in dorsal root ganglia neurons of experimental diabetic peripheral neuropathy. *Neuroscience* **2014**, *259*, 155–163. [CrossRef]
77. Wang, X.; Zhou, Y.; Gao, Q.; Ping, D.; Wang, Y.; Wu, W.; Lin, X.; Fang, Y.; Zhang, J.; Shao, A. The Role of Exosomal microRNAs and Oxidative Stress in Neurodegenerative Diseases. *Oxid. Med. Cell. Longev.* **2020**, *2020*, 3232869. [CrossRef]
78. Yu, Y.; Hou, K.; Ji, T.; Wang, X.; Liu, Y.; Zheng, Y.; Xu, J.; Hou, Y.; Chi, G. The role of exosomal microRNAs in central nervous system diseases. *Mol. Cell. Biochem.* **2021**, *476*, 2111–2124. [CrossRef]
79. Bolukbasi, M.F.; Mizrak, A.; Ozdener, G.B.; Madlener, S.; Ströbel, T.; Erkan, E.P.; Fan, J.B.; Breakefield, X.O.; Saydam, O. miR-1289 and "Zipcode"-like Sequence Enrich mRNAs in Microvesicles. *Mol. Ther. Nucleic Acids* **2012**, *1*, e10. [CrossRef]
80. Hooper, C.; Sainz-Fuertes, R.; Lynham, S.; Hye, A.; Killick, R.; Warley, A.; Bolondi, C.; Pocock, J.; Lovestone, S. Wnt3a induces exosome secretion from primary cultured rat microglia. *BMC Neurosci.* **2012**, *13*, 144. [CrossRef]
81. Soares Martins, T.; Trindade, D.; Vaz, M.; Campelo, I.; Almeida, M.; Trigo, G.; da Cruz, E.S.O.A.B.; Henriques, A.G. Diagnostic and therapeutic potential of exosomes in Alzheimer's disease. *J. Neurochem.* **2021**, *156*, 162–181. [CrossRef] [PubMed]
82. Cui, G.-H.; Wu, J.; Mou, F.-F.; Xie, W.-H.; Wang, F.-B.; Wang, Q.-L.; Fang, J.; Xu, Y.-W.; Dong, Y.-R.; Liu, J.-R.; et al. Exosomes derived from hypoxia-preconditioned mesenchymal stromal cells ameliorate cognitive decline by rescuing synaptic dysfunction and regulating inflammatory responses in APP/PS1 mice. *FASEB J.* **2017**, *32*, 654–668. [CrossRef] [PubMed]
83. Cai, Z.Y.; Xiao, M.; Quazi, S.H.; Ke, Z.Y. Exosomes: A novel therapeutic target for Alzheimer's disease? *Neural Regen. Res.* **2018**, *13*, 930–935. [CrossRef]
84. Katsuda, T.; Tsuchiya, R.; Kosaka, N.; Yoshioka, Y.; Takagaki, K.; Oki, K.; Takeshita, F.; Sakai, Y.; Kuroda, M.; Ochiya, T. Human adipose tissue-derived mesenchymal stem cells secrete functional neprilysin-bound exosomes. *Sci. Rep.* **2013**, *3*, 1197. [CrossRef]
85. Shen, Y.; Shen, Z.; Guo, L.; Zhang, Q.; Wang, Z.; Miao, L.; Wang, M.; Wu, J.; Guo, W.; Zhu, Y. MiR-125b-5p is involved in oxygen and glucose deprivation injury in PC-12 cells via CBS/H(2)S pathway. *Nitric Oxide* **2018**, *78*, 11–21. [CrossRef]
86. Sharples, R.A.; Vella, L.J.; Nisbet, R.M.; Naylor, R.; Perez, K.; Barnham, K.J.; Masters, C.L.; Hill, A.F. Inhibition of gamma-secretase causes increased secretion of amyloid precursor protein C-terminal fragments in association with exosomes. *FASEB J.* **2008**, *22*, 1469–1478. [CrossRef]
87. Yuyama, K.; Sun, H.; Sakai, S.; Mitsutake, S.; Okada, M.; Tahara, H.; Furukawa, J.; Fujitani, N.; Shinohara, Y.; Igarashi, Y. Decreased amyloid-β pathologies by intracerebral loading of glycosphingolipid-enriched exosomes in Alzheimer model mice. *J. Biol. Chem.* **2014**, *289*, 24488–24498. [CrossRef]

88. De Godoy, M.A.; Saraiva, L.M.; de Carvalho, L.R.P.; Vasconcelos-Dos-Santos, A.; Beiral, H.J.V.; Ramos, A.B.; Silva, L.R.P.; Leal, R.B.; Monteiro, V.H.S.; Braga, C.V.; et al. Mesenchymal stem cells and cell-derived extracellular vesicles protect hippocampal neurons from oxidative stress and synapse damage induced by amyloid-β oligomers. *J. Biol. Chem.* **2018**, *293*, 1957–1975. [CrossRef]
89. Falker, C.; Hartmann, A.; Guett, I.; Dohler, F.; Altmeppen, H.; Betzel, C.; Schubert, R.; Thurm, D.; Wegwitz, F.; Joshi, P.; et al. Exosomal cellular prion protein drives fibrillization of amyloid beta and counteracts amyloid beta-mediated neurotoxicity. *J. Neurochem.* **2016**, *137*, 88–100. [CrossRef]
90. Xin, H.; Li, Y.; Buller, B.; Katakowski, M.; Zhang, Y.; Wang, X.; Shang, X.; Zhang, Z.G.; Chopp, M. Exosome-mediated transfer of miR-133b from multipotent mesenchymal stromal cells to neural cells contributes to neurite outgrowth. *Stem Cells* **2012**, *30*, 1556–1564. [CrossRef]
91. Ba, Q.; Cui, C.; Wen, L.; Feng, S.; Zhou, J.; Yang, K. Schisandrin B shows neuroprotective effect in 6-OHDA-induced Parkinson's disease via inhibiting the negative modulation of miR-34a on Nrf2 pathway. *Biomed. Pharm.* **2015**, *75*, 165–172. [CrossRef] [PubMed]
92. Narbute, K.; Piļipenko, V.; Pupure, J.; Dzirkale, Z.; Jonavičė, U.; Tunaitis, V.; Kriaučiūnaitė, K.; Jarmalavičiūtė, A.; Jansone, B.; Kluša, V.; et al. Intranasal Administration of Extracellular Vesicles Derived from Human Teeth Stem Cells Improves Motor Symptoms and Normalizes Tyrosine Hydroxylase Expression in the Substantia Nigra and Striatum of the 6-Hydroxydopamine-Treated Rats. *Stem Cells Transl. Med.* **2019**, *8*, 490–499. [CrossRef]
93. Mao, S.; Sun, Q.; Xiao, H.; Zhang, C.; Li, L. Secreted miR-34a in astrocytic shedding vesicles enhanced the vulnerability of dopaminergic neurons to neurotoxins by targeting Bcl-2. *Protein Cell* **2015**, *6*, 529–540. [CrossRef]
94. Chen, P.; Chen, F.; Lei, J.; Li, Q.; Zhou, B. Activation of the miR-34a-Mediated SIRT1/mTOR Signaling Pathway by Urolithin A Attenuates D-Galactose-Induced Brain Aging in Mice. *Neurotherapeutics* **2019**, *16*, 1269–1282. [CrossRef]
95. Jiang, Y.; Liu, J.; Chen, L.; Jin, Y.; Zhang, G.; Lin, Z.; Du, S.; Fu, Z.; Chen, T.; Qin, Y.; et al. Serum secreted miR-137-containing exosomes affects oxidative stress of neurons by regulating OXR1 in Parkinson's disease. *Brain Res.* **2019**, *1722*, 146331. [CrossRef]
96. Oh, S.H.; Kim, H.N.; Park, H.J.; Shin, J.Y.; Kim, D.Y.; Lee, P.H. The Cleavage Effect of Mesenchymal Stem Cell and Its Derived Matrix Metalloproteinase-2 on Extracellular α-Synuclein Aggregates in Parkinsonian Models. *Stem Cells Transl. Med.* **2017**, *6*, 949–961. [CrossRef]
97. Lee, M.; Im, W.; Kim, M. Exosomes as a potential messenger unit during heterochronic parabiosis for amelioration of Huntington's disease. *Neurobiol. Dis.* **2021**, *155*, 105374. [CrossRef]
98. Lee, M.; Liu, T.; Im, W.; Kim, M. Exosomes from adipose-derived stem cells ameliorate phenotype of Huntington's disease in vitro model. *Eur. J. Neurosci.* **2016**, *44*, 2114–2119. [CrossRef]
99. Jeon, I.; Cicchetti, F.; Cisbani, G.; Lee, S.; Li, E.; Bae, J.; Lee, N.; Li, L.; Im, W.; Kim, M.; et al. Human-to-mouse prion-like propagation of mutant huntingtin protein. *Acta Neuropathol.* **2016**, *132*, 577–592. [CrossRef]
100. Das, E.; Jana, N.R.; Bhattacharyya, N.P. MicroRNA-124 targets CCNA2 and regulates cell cycle in STHdh(Q111)/Hdh(Q111) cells. *Biochem. Biophys. Res. Commun.* **2013**, *437*, 217–224. [CrossRef]
101. Lee, S.T.; Im, W.; Ban, J.J.; Lee, M.; Jung, K.H.; Lee, S.K.; Chu, K.; Kim, M. Exosome-Based Delivery of miR-124 in a Huntington's Disease Model. *J. Mov. Disord.* **2017**, *10*, 45–52. [CrossRef] [PubMed]
102. Ananbeh, H.; Vodicka, P.; Kupcova Skalnikova, H. Emerging Roles of Exosomes in Huntington's Disease. *Int. J. Mol. Sci.* **2021**, *22*, 4085. [CrossRef]
103. Rizzuti, M.; Filosa, G.; Melzi, V.; Calandriello, L.; Dioni, L.; Bollati, V.; Bresolin, N.; Comi, G.P.; Barabino, S.; Nizzardo, M.; et al. MicroRNA expression analysis identifies a subset of downregulated miRNAs in ALS motor neuron progenitors. *Sci. Rep.* **2018**, *8*, 10105. [CrossRef] [PubMed]
104. Pusic, A.D.; Pusic, K.M.; Clayton, B.L.; Kraig, R.P. IFNγ-stimulated dendritic cell exosomes as a potential therapeutic for remyelination. *J. Neuroimmunol.* **2014**, *266*, 12–23. [CrossRef]
105. Derkus, B.; Emregul, K.C.; Emregul, E. A new approach in stem cell research—Exosomes: Their mechanism of action via cellular pathways. *Cell Biol. Int.* **2017**, *41*, 466–475. [CrossRef]
106. Lugli, G.; Cohen, A.M.; Bennett, D.A.; Shah, R.C.; Fields, C.J.; Hernandez, A.G.; Smalheiser, N.R. Plasma Exosomal miRNAs in Persons with and without Alzheimer Disease: Altered Expression and Prospects for Biomarkers. *PLoS ONE* **2015**, *10*, e0139233. [CrossRef]
107. Barbagallo, C.; Mostile, G.; Baglieri, G.; Giunta, F.; Luca, A.; Raciti, L.; Zappia, M.; Purrello, M.; Ragusa, M.; Nicoletti, A. Specific Signatures of Serum miRNAs as Potential Biomarkers to Discriminate Clinically Similar Neurodegenerative and Vascular-Related Diseases. *Cell. Mol. Neurobiol.* **2020**, *40*, 531–546. [CrossRef]
108. Yang, T.T.; Liu, C.G.; Gao, S.C.; Zhang, Y.; Wang, P.C. The Serum Exosome Derived MicroRNA−135a, −193b, and −384 Were Potential Alzheimer's Disease Biomarkers. *Biomed. Environ. Sci.* **2018**, *31*, 87–96.
109. Liu, C.-G.; Song, J.; Zhang, Y.-Q.; Wang, P.-C. MicroRNA-193b is a regulator of amyloid precursor protein in the blood and cerebrospinal fluid derived exosomal microRNA-193b is a biomarker of Alzheimer's disease. *Mol. Med. Rep.* **2014**, *10*, 2395–2400. [CrossRef]
110. Riancho, J.; Vázquez-Higuera, J.L.; Pozueta, A.; Lage, C.; Kazimierczak, M.; Bravo, M.; Calero, M.; Gonalezález, A.; Rodríguez, E.; Lleó, A.; et al. MicroRNA Profile in Patients with Alzheimer's Disease: Analysis of miR-9–5p and miR-598 in Raw and Exosome Enriched Cerebrospinal Fluid Samples. *J. Alzheimer's Dis.* **2017**, *57*, 483–491. [CrossRef]

111. Yao, Y.F.; Qu, M.W.; Li, G.C.; Zhang, F.B.; Rui, H.C. Circulating exosomal miRNAs as diagnostic biomarkers in Parkinson's disease. *Eur. Rev. Med. Pharmacol. Sci.* **2018**, *22*, 5278–5283. [PubMed]
112. Gui, Y.; Liu, H.; Zhang, L.; Lv, W.; Hu, X. Altered microRNA profiles in cerebrospinal fluid exosome in Parkinson disease and Alzheimer disease. *Oncotarget* **2015**, *6*, 37043–37053. [CrossRef] [PubMed]
113. Xu, Q.; Zhao, Y.; Zhou, X.; Luan, J.; Cui, Y.; Han, J. Comparison of the extraction and determination of serum exosome and miRNA in serum and the detection of miR-27a-3p in serum exosome of ALS patients. *Intractable Rare Dis. Res.* **2018**, *7*, 13–18. [CrossRef]
114. Freischmidt, A.; Müller, K.; Ludolph, A.C.; Weishaupt, J.H. Systemic dysregulation of TDP-43 binding microRNAs in amyotrophic lateral sclerosis. *Acta Neuropathol. Commun.* **2013**, *1*, 42. [CrossRef]
115. Toh, W.S.; Lai, R.C.; Zhang, B.; Lim, S.K. MSC exosome works through a protein-based mechanism of action. *Biochem. Soc. Trans.* **2018**, *46*, 843–853. [CrossRef]
116. Albanese, M.; Chen, Y.A.; Hüls, C.; Gärtner, K.; Tagawa, T.; Mejias-Perez, E.; Keppler, O.T.; Göbel, C.; Zeidler, R.; Shein, M.; et al. MicroRNAs are minor constituents of extracellular vesicles that are rarely delivered to target cells. *PLoS Genet.* **2021**, *17*, e1009951. [CrossRef]
117. Chevillet, J.R.; Kang, Q.; Ruf, I.K.; Briggs, H.A.; Vojtech, L.N.; Hughes, S.M.; Cheng, H.H.; Arroyo, J.D.; Meredith, E.K.; Gallichotte, E.N.; et al. Quantitative and stoichiometric analysis of the microRNA content of exosomes. *Proc. Natl. Acad. Sci. USA* **2014**, *111*, 14888–14893. [CrossRef]
118. Song, Y.; Dou, H.; Li, X.; Zhao, X.; Li, Y.; Liu, D.; Ji, J.; Liu, F.; Ding, L.; Ni, Y.; et al. Exosomal miR-146a Contributes to the Enhanced Therapeutic Efficacy of Interleukin-1β-Primed Mesenchymal Stem Cells Against Sepsis. *Stem Cells* **2017**, *35*, 1208–1221. [CrossRef]
119. Tejeda-Mora, H.; Leon, L.G.; Demmers, J.; Baan, C.C.; Reinders, M.E.J.; Bleck, B.; Lombardo, E.; Merino, A.; Hoogduijn, M.J. Proteomic Analysis of Mesenchymal Stromal Cell-Derived Extracellular Vesicles and Reconstructed Membrane Particles. *Int. J. Mol. Sci.* **2021**, *22*, 12935. [CrossRef]
120. Akbari, A.; Jabbari, N.; Sharifi, R.; Ahmadi, M.; Vahhabi, A.; Seyedzadeh, S.J.; Nawaz, M.; Szafert, S.; Mahmoodi, M.; Jabbari, E.; et al. Free and hydrogel encapsulated exosome-based therapies in regenerative medicine. *Life Sci.* **2020**, *249*, 117447. [CrossRef]
121. Cui, G.H.; Guo, H.D.; Li, H.; Zhai, Y.; Gong, Z.B.; Wu, J.; Liu, J.S.; Dong, Y.R.; Hou, S.X.; Liu, J.R. RVG-modified exosomes derived from mesenchymal stem cells rescue memory deficits by regulating inflammatory responses in a mouse model of Alzheimer's disease. *Immun. Ageing* **2019**, *16*, 10. [CrossRef] [PubMed]
122. Haney, M.J.; Klyachko, N.L.; Zhao, Y.; Gupta, R.; Plotnikova, E.G.; He, Z.; Patel, T.; Piroyan, A.; Sokolsky, M.; Kabanov, A.V.; et al. Exosomes as drug delivery vehicles for Parkinson's disease therapy. *J. Control. Release* **2015**, *207*, 18–30. [CrossRef]
123. Liu, X.; Yang, Y.; Li, Y.; Niu, X.; Zhao, B.; Wang, Y.; Bao, C.; Xie, Z.; Lin, Q.; Zhu, L. Integration of stem cell-derived exosomes with in situ hydrogel glue as a promising tissue patch for articular cartilage regeneration. *Nanoscale* **2017**, *9*, 4430–4438. [CrossRef]
124. Tejedor, L.S.; Wostradowski, T.; Gingele, S.; Skripuletz, T.; Gudi, V.; Stangel, M. The Effect of Stereotactic Injections on Demyelination and Remyelination: A Study in the Cuprizone Model. *J. Mol. Neurosci.* **2017**, *61*, 479–488. [CrossRef]
125. Neffendorf, J.E.; Jackson, T.L. Stereotactic radiotherapy for wet age-related macular degeneration: Current perspectives. *Clin. Ophthalmol.* **2015**, *9*, 1829–1834.
126. Kim, H.J.; Seo, S.W.; Chang, J.W.; Lee, J.I.; Kim, C.H.; Chin, J.; Choi, S.J.; Kwon, H.; Yun, H.J.; Lee, J.M.; et al. Stereotactic brain injection of human umbilical cord blood mesenchymal stem cells in patients with Alzheimer's disease dementia: A phase 1 clinical trial. *Alzheimers Dement.* **2015**, *1*, 95–102. [CrossRef]
127. Erdő, F.; Bors, L.A.; Farkas, D.; Bajza, Á.; Gizurarson, S. Evaluation of intranasal delivery route of drug administration for brain targeting. *Brain Res. Bull.* **2018**, *143*, 155–170. [CrossRef]
128. Matsumoto, A.; Takahashi, Y.; Nishikawa, M.; Sano, K.; Morishita, M.; Charoenviriyakul, C.; Saji, H.; Takakura, Y. Accelerated growth of B16BL6 tumor in mice through efficient uptake of their own exosomes by B16BL6 cells. *Cancer Sci.* **2017**, *108*, 1803–1810. [CrossRef]
129. Kodali, M.; Castro, O.W.; Kim, D.K.; Thomas, A.; Shuai, B.; Attaluri, S.; Upadhya, R.; Gitai, D.; Madhu, L.N.; Prockop, D.J.; et al. Intranasally Administered Human MSC-Derived Extracellular Vesicles Pervasively Incorporate into Neurons and Microglia in both Intact and Status Epilepticus Injured Forebrain. *Int. J. Mol. Sci.* **2019**, *21*, 181. [CrossRef]
130. Perets, N.; Betzer, O.; Shapira, R.; Brenstein, S.; Angel, A.; Sadan, T.; Ashery, U.; Popovtzer, R.; Offen, D. Golden Exosomes Selectively Target Brain Pathologies in Neurodegenerative and Neurodevelopmental Disorders. *Nano Lett.* **2019**, *19*, 3422–3431. [CrossRef]
131. Wu, H.; Hu, K.; Jiang, X. From nose to brain: Understanding transport capacity and transport rate of drugs. *Expert Opin. Drug Deliv.* **2008**, *5*, 1159–1168. [CrossRef] [PubMed]
132. Wei, W.; Ao, Q.; Wang, X.; Cao, Y.; Liu, Y.; Zheng, S.G.; Tian, X. Mesenchymal Stem Cell–Derived Exosomes: A Promising Biological Tool in Nanomedicine. *Front. Pharmacol.* **2021**, *11*, 590470. [CrossRef]
133. Shi, Q.; Huo, N.; Wang, X.; Yang, S.; Wang, J.; Zhang, T. Exosomes from oral tissue stem cells: Biological effects and applications. *Cell Biosci.* **2020**, *10*, 108. [CrossRef] [PubMed]
134. Munir, J.; Yoon, J.K.; Ryu, S. Therapeutic miRNA-Enriched Extracellular Vesicles: Current Approaches and Future Prospects. *Cells* **2020**, *9*, 2271. [CrossRef]

135. Luarte, A.; Bátiz, L.F.; Wyneken, U.; Lafourcade, C. Potential Therapies by Stem Cell-Derived Exosomes in CNS Diseases: Focusing on the Neurogenic Niche. *Stem Cells Int.* **2016**, *2016*, 5736059. [CrossRef]
136. Chen, C.C.; Liu, L.; Ma, F.; Wong, C.W.; Guo, X.E.; Chacko, J.V.; Farhoodi, H.P.; Zhang, S.X.; Zimak, J.; Ségaliny, A. Elucidation of exosome migration across the blood–brain barrier model in vitro. *Cell. Mol. Bioeng.* **2016**, *9*, 509–529. [CrossRef]
137. Banks, W.A.; Sharma, P.; Bullock, K.M.; Hansen, K.M.; Ludwig, N.; Whiteside, T.L. Transport of extracellular vesicles across the blood-brain barrier: Brain pharmacokinetics and effects of inflammation. *Int. J. Mol. Sci.* **2020**, *21*, 4407. [CrossRef]
138. Jeske, R.; Bejoy, J.; Marzano, M.; Li, Y. Human Pluripotent Stem Cell-Derived Extracellular Vesicles: Characteristics and Applications. *Tissue Eng. Part B Rev.* **2020**, *26*, 129–144. [CrossRef]
139. Araldi, R.P.; D'Amelio, F.; Vigerelli, H.; de Melo, T.C.; Kerkis, I. Stem Cell-Derived Exosomes as Therapeutic Approach for Neurodegenerative Disorders: From Biology to Biotechnology. *Cells* **2020**, *9*, 2663. [CrossRef]
140. Joo, H.S.; Suh, J.H.; Lee, H.J.; Bang, E.S.; Lee, J.M. Current Knowledge and Future Perspectives on Mesenchymal Stem Cell-Derived Exosomes as a New Therapeutic Agent. *Int. J. Mol. Sci.* **2020**, *21*, 727. [CrossRef]
141. Rezaie, J.; Ajezi, S.; Avci, Ç.B.; Karimipour, M.; Geranmayeh, M.H.; Nourazarian, A.; Sokullu, E.; Rezabakhsh, A.; Rahbarghazi, R. Exosomes and their Application in Biomedical Field: Difficulties and Advantages. *Mol. Neurobiol.* **2018**, *55*, 3372–3393. [CrossRef] [PubMed]
142. Vinaiphat, A.; Sze, S.K. Clinical implications of extracellular vesicles in neurodegenerative diseases. *Expert Rev. Mol. Diagn.* **2019**, *19*, 813–824. [CrossRef]
143. Jarmalavičiūtė, A.; Pivoriūnas, A. Exosomes as a potential novel therapeutic tools against neurodegenerative diseases. *Pharmacol. Res.* **2016**, *113*, 816–822. [CrossRef]
144. Momin, M.Y.; Gaddam, R.R.; Kravitz, M.; Gupta, A.; Vikram, A. The Challenges and Opportunities in the Development of MicroRNA Therapeutics: A Multidisciplinary Viewpoint. *Cells* **2021**, *10*, 3097. [CrossRef]
145. Kalavrizioti, D.; Vourekas, A.; Stamatopoulou, V.; Toumpeki, C.; Giannouli, S.; Stathopoulos, C.; Drainas, D. RNA-mediated therapeutics: From gene inactivation to clinical application. *Curr. Top. Med. Chem.* **2006**, *6*, 1737–1758. [CrossRef]
146. Qiu, L.; Tan, E.K.; Zeng, L. microRNAs and neurodegenerative diseases. In *microRNA: Medical Evidence: From Molecular Biology to Clinical Practice*; Springer: Berlin/Heidelberg, Germany, 2015; pp. 85–105.
147. Li, Z.; Rana, T.M. Therapeutic targeting of microRNAs: Current status and future challenges. *Nat. Rev. Drug Discov.* **2014**, *13*, 622–638. [CrossRef]
148. O'Brien, J.; Hayder, H.; Zayed, Y.; Peng, C. Overview of MicroRNA Biogenesis, Mechanisms of Actions, and Circulation. *Front. Endocrinol.* **2018**, *9*, 402. [CrossRef]
149. Wiklander, O.P.; Nordin, J.Z.; O'Loughlin, A.; Gustafsson, Y.; Corso, G.; Mäger, I.; Vader, P.; Lee, Y.; Sork, H.; Seow, Y. Extracellular vesicle in vivo biodistribution is determined by cell source, route of administration and targeting. *J. Extracell. Vesicles* **2015**, *4*, 26316. [CrossRef]
150. Choo, Y.W.; Kang, M.; Kim, H.Y.; Han, J.; Kang, S.; Lee, J.-R.; Jeong, G.-J.; Kwon, S.P.; Song, S.Y.; Go, S. M1 macrophage-derived nanovesicles potentiate the anticancer efficacy of immune checkpoint inhibitors. *ACS Nano* **2018**, *12*, 8977–8993. [CrossRef]
151. Pulliam, L.; Liston, M.; Sun, B.; Narvid, J. Using neuronal extracellular vesicles and machine learning to predict cognitive deficits in HIV. *J. Neurovirol.* **2020**, *26*, 880–887. [CrossRef]
152. Yee, J.; Oh, K.-W.; Kim, S. Stem Cell Therapy for Neurodegenerative Diseases. *Hanyang Med. Rev.* **2015**, *35*, 229. [CrossRef]
153. Smyth, T.; Kullberg, M.; Malik, N.; Smith-Jones, P.; Graner, M.W.; Anchordoquy, T.J. Biodistribution and delivery efficiency of unmodified tumor-derived exosomes. *J. Control. Release* **2015**, *199*, 145–155. [CrossRef] [PubMed]
154. Takakura, Y.; Matsumoto, A.; Takahashi, Y. Therapeutic application of small extracellular vesicles (sEVs): Pharmaceutical and pharmacokinetic challenges. *Biol. Pharm. Bull.* **2020**, *43*, 576–583. [CrossRef] [PubMed]
155. Maciotta, S.; Meregalli, M.; Torrente, Y. The involvement of microRNAs in neurodegenerative diseases. *Front. Cell. Neurosci.* **2013**, *7*, 265. [CrossRef]
156. Junn, E.; Mouradian, M.M. MicroRNAs in neurodegenerative diseases and their therapeutic potential. *Pharmacol. Ther.* **2012**, *133*, 142–150. [CrossRef]

pharmaceutics

MDPI

Review

Membrane Vesicles Derived from Gut Microbiota and Probiotics: Cutting-Edge Therapeutic Approaches for Multidrug-Resistant Superbugs Linked to Neurological Anomalies

Prakhar Srivastava and Kwang-sun Kim *

Department of Chemistry and Chemistry Institute of Functional Materials, Pusan National University, Busan 46241, Korea
* Correspondence: kwangsun.kim@pusan.ac.kr; Tel.: +82-51-510-2241

Abstract: Multidrug-resistant (MDR) superbugs can breach the blood–brain barrier (BBB), leading to a continuous barrage of pro-inflammatory modulators and induction of severe infection-related pathologies, including meningitis and brain abscess. Both broad-spectrum or species-specific antibiotics (β-lactamase inhibitors, polymyxins, vancomycin, meropenem, plazomicin, and sarecycline) and biocompatible poly (lactic-co-glycolic acid) (PLGA) nanoparticles have been used to treat these infections. However, new therapeutic platforms with a broad impact that do not exert off-target deleterious effects are needed. Membrane vesicles or extracellular vesicles (EVs) are lipid bilayer-enclosed particles with therapeutic potential owing to their ability to circumvent BBB constraints. Bacteria-derived EVs (bEVs) from gut microbiota are efficient transporters that can penetrate the central nervous system. In fact, bEVs can be remodeled via surface modification and CRISPR/Cas editing and, thus, represent a novel platform for conferring protection against infections breaching the BBB. Here, we discuss the latest scientific research related to gut microbiota- and probiotic-derived bEVs, and their therapeutic modifications, in terms of regulating neurotransmitters and inhibiting quorum sensing, for the treatment of neurodegenerative diseases, such as Parkinson's and Alzheimer's diseases. We also emphasize the benefits of probiotic-derived bEVs to human health and propose a novel direction for the development of innovative heterologous expression systems to combat BBB-crossing pathogens.

Keywords: blood–brain barrier; extracellular vesicles; gut microbiota; membrane vesicles; meningitis; probiotics; superbugs

Citation: Srivastava, P.; Kim, K.-s. Membrane Vesicles Derived from Gut Microbiota and Probiotics: Cutting-Edge Therapeutic Approaches for Multidrug-Resistant Superbugs Linked to Neurological Anomalies. *Pharmaceutics* **2022**, *14*, 2370. https://doi.org/10.3390/pharmaceutics14112370

Academic Editor: Yong Chen

Received: 22 September 2022
Accepted: 2 November 2022
Published: 3 November 2022

1. Introduction

The blood–brain barrier (BBB) plays a central role in the unique and complex microenvironment of the central nervous system (CNS) [1]. In particular, it restricts the entry of drugs and other exogenous molecules, including host immune cells [2] and infectious pathogens [3]. Nevertheless, opportunistic pathogens can occasionally breach the BBB and cause serious illnesses, including meningitis and brain abscess [4]. Although the occurrence of CNS infection is relatively rare, chronic malignancies can result in serious neurological disorders [5]. Drug-resistant pathogens, including *Acinetobacter baumannii*, *Escherichia coli*, *Listeria monocytogenes*, *Staphylococcus aureus*, and *Streptococcus* spp. can enter via the respiratory tract and mucosa and breach the BBB [6]. In the BBB, pathogens tightly regulate intrinsic virulence mechanisms via drug-resistance pumps [7] and biofilm formation [8]. *Acinetobacter* spp., *Klebsiella*, and *S. aureus* further modulate the expression of proinflammatory cytokines [9] and movement of immune cells, thereby destabilizing the endothelial lining and tight junctions of the BBB [10]. However, due to the complexity of the brain microenvironment and its associated endothelial tight junctions, transport of effective antimicrobials and therapies is challenging [11]. In fact, the physiological nature of the CNS environment prevents 90–95% of antimicrobials from progressing toward drug development [12]. Various nanoparticles (NPs), especially liposomal NPs [13,14], and their derivatives (e.g., polysaccharide and polyester NPs) [15,16] are considered effective and innovative drugs against pathogens that invade the BBB. However, NP-associated toxicity [17] and dose-dependent mortality [18] seriously limit their application. It is, therefore, necessary to consider alternatives, particularly those that can mimic non-immunogenic biological entities [19].

Membrane vesicles or extracellular vesicles (EVs) play crucial roles in polymicrobial interkingdom communication [20]. Microbial evolution involves the continuous transfer of metabolites via nanosized vesicles that carry important biomolecules, virulence factors, and membrane receptors of the cells from which they originate [21] to proximal and distant cells via blood and lymphatic systems. These vesicles range in size from 20 to 400 nm. The release of EVs is a general phenomenon performed by many cell types, including those of eukaryotes, Gram-negative/-positive bacteria, and archaea [22], as a means of communicating with other cells. In particular, bEVs have been characterized as the delivery vehicles of host–microbe interactions, responsible for the delivery of signaling molecules, such as autoinducers, virulence factors [23,24], and antibiotic genes [25,26]. In contrast to pathogen–host interactions, mucosal- or gut microbiota-derived bEVs contribute to homeostasis, immune system regulation, bowel movements, and the gut–brain axis [27]. Based on their immunomodulatory properties, gut microbiota-derived bEVs are currently employed in therapies aimed at promoting both humoral and cell-mediated responses [28]. Among them, tuning probiotic-derived bEVs, for interactions between interstitial cells and the gut–brain axis, represents a novel strategy for promoting immune responses during infectious disease [29]. Furthermore, this strategy can benefit from the ease of fermentation culture techniques, potential application of probiotics, and mucoadhesive encapsulation [30,31]. Moreover, combining functional biomaterials with active bEVs has the potential to target autoimmune inflammatory dispositions and treat severe chronic infections [32]. More specifically, beneficial gut microbiota-derived bEVs are a promising tool to regulate the gut–brain axis by reducing inflammation and restoring immunity [33], creating a benchmark for the targeted delivery of drugs to the CNS. However, currently, most EV-based drugs are derived from eukaryotic systems, including those for cancer [34], gastric disorders, and polymicrobial infections, due to the various challenges related to bEVs [35]. Nevertheless, genetically modifying bEVs via surface remodeling [36] to target neurotransmitters and quorum sensing (QS) inhibitors, and through CRISPR/Cas system-based modifications [37], has the potential to provide novel noninvasive therapies against BBB infections [38].

In this review, we introduce cutting-edge research on the mechanism of action and production of gut microbiota- and probiotic-derived bEVs against pathogens crossing the BBB. Hence, this article will serve as a valuable resource for future research aimed at enhancing the production of probiotic-derived bEVs in the context of antimicrobial research and designing novel heterologous expression systems.

2. Blood–Brain Barrier (BBB): A Roadblock to Invading Pathogens

The endothelial layer of the BBB selectively transports immune cells and other metabolites involved in maintaining the functional stability of the nervous system [39]. However, during the neonatal period, in some cases, the BBB can shield pathogens, resulting in a breach of the protective layer and subsequent serious disorders and infection [40]. Endogenous markers, such as pathogen-associated molecular patterns and small molecular motifs conserved within a class of microbes [41], are recognized by endothelial receptors of the BBB. This recognition results in an immunological burst at the target site [42] that can breach the endothelial lining. Moreover, the complicated structure of the CNS limits the access of several antimicrobial agents to the nervous system [43], however, facilitating the transport of lipophilic drugs with a molecular weight <400 Da [44] that form fewer than eight hydrogen bonds via lipid-mediated free diffusion [45], into the bloodstream via the transcellular route [46]. As efficient drugs, antiepileptics (e.g., diazepam and phenytoin) [47,48], PLGA-coated nanoparticles, and laser-assisted therapies (e.g., focused ultrasound and interstitial thermal therapy) are commercially available [49,50]. However, these therapies do not guarantee the long-term potency of drugs because the microbial flora is constantly evolving, either through horizontal gene transfer or cell-to-cell communication, resulting in reduced susceptibility to certain drugs [51].

3. Multidrug-Resistant (MDR) Superbugs: A Prominent Case Involving the BBB

Infections caused by MDR superbugs have emerged as a major threat to global health in the post-antibiotic era, especially in the 21st century [52]. The Centre for Disease Control and World Health Organization have predicted that there will be ~2 million cases of MDR infections and 27,000 related deaths per year by 2050 in Asia, Africa, and North America [53]. Carbapenem and colistin are the most widely used last-resort antibiotics against bacterial infections [54]; however, by the late 2000s, drug resistance exhibited an unexpected increase in mortality associated with hospital-acquired infections by 40–60% [55]. Pan-drug resistant *A. baumannii* is routinely reported in patients with meningitis [56–58] and has acquired resistance to most antibiotic therapies, including colistin and tetracycline [59,60]. Although combined treatment with gentamicin and meropenem is efficient, the reduction rate of infection is <17–19% [61] given that the BBB limits the permeability of drugs and the continuous administration of drugs further increases the probability of resistance [62,63]. Moreover, frequently screened drug-resistant pathogens (*A. baumannii* [64] and *E. coli* [65]), few routinely screened pathogens (*N. meningitidis* and *Streptococcus* spp.) [66,67], other neuroinvasive pathogens (*Haemophilus influenzae*) [68], and *Chlamydophila pneumoniae* [69] not only disrupt the tight junctions of the BBB but also induce leakage between tight junctions and vascular endothelial cells [70]. For example, Gram-positive *L. monocytogenes*, *Staphylococcus* spp., and *Streptococcus pneumoniae* elevate the levels of proinflammatory cytokines and disrupt the endothelial lining in the CNS [71], thus creating a path of invasion for opportunistic pathogens.

4. Bacteria-Derived EVs (bEVs): Nanoscale Vesicles

bEVs have been studied since the early 1960s when lipid-like structures released from *E. coli* were discovered as a means to transport secondary metabolites and intrinsic biomolecules to the communicating host [72]. After the discovery of bEV production from Gram-positive bacteria, such as *Bacillus subtilis*, *Mycobacterium tuberculosis*, *S. aureus*, and *Streptococcus* spp., bEV release is regarded as a general phenomenon carried out by bacteria that has an important role in cell-to-cell communication and disease progression during gastric cancers and tuberculosis [73,74]. Cell-to-cell communication by bEVs involves internalization via the endothelial layer, micropinocytosis, and endocytosis by utilizing invasion proteins at the host–pathogen interface [75]. Certain pathways, such as the stress induced network, cause bEVs to function as anti-phagocytosis bodies, evading phagocytosis and weakening the clearing mechanism via the host immune response [76]. *M. tuberculosis* is a classic example of pathogen evasion of the innate immune responses; that is, it infects phagocytic and inhibits phagosome maturation. Moreover, Athman et al. [77] discovered that *Mycobacterium* bEVs produce lipoglycans and lipoproteins that play an important role in regulating the host immune response and facilitating persistent infection. Further, it was found that *S. aureus*-derived bEVs contain super-antigens (protein A and lipase) that aid cells in phagocytosis evasion. Meanwhile, a proteomics study [78] found that immunoglobulin (IgG)-bound lipase and super-antigen (hydrogenated form of squalene; SQA) are presented in bEVs, thus highlighting the potential role of *S. aureus* in evading anti-phagocytic activity via super-antigens and lipase production. bEVs also have a basic role in exchange of genetic materials (DNA and RNA) through horizontal gene transfer, during which bEVs serve as a means of cell-to-cell communication within the same bacterial species [79]. Additionally, a study conducted on bEV cargo of *A. baumannii* reported the presence of a carbapenamse gene (*bla*$_{OXA-24}$) that increases the antibiotic susceptibility pattern against β-lactam antibiotics [80]. Similar studies on bEVs derived from *N. gonorrhoeae* [81] and *S. aureus* [82] have identified the presence of the outer membrane (OM) protein PorB and alpha toxins that transfer genetic materials, inducing apoptosis and host cell death.

bEVs released from the cell envelope of Gram-negative bacteria are so-called outer membrane vesicles (OMVs). The envelope is made up of three layers: the OM, cytoplasmic membrane, and the periplasmic space in between, which contains a layer of peptidoglycan (PG) [83]. An inside leaflet of phospholipids and an outer leaflet of lipopolysaccharide (LPS; also known as endotoxin) constitute the OM. LPS causes inflammatory responses in host cells [84], whereas the OM has a porous structure that aids in waste removal and nutrition uptake, and the peptidoglycan (PG) layer maintains the osmotic pressure of the cell and regulates the hostile environment (antibiotic stress) [85]. Gram-positive, unlike Gram-negative, bEVs are produced from cytoplasmic constituents via a blebbing mechanism; their genetic composition is comparable to that of Gram-negative bEVs, with the exception of the lipoprotein structure [86]. Apart from the normal mechanism of blebbing, prophage-encoded endolysins have also facilitated bEV release from Gram-negative and -positive bacteria. Studies on *Bacillus* spp. and *Staphylococcus* spp. have revealed that the prophage-encoded endolysin generates holes in the peptidoglycan cell wall, thus highlighting the potential role of these enzymes in bacterial cell wall lysis during mass production of bEVs [87,88].

5. Nanoscale bEVs as Potential Therapeutic Platforms

Recently, bioinspired NPs such as host (eukaryotic) EVs (hEV) and bEVs have shown promising effects against chronic infections [89,90]. Compared with their nanomaterial counterparts (liposomal NPs), bEVs provide increased drug delivery and efficient antigen-presenting properties [91–93]. Various microbes including *Helicobacter* spp., *Klebsiella pneumoniae*, *Lactobacillus* spp., *P. aeruginosa*, *S. aureus*, and *Streptococcus* spp. are involved in the transfer of metabolites between species for intracellular communication and are used in novel adjuvant-associated therapeutics as well as nano-sized vaccine delivery platforms for various infections [94,95] (Table 1).

Table 1. bEVs involved in the pathogenic infections and their roles.

Origin of bEV	Infecting Pathogens	Role of bEV	Reference
Gram-positive bacteria			
Bifidobacterium longum	Food-borne infections	Induction of progenitor cells	[96]
Burkholderia spp.	Activity against *A. baumannii* and *S. aureus*	N.D.	[97]
L. gasseri	Human Immunodeficiency Virus (HIV)	Change in susceptibility pattern of viral infection by regulation of toll-like receptor (TLR)-2 signaling	[98]
L. rhamnosus	Superficial infections	M2 Macrophage	[99]
S. aureus	*Pneumococcal* infection	TH1-mediated cell immunity	[100]
Streptococcus spp.	*Streptococcal* infection	Induction of dendritic cells	[101]
Tetragenococcus halophilus	Opportunistic pathogens	Anti-inflammatory factor interferon beta (IFN-β)	[102]
Gram-negative bacteria			
Acinetobacter spp.	Pan-drug resistant *A. baumannii*	Activation of IgG and IgM	[103]
Borrelia burgdorferi	*B. burgdorferi* colonization	Stabilizing superoxide	[104]
Helicobacter pylori	*H. pylori* infection	Induction of TH2 immune cells	[105]
K. pneumoniae	*K. pneumoniae* infection	Humoral and cellular immunity	[106]
N. meningitis	Meningococcal disease	IgG-mediated response	[107]
Pertussis A	*Bordetella pertussis* infection	Induction of CD4 cells	[108]
P. aeruginosa	Lethal dose of *P. aeruginosa*	Mixed cellular response	[109]

hEVs have shown complexity of the yield coefficient, a high production cost, and limited downstream process, all of which limit their biomedical applications [110,111] (Table 2). The continuous evaluation of EVs as potential tools against chronic infection has led to the development of bEVs derived from *Clostridium butyricum* [112] and *L. paracasei* [113]. Given that most chronic illnesses involve 'dysbiosis' of the gut microbiota, tuning the absorption capacity and nutrition digestion factors of the microbiome might influence the host–microbe physiological imbalance.

Table 2. Current limitations of eukaryotic and bacterial EVs in biomedical applications.

Eukaryotic (hEVs)	Bacterial (bEVs)	Common Limitations
Differentiation between cell surface markers	Lipopolysaccharide (LPS) toxicity	Immunomodulators outburst
Inefficient purification of vesicles	High inflammatory responses	Low viability and inefficient growth conditions
Lack of heterogeneity	High chance of infection (pathogen-derived bEVs)	High cellular toxicity

6. Unresolved Issues with Gut Microbiota-Derived bEVs in Modulating the Gut–Brain Axis: *Old Is Gold*

The continuous usage of antibiotics during BBB infections leads to prognosis of early psychosis and neurotoxicity [114]. Gut microbiota dysbiosis, a state where the physiological combinations of flora are transformed into pathological combinations [115] via continuous antibiotic administration, has been linked to neural abnormalities. This link is via the vagal nerve, which is associated with a lower response of neurotransmitters inducing systemic inflammation in the CNS [116]. These features highlight the importance of the gut–brain axis in modulating CNS homeostasis.

6.1. Gut–Brain Axis

The term '*Gut–Brain axis*' refers to a bidirectional network that includes multiple connections such as the vagus nerve (nervous control), immune coordination (epithelial and mucosal barrier), and secondary metabolite generation from microbes [117]. The complex architecture of the gut–brain axis entails the constant transit of neurotransmitters within the gastrointestinal (GI) tract, which, in turn, modulates the immune system, including macrophages and mast cells [118]. These immune cells boost neuron excitability and regulate the host's behavioral response. A recent study found that gut dysbiosis caused by a broad-spectrum antibiotic during traumatic brain injury (TBI) resulted in increased neuronal loss, suppressed neurogenesis, altered microglia and peripheral immune response, and modulated fear memory response, suggesting a role of gut microbiota in the recovery from TBI [119].

6.2. Gut Microbiota-Derived bEVs vs. Eukaryotic-Derived hEVs (Physiological Counterpart)

Generally, the use of hEVs is significantly limited by the yield coefficient and high-throughput screening. In addition, the current scenario for combating antibiotic resistance with chronic illness is not favored by the use of pathogen-derived bEVs, because the sudden release of pro-inflammatory factors by bacteria cannot be controlled [120]. In contrast, beneficial gut microbiota have shown the effective immune responses and efficient pathogen inhibition activity [121]. Moreover, bEVs from beneficial gut microbiota take a role in triggering inflammatory responses through LPS and lipoteichoic acid [122] and can cross the intestinal barrier, and have effective anti-inflammatory properties against chronic infections and gut dysbiosis [123]. The physiological features of hEVs differ significantly from gut microbiota-derived bEVs, as shown in Table 3.

Table 3. Difference between eukaryotic-derived hEVs and gut-microbiota-derived bEVs.

Category	Eukaryotic-Derived hEVs	Gut-Microbiota-Derived bEVs
Biogenesis	Generally produced from plasma membrane except exosomes, which originate from endocytic pathway	Gram-negative bacteria: decreased protein linkages between the OM and peptidoglycan, accumulation of unfolded proteins and/or peptidoglycan in the periplasmic space, and explosive cell lysis Gram-positive bacteria: turgor pressure by accumulation of bEVs and the action of cell-wall-degrading enzymes
Composition (Cargo)	Multivesicular bodies composed of endosomal proteins; RNA and miRNA are regularly incorporated	Proteins, peptidoglycans, lipids, LPS, lipoteichoic acids (LTA), nucleic acids, and metabolites
Major functions	Intercellular communications (cell proliferation, matrix formation, and phagocytosis)	Innate and adaptive immunity, bacterial communications, interaction with host miRNA for movement across intestinal barrier
Size	40–100 nm (exosomes) [124]; 500–2000 nm (apoptotic bodies) and 100–500 nm (microvesicles) [125]	10–300 nm [126]

6.3. Problems Related to Gut Microbiota-Derived bEVs on BBB-Associated Diseases

The 'dysbiosis' condition in the gut microbiota environment by antibiotic usage has also shown certain detrimental impacts such as Alzheimer's disease, autism, and arthritis, all of which clearly demonstrate the mechanistic behavior and coordinated axis of mental health and intestinal mucosa [127]. A study by Lee et al. [128] showed that the release of bEVs from a gut pathogen *Paenalcaligenes hominis*, revealed movement of bEVs via the vagus nerve, producing cognitive impairment in the nervous system. Another study using *Porphyromonas gingivalis*, an oral pathogen, demonstrated the importance of LPS-coated bEVs in the onset of Alzheimer's disease, emphasizing the role of protease and LPS in triggering the damage of collagen fibers, fibrinogen connective tissues, and induction of proinflammatory mediators in the transfer of bEVs that alter brain cognitive function [129]. The main drawback of bEVs derived from the gut microbiota is that they have a negative impact on memory, cognition, and neuroinflammation. Therefore, direct application of such bEVs may have both adverse and beneficial neurologic effects on CNS homeostasis.

6.4. Beneficial Roles of Probiotic-Derived bEVs on Gut–Brain-Axis Control

Considering the diverse array of gut microbiota from intestinal niches, probiotics including *Bifidobacterium* spp. and *Lactobacillus* spp. have been identified to create neurotransmitters (acetylcholine, gamma-aminobutyric acid (GABA), and serotonin), which continually control CNS homeostasis [130,131]. Overall, probiotics not only govern the bidirectional transit of biochemical signals, but also improve the host's behavioral response such as anxiety [132], depression, and stroke [133]. Apart from periodontal and gut pathogens, probiotics such as *Lactobacillus* spp. have influence on the motor neuron complex (M-N complex). This M-N complex includes the enteric nervous system (endocrine functions and secretion from intestinal mucosa) and the vagus nerve. *Lactobacillus* spp. normally modulates the neurotransmitter signals via the vagus nerve (intestinal nerve), involving sensory transmission of neuronal signals via the enteric nervous system to the CNS [131]. Few bEVs derived from *Lactobacillus* spp. have also demonstrated the direct regulation of the gut–brain axis in CNS homeostasis (Table 4).

Table 4. Beneficial roles of probiotic-derived bEVs on gut–brain-axis control.

Origin of bEVs	Roles of bEVs	References
L. acidophilus	Changes in complex microbial communities	[134]
L. plantarum	Enhance the action of brain-derived neurotropic factor (BDNF), lowering the stress level in hippocampus neuron	[135]
L. reuteri DSM 17938	Modulate intestinal and colon motility and enhance gut–brain intercommunication for CNS homeostasis	[136]
L. rhamnosus	Reduce the behavioral changes including anxiety and depression	[137]

7. Filling Gaps with Probiotic-Derived bEVs against BBB-Breaching Pathogens

The fundamental issue with antibiotic therapy is the associated drug resistance, which causes a widespread distribution of MDR BBB-breaching bacteria, causing secondary neurological disorders that impair CNS homeostasis [138]. Moreover, the risks associated with the continuous use of antibiotics include seizure, neuromuscular blockade, cranial nerve toxicity, and intracranial hypertension [139]. Conventional therapeutic options for the treatment of MDR bacterial infections include β-lactamase inhibitors, aminoglycosides, fluoroquinolones, and last-resort polymyxins [140,141]. However, such therapies have limited efficacy in CNS infections caused by MDR bacteria, such as *A. baumannii*, *K. pneumoniae*, *M. tuberculosis*, *L. monocytogenes*, *N. meningitidis*, and *Streptococcus* spp. (Table 5). This is due to the BBB integrity as well as severe side-effects such as neurotoxicity and nonspecific targeting. The continuous administration of antibiotics, and its associated risk factors, often creates dysregulation between the gut microbiota and the cerebrospinal fluid of the CNS. Mucosal bacteria regulate the communication between the enteric nervous system and peripheral intestinal regulation. Meanwhile, the constant dysregulation caused by antibiotic overuse has created a gap between efficient metabolism of intestinal regulation and CNS modulation.

Table 5. BBB-breaching pathogenic infections and associated immunomodulatory activity.

Pathogen	Mode of Pathogenesis	Immunological Factors Contributing BBB Infection	References
A. baumannii	-Meningitis -Catheter-associated infection	Increased inflammatory cell response, toll-like receptor (TLR) altered expression, and proinflammatory cytokine burst within 24 h of infection	[142,143]
E. coli	-Endothelial cells -Attenuation of transforming growth factor (TGF)-β 1 signaling	Increased expression of endothelial-derived platelet-derived growth factor receptor (PDFGR) and intercellular adhesion molecule (ICAM), resulting in inflammation	[144]
H. influenzae	-Large amount of vascular endothelial growth factor receptor (VEGFR) -Adenosine receptor dysfunction	Endothelial disruption and tight junction altered expression: downregulation of tumor necrosis factor (TNF-α); endothelial proliferation	[145,146]
K. pneumoniae	-Cerebrospinal infection -Intracranial infection	Increased production of proinflammatory cytokines and chemokines; induction of hypoxia inducible factor (HIF)-1α	[147]
L. monocytogenes	-Vimentin-mediated infection Neuroinflammation	In1F virulent factor-associated downregulation of tight junction and overexpression of PDFGR and ICAM, resulting in inflammation	[148]
N. meningitidis	-Secretion of IgA protease -Evasion of immune response	Deformation of adherence junction, triggering IL-6 and IL-8 expression: leukocyte infiltration and infected phagocyte movement	[149,150]
P. aeruginosa	-Cerebrospinal infection -Meningitis	Increased production of inflammatory cell response; overproduction of IL-1β and IL-6	[151]

Table 5. *Cont.*

Pathogen	Mode of Pathogenesis	Immunological Factors Contributing BBB Infection	References
S. aureus	-Brain abscesses and endocarditis -Cytokine burst	Stimulate immune invasion, T cell activation: burst of proinflammatory cytokines; TNF-α, IL-6, and IL-10 overproduction	[152]
S. pneumoniae	-Neonatal meningitis -Laminin receptor transcytosis	TNF-α, IL-6, and IL-10 overproduction and increased permeability through anchored tight junction; cleavage of IgA through *pneumococci* IgA protease	[153,154]

Several probiotics such as *Bifidobacterium* spp., *L. lactis*, and *L. rhamanosus* are being actively investigated for their therapeutic potential and are in the final stage of clinical trials [155]. bEVs originated from such species have gained attention as effective therapeutic platforms owing to their natural immunogenicity and self-adjuvating properties [156], which induce a better adaptive immune response and can transport diverse cargos across various cell types. In addition, such therapeutic platforms against antibiotic-resistance-related neurological disorders could be improved using genetic modification of gut microbiota with the CRISPR/Cas9 system [157]. The antimicrobial activity of probiotic-derived bEVs against pathogens has revealed a broader role of probiotics in enhancing the anti-inflammatory response during pathogen invasion (Table 6).

Table 6. Probiotic-derived bEVs against BBB-invading pathogens.

Origin of bEV	Physiological Roles	Invading Pathogen(s)	References
Burkholderia thailandensis with quinolone	Synergistic antibiofilm activity	*Streptococcus* spp.	[158]
E. coli Nissle 1917	Increased anti-inflammatory properties, such as IL-10 and T helper (T_H) cell-mediated cytotoxicity	*E. coli* and *S. aureus*	[159]
L. crispatus and *L. jensenii*	Antibiofilm and anti-inflammatory effect	*Candida albicans*	[160]
L. paracasei and *L. plantarum*	Decrease pro-inflammatory cytokine production	Enteroinvasive *E. coli*	[161]

A proteomics study of probiotic *L. plantarum* BGAN8-derived bEVs that regulate brain function [136] revealed the enrichment in enzymes involved in central metabolic pathways and in membrane components with transporters [162]. Because such proteins are associated with transferring beneficial metabolites to pathogens or hosts, proteomics of probiotic-derived bEVs appears to be a potential tool to reveal underlying mechanisms of bEVs on escaping pathogen infection and the beneficial effect on brain function.

Vaccine-antigen-presenting probiotic-derived bEVs can also be employed as vehicles to transport antigens and potent antimicrobial agents to specific targets. Moreover, given that probiotics regulate various intrinsic signals, such as regulation of active short chain fatty acids, hormone metabolism, and neurotransmitters signaling and expression, they can also facilitate a wide range of interactions between the normal flora and host cognitive behavior [163]. Moreover, their role in regulating the gut–brain axis has highlighted the potential application of probiotic-derived bEVs for enhancing the neurodevelopment process [164]. For instance, studies with *L. plantarum* JB-1-derived bEVs highlighted the role of bEVs in regulating the neuron signaling system [165], demonstrating the direct role that probiotic-derived bEVs have in CNS development [166] (Figure 1). Moreover, unlike host immune cells, bEVs derived from immune cells can pass though the BBB and, thus, participate in the immunological regulation of the CNS.

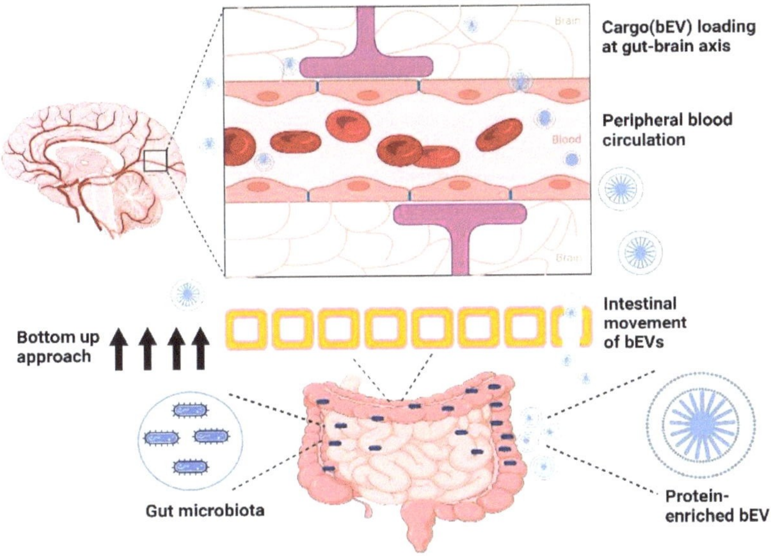

Figure 1. Bottom-up approach for the transport of probiotic-derived extracellular vesicles (bEVs). The figure was created using BioRender.com (https://app.biorender.com; accessed on 2 November 2022).

8. Remodeling of Probiotic-Derived bEVs against BBB-Invading Pathogens

NP-derived therapeutics show high efficacy against pathogens [167]. As it is possible to control the size and release of NP-derived therapeutics, modified NPs are potential candidates for conferring protection against drug-resistant pathogens [168]. Combination therapies with commercial antibiotics also exert beneficial effects against antibiotic-resistant pathogens; however, their selectivity and toxicity remain major concerns [169]. The modification of NPs with EVs has been driven by the aim to increase yield and reduce toxicity [170,171]. For instance, amalgamated nanocarriers with hEVs have shown promising results in cancer therapy [172]. However, to induce an efficient immunogenic response with low toxicity, bEVs from probiotics should be used in native or genetically modified form to protect against hospital-acquired infections [173]. Such an engineered, or remodeled, probiotic-derived bEV will have advantages over conventional drug delivery systems in terms of their bioavailability and targeted drug distribution.

8.1. Surface-Modified Proteins in Probiotic-Derived bEVs

Exosome-associated transmembrane proteins and their fusion to peptide domains have been investigated for their ability to confer protection against various pathological conditions in eukaryotes. For example, their role in tumor therapy, and the delivery of siRNAs and miRNAs targeting immune cells and neuronal junctions of the brain, have been evaluated [174]. However, targeting the efficiency of surface-modified probiotic-derived bEVs has not been evaluated in infections involving BBB breach. Among prokaryotes, a two-component signaling system in Gram-positive bacteria regulates diverse intracellular signals, including genetic transduction and bacteriocin production [175]. Studies conducted on *Bifidobacterium* spp., *L. gasseri*, and *L. plantarum* have demonstrated the role of the two-component system in the regulation of bacteriocin production [176]. For instance, surface-associated proteins of *Lactobacillus* spp., such as histidine protein kinase (HPK), and S-layer proteins (SlpA, B, and X) [177], have been explored in bEV studies for evaluating heterologous gene expression and enhancement of host–microbe interactions. HPK-associated recombinant protein expression is a novel approach for biotherapeutic delivery. Previous studies on bEVs revealed that the expression of heterologous antigens such as OmpA was in response to infection severity. The production of fusion proteins and hemolysin ClyA in *E. coli* bEVs elicited an immune response against green fluorescent (GFP) protein [178]. The concept may involve the association of a signal peptide with a reporter system that can trigger the robust secretion of target molecules for cell surface display. Similarly, the Slp system has been studied extensively in *L. acidophilus* and *L. brevis* against diarrhea and skin infections [179]. A system with strong transcription facilitated by promoter fusion [180] could increase protein production and provide a useful vaccine delivery platform. Strategies for protection against infections crossing the BBB may involve the addition of the Slp short peptide region to the upstream region of the targeted antigen or therapeutic gene, which can increase the secretion and efficacy of the therapeutic protein against infectious agents [181].

8.2. Regulation of Neurotransmitters across the BBB

BBB-associated infections are related to Parkinson's and Alzheimer's diseases, in which direct correlations between pathogens such as *Staphylococcus* spp. have been demonstrated to regulate the neurotransmitter-serotonin signaling mechanism [182]. To date, the interaction of probiotics with host miRNAs in regulating host cerebral inflammatory signaling is rare. Instead, the regulation of the bidirectional movement of miRNA by probiotic-derived bEVs in regulating the neuro-immune endocrine regulation was reported [183].

Only a few studies examining the relationship between probiotics and the serotonergic system, as well as the role of the GI tract in managing neuropsychotic disorders, have been reported. For instance, a previous study [30] reported that *Akkermansia muciniphila*, an intestinal symbiont colonizing the mucosal layer, increases the serotonin signaling pathway via the gut–brain axis in mice. More specifically, they showed that downregulation of *Htr* mediators (secreted metabolites in the colon) in the intestinal mucosa activates the bacterial colonization and, hence, increases the serotonin level and enteric neuronal activity. One classic study on probiotic supplements, including short-chain and long-chain oligosaccharides, showed that lower expression of *Htr* reduces anxiety behavior in mice, thus demonstrating the possible significance of probiotics in maintaining neurotransmitter signaling [184].

8.3. Quorum-Quenching Proteins

Studies of microbiome-associated neurological disorders have supported the systemic movement of quorum-sensing molecules [185] and their associated virulence factors. These factors penetrate tight junctions using the Trojan horse method and trigger nervous system connections [186]. Pathogens (e.g., *Clostridium* and *Streptomyces* species) can induce nervous system dysregulation and result in anxiety and stress-associated disorders [187]. The association between polymicrobial infections and common neurological disorders has been clarified; however, well-established tools to overcome chronic-infection-associated neurological disorders, such as bacterial meningitis and polymicrobial-associated multiple sclerosis, are needed [185]. Most neurological disorders are accompanied by a decreased abundance of beneficial, as well as commensal, microbes. Accordingly, it may be possible to express quorum-quenching-related proteins on the surface of probiotic-derived bEVs, as a targeted approach against microbes to reduce their virulence and chronicity.

8.4. bEVs as a Drug Delivery Platform to Prevent Degradation and Immune Elimination of Antimicrobials

Regarding CNS infections, most CNS-associated drugs have side-effects and lack the potential to cross the BBB. Additionally, the inefficient movement of neurotherapeutic drugs requires them to remain in the neural environment for a sufficient duration to exert the desired effect. The presence of phosphorylated glycoprotein (P-gp) in the endothelial lining of the BBB undoubtedly limits the entry of lipophilic drugs, thus increasing the risk of meningococcal infections [188]. Antibiotics such as vancomycin, meropenem, fluoroquinolones, β-lactams (occasionally), and cephalosporins are thought to be effective against CNS infection. However, inefficient administration and toxicity levels limit their usage [189]. In this case, bEVs can act as high specific loading cargos for antibiotics to provide a shielding effect [190], which will protect the antibiotics against various pathogen-derived enzymes and multi-antigen determinants on the surface will specifically target meningococcal infections [191].

8.5. CRISPR/Cas-Modified bEVs as Biotherapeutic Agents against BBB-Breach-Related Infections

The CRISPR/Cas system is a novel gene editing approach that has been successfully employed to make opportunistic pathogens (e.g., *E. coli* and *S. aureus*) vulnerable to commercially available antibiotics, or to reverse their drug resistance [192] (Figure 2).

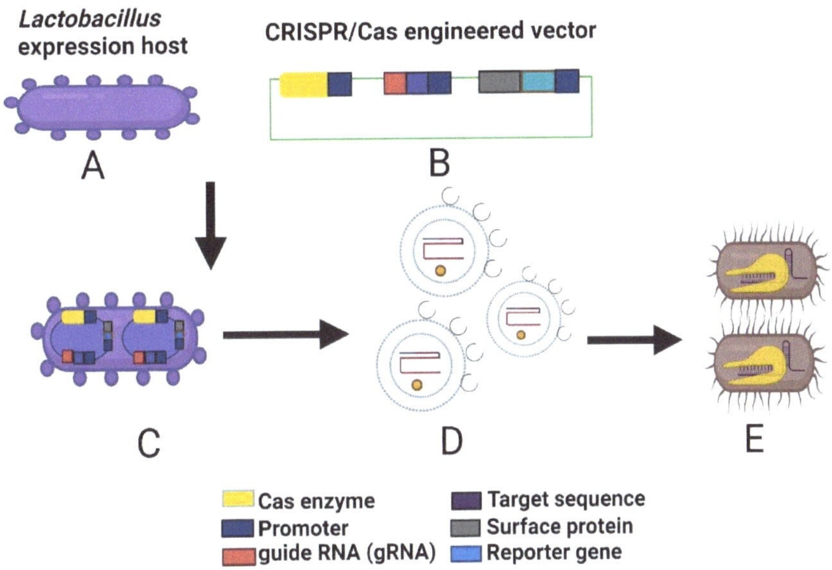

Figure 2. Application of the CRISPR/Cas system for the development of biotherapeutic tools against infections crossing the BBB. (**A**) *Lactobacillus* expression host, (**B**) CRISPR/Cas expression vector, (**C**) expression of the engineered vector in *Lactobacillus*, (**D**) CRISPR/Cas-enriched *Lactobacillus* bEV, and (**E**) targeted therapy against pathogenic bacteria via surface protein receptors. The figure was created using BioRender.com (https://app.biorender.com; accessed on 2 November 2022).

This approach involves identification of the Cas system from *Lactobacillus* species (Type I or Type II system), constructing an engineered vector model and designing an expression system based on the surface modification of a targeted ligand using a reporter system [191] comprising an inducible promoter sequence, guide RNA, Cas9, selectable marker, surface protein with a reporter gene, and target DNA sequence. Using this approach, the entire vector can be transformed into the *Lactobacillus* via electroporation or microfluidic injection. bEVs from transformed *Lactobacillus* contain surface-expressed heterologous proteins that can be targeted to the specific host cell receptors for vaccine therapy. Studies on *L. reuteri* and *L. sakei* [193,194] have identified the presence of 20–25 CRISPR systems with varying degrees of polymorphism, conferring an evolutionary advantage against invasive pathogens. Recent examples of *L. acidophilus* and *L. crispatus* delivery mechanisms using the Slp system (S-layer membrane protein) (see Section 8.1) [180] have highlighted the utility of genome editing tools in probiotic species. Therefore, the CRISPR/Cas system can facilitate development of tools targeting drug-resistant pathogens and create avenues for designing potent and targeted therapeutic strategies against infections crossing the BBB.

The potential role of probiotic-derived bEVs can provide numerous benefits against hospital-acquired infections. The fine tuning of probiotic-derived bEVs on parameters such as quorum-quenching enzymes and the CRISPR/Cas mechanism can provide a possible strategy to target secondary risk factors associated with dysbiosis in the gut–brain axis (Figure 3).

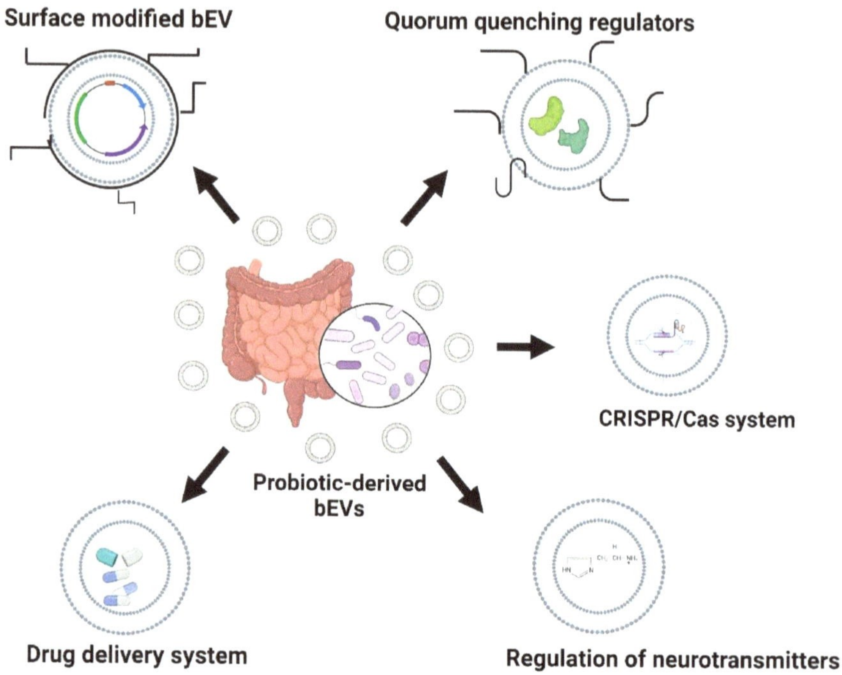

Figure 3. Remodeling of probiotic-derived bEVs against BBB related anomalies. The figure was created using BioRender.com (https://app.biorender.com; accessed on 2 November 2022).

9. Potential for Application of Probiotic-Derived bEV Platforms against BBB-Associated CNS Infections

Infections with MDR bacteria, which secrete various virulence factors and toxic proteins that target sensitive regions of the brain, can readily cross the BBB's endothelial barrier and cause serious neurological disorders. Furthermore, the robust movement of various immune cells at the site of injury promotes localized inflammatory responses and results in cytokine bursts, thus affecting CNS permeability and causing neurological imbalance.

Probiotic-derived bEVs represent safe therapeutic agents against a variety of infections and outperform conventional antibiotic therapy for BBB-associated CNS infections. However, the efficacy of bEVs derived from probiotics other than *L. paracasei*, in the treatment of CNS infections, is currently under evaluation in ongoing clinical trials [195]. Indeed, the presence of CNS inflammation can significantly impact bEV efficacy as it reduces the amount of drug crossing the CNS barrier, which is impeded by BBB-mediated exclusion. Nevertheless, certain drugs, including citalopram, doxepin, erythropoietin, and fluvoxamine, have demonstrated significant anti-neural anomaly activity [196]. However, these drugs are limited by their low membrane permeability, rapid clearance, and rapid degradation. Therefore, additional treatments are now being developed, such as nano-based drug delivery agents, liposomal NPs, and biomimetic NPs or nanocomposites with the potential to penetrate the BBB. However, studies using anti-seizure drug-loaded gold NPs revealed increased oxidative stress [195], necessitating a re-evaluation of the associated dosing regimen. Similarly, chitosan-based NPs exhibit minimal BBB absorption and are not currently used in clinical practice [196]. Meanwhile, for extended periods of usage, liposomal NPs outperformed metallic counterparts in post-stroke inflammatory responses.

However, their instability, shorter lifetime, and restricted drug encapsulation capability limit their use as a drug delivery vehicle for nondegenerative disorders.

In contrast, bEVs outperform lipophilic and hydrophilic/hydrophobic drugs. In fact, a bEV derived from *Chromobacterium violaceum*—a facultative anaerobic, oxidase-positive, glucose-fermenting, non-lactose-fermenting, Gram-negative *Bacillus*—was successfully used to encapsulate violacein by enhancing its absorption coefficient [197]. Hence, due to their direct linkage with the gut–brain axis, as well as their movement via the autonomic nervous system, bEVs might represent an alternative drug-encapsulating vehicle for treatment of BBB infections; however, it is necessary to first address the issues regarding their bioavailability and surface modifications. In fact, probiotic-derived bEVs represent a useful platform for the development of new treatments as they have been shown to improve immunogenic responses to numerous pathogens that affect the gut–brain-axis function.

Genetic engineering of hEVs has recently been recognized as a paradigm shift in the treatment of CNS infections. Therefore, modified eukaryotic hEVs are regarded as effective delivery vehicles for hydrophobic and hydrophilic medicines. However, improving the ability of hEVs to invade the BBB has proven challenging. In this regard, probiotics with enhanced invading BBB activity might be viable therapeutic options against BBB-associated MDR pathogen infections. Most microbiota-related neurological disorders are associated with an imbalance of intestinal commensal bacteria, and probiotic-derived bEV-based platforms provide a successful therapy against CNS infections.

10. Future Research and Perspective

Strong efforts are required to improve the design of therapeutic agents that target MDR superbugs associated with the BBB. Unlike eukaryotic hEV biomarkers, proteins of probiotic-derived bEVs remain unidentified, thus limiting the utility of bEVs in BBB-associated therapy. Therefore, multiple omics approaches and in silico analysis are warranted. Additional high-throughput-scale functional analysis is required to identify potential therapeutic proteins of bEVs and design novel platforms for the selective and efficient targeting of BBB-associated infections that also elicit memory T cell responses to establish long-term immunity. Notably, most probiotic-derived bEVs exhibit antibacterial activity and enrichment of antibacterial metabolites. Thus, probiotic-derived bEVs can be used in combination with commercial antibiotics or repurposed drugs to increase their therapeutic efficacy against pathogens. With the aid of cheminformatics [197], formulated antimicrobial analogs can be designed to target pathogenic microbial factors. Indeed, this approach is expected to expand the current scope of antimicrobial use by generating probiotic-derived bEVs to effectively treat BBB-breaching infections.

11. Conclusions

The recent literature has demonstrated the effectiveness of EVs against various infectious pathogens. However, most research has largely focused on developing therapeutics or drug delivery vehicles by utilizing either NPs or hEVs (exosomes). Although these agents are clinically significant, their utilization is limited by long-term toxicity and the related mortality, low immunogenic response, stability issues, cost of scaling up, fermentation culture conditions, and downstream processing. In contrast to hEVs, there are only a few FDA-approved therapeutic bEVs, including a bEV vaccine (MeNZB) cleared for use against *N. meningitidis*. This is due to either failed trials or a low therapeutic efficiency. The concept of 'postbiotics' has recently been evaluated as a source of nonviable bacterial supplements capable of regulating the gut–brain axis. That is, the use of probiotics alone may be limited in scope; however, it can be enhanced by tuning the active components of postbiotics to initiate the release of probiotics-derived bEVs or -enriched bEVs. Meanwhile, limitations of combining NPs with antimicrobial compounds have hampered their application for the treatment of infections; moreover, this strategy does not address safety issues related to BBB breach. Collectively, the work summarized in this review provides insights into the efficacy of probiotic-derived bEVs and the novel concept of 'postbiotics' as a potential tool for the development of therapeutic platforms to overcome drug resistance in pathogens causing neurological disorders.

Author Contributions: P.S.: conceptualization, investigation, data collection, formal analysis, writing—original draft; K.-s.K.: conceptualization, supervision, writing—reviewing and editing. All authors have read and agreed to the published version of the manuscript.

Funding: This research was funded by a National Research Foundation of Korea (NRF) grant funded by the Korean government (MSIT) (grant number NRF-2021R1A2C1007413).

Institutional Review Board Statement: Not applicable.

Informed Consent Statement: Not applicable.

Data Availability Statement: Not applicable.

Conflicts of Interest: The authors declare no conflict of interest.

References

1. Gosselet, F.; Loiola, R.A.; Roig, A.; Rosell, A.; Culot, M. Central nervous system delivery of molecules across the blood-brain barrier. *Neurochem. Int.* **2021**, *144*, 104952. [CrossRef] [PubMed]
2. Muldoon, L.L.; Alvarez, J.I.; Begley, D.J.; Boado, R.J.; Del Zoppo, G.J.; Doolittle, N.D.; Engelhardt, B.; Hallenbeck, J.M.; Lonser, R.R.; Ohlfest, J.R.; et al. Immunologic privilege in the central nervous system and the blood-brain barrier. *J. Cereb. Blood Flow Metab.* **2013**, *33*, 13–21. [CrossRef] [PubMed]
3. Miner, J.J.; Diamond, M.S. Mechanisms of restriction of viral neuroinvasion at the blood-brain barrier. *Curr. Opin. Immunol.* **2016**, *38*, 18–23. [CrossRef]
4. Cain, M.D.; Salimi, H.; Diamond, M.S.; Klein, R.S. Mechanisms of Pathogen Invasion into the Central Nervous System. *Neuron* **2019**, *103*, 771–783. [CrossRef]
5. Li, S.; Nguyen, I.P.; Urbanczyk, K. Common infectious diseases of the central nervous system-clinical features and imaging characteristics. *Quant. Imaging Med. Surg.* **2020**, *10*, 2227–2259. [CrossRef]
6. Sousa, S.A.; Feliciano, J.R.; Pita, T.; Soeiro, C.F.; Mendes, B.L.; Alves, L.G.; Leitao, J.H. Bacterial Nosocomial Infections: Multidrug Resistance as a Trigger for the Development of Novel Antimicrobials. *Antibiotics* **2021**, *10*, 942. [CrossRef]
7. Loscher, W.; Potschka, H. Drug resistance in brain diseases and the role of drug efflux transporters. *Nat. Rev. Neurosci.* **2005**, *6*, 591–602. [CrossRef]
8. Gaddy, J.A.; Actis, L.A. Regulation of *Acinetobacter baumannii* biofilm formation. *Future Microbiol.* **2009**, *4*, 273–278. [CrossRef]
9. Galea, I. The blood-brain barrier in systemic infection and inflammation. *Cell. Mol. Immunol.* **2021**, *18*, 2489–2501. [CrossRef] [PubMed]
10. Huang, X.; Hussain, B.; Chang, J. Peripheral inflammation and blood-brain barrier disruption: Effects and mechanisms. *CNS Neurosci. Ther.* **2021**, *27*, 36–47. [CrossRef]
11. Teleanu, R.I.; Preda, M.D.; Niculescu, A.G.; Vladacenco, O.; Radu, C.I.; Grumezescu, A.M.; Teleanu, D.M. Current Strategies to Enhance Delivery of Drugs across the Blood-Brain Barrier. *Pharmaceutics* **2022**, *14*, 987. [CrossRef] [PubMed]
12. Bhowmik, A.; Khan, R.; Ghosh, M.K. Blood brain barrier: A challenge for effectual therapy of brain tumors. *BioMed Res. Int.* **2015**, *2015*, 320941. [CrossRef]
13. Morse, S.V.; Mishra, A.; Chan, T.G.; de Rosales, R.T.M.; Choi, J.J. Liposome delivery to the brain with rapid short-pulses of focused ultrasound and microbubbles. *J. Control. Release* **2022**, *341*, 605–615. [CrossRef] [PubMed]
14. Juhairiyah, F.; de Lange, E.C.M. Understanding Drug Delivery to the Brain Using Liposome-Based Strategies: Studies that Provide Mechanistic Insights Are Essential. *AAPS J.* **2021**, *23*, 114. [CrossRef] [PubMed]
15. Curcio, M.; Cirillo, G.; Rouaen, J.R.C.; Saletta, F.; Nicoletta, F.P.; Vittorio, O.; Iemma, F. Natural Polysaccharide Carriers in Brain Delivery: Challenge and Perspective. *Pharmaceutics* **2020**, *12*, 1183. [CrossRef]
16. Zhang, W.; Mehta, A.; Tong, Z.; Esser, L.; Voelcker, N.H. Development of Polymeric Nanoparticles for Blood-Brain Barrier Transfer-Strategies and Challenges. *Adv. Sci.* **2021**, *8*, 2003937. [CrossRef]
17. Boyes, W.K.; van Thriel, C. Neurotoxicology of Nanomaterials. *Chem. Res. Toxicol.* **2020**, *33*, 1121–1144. [CrossRef]
18. Daraee, H.; Etemadi, A.; Kouhi, M.; Alimirzalu, S.; Akbarzadeh, A. Application of liposomes in medicine and drug delivery. *Artif. Cells Nanomed. Biotechnol.* **2016**, *44*, 381–391. [CrossRef]
19. Fikatas, A.; Dehairs, J.; Noppen, S.; Doijen, J.; Vanderhoydonc, F.; Meyen, E.; Swinnen, J.V.; Pannecouque, C.; Schols, D. Deciphering the Role of Extracellular Vesicles Derived from ZIKV-Infected hcMEC/D3 Cells on the Blood-Brain Barrier System. *Viruses* **2021**, *13*, 2363. [CrossRef]
20. Correa, R.; Caballero, Z.; De Leon, L.F.; Spadafora, C. Extracellular Vesicles Could Carry an Evolutionary Footprint in Interkingdom Communication. *Front. Cell. Infect. Microbiol.* **2020**, *10*, 76. [CrossRef]
21. Hendrix, A.; De Wever, O. Systemically circulating bacterial extracellular vesicles: Origin, fate, and function. *Trends Microbiol.* **2022**, *30*, 213–216. [CrossRef] [PubMed]

22. Fang, Y.; Wang, Z.; Liu, X.; Tyler, B.M. Biogenesis and Biological Functions of Extracellular Vesicles in Cellular and Organismal Communication with Microbes. *Front. Microbiol.* **2022**, *13*, 817844. [CrossRef] [PubMed]
23. Van Beek, L.F.; Surmann, K.; van den Berg van Saparoea, H.B.; Houben, D.; Jong, W.S.P.; Hentschker, C.; Ederveen, T.H.A.; Mitsi, E.; Ferreira, D.M.; van Opzeeland, F.; et al. Exploring metal availability in the natural niche of *Streptococcus pneumoniae* to discover potential vaccine antigens. *Virulence* **2020**, *11*, 1310–1328. [CrossRef] [PubMed]
24. Malekan, M.; Siadat, S.D.; Aghasadeghi, M.; Shahrokhi, N.; Afrough, P.; Behrouzi, A.; Ahmadi, K.; Mousavi, S.F. Evaluation of protective immunity responses against *pneumococcal* PhtD and its C-terminal in combination with outer-membrane vesicles as adjuvants. *J. Med. Microbiol.* **2020**, *69*, 465–477. [CrossRef] [PubMed]
25. Guerrero-Mandujano, A.; Hernandez-Cortez, C.; Ibarra, J.A.; Castro-Escarpulli, G. The outer membrane vesicles: Secretion system type zero. *Traffic* **2017**, *18*, 425–432. [CrossRef]
26. Schaar, V.; Nordstrom, T.; Morgelin, M.; Riesbeck, K. Moraxella catarrhalis outer membrane vesicles carry beta-lactamase and promote survival of *Streptococcus pneumoniae* and *Haemophilus influenzae* by inactivating amoxicillin. *Antimicrob. Agents Chemother.* **2011**, *55*, 3845–3853. [CrossRef]
27. Cuesta, C.M.; Guerri, C.; Urena, J.; Pascual, M. Role of Microbiota-Derived Extracellular Vesicles in Gut-Brain Communication. *Int. J. Mol. Sci.* **2021**, *22*, 4235. [CrossRef]
28. Kato, T.; Fahrmann, J.F.; Hanash, S.M.; Vykoukal, J. Extracellular Vesicles Mediate B Cell Immune Response and Are a Potential Target for Cancer Therapy. *Cells* **2020**, *9*, 1518. [CrossRef]
29. Rubio, A.P.D.; D'Antoni, C.L.; Piuri, M.; Perez, O.E. Probiotics, Their Extracellular Vesicles and Infectious Diseases. *Front. Microbiol.* **2022**, *13*, 864720. [CrossRef]
30. Yaghoubfar, R.; Behrouzi, A.; Ashrafian, F.; Shahryari, A.; Moradi, H.R.; Choopani, S.; Hadifar, S.; Vaziri, F.; Nojoumi, S.A.; Fateh, A.; et al. Modulation of serotonin signaling/metabolism by *Akkermansia muciniphila* and its extracellular vesicles through the gut-brain axis in mice. *Sci. Rep.* **2020**, *10*, 22119. [CrossRef]
31. Heavey, M.K.; Durmusoglu, D.; Crook, N.; Anselmo, A.C. Discovery and delivery strategies for engineered live biotherapeutic products. *Trends Biotechnol.* **2022**, *40*, 354–369. [CrossRef]
32. Kuhn, T.; Koch, M.; Fuhrmann, G. Probiomimetics-Novel Lactobacillus-Mimicking Microparticles Show Anti-Inflammatory and Barrier-Protecting Effects in Gastrointestinal Models. *Small* **2020**, *16*, e2003158. [CrossRef]
33. Shandilya, S.; Kumar, S.; Jha, N.K.; Kesari, K.K.; Ruokolainen, J. Interplay of gut microbiota and oxidative stress: Perspective on neurodegeneration and neuroprotection. *J. Adv. Res.* **2022**, *38*, 223–244. [CrossRef] [PubMed]
34. Jahan, S.; Mukherjee, S.; Ali, S.; Bhardwaj, U.; Choudhary, R.K.; Balakrishnan, S.; Naseem, A.; Mir, S.A.; Banawas, S.; Alaidarous, M.; et al. Pioneer Role of Extracellular Vesicles as Modulators of Cancer Initiation in Progression, Drug Therapy, and Vaccine Prospects. *Cells* **2022**, *11*, 490. [CrossRef] [PubMed]
35. Elsharkasy, O.M.; Nordin, J.Z.; Hagey, D.W.; de Jong, O.G.; Schiffelers, R.M.; Andaloussi, S.E.; Vader, P. Extracellular vesicles as drug delivery systems: Why and how? *Adv. Drug Deliv. Rev.* **2020**, *159*, 332–343. [CrossRef] [PubMed]
36. Armstrong, J.P.; Holme, M.N.; Stevens, M.M. Re-Engineering Extracellular Vesicles as Smart Nanoscale Therapeutics. *ACS Nano* **2017**, *11*, 69–83. [CrossRef]
37. Loureiro, A.; da Silva, G.J. CRISPR-Cas: Converting A Bacterial Defence Mechanism into A State-of-the-Art Genetic Manipulation Tool. *Antibiotics* **2019**, *8*, 18. [CrossRef]
38. Gao, Y.; Gao, K.; Yang, H. CRISPR/Cas: A potential gene-editing tool in the nervous system. *Cell Regen.* **2020**, *9*, 12. [CrossRef]
39. Rhea, E.M.; Banks, W.A. Role of the Blood-Brain Barrier in Central Nervous System Insulin Resistance. *Front. Neurosci.* **2019**, *13*, 521. [CrossRef]
40. Le Govic, Y.; Demey, B.; Cassereau, J.; Bahn, Y.S.; Papon, N. Pathogens infecting the central nervous system. *PLoS Pathog.* **2022**, *18*, e1010234. [CrossRef]
41. Festoff, B.W.; Sajja, R.K.; Cucullo, L. Proximate Mediators of Microvascular Dysfunction at the Blood-Brain Barrier: Neuroinflammatory Pathways to Neurodegeneration. *BioMed Res. Int.* **2017**, *2017*, 1549194. [CrossRef] [PubMed]
42. Shaheryar, Z.A.; Khan, M.A.; Adnan, C.S.; Zaidi, A.A.; Hanggi, D.; Muhammad, S. Neuroinflammatory Triangle Presenting Novel Pharmacological Targets for Ischemic Brain Injury. *Front. Immunol.* **2021**, *12*, 748663. [CrossRef] [PubMed]
43. Connell, J.J.; Chatain, G.; Cornelissen, B.; Vallis, K.A.; Hamilton, A.; Seymour, L.; Anthony, D.C.; Sibson, N.R. Selective permeabilization of the blood-brain barrier at sites of metastasis. *J. Natl. Cancer Inst.* **2013**, *105*, 1634–1643. [CrossRef]
44. Banks, W.A. Characteristics of compounds that cross the blood-brain barrier. *BMC Neurol.* **2009**, *9* (Suppl. 1), S3. [CrossRef]
45. Pardridge, W.M. Drug transport across the blood-brain barrier. *J. Cereb. Blood Flow Metab.* **2012**, *32*, 1959–1972. [CrossRef] [PubMed]
46. Dando, S.J.; Mackay-Sim, A.; Norton, R.; Currie, B.J.; John, J.A.S.; Ekberg, J.A.; Batzloff, M.; Ulett, G.C.; Beacham, I.R. Pathogens penetrating the central nervous system: Infection pathways and the cellular and molecular mechanisms of invasion. *Clin. Microbiol. Rev.* **2014**, *27*, 691–726. [CrossRef]
47. Novakova, I.; Subileau, E.A.; Toegel, S.; Gruber, D.; Lachmann, B.; Urban, E.; Chesne, C.; Noe, C.R.; Neuhaus, W. Transport rankings of non-steroidal antiinflammatory drugs across blood-brain barrier in vitro models. *PLoS ONE* **2014**, *9*, e86806. [CrossRef]
48. Marchi, N.; Betto, G.; Fazio, V.; Fan, Q.; Ghosh, C.; Machado, A.; Janigro, D. Blood-brain barrier damage and brain penetration of antiepileptic drugs: Role of serum proteins and brain edema. *Epilepsia* **2009**, *50*, 664–677. [CrossRef]

49. Appelboom, G.; Detappe, A.; LoPresti, M.; Kunjachan, S.; Mitrasinovic, S.; Goldman, S.; Chang, S.D.; Tillement, O. Stereotactic modulation of blood-brain barrier permeability to enhance drug delivery. *Neuro-Oncology* **2016**, *18*, 1601–1609. [CrossRef]
50. Salehi, A.; Paturu, M.R.; Patel, B.; Cain, M.D.; Mahlokozera, T.; Yang, A.B.; Lin, T.H.; Leuthardt, E.C.; Yano, H.; Song, S.K.; et al. Therapeutic enhancement of blood-brain and blood-tumor barriers permeability by laser interstitial thermal therapy. *Neurooncol. Adv.* **2020**, *2*, vdaa071. [CrossRef]
51. Karmur, B.S.; Philteos, J.; Abbasian, A.; Zacharia, B.E.; Lipsman, N.; Levin, V.; Grossman, S.; Mansouri, A. Blood-Brain Barrier Disruption in Neuro-Oncology: Strategies, Failures, and Challenges to Overcome. *Front. Oncol.* **2020**, *10*, 563840. [CrossRef] [PubMed]
52. Hoffman, P.S. Antibacterial Discovery: 21st Century Challenges. *Antibiotics* **2020**, *9*, 213. [CrossRef]
53. Saha, M.; Sarkar, A. Review on Multiple Facets of Drug Resistance: A Rising Challenge in the 21st Century. *J. Xenobiotics* **2021**, *11*, 197–214. [CrossRef]
54. Sun, H.; Zhang, Q.; Wang, R.; Wang, H.; Wong, Y.T.; Wang, M.; Hao, Q.; Yan, A.; Kao, R.Y.; Ho, P.L.; et al. Resensitizing carbapenem- and colistin-resistant bacteria to antibiotics using auranofin. *Nat. Commun.* **2020**, *11*, 5263. [CrossRef] [PubMed]
55. Nation, R.L.; Li, J. Colistin in the 21st century. *Curr. Opin. Infect. Dis.* **2009**, *22*, 535–543. [CrossRef]
56. Kim, B.-N.; Peleg, A.Y.; Lodise, T.P.; Lipman, J.; Li, J.; Nation, R.; Paterson, D.L. Management of meningitis due to antibiotic-resistant *Acinetobacter* species. *Lancet Infect. Dis.* **2009**, *9*, 245–255. [CrossRef]
57. Huang, Q.; Zhang, X.; Jia, A.; Huang, Q.; Jiang, Y.; Xie, L. The Pharmacokinetics/Pharmacodynamics and Neurotoxicity of Tigecycline Intraventricular Injection for the Treatment of Extensively Drug-Resistant *Acinetobacter baumannii* Intracranial Infection. *Infect. Drug Resist.* **2022**, *15*, 4809–4817. [CrossRef]
58. Yu, X.B.; Huang, Y.Y.; Zhang, X.S.; Wang, Y.Z.; Shi, D.W.; Zhang, C.H.; Chen, J.; Wang, X.R.; Lin, G.Y. Intraventricular colistin sulphate as a last resort therapy in a patient with multidrug-resistant *Acinetobacter baumannii* induced post-neurosurgical ventriculitis. *Br. J. Clin. Pharmacol.* **2022**, *88*, 3490–3494. [CrossRef]
59. Lin, M.F.; Lan, C.Y. Antimicrobial resistance in *Acinetobacter baumannii*: From bench to bedside. *World J. Clin. Cases* **2014**, *2*, 787–814. [CrossRef]
60. Wu, X.; Wang, L.; Ye, Y.Z.; Yu, H. Postoperative multidrug-resistant *Acinetobacter baumannii* meningitis successfully treated with intravenous doxycycline and intraventricular gentamicin: A case report. *World J. Clin. Cases* **2019**, *7*, 4342–4348. [CrossRef]
61. Schneider, F.; Gessner, A.; El-Najjar, N. Efficacy of Vancomycin and Meropenem in Central Nervous System Infections in Children and Adults: Current Update. *Antibiotics* **2022**, *11*, 173. [CrossRef] [PubMed]
62. Pimentel, E.; Sivalingam, K.; Doke, M.; Samikkannu, T. Effects of Drugs of Abuse on the Blood-Brain Barrier: A Brief Overview. *Front. Neurosci.* **2020**, *14*, 513. [CrossRef] [PubMed]
63. Fang, Y.-Q.; Zhan, R.-C.; Jia, W.; Zhang, B.-Q.; Wang, J.-J. A case report of intraventricular tigecycline therapy for intracranial infection with extremely drug resistant *Acinetobacter baumannii*. *Medicine* **2017**, *96*, e7703. [CrossRef] [PubMed]
64. Li, Z.; An, Y.; Li, L.; Yi, H. Intrathecal Injection of Tigecycline and Polymyxin B in the Treatment of Extensively Drug-Resistant Intracranial *Acinetobacter baumannii* Infection: A Case Report and Review of the Literature. *Infect. Drug Resist.* **2022**, *15*, 1411–1423. [CrossRef]
65. Zhong, Y.M.; Zhang, X.H.; Ma, Z.; Liu, W.E. Prevalence of *Escherichia coli* ST1193 Causing Intracranial Infection in Changsha, China. *Trop. Med. Infect. Dis.* **2022**, *7*, 217. [CrossRef]
66. Coureuil, M.; Join-Lambert, O.; Lécuyer, H.; Bourdoulous, S.; Marullo, S.; Nassif, X. Mechanism of meningeal invasion by *Neisseria meningitidis*. *Virulence* **2014**, *3*, 164–172. [CrossRef]
67. Cutting, A.S.; Del Rosario, Y.; Mu, R.; Rodriguez, A.; Till, A.; Subramani, S.; Gottlieb, R.A.; Doran, K.S. The Role of Autophagy during Group B *Streptococcus* Infection of Blood-Brain Barrier Endothelium. *J. Biol. Chem.* **2014**, *289*, 35711–35723. [CrossRef]
68. Parisi, D.N.; Martinez, L.R. Intracellular *Haemophilus influenzae* invades the brain. *Virulence* **2014**, *5*, 645–647. [CrossRef]
69. Chacko, A.; Delbaz, A.; Walkden, H.; Basu, S.; Armitage, C.W.; Eindorf, T.; Trim, L.K.; Miller, E.; West, N.P.; John, J.A.S.; et al. *Chlamydia pneumoniae* can infect the central nervous system via the olfactory and trigeminal nerves and contributes to Alzheimer's disease risk. *Sci. Rep.* **2022**, *12*, 2759. [CrossRef]
70. Guttman, J.A.; Samji, F.N.; Li, Y.; Vogl, A.W.; Finlay, B.B. Evidence that Tight Junctions Are Disrupted Due to Intimate Bacterial Contact and Not Inflammation during Attaching and Effacing Pathogen Infection In Vivo. *Infect. Immun.* **2006**, *74*, 6075–6084. [CrossRef]
71. Doran, K.S.; Engelson, E.J.; Khosravi, A.; Maisey, H.C.; Fedtke, I.; Equils, O.; Michelsen, K.S.; Arditi, M.; Peschel, A.; Nizet, V. Blood-brain barrier invasion by group B *Streptococcus* depends upon proper cell-surface anchoring of lipoteichoic acid. *J. Clin. Investig.* **2005**, *115*, 2499–2507. [CrossRef] [PubMed]
72. Deatherage, B.L.; Cookson, B.T. Membrane vesicle release in bacteria, eukaryotes, and archaea: A conserved yet underappreciated aspect of microbial life. *Infect. Immun.* **2012**, *80*, 1948–1957. [CrossRef] [PubMed]
73. Turkina, M.V.; Olofsson, A.; Magnusson, K.E.; Arnqvist, A.; Vikstrom, E. *Helicobacter pylori* vesicles carrying CagA localize in the vicinity of cell-cell contacts and induce histone H1 binding to ATP in epithelial cells. *FEMS Microbiol. Lett.* **2015**, *362*, fnv076. [CrossRef] [PubMed]
74. Prados-Rosales, R.; Baena, A.; Martinez, L.R.; Luque-Garcia, J.; Kalscheuer, R.; Veeraraghavan, U.; Camara, C.; Nosanchuk, J.D.; Besra, G.S.; Chen, B.; et al. *Mycobacteria* release active membrane vesicles that modulate immune responses in a TLR2-dependent manner in mice. *J. Clin. Investig.* **2011**, *121*, 1471–1483. [CrossRef]

75. Volgers, C.; Savelkoul, P.H.M.; Stassen, F.R.M. Gram-negative bacterial membrane vesicle release in response to the host-environment: Different threats, same trick? *Crit. Rev. Microbiol.* **2018**, *44*, 258–273. [CrossRef]
76. de Figueiredo, P.; Ficht, T.A.; Rice-Ficht, A.; Rossetti, C.A.; Adams, L.G. Pathogenesis and immunobiology of brucellosis: Review of Brucella-host interactions. *Am. J. Pathol.* **2015**, *185*, 1505–1517. [CrossRef]
77. Athman, J.J.; Wang, Y.; McDonald, D.J.; Boom, W.H.; Harding, C.V.; Wearsch, P.A. Bacterial Membrane Vesicles Mediate the Release of *Mycobacterium tuberculosis* Lipoglycans and Lipoproteins from Infected Macrophages. *J. Immunol.* **2015**, *195*, 1044–1053. [CrossRef]
78. Lee, E.Y.; Choi, D.Y.; Kim, D.K.; Kim, J.W.; Park, J.O.; Kim, S.; Kim, S.H.; Desiderio, D.M.; Kim, Y.K.; Kim, K.P.; et al. Gram-positive bacteria produce membrane vesicles: Proteomics-based characterization of *Staphylococcus aureus*-derived membrane vesicles. *Proteomics* **2009**, *9*, 5425–5436. [CrossRef]
79. Domingues, S.; Nielsen, K.M. Membrane vesicles and horizontal gene transfer in prokaryotes. *Curr. Opin. Microbiol.* **2017**, *38*, 16–21. [CrossRef]
80. Rumbo, C.; Fernandez-Moreira, E.; Merino, M.; Poza, M.; Mendez, J.A.; Soares, N.C.; Mosquera, A.; Chaves, F.; Bou, G. Horizontal transfer of the OXA-24 carbapenemase gene via outer membrane vesicles: A new mechanism of dissemination of carbapenem resistance genes in *Acinetobacter baumannii*. *Antimicrob. Agents Chemother.* **2011**, *55*, 3084–3090. [CrossRef]
81. Deo, P.; Chow, S.H.; Hay, I.D.; Kleifeld, O.; Costin, A.; Elgass, K.D.; Jiang, J.H.; Ramm, G.; Gabriel, K.; Dougan, G.; et al. Outer membrane vesicles from *Neisseria gonorrhoeae* target PorB to mitochondria and induce apoptosis. *PLoS Pathog.* **2018**, *14*, e1006945. [CrossRef] [PubMed]
82. Thay, B.; Wai, S.N.; Oscarsson, J. *Staphylococcus aureus* alpha-toxin-dependent induction of host cell death by membrane-derived vesicles. *PLoS ONE* **2013**, *8*, e54661. [CrossRef] [PubMed]
83. Wang, S.; Gao, J.; Wang, Z. Outer membrane vesicles for vaccination and targeted drug delivery. *Wiley Interdiscip. Rev. Nanomed. Nanobiotechnol.* **2019**, *11*, e1523. [CrossRef]
84. Jones, L.B.; Kumar, S.; Bell, C.R.; Crenshaw, B.J.; Coats, M.T.; Sims, B.; Matthews, Q.L. Lipopolysaccharide Administration Alters Extracellular Vesicles in Cell Lines and Mice. *Curr. Microbiol.* **2021**, *78*, 920–931. [CrossRef] [PubMed]
85. Fabrega, M.J.; Aguilera, L.; Gimenez, R.; Varela, E.; Canas, M.A.; Antolin, M.; Badia, J.; Baldoma, L. Activation of Immune and Defense Responses in the Intestinal Mucosa by Outer Membrane Vesicles of Commensal and Probiotic *Escherichia coli* Strains. *Front. Microbiol.* **2016**, *7*, 705. [CrossRef] [PubMed]
86. Dean, S.N.; Thakur, M.; Spangler, J.R. Extracellular vesicle production in Gram-positive bacteria. *Microb. Biotechnol.* **2022**, *15*, 1055–1057. [CrossRef]
87. Wang, X.; Thompson, C.D.; Weidenmaier, C.; Lee, J.C. Release of *Staphylococcus aureus* extracellular vesicles and their application as a vaccine platform. *Nat. Commun.* **2018**, *9*, 1379. [CrossRef]
88. Toyofuku, M.; Carcamo-Oyarce, G.; Yamamoto, T.; Eisenstein, F.; Hsiao, C.C.; Kurosawa, M.; Gademann, K.; Pilhofer, M.; Nomura, N.; Eberl, L. Prophage-triggered membrane vesicle formation through peptidoglycan damage in *Bacillus subtilis*. *Nat. Commun.* **2017**, *8*, 481. [CrossRef]
89. Raghav, A.; Jeong, G.B. A systematic review on the modifications of extracellular vesicles: A revolutionized tool of nano-biotechnology. *J. Nanobiotechnol.* **2021**, *19*, 459. [CrossRef]
90. Zou, C.; Zhang, Y.; Liu, H.; Wu, Y.; Zhou, X. Extracellular Vesicles: Recent Insights into the Interaction Between Host and Pathogenic Bacteria. *Front. Immunol.* **2022**, *13*, 840550. [CrossRef]
91. Pant, S.; Hilton, H.; Burczynski, M.E. The multifaceted exosome: Biogenesis, role in normal and aberrant cellular function, and frontiers for pharmacological and biomarker opportunities. *Biochem. Pharmacol.* **2012**, *83*, 1484–1494. [CrossRef] [PubMed]
92. Robbins, P.D.; Morelli, A.E. Regulation of immune responses by extracellular vesicles. *Nat. Rev. Immunol.* **2014**, *14*, 195–208. [CrossRef] [PubMed]
93. Brakhage, A.A.; Zimmermann, A.-K.; Rivieccio, F.; Visser, C.; Blango, M.G. Host-derived extracellular vesicles for antimicrobial defense. *microLife* **2021**, *2*, uqab003. [CrossRef]
94. Seo, M.K.; Park, E.J.; Ko, S.Y.; Choi, E.W.; Kim, S. Therapeutic effects of kefir grain *Lactobacillus*-derived extracellular vesicles in mice with 2,4,6-trinitrobenzene sulfonic acid-induced inflammatory bowel disease. *J. Dairy Sci.* **2018**, *101*, 8662–8671. [CrossRef]
95. Morishita, M.; Horita, M.; Higuchi, A.; Marui, M.; Katsumi, H.; Yamamoto, A. Characterizing Different Probiotic-Derived Extracellular Vesicles as a Novel Adjuvant for Immunotherapy. *Mol. Pharm.* **2021**, *18*, 1080–1092. [CrossRef]
96. Kim, J.H.; Jeun, E.J.; Hong, C.P.; Kim, S.H.; Jang, M.S.; Lee, E.J.; Moon, S.J.; Yun, C.H.; Im, S.H.; Jeong, S.G.; et al. Extracellular vesicle-derived protein from *Bifidobacterium longum* alleviates food allergy through mast cell suppression. *J. Allergy Clin. Immunol.* **2016**, *137*, 507–516.e8. [CrossRef]
97. Wang, Y.; Hoffmann, J.P.; Chou, C.-W.; Bentrup, K.H.Z.; Fuselier, J.A.; Bitoun, J.P.; Wimley, W.C.; Morici, L.A. *Burkholderia thailandensis* outer membrane vesicles exert antimicrobial activity against drug-resistant and competitor microbial species. *J. Microbiol.* **2020**, *58*, 550–562. [CrossRef]
98. Costantini, P.E.; Vanpouille, C.; Firrincieli, A.; Cappelletti, M.; Margolis, L.; Palomino, R.A.N. Extracellular Vesicles Generated by Gram-Positive Bacteria Protect Human Tissues Ex Vivo From HIV-1 Infection. *Front. Cell. Infect. Microbiol.* **2021**, *11*, 822882. [CrossRef]

99. Kim, W.; Lee, E.J.; Bae, I.H.; Myoung, K.; Kim, S.T.; Park, P.J.; Lee, K.H.; Pham, A.V.Q.; Ko, J.; Oh, S.H.; et al. *Lactobacillus plantarum*-derived extracellular vesicles induce anti-inflammatory M2 macrophage polarization in vitro. *J. Extracell. Vesicles* **2020**, *9*, 1793514. [CrossRef]
100. Tartaglia, N.R.; Breyne, K.; Meyer, E.; Cauty, C.; Jardin, J.; Chretien, D.; Dupont, A.; Demeyere, K.; Berkova, N.; Azevedo, V.; et al. *Staphylococcus aureus* Extracellular Vesicles Elicit an Immunostimulatory Response in vivo on the Murine Mammary Gland. *Front. Cell. Infect. Microbiol.* **2018**, *8*, 277. [CrossRef]
101. Lee, H.; Yun, S.H.; Hyon, J.Y.; Lee, S.Y.; Yi, Y.S.; Choi, C.W.; Jun, S.; Park, E.C.; Kim, S.I. *Streptococcus equi*-derived extracellular vesicles as a vaccine candidate against *Streptococcus equi* infection. *Vet. Microbiol.* **2021**, *259*, 109165. [CrossRef] [PubMed]
102. Islam, S.M.S.; Ryu, H.M.; Sohn, S. *Tetragenococcus halophilus* Alleviates Intestinal Inflammation in Mice by Altering Gut Microbiota and Regulating Dendritic Cell Activation via CD83. *Cells* **2022**, *11*, 1903. [CrossRef] [PubMed]
103. Huang, W.; Zhang, Q.; Li, W.; Chen, Y.; Shu, C.; Li, Q.; Zhou, J.; Ye, C.; Bai, H.; Sun, W.; et al. Anti-outer Membrane Vesicle Antibodies Increase Antibiotic Sensitivity of Pan-Drug-Resistant *Acinetobacter baumannii*. *Front. Microbiol.* **2019**, *10*, 1379. [CrossRef] [PubMed]
104. Wawrzeniak, K.; Gaur, G.; Sapi, E.; Senejani, A.G. Effect of *Borrelia burgdorferi* Outer Membrane Vesicles on Host Oxidative Stress Response. *Antibiotics* **2020**, *9*, 275. [CrossRef]
105. Gonzalez, M.F.; Diaz, P.; Sandoval-Borquez, A.; Herrera, D.; Quest, A.F.G. Helicobacter pylori Outer Membrane Vesicles and Extracellular Vesicles from *Helicobacter pylori*-Infected Cells in Gastric Disease Development. *Int. J. Mol. Sci.* **2021**, *22*, 4823. [CrossRef]
106. Lee, W.H.; Choi, H.I.; Hong, S.W.; Kim, K.S.; Gho, Y.S.; Jeon, S.G. Vaccination with *Klebsiella pneumoniae*-derived extracellular vesicles protects against bacteria-induced lethality via both humoral and cellular immunity. *Exp. Mol. Med.* **2015**, *47*, e183. [CrossRef]
107. Cai, W.; Kesavan, D.K.; Wan, J.; Abdelaziz, M.H.; Su, Z.; Xu, H. Bacterial outer membrane vesicles, a potential vaccine candidate in interactions with host cells based. *Diagn. Pathol* **2018**, *13*, 95. [CrossRef]
108. Bottero, D.; Gaillard, M.E.; Errea, A.; Moreno, G.; Zurita, E.; Pianciola, L.; Rumbo, M.; Hozbor, D. Outer membrane vesicles derived from *Bordetella parapertussis* as an acellular vaccine against *Bordetella parapertussis* and *Bordetella pertussis* infection. *Vaccine* **2013**, *31*, 5262–5268. [CrossRef]
109. Armstrong, D.A.; Lee, M.K.; Hazlett, H.F.; Dessaint, J.A.; Mellinger, D.L.; Aridgides, D.S.; Hendricks, G.M.; Abdalla, M.A.K.; Christensen, B.C.; Ashare, A. Extracellular Vesicles from *Pseudomonas aeruginosa* Suppress MHC-Related Molecules in Human Lung Macrophages. *Immunohorizons* **2020**, *4*, 508–519. [CrossRef]
110. Ramirez, M.I.; Amorim, M.G.; Gadelha, C.; Milic, I.; Welsh, J.A.; Freitas, V.M.; Nawaz, M.; Akbar, N.; Couch, Y.; Makin, L.; et al. Technical challenges of working with extracellular vesicles. *Nanoscale* **2018**, *10*, 881–906. [CrossRef]
111. Turturici, G.; Tinnirello, R.; Sconzo, G.; Geraci, F. Extracellular membrane vesicles as a mechanism of cell-to-cell communication: Advantages and disadvantages. *Am. J. Physiol. Cell Physiol.* **2014**, *306*, C621–C633. [CrossRef] [PubMed]
112. Wang, Y.; Xie, Q.; Zhang, Y.; Ma, W.; Ning, K.; Xiang, J.Y.; Cui, J.; Xiang, H. Combination of probiotics with different functions alleviate DSS-induced colitis by regulating intestinal microbiota, IL-10, and barrier function. *Appl. Microbiol. Biotechnol.* **2020**, *104*, 335–349. [CrossRef] [PubMed]
113. Choi, J.H.; Moon, C.M.; Shin, T.S.; Kim, E.K.; McDowell, A.; Jo, M.K.; Joo, Y.H.; Kim, S.E.; Jung, H.K.; Shim, K.N.; et al. *Lactobacillus paracasei*-derived extracellular vesicles attenuate the intestinal inflammatory response by augmenting the endoplasmic reticulum stress pathway. *Exp. Mol. Med.* **2020**, *52*, 423–437. [CrossRef] [PubMed]
114. Hurkacz, M.; Dobrek, L.; Wiela-Hojenska, A. Antibiotics and the Nervous System-Which Face of Antibiotic Therapy Is Real, Dr. Jekyll (Neurotoxicity) or Mr. Hyde (Neuroprotection)? *Molecules* **2021**, *26*, 7456. [CrossRef]
115. Ou, J.; Wang, Z.; Liu, X.; Song, B.; Chen, J.; Li, R.; Jia, X.; Huang, R.; Xiang, W.; Zhong, S. Regulatory effects of marine polysaccharides on gut microbiota dysbiosis: A review. *Food Chem. X* **2022**, *15*, 100444. [CrossRef]
116. Shaik, L.; Kashyap, R.; Thotamgari, S.R.; Singh, R.; Khanna, S. Gut-Brain Axis and its Neuro-Psychiatric Effects: A Narrative Review. *Cureus* **2020**, *12*, e11131. [CrossRef]
117. Rutsch, A.; Kantsjo, J.B.; Ronchi, F. The Gut-Brain Axis: How Microbiota and Host Inflammasome Influence Brain Physiology and Pathology. *Front. Immunol.* **2020**, *11*, 604179. [CrossRef]
118. McVey Neufeld, K.A.; Mao, Y.K.; Bienenstock, J.; Foster, J.A.; Kunze, W.A. The microbiome is essential for normal gut intrinsic primary afferent neuron excitability in the mouse. *Neurogastroenterol. Motil.* **2013**, *25*, 183-e88. [CrossRef]
119. Celorrio, M.; Abellanas, M.A.; Rhodes, J.; Goodwin, V.; Moritz, J.; Vadivelu, S.; Wang, L.; Rodgers, R.; Xiao, S.; Anabayan, I.; et al. Gut microbial dysbiosis after traumatic brain injury modulates the immune response and impairs neurogenesis. *Acta Neuropathol. Commun.* **2021**, *9*, 40. [CrossRef]
120. Palomino, R.A.N.; Vanpouille, C.; Costantini, P.E.; Margolis, L. Microbiota-host communications: Bacterial extracellular vesicles as a common language. *PLoS Pathog.* **2021**, *17*, e1009508. [CrossRef]
121. Cheng, H.Y.; Ning, M.X.; Chen, D.K.; Ma, W.T. Interactions Between the Gut Microbiota and the Host Innate Immune Response Against Pathogens. *Front. Immunol.* **2019**, *10*, 607. [CrossRef] [PubMed]
122. Kaparakis-Liaskos, M.; Ferrero, R.L. Immune modulation by bacterial outer membrane vesicles. *Nat. Rev. Immunol.* **2015**, *15*, 375–387. [CrossRef] [PubMed]

123. Shen, Q.; Huang, Z.; Yao, J.; Jin, Y. Extracellular vesicles-mediated interaction within intestinal microenvironment in inflammatory bowel disease. *J. Adv. Res.* **2022**, *37*, 221–233. [CrossRef] [PubMed]
124. Doyle, L.M.; Wang, M.Z. Overview of Extracellular Vesicles, Their Origin, Composition, Purpose, and Methods for Exosome Isolation and Analysis. *Cells* **2019**, *8*, 727. [CrossRef] [PubMed]
125. Battistelli, M.; Falcieri, E. Apoptotic Bodies: Particular Extracellular Vesicles Involved in Intercellular Communication. *Biology* **2020**, *9*, 21. [CrossRef]
126. Wu, Q.Y.; Liu, B.C.; Ruan, X.Z.; Ma, K.L. Intestinal microbiota-derived membrane vesicles and their role in chronic kidney disease. *Biochim. Biophys. Acta Mol. Basis Dis.* **2022**, *1868*, 166478. [CrossRef]
127. Liu, S.; Gao, J.; Zhu, M.; Liu, K.; Zhang, H.L. Gut Microbiota and Dysbiosis in Alzheimer's Disease: Implications for Pathogenesis and Treatment. *Mol. Neurobiol.* **2020**, *57*, 5026–5043. [CrossRef]
128. Lee, K.E.; Kim, J.K.; Han, S.K.; Lee, D.Y.; Lee, H.J.; Yim, S.V.; Kim, D.H. The extracellular vesicle of gut microbial *Paenalcaligenes hominis* is a risk factor for vagus nerve-mediated cognitive impairment. *Microbiome* **2020**, *8*, 107. [CrossRef]
129. Singhrao, S.K.; Olsen, I. Are *Porphyromonas gingivalis* Outer Membrane Vesicles Microbullets for Sporadic Alzheimer's Disease Manifestation? *J. Alzheimer's Dis. Rep.* **2018**, *2*, 219–228. [CrossRef]
130. Pokusaeva, K.; Johnson, C.; Luk, B.; Uribe, G.; Fu, Y.; Oezguen, N.; Matsunami, R.K.; Lugo, M.; Major, A.; Mori-Akiyama, Y.; et al. GABA-producing *Bifidobacterium dentium* modulates visceral sensitivity in the intestine. *Neurogastroenterol. Motil.* **2017**, *29*, e12904. [CrossRef]
131. Bravo, J.A.; Forsythe, P.; Chew, M.V.; Escaravage, E.; Savignac, H.M.; Dinan, T.G.; Bienenstock, J.; Cryan, J.F. Ingestion of *Lactobacillus* strain regulates emotional behavior and central GABA receptor expression in a mouse via the vagus nerve. *Proc. Natl. Acad. Sci. USA* **2011**, *108*, 16050–16055. [CrossRef] [PubMed]
132. Neufeld, K.-A.M.; Kang, N.; Bienenstock, J.; Foster, J.A. Effects of intestinal microbiota on anxiety-like behavior. *Commun. Integr. Biol.* **2014**, *4*, 492–494. [CrossRef]
133. Derrien, M.; van Hylckama Vlieg, J.E. Fate, activity, and impact of ingested bacteria within the human gut microbiota. *Trends Microbiol.* **2015**, *23*, 354–366. [CrossRef] [PubMed]
134. Dean, S.N.; Rimmer, M.A.; Turner, K.B.; Phillips, D.A.; Caruana, J.C.; Hervey, W.J.T.; Leary, D.H.; Walper, S.A. *Lactobacillus acidophilus* Membrane Vesicles as a Vehicle of Bacteriocin Delivery. *Front. Microbiol.* **2020**, *11*, 710. [CrossRef]
135. Choi, J.; Kim, Y.K.; Han, P.L. Extracellular Vesicles Derived from *Lactobacillus plantarum* Increase BDNF Expression in Cultured Hippocampal Neurons and Produce Antidepressant-like Effects in Mice. *Exp. Neurobiol.* **2019**, *28*, 158–171. [CrossRef] [PubMed]
136. West, C.L.; Stanisz, A.M.; Mao, Y.K.; Champagne-Jorgensen, K.; Bienenstock, J.; Kunze, W.A. Microvesicles from *Lactobacillus reuteri* (DSM-17938) completely reproduce modulation of gut motility by bacteria in mice. *PLoS ONE* **2020**, *15*, e0225481. [CrossRef]
137. Haas-Neill, S.; Iwashita, E.; Dvorkin-Gheva, A.; Forsythe, P. Effects of Two Distinct Psychoactive Microbes, *Lacticaseibacillus rhamnosus* JB-1 and *Limosilactobacillus reuteri* 6475, on Circulating and Hippocampal mRNA in Male Mice. *Int. J. Mol. Sci.* **2022**, *23*, 9653. [CrossRef]
138. Xiao, M.; Huang, X. Unmasking antibiotic-associated neurological disorders: The underminer in Intensive Care Unit. *J. Clin. Neurosci.* **2021**, *91*, 131–135. [CrossRef]
139. Wanleenuwat, P.; Suntharampillai, N.; Iwanowski, P. Antibiotic-induced epileptic seizures: Mechanisms of action and clinical considerations. *Seizure* **2020**, *81*, 167–174. [CrossRef]
140. Kim, K.S. Investigating Bacterial Penetration of the Blood-Brain Barrier for the Pathogenesis, Prevention, and Therapy of Bacterial Meningitis. *ACS Infect. Dis.* **2020**, *6*, 34–42. [CrossRef]
141. Nau, R.; Sorgel, F.; Eiffert, H. Penetration of drugs through the blood-cerebrospinal fluid/blood-brain barrier for treatment of central nervous system infections. *Clin. Microbiol. Rev.* **2010**, *23*, 858–883. [CrossRef] [PubMed]
142. Jimenez-Mejias, M.E.; Pichardo-Guerrero, C.; Marquez-Rivas, F.J.; Martin-Lozano, D.; Prados, T.; Pachon, J. Cerebrospinal fluid penetration and pharmacokinetic/pharmacodynamic parameters of intravenously administered colistin in a case of multidrug-resistant *Acinetobacter baumannii* meningitis. *Eur. J. Clin. Microbiol. Infect. Dis.* **2002**, *21*, 212–214. [CrossRef] [PubMed]
143. Cascio, A.; Conti, A.; Sinardi, L.; Iaria, C.; Angileri, F.F.; Stassi, G.; David, T.; Versaci, A.; Iaria, M.; David, A. Post-neurosurgical multidrug-resistant *Acinetobacter baumannii* meningitis successfully treated with intrathecal colistin. A new case and a systematic review of the literature. *Int. J. Infect. Dis.* **2010**, *14*, e572–e579. [CrossRef] [PubMed]
144. Fu, J.; Li, L.; Huo, D.; Yang, R.; Yang, B.; Xu, B.; Yang, X.; Dai, M.; Tan, C.; Chen, H.; et al. Meningitic *Escherichia coli* alpha-hemolysin aggravates blood-brain barrier disruption via targeting TGFbeta1-triggered hedgehog signaling. *Mol. Brain* **2021**, *14*, 116. [CrossRef]
145. Caporarello, N.; Olivieri, M.; Cristaldi, M.; Scalia, M.; Toscano, M.A.; Genovese, C.; Addamo, A.; Salmeri, M.; Lupo, G.; Anfuso, C.D. Blood-Brain Barrier in a *Haemophilus influenzae* Type a In Vitro Infection: Role of Adenosine Receptors A2A and A2B. *Mol. Neurobiol.* **2018**, *55*, 5321–5336. [CrossRef] [PubMed]
146. Wegele, C.; Stump-Guthier, C.; Moroniak, S.; Weiss, C.; Rohde, M.; Ishikawa, H.; Schroten, H.; Schwerk, C.; Karremann, M.; Borkowski, J. Non-Typeable *Haemophilus influenzae* Invade Choroid Plexus Epithelial Cells in a Polar Fashion. *Int. J. Mol. Sci.* **2020**, *21*, 5739. [CrossRef]
147. Ku, Y.H.; Chuang, Y.C.; Chen, C.C.; Lee, M.F.; Yang, Y.C.; Tang, H.J.; Yu, W.L. *Klebsiella pneumoniae* Isolates from Meningitis: Epidemiology, Virulence and Antibiotic Resistance. *Sci. Rep.* **2017**, *7*, 6634. [CrossRef]

148. Cassidy, B.R.; Zhang, M.; Sonntag, W.E.; Drevets, D.A. Neuroinvasive *Listeria monocytogenes* infection triggers accumulation of brain CD8+ tissue-resident memory T cells in a miR-155-dependent fashion. *J. Neuroinflammation* **2020**, *17*, 259. [CrossRef]
149. Schubert-Unkmeir, A.; Konrad, C.; Slanina, H.; Czapek, F.; Hebling, S.; Frosch, M. *Neisseria meningitidis* induces brain microvascular endothelial cell detachment from the matrix and cleavage of occludin: A role for MMP-8. *PLoS Pathog.* **2010**, *6*, e1000874. [CrossRef]
150. Orihuela, C.J.; Mahdavi, J.; Thornton, J.; Mann, B.; Wooldridge, K.G.; Abouseada, N.; Oldfield, N.J.; Self, T.; Ala'Aldeen, D.A.; Tuomanen, E.I. Laminin receptor initiates bacterial contact with the blood brain barrier in experimental meningitis models. *J. Clin. Investig.* **2009**, *119*, 1638–1646. [CrossRef]
151. Chen, H.; Guo, X.; Xie, D.; Dong, X.; Niu, J.; Chen, G. A Clinical Study on the Use of Intraventricular Polymyxin B Supplemented by Continuous External Ventricular Drainage in the Treatment of Drug-Resistant Gram-Negative Bacilli Intracranial Infection. *Infect. Drug Resist.* **2020**, *13*, 2963–2970. [CrossRef] [PubMed]
152. McLoughlin, A.; Rochfort, K.D.; McDonnell, C.J.; Kerrigan, S.W.; Cummins, P.M. *Staphylococcus aureus*-mediated blood-brain barrier injury: An in vitro human brain microvascular endothelial cell model. *Cell. Microbiol.* **2017**, *19*, e12664. [CrossRef] [PubMed]
153. Anil, A.; Banerjee, A. Pneumococcal Encounter with the Blood-Brain Barrier Endothelium. *Front. Cell. Infect. Microbiol.* **2020**, *10*, 590682. [CrossRef] [PubMed]
154. Iovino, F.; Seinen, J.; Henriques-Normark, B.; van Dijl, J.M. How Does *Streptococcus pneumoniae* Invade the Brain? *Trends Microbiol.* **2016**, *24*, 307–315. [CrossRef] [PubMed]
155. Zocco, M.A.; dal Verme, L.Z.; Cremonini, F.; Piscaglia, A.C.; Nista, E.C.; Candelli, M.; Novi, M.; Rigante, D.; Cazzato, I.A.; Ojetti, V.; et al. Efficacy of *Lactobacillus* GG in maintaining remission of ulcerative colitis. *Aliment. Pharmacol. Ther.* **2006**, *23*, 1567–1574. [CrossRef]
156. Tsai, Y.-L.; Tsai, W.-C.; Qing, Z.; Chang, C.-J. Dichotomous effects of microbial membrane vesicles on the regulation of immunity. *Med. Microecol.* **2020**, *3*, 100009. [CrossRef]
157. Ramachandran, G.; Bikard, D. Editing the microbiome the CRISPR way. *Philos. Trans. R. Soc. Lond. B Biol. Sci.* **2019**, *374*, 20180103. [CrossRef]
158. Wang, Y.; Hoffmann, J.P.; Baker, S.M.; Bentrup, K.H.Z.; Wimley, W.C.; Fuselier, J.A.; Bitoun, J.P.; Morici, L.A. Inhibition of *Streptococcus mutans* biofilms with bacterial-derived outer membrane vesicles. *BMC Microbiol.* **2021**, *21*, 234. [CrossRef]
159. Hu, R.; Lin, H.; Li, J.; Zhao, Y.; Wang, M.; Sun, X.; Min, Y.; Gao, Y.; Yang, M. Probiotic *Escherichia coli* Nissle 1917-derived outer membrane vesicles enhance immunomodulation and antimicrobial activity in RAW264.7 macrophages. *BMC Microbiol.* **2020**, *20*, 268. [CrossRef]
160. Chee, W.J.Y.; Chew, S.Y.; Than, L.T.L. Vaginal microbiota and the potential of *Lactobacillus* derivatives in maintaining vaginal health. *Microb. Cell Fact.* **2020**, *19*, 203. [CrossRef]
161. Qin, H.; Zhang, Z.; Hang, X.; Jiang, Y.L. *plantarum* prevents enteroinvasive *Escherichia coli*-induced tight junction proteins changes in intestinal epithelial cells. *BMC Microbiol.* **2009**, *9*, 63. [CrossRef] [PubMed]
162. Bajic, S.S.; Canas, M.A.; Tolinacki, M.; Badia, J.; Sanchez, B.; Golic, N.; Margolles, A.; Baldoma, L.; Ruas-Madiedo, P. Proteomic profile of extracellular vesicles released by *Lactiplantibacillus plantarum* BGAN8 and their internalization by non-polarized HT29 cell line. *Sci. Rep.* **2020**, *10*, 21829. [CrossRef] [PubMed]
163. Zheng, D.; Liwinski, T.; Elinav, E. Interaction between microbiota and immunity in health and disease. *Cell Res.* **2020**, *30*, 492–506. [CrossRef] [PubMed]
164. Han, E.C.; Choi, S.Y.; Lee, Y.; Park, J.W.; Hong, S.H.; Lee, H.J. Extracellular RNAs in periodontopathogenic outer membrane vesicles promote TNF-α production in human macrophages and cross the blood–brain barrier in mice. *FASEB J.* **2019**, *33*, 13412. [CrossRef]
165. Al-Nedawi, K.; Mian, M.F.; Hossain, N.; Karimi, K.; Mao, Y.K.; Forsythe, P.; Min, K.K.; Stanisz, A.M.; Kunze, W.A.; Bienenstock, J. Gut commensal microvesicles reproduce parent bacterial signals to host immune and enteric nervous systems. *FASEB J.* **2015**, *29*, 684–695. [CrossRef]
166. Haas-Neill, S.; Forsythe, P. A Budding Relationship: Bacterial Extracellular Vesicles in the Microbiota-Gut-Brain Axis. *Int. J. Mol. Sci.* **2020**, *21*, 8899. [CrossRef]
167. Mba, I.E.; Nweze, E.I. Nanoparticles as therapeutic options for treating multidrug-resistant bacteria: Research progress, challenges, and prospects. *World J. Microbiol. Biotechnol.* **2021**, *37*, 108. [CrossRef]
168. Rudramurthy, G.R.; Swamy, M.K.; Sinniah, U.R.; Ghasemzadeh, A. Nanoparticles: Alternatives Against Drug-Resistant Pathogenic Microbes. *Molecules* **2016**, *21*, 836. [CrossRef]
169. Khan, I.; Saeed, K.; Khan, I. Nanoparticles: Properties, applications and toxicities. *Arab. J. Chem.* **2019**, *12*, 908–931. [CrossRef]
170. Van de Waterbeemd, B.; Streefland, M.; van der Ley, P.; Zomer, B.; van Dijken, H.; Martens, D.; Wijffels, R.; van der Pol, L. Improved OMV vaccine against *Neisseria meningitidis* using genetically engineered strains and a detergent-free purification process. *Vaccine* **2010**, *28*, 4810–4816. [CrossRef]
171. Van der Pol, L.; Stork, M.; van der Ley, P. Outer membrane vesicles as platform vaccine technology. *Biotechnol. J.* **2015**, *10*, 1689–1706. [CrossRef] [PubMed]
172. Meng, W.; He, C.; Hao, Y.; Wang, L.; Li, L.; Zhu, G. Prospects and challenges of extracellular vesicle-based drug delivery system: Considering cell source. *Drug Deliv.* **2020**, *27*, 585–598. [CrossRef] [PubMed]

173. Zhu, Z.; Antenucci, F.; Villumsen, K.R.; Bojesen, A.M. Bacterial Outer Membrane Vesicles as a Versatile Tool in Vaccine Research and the Fight against Antimicrobial Resistance. *mBio* **2021**, *12*, e0170721. [CrossRef] [PubMed]
174. Xu, M.; Feng, T.; Liu, B.; Qiu, F.; Xu, Y.; Zhao, Y.; Zheng, Y. Engineered exosomes: Desirable target-tracking characteristics for cerebrovascular and neurodegenerative disease therapies. *Theranostics* **2021**, *11*, 8926–8944. [CrossRef]
175. Tiwari, S.; Jamal, S.B.; Hassan, S.S.; Carvalho, P.; Almeida, S.; Barh, D.; Ghosh, P.; Silva, A.; Castro, T.L.P.; Azevedo, V. Two-Component Signal Transduction Systems of Pathogenic Bacteria as Targets for Antimicrobial Therapy: An Overview. *Front. Microbiol.* **2017**, *8*, 1878. [CrossRef] [PubMed]
176. Dobson, A.; Cotter, P.D.; Ross, R.P.; Hill, C. Bacteriocin production: A probiotic trait? *Appl. Environ. Microbiol.* **2012**, *78*, 1–6. [CrossRef]
177. Jakava-Viljanen, M.; Avall-Jaaskelainen, S.; Messner, P.; Sleytr, U.B.; Palva, A. Isolation of three new surface layer protein genes (slp) from *Lactobacillus brevis* ATCC 14869 and characterization of the change in their expression under aerated and anaerobic conditions. *J. Bacteriol.* **2002**, *184*, 6786–6795. [CrossRef]
178. Kim, J.Y.; Doody, A.M.; Chen, D.J.; Cremona, G.H.; Shuler, M.L.; Putnam, D.; DeLisa, M.P. Engineered bacterial outer membrane vesicles with enhanced functionality. *J. Mol. Biol.* **2008**, *380*, 51–66. [CrossRef]
179. Uchida, H.; Kinoshita, H.; Kawai, Y.; Kitazawa, H.; Miura, K.; Shiiba, K.; Horii, A.; Kimura, K.; Taketomo, N.; Oda, M.; et al. *Lactobacilli* binding human A-antigen expressed in intestinal mucosa. *Res. Microbiol.* **2006**, *157*, 659–665. [CrossRef]
180. Klotz, C.; Barrangou, R. Engineering Components of the *Lactobacillus* S-Layer for Biotherapeutic Applications. *Front. Microbiol.* **2018**, *9*, 2264. [CrossRef]
181. Lee, S.H.; Kim, M.S.; Jung, H.C.; Lee, J.; Lee, J.H.; Lee, H.S.; Kang, S.G. Screening of a novel strong promoter by RNA sequencing and its application to H2 production in a hyperthermophilic archaeon. *Appl. Microbiol. Biotechnol.* **2015**, *99*, 4085–4092. [CrossRef] [PubMed]
182. Parker, A.; Fonseca, S.; Carding, S.R. Gut microbes and metabolites as modulators of blood-brain barrier integrity and brain health. *Gut Microbes* **2020**, *11*, 135–157. [CrossRef] [PubMed]
183. Zhao, L.; Ye, Y.; Gu, L.; Jian, Z.; Stary, C.M.; Xiong, X. Extracellular vesicle-derived miRNA as a novel regulatory system for bi-directional communication in gut-brain-microbiota axis. *J. Transl. Med.* **2021**, *19*, 202. [CrossRef] [PubMed]
184. Layunta, E.; Buey, B.; Mesonero, J.E.; Latorre, E. Crosstalk Between Intestinal Serotonergic System and Pattern Recognition Receptors on the Microbiota-Gut-Brain Axis. *Front. Endocrinol.* **2021**, *12*, 748254. [CrossRef] [PubMed]
185. Wynendaele, E.; Verbeke, F.; Stalmans, S.; Gevaert, B.; Janssens, Y.; Van De Wiele, C.; Peremans, K.; Burvenich, C.; De Spiegeleer, B. Quorum Sensing Peptides Selectively Penetrate the Blood-Brain Barrier. *PLoS ONE* **2015**, *10*, e0142071. [CrossRef]
186. Abib, R.T.; Gaman, A.; Dargel, A.A.; Tamouza, R.; Kapczinski, F.; Gottfried, C.; Leboyer, M. Intracellular Pathogen Infections and Immune Response in Autism. *Neuroimmunomodulation* **2018**, *25*, 271–279. [CrossRef]
187. Garcia-Gutierrez, E.; Narbad, A.; Rodriguez, J.M. Autism Spectrum Disorder Associated with Gut Microbiota at Immune, Metabolomic, and Neuroactive Level. *Front. Neurosci.* **2020**, *14*, 578666. [CrossRef]
188. Jodoin, J.; Demeule, M.; Fenart, L.; Cecchelli, R.; Farmer, S.; Linton, K.J.; Higgins, C.F.; Beliveau, R. P-glycoprotein in blood-brain barrier endothelial cells: Interaction and oligomerization with caveolins. *J. Neurochem.* **2003**, *87*, 1010–1023. [CrossRef]
189. Grill, M.F.; Maganti, R.K. Neurotoxic effects associated with antibiotic use: Management considerations. *Br. J. Clin. Pharmacol.* **2011**, *72*, 381–393. [CrossRef]
190. Fazal, S.; Lee, R. Biomimetic Bacterial Membrane Vesicles for Drug Delivery Applications. *Pharmaceutics* **2021**, *13*, 1430. [CrossRef]
191. Chen, G.; Bai, Y.; Li, Z.; Wang, F.; Fan, X.; Zhou, X. Bacterial extracellular vesicle-coated multi-antigenic nanovaccines protect against drug-resistant *Staphylococcus aureus* infection by modulating antigen processing and presentation pathways. *Theranostics* **2020**, *10*, 7131–7149. [CrossRef] [PubMed]
192. Wu, Y.; Battalapalli, D.; Hakeem, M.J.; Selamneni, V.; Zhang, P.; Draz, M.S.; Ruan, Z. Engineered CRISPR-Cas systems for the detection and control of antibiotic-resistant infections. *J. Nanobiotechnol.* **2021**, *19*, 401. [CrossRef] [PubMed]
193. Oh, J.H.; van Pijkeren, J.P. CRISPR-Cas9-assisted recombineering in *Lactobacillus reuteri*. *Nucleic Acids Res.* **2014**, *42*, e131. [CrossRef] [PubMed]
194. Schuster, J.A.; Vogel, R.F.; Ehrmann, M.A. Characterization and distribution of CRISPR-Cas systems in *Lactobacillus sakei*. *Arch. Microbiol.* **2019**, *201*, 337–347. [CrossRef] [PubMed]
195. Loo, Y.S.; Bose, R.J.; McCarthy, J.R.; Azmi, I.D.M.; Madheswaran, T. Biomimetic bacterial and viral-based nanovesicles for drug delivery, theranostics, and vaccine applications. *Drug Discov. Today* **2021**, *26*, 902–915. [CrossRef] [PubMed]
196. Zambrowicz, B.P.; Sands, A.T. Knockouts model the 100 best-selling drugs—Will they model the next 100? *Nat. Rev. Drug Discov.* **2003**, *2*, 38–51. [CrossRef]
197. Choi, S.Y.; Lim, S.; Cho, G.; Kwon, J.; Mun, W.; Im, H.; Mitchell, R.J. *Chromobacterium violaceum* delivers violacein, a hydrophobic antibiotic, to other microbes in membrane vesicles. *Environ. Microbiol.* **2020**, *22*, 705–713. [CrossRef]

pharmaceutics

MDPI

Review

Bacterial Membrane Vesicles as Smart Drug Delivery and Carrier Systems: A New Nanosystems Tool for Current Anticancer and Antimicrobial Therapy

Pınar Aytar Çelik [1,2,*], Kubra Erdogan-Gover [2], Dilan Barut [2], Blaise Manga Enuh [2], Gülin Amasya [3], Ceyda Tuba Sengel-Türk [3], Burak Derkus [4] and Ahmet Çabuk [2,5]

1 Environmental Protection and Control Program, Eskisehir Osmangazi University, Eskisehir 26110, Turkey
2 Department of Biotechnology and Biosafety, Graduate School of Natural and Applied Science, Eskisehir Osmangazi University, Eskisehir 26040, Turkey
3 Department of Pharmaceutical Technology, Faculty of Pharmacy, Ankara University, Ankara 06100, Turkey
4 Department of Chemistry, Faculty of Science, Ankara University, Ankara 06560, Turkey
5 Department of Biology, Faculty of Science, Eskisehir Osmangazi University, Eskisehir 26040, Turkey
* Correspondence: paytar@ogu.edu.tr

Abstract: Bacterial membrane vesicles (BMVs) are known to be critical communication tools in several pathophysiological processes between bacteria and host cells. Given this situation, BMVs for transporting and delivering exogenous therapeutic cargoes have been inspiring as promising platforms for developing smart drug delivery systems (SDDSs). In the first section of this review paper, starting with an introduction to pharmaceutical technology and nanotechnology, we delve into the design and classification of SDDSs. We discuss the characteristics of BMVs including their size, shape, charge, effective production and purification techniques, and the different methods used for cargo loading and drug encapsulation. We also shed light on the drug release mechanism, the design of BMVs as smart carriers, and recent remarkable findings on the potential of BMVs for anticancer and antimicrobial therapy. Furthermore, this review covers the safety of BMVs and the challenges that need to be overcome for clinical use. Finally, we discuss the recent advancements and prospects for BMVs as SDDSs and highlight their potential in revolutionizing the fields of nanomedicine and drug delivery. In conclusion, this review paper aims to provide a comprehensive overview of the state-of-the-art field of BMVs as SDDSs, encompassing their design, composition, fabrication, purification, and characterization, as well as the various strategies used for targeted delivery. Considering this information, the aim of this review is to provide researchers in the field with a comprehensive understanding of the current state of BMVs as SDDSs, enabling them to identify critical gaps and formulate new hypotheses to accelerate the progress of the field.

Keywords: bacterial membrane vesicle; smart drug delivery systems; carrier adjuvant systems

Citation: Aytar Çelik, P.; Erdogan-Gover, K.; Barut, D.; Enuh, B.M.; Amasya, G.; Sengel-Türk, C.T.; Derkus, B.; Çabuk, A. Bacterial Membrane Vesicles as Smart Drug Delivery and Carrier Systems: A New Nanosystems Tool for Current Anticancer and Antimicrobial Therapy. *Pharmaceutics* **2023**, *15*, 1052. https://doi.org/10.3390/pharmaceutics15041052

Academic Editor: Yong Chen

Received: 19 February 2023
Revised: 19 March 2023
Accepted: 21 March 2023
Published: 24 March 2023

1. Introduction

Considering that the discovery of a new drug molecule is both costly and time-consuming, the use of state-of-art drug delivery systems is the most up-to-date approach in the pharmaceutical sciences to increase therapeutic efficacy as well as reduce the side-effect profile of currently used active molecules. Therefore, the concept of a drug delivery system keeps up with technological advances. It has also become inevitable for drug delivery systems to become smarter in today's world, as everything from the watch to the phone has become smart.

In the classical sense, "drug delivery system" refers to the technologies that carry the active ingredients used for the treatment of any disease into the body. The principal purpose of conventional drug delivery systems is to transport the active molecule in the optimal dose and in a convenient way as well as to facilitate patient compliance and to maintain the stability of the active substance. However, the most notable drawback of conventional systems is that they offer low bioavailability due to the physicochemical properties of the active molecule and they may cause fluctuations in plasma drug level. Drug release from these systems cannot be controlled either [1]. The low water solubility and poor permeability of active molecules as well as rapid metabolization and elimination are associated with their bioavailability, and these features largely limit the pharmacological potential of the active molecules. Therefore, advances in the development of drug delivery systems have always been aimed to increase bioavailability. While we cannot intervene in the physical properties of active molecules, all therapeutic functions can be controlled with the construction of an effective delivery system [2,3].

Since the rise of nanotechnology in the early 2000s and its relationship with drug release technologies, the advantages of "nano-size" over bioavailability have been exploited and many studies have been conducted on nanoscale drug release strategies and their PEGylated derivatives. Today, many commercial examples of "nanocarriers" appear in the world pharmaceutical market. This is simply reasoned by the unique advantages of adaptation of nanotechnology to drug delivery systems, such as the increased release of drugs with low water solubility, facilitated access of the active substance to cells or tissues, efficient passage through epithelial and endothelial barriers, the acquired potential of simultaneous application of multiple substances, and the enabled ability to develop theranostic systems by combining the active substances with imaging agents [4].

The expectation from a novel drug delivery system involves a specific delivery of the loaded active molecule only to the damaged/diseased tissues and cells where a pharmacological activity is needed. Beyond any doubt, the aim of this approach is strictly to maximize treatment response and minimize side effects. Thus, besides basic concepts such as drug delivery systems, controlled release, and nanotechnology, materials science also comes into play and contributes to emerging smart drug systems strategies. The smart drug delivery phenomenon is mostly based on materials; in many cases polymers with unique properties that sense a change upon external exposure. Later, they initiate a response to the stimuli via different mechanisms depending on the chemical bases of the building-blocks, in other words, they exhibit stimuli-responsive features. This phenomenon can be adapted to the macro, micro, or nanoscales [5]. Stimuli-responsive drug delivery systems can be created in various organic architectures such as vesicles, polymeric nanoparticles, micelles, dendrimers, or hydrogels as well as inorganic metal oxide frameworks, quantum dots, and mesoporous silica nanoparticles. Basically, the reason why the carrier system is called "smart" is that it reveals the active component it carries as a result of the system's response to various stimuli. Depending on the source of the stimulus, as endogenous or exogenous, stimuli-responsive materials can be used to effectively deliver the drug of interest [6–9].

Bacterial membrane vesicles (BMVs) derived from bacteria have also been recognized as smart drug delivery systems due to their biomimetic properties and versatile functions, as well as the nature of the vesicles, which are important in intercellular communication [10]. They are distinguished from other nano-sized drug delivery systems as next-generation biomimetic vehicles that can be produced on a large scale at lower costs. Another advantage they provide is that isolated BMVs are amenable to surface modification and allow active targeting via specific ligands, or it is possible to obtain tailor-made BMVs by genetic manipulation on vesicle source strains. Moreover, the most fundamental feature of BMVs that enable them to be used as smart drug delivery systems is their ability to evade the host immune system and maintain the stability of the therapeutic agent [11].

Herein, we have focused on the roles and potentials of BMVs in smart delivery systems; additionally, the fabrication principles, characterizations, and applications of BMVs have been covered.

2. Design and Classification of Smart Drug Delivery Systems

2.1. Design

The main purpose of drug delivery systems is to deliver and target drugs to tissues in a protected manner. The drug given with traditional systems is quickly eliminated from the body. In these cases, regular multiple doses seem to be an alternative, but toxic levels can be observed as a result of overdosing, resulting in poor patient compliance. Smart drug delivery systems (SDDSs) are required to obtain a steady-state concentration in targeted tissues to provide a prolonged effect and eliminate side effects. While designing these systems, there are important parameters such as biomaterial properties, stability, and stimulants. Delivery systems sensitive to stimuli are grouped into two categories: those sensitive to internal and external stimuli [2].

2.1.1. Internal

Among the internal stimulants, there are pH-responsive, redox-responsive, enzyme-responsive, and ionic microenvironment-responsive systems. In SDDSs designed for stimulation by internal stimuli, drug release occurs with the deterioration of the physicochemical structure of the materials suitable for these stimuli [12].

pH-responsive. Among the internal stimulants, the pH factor is frequently used [13]. In pH-responsive biomaterials, deterioration occurs that triggers drug release according to the difference in pH. While in the normal pH range, pH-responsive carriers keep the drug stable and release it with the changing pH in the therapeutic tissues after depots [2]. Ionizing polymers such as polyacrylic acid and polymethacrylic acid can be used to design pH-responsive carriers. These pH-responsive polymers are categorized as polyacids and poly basics [14,15].

Redox-responsive. While the intracellular reduced glutathione (GSH) concentration is between 2 and 10 mM, this ratio is 1/1000 outside the cell. Thus, a redox gradient is formed between the extracellular and the intracellular. The disulfide bond has been recognized as the main binding agent for redox-sensitive systems. While the disulfide bonds in the transporters are stable at low GSH levels in the extracellular environment, they are reduced to thiol groups at high GSH levels inside the cell, and the transporters are disrupted resulting in drug release [14]. In addition, considering the high accumulation of reactive oxygen species (ROS) in some therapeutic situations, carrier systems have been developed to respond to ROS [13,16].

Enzyme-responsive. In certain therapeutic situations, some enzymes are specifically produced at high levels. By using these specific enzymes, SDDSs with high substrate specificity and selectivity have been developed [13,17,18].

Ionic microenvironment-responsive. Ionic microenvironment-responsive carriers are designed by adding acidic and basic functional molecules that affect the ionization power. The presence of highly acidic groups in the carriers creates increased electrostatic repulsion between the negatively charged groups, and at high pH, the physiology of the carrier changes. Thus, drug release is triggered [12].

2.1.2. External

In the class of external stimulants, some systems are temperature-responsive, light-responsive, electrical field-responsive, magnetic field-responsive, and ultrasound-responsive systems.

Temperature-responsive. Among carriers sensitive to external stimuli, temperature-responsive ones are preferred as a more common strategy. The applicability of naturally occurring and easily generated temperature differences is the main reason for this [16]. The presence of high temperatures in therapeutic tissues, ranging from 40 to 45 °C, makes the use of temperature-responsive carriers important [19]. Basically, temperature-responsive carriers retain the drug at a normal temperature and release it when exposed to the high temperature of the therapeutic tissue [12]. There are two types of temperature-responsive carrier systems. These are the low critical solution temperature (LCST) and the upper critical solution temperature (UCST). In the LCST type, the carrier physiology is triggered at temperatures below the LCST; in the same way, in the UCST type, the carrier physical chemistry is triggered at temperatures above the UCST and directs the drug release [12,18].

Light-responsive. Ultraviolet light, visible light, and near-infrared light (NIR) are external stimuli used for photosensitive carriers. NIR, with its advantages such as high biocompatibility and in situ polymerization, is an effective stimulant as a photosensitive drug carrier. Different mechanisms have been reported for drug release by systems that respond to NIR: the photo-thermal effect and two-photon activation [12,16,19].

Electrical field-responsive. Heat generation and redox reactions occur as a result of the electrical application in drug delivery systems designed as sensitive to an electric field. In this way, different drug-release pathways are activated by electrical stimulation. Electrical field-responsive polymers such as polypyrrole, polyaniline, and graphene are examples of this system [2,12].

Magnetic field-responsive. The magnetic field can penetrate tissues and is frequently used in imaging. Apart from imaging, it has potential as an effective external stimulant for drug delivery systems. Magnetic field-responsive drug delivery systems have magnetic field-induced hyperthermia and magnetic field-directed drug targeting mechanisms. When a magnetic field is applied, heat is generated. Therefore, magnetic nanoparticles are encapsulated in colloidal carriers that trigger drug release in the case of hyperthermia in magnetic field-responsive systems [2,12].

Ultrasound-responsive. Ultrasound waves are used as external stimulants in drug release because of their tissue penetration and good spatio-temporal control properties. Ultrasound waves create thermal, mechanical, and radiation forces and these effects trigger drug release in carrier systems [12].

Dual/Multi-responsive. In addition to drug delivery systems responsive to a single stimulant, combinations of multiple internal or external stimulators can be used to increase efficiency. Among systems responsive to dual stimuli, pH/temperature-responsive systems have been extensively studied. These systems are used in situations that are difficult to target when only temperature-responsive systems are used [15,16].

2.2. Classification

There are three main release mechanisms for drug delivery systems: diffusion controlled, osmotically controlled, and chemically controlled. In diffusion-controlled systems, the drug is retained in water-insoluble polymeric membranes or matrices and released by diffusion. Biocompatible membranes with water permeability are used in osmotically controlled systems. In these systems, osmotic pressure is created by the use of NaCl or formulation with an osmogenic effect. Polymers such as cellulose acetate and ethyl cellulose are widely used in osmotically controlled systems. In chemically controlled systems or, in other words, erosion-controlled systems, materials that can degrade in a biological environment are used. There are two types of mechanisms in these systems: polymer-drug dispersion and polymer-drug conjugation. In polymer-drug dispersion, the drug is dispersed into the biodegradable polymer, and drug release occurs with the degradation of the polymer under therapeutic conditions. In the polymer-drug conjugate, the drug is conjugated to the polymer surface by covalent bonds, and drug release occurs by breaking the polymer-drug bonds under therapeutic conditions [2].

Nanosized drug carriers have a high loading capacity, increase bioavailability by keeping the drug in circulation for longer periods, and are advantageous for targeted delivery as their surface is easy to modify [2]. Many nanosized carriers are available for SDDSs.

Mesoporous silica systems. Mesoporous silica systems range in size from 50 to 300 nm. Endocytosis allows them to enter the cell without causing cytotoxicity. It has inner and outer surfaces, and these surfaces can be modified to make it functional [20].

Hydrogels. Hydrogel structures are frequently used in drug delivery. They consist of water-soluble polymers with cross-linked networks. The release of the drug embedded in the hydrogel occurs by the swelling of the polymer in the aqueous medium. Temperature, pH, and the ionic environment are effective in swelling the hydrogel [18].

Dendrimers. Dendrimers are less common as carrier systems. They have a central core, an inner layer of blocks, and a peripheral region consisting of hyperbranched chains. They can be functionalized with specific ligands to form SDDSs. Its advantages include providing controllable size and molecular weight [20,21].

Liposomes. Liposomes are composed of phospholipids arranged in vesicle form. Their size ranges from nanometer sizes to micrometer sizes. Vesicular systems inspired by liposomes can be categorized as niosomes, transfersomes, etosomes, and phytosomes. Niosomes have a non-ionic surface containing low concentrations of phospholipids. Transfersomes are liposomes that have increased flexibility by adding a single chain activator to the surface. If ethanol is used in the preparation of liposomes, they are called etosomes. Finally, if the phospholipids used in the composition are obtained from plants, the structures formed are called phytosomes. The liposome core is suitable for encapsulating hydrophilic drugs, while the peripheral region between the lipid and phospholipid layers encapsulates hydrophobic drugs [2,21].

Metal nanoparticles. Metal nanoparticles can be used in the visualization and diagnosis of cellular components as well as in drug delivery. Gold and silver nanoparticles are the most popular. They can be functionalized with bioactive molecules such as antibodies and enzymes. These structures can be included in SDDSs by adding hybrid features [20].

Polymeric nanoparticles. Polymeric nanoparticles are usually 100–700 nm in size and consist of biodegradable polymer/copolymer structures. Drugs can be encapsulated in these structures, physically absorbed at the surface, or chemically bound to the surface [20].

Solid-lipid nanoparticles (SLN). Solid lipid nanoparticles have emerged by combining polymeric nanoparticles and liposomes. They can be defined as particles in the nanometer range consisting of biocompatible lipids in solid form at room/body temperature [2].

Carbon nanotubes (CNT). Carbon nanotubes consist of spherical graphene layers that can be sealed with fullerene. CNTs must be functionalized in order to be used in biological systems; otherwise, they may show cytotoxic effects. Bioactive agents can be conjugated or coated with biodegradable agents to functionalize them [2,20].

Polymeric carbon nanoparticles. These are formed by modifying carbon nanotubes with polymers. Polymer wrapping or polymer adsorption can occur based on weak wave-like interactions between carbon nanotubes and polymers, or polymers can be integrated into the carbon nanotube surface by chemical bonds [20].

Exosomes. Exosomes are vesicles derived from eukaryotic cells that range in size from 30 to 100 nm. It is a biological material and has been frequently studied in recent years due to its ability to enter cells. The advantages of exosomes are their non-cytotoxic, natural targeting abilities and high drug-loading capacity. The disadvantages of exosomes are the difficulty in their large-scale production and purification without losing their biological properties in clinical use [2,13,22].

Bacterial membrane vesicles (BMVs). BMVs are vesicles derived from bacterial cells. BMVs have certain advantages over existing carrier vehicles: they are more stable against leakage and deterioration by keeping the drug more stable in circulation. They can increase the effect of the drug with their immunogenic effects due to the presence of antigen and LPS on their surface. They are highly suitable for surface modification and genetic engineering regulations that will increase targeting efficiency [23].

Exosomes from eukaryotic cells and membrane vesicles from bacteria have numerous structural and biologically functional similarities [24]. Although exosomes are being investigated more and more as carrier systems with high biocompatibility and translation ability around the world, their manufacture is challenging and costly, especially in large-scale mammalian cultures, when compared to BMVs. On the other hand, the production of BMVs in bacterial cultures is faster, simpler, and relatively cheaper. In addition, BMVs are nanostructures specifically suitable for design and production, where genetic engineering is more convenient [11]. Although research on exosomes in biological applications is intense, investigations in this field have increased steadily in recent years after the discovery of BMVs [25].

The basic features of BMVs, their production and purification techniques, and their use as SDDSs in the biomedical field will be explained in detail in the chapters of this review paper. The classification of SDDSs as well as their advantages and disadvantages are presented in Table 1 [22,26–45].

Table 1. The classification of SDDSs as well as their advantages and disadvantages.

Classification of SDDS		Advantages	Disadvantages
Organic	Polymeric nanoparticles	Controllable particle and surface properties Enhanced stability of API Tunable release properties API encapsulation both hydrophilic and lipophilic character	Difficulty in adapting production processes on an industrial scale Residual material associated with production process
	Hydrogels	Ability to absorb water or biological fluids Capacity to mimic biological structures with 3D structure Biodegradable and nontoxic nature Site-specific application	Possibility of drug deactivation during production Limited hydrophobic drug delivery Difficulty in sterilization Mechanically unstable High production costs
	Dendrimers	Increased drug solubility High loading efficiency through internal cavities Surface modification with terminal functional groups Enhanced permeation effects and long in vivo circulation lifetime	High nonspecific toxicity Increased cytotoxicity due to an increase in the number of generations Possible hemolytic activity Relatively expensive raw material requirement
	Liposomes	Nontoxic, biodegradable, and flexible vesicles cell membrane-like structure Simultaneous entrapment of hydrophilic and lipophilic API prolonging circulation time Possible to formulate sterically stabilized liposomes	Possibility of organic solvent residue Lipid oxidation/hydrolysis problem during shelf life
	Lipid nanoparticles	Safe composition of physiological lipids Avoiding the use of organic solvents Economical and low-cost production Possible to scale up Site-specific drug delivery	Low drug-loading capacity for hydrophilic molecules Expulsion of API due to polymorphic transitions during storage Burst release

Table 1. *Cont.*

Classification of SDDS		Advantages	Disadvantages
Inorganic	Carbon nanotubes	Easy to modify and functionalize Sequential structure High mechanical strength Effective for molecules to enter cells	Highly hydrophobic nature The lack of solubility in solvents compatible with biological fluid Biodegradation problem
	Mesoporous silica system	High surface–volume ratio Presence of nanopores Low-cost complex system design Avoiding the early drug release	Solubility and biodegradability characteristics Presence of silanol groups and their interaction with membrane lipids
	Metal nanoparticles	Availability of green synthesis Tunable size, geometry, and surface Suitable for large-scale production Unique optical, electronic physicochemical features Can be used as a diagnostic tool	Not biodegradable Tendency to accumulate non-specifically in the body Environmental toxicity risk
Biologic	Exosomes	Ability to mediate intercellular communication Resistant to digestive enzymes	Challenges related to the isolation and purity Rapid elimination from the bloodstream Limited large-scale production
	Bacterial membrane vesicles	Easy-to-access raw material source Able to be designed with the help of genetic engineering Surface modification with biological ligands	Limited scalable manufacturing Relatively low BMV yield Lack of standardization in production

3. BMVs as Smart Drug Delivery Systems

The history and timeline of milestones of BMVs and their applications in drug delivery can be traced back to the late 1970s and early 1980s when the concept of using BMVs as drug carriers was first proposed. A general timeline of key events and milestones in the history of BMVs and their applications in drug delivery is shown in Figure 1. While BMVs show great promise as drug delivery systems, there are still concerns about their stability and toxicity. However, one novel angle to consider is the potential for BMVs to be modified to respond to specific environmental cues within the body, such as pH or temperature changes, to release their contents. This "smart" approach could increase drug efficacy while reducing potential side effects.

3.1. Fabrications of BMVs

The release of extracellular vesicles is an evolutionarily conserved feature. They are produced from the cells of all organisms, including prokaryotes and eukaryotes. The vesicles produced by bacteria are generally referred to as "bacterial membrane vesicles". BMVs are defined as non-replicative spherical nanostructures with a lipid bilayer about 100–400 nm in diameter [46]. The discovery of BMVs dates back to the 1960s with the development of the electron microscope [47].

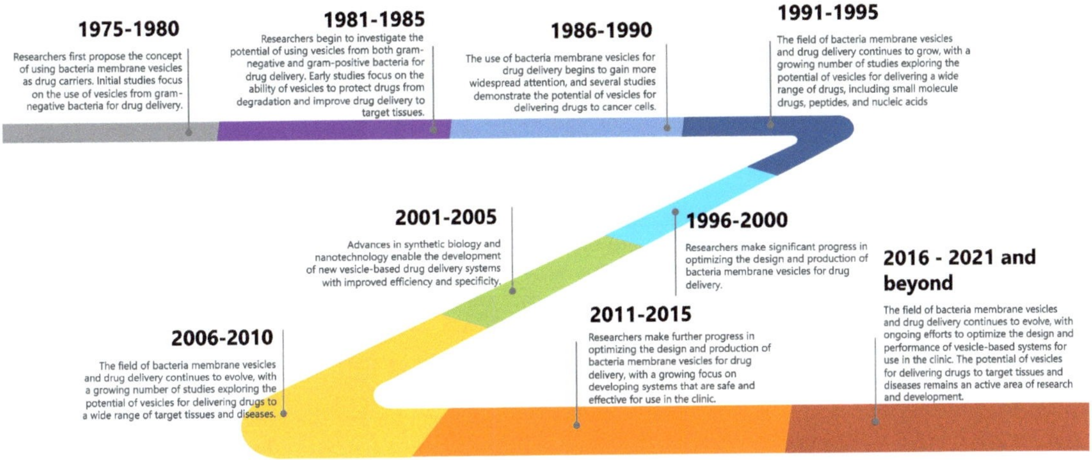

Figure 1. A general timeline of key events and milestones in the history of BMVs and their applications in drug delivery.

BMVs are released from both Gram-negative and Gram-positive bacteria. Basically, three models are presented for BMV biogenesis. The first is through the loss of outer membrane and peptidoglycan layer connectivity by the deposition of outer membrane proteins in the periplasmic space. Evidence for this model is the reduction of outer membrane proteins in vesicle-producing bacteria. In the second model, it is assumed that the turgor pressure created by the accumulation of periplasmic proteins and peptidoglycan fragments in the periplasmic space may cause vesicle formation. Finally, vesicle formation is believed to be facilitated by the conformational change of phospholipids on the membrane, leading to a curvature in the membrane [48].

BMV production has been shown to be impacted by various stress factors, including the growth environment, oxidative stress, and temperature. Studies have revealed an increase in the number of BMVs when bacteria are grown in nutrient-enhanced environments and acidified growth media. Similarly, when oxidative stress was introduced through a non-lethal dose of hydrogen peroxide to *Pseudomonas aeruginosa*, an increase in the number of BMVs was observed. Heat shock, which causes protein denaturation, has also been shown to increase the production of BMVs as these vesicles act to remove these denatured proteins. Furthermore, genetic modifications besides stress factors have also been reported to augment BMV production [48].

3.2. Purification and Characterization Techniques of BMVs

BMVs for biotechnological uses must be obtained in high purity and be well characterized. So far, there has not been described a standard method for BMV isolation. Hence, researchers mostly combine multiple methods. Centrifugation and filtration of bacterial cultures is the first step for the isolation of BMVs.

Serial ultracentrifugation is the most widely utilized method for BMV isolation. This approach involves multiple steps to reach BMVs with the highest purity. First, the bacterial culture is centrifuged at approximately 10,000× *g* to remove bacterial cell debris. The resulting supernatant is then filtered through a 0.22–0.45 μm filter, and cellular debris is completely removed. Afterward, the cell-free supernatant is ultracentrifuged at 100,000–200,000× g for 1–4 h to obtain BMVs [49]. The disadvantages of this method include long processing times and a loss of integrity in BMVs. In addition, different centrifugal forces and times need to be standardized for this method [50].

Ultrafiltration is another frequently used method in BMV isolation. It is also used to concentrate BMVs following the centrifugation step. This technique provides various advantages such as fast and easy operation, yet it cannot purify the vesicles from other structures with similar size, depending on the pore size of the filter, and therefore may cause contamination. In addition, vesicles may be deformed by the force applied during ultrafiltration [25].

The precipitation method is a reliable technique for removing macromolecules in solution, and it can also be used for purifying BMVs. To achieve optimal results, precipitation is often combined with ultracentrifugation and ultrafiltration methods. Although the precipitation procedure for BMVs requires multiple steps and additional purification due to the saturation concentration, it is still a cost-effective and efficient option thanks to commercially available precipitation reagents. In fact, a commercial kit specifically designed for BMV isolation is now available [51].

The ultracentrifugation method is another of the techniques widely used for the purification and isolation of BMVs. The process involves density gradient centrifugation (DGC), where the samples are loaded into a density gradient medium and subjected to centrifugation. This allows for the separation of BMVs based on their density, making it easier to isolate the vesicles through fraction collection. Iodixanol solution is commonly used in this method as it helps preserve the size and shape of the vesicles. However, the DGC method also has its limitations, such as the potential for compromising vesicle integrity due to changing osmotic conditions and the cost of equipment, which may limit its sustainability [52,53].

Size exclusion chromatography is another alternative method used in the purification of BMVs. This method is based on the collection of particles of varying sizes as they pass through the porous material within the column. As BMVs are too large to interact with the column material, they are isolated quickly and easily. Compared to centrifugation-based methods, the size exclusion method is faster and simpler, and it also preserves the integrity of the vesicles as it does not involve any physical force. However, its disadvantage lies in the limited amount of sample that can be processed due to the column volume, which is why it is often combined with other isolation methods [52,53].

The next important step is their characterization after the pure and efficient isolation of BMVs. The characterization of BMVs can be basically divided into three categories: size, morphology, and composition. For dimensional analysis of BMVs, dynamic light scattering (DLS) and nanoparticle tracking analysis (NTA) are mostly utilized. The diameter, size distribution, and zeta potential of BMVs can be measured simultaneously with DLS analysis. DLS analysis is advantageous in terms of measurement speed and repeatability. With NTA analysis, both the size characterization of BMVs and the number of particles that reflect the yield capacity can be calculated. The advantage of this analysis is that it can measure even small (50 nm) vesicles [54,55].

The structures of BMVs can be investigated using various microscopic techniques. Scanning electron microscopy and transmission electron microscopy are common methods; however, staining and fixation during imaging can alter the morphology of BMVs. Cryo-electron microscopy is an alternative technique that enables the preservation of the BMV structure and the determination of its total number. BMVs can also be visualized using atomic force microscopy (AFM), which does not require additional imaging but has a limited imaging range [55,56].

Identifying the biomolecules involved in the BMV's structure is the final step in their characterization. The presence of proteins in BMVs can be identified through qualitative and quantitative analyses, including bicinchoninic acid assay (BCA), sodium dodecyl sulfate-polyacrylamide gel electrophoresis (SDS-PAGE), Western blotting, and mass spectrometry.

The BCA is used to determine the total amount of protein, while SDS-PAGE provides a qualitative analysis. Western blotting is employed to detect the presence of specific desired proteins in BMVs. Mass spectrometry, with its high efficiency in proteomic analysis, is utilized to examine the biogenesis and physiological functions of BMVs [57,58]. Moreover, using a matrix-assisted laser desorption ionization (MALDI) based mass spectrometry approach, various fatty acids contained in BMVs can also be characterized under lipidomics studies [59].

3.3. *Properties of BMVs*

BMVs are classified based on the gram characteristics of the bacteria from which they are released. Outer membrane vesicles (OMVs) refer to vesicles produced by Gram-negative bacteria, while membrane vesicles (MVs) refer to those produced by Gram-positive bacteria. OMVs range from 30 to 250 nm in diameter and share components with the bacterial outer membrane. OMVs have been found to contain proteins, nucleic acids, and lipids, with various functions attributed to the identified proteins [60,61]. On the other hand, MVs range in size from 10 to 500 nm and contain proteins, nucleic acids, and lipids, similar to OMVs [59,62].

BMVs have a wide range of functions, which depend on the biomolecules they carry, including adaptation to the environment and pathogenesis. They play a role in transport systems, biofilm formation, antibiotic resistance, phage removal, microbiota protection, gene transfer, pathogenesis, and immune modulation [59,62] and also are known to transport various biomolecules, including proteins and virulence factors, between cells. One of the most important advantages over other transport systems is their ability to transport more than one type of biomolecule simultaneously and to transmit these molecules over long distances by protecting them from lytic enzymes [63]. This property of BMVs makes them particularly effective in the transmission of toxins and virulence factors, which are key factors in bacterial pathogenesis [64]. The ability of BMVs to carry enzymes such as β-lactamase and drug-binding proteins, and to bind antibiotics outside the cell also contributes to antibiotic resistance in bacteria [65]. Moreover, BMVs can protect bacteria from phage infection by irreversibly binding phage receptors to their surfaces, thus preventing the phages from reaching the bacterial cells [66]. Overall, BMVs play a critical role in bacterial pathogenesis and antibiotic resistance, and, in a way, these mechanisms can be harnessed for the development of novel antimicrobial therapies. BMVs are known to contain both chromosomal and plasmid DNA, which they can protect and transfer against thermal and enzymatic denaturation [67]. These vesicles also play a crucial role in biofilm formation by facilitating interactions between bacterial cells, delivering nutrients, and dispersing on biofilm surfaces [68]. Interestingly, studies have also shown that BMVs belonging to biofilm-forming bacteria can trigger biofilm formation in non-biofilm-forming bacteria [69,70]. Moreover, BMVs can initiate signaling within the host cell through the molecules they carry and contain on their surfaces, creating an immune response. The specific immune response elicited depends on the bacteria from which the BMVs are obtained and the molecules they carry [71]. Finally, it is worth noting that the microbiota, the bacteria that make up the body's natural microbial community, also produce BMVs. These vesicles have been implicated in the protection of microbiota homeostasis against inflammatory bowel diseases [72].

3.4. *Cargo Loading or/and Drug Encapsulation Techniques into BMVs*

There are two main encapsulation approaches for loading cargo into BMVs. These are energy-dependent (active loading) and energy-independent (passive loading) techniques developed based on the energy requirement principle (Figure 2). The application fundamentals of these different drug-loading techniques are discussed in detail below with specific examples.

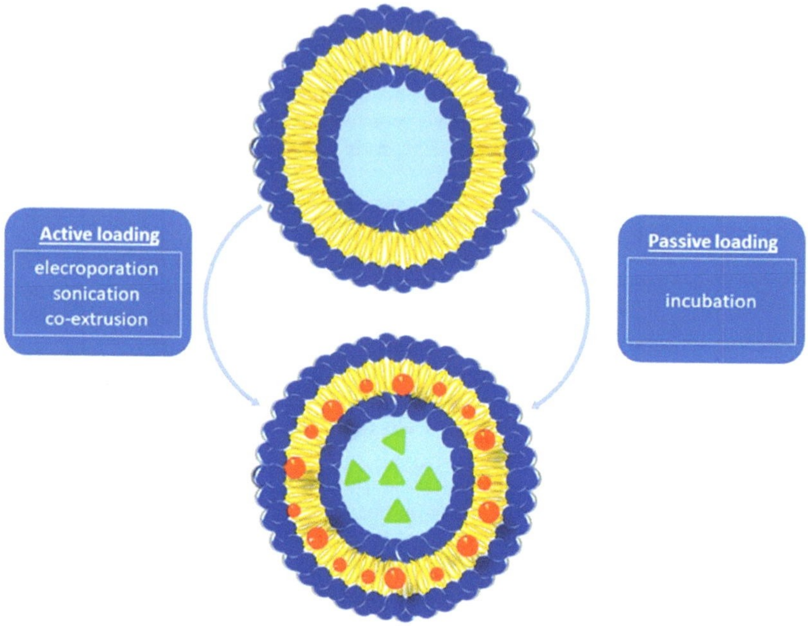

Figure 2. Drug loading approaches into BMVs.

3.4.1. Active Cargo Loading

The active cargo loading principle is an energy-requiring approach and is implemented by electroporation, co-extrusion, and sonication methods. Among these techniques, electroporation is based on the principle of creating pores by breaking the integrity of the membrane in order to create a temporary permeability state in the bacterial cell membrane. For this purpose, short-term electrical voltage pulses are applied to the bacteria cells [73,74]. The pores formed in the cell membrane allow the loading of various chemically synthetic drug compounds. By changing the duration and intensity of electrical voltage pulses applied to the cell membrane, low molecular weight synthetic agents, as well as high molecular weight compounds such as nucleotides, can be introduced into the vehicles. After a certain time, the cell membrane returns to its original structure without any damage. This process has also been utilized to entrap active molecules into other vehicles such as exosomes that have a lipid bilayer membrane structure similar to BMVs [75,76].

The electroporation technique was utilized by Gujrati and his co-workers [77] for the purpose of loading cargoes into Gram-negative *Escherichia coli* OMVs. They accomplished inserting fluorescent dye-labeled siRNAs into BMVs by using 50 μF and 700 V electroporation conditions, and without causing permanent damage to the cell membrane integrity. Such probes demonstrate the feasibility of BMVs as theranostic agents in cancer diagnosis and treatment. It is also possible to load nanoparticles such as quantum dots, silver or gold nanoparticles, and iron oxides into BMVs by using electroporation for different therapeutic indications. The prominent need is to optimize the applied electroporation voltage to reach high encapsulation efficiency, optimum vesicle diameter, and stability of the system during the loading of cargo molecules into BMVs [78].

The ultrasonication method, which is another technique utilized for loading cargo molecules into BMVs, is based on the reversible disruption of cell membrane integrity through ultrasonic frequencies, and, thereby, the realization of drug loading [10]. This technique also enables coating the surfaces of conventional polymeric nanoparticles with BMVs to gain biomimetic character [79]. In 2019, Gao and his colleagues coated vancomycin and rifampicin-encapsulated poly(lactic-co-glycolic acid) (PLGA) nanoparticles with BMVs isolated from *Streptococcus aureus* or *E. coli* bacteria by using the ultrasonication technique to impart active targeting ability to the vehicle. Herewith, the researchers improved the in vivo antibacterial activities of the polymeric nanocarriers [80].

The co-extrusion technique is a relatively current method among the active cargo loading approaches. This technique uses the cell membrane supplied by the host and follows a repeated mechanical extrusion process through polycarbonate filter membranes with different pore sizes [10]. Similar to the ultrasonication technique, this drug encapsulation approach is also preferred for the surface modification of various nanosized drug carriers to obtain biomimetic structures. For example, Chen and co-workers modified the surface of tegafur-loaded polymeric micelles with OMVs isolated from *Salmonella typhimurium* to bring efficacy for cancer immunotherapy and to alleviate metastasis. To this goal, they applied two different extrusion steps; in the first step, the immunogenicity of the BMVs was reduced by modification with polyethylene glycol (PEG) and Arg-Gly-Asp peptide (RGD) through the polycarbonate membrane extrusion technique. This step was followed by a second extrusion step which was implemented to coat the micelle surface with BMVs to depress immunogenic activity [81].

3.4.2. Passive Cargo Loading

Another approach harnessed to load cargo molecules into BMVs is the incubation of drugs with BMVs under appropriate conditions. Kuerban et al. (2020) developed an effective strategy for the treatment of non-small-cell lung cancer with this technique. They aimed to encapsulate doxorubicin hydrochloride (DOX), which is a broad-spectrum antineoplastic agent, into OMVs derived from Gram-negative *Klebsiella pneumoniae*. The incubation procedure for loading the active agent in phosphate-buffered saline (PBS) solution into OMVs was performed at 37 °C for a period of 4 h. To remove the unloaded DOX from the incubation medium, an ultrafiltration step was performed through 100 kDa membranes. The DOX:OMV mass ratio of 1:45 was determined as the optimum ratio to obtain the highest encapsulation efficiency. Particle size analysis demonstrated that the mean size of DOX-loaded OMVs was approximately 93 nm. In vitro dissolution studies depicted that DOX was released from OMVs by 30% over 48 h, exhibiting an extended-release profile [82]. In a study conducted by our research group, Capacitabine-loaded MVs were produced to investigate the anti-apoptotic effects of vehicles derived from Gram-positive *Enterococcus faecalis* on HT-29 colon cancer cell lines. Among the evaluated drug:MV mass ratios of 1:20, 1:40, and 1:60, a maximum loading efficiency of 54% was obtained with a drug:MV ratio of 1:60. Particle size of the optimum formulation was determined as 193.3 nm with a −22.4 mV surface charge. Cell culture studies proved that the drug-loaded MVs increase the apoptosis of cancer cells [83].

Another incubation-based strategy utilized for the loading of cargo molecules into BMVs is to incorporate drugs into BMVs during their biogenesis by the parent bacteria. This technique is mostly preferred for loading mRNA-type genetic materials or aminoglycoside-structured antibiotics that cannot be successfully encapsulated into BMVs after their isolation due to their high molecular weight [10]. Gentamicin was successfully loaded into the OMVs during the growth of *P. aeruginosa* PAO1 by using this technique [84]. However, the major limitation of this approach is the co-transfer of genetic material during the encapsulation process of the antibiotics. Essential purification steps and quality controls have to be carried out after the cargo loading procedure to make sure that genetic material is not entrapped simultaneously with cargo molecules.

3.5. *Drug Release Mechanisms from BMVs*

The main release mechanisms by which the release of the active molecule can occur in drug delivery vehicles are diffusion, dissolution, or erosion. It is important to know the mechanism of drug release from BMVs in order to maximize the expected therapeutic response from the carriers and to expand their clinical use. "*Drug release*" describes the process by which active molecule solutes can pass the membranes of the BMVs to the dissolution medium or biological fluid. Since the outer membrane structures of BMVs contain lipopolysaccharides, proteins, and lipids, the essential mechanism underlying the release of drugs from BMVs is the diffusion mechanism [85]. Huang et al. (2020) produced levofloxacin-loaded BMVs and examined the therapeutic efficacy of these drug-delivery vehicles in a mouse model of intestinal bacterial infection. The diffusion rate of the levofloxacin from orally administered drug-loaded BMVs was observed to be slower than the free molecule. Due to this situation, the drug concentration in plasma was obtained at a lower level but in a more prolonged release type compared to free levofloxacin [86]. However, more research needs to be conducted to elucidate the release kinetics and mechanisms of active molecules from BMVs.

3.6. Strategies Used in BMVs for Targeting

As can be seen from the studies in the literature, we will mention two main targeting strategies using BMVs. These are static and dynamic targeting strategies (Figure 3), which will be explained in detail below.

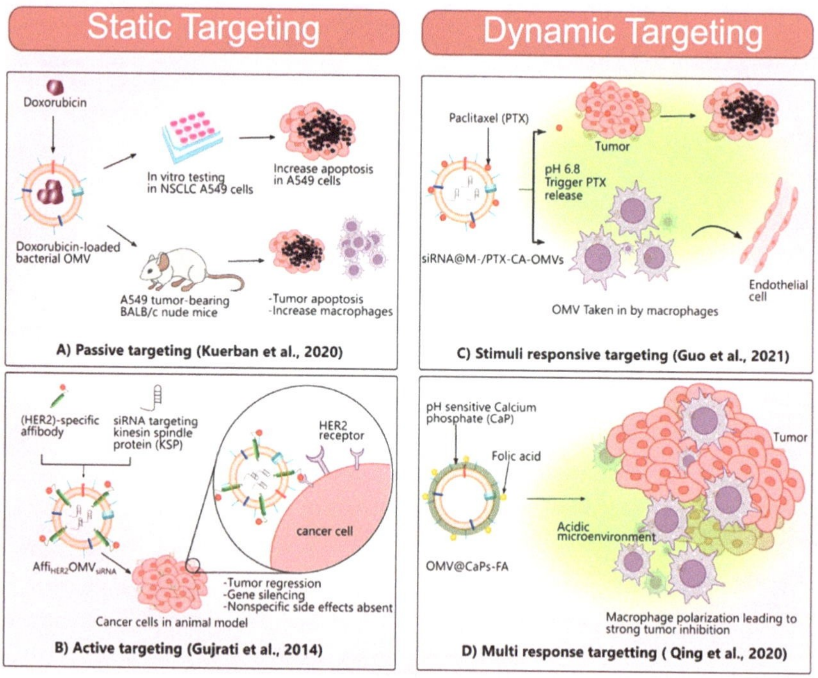

Figure 3. Static and dynamic targeting strategies of BMVs used as carrier systems [77,82,87,88].

3.6.1. Static Targeting

In this section, we describe passive and active transport, which are among the targeting strategies of tumor tissues. These are referred "*static targeting*" since the operator has no control over the nanosystems injected using these targeting strategies.

Passive Targeting

The process of angiogenesis which is necessary for metastasis to occur in tumor development is critical. The development of this process in tumor cells is quite rapid. The endothelial cells of the tumor tissues are not wrapped by pericytes, which ensures the preservation of normal blood vessels, and there is no smooth layer of muscle on the edges of the vessels. Because of this, tumor tissues contain extremely permeable vascular structures also called *"leaky vessels"* [89]. Many solid tumors have excessively permeable vasculature and less lymphatic drainage compared to normal tissues [90]. Enhanced permeability and retention effect (EPR) which is commonly seen in tumorous areas is characterized by increased capillary permeability in affected tissues with much less return of fluids to the lymphatic circulation and is the main driving power of *"passive targeting"* [91]. While free therapeutic agents can spread non-specifically, a nanocarrier system can accumulate in tumor tissues thanks to leaking vessels with EPR [92]. Due to the lack of a functional lymphatic drainage system, nanocarriers cannot be efficiently cleared from the bloodstream, so their circulation in the bloodstream is prolonged [89].

Researchers have used BMVs to deploy therapeutic agents through passive targeting. Kuerban et al. showed that DOX-loaded OMVs, due to their nano size, can passively accumulate in lung cancer cells via the EPR effect and then be rapidly internalized by recipient cells by endocytosis. Thanks to the rapid entry of doxorubicin into cells, drug loaded OMVs caused intense cytotoxic effects [82]. In another study, it was emphasized that optoacoustic signals increased significantly in tumor cells due to melanin-loaded OMVs, and this increase was thought to be due to the accumulation of melanin-loaded OMVs in tumor cells via the EPR effect [93].

Although EPR through passive targeting provides an advantage for accumulation in tumor tissues, it is significantly affected due to the heterogeneous nature of tumor tissues, and vascular permeability may not be the same throughout a single tumor [92,94]. To overcome this limitation, BMVs need to be designed to actively bind to specific cells.

Active Targeting

Since the application site of therapeutics is usually distant from the sites where the therapeutic agent will be affected, the development of effective targeting strategies is critical to therapeutic effectiveness [95]. In this regard, the research focused on the surface modification of BMVs has opened a new era in SDDSs using biological ligands [77,96,97]. Modified BMVs increase affinity and facilitate the internalization of therapeutic cargo by target cells via receptor-mediated endocytosis and/or disruption of cellular function thanks to an *"active targeting"* strategy based on the biological interaction between ligands and the target cell [98].

Even if the nanosystems are intended for active targeting, a passive accumulation occurs first followed by target-specific binding as a complementary strategy [99]. Active targeting increases the effectiveness of cargoes loaded into nanosystems and makes therapeutic cargoes more specific to the target area [100]. Thus, undesirable, non-specific interactions and localization of therapeutic cargo in peripheral tissues are reduced [101]. Herein, the key challenge is to identify the most appropriate targeting ligand for the selective and successful delivery of nanosystems to the target tissue or cell and to minimize or prevent the toxicity that may result [101]. At this point, in the design of the SDDS, the target ligands are selected to bind to a receptor that is overexpressed by the target cell but not by normal cells. Moreover, these targeted receptors must be expressed homogeneously in all targeted cells [102].

Biological ligands such as proteins, carbohydrates, nucleic acids, and peptides have been used to facilitate the active targeting of BMVs [87,96,97,103] (Table 2). Human epidermal receptor 2 (HER2) has been found to be expressed in 14–91% of breast cancer patients [102]. Gujrati et al. modified the surface of OMVs obtained from *E. coli* with the HER2 affibody by fusion with the ClyA protein. It showed high specificity of modified OMVs in HER2-overexpressing ovarian (SKOV3) and breast cancer (BT474 and HC1954) cells compared with HER2-negative breast cancer (MDA-MB-231) cells. They also reported that the siRNA molecule transported by this active targeting is effectively transported to the target site and causes more cytotoxicity in cancer cells [77]. Guo and colleagues modified the surface of the OMVs with mannose to target M2 macrophages. They reported increased secretion of recruited tumor-associated macrophages (TAMs) in 4T1 breast cancer cells thanks to increased macrophage affinity compared to native OMVs as the modification rate of mannose-OMVs increases [87]. Aptamers are short chains of nucleic acids consisting of several nucleotides. Due to their small and sensitive structure, biodegradability, and immunogenic effect, they are very good candidates as active targeting ligands for BMVs. AS-1411 is a Guanine-rich DNA aptamer that specifically recognizes the nucleolin that is upregulated in many cancer cells [95]. In a recent study, AS-1411 aptamer was modified by adding to the surface of *E. coli* OMVs and by specifically targeting cancer cells. They also reported that modified OMVs accumulated in tumor tissues and inhibited tumor growth [103].

Table 2. Ligands used for active targeting of BMVs in cancer research.

Class	Indication	Ligand	Target	References
Aptamer	Breast cancer	AS-1411	Nucleolin	[103]
Carbohydrate	M2 macrophages	Mannose	Mannose receptor (MR, CD206+)	[87]
Peptide	Melanoma	RGP and RGD	αvβ3 integrin	[96]
		RGP		[104]
	Breast cancer Melanoma Colon cancer	LyP1	p32/gC1qR	[105,106]
Protein	Breast cancer Ovarian cancer	HER2 affibody	HER2 receptor	[77]
	Breast cancer	EGFR affibody	EGFR	[107]
	Colon cancer	PD1	PD-L1	[108]
Small molecule	Breast cancer	Folic acid (FA)	Folate receptor (FR)	[88]

3.6.2. Dynamic Targeting

To increase therapeutic efficacy and reduce or avoid adverse effects, drugs must be administered to target sites in a controlled manner. Stimuli-based drug delivery systems have demonstrated significant potential for the effective targeting of active drug moieties in this approach [109].

In this section, we will provide insights into dynamic simulations in BMVs used as stimuli-triggered drug delivery systems for cancer therapy through active and passive targeting.

Stimuli-Responsive Targeting

To improve drug delivery specificity, efficacy, and biological activities, stimuli-responsive nanocarriers were rationally designed and developed by considering different pathological profiles in normal tissues, intracellular compartments, and tumor microenvironments. Furthermore, it has been reported that stimuli-responsive nanocarriers can overcome multidrug resistance in cancer treatment [110]. Starting from this, research with BMVs has focused on different internal and external stimuli to trigger drug and/or cargo release.

pH. Among the internal stimuli, pH is one of the most used to reduce drug toxicity and provide targeted drug release, especially in oncology and inflammation treatments [19,111]. Tumor cells have an acidic environment due to hypoxia and lactic acid accumulation than normal cells [112]. Based on this feature of tumor cells, pH has been used as an effective stimulus in the controlled release of BMVs.

A new drug delivery system that uses OMVs derived from Gram-negative bacteria to co-deliver paclitaxel (PTX) and regulate the tumor metabolism microenvironment was described. The OMVs were pH-sensitive and released PTX when the tumor pH was at 6.8. The system was also designed to deliver a regulated development and DNA damage response 1 (Redd1)-siRNA. The delivery system was shown to successfully regulate tumor metabolism and suppress tumor growth. The OMVs have the potential for use in establishing a co-delivery platform for chemical drugs and genetic medicines. The study emphasizes the pH-sensitivity of the OMV and its ability to target different cells in the tumor microenvironment successively [87].

Light. Light-responsive drug delivery systems that use photosensitive carriers exhibit an on/off drug release mechanism when stimulated with light. Various light wavelengths (ultraviolet, near-infrared, visible) have been reported and discussed for controlled drug delivery. Because of their low penetration, visible and UV light were deemed unsuitable for clinical purposes in vivo, whereas the NIR spectrum is regarded as an ideal light source for monitoring drug release due to its safety and enhanced tissue penetration [109].

A recent study has focused on loading biomimetic copper sulfide nanoparticles (CuS-OMVs) into OMVs derived from *E. coli* Nissle 1917 for systemic photothermal-immunotherapeutic synergy. CuS-OMVs have high photothermal conversion efficacy, good photostability, and significant tumor targeting capacity, resulting in visible hyperthermia and subsequent distinct suppression of tumor cells when exposed to second near-infrared (NIR-II) light. CuS-OMVs-induced cytotoxicity induces strong immunogenic cell death (ICD) in tumor cells while also promoting dendritic cell (DC) maturation and subsequent $CD8^+$ T cell activation [113].

Dual/Multi-Responsive Targeting

Dual/multi-responsive targeting of BMVs involves the use of targeting moieties that respond to multiple signals, such as pH, temperature, or enzymes, to achieve selective targeting of BMVs. This strategy has the advantage of allowing for multiple triggers to control the release of drugs from BMVs, thereby increasing the level of control and specificity in drug delivery.

One example of a dual/multi-responsive targeting strategy is the combined use of molecules and light-sensitive molecules that will promote the production of ROS as a result of redox reactions as targeting moieties for BMVs. These molecules can be incorporated into the BMVs, and their response to changes in the redox and light of the environment can be used to trigger the release of drugs from BMVs. This allows for a high degree of control over the timing and location of drug release [114]. A new drug delivery system has been designed that uses αPD-L1-modified OMVs derived from Gram-negative bacteria to deliver the enzyme catalase which breaks down H_2O_2 into O_2, and the photo-sensitive Ce6 molecule together. This nanosystem relieved hypoxia for a long time in vivo by attenuating the hypoxic feature of solid tumors, which inhibited their photodynamic activity. On the other hand, it has been reported that bacterial-based SDDSs developed due to stimuli induces greater DC and $CD8^+$ T cell migration into tumor tissues and improves immune memory in treated mice [114].

A study focused on the use of OMVs for TME reprogramming in solid tumors. To overcome the issues of antibody-dependent clearance and high toxicity caused by OMVs upon intravenous injection, the OMVs were covered with pH-sensitive calcium phosphate (CaP) shells. These CaP shells were able to neutralize the acidic TME and reprogram macrophages from the M2-to-M1 phenotype, resulting in an improved antitumor effect. Additionally, the CaP shells could be functionalized with folic acid or photosensitizer agents, allowing for the use of OMVs in combination therapies to achieve a synergistic therapeutic effect. The pH-sensitivity of the CaP shells is emphasized as a crucial feature in the effects delivered by the OMVs [88].

Another example of dual/multi-responsive targeting is the use of enzymes as triggers for drug release. For instance, enzymes that are expressed in diseased tissues can be used to trigger the release of drugs to those tissues. This allows for the targeted delivery of drugs to specific regions of the body while avoiding systemic toxicity. It is a promising strategy for achieving selective and controlled drug delivery, and further research is needed to fully understand the potential of this approach.

In terms of recent discoveries in the field of dual/multi-responsive targeting of BMVs, one notable example is the use of dual-responsive polymers for the targeted delivery of drugs to cancer cells. Researchers have developed a dual-responsive polymer that can respond to both pH and temperature, and that can be used to achieve targeted delivery of drugs to cancer cells. The polymer is capable of triggering the release of drugs from nanostructures in response to changes in the pH or temperature of the microenvironment of cancer cells, which allows for precise and controlled delivery of drugs to these cells [115,116]. These approaches have been more extensively investigated with liposomes but studies examining their applications in BMVs are lacking.

Inverse Targeting

Inverse targeting of BMVs involves the use of targeting moieties that actively avoid specific regions or conditions, rather than being attracted to them. This strategy is useful for avoiding unwanted toxicity or interactions with non-target cells and could be used to improve the specificity and safety of BMV-based drug delivery.

For example, inverse targeting can be achieved using magnetic nanoparticles that are coated with targeting moieties that bind to vesicles. The magnetic nanoparticles are then functionalized with drugs, and their magnetic properties can be used to direct them away from specific regions or conditions. This allows for targeted delivery of drugs to specific regions of the body while avoiding systemic toxicity. Another example of inverse targeting is the use of light-sensitive polymers as targeting moieties. These polymers can be triggered to release drugs upon exposure to specific wavelengths of light. This allows for the precise and controlled release of drugs and can be used to improve the safety and specificity of drug delivery [117]. However, it is important to note that the field of inverse targeting in bacterial membrane vesicles is still in its infancy, and much more research is needed to fully understand its potential benefits and drawbacks.

4. The Role of BMV-Based Smart Drug Delivery Systems in Diagnosis

BMVs are candidates with the potential to be used for bioimaging in the early diagnosis of cancer and evaluation of treatment efficacy due to their ability to encapsulate imaging reporters and target ligands. In this regard, Gujrati and colleagues engineered *E. coli* cells to overexpress the tyrosine enzyme, resulting in melanin that was contrast-enhancing by optimizing it as a natural light absorber accumulating in the bacteria's cytosol and packaged in OMVs released from *E. coli*. Melanin-containing OMVs (OMVMel) capable of generating optoacoustic signals under infrared light induced apoptosis in 4T1 breast cancer cells. In the murine orthotopic breast cancer model, OMVMel exhibited strong necrotic activity by accumulating in tumor tissues with the effect of EPR. These locations have been non-invasively monitored utilizing OMVMel as multispectral optoacoustic tomography (MSOT) probes. Moreover, OMVMel have been demonstrated to be biocompatible without causing any organ damage. As a consequence, when exposed to pulsed near-infrared radiation, OMVMel displayed a theranostic potential by boosting localized heat generation, enabling the suppression of tumor development as well as tumor visualization [93].

Fusion proteins can be attached to membrane-associated proteins on BMVs through genetic modification and serve many different purposes such as protein transport, fluorescent molecular labeling, tumor therapy, and cell bioimaging [118]. The OMV-based multifunctional biosensor platform for both antigen targeted, and signal generation developed by Chen et al. (2017) is notable for its simultaneous functionalization of both the interior and exterior of the OMV. To achieve this, the researchers used SlyB lipoprotein as an anchor to direct nanoluciferase (Nluc) interior *E. coli* OMVs. The choice of Nluc as a fusion partner was based on its small size of 19 kDa and highly sensitive luminescence signaling. In a novel strategy, the OMVs were operationalized with a target-specific antibody using the ice nucleation protein (INP)-Scaf3 surface scaffolding and the small antibody-binding Z domain on the OMV surface. To test the biosensor's ability to target cancer cells, the researchers chose the cancer-specific surface marker Mucin-1 (MUC1). They further modified the OMVs by mounting dockerin-labeled green fluorescent protein (GFP) for immunofluorescence imaging on the INP-Scaf3-Z scaffold. When GFP-OMVs were added to HeLa cells stained with anti-MUC1 antibody, bright green fluorescence was detected in cells, demonstrating the OMVs' ability to detect cancer cells. Overall, this study shows that OMVs can be used for immunofluorescence imaging with target-specific antibodies [119]. Another study evaluated the bioluminescence kinetics of OMVs generated from modified *E. coli* using the same genetic alteration method. A theoretical model was developed to simulate the enzyme-substrate reaction kinetics by mixing these OMVs with the substrate furimazine, which could potentially be used for bioluminescence-based optical imaging. OMVs were injected subcutaneously in a mouse model to investigate the local absorption of substrate and OMVs and bioluminescence kinetics. The bioluminescence signal produced by these OMVs was tracked using non-invasive optical imaging. Strong signals from experimental animals indicated that these vesicles have great potential as a class of functional nanomaterials for imaging-related biomedical applications [120].

Presently, there has been limited focus on biosensing and bioimaging utilizing modified BMVs. Because of the increased interest in this topic, numerous OMVs or MVs will be created in the future to be utilized as customized imaging tools with the needed properties through genetic engineering.

5. The Potential Role of BMV-Based Smart Drug Delivery Systems in Therapy

5.1. Cancer Therapy

The potential use of BMVs as immunomodulatory candidates in cancer treatment is of great interest because of their multi-antigenic nature [121]. While many studies have reported the anti-tumor effects of OMVs derived from Gram-negative bacteria [113,122,123], there are only a few cancer studies related to MVs obtained from Gram-positive bacteria [83,124,125]. Therefore, this section will mainly focus on the latest research on the use of OMVs in cancer immunotherapy.

According to our literature knowledge, OMVs are utilized in cancer therapy with four different approaches; natural OMVs, cargo and drug-loading OMVs, modified OMVs, and OMVs created with hybrid membrane technology or designed with a coating (Figure 4). Herein, we will examine these nanoscale biomaterial-based carrier systems applied with different strategies as therapeutic and SDDSs and analyze their advantages by summarizing their designs.

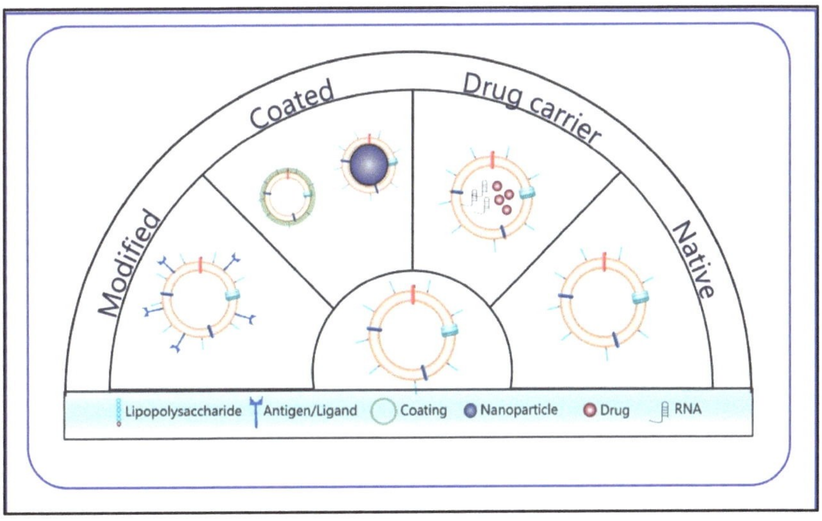

Figure 4. Different OMV approaches used in cancer therapy.

5.1.1. Native OMVs

In oncology applications, BMVs offer several advantages. Firstly, their nano sizes ranging from 20 to 200 nm allow for enhanced localization to solid tumors with passive targeting and lymphatic drainage [126]. Secondly, their EPR properties enable them to accumulate in tumor tissue, triggering local immunity [127]. Thirdly, BMVs are enriched in pathogen-associated molecular patterns (PAMPs), such as lipopolysaccharide (LPS), found on their surface and originating from the parent bacteria. This natural adjuvant effect activates various toll-like receptor (TLR) signaling pathways, triggering an inflammatory response associated with the activation of the complement system [48]. Fourthly, BMVs can be genetically engineered through modification of the parent bacteria [93] with molecular techniques and bioconjugation methods for cell targeting and recognition [81,128]. Finally, BMVs cannot reproduce themselves, making them a safer vehicle compared to bacteria [129,130].

According to Kim et al. (2017), membrane vesicles released by different types of bacteria can potentially be utilized for immunotherapy in various types of cancer. *E. coli*-derived OMVs were found to accumulate in tumor tissues via EPR, affecting antigen-presenting cells (APCs) and adaptive immunity, which facilitated the infiltration and accumulation of natural killer (NK) and T cells in tumor tissues. The study further revealed that the antitumor mechanism of OMVs is reliant on interferon-gamma (IFN-γ) production in the tumor microenvironment and CXCL10 expression to attract effector T cells. Additionally, the study was the first to exhibit the substantial anti-tumor effects of MVs produced by Gram-positive bacteria, *Lactobacillus acidophilus* and *S. aureus*, which demonstrates the feasibility of using Gram-positive bacteria for clinical applications [125].

Another study by Aly et al. (2021) found that OMVs obtained from *Salmonella typhimurium* exhibited higher cytotoxicity in cancer cells than paclitaxel (PTX). The researchers utilized OMVs as an adjuvant to enhance the effect of a chemotherapy agent and evidenced that combining OMVs and paclitaxel treatment resulted in a significant reduction in tumor volume and the greatest tumor inhibitory ability at a rate of 94.7% [122].

5.1.2. Cargo or Drug Loading OMVs

OMVs appear to be magnificent platforms in bio-applications due to their unique biological properties; even so, more efforts are needed to take them one step further and improve their functionality for practical use. Long-distance transportation and communication are some core functions of OMVs in biological systems [131,132]. With the aim of improving their therapeutic functions, research has currently focused on their potential as drug-delivery systems [87,133]. OMVs efficiently protect their cargoes against DNase, RNase, protease, and extracellular degradation caused by extreme conditions, such as extreme pH [134]. Additionally, they can carry both hydrophobic and hydrophilic components owing to their lipid bilayer structure [135]. They not only improve drug delivery inside tumor cells but also stimulate immune responses, which boost the effectiveness of anticancer drugs [82,122]. Moreover, OMVs are used in combination with photothermal therapy or photosensitive agents to enhance their immunotherapeutic role to completely eradicate the tumor, prevent recurrence and metastasis [113].

Recent studies have shown promising results in enhancing the antitumor effects against cancer cells by loading the antineoplastic agent DOX into OMVs [82,133]. Li et al. (2023) developed a new smart drug delivery therapeutic platform that co-loaded photosensitizer chlorin e6 (Ce6) and DOX into OMVs for combined photodynamic/chemo/immunotherapy. Then, they loaded the OMVs into macrophages to improve their safety and antitumor effects. The researchers reported that the developed Ce6/DOX-OMVs@M nanoplatform destroyed orthotopic triple-negative breast cancer (TNBC) and prevented lung metastasis in mice with no side effects. The study also demonstrated that laser light could induce ICD by effectively generating ROS, shifting polarization from tumor-associated macrophage M2 to M1, and activating pyroptosis-related pathways to activate antitumor immune responses [133].

5.1.3. Modification of OMVs

Although OMVs play an important role in transporting biomolecules to distant sites, targeting and processing immunomodulatory agents into the tumor microenvironment remains a major challenge. One of the major advantages of using OMVs in cancer therapy is their flexibility to be modified by genetic engineering [127,131]. Modifying them is an excellent strategy to improve the expression of specific peptides and the presentation of multiple antigens in targeting cancer cells and forming the tumor-associated immune response.

The functionalization of OMVs with different biomolecules through genetic engineering has several advantages over other methods: (1) There is no need for decoration material because it is created by introducing heterologous DNA into bacteria. (2) Large-scale production of functionalized OMVs can be achieved at a low cost with simple bacterial cultures. As a result, no further purification steps are required after collection. (3) Finally, this method allows the placement of desired biomolecules inside or outside the OMVs according to different application strategies.

Researchers have explored using various proteins and ligands to enhance the ability of OMVs to target cancer cells. For example, HER2 and peptides (e.g., RGD and RGP) have been investigated as potential targeting moieties [77,96,104]. In one study, tumor necrosis factor-related apoptosis-inducing ligand (TRAIL) protein overexpressing OMVs were produced using recombinant *E. coli* cells, and these vesicles were bonded with RGD peptide which shows high affinity for the most integrin avβ3 that is specifically overexpressed in melanoma cells across the other types of cancers. These nanoplatforms showed strong binding affinity to the integrin receptor, increasing tumor-targeting ability and accumulation in melanoma cells [96].

Recently, OMVs derived from genetically modified basic fibroblast growth factor (BFGF) overexpressing *E. coli* have been shown to be enriched in the BFGF protein [128]. Thus, the immunoadjuvant potential of BFGF-loaded OMVs (BFGF-OMVs) was investigated by their administration to tumor-bearing mice. It was reported that the production of anti-BFGF autoantibodies was induced, tumor metastasis and angiogenesis were inhibited, and a tumor antigen-specific cellular immune response was promoted. Pan et al. (2022) produced OMVs (LOMV@PD-1) that were loaded with plasmids carrying the programmed death-1 (PD-1) and modified with LyP1 polypeptide to induce PD-1 expression in tumor cells. Upon intravenous injection, the LOMV@PD-1 nanostructures were effectively internalized by tumor cells through LyP1 peptide-mediated targeting, and PD-1 expression was observed in tumor cells by transmitting the PD-1 plasmid to the nucleus. The overexpression of PD-1 on the surface of tumor cells inhibited the PD-1/PD-L1 pathway and prevented tumor cells from escaping immunity. Furthermore, OMVs induced IFN-γ secretion, enhancing antitumor immune responses in tumor tissues. The LOMV@PD-1 nanocarrier system exhibited the strongest anti-tumor effect in melanoma cells, with a tumor inhibition rate of 94.21% [105].

Studies on the use of OMVs as carrier adjuvant systems in cancer therapy are summarized in detail in Table 3.

Table 3. Application of OMVs as smart delivery systems in cancer therapy.

Bacterial Source of OMVs	Modification and/or Guest Molecules	Particle Size (nm)	Modification or Loading Method	Stimulating Factor	Therapy Strategy	Outcomes	References
E. coli DH5α	Ce6 DOX	70–140	Co-incubation	Photodynamic	- trigger drug release with laser irrigation - achieve effective antitumoral effects with combined photo/-chemo/immunotherapy	- decreased cell viability - induced ROS generation - suppression of tumor growth and eradication of tumor tissues - shifting macrophages M2-to-M1 polarization in 4T1 breast cancer-bearing mice in vivo	[133]
E. coli BL21 (ΔmsbB)	tRNALys-pre-miRNA-126 aptamer AS1411	108.2	Genetic engineering Incubation	-	Targeting breast cancer cells by specific binding of the aptamer to nucleolus proteins on the surface of breast cancer cell membranes.	- inhibition of cell proliferation - decreased expression of target genes corresponding to invasion miRNA - accumulation in tumor tissues - inhibition of tumor growth	[103]
Attenuated *Salmonella*	αPD-L1 Catalase-Ce6	140.907	Extrusion Co-extrusion	Photodynamic	To increase the amount of O_2 in tumor cells by means of negatively charged catalase and Ce-6, thus overcoming the hypoxia barrier in front of the photodynamic effect and obtaining an effective antitumoral effect.	- accumulation in tumor tissues - decreased cell viability - decreased HIF-1α expression - induced ROS generation and increased dissolved O_2 - maturation of dendritic cells - increase in effector T cells population in 4T1 breast cancer-bearing mice in vivo	[114]

Table 3. *Cont.*

Bacterial Source of OMVs	Modification and/or Guest Molecules	Particle Size (nm)	Modification or Loading Method	Stimulating Factor	Therapy Strategy	Outcomes	References
E. coli K12 (ΔmsbB)	LyP1 polypeptide	~136.9	Genetic engineering	-	- effective tumor targeting and increased internalization rate through the LyP1 polypeptide - ensuring the expression of PD1 in tumor cell membranes and self-blocking of the PD1/PD-L1 axis in tumor cells	- inhibition of tumor growth inhibition - decrease in Ki-67+ cell populations - increase of apoptotic cells in tumor tissues - increase of NK cells and CTLs population - maturation of dendritic cells - increase of TCM cells	[105]
	PD1 plasmid		Electroporation				
E. coli Nissle 1917	CuS	170.2 ± 0.2	Incubation	Photothermal	Generating strong hyperthermia in tumors through the photothermal effect.	- effective photothermal conversion - induce stronger cytotoxicity - effectively accumulate in tumor tissues - induce ICD of tumor cells - remarkable tumor growth inhibition - maturation of dendritic cells - decrease in Ki-67+ cell populations - activation of cytotoxic T cells in 4T1 breast cancer-bearing mice in vivo	[113]

Table 3. *Cont.*

Bacterial Source of OMVs	Modification and/or Guest Molecules	Particle Size (nm)	Modification or Loading Method	Stimulating Factor	Therapy Strategy	Outcomes	References
E. coli BL21 (ΔmsbB)	Redd1 siRNA	130 ± 15.16	Electroporation	pH-sensitive	- siRNA-mediated silencing of key genes in cancer cells - ensuring the pre-release of the therapeutic agent paclitaxel by triggering pH-sensitive CA	- downregulated the mRNA expression level of Redd1 - inhibition of malignant cell proliferation - effective metastasis inhibition capacity - increased cleaved caspase-3 - decreased Ki-67+ cell populations - increased effector T cells and decreased Treg cell population in 4T1 breast cancer-bearing mice in vivo - maturation of dendritic cells	[87]
	DSPE-PEG-CA-PTX		Co-incubation				
E. coli (ΔmsbB/ΔpagP)	GALA	135.76 ± 30.33	Genetic engineering		Ensuring targeted binding, specifically to cancer cells overexpressing the EGF receptor through expressed affi-EGFR proteins.	- specific binding to EGFR-overexpressing breast cancer cells - no cytotoxicity - no immunogenicity	[107]
	EGFR						

Table 3. *Cont.*

Bacterial Source of OMVs	Modification and/or Guest Molecules	Particle Size (nm)	Modification or Loading Method	Stimulating Factor	Therapy Strategy	Outcomes	References
E. coli DH5α	BFGF	166.9	Genetic engineering	-	To achieve a lasting and effective antitumor effect by inducing the production of anti-BFGF autoantibodies.	- best tumor suppression function because of induction of anti-BFGF autoantibodies - decreased tumor volume and inhibition of tumor growth - inhibition of FGFR1 phosphorylation level - reduction of lung metastasis - increased caspase-3 expression - decreased Treg cells and increased Th1 and CTLs in the mouse B16F10 xenograft model	[128]
E. coli	TRAIL	94.46 ± 5.22	Genetic engineering	Photothermal	- specific tumor targeting by the ligand RGP or RGD peptides - increasing the synergistic anti-tumor therapeutic effect by combining photothermal therapy	- effective transdermal efficiency - effective tumor targeting by peptide ligand - accumulation in melanoma spheroids - induction of apoptosis in tumor cells	[96]
	ICG		Incubation				
	RGP or RGD peptide		Incubation				

Table 3. *Cont.*

Bacterial Source of OMVs	Modification and/or Guest Molecules	Particle Size (nm)	Modification or Loading Method	Stimulating Factor	Therapy Strategy	Outcomes	References
E. coli (ΔmsbB)	PD1	32.7 ± 10.6	Genetic engineering	-	Enabling both internalizations of OMVs by binding of PD1 to PD-L1 on the surface of tumor cells as well as preventing inhibition of T cell proliferation by tumor cells through inhibition of PD-L1.	- maturation of dendritic cells - accumulate in tumor tissues - induction of apoptosis and necrosis in tumor cells - increase of effector memory T cells, NK cells and macrophages population in CT-26 colon cancer-bearing mice in vivo	[108]
Attenuated *K. pneumonia* ATCC 60095	DOX	93.09	Incubation	-	Enabling the generation of chemoimmunotherapeutic responses by using OMVs as drug delivery systems for chemotherapeutic agents.	- cytotoxic effect on lung cancer cells - increased cleaved caspase-3 and PARP - triggering extensive tumor necrosis - increase in tumor growth inhibition - increased serum TNF-α and IL-6 levels	[82]

Table 3. *Cont.*

Bacterial Source of OMVs	Modification and/or Guest Molecules	Particle Size (nm)	Modification or Loading Method	Stimulating Factor	Therapy Strategy	Outcomes	References
E. coli	TRAIL ICG RGP peptide	94.54 ± 1.46	Genetic engineering Electrostatic interaction Incubation	Photothermal	- specific tumor targeting by the ligand RGP peptide - increasing the synergistic anti-tumor therapeutic effect by combining photothermal therapy	- infiltration and accumulation of OMVs in tumor spheroid - inhibition of tumor cell proliferation and invasion - induction of apoptosis in tumor cells - decrease in c-FLIP and survivin protein expression - increase in cleaved caspase-3 and caspase-8 protein expression - effective skin penetration - increase in temperature of tumor sites	[104]
E. coli BL21	Calcium phosphate (CaP) shells ICG	100–150	Incubation	pH-sensitive Photothermal	- providing tumor inhibition by dissolving CaP shells in the tumor environment with a slightly acidic pH - increasing the synergistic anti-tumor therapeutic effect by combining photothermal with immunotherapy	- accumulate in tumor tissues - pronounced tumor inhibition - increased effector T lymphocyte and decreased Treg cell population in CT-26 colon cancer-bearing mice in vivo - increased cytokine secretion levels in CT-26 colon cancer-bearing mice in vivo - induced ICD of tumor cells - maturation of dendritic cells	[88]

Table 3. *Cont.*

Bacterial Source of OMVs	Modification and/or Guest Molecules	Particle Size (nm)	Modification or Loading Method	Stimulating Factor	Therapy Strategy	Outcomes	References
E. coli K12 (ΔmsbB)	Melanin	20–100	Genetic engineering	Photothermal	Both to create contrast for optoacoustic imaging on cancer cells and to achieve an anti-tumoral effect benefiting from the high photothermal conversion effect of melanin.	- effective photothermal conversion - accumulation of tumor tissues via the EPR effect - increased tumor surface temperature - decreased tumor growth - necrosis in tumor tissues	[93]
E. coli DH5α	Protein E7 (HPV16E7)	20–200	Genetic engineering	-	Enabling antitumoral effects to occur by stimulating cellular immune responses of antigen-presenting recombinant OMVs.	- maturation of dendritic cells - significant suppression of tumor growth	[97]
E. coli K12 (ΔmsbB)	HER2	30–250	Genetic engineering	-	- specific tumor targeting by the HER2 affibody - siRNA-mediated silencing of key genes in cancer cells	- inhibition of cell proliferation through siRNA-mediated degradation of KSP mRNA - large accumulation in tumor tissues	[77]
	KSP siRNA		Electroporation				

5.1.4. OMVs Designed with Coated and Hybrid Membrane Technology

Nanoparticles (NPs) have gained significant attention as a promising drug delivery system due to their simple design, low toxicity, and in vivo potency enhancement. However, as exogenous substances, they can be efficiently identified and eliminated by the mononuclear phagocyte system (MPS) in the bloodstream, while their nonspecific distribution can lead to increased toxic effects [136]. To overcome these limitations, modified NPs in engineered systems have been proposed as a promising strategy.

In recent years, nanoparticle cell membrane coating technology has emerged as a sophisticated and powerful approach to functionalizing NPs [137]. The approach was initially designed using red blood cell (RBC) membranes to coat polymeric nanoparticles. Subsequently, a broad range of existing cell membrane types such as RBCs, platelets, leukocytes, cancer cells, stem cells, dendritic cells, natural killer cells, and cell membrane-derived structures including exosomes and extracellular vesicles have been comprehensively investigated as nanoparticle coating structures [138].

Researchers are increasingly interested in using OMVs for making NPs more functional in biomedical applications. The coating of NPs with OMVs, referred to as NP-OMVs, preserves the physicochemical properties of synthetic NPs and enhances the biological functions of OMVs [24]. While OMVs have a membrane barrier, which results in low drug-loading efficiency, NPs have a high drug-loading capacity. When coated with membrane vesicles, nanoparticles exhibit an enhanced drug-loading capacity for cancer therapy [135]. Moreover, membrane vesicle-coated camouflaged NPs can evade the immune system, allowing them to remain in circulation for an extended period. Compared to traditional surface modification of OMVs, this soft modification process is simple and does not require the use of organic solvents, reducing potential limitations and improving biocompatibility [24].

Shi et al. (2020), loaded mesoporous silica nanoparticles (MSNPs) with 5-fluorouracil (5-FU) and camouflaged these drug-loaded nanoparticles with *E. coli*-derived OMVs to improve the ability of MSNPs to target colon cancer. Following oral administration, they observed that this composite delivery system increased cellular uptake by virtue of the mechanism of specific hyaluronic acid receptor-mediated endocytosis and caused a strong cytotoxic effect on cancer cells [139]. This study is a good example that reveals the synergistic effects of a combined OMV-NPs strategy.

A new class of biocompatible hybrid eukaryotic-prokaryotic nanovesicles (EPVs) has been developed, which combines melanoma cytomembrane vesicles for immunotherapy with attenuated *Salmonella* OMVs due to their natural adjuvant properties [140]. The hybrid EPVs were found to trigger a tumor-specific immune response by enhancing DC maturation and T-cell proliferation in melanoma cells. Subsequently, a PLGA-indocyanine green (ICG) core was implanted into EPVs to construct PI@EPV nanoplatforms for photothermal core structure. Under NIR laser irradiation, the PI@EPV surface temperature increased, which facilitated the spread of tumor-specific antigens and adjuvant components as a result of the inducing and photothermal conversion of ICG. This supported the further enhancement of EPV's anti-tumor immune effects. They found that the PI@EPV and laser combined group exhibited the strongest tumor inhibition activity compared to the control group and other treatment groups. Moreover, the treated mice survived for up to 60 days after the tumor formation.

Zhuang et al. (2022) successfully created new bacteria-plant hybrid nanoplatforms (called BPNs) by integrating thylakoid membranes with OMVs obtained from *E. coli* due to their ability to enhance the antitumor immunity of thylakoid membranes. The effect of OMV-based immunoregulation with photodynamic effects from the thylakoid membrane under laser irradiation provided a strong therapeutic efficacy in colon cancer cells by repolarizing M2 macrophages and increasing the release of tumor-associated antigens presented by dendritic cells, especially effector T lymphocytes that infiltrated the tumor. The combined use of the hybrid structure BPNs and laser irradiation suppressed tumor growth by 94.33% and strongly inhibited tumor metastasis. Furthermore, mice had a 90% survival rate after thirty-six days [123].

Recent research has shown that cancer cell membranes alone are not enough to trigger an antitumor immune response. To address this issue, hybrid membranes have been created by fusing OMVs with cancer cell membranes to facilitate cancer targeting and immunotherapy. Wang et al. (2020) developed a hybrid membrane model (OMV-CC) by fusing cell membranes derived from B16F10 melanoma cells with OMVs derived from *E. coli*, resulting in the specific targeting of melanoma cells in vivo. The researchers further coated hollow polydopamine nanoparticles with this hybrid membrane to form the HPDA@[OMV-CC] structure, which demonstrated selective tumor recognition ability by highly accumulating more in melanoma cells. The structure activated an antitumor immune response by rapidly triggering DC maturation in treated mice, and HPDA-mediated photothermal therapy completely reversed melanoma formation in mice without significant side effects [141]. This study is a useful example of combining the coating- and hybrid-membrane technologies to be used in cancer treatment.

In cancer therapy, the targeted delivery of therapeutics is crucial for effectiveness. To achieve this, microrobots have been engineered for their mobility, functionality, and ability to penetrate tissues and reach cancerous cells [142]. Zhou et al. (2021) developed a combinatorial microrobot system (Motor-OMV) by loading OMVs obtained from *E. coli* onto self-propelled Mg-based micromotors. Intratumoral injection of Motor-OMVs caused significant deterioration of colorectal cancer and melanoma tumor tissues synergistically with tumor tissue destruction caused by the micromotor system and the immuno-stimulating effect of OMVs [143].

5.2. Antimicrobial Therapy

5.2.1. Antibacterial Activity

The most common approach to recovering bacterial infections is antibiotic therapy. However, antibiotic treatment cannot be efficient in some cases, e.g., in the case of misuse and self-medication; moreover, it may lead to drug resistance. In this context, the discovery of different antibiotic delivery systems and antibacterial agents is of great importance. The administration of antibiotic therapy is particularly challenging for Gram-negative bacteria due to their double-membrane cell envelope. The ability of BMVs to deliver molecules across the cell envelope of Gram-negative bacteria reveals their antibiotic transport potential [144,145].

The antibacterial effects of OMVs have been documented, with initial evidence provided by Kadurugamuwa and Beveridge in 1996 for lysines in *P. aeruginosa*-derived vesicles [146]. Subsequent studies have identified several other naturally occurring antibacterial molecules in BMVs from different bacteria (Table 4). In *L. acidophilus*, increased amounts of lactacin B in MVs were shown to inhibit the growth of *Lactobacillus delbrueckii* [147]. Moreover, the potential of BMVs as a delivery system for antibacterial agents has been explored as a promising alternative to address the limited availability of such agents at the site of infection [148]. Huang et al. (2020) demonstrated that levofloxacin-loaded OMVs (LEV-OMV) produced by *Acinetobacter baumanii* retained their structure and exhibited a stronger antibacterial effect in mice with an intestinal bacterial infection compared to freely administered levofloxacin [86]. Similarly, BMV-coated nanoparticles (NP-BMV) have been shown to possess antibacterial properties due to the natural immunogenicity of BMVs, as well as providing structural stability and homogeneity. Wu et al. reported high cytokine levels and CRKP-specific antibody production in mice administered with nanoparticles coated with OMVs obtained from carbapenem-resistant *K. pneumoniae* (CRKP) [149]. In a different NP-MV study, Gao et al. showed that antibiotic-loaded PLGA nanoparticles coated with MVs obtained from *S. aureus* were taken up by infected macrophage cells, resulting in antibiotic release and a decrease in the number of *S. aureus* [80].

Table 4. Antibacterial effect studies of BMVs.

BMV Source	Application Type of BMVs	Active Ingredient	Target Bacteria	References
P.aeruginosa	Natural Drug delivery	Autolysin Gentamicin	*S. aureus* *E. coli*	[150,151]
Lysobacter sp. XL1	Natural	Endopeptidase L5	*S. aureus* *Erwinia marcescens*	[152]
Myxococcus xanthus	Natural	Hydrolase content	*E. coli*	[153]
Cystobacter velatus Cbv34, *Cystobacter ferrugineus* Cbfe23	Natural	Cystobactamid	*S. aureus* *E. coli*	[154,155]
Lysobacter capsici	Natural	Bacteriolytic enzymes	*Micrococcus roseus* *S. aureus* *Micrococcus luteus* *Bacillus cereus*	[156]
Burkholderia thailandensis E264	Natural	Peptidoglycan hydrolases, 4-hydroxy-3-methyl-2-(2-non-enyl)-quinoline (HMNQ), long-chain rhamnolipid	*A. baumannii* *S. aureus*	[157]
L. acidophilus	Natural	lactacin B	*L. delbrueckii*	[147]
Lacticaseibacillus casei BL23	Natural	Antibofilm agent peptidoglycan hydrolases	*Salmonella enterica*	[158]
Buttiauxella agrestis	Drug delivery	Gentamicin	*Buttiauxella agrestis*	[159]
A. baumannii	Drug delivery	Levofloxacin, Amikacin Ciprofloxacin, Norfloxacin	*K. pneumoniae* *E. coli* *P. aeruginosa*	[86]
Shigella flexneri	NP-OMV	Poly(anhydride) NP-OMV	*Shigella flexneri*	[160]
E. coli	NP-OMV	Gold nanoparticles (AuNPs)-OMV	Unknown	[161]
Vibrio cholerae	NP-OMV	Chitosan-tripolyphosphate NP-OMV	*Vibrio cholerae*	[162]
Helicobacter pylori	NP-OMV	PLGA NP-OMV	*Helicobacter pylori*	[163]
S. aureus	NP-MV	PLGA NP-MV	*S. aureus*	[80]
K. pneumoniae	NP-OMV	-	carbapenem-resistant *K. pneumoniae*	[149]
Bordetella bronchiseptica	NP-OMV	Glycyrrhizic acid-NP	*Bordetella bronchiseptica*	[164]

5.2.2. Antifungal Activity

Recent studies have shown that, besides their antibacterial properties, BMVs naturally carry antifungal compounds that exhibit antifungal activity. In *Streptomyces albus*, genes encoding the synthesis of antifungal compounds, candicidin and antimycin were identified. The production and secretion of these antifungals were observed in the wild-type and mutant strains of *S. albus*, and it was discovered that *S. albus* MVs carry candicidine [165]. *Lysobacter enzymogenes* produces thermostable antifungal factors (HSAF) and their analogs that are induced by fungal mycelia or chitin-enriched media. The LeLPMO1A gene, which encodes a chitin-binding protein, was identified in the genome analysis of *L. enzymogenes*. Its deletion reduced HSAF production by chitin, indicating the gene's role in antifungal compound synthesis. In the study on *L. enzymogenes* OMVs, the colocalization of antifungal compounds and the LeLPMO1A gene was established by metabolic and proteomic analyses [166]. Furthermore, OMVs obtained from another strain of *L. enzymogenes* exhibited chitinase and antifungal activity, inhibiting the growth of *Saccharomyces cerevisiae* and *Fusarium subglutinacin* [167]. These findings indicate the potential of BMVs as natural sources of antifungal compounds for the development of antifungal therapeutics.

5.2.3. Antiviral Activity

BMVs can be an intriguing vaccine delivery vehicle for viral antigens because of their self-adjuvant properties and capacity to be adorned with antigens. Finally, studies have evaluated the antiviral abilities of BMVs and their potential as a vaccine platform against viruses. In particular, they have shown promise in protecting against lethal doses of influenza viruses. In a study using BMVs with attenuated lipopolysaccharide content, protection was observed against pandemic H1N1, PR8, and H5N1 virus types, and this antiviral activity was dependent on macrophages, which were induced to produce IFN after BMV administration [168]. Although the immune response generated by BMVs is temporary, a subsequent study applied BMVs with attenuated lipopolysaccharide content and influenza infections consecutively. This resulted in the induction of virus-specific antibodies in mice, and a second infection at week 4 provided complete protection against viral loading in BMV-treated mice for up to 18 weeks [169]. These findings demonstrate the potential of BMVs as a vaccine platform against influenza viruses.

Other studies have shown that OMVs have potential as a vaccine platform against various viruses, including the Zika virus and severe acute respiratory syndrome coronavirus 2 (SARS-CoV-2). Martins et al. (2018) demonstrated that the administration of OMVs isolated from *Neisseria meningitidis* fused with a Zika virus-infected cell line led to higher antibody production in mice than in non-treated mice [170]. With the increasing course of the COVID-19 epidemic and the formation of variants, alternative vaccine platforms are necessary. The current SARS-CoV-2 vaccines have limitations, and BMVs offer potential advantages. Thapa et al. showed that *Vibrio cholerae* and *E. coli* cells can be genetically modified to secrete OMVs decorated with the receptor binding domain (RBD) of the SARS-CoV-2 spike protein. Mice administered with RBD-decorated OMVs produced antibodies against the spike protein [171]. In another study, BMVs decorated with RBD and loaded with siRNAs against SARS-CoV-2 were shown to suppress infection by specifically targeting lung tissues [172]. Jiang et al. (2022) investigated the efficacy of OMVs against SARS-CoV-2 variants. They administered RBD-decorated OMVs from *S. typhimurium* to mouse models infected with wild-type and delta variants and reported high anti-RBD IgG levels in the blood of all subjects [173].

The use of BMVs as smart drug delivery systems in antimicrobial and anticancer therapies is presented in Figure 5.

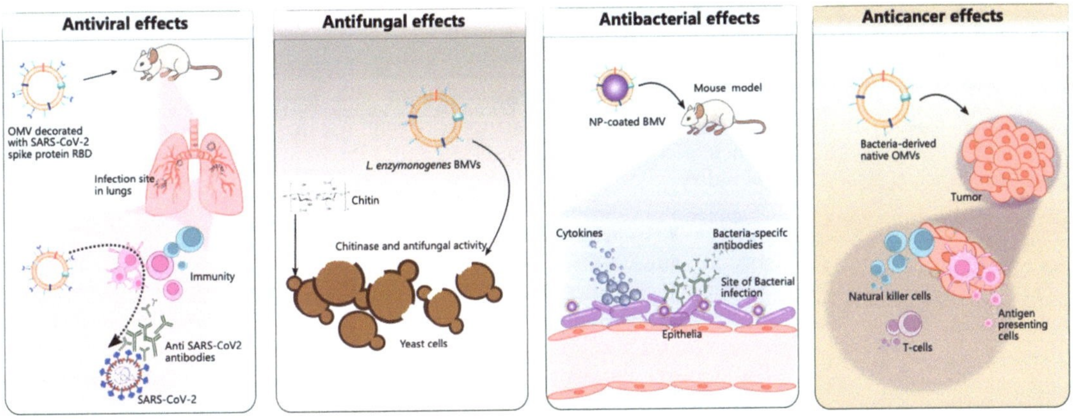

Figure 5. Potential uses of BMVs in antimicrobial and anticancer therapy.

6. Safety of BMVs as Smart Drug Delivery Systems

The lack of replicative abilities in BMVs makes them less virulent, yet still potentially harmful due to the presence of virulence factors and toxic components [148]. A crucial step for BMV applications is the detoxification of toxic components, particularly LPS found on the surface of BMVs [174]. The LPS consists of acyl chains, core oligosaccharides, lipid A moieties, and O-antigen, with the lipid A moiety being the primary contributor to LPS toxicity [144]. Detergents are often used to remove LPS from BMVs, which reduces their toxicity. Another approach involves editing genes in bacterial cells to reduce toxicity, such as inactivating the msbB gene or modifying operon genes involved in core oligosaccharide and O-antigen synthesis [93,125]. However, genetic modification can also result in decreased BMV yield and needs optimization. An alternative approach is modifying the phosphorylation of the lipid A portion, such as expressing the Hp0021 gene in *E. coli* to obtain monophosphorylated lipid A. While promising, this approach has yet to be used in BMV biotechnological applications [144,175]. Additionally, selecting non-pathogenic bacteria to obtain BMVs with low toxicity is an alternative approach. For instance, BMVs from symbiotic bacteria can stimulate immune regulation and prevent colitis [176].

Apart from LPS, many virulence factors, such as cytotoxins and adhesins carried by BMVs, also cause toxicity. In a study conducted to eliminate this toxicity, a mutant strain was created by deleting 14 genes encoding virulence factors in *P. aeruginosa*. BMVs produced from the mutant strain did not cause any death when administered to mice. Time and applicability are limiting factors in this detoxification approach [177].

7. Obstacles of BMVs for Clinical Use as Smart Drug Delivery Systems

We have reviewed the properties of BMVs and their various applications. While BMVs have demonstrated their effectiveness against cancer and infectious diseases in both in vitro and in vivo studies, there are still unresolved practical issues in their clinical use as potential smart delivery vehicles. It is crucial to address these issues to bridge the gap between laboratory research and clinical applications of BMVs [60].

Biosafety. The use of BMVs in clinical practice faces a major obstacle, which is safety. OMVs are typically derived from Gram-negative bacteria and contain endotoxins and virulence factors such as LPS that can elicit immune responses and toxicity. To address this challenge, genetic engineering has been used to develop OMVs with reduced/attenuated endotoxins by deleting the msbA, msbB, lpxM, and lpxL1 genes [55]. LPS-deficient OMVs exhibit lower immunogenicity than those with normal LPS levels [178], but the optimal balance between low toxicity and high immunogenicity remains a challenge. Additionally, to ensure safety in clinical trials, OMVs' endotoxin levels should be as low as possible, and further in vivo studies are necessary to expedite OMV applications in humans.

Strain selection. OMVs obtained from *E. coli* are widely used in cancer therapy (Table 2). However, in using BMVs for these purposes, the identification and selection of specific strains can provide a better balance between the safety and immunogenicity of BMVs. Thus, there is a need for methods to control the immunotoxicity of BMVs to increase their biosafety.

Biogenesis. Literature reports suggest that information on MVs is relatively limited compared to OMVs [48]. Consequently, the mechanisms of BMV biogenesis remain poorly understood. Further research into the underlying biogenesis mechanisms will aid in discovering and characterizing membrane vesicles from other bacterial species. This will also facilitate the development of improved bacterial-based nanoplatforms for biomedical applications through more in vivo and in vitro studies.

Standardized Production. Obtaining BMVs involves many methods, and there is no standardized analytical protocol. Different production and isolation techniques result in a large heterogeneity of the obtained BMV populations due to the characteristics of BMVs, such as their size and components. This makes it difficult to achieve reproducibility and consistency of results in clinical applications. The interaction of heterogeneous BMVs with target cells and their intracellular fate is unpredictable. Therefore, the development of methods like proteomics and lipidomics to produce homogeneous BMV structures and analyze their composition is critical for their use in clinical applications [135]. These methods will pave the way for the successful use of BMVs for clinical purposes.

Scalability. The collection and purification of BMVs using the ultracentrifugation method require advanced equipment and qualified personnel, making it time-consuming and costly [131]. Furthermore, commercial kits available for BMV purification suffer from low yield and purity issues, thereby causing high prices [179]. Thus, there is an urgent need to develop new and scalable BMV separation/purification methods that can continuously separate BMVs from the culture medium with high yield and purity. Although bacteria can be easily produced in large quantities using large fermentation vessels, the amount of BMVs released from bacteria is not sufficient for their mass production to be cost-effective. Therefore, there is a requirement for high-efficiency production of BMVs to be scalable for clinical applications. To achieve this, different cultural conditions and systems must be explored to optimize BMV production and lay the foundation for BMV industrialization.

Drug-loading. One of the challenges of loading therapeutics into BMVs is the bilayer lipid membrane, which makes it difficult despite various drug-loading strategies. This low loading rate has hindered the clinical application of BMVs. Although Gao et al. performed drug loading with a pH gradient to overcome this situation, they were only able to increase drug loading to 12% [180]. As a result, new approaches and methods should be developed to increase drug loading to BMVs.

The limitations of using BMVs in clinical practice as previously mentioned are concerning. To address this limitation, an alternative method is the development of controllable artificial BMVs that enable a more comprehensive understanding of their active ingredients. This can be achieved by obtaining detoxified BMVs, which can be exploited for their unique biological properties in biomedical applications [130].

8. Outlook and Conclusions

With the publication of research over the last two decades, our knowledge of the biogenesis and function of BMVs has advanced rapidly. BMVs are among the most extensively studied bacterial strategies in the fight against infectious and non-infectious diseases. In this review, we discussed the many unique properties of BMVs, especially OMVs generated from Gram-negative bacteria, their current production and purification procedures, characterization methods, and their functions in biomedical applications. In addition to their direct production by bacterial cell culture, biotechnological developments have enabled OMVs to be customized to contain various proteins and ligands using recombinant

DNA technology to produce them in accordance with the desired purpose, and thus their usability as carrier systems for antigens and therapeutic agents. We have clarified in detail the strengths and weaknesses of smart drug delivery systems in this review, which serve as the foundation for the use of BMVs in biomedical applications. In addition, OMVs can be functionalized not only as targeted drug delivery systems but also as bioimaging platforms using protein–protein binding pairs and multi-domain scaffold structures through genetic modification.

To date, BMVs have been researched and encouraging advances have been made for the transmission of many therapeutic cargoes (chemotherapeutic drugs, therapeutic nucleic acids, antibiotics, nanoparticles, proteins, etc.). However, despite the many notable studies that have been successful in vitro and in vivo with sophisticated approaches to smart drug and/or cargo delivery, the critical limitations detailed here need to be overcome in order to pave the way for their clinical use, and more studies are needed to do so. Limited research is available on the biogenesis of BMVs and, in particular, MVs from Gram-positive bacteria, and future studies in this field will aid discovery and characterization of membrane vesicles from bacterial species. The fact that researchers will utilize multiomic techniques to disclose the composition variety and diverse nature of BMVs using distinct datasets will provide us greater insight into their diversity of functions. In particular, the safety of OMVs is a major issue and the identification of different strains from *E. coli* and new ways of weakening endotoxin content are critical to achieving a balance in terms of immunogenicity and the safe use of OMVs. In this context, more clinical and in vivo research are needed to investigate bacterial strains and evaluate immunogenicity. Moreover, the optimization and development of standard and repeatable protocols in the production and purification of BMVs are crucial both for their production and for their functionalization on a large scale. The main problem as carrier systems is the low loading rate of therapeutical agents, since BMVs contain bilayer lipid barriers. In order to overcome this, researchers turn to the BMV's production strategy designed with stimuli, but it is thought that studies on the production and design of controllable artificial BMVs will be more solution-oriented in order to increase the loading capacity of the therapeutic agent.

Overall, the door to a new era has been opened in the use of bacteria-based nanotechnology for the treatment of diseases. The use and development of BMVs as nanocarrier smart systems in the treatment and diagnosis of target cells is the focus of studies that will contribute to the development of new bacterial-based nanovesicle technology.

Author Contributions: Conceptualization, all authors contributed equally; resources, A.Ç. and P.A.Ç.; writing—original draft preparation, all authors; writing—review and editing, all authors; visualization, B.M.E.; supervision, P.A.Ç.; B.D., C.T.S.-T., G.A. and A.Ç. All authors have read and agreed to the published version of the manuscript.

Funding: This research received no external funding.

Institutional Review Board Statement: Not applicable.

Informed Consent Statement: Not applicable.

Data Availability Statement: Not applicable.

Conflicts of Interest: The authors declare no conflict of interest.

References

1. Zhu, H.; Li, B.V.; Uppoor, R.S.; Mehta, M.; Yu, L.X. Pharmaceutical Theory and Practice. In *Developing Solid Oral Dosage Forms*, 2nd ed.; Bioavailability and Bioequivalence; Academic Press: Cambridge, MA, USA, 2017; pp. 381–397. [CrossRef]
2. Adepu, S.; Ramakrishna, S. Controlled Drug Delivery Systems: Current Status and Future Directions. *Molecules* **2021**, *26*, 5905. [CrossRef] [PubMed]
3. Park, H.; Otte, A.; Park, K. Evolution of drug delivery systems: From 1950 to 2020 and beyond. *J. Control. Release* **2022**, *342*, 53–65. [CrossRef] [PubMed]
4. Calis, S.; Ozturk Atar, K.; Arslan, F.B.; Eroglu, H.; Capan, Y. Nanopharmaceuticals as Drug-Delivery Systems. In *Nanocarriers for Drug Delivery*; Elsevier: Amsterdam, The Netherlands, 2019; pp. 133–154. [CrossRef]

5. Alvarez-Lorenzo, C.; Concheiro, A. Smart drug delivery systems: From fundamentals to the clinic. *Chem. Commun.* **2014**, *50*, 7743–7765. [CrossRef]
6. Siddique, S.; Chow, J.C.L. Application of Nanomaterials in Biomedical Imaging and Cancer Therapy. *Nanomaterials* **2020**, *10*, 1700. [CrossRef] [PubMed]
7. Siddique, S.; Chow, J.C.L. Recent Advances in Functionalized Nanoparticles in Cancer Theranostics. *Nanomaterials* **2022**, *12*, 2826. [CrossRef]
8. Khizar, S.; Alrushaid, N.; Alam Khan, F.; Zine, N.; Jaffrezic-Renault, N.; Errachid, A.; Elaissari, A. Nanocarriers based novel and effective drug delivery system. *Int. J. Pharm.* **2023**, *632*, 122570. [CrossRef]
9. Wen, J.; Lv, Y.; Xu, Y.; Zhang, P.; Li, H.; Chen, X.; Li, X.; Zhang, L.; Liu, F.; Zeng, W.; et al. Construction of a biodegradable, versatile nanocarrier for optional combination cancer therapy. *Acta Biomater.* **2019**, *83*, 359–371. [CrossRef]
10. Jain, S.; Pillai, J. Bacterial membrane vesicles as novel nanosystems for drug delivery. *Int. J. Nanomed.* **2017**, *12*, 6329–6341. [CrossRef]
11. Fazal, S.; Lee, R. Biomimetic Bacterial Membrane Vesicles for Drug Delivery Applications. *Pharmaceutics* **2021**, *13*, 1430. [CrossRef]
12. Raza, A.; Rasheed, T.; Nabeel, F.; Hayat, U.; Bilal, M.; Iqbal, H.M.N. Endogenous and Exogenous Stimuli-Responsive Drug Delivery Systems for Programmed Site-Specific Release. *Molecules* **2019**, *24*, 1117. [CrossRef]
13. Liu, D.; Yang, F.; Xiong, F.; Gu, N. The Smart Drug Delivery System and Its Clinical Potential. *Theranostics* **2016**, *6*, 1306–1323. [CrossRef] [PubMed]
14. Liu, M.; Du, H.; Zhang, W.; Zhai, G. Internal stimuli-responsive nanocarriers for drug delivery: Design strategies and applications. *Mater. Sci. Eng. C Mater. Biol. Appl.* **2017**, *71*, 1267–1280. [CrossRef] [PubMed]
15. Jha, A.; Rama, A.; Ladani, B.; Verma, N.; Kannan, S.; Naha, A. Temperature and pH-responsive nanogels as intelligent drug delivery systems: A comprehensive review. *J. Appl. Pharm. Sci.* **2021**, *11*, 1–16. [CrossRef]
16. Chen, Y.; Chen, N.; Feng, X. The role of internal and external stimuli in the rational design of skin-specific drug delivery systems. *Int. J. Pharm.* **2021**, *592*, 120081. [CrossRef] [PubMed]
17. Zhao, Z.; Shen, J.; Zhang, L.; Wang, L.; Xu, H.; Han, Y.; Jia, J.; Lu, Y.; Yu, R.; Liu, H. Injectable postoperative enzyme-responsive hydrogels for reversing temozolomide resistance and reducing local recurrence after glioma operation. *Biomater. Sci.* **2020**, *8*, 5306–5316. [CrossRef]
18. Bordbar-Khiabani, A.; Gasik, M. Smart Hydrogels for Advanced Drug Delivery Systems. *Int. J. Mol. Sci.* **2022**, *23*, 3365. [CrossRef]
19. Hajebi, S.; Rabiee, N.; Bagherzadeh, M.; Ahmadi, S.; Rabiee, M.; Roghani-Mamaqani, H.; Tahriri, M.; Tayebi, L.; Hamblin, M.R. Stimulus-responsive polymeric nanogels as smart drug delivery systems. *Acta Biomater.* **2019**, *92*, 1–18. [CrossRef]
20. Safari, J.; Zarnegar, Z. Advanced drug delivery systems: Nanotechnology of health design A review. *J. Saudi Chem. Soc.* **2014**, *18*, 85–99. [CrossRef]
21. Faheem, A.M.; Abdelkader, D.H. Novel drug delivery systems. In *Engineering Drug Delivery Systems*; Woodhead Publishing: Sawston, UK, 2020; pp. 1–16. [CrossRef]
22. Wang, J.; Chen, D.; Ho, E.A. Challenges in the development and establishment of exosome-based drug delivery systems. *J. Control. Release* **2021**, *329*, 894–906. [CrossRef]
23. Wang, S.; Gao, J.; Wang, Z. Outer membrane vesicles for vaccination and targeted drug delivery. *Wiley Interdiscip. Rev. Nanomed. Nanobiotechnol.* **2019**, *11*, e1523. [CrossRef] [PubMed]
24. Naskar, A.; Cho, H.; Lee, S.; Kim, K.S. Biomimetic Nanoparticles Coated with Bacterial Outer Membrane Vesicles as a New-Generation Platform for Biomedical Applications. *Pharmaceutics* **2021**, *13*, 1887. [CrossRef]
25. Liu, H.; Zhang, Q.; Wang, S.; Weng, W.; Jing, Y.; Su, J. Bacterial extracellular vesicles as bioactive nanocarriers for drug delivery: Advances and perspectives. *Bioact. Mater.* **2022**, *14*, 169–181. [CrossRef] [PubMed]
26. Wibowo, D.; Jorritsma, S.H.T.; Gonzaga, Z.J.; Evert, B.; Chen, S.; Rehm, B.H.A. Polymeric nanoparticle vaccines to combat emerging and pandemic threats. *Biomaterials* **2021**, *268*, 120597. [CrossRef]
27. El-Say, K.M.; El-Sawy, H.S. Polymeric nanoparticles: Promising platform for drug delivery. *Int. J. Pharm.* **2017**, *528*, 675–691. [CrossRef]
28. Lee, S.C.; Kwon, I.K.; Park, K. Hydrogels for delivery of bioactive agents: A historical perspective. *Adv. Drug. Deliv. Rev.* **2013**, *65*, 17–20. [CrossRef]
29. Caló, E.; Khutoryanskiy, V.V. Biomedical applications of hydrogels: A review of patents and commercial products. *Eur. Polym. J.* **2015**, *65*, 252–267. [CrossRef]
30. Jain, K.; Kesharwani, P.; Gupta, U.; Jain, N.K. Dendrimer toxicity: Let's meet the challenge. *Int. J. Pharm.* **2010**, *394*, 122–142. [CrossRef] [PubMed]
31. Chis, A.A.; Dobrea, C.; Morgovan, C.; Arseniu, A.M.; Rus, L.L.; Butuca, A.; Juncan, A.M.; Totan, M.; Vonica-Tincu, A.L.; Cormos, G.; et al. Applications and Limitations of Dendrimers in Biomedicine. *Molecules* **2020**, *25*, 3982. [CrossRef] [PubMed]
32. Santos, A.; Veiga, F.; Figueiras, A. Dendrimers as Pharmaceutical Excipients: Synthesis, Properties, Toxicity and Biomedical Applications. *Materials* **2019**, *13*, 65. [CrossRef] [PubMed]
33. Guimaraes, D.; Cavaco-Paulo, A.; Nogueira, E. Design of liposomes as drug delivery system for therapeutic applications. *Int. J. Pharm.* **2021**, *601*, 120571. [CrossRef]
34. Dymek, M.; Sikora, E. Liposomes as biocompatible and smart delivery systems—The current state. *Adv. Colloid. Interface Sci.* **2022**, *309*, 102757. [CrossRef] [PubMed]

35. Amasya, G.; Bakar-Ates, F.; Wintgens, V.; Amiel, C. Layer by layer assembly of core-corona structured solid lipid nanoparticles with beta-cyclodextrin polymers. *Int. J. Pharm.* **2021**, *592*, 119994. [CrossRef] [PubMed]
36. Das, S.; Chaudhury, A. Recent advances in lipid nanoparticle formulations with solid matrix for oral drug delivery. *AAPS PharmSciTech* **2011**, *12*, 62–76. [CrossRef] [PubMed]
37. Lacerda, L.; Bianco, A.; Prato, M.; Kostarelos, K. Carbon nanotubes as nanomedicines: From toxicology to pharmacology. *Adv. Drug. Deliv. Rev.* **2006**, *58*, 1460–1470. [CrossRef] [PubMed]
38. Vallet-Regi, M.; Colilla, M.; Izquierdo-Barba, I.; Manzano, M. Mesoporous Silica Nanoparticles for Drug Delivery: Current Insights. *Molecules* **2017**, *23*, 47. [CrossRef]
39. Bharti, C.; Nagaich, U.; Pal, A.K.; Gulati, N. Mesoporous silica nanoparticles in target drug delivery system: A review. *Int. J. Pharm. Investig.* **2015**, *5*, 124–133. [CrossRef]
40. Jamkhande, P.G.; Ghule, N.W.; Bamer, A.H.; Kalaskar, M.G. Metal nanoparticles synthesis: An overview on methods of preparation, advantages and disadvantages, and applications. *J. Drug. Deliv. Sci. Technol.* **2019**, *53*, 101174. [CrossRef]
41. Khursheed, R.; Dua, K.; Vishwas, S.; Gulati, M.; Jha, N.K.; Aldhafeeri, G.M.; Alanazi, F.G.; Goh, B.H.; Gupta, G.; Paudel, K.R.; et al. Biomedical applications of metallic nanoparticles in cancer: Current status and future perspectives. *Biomed. Pharmacother.* **2022**, *150*, 112951. [CrossRef]
42. Kuchur, O.A.; Tsymbal, S.A.; Shestovskaya, M.V.; Serov, N.S.; Dukhinova, M.S.; Shtil, A.A. Metal-derived nanoparticles in tumor theranostics: Potential and limitations. *J. Inorg. Biochem.* **2020**, *209*, 111117. [CrossRef]
43. Smyth, T.; Kullberg, M.; Malik, N.; Smith-Jones, P.; Graner, M.W.; Anchordoquy, T.J. Biodistribution and delivery efficiency of unmodified tumor-derived exosomes. *J. Control. Release* **2015**, *199*, 145–155. [CrossRef]
44. Mitchell, M.J.; Billingsley, M.M.; Haley, R.M.; Wechsler, M.E.; Peppas, N.A.; Langer, R. Engineering precision nanoparticles for drug delivery. *Nat. Rev. Drug. Discov.* **2021**, *20*, 101–124. [CrossRef]
45. Campora, S.; Ghersi, G. Recent developments and applications of smart nanoparticles in biomedicine. *Nanotechnol. Rev.* **2022**, *11*, 2595–2631. [CrossRef]
46. Castillo-Romero, K.F.; Santacruz, A.; Gonzalez-Valdez, J. Production and purification of bacterial membrane vesicles for biotechnology applications: Challenges and opportunities. *Electrophoresis* **2023**, *44*, 107–124. [CrossRef] [PubMed]
47. De, S.N. Enterotoxicity of Bacteria-free Culture-filtrate of Vibrio cholerae. *Nature* **1959**, *183*, 1533–1534. [CrossRef]
48. Aytar Celik, P.; Derkus, B.; Erdogan, K.; Barut, D.; Blaise Manga, E.; Yildirim, Y.; Pecha, S.; Cabuk, A. Bacterial membrane vesicle functions, laboratory methods, and applications. *Biotechnol. Adv.* **2022**, *54*, 107869. [CrossRef] [PubMed]
49. Wu, J.; An, M.; Zhu, J.; Tan, Z.; Chen, G.Y.; Stidham, R.W.; Lubman, D.M. A Method for Isolation and Proteomic Analysis of Outer Membrane Vesicles from Fecal Samples by LC-MS/MS. *J. Proteom. Bioinform.* **2019**, *12*, 38–42. [CrossRef] [PubMed]
50. Torres Crigna, A.; Fricke, F.; Nitschke, K.; Worst, T.; Erb, U.; Karremann, M.; Buschmann, D.; Elvers-Hornung, S.; Tucher, C.; Schiller, M.; et al. Inter-Laboratory Comparison of Extracellular Vesicle Isolation Based on Ultracentrifugation. *Transfus. Med. Hemother* **2021**, *48*, 48–59. [CrossRef]
51. Qing, G.; Gong, N.; Chen, X.; Chen, J.; Zhang, H.; Wang, Y.; Wang, R.; Zhang, S.; Zhang, Z.; Zhao, X.; et al. Natural and engineered bacterial outer membrane vesicles. *Biophys. Rep.* **2019**, *5*, 184–198. [CrossRef]
52. Klimentova, J.; Stulik, J. Methods of isolation and purification of outer membrane vesicles from gram-negative bacteria. *Microbiol. Res.* **2015**, *170*, 1–9. [CrossRef]
53. Li, R.; Liu, Q. Engineered Bacterial Outer Membrane Vesicles as Multifunctional Delivery Platforms. *Front. Mater.* **2020**, *7*, 202. [CrossRef]
54. De Benedetto, G.; Cescutti, P.; Giannelli, C.; Rizzo, R.; Micoli, F. Multiple Techniques for Size Determination of Generalized Modules for Membrane Antigens from *Salmonella typhimurium* and *Salmonella enteritidis*. *ACS Omega* **2017**, *2*, 8282–8289. [CrossRef] [PubMed]
55. Chen, H.; Zhou, M.; Zeng, Y.; Lv, Z.; Wang, P.; Han, L. Recent advances in biomedical applications of bacterial outer membrane vesicles. *J. Mater. Chem. B* **2022**, *10*, 7384–7396. [CrossRef] [PubMed]
56. Tiwari, S.; Kumar, V.; Randhawa, S.; Verma, S.K. Preparation and characterization of extracellular vesicles. *Am. J. Reprod. Immunol.* **2021**, *85*, e13367. [CrossRef] [PubMed]
57. Tiku, V.; Kofoed, E.M.; Yan, D.; Kang, J.; Xu, M.; Reichelt, M.; Dikic, I.; Tan, M.W. Outer membrane vesicles containing OmpA induce mitochondrial fragmentation to promote pathogenesis of *Acinetobacter baumannii*. *Sci. Rep.* **2021**, *11*, 618. [CrossRef]
58. Barut, D.; Enuh, B.M.; Derkuş, B.; Güler, B.; Salih, B.; Çelik, P.A. The relationship between bacterial outer membrane vesicles and halophilic adaptation. *Mol. Omics* **2023**, *19*, 174–181. [CrossRef]
59. Yu, Y.J.; Wang, X.H.; Fan, G.C. Versatile effects of bacterium-released membrane vesicles on mammalian cells and infectious/inflammatory diseases. *Acta Pharmacol. Sin.* **2018**, *39*, 514–533. [CrossRef]
60. Kulkarni, H.M.; Jagannadham, M.V. Biogenesis and multifaceted roles of outer membrane vesicles from Gram-negative bacteria. *Microbiology* **2014**, *160*, 2109–2121. [CrossRef]
61. Jan, A.T. Outer Membrane Vesicles (OMVs) of Gram-negative Bacteria: A Perspective Update. *Front. Microbiol.* **2017**, *8*, 1053. [CrossRef]
62. Briaud, P.; Carroll, R.K. Extracellular Vesicle Biogenesis and Functions in Gram-Positive Bacteria. *Infect. Immun.* **2020**, *88*, e00433-20. [CrossRef]

63. Lima, S.; Matinha-Cardoso, J.; Tamagnini, P.; Oliveira, P. Extracellular Vesicles: An Overlooked Secretion System in Cyanobacteria. *Life* **2020**, *10*, 129. [CrossRef]
64. Haurat, M.F.; Elhenawy, W.; Feldman, M.F. Prokaryotic membrane vesicles: New insights on biogenesis and biological roles. *Biol. Chem.* **2015**, *396*, 95–109. [CrossRef] [PubMed]
65. Chattopadhyay, M.K.; Jaganandham, M.V. Vesicles-mediated resistance to antibiotics in bacteria. *Front. Microbiol.* **2015**, *6*, 758. [CrossRef]
66. Azam, A.H.; Tanji, Y. Bacteriophage-host arm race: An update on the mechanism of phage resistance in bacteria and revenge of the phage with the perspective for phage therapy. *Appl. Microbiol. Biotechnol.* **2019**, *103*, 2121–2131. [CrossRef]
67. Tran, F.; Boedicker, J.G. Plasmid Characteristics Modulate the Propensity of Gene Exchange in Bacterial Vesicles. *J. Bacteriol.* **2019**, *201*, e00430-18. [CrossRef]
68. Cao, Y.; Lin, H. Characterization and function of membrane vesicles in Gram-positive bacteria. *Appl. Microbiol. Biotechnol.* **2021**, *105*, 1795–1801. [CrossRef]
69. Seike, S.; Kobayashi, H.; Ueda, M.; Takahashi, E.; Okamoto, K.; Yamanaka, H. Outer Membrane Vesicles Released From Aeromonas Strains Are Involved in the Biofilm Formation. *Front. Microbiol.* **2020**, *11*, 613650. [CrossRef] [PubMed]
70. Wu, R.; Tao, Y.; Cao, Y.; Zhou, Y.; Lin, H. Streptococcus mutans Membrane Vesicles Harboring Glucosyltransferases Augment Candida albicans Biofilm Development. *Front. Microbiol.* **2020**, *11*, 581184. [CrossRef] [PubMed]
71. Mancini, F.; Rossi, O.; Necchi, F.; Micoli, F. OMV Vaccines and the Role of TLR Agonists in Immune Response. *Int. J. Mol. Sci.* **2020**, *21*, 4416. [CrossRef]
72. Chelakkot, C.; Choi, Y.; Kim, D.K.; Park, H.T.; Ghim, J.; Kwon, Y.; Jeon, J.; Kim, M.S.; Jee, Y.K.; Gho, Y.S.; et al. Akkermansia muciniphila-derived extracellular vesicles influence gut permeability through the regulation of tight junctions. *Exp. Mol. Med.* **2018**, *50*, e450. [CrossRef]
73. Fuhrmann, G.; Serio, A.; Mazo, M.; Nair, R.; Stevens, M.M. Active loading into extracellular vesicles significantly improves the cellular uptake and photodynamic effect of porphyrins. *J. Control. Release* **2015**, *205*, 35–44. [CrossRef]
74. Young, J.L.; Dean, D.A. Electroporation-mediated gene delivery. *Adv. Genet.* **2015**, *89*, 49–88. [CrossRef] [PubMed]
75. Lamichhane, T.N.; Raiker, R.S.; Jay, S.M. Exogenous DNA Loading into Extracellular Vesicles via Electroporation is Size-Dependent and Enables Limited Gene Delivery. *Mol. Pharm.* **2015**, *12*, 3650–3657. [CrossRef] [PubMed]
76. Pomatto, M.A.C.; Bussolati, B.; D'Antico, S.; Ghiotto, S.; Tetta, C.; Brizzi, M.F.; Camussi, G. Improved Loading of Plasma-Derived Extracellular Vesicles to Encapsulate Antitumor miRNAs. *Mol. Ther. Methods Clin. Dev.* **2019**, *13*, 133–144. [CrossRef] [PubMed]
77. Gujrati, V.; Kim, S.; Kim, S.H.; Min, J.J.; Choy, H.E.; Kim, S.C.; Jon, S. Bioengineered Bacterial Outer Membrane Vesicles as Cell-Specific Drug-Delivery Vehicles for Cancer Therapy. *ACS Nano* **2014**, *8*, 1525–1537. [CrossRef]
78. Ayed, Z.; Cuvillier, L.; Dobhal, G.; Goreham, R.V. Electroporation of outer membrane vesicles derived from Pseudomonas aeruginosa with gold nanoparticles. *SN Appl. Sci.* **2019**, *1*, 1600. [CrossRef]
79. Zhang, Q.; Fang, R.H.; Gao, W.; Zhang, L. A Biomimetic Nanoparticle to "Lure and Kill" Phospholipase A2. *Angew. Chem. Int. Ed. Engl.* **2020**, *59*, 10461–10465. [CrossRef]
80. Gao, F.; Xu, L.; Yang, B.; Fan, F.; Yang, L. Kill the Real with the Fake: Eliminate Intracellular Staphylococcus aureus Using Nanoparticle Coated with Its Extracellular Vesicle Membrane as Active-Targeting Drug Carrier. *ACS Infect. Dis.* **2019**, *5*, 218–227. [CrossRef]
81. Chen, Q.; Bai, H.; Wu, W.; Huang, G.; Li, Y.; Wu, M.; Tang, G.; Ping, Y. Bioengineering Bacterial Vesicle-Coated Polymeric Nanomedicine for Enhanced Cancer Immunotherapy and Metastasis Prevention. *Nano Lett.* **2020**, *20*, 11–21. [CrossRef]
82. Kuerban, K.; Gao, X.; Zhang, H.; Liu, J.; Dong, M.; Wu, L.; Ye, R.; Feng, M.; Ye, L. Doxorubicin-loaded bacterial outer-membrane vesicles exert enhanced anti-tumor efficacy in non-small-cell lung cancer. *Acta Pharm. Sin. B* **2020**, *10*, 1534–1548. [CrossRef]
83. Erdogan Gover, K.; Isik, M.; Barut, D.; Sengel-Turk, C.T.; Amasya, G.; Derkus, B.; Cabuk, A.; Aytar Celik, P. Capecitabine-loaded bacterial membrane vesicles derived from Enterococcus faecalis promotes apoptosis in HT-29 colon cancer cells. *Biochem. Eng. J.* **2022**, *189*, 108722. [CrossRef]
84. Allan, N.D.; Beveridge, T.J. Gentamicin delivery to Burkholderia cepacia group IIIa strains via membrane vesicles from *Pseudomonas aeruginosa* PAO1. *Antimicrob. Agents Chemother.* **2003**, *47*, 2962–2965. [CrossRef] [PubMed]
85. Jang, S.C.; Kim, S.R.; Yoon, Y.J.; Park, K.S.; Kim, J.H.; Lee, J.; Kim, O.Y.; Choi, E.J.; Kim, D.K.; Choi, D.S.; et al. In vivo kinetic biodistribution of nano-sized outer membrane vesicles derived from bacteria. *Small* **2015**, *11*, 456–461. [CrossRef] [PubMed]
86. Huang, W.; Zhang, Q.; Li, W.; Yuan, M.; Zhou, J.; Hua, L.; Chen, Y.; Ye, C.; Ma, Y. Development of novel nanoantibiotics using an outer membrane vesicle-based drug efflux mechanism. *J. Control. Release* **2020**, *317*, 1–22. [CrossRef] [PubMed]
87. Guo, Q.; Li, X.; Zhou, W.; Chu, Y.; Chen, Q.; Zhang, Y.; Li, C.; Chen, H.; Liu, P.; Zhao, Z.; et al. Sequentially Triggered Bacterial Outer Membrane Vesicles for Macrophage Metabolism Modulation and Tumor Metastasis Suppression. *ACS Nano* **2021**, *15*, 13826–13838. [CrossRef] [PubMed]
88. Qing, S.; Lyu, C.; Zhu, L.; Pan, C.; Wang, S.; Li, F.; Wang, J.; Yue, H.; Gao, X.; Jia, R.; et al. Biomineralized Bacterial Outer Membrane Vesicles Potentiate Safe and Efficient Tumor Microenvironment Reprogramming for Anticancer Therapy. *Adv. Mater.* **2020**, *32*, e2002085. [CrossRef]
89. Elkhodiry, M.A.; Momah, C.C.; Suwaidi, S.R.; Gadalla, D.; Martins, A.M.; Vitor, R.F.; Husseini, G.A. Synergistic Nanomedicine: Passive, Active, and Ultrasound-Triggered Drug Delivery in Cancer Treatment. *J. Nanosci. Nanotechnol.* **2016**, *16*, 1–18. [CrossRef]

90. Dutta, B.; Barick, K.C.; Hassan, P.A. Recent advances in active targeting of nanomaterials for anticancer drug delivery. *Adv. Colloid Interface Sci.* **2021**, *296*, 102509. [CrossRef]
91. Alavi, M.; Hamidi, M. Passive and active targeting in cancer therapy by liposomes and lipid nanoparticles. *Drug. Metab. Pers. Ther.* **2019**, *34*, 20180032. [CrossRef]
92. Dadwal, A.; Baldi, A.; Kumar Narang, R. Nanoparticles as carriers for drug delivery in cancer. *Artif. Cells Nanomed. Biotechnol.* **2018**, *46*, 295–305. [CrossRef]
93. Gujrati, V.; Prakash, J.; Malekzadeh-Najafabadi, J.; Stiel, A.; Klemm, U.; Mettenleiter, G.; Aichler, M.; Walch, A.; Ntziachristos, V. Bioengineered bacterial vesicles as biological nano-heaters for optoacoustic imaging. *Nat. Commun.* **2019**, *10*, 1114. [CrossRef]
94. Dai, L.; Liu, J.; Luo, Z.; Li, M.; Cai, K. Tumor therapy: Targeted drug delivery systems. *J. Mater. Chem. B.* **2016**, *4*, 6758–6772. [CrossRef]
95. Yoo, J.; Park, C.; Yi, G.; Lee, D.; Koo, H. Active Targeting Strategies Using Biological Ligands for Nanoparticle Drug Delivery Systems. *Cancers* **2019**, *11*, 640. [CrossRef]
96. Gu, T.W.; Wang, M.Z.; Niu, J.; Chu, Y.; Guo, K.R.; Peng, L.H. Outer membrane vesicles derived from E. coli as novel vehicles for transdermal and tumor targeting delivery. *Nanoscale* **2020**, *12*, 18965–18977. [CrossRef]
97. Wang, S.; Huang, W.; Li, K.; Yao, Y.; Yang, X.; Bai, H.; Sun, W.; Liu, C.; Ma, Y. Engineered outer membrane vesicle is potent to elicit HPV16E7-specific cellular immunity in a mouse model of TC-1 graft tumor. *Int. J. Nanomed.* **2017**, *12*, 6813–6825. [CrossRef]
98. Hirsjärvi, S.; Passirani, C.; Benoit, J.P. Passive and Active Tumour Targeting with Nanocarriers. *Curr. Drug. Discov. Technol.* **2011**, *8*, 188–196. [CrossRef]
99. Biffi, S.; Voltan, R.; Bortot, B.; Zauli, G.; Secchiero, P. Actively targeted nanocarriers for drug delivery to cancer cells. *Expert. Opin. Drug. Deliv.* **2019**, *16*, 481–496. [CrossRef]
100. Behera, A.; Padhi, S. Passive and active targeting strategies for the delivery of the camptothecin anticancer drug: A review. *Environ. Chem. Lett.* **2020**, *18*, 1557–1567. [CrossRef]
101. Wakaskar, R.R. Passive and Active Targeting in Tumor Microenvironment. *Int. J. Drug. Dev. Res.* **2017**, *9*, 37–41.
102. Danhier, F.; Feron, O.; Preat, V. To exploit the tumor microenvironment: Passive and active tumor targeting of nanocarriers for anti-cancer drug delivery. *J. Control. Release* **2010**, *148*, 135–146. [CrossRef]
103. Cui, C.; Guo, T.; Zhang, S.; Yang, M.; Cheng, J.; Wang, J.; Kang, J.; Ma, W.; Nian, Y.; Sun, Z.; et al. Bacteria-derived outer membrane vesicles engineered with over-expressed pre-miRNA as delivery nanocarriers for cancer therapy. *Nanomedicine* **2022**, *45*, 102585. [CrossRef]
104. Peng, L.; Wang, M.; Chu, Y.; Zhang, L.; Niu, J.; Shao, H.; Yuan, T.; Jiang, Z.; Gao, J.; Ning, X. Engineering bacterial outer membrane vesicles as transdermal nanoplatforms for photo-TRAIL–programmed therapy against melanoma. *Sci. Adv.* **2020**, *6*, eaba2735. [CrossRef] [PubMed]
105. Pan, J.; Li, X.; Shao, B.; Xu, F.; Huang, X.; Guo, X.; Zhou, S. Self-Blockade of PD-L1 with Bacteria-Derived Outer-Membrane Vesicle for Enhanced Cancer Immunotherapy. *Adv. Mater.* **2022**, *34*, e2106307. [CrossRef]
106. Jiang, Z.; Guan, J.; Qian, J.; Zhan, C. Peptide ligand-mediated targeted drug delivery of nanomedicines. *Biomater. Sci.* **2019**, *7*, 461–471. [CrossRef]
107. Sepahdar, Z.; Miroliaei, M.; Bouzari, S.; Khalaj, V.; Salimi, M. Surface Engineering of Escherichia coli-Derived OMVs as Promising Nano-Carriers to Target EGFR-Overexpressing Breast Cancer Cells. *Front. Pharmacol.* **2021**, *12*, 719289. [CrossRef]
108. Li, Y.; Zhao, R.; Cheng, K.; Zhang, K.; Wang, Y.; Zhang, Y.; Li, Y.; Liu, G.; Xu, J.; Xu, J.; et al. Bacterial Outer Membrane Vesicles Presenting Programmed Death 1 for Improved Cancer Immunotherapy via Immune Activation and Checkpoint Inhibition. *ACS Nano* **2020**, *14*, 16698–16711. [CrossRef]
109. Das, S.S.; Bharadwaj, P.; Bilal, M.; Barani, M.; Rahdar, A.; Taboada, P.; Bungau, S.; Kyzas, G.Z. Stimuli-Responsive Polymeric Nanocarriers for Drug Delivery, Imaging, and Theragnosis. *Polymers* **2020**, *12*, 1397. [CrossRef]
110. Mi, P. Stimuli-responsive nanocarriers for drug delivery, tumor imaging, therapy and theranostics. *Theranostics* **2020**, *10*, 4557–4588. [CrossRef]
111. Castillo, R.R.; Lozano, D.; Gonzalez, B.; Manzano, M.; Izquierdo-Barba, I.; Vallet-Regi, M. Advances in mesoporous silica nanoparticles for targeted stimuli-responsive drug delivery: An update. *Expert. Opin. Drug. Deliv.* **2019**, *16*, 415–439. [CrossRef]
112. Moradi Kashkooli, F.; Soltani, M.; Souri, M. Controlled anti-cancer drug release through advanced nano-drug delivery systems: Static and dynamic targeting strategies. *J. Control. Release* **2020**, *327*, 316–349. [CrossRef]
113. Qin, J.; Yang, T.; Li, J.; Zhan, G.; Li, X.; Wei, Z.; Chen, Z.; Zheng, W.; Chen, H.; Yang, X.; et al. Bacterial outer membrane vesicle-templated biomimetic nanoparticles for synergistic photothermo-immunotherapy. *Nano Today* **2022**, *46*, 101591. [CrossRef]
114. Zhang, J.; Li, Z.; Liu, L.; Li, L.; Zhang, L.; Wang, Y.; Zhao, J. Self-Assembly Catalase Nanocomplex Conveyed by Bacterial Vesicles for Oxygenated Photodynamic Therapy and Tumor Immunotherapy. *Int. J. Nanomed.* **2022**, *17*, 1971–1985. [CrossRef]
115. Shahriari, M.; Zahiri, M.; Abnous, K.; Taghdisi, S.M.; Ramezani, M.; Alibolandi, M. Enzyme responsive drug delivery systems in cancer treatment. *J. Control. Release* **2019**, *308*, 172–189. [CrossRef]
116. Wells, C.M.; Harris, M.; Choi, L.; Murali, V.P.; Guerra, F.D.; Jennings, J.A. Stimuli-Responsive Drug Release from Smart Polymers. *J. Funct. Biomater.* **2019**, *10*, 34. [CrossRef]
117. Shukla, T.; Upmanyu, N.; Pandey, S.P.; Sudheesh, M.S. Site-specific drug delivery, targeting, and gene therapy. In *Nanoarchitectonics in Biomedicine*; William Andrew: Norwich, NY, USA, 2019; pp. 473–505. [CrossRef]

118. Jahromi, L.P.; Fuhrmann, G. Bacterial extracellular vesicles: Understanding biology promotes applications as nanopharmaceuticals. *Adv. Drug. Deliv. Rev.* **2021**, *173*, 125–140. [CrossRef] [PubMed]
119. Chen, Q.; Rozovsky, S.; Chen, W. Engineering multi-functional bacterial outer membrane vesicles as modular nanodevices for biosensing and bioimaging. *Chem. Commun.* **2017**, *53*, 7569–7572. [CrossRef]
120. Huang, Y.; Beringhs, A.O.; Chen, Q.; Song, D.; Chen, W.; Lu, X.; Fan, T.H.; Nieh, M.P.; Lei, Y. Genetically Engineered Bacterial Outer Membrane Vesicles with Expressed Nanoluciferase Reporter for in Vivo Bioluminescence Kinetic Modeling through Noninvasive Imaging. *ACS Appl. Bio Mater.* **2019**, *2*, 5608–5615. [CrossRef] [PubMed]
121. Zhou, J.; Kroll, A.V.; Holay, M.; Fang, R.H.; Zhang, L. Biomimetic Nanotechnology toward Personalized Vaccines. *Adv. Mater.* **2020**, *32*, e1901255. [CrossRef]
122. Aly, R.G.; El-Enbaawy, M.I.; Abd El-Rahman, S.S.; Ata, N.S. Antineoplastic activity of Salmonella Typhimurium outer membrane nanovesicles. *Exp. Cell Res.* **2021**, *399*, 112423. [CrossRef]
123. Zhuang, W.R.; Wang, Y.; Lei, Y.; Zuo, L.; Jiang, A.; Wu, G.; Nie, W.; Huang, L.L.; Xie, H.Y. Phytochemical Engineered Bacterial Outer Membrane Vesicles for Photodynamic Effects Promoted Immunotherapy. *Nano Lett.* **2022**, *22*, 4491–4500. [CrossRef]
124. Behzadi, E.; Mahmoodzadeh Hosseini, H.; Imani Fooladi, A.A. The inhibitory impacts of Lactobacillus rhamnosus GG-derived extracellular vesicles on the growth of hepatic cancer cells. *Microb. Pathog.* **2017**, *110*, 1–6. [CrossRef]
125. Kim, O.Y.; Park, H.T.; Dinh, N.T.H.; Choi, S.J.; Lee, J.; Kim, J.H.; Lee, S.W.; Gho, Y.S. Bacterial outer membrane vesicles suppress tumor by interferon-gamma-mediated antitumor response. *Nat. Commun.* **2017**, *8*, 626. [CrossRef]
126. Zhang, Y.; Fang, Z.; Li, R.; Huang, X.; Liu, Q. Design of Outer Membrane Vesicles as Cancer Vaccines: A New Toolkit for Cancer Therapy. *Cancers* **2019**, *11*, 1314. [CrossRef]
127. Long, Q.; Zheng, P.; Zheng, X.; Li, W.; Hua, L.; Yang, Z.; Huang, W.; Ma, Y. Engineered bacterial membrane vesicles are promising carriers for vaccine design and tumor immunotherapy. *Adv. Drug. Deliv. Rev.* **2022**, *186*, 114321. [CrossRef] [PubMed]
128. Huang, W.; Shu, C.; Hua, L.; Zhao, Y.; Xie, H.; Qi, J.; Gao, F.; Gao, R.; Chen, Y.; Zhang, Q.; et al. Modified bacterial outer membrane vesicles induce autoantibodies for tumor therapy. *Acta Biomater.* **2020**, *108*, 300–312. [CrossRef]
129. Gao, X.; Feng, Q.; Wang, J.; Zhao, X. Bacterial outer membrane vesicle-based cancer nanovaccines. *Cancer Biol. Med.* **2022**, *19*, 1290–1300. [CrossRef]
130. Li, M.; Zhou, H.; Yang, C.; Wu, Y.; Zhou, X.; Liu, H.; Wang, Y. Bacterial outer membrane vesicles as a platform for biomedical applications: An update. *J. Control. Release* **2020**, *323*, 253–268. [CrossRef] [PubMed]
131. Huang, Y.; Nieh, M.P.; Chen, W.; Lei, Y. Outer membrane vesicles (OMVs) enabled bio-applications: A critical review. *Biotechnol. Bioeng.* **2022**, *119*, 34–47. [CrossRef]
132. Yang, J.; Kim, E.K.; McDowell, A.; Kim, Y.K. Microbe-derived extracellular vesicles as a smart drug delivery system. *Transl. Clin. Pharmacol.* **2018**, *26*, 103–110. [CrossRef]
133. Li, Y.; Wu, J.; Qiu, X.; Dong, S.; He, J.; Liu, J.; Xu, W.; Huang, S.; Hu, X.; Xiang, D.X. Bacterial outer membrane vesicles-based therapeutic platform eradicates triple-negative breast tumor by combinational photodynamic/chemo-/immunotherapy. *Bioact. Mater.* **2023**, *20*, 548–560. [CrossRef]
134. Xie, Y.J.; Huang, M.; Li, D.; Hou, J.C.; Liang, H.H.; Nasim, A.A.; Huang, J.M.; Xie, C.; Leung, E.L.; Fan, X.X. Bacteria-based nanodrug for anticancer therapy. *Pharmacol. Res.* **2022**, *182*, 106282. [CrossRef]
135. Gao, J.; Su, Y.; Wang, Z. Engineering bacterial membrane nanovesicles for improved therapies in infectious diseases and cancer. *Adv. Drug. Deliv. Rev.* **2022**, *186*, 114340. [CrossRef]
136. Zeng, Y.; Li, S.; Zhang, S.; Wang, L.; Yuan, H.; Hu, F. Cell membrane coated-nanoparticles for cancer immunotherapy. *Acta Pharm. Sin. B* **2022**, *12*, 3233–3254. [CrossRef]
137. Krishnan, N.; Kubiatowicz, L.J.; Holay, M.; Zhou, J.; Fang, R.H.; Zhang, L. Bacterial membrane vesicles for vaccine applications. *Adv. Drug. Deliv. Rev.* **2022**, *185*, 114294. [CrossRef] [PubMed]
138. Zhao, Y.; Li, A.; Jiang, L.; Gu, Y.; Liu, J. Hybrid Membrane-Coated Biomimetic Nanoparticles (HM@BNPs): A Multifunctional Nanomaterial for Biomedical Applications. *Biomacromolecules* **2021**, *22*, 3149–3167. [CrossRef] [PubMed]
139. Shi, J.; Ma, Z.; Pan, H.; Liu, Y.; Chu, Y.; Wang, J.; Chen, L. Biofilm-encapsulated nano drug delivery system for the treatment of colon cancer. *J. Microencapsul.* **2020**, *37*, 481–491. [CrossRef] [PubMed]
140. Chen, Q.; Huang, G.; Wu, W.; Wang, J.; Hu, J.; Mao, J.; Chu, P.K.; Bai, H.; Tang, G. A Hybrid Eukaryotic-Prokaryotic Nanoplatform with Photothermal Modality for Enhanced Antitumor Vaccination. *Adv. Mater.* **2020**, *32*, e1908185. [CrossRef]
141. Wang, D.; Liu, C.; You, S.; Zhang, K.; Li, M.; Cao, Y.; Wang, C.; Dong, H.; Zhang, X. Bacterial Vesicle-Cancer Cell Hybrid Membrane-Coated Nanoparticles for Tumor Specific Immune Activation and Photothermal Therapy. *ACS Appl. Mater. Interfaces* **2020**, *12*, 41138–41147. [CrossRef]
142. Schmidt, C.K.; Medina-Sanchez, M.; Edmondson, R.J.; Schmidt, O.G. Engineering microrobots for targeted cancer therapies from a medical perspective. *Nat. Commun.* **2020**, *11*, 5618. [CrossRef]
143. Zhou, J.; Karshalev, E.; Mundaca-Uribe, R.; Esteban-Fernandez de Avila, B.; Krishnan, N.; Xiao, C.; Ventura, C.J.; Gong, H.; Zhang, Q.; Gao, W.; et al. Physical Disruption of Solid Tumors by Immunostimulatory Microrobots Enhances Antitumor Immunity. *Adv. Mater.* **2021**, *33*, e2103505. [CrossRef]
144. Collins, S.M.; Brown, A.C. Bacterial Outer Membrane Vesicles as Antibiotic Delivery Vehicles. *Front. Immunol.* **2021**, *12*, 733064. [CrossRef]

145. Huang, W.; Meng, L.; Chen, Y.; Dong, Z.; Peng, Q. Bacterial outer membrane vesicles as potential biological nanomaterials for antibacterial therapy. *Acta Biomater.* **2022**, *140*, 102–115. [CrossRef]
146. Kadurugamuwa, J.L.; Beveridge, T.J. Bacteriolytic effect of membrane vesicles from Pseudomonas aeruginosa on other bacteria including pathogens: Conceptually new antibiotics. *J. Bacteriol.* **1996**, *178*, 2767–2774. [CrossRef] [PubMed]
147. Dean, S.N.; Rimmer, M.A.; Turner, K.B.; Phillips, D.A.; Caruana, J.C.; Hervey, W.J.t.; Leary, D.H.; Walper, S.A. Lactobacillus acidophilus Membrane Vesicles as a Vehicle of Bacteriocin Delivery. *Front. Microbiol.* **2020**, *11*, 710. [CrossRef] [PubMed]
148. Gan, Y.; Li, C.; Peng, X.; Wu, S.; Li, Y.; Tan, J.P.K.; Yang, Y.Y.; Yuan, P.; Ding, X. Fight bacteria with bacteria: Bacterial membrane vesicles as vaccines and delivery nanocarriers against bacterial infections. *Nanomedicine* **2021**, *35*, 102398. [CrossRef] [PubMed]
149. Wu, G.; Ji, H.; Guo, X.; Li, Y.; Ren, T.; Dong, H.; Liu, J.; Liu, Y.; Shi, X.; He, B. Nanoparticle reinforced bacterial outer-membrane vesicles effectively prevent fatal infection of carbapenem-resistant Klebsiella pneumoniae. *Nanomedicine* **2020**, *24*, 102148. [CrossRef]
150. Cooke, A.C.; Nello, A.V.; Ernst, R.K.; Schertzer, J.W. Analysis of *Pseudomonas aeruginosa* biofilm membrane vesicles supports multiple mechanisms of biogenesis. *PLoS ONE* **2019**, *14*, e0212275. [CrossRef]
151. Kadurugamuwa, J.L.; Beveridge, T.J. Delivery of the Non-Membrane-Permeative Antibiotic Gentamicin into Mammalian Cells by Using Shigella flexneri Membrane Vesicles. *Antimicrob. Agents Chemother.* **1998**, *42*, 1476–1483. [CrossRef]
152. Vasilyeva, N.V.; Tsfasman, I.M.; Suzina, N.E.; Stepnaya, O.A.; Kulaev, I.S. Secretion of bacteriolytic endopeptidase L5 of Lysobacter sp. XL1 into the medium by means of outer membrane vesicles. *FEBS J.* **2008**, *275*, 3827–3835. [CrossRef]
153. Evans, A.G.L.; Davey, H.M.; Cookson, A.; Currinn, H.; Cooke-Fox, G.; Stanczyk, P.J.; Whitworth, D.E. Predatory activity of Myxococcus xanthus outer-membrane vesicles and properties of their hydrolase cargo. *Microbiology* **2012**, *158*, 2742–2752. [CrossRef]
154. Schulz, E.; Goes, A.; Garcia, R.; Panter, F.; Koch, M.; Muller, R.; Fuhrmann, K.; Fuhrmann, G. Biocompatible bacteria-derived vesicles show inherent antimicrobial activity. *J. Control. Release* **2018**, *290*, 46–55. [CrossRef]
155. Goes, A.; Lapuhs, P.; Kuhn, T.; Schulz, E.; Richter, R.; Panter, F.; Dahlem, C.; Koch, M.; Garcia, R.; Kiemer, A.K.; et al. Myxobacteria-Derived Outer Membrane Vesicles: Potential Applicability Against Intracellular Infections. *Cells* **2020**, *9*, 194. [CrossRef] [PubMed]
156. Afoshin, A.S.; Kudryakova, I.V.; Borovikova, A.O.; Suzina, N.E.; Toropygin, I.Y.; Shishkova, N.A.; Vasilyeva, N.V. Lytic potential of Lysobacter capsici VKM B-2533(T): Bacteriolytic enzymes and outer membrane vesicles. *Sci. Rep.* **2020**, *10*, 9944. [CrossRef] [PubMed]
157. Wang, Y.; Hoffmann, J.P.; Chou, C.W.; Honer Zu Bentrup, K.; Fuselier, J.A.; Bitoun, J.P.; Wimley, W.C.; Morici, L.A. Burkholderia thailandensis outer membrane vesicles exert antimicrobial activity against drug-resistant and competitor microbial species. *J. Microbiol.* **2020**, *58*, 550–562. [CrossRef] [PubMed]
158. da Silva Barreira, D.; Laurent, J.; Lourenco, J.; Novion Ducassou, J.; Coute, Y.; Guzzo, J.; Rieu, A. Membrane vesicles released by Lacticaseibacillus casei BL23 inhibit the biofilm formation of Salmonella Enteritidis. *Sci. Rep.* **2023**, *13*, 1163. [CrossRef]
159. Tashiro, Y.; Hasegawa, Y.; Shintani, M.; Takaki, K.; Ohkuma, M.; Kimbara, K.; Futamata, H. Interaction of Bacterial Membrane Vesicles with Specific Species and Their Potential for Delivery to Target Cells. *Front. Microbiol.* **2017**, *8*, 571. [CrossRef] [PubMed]
160. Camacho, A.I.; Irache, J.M.; de Souza, J.; Sanchez-Gomez, S.; Gamazo, C. Nanoparticle-based vaccine for mucosal protection against Shigella flexneri in mice. *Vaccine* **2013**, *31*, 3288–3294. [CrossRef]
161. Gao, W.; Fang, R.H.; Thamphiwatana, S.; Luk, B.T.; Li, J.; Angsantikul, P.; Zhang, Q.; Hu, C.M.; Zhang, L. Modulating antibacterial immunity via bacterial membrane-coated nanoparticles. *Nano Lett.* **2015**, *15*, 1403–1409. [CrossRef]
162. Adriani, R.; Mousavi Gargari, S.L.; Nazarian, S.; Sarvary, S.; Noroozi, N. Immunogenicity of Vibrio cholerae outer membrane vesicles secreted at various environmental conditions. *Vaccine* **2018**, *36*, 322–330. [CrossRef]
163. Zhang, Y.; Chen, Y.; Lo, C.; Zhuang, J.; Angsantikul, P.; Zhang, Q.; Wei, X.; Zhou, Z.; Obonyo, M.; Fang, R.H.; et al. Inhibition of Pathogen Adhesion by Bacterial Outer Membrane-Coated Nanoparticles. *Angew. Chem. Int. Ed. Engl.* **2019**, *58*, 11404–11408. [CrossRef]
164. Huang, Y.; Nan, L.; Xiao, C.; Dong, J.; Li, K.; Cheng, J.; Ji, Q.; Wei, Q.; Bao, G.; Liu, Y. Outer Membrane Vesicles Coating Nano-Glycyrrhizic Acid Confers Protection Against Borderella bronchiseptica Through Th1/Th2/Th17 Responses. *Int. J. Nanomed.* **2022**, *17*, 647–663. [CrossRef]
165. Blackburn, S.A.; Shepherd, M.; Robinson, G.K. The polyene antifungal candicidin is selectively packaged into membrane vesicles in Streptomyces S4. *Arch. Microbiol.* **2022**, *204*, 289. [CrossRef] [PubMed]
166. Yue, H.; Jiang, J.; Taylor, A.J.; Leite, A.L.; Dodds, E.D.; Du, L. Outer Membrane Vesicle-Mediated Codelivery of the Antifungal HSAF Metabolites and Lytic Polysaccharide Monooxygenase in the Predatory Lysobacter enzymogenes. *ACS Chem. Biol.* **2021**, *16*, 1079–1089. [CrossRef]
167. Meers, P.R.; Liu, C.; Chen, R.; Bartos, W.; Davis, J.; Dziedzic, N.; Orciuolo, J.; Kutyla, S.; Pozo, M.J.; Mithrananda, D.; et al. Vesicular Delivery of the Antifungal Antibiotics of Lysobacter enzymogenes C3. *Appl. Environ. Microbiol.* **2018**, *84*, e01353-18. [CrossRef] [PubMed]
168. Bae, E.H.; Seo, S.H.; Kim, C.U.; Jang, M.S.; Song, M.S.; Lee, T.Y.; Jeong, Y.J.; Lee, M.S.; Park, J.H.; Lee, P.; et al. Bacterial Outer Membrane Vesicles Provide Broad-Spectrum Protection against Influenza Virus Infection via Recruitment and Activation of Macrophages. *J. Innate Immun.* **2019**, *11*, 316–329. [CrossRef] [PubMed]

169. Kim, C.U.; Eo, S.; Lee, P.; Kim, S.H.; Kim, Y.S.; Kim, D.J. Pretreatment of outer membrane vesicle and subsequent infection with influenza virus induces a long-lasting adaptive immune response against broad subtypes of influenza virus. *Microbes Infect.* **2022**, *24*, 104878. [CrossRef] [PubMed]
170. Martins, P.; Machado, D.; Theizen, T.H.; Guarnieri, J.P.O.; Bernardes, B.G.; Gomide, G.P.; Corat, M.A.F.; Abbehausen, C.; Modena, J.L.P.; Melo, C.; et al. Outer Membrane Vesicles from Neisseria Meningitidis (Proteossome) Used for Nanostructured Zika Virus Vaccine Production. *Sci. Rep.* **2018**, *8*, 8290. [CrossRef]
171. Thapa, H.B.; Muller, A.M.; Camilli, A.; Schild, S. An Intranasal Vaccine Based on Outer Membrane Vesicles Against SARS-CoV-2. *Front. Microbiol.* **2021**, *12*, 752739. [CrossRef]
172. Fu, Y.; Xiong, S. Tagged extracellular vesicles with the RBD of the viral spike protein for delivery of antiviral agents against SARS-COV-2 infection. *J. Control. Release* **2021**, *335*, 584–595. [CrossRef]
173. Jiang, L.; Driedonks, T.A.P.; Jong, W.S.P.; Dhakal, S.; Bart van den Berg van Saparoea, H.; Sitaras, I.; Zhou, R.; Caputo, C.; Littlefield, K.; Lowman, M.; et al. A bacterial extracellular vesicle-based intranasal vaccine against SARS-CoV-2 protects against disease and elicits neutralizing antibodies to wild-type and Delta variants. *J. Extracell. Vesicles* **2022**, *11*, e12192. [CrossRef]
174. Qiao, L.; Rao, Y.; Zhu, K.; Rao, X.; Zhou, R. Engineered Remolding and Application of Bacterial Membrane Vesicles. *Front. Microbiol.* **2021**, *12*, 729369. [CrossRef]
175. Tran, A.X.; Karbarz, M.J.; Wang, X.; Raetz, C.R.; McGrath, S.C.; Cotter, R.J.; Trent, M.S. Periplasmic cleavage and modification of the 1-phosphate group of Helicobacter pylori lipid A. *J. Biol. Chem.* **2004**, *279*, 55780–55791. [CrossRef] [PubMed]
176. Carvalho, A.L.; Fonseca, S.; Miquel-Clopes, A.; Cross, K.; Kok, K.S.; Wegmann, U.; Gil-Cordoso, K.; Bentley, E.G.; Al Katy, S.H.M.; Coombes, J.L.; et al. Bioengineering commensal bacteria-derived outer membrane vesicles for delivery of biologics to the gastrointestinal and respiratory tract. *J. Extracell. Vesicles* **2019**, *8*, 1632100. [CrossRef] [PubMed]
177. Li, P.; Wang, X.; Sun, X.; Cimino, J.; Guan, Z.; Sun, W. Recombinant Pseudomonas Bionanoparticles Induce Protection against Pneumonic Pseudomonas aeruginosa Infection. *Infect. Immun.* **2021**, *89*, e00396-21. [CrossRef]
178. Gnopo, Y.M.D.; Watkins, H.C.; Stevenson, T.C.; DeLisa, M.P.; Putnam, D. Designer outer membrane vesicles as immunomodulatory systems–Reprogramming bacteria for vaccine delivery. *Adv. Drug. Deliv. Rev.* **2017**, *114*, 132–142. [CrossRef]
179. Liu, H.; Li, M.; Zhang, T.; Liu, X.; Zhang, H.; Geng, Z.; Su, J. Engineered bacterial extracellular vesicles for osteoporosis therapy. *Chem. Eng. J.* **2022**, *450*, 138309. [CrossRef]
180. Gao, J.; Wang, S.; Dong, X.; Wang, Z. RGD-expressed bacterial membrane-derived nanovesicles enhance cancer therapy via multiple tumorous targeting. *Theranostics* **2021**, *11*, 3301–3316. [CrossRef] [PubMed]

pharmaceutics

Review

Extracellular Vesicle-Based Drug Delivery Systems for Head and Neck Squamous Cell Carcinoma: A Systematic Review

Karolina Dżaman * and Katarzyna Czerwaty

Department of Otolaryngology, Centre of Postgraduate Medical Education, Marymoncka 99/103, 01-813 Warsaw, Poland

* Correspondence: kfrydel@poczta.onet.pl

Abstract: It is estimated that there are over 890,000 new cases of head and neck squamous cell carcinoma (HNSCC) worldwide each year, accounting for approximately 5% of all cancer cases. Current treatment options for HNSCC often cause significant side effects and functional impairments, thus there is a challenge to discover more acceptable treatment technologies. Extracellular vesicles (EVs) can be utilized for HNSCC treatment in several ways, for example, for drug delivery, immune modulation, as biomarkers for diagnostics, gene therapy, or tumor microenvironment modulation. This systematic review summarizes new knowledge regarding these options. Articles published up to 11 December 2022, were identified by searching the electronic databases PubMed/MEDLINE, Scopus, Web of Science, and Cochrane. Only full-text original research papers written in English were considered eligible for analysis. The quality of studies was assessed using the Office of Health Assessment and Translation (OHAT) Risk of Bias Rating Tool for Human and Animal Studies, modified for the needs of this review. Of 436 identified records, 18 were eligible and included. It is important to note that the use of EVs as a treatment for HNSCC is still in the early stages of research, so we summarized information on challenges such as EV isolation, purification, and standardization of EV-based therapies in HNSCC.

Keywords: drug delivery systems; head and neck squamous cell carcinoma; exosomes; extracellular vesicles; nanoparticles

Citation: Dżaman, K.; Czerwaty, K. Extracellular Vesicle-Based Drug Delivery Systems for Head and Neck Squamous Cell Carcinoma: A Systematic Review. *Pharmaceutics* **2023**, *15*, 1327. https://doi.org/10.3390/pharmaceutics15051327

Academic Editor: Yong Chen

Received: 19 February 2023
Revised: 7 April 2023
Accepted: 21 April 2023
Published: 24 April 2023

1. Introduction

It is estimated that there are over 890,000 new cases of head and neck squamous cell carcinoma (HNSCC) worldwide each year, accounting for approximately 5% of all cancer cases [1]. HNSCC is a complex and challenging cancer to treat, due to its anatomical location. Current treatment options for HNSCC often cause significant side effects and functional impairments, thus the challenge is to discover more acceptable treatment technologies [2,3]. Extracellular vesicles (EVs) carry biological information [4] and can be utilized for HNSCC treatment in several ways, for example for drug delivery, immune modulation, as biomarkers for diagnostics, gene therapy, or tumor microenvironment modulation.

EVs are nanoparticles released by most cell types and play an important role in cell-to-cell communication. According to current research, signals from EVs are transmitted to the target cell through receptor interaction, membrane fusion, and endocytosis/phagocytosis. Based on their origin and size, EVs can be classified into three groups: (a) exosomes (diameter in the range of 30–150 nm), (b) microparticles, micro-vesicles, or ectosomes (50 nm–1 μm), and (c) apoptotic bodies (50 nm–5 μm) [5]. Among the most widely studied EVs are exosomes. EVs are membranous vesicles that are secreted by various cells, such as dendritic cells, macrophages, mesenchymal stem cells, and endothelial and epithelial cells, into the extracellular space. Many studies indicate that EVs can efficiently provide many distinct sorts of cargo to the recipient cell and can be altered to carry specific proteins, lipids and genetic materials, including messenger RNA (mRNA), microRNA (miRNA, miR), and other small non-coding RNAs and genomic DNA (gDNA), from their progenitor cell [6–8]. Therefore, EVs are excellent vehicles for the natural targeting and delivery of therapeutics with unique properties. Engineered EVs containing therapeutic agents can modify the activity of cancer cells. These characteristics have led recent studies to analyse EVs, both unmodified and modified or loaded with drugs, for targeted cancer therapy [9].

This review article summarizes the current state of knowledge regarding the possibility of using EVs as drug delivery systems (DDS) in the treatment of HNSCC. We hope that the information obtained, through a comprehensive search of the literature, will contribute to further development and research in this field.

2. Materials and Methods

This systematic review follows the Preferred Reporting Items for Systematic Reviews and Meta-Analyses Statement (PRISMA) [10].

2.1. Search Strategy and Eligibility Criteria

The literature search for articles regarding membrane vesicle-based DDS for HNSCC was performed using the four following databases: Scopus, Web of Science, MEDLINE (through PubMed), and Cochrane. The search strategies for each database were properly adapted to each database and are presented in Table 1. The last search was conducted on 11 December 2022, in each of the databases. It was not necessary to contact the authors of the retrieved research articles for additional information.

Table 1. Search strategy for the databases used.

Database	Number of Results	Search Strategy
Scopus	428	TITLE-ABS-KEY ((extracellular vesicle *) OR (multivesicular bodies) OR (exosome *)) AND ((squamous cell carcinoma *) AND ((head and neck) OR (larynx) OR (laryngeal) OR (nasal cavity) OR (oral) OR (pharyngeal) OR (hypopharyngeal) OR (nasopharyngeal) OR (oropharyngeal) OR (mouth))) AND ((delivery system *) AND (drug *)) Limited to: Article
Web of Science	6	AB = (((extracellular vesicle *) OR (multivesicular bodies) OR (exosome *)) AND ((squamous cell carcinoma *) AND ((head and neck) OR (larynx) OR (laryngeal) OR (nasal cavity) OR (oral) OR (pharyngeal) OR (hypopharyngeal) OR (nasopharyngeal) OR (oropharyngeal) OR (mouth))) AND ((delivery system *) AND (drug *)))
Pubmed	2	((“Extracellular Vesicles”[Mesh]) OR (“Multivesicular Bodies”[Mesh]) OR (“Exosomes”[Mesh)) AND (“Squamous Cell Carcinoma of Head and Neck”[Mesh]) AND (“Drug Delivery Systems”[Mesh])
Cochrane	0	#1 MeSH descriptor: [Extracellular Vesicles] explode all trees #2 MeSH descriptor: [Multivesicular Bodies] explode all trees #3 MeSH descriptor: [Exosomes] explode all trees #4 MeSH descriptor: [Drug Delivery Systems] explode all trees #5 MeSH descriptor: [Squamous Cell Carcinoma of Head and Neck] explode all trees #6 (#1 OR #2 OR #3) AND #4 AND #5

A systematic literature search identified 436 studies. Duplicates were discarded using the automatic EndNote 10 (Clarivate Analytics, Philadelphia, Pennsylvania, United States) duplicate finder, and then searched manually. Two authors of the study independently screened the records sequentially by titles, abstracts and full-text versions. This systematic review included only English-written, full-text, original research studies regarding membrane vesicle-based DDSs for HNSCC. Figure 1 shows the selection process summarized in a custom-built PRISMA flow chart.

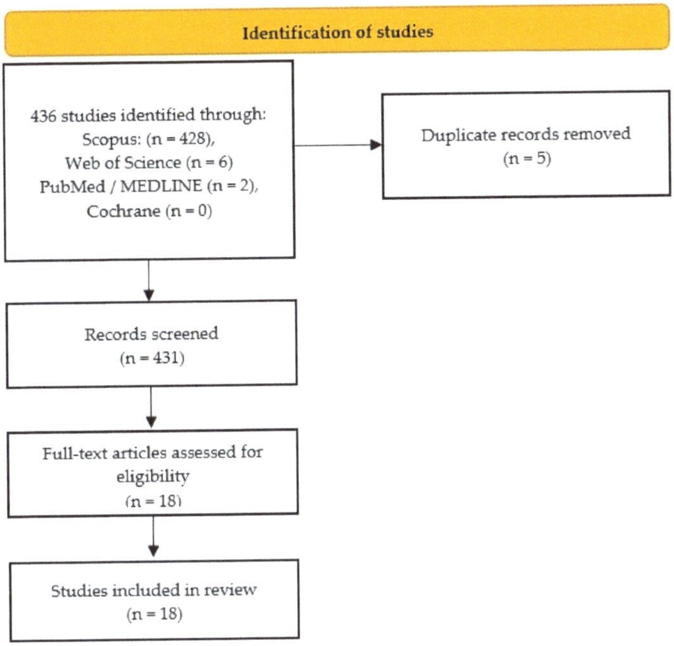

Figure 1. Flow diagram of the systematic literature search.

2.2. Data Extraction

After evaluation of the eligibility of all included studies, the data for each study were retrieved individually by two reviewers. The following outcomes were taken into account and are presented in this review: baseline information (the first author's name, year of publication), study design, study and control group, main results, HNSCC model, source of EVs, methods of EVs: purification, isolation, characterization, labelling, tracking, loading, modification for DDS and, finally, therapeutic effects of membrane vesicle-based DDS for HNSCC.

2.3. Assessment of Quality of Studies

The risk of bias in data interpretation was assessed using the Office of Health Assessment and Translation (OHAT) [11] and evaluated independently by two investigators. Any discrepancies in judgments regarding the risk of bias were resolved by discussion to reach a consensus between the two review authors. The summarised quality assessment for all studies is reported in Table S1.

3. Results

3.1. Search Results, Study Characteristics and Study Quality

Details of the selection process are summarized in a custom-built PRISMA flow chart (Figure 1). Upon implementing the search strategy outlined above, a total of 18 articles were identified that met all the inclusion criteria [12–29]. The articles were analyzed for their basic data and the main results are described in Table 2, though more detailed information is also presented in Table S2.

Table 2. Main data from the included studies.

	Type of Study	Type of EVs	EVs Cargo	Main Results
Cohen [12]	in vitro–A431 cell line in vivo–mice model (xenograft HNSCC)	Human MSC-EVs, A431-EVs	GNPs as labeling	1. The EVs origin has a direct impact on the tumor targeting and penetration ability. 2. MSC-EVs had superior tumor accumulation when compared to A431-EVs. 3. The use of biocompatible GNP-labeled EVs, combined with CT imaging, has the potential for application in cancer therapy.
Cui [13]	in vitro–HSC-3 cell line in vivo–mice model (xenograft TSCC)	NTECs-EVs	miR-200c	1. HSC-3DR cells showed downregulation of miR-200c. 2. The level of miR-200c was lower in TSCC lines relative to NTECs. 3. MiR-200c delivered by EVs to carcinoma cells decreased DTX resistance by targeting TUBB3 and PPP2R1B both in vitro and in vivo.
Deng [14]	in vitro–HN6 cells	HEK293T c-EVs	miR-34a	MiR-34a-EVs led to significant inhibition of HN6 cell proliferation, migration, and invasion by down-regulating SATB2 expression.
Kase [15]	in vitro–cell lines (OSCC-derived) in vivo–mice model (xenograft OSCC)	Oct-EVs	siLCP1	The silencing of LCP1 by siRNA-suppressed OSCC tumor.
Li [17]	in vitro–CAL27 in vivo–mice model (xenograft OSCC)	$\gamma\delta$ Tcell-EVs	miR-138	1. MiR-138—$\gamma\delta$ Tcell-EVs increased expansion and cytotoxicity of $\gamma\delta$ Tcells resulting in inhibition of OSCC both in vitro and in vivo. 2. MiR-138—$\gamma\delta$ Tcell-EVs were more effective than liposome transfected miR-138 and scramble-cargo $\gamma\delta$ Tcell- EVs.
Li [16]	in vitro–UM-SCC083A, UPCI-SCC029B	M-EVs	CA-miR-144/451a	M-EVs/CA-miR-144/451a biomimetic system effectively reduced the migration, invasion, and viability of OSCC cells and was more effective than free miR-144/451a.
Liu [18]	in vitro–HUVEC in vivo–mice model (xenograft OSCC)	SHED-EVs	miR-100-5p miR-1246	1. SHED-EVs inhibited cell proliferation and migration and induced apoptosis in HUVECs. 2. SHED-EVs downregulated several angiogenesis-related factors, (VEGFA, MMP-9, and ANGPT) and inhibited micro-vascular formation in OSCC tumor.
Liu [19]	in vitro–SCC25	MSCT-EVs	SNS032	SNS032/TRAIL delivered by gelatin biomimetic system can effectively induce apoptosis of tumor cells, reduces the dosage of free drugs, and shows a high inhibitory effect on OSCC.
Qiu [20]	in vitro–SCC25 in vivo–mice model (xenograft OSCC)	MSCT-EVs	CTX/TRAIL	1. The antitumor effect of MSCT-EVs/CTX was confirmed in vitro and in vivo. 2. MSCT-EVs/CTX inhibited cell proliferation and migration and induced apoptosis in SCC cell lines and mice models.
Sayyed [21]	ex vivo–3D tumor spheroids model of UPCI-SCC-131 in vivo–mice model (xenograft OSCC)	UPCI-SCC-131-EVs	miR-155 inhibitor	1. Cisplatin-resistant OSCC tumors showed a more malignant phenotype and elevated miR-155 level. 2. Treatment with miR-155 inhibitor-loaded EVs caused chemosensitization toward cisplatin via upregulation of FOXO3a and reducing EMT.
Tong [22]	human HNSCC cell lines: SCC90, SCC47, SCC104, SAS, CAL33 HPV- cell line CAL27	HPV + HNSCC-EVs	miR-9-5p	1. HPV + HNSCC-EVs were rich in miR-9-5p. 2. HPV + HNSCC-EVs miR-9 increased the radiosensitivity of HNSCC cells by polarizing macrophages into the M1 phenotypes which produce iNOS.
Wang [23]	in vitro–FaDu cells	HEK293T cells-EVs	TRPP2 siRNA	EV/TRPP2 siRNA complexes reduced EMT in FaDu cells and inhibited FaDu cell migration and invasion.

Table 2. *Cont.*

	Type of Study	Type of EVs	EVs Cargo	Main Results
Wang [24]	in vitro–EBV-negative and positive NPC cell lines in vivo–NPC mice model	HUVEC–EVs	antagomiR-BART10-5p; antagomiR-18a	1. IRGD-EVs-antagomiRs that contained both antagomiR-BART10-5p and antagomiR-18a attenuated the angiogenesis and growth of NPC with greater efficiency than a single treatment. 2. The findings established a synergistic role for virus and host miRs in the regulation of virus-associated tumor angiogenesis.
Wang [25]	in vitro–EBV-negative and positive NPC cell lines, radioresistant CSCs in vivo–NPC mice model	γδ TD-EVs	-	1. γδ-T-EVs can effectively interact with and kill both EBV-positive and negative NPC cells. 2. The combination therapy of radiotherapy and γδ-T-EVs was more efficient because γδ-T-EVs improved radiosensitivity by eradicating the NPC CSCs.
Yakavets [26]	ex vivo–3D tumor spheroids model of PSCC (FaDu cells)	HUVEC–EVs	mTHPC	MTHPC—EVs most effectively improved the drug delivery to PSCC due to extremely high loading capacity.
Yamayoshi [27]	in vitro–CAL27 in vivo–hind model	CAL27-EVs	ExomiR-Tracker	ExomiR-Tracker successfully inhibited the function of miR-21 and the Cal27cells growth but also inhibited tumorigenesis in vivo.
Yang [28]	in vitro – CAL 27, WSU-HN6 ex vivo–3D spheroid-model of OSCC in vivo–mice model	BMEVs	24 miRs identified in BMEVs	1. BMEVs had a synergistic therapeutic effect of 5-FU against OSCC both in vitro and in vivo. 2. BMEVs significantly downregulated NLRP3 expression. 3. BMEVs suppressed OSCC proliferation and induced apoptosis by the generation of reactive oxygen species (ROS).
Zhang [29]	in vitro–HSC-3, SCC-9, CAL-27), HCM cell line in vivo–mice model	Milk- EVs	EV@Dox loaded with EPT1 and Ce6	1. EV@Dox–EPT1 caused significantly more cytotoxicity in cancer cells under 808 nm laser irradiation than free Dox. 2. NPs produced synergistic effects of photochemistry triggered by acid TME and NIR.

BMEVs—bitter melon-derived EVs, CAL 27—an oral adeno-squamous carcinoma cell line, CAs—miR-144/451a (chitosan NPs complex with miR), Ce6—chlorin e6, CSCs—cancer stem-like cells, CTX—cabazitaxel, Dox—doxorubicin, DTX—docetaxel, EMT—epithelial to mesenchymal transition, EPT1—anthracene endoperoxide derivative, ExomiR-Tracker—anti-miR oligonucleotides+ anty CD63 antibody binds onto the surface of EVs, FaDu cells—a cell line originating from human PSCC, GNPs—gold NPs, G-SNS032—SNS032 loaded gelatin NPs, HCM—a human cardiac muscle cell line, HN6 cells—OSCC cell line, HSC-3—human TSCC cell line, MSCT-EVs—transfected MSC-EVs, MSCT-EVs/CTX—MSC-derived EVs containing TRAIL and CTX combination, mTHPC—temoporfin meta-tetra (hydroxyphenyl) chlorin, NPC—nasopharyngeal carcinoma, OSCC—oral SCC, PSCC—pharyngeal SCC, SATB2—the special AT-rich sequence-binding protein 2, SCC—squamous cell carcinoma, siLCP1—small interfering RNA of lymphocyte cytoplasmic protein 1, siRNA—small interfering RNA, TRAIL—tumour necrosis factor-related apoptosis-inducing ligand, TRPP2—transient receptor potential polycystic 2, TSCC—tongue SCC, UPCI-SCC-131—human OSCC cell lines.

The articles included in this systematic review consist of original studies that were published between 2019–2022, reflecting the recent advancements in this field. Among the selected papers, the majority (13) were conducted in China, while two studies were conducted in Japan, and one each in Israel, France and India. The studies primarily utilized in vivo models, predominantly mice models [12,13,15,17,18,20,21,24,25,27–29], in vitro [12–20,22–25,27–29], and ex vivo studies [21,26,28].

The risk of bias in the retrieved studies was assessed using the OHAT Tool adopted by the authors for the needs of this review [11]. All included studies had a low to moderate risk of overall bias. The evaluation results are presented in Table S1.

3.2. Uniqueness of HNSCC

The vast majority of cancers in the head and neck are HNSCCs originating in the mucosa of the mouth, pharynx and larynx. Unlike other cancers, despite developments in medicine, there is an upward trend in the incidence of these cancers [30].

A. Unique risk factors—Cancers for Which a Vaccine Has Been Discovered.

Main risk factors for these cancers include smoking, alcohol abuse, and oncogenic viruses such as Epstein-Barr virus (EBV) and human papillomavirus (HPV), whose role in this disease has been gaining importance in recent years [31,32] (Figure 2). Because HPV is mainly transmitted to the upper airway through oral sex, the unique feature of HNSCC is an association with sexual behavior. The most oncogenic types are HPV-16 and HPV-18. The importance of HPV is increasing, especially in populations where HPV vaccination has not been introduced [33]. To date, the FDA has approved three prophylactic vaccines against HPV—bivalent, quadrivalent and non-valent, designed for specific age groups and genders. Unfortunately, they are only effective for primary prevention.

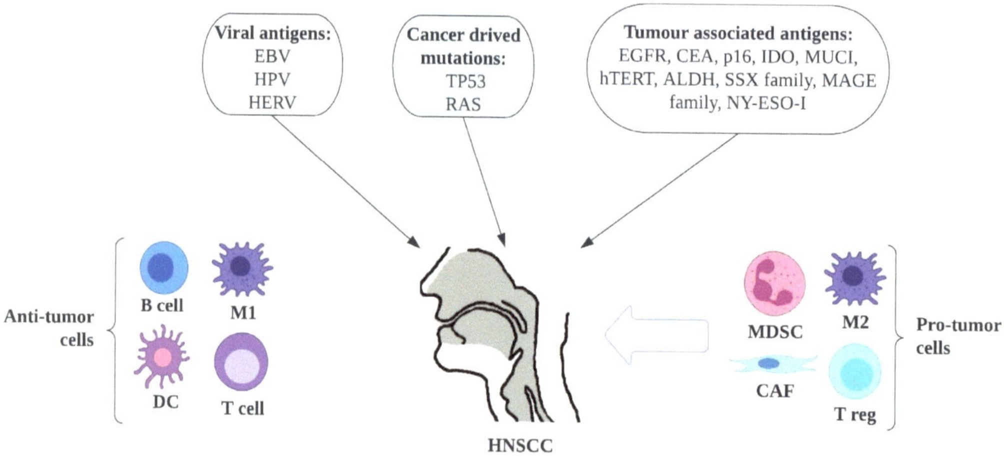

Figure 2. Overview of cancer antigens, immunosuppressive and anti-tumour immune cells in HNSCC. ALDH—aldehyde dehydrogenase, CAF—cancer-associated fibroblast, CEA—carcinoembryonic antigen, DC—dendritic cell, EBV—Epstein-Barr virus, EGFR—epithelial growth factor receptor, HERV—human endogenous retroviruses, HNSCC—head and neck squamous cell carcinoma, HPV—human papillomavirus, hTERT—human telomerase reverse transcriptase, IDO—indoleamine-2,3-dioxygenase, M1—macrophage 1, MAGE—melanoma-associated antigen, MDSC—myeloid-derived suppressor cell, MUCI—mucin-1, NK—natural killer cell, NY-ESO-I—New York esophageal squamous cell carcinoma-1, SSX—synovial sarcoma X, T reg—T regulatory cell.

Genetic factors are also important in the development of HNSCC. A highly increased risk of developing HNSCC is observed in patients with Fanconi anemia (associated with mutations in the FANC genes) [34]. Additionally, polymorphisms of other genes, e.g., in CTLA4 [35] or CYP1A1 [36], cause an increased incidence of these cancers.

It has also been observed that there is an increased incidence of these cancers in certain geographic areas, which is associated with cultural factors very specific to HNSCC, such as the chewing of areca nut products in the Asia-Pacific region [1]. Another important risk factor for HNSCC is exposure to air pollution, which is particularly intense in Asia [37].

B. Specific Biomarkers for HNSCC and Second Primary Tumors.

To date, many biomarkers with prognostic significance in HNSCC have been discovered. Among the most important are CD44, CD133 and ALDH1, high levels of which are associated with metastasis, invasiveness and poor prognosis [38,39].

A huge problem concerning patients with HNSCC is that the diagnosis of this disease is most often made at a late stage, with a high local stage of the disease and the presence of metastases to regional lymph nodes [40]. Moreover, a very distinctive feature of HNSCC is an association with the development of second (or even third or fourth) primary tumors, which are most often located in the head and neck, lung and esophageal regions [41], that has to be considered during diagnosis.

C. High Suicide Rate and Poor Quality of Life.

However, the most important distinguishing factor of HNSCCs is their critical location. The head and neck region is responsible for the most important life functions such as eating, breathing, communication and social relations. There, all sense organs responsible for receiving stimuli from the outside world are situated. So, HNSCC diagnosis and treatment are most likely to be related to the significantly reduced quality of life. Therefore, unfortunately, patients with HNSCC, after pancreatic cancer patients, have the highest suicide rate (63.4 suicides per 100,000 patients) among oncology patients [42].

When treating patients with HNSCC, special attention should be paid to the possibility of preserving the function of affected organs. Patients after surviving this disease complain of a significantly reduced quality of life and disabilities such as swallowing, speech and voice problems [43–45].

3.3. Head and Neck Squamous Cell Carcinoma Model

Several authors have demonstrated EVs potential for therapeutic drug delivery in HNSCC. The majority of these studies focussed on oral squamous cell carcinoma (OSSC) (Table S2) and were based on both in vitro and in vivo models. In three research papers, only in vitro analysis was performed, using cell lines transfected with specific EVs [14,19,23].

In most publications, the xenograft OSSC mice model was used to design the in vivo study, and in one article the hind model [27].

Interestingly, some investigators also performed ex vivo studies and developed an ex vivo tumour spheroid model to check the efficacy of the proposed therapeutic approach [21,26,28]. The 3D tumour spheroid models have changed the typical processes of cancer research. The engineered 3D human tumour models using carcinoma cells in polymeric scaffolds recreate microenvironmental characteristics representative of tumours in vivo [5]. They recapitulate several aspects of the tumour microenvironment (TME), especially critical stroma components, and provide better predictive results than 2D culture monolayers used in in vitro studies. Thus some researchers treat 3D ex vivo models as in vivo models. Using a 3D model, the authors demonstrated that the presence of stroma content in 3D HNSCC spheroids strongly affected the uptake of NPs (nanoparticles), while penetration and photodynamic therapy (PDT) efficacy were less sensitive to the presence of stromal components. To sum up, the 3D tumour models mimic heterogeneity and tumour pathophysiology, bridging the gap between 2D cultures and in vivo testing [9].

3.4. Carriers for Head and Neck Squamous Cell Carcinoma Drug Delivery Systems

The use of nanotechnology and, more specifically, drug delivery is a growing field of medicine and biotechnology. Despite convenience for the patient, traditional oral administration of anticancer drugs is often impossible due to their poor water solubility, so they are delivered intravenously. Most anticancer agents can also be administered via other means of delivery when incorporated in suitable carrier (bio)materials. Carrier-based DDSs allow for the controlled release of drugs, enhance selectivity and effectiveness, and reduce the side effects of chemotherapy. Currently, there are DDSs based on NPs, nano lipids, hydrogels and, recently, widely investigated EVs. Here, we focus on membrane vesicle-based DDS for HNSCC and the application of different types of cell-derived EVs for cancer therapy.

3.5. Membrane Vesicles for Drug Delivery Systems

3.5.1. Source of Extracellular Vesicles

Membrane vesicles for DDS can come from various types or parts of cells, including EVs. The membrane vesicles for DDS encompass a variety of types, such as apoptotic bodies, exosomes, microparticles, outer membrane vesicles, or cell-bound membrane vesicles isolated from cell surfaces.

EVs have been identified from several sources [12,28,29,46,47]. However, it is important to consider that EVs derived from different sources have diverse applications in EV-based cancer treatment, because they reflect the functional status of their parent cells. The EVs' parent cell origin determines membrane composition and bioactive cargo.

$\gamma\delta$T Cell-Derived Extracellular Vesicles ($\gamma\delta$TDEVs)

It is reasonable to assume that EVs derived from $\gamma\delta$T cells, dendritic cells (DCs) and natural killer (NK) cells could inherit the direct cytotoxicity and antigen-presenting role and be considered for cancer therapy [46–48]. The $\gamma\delta$T cells represent a minor lymphocyte population (about 0.5–16% of total CD3+ cells) and, when isolated from patients with cancers, efficiently killed tumour cell lines, played a role at antigen-presenting cells (APCs) and induced CD4+ and CD8+ T cell proliferation and cytotoxicity. Two included studies [17,25] reported $\gamma\delta$Tcell-derived EVs' ($\gamma\delta$TDEVs') advantages mentioned above, such as direct cytotoxicity against cancer cells and antigen-presenting function, but also adopted a large-scale expansion protocol for $\gamma\delta$ T cell production [49]. The authors confirmed that the specific features of $\gamma\delta$-T-EVs may potentially play a role in nasopharyngeal carcinoma (NPC) therapy [25]. As demonstrated previously, NPC cells secrete abundant CCR5 chemokine ligands and TGFβ in order to suppress T-cell responses [50]. The authors revealed that $\gamma\delta$-T-EVs promoted T-cell migration into NPC by upregulating CCR5 on T cells. In consequence, $\gamma\delta$ T cells were chemoattracted by CCR5 ligands in TME. Moreover, $\gamma\delta$-T-EVs preserved T-cells' direct antitumor activity in NPC and effectively killed both NPC EBV positive and negative cells and reduced the tumour size by around 80%. This reaction was mediated by Fas ligand (FasL) and DR5/TRAIL pathways (DR 5—death receptor 5, TRAIL—tumour necrosis factor-related apoptosis-inducing ligand).

Additionally, they demonstrated that $\gamma\delta$-T-EVs induced significant cell apoptosis and selectively targeted radioresistant CD44+/high cancer stem-like cells (CSCs) [50]. Thus, combined therapy using irradiation and $\gamma\delta$-T- EVs increased NPC cell apoptosis when compared with monotherapies.

In another study, $\gamma\delta$-T-EVs used in OSSC therapy [17] were additionally loaded with miR-138 and had dual anti-tumoral functions. They immune-stimulated both CD3+T and CD8+ T cells and impacted cell cycle and proliferation by gene regulation. Furthermore, the researchers revealed that miR-138 $\gamma\delta$ Tcell-derived EVs were more effective than miR-138-transfected liposomes.

Taken together, these data indicate that $\gamma\delta$-T-EVs can promote T-cell migration into the TME of HNSCCs, preserve their tumour-killing activities, and overcome their radioresistance.

Macrophage-Derived Extracellular Vesicles (M-EVs)

Recent studies have shown that macrophages are fundamental for promoting tumour genesis, development, metastasis and chemoresistance through modulating TEM and cancer cells. Macrophages are the most infiltrative immune-related stromal cells [51] and can be polarized into classical M1 or M2. Some authors noticed that HPV + HNSCC-EVs were able to transform macrophages into the M1 phenotype, which subsequently increased the radiosensitivity of HNSCC [22].

Moreover, M-EVs show heterogeneity in various cancers and play paradoxical roles in tumour-suppression and promotion, mainly through post-transcriptional control and regulation of protein phosphorylation in the recipient cells [52]. Li [16] used M-EVs as a biomimetic strategy to coat and protect the miR-144/451a cluster from the immunological system, and improved its delivery to OSCC cells.

Mesenchymal Stem Cell-Derived Extracellular Vesicles

The most common sources of EVs are mesenchymal stem cells (MSCs), due to their multipotential in differentiating into several cell types. MSC-EVs are involved in intercellular communication through the transfer of proteins, RNA, DNA and bioactive lipids, and thus are implicated as the mediator of many therapeutic potencies. Both natural or engineered EVs derived from MSCs or tumour cells with different origins have been previously investigated in cancers such as pancreatic cancer or breast cancer and used as DDS [53,54]. MSCs have been successfully isolated from numerous tissues, including bone marrow, adipose, peripheral blood, skin, brain, dental tissues and endometrium. In this systematic review, some authors explored the therapeutic potential of MSC-EVs derived from human umbilical cord MSCs [12,26,28], but also the subtypes of immature MSC—SHED cells (stem cells of deciduous exfoliated teeth) [18].

Compared to other EV sources, MSCs are characterized by higher EV production, good stability in vivo, high targeting specificity, strong ability to proliferate and easy accessibility as a source of stem cells [55].

Moreover, MSCs have been genetically engineered using viral and nonviral vectors to improve host immune response against cancer cells and to carry traditional anticancer cytotoxic drugs. The viral vector-lentivirus expressing human TRIAL was used in two included studies to engineering transfected MSC (MSCT) [18,20].

Carcinoma Cell and Normal Cell Lines—Derived Extracellular Vesicles

Recently, several studies have demonstrated that tumour-derived EVs (TEVs) have potential in immunomodulation and play an important role in the escape of tumour cells from immune surveillance. It has been observed that TEVs can activate CD4+ T cells to promote the mitochondrial apoptotic pathway [56].

In revised in vitro studies, the investigators used EVs derived from several carcinoma cells, such as the human epidermal carcinoma cell line (A431-exo) [12], the oral adenosquamous carcinoma cell line (CAL 27) [27], the human cisplatin-resistant and cisplatin-sensitive OSCC cell lines (UPCI-SCC-131) [21], and the HPV positive HNSCC (HPV + HNSCC-EVs) [22].

Other authors have explored EVs derived from normal tongue epithelial cells (NTECs –exo) [13], human embryonic kidney cells (HEK293T cells) [14,23], or octEVs—engineered OSCC-targeted EVs which were constructed based on human skin-derived fibroblasts transfected with EBV [48].

Plant-Derived Extracellular Vesicles

EVs are present in biological fluids from mammals, such as blood, urine and plasma. However, many disadvantages slow down the translation of autologous EVs, such as limited yields, longer drug preparation time, cancer-stimulating risk and ethical problems. Therefore, techniques for obtaining EVs from other sources are being developed [28,29].

For example, it has been found that plant–derived EVs play a role in regulating intestinal homeostasis and cell-to-cell communication, but also may exhibit anti-inflammatory and anti-cancerous effects [57]. Furthermore, some data suggest that other tissues in the body may be affected by dietary PDEVs. It has been noticed that a clear preference for specific organs depends on the source of the PDEV [58]. While plant-derived EVs have been shown to have numerous benefits, they also have some limitations. The main challenges are the protocol standardization and characterization of PDEVs [59]. Only one reviewed study explored the potential of plant-derived EVs for HNSCC treatment [28]. The authors revealed that bitter melon-derived EVs (BMEVs) suppressed OSCC proliferation, induced S phase arrest, and persuaded apoptosis via ROS-mediated mitochondrial injury (ROS—reactive oxygen species). BMEVs significantly downregulated NLRP3 (NOD-like receptor family pyrin domain containing 3) expression. The NLRP3 activation contributed to the resistance of OSCC cells to 5-FU. Therefore, BMEVs demonstrated the synergistic therapeutic effects of 5-FU against OSCC, both in vitro and in vivo. Twenty-four kinds of miRs were detected in BMEVs and 11 had the potential to regulate the expression of NLRP3 mRNA.

Bovine Milk-Derived Extracellular Vesicles

Bovine milk-derived EVs were firstly isolated in 2010 [60]. These EVs have been proven to reduce the systemic toxicity of free chemotherapeutics and improve antitumor effects against lung and breast cancers. Moreover, they have been orally administered, because bovine milk-derived EVs can pass through the gastrointestinal barrier. Interestingly, despite the reduction in primary tumour growth, milk-derived EVs accelerate metastasis in breast and pancreatic cancer mouse models. Surprisingly, the timing of EV administration after resection of the primary tumour was critical in reversing their pro-metastatic effects [61]. Bovine milk-derived EVs have the advantages of both synthetic and cell-mediated nanocarriers. Zhang [29] used milk-EVs to develop a new sensitive DDS loaded with doxorubicin (Dox) for photochemistry therapy against OSCC. Milk-EV technology has been proven to reduce normal tissue toxicity from Dox.

To sum up, it needs to be highlighted that the EVs' source impacts their targeting abilities, EV migration, biodistribution and tumour accumulation. Thus, before EV engineering, it is crucial to choose the appropriate EV source as a starting point. The most common sources of EVs in the research field are MSCs, due to their multipotent nature and their ability to differentiate into various cell types. From this point of view, they are excellent candidates for cell-based therapy. On the other hand, their expression in tumour cells and promotion of tumour growth in vivo could be controversial in their usage as EV source. Therefore, some researchers indicate that the best sources of EV are cytotoxic cells against cancer cells, such as $\gamma\delta$ T cells or macrophages. Recently, more attention has been paid to new EV sources, such as plants.

3.5.2. Extracellular Vesicles—Purification and Isolation

One of the basic conditions for the clinical use of EVs is the standardization of the isolation process, increasing its efficiency, repeatability and purity. In the case of large-scale EV production, the production process sequentially involves the expansion of the donor cell line, collection of the conditioned medium and EV purification [62]. To date, several approaches to EV isolation have been reported: differential centrifugation (ultracentrifugation, UCG), precipitation, flushing separation, ultrafiltration, antibody affinity capture, microfluidic separation and mass spectrometry. The UCG is currently the most available method, considered the "gold standard" for EV isolation, and was used in almost all studies included in the review (Table S2). While UCG is the most popular and cost-effective procedure, there is a risk of disrupting EVs beyond a certain speed and force, which must be taken into account [63]. The latest evidence has shown that, compared to other methods, three-time UCG is a time-consuming procedure, may result in a lower yield of vesicles, and raises the problem of co-contamination with unwanted proteins [64]. Therefore, a double

UCG scheme has been proposed that involves the addition of 30% sucrose buffer solution during the first centrifugation step [65]. Summarizing, the final result of UCG may be affected by centrifugation speed, force, and type of rotor.

Only in one study [18] was the precipitation method applied, based on the EV isolation kit and addressing EVs. EV purification kits enable the isolation of EVs from all major biofluids, including plasma, and are considered as simple methods for EV isolation This method delivers comparable results to UCG without the necessity for specialized equipment.

3.5.3. Extracellular Vesicles' Characterization

As mentioned above, EVs can be divided into three types, depending on their size. To clearly understand the role of EVs, it is essential to assess their physical and chemical properties, such as shape, size, surface charge and density. Characterization of EVs to establish their role in physiological and/or pathological processes is one of the major challenges in the EV field. Many technologies are frequently applied to characterize EVs, among them dynamic light scattering (DLS), transmission electron microscopy (TEM), scanning electron microscopy (SEM), atomic force microscopy (AFM), tuneable resistance pulse sensing (TRPS), nanoparticle tracking analysis (NTA), flow cytometry (FCM), and confocal microscopy (LSM—confocal laser scanning) [66]. Most of those techniques were used in the reviewed studies (Table S2).

In the majority of articles, the size and structural morphology of EVs were confirmed by TEM and showed a typical bilayer membrane. Exosomes, which have a uniform round cup shape and a diameter of 30–150 nm, can also be observed by SEM. These features distinguish them from apoptotic bodies and micro-vesicles. The major distinction between SEM and TEM technology is that SEM generates an image by detecting reflected or knocked-off electrons, whereas TEM uses transmitted electrons (electrons that are passing through the sample) to create an image. As a consequence, TEM provides precious details regarding the internal structure of the sample, such as crystal structure, morphology and stress state information, while SEM delivers information on the surface of the sample and its composition [67]. Few researchers have assessed the particle size of EVs using DLS [24,29] or LSM [24,27].

In addition, in all studies, the western blotting analysis confirmed the existence of typical membrane proteins of the EVs, including well-known markers. In mammalian cells, CD63, CD81 and CD9 are among the most common positive markers, and they were the most frequently used in the reviewed studies, and also TSG101, while negative exo-somal markers were, unfortunately, reported only in four papers pointing to calnexin [14,17,22] and GM130 [13].

It has to be mentioned that, depending on the origin cells, the markers for detection may vary, therefore for PDEV identification authors [28] used other specific markers, such as heat shock protein 70 (HSP70), S-adenosyl-homocysteinase and glyceraldehyde 3 phosphate dehydrogenase.

3.5.4. Extracellular Vesicles' Labeling and Tracking

EV labelling is a novel strategy for monitoring EV distribution in vivo, which contributes to optimizing EV-based diagnosis and treatment. EV tracking helps in determining their applicability as site-specific delivery vesicles and their half-life, biodistribution and migration abilities, but also to understanding their role in intercellular communication [68]. Recent studies have developed different methods for EV labelling and imaging. Simple and widely used tracking is performed by lipophilic labelling of EVs, either using fluorescent dyes or radiolabelled dyes [69,70].

Direct fluorescence tagging of EVs is extensively used to study the in vivo behaviour of exogenous EVs. Fluorescence labelling can provide whole-body images in highly sensitive optical cameras, as well as fluorescence microscopic images [71]. Fluorescence dyes including green fluorescent protein (GFP), or lipophilic substances like PKH, DiI, and

DiR are simply and commonly used to track EVs [72], and this is the most commonly applied strategy in the reviewed studies (Table S2). The marking procedure is quite simple and no genetically modified EVs are needed. Nevertheless, optical imaging is restricted to exogenous EVs, and fluorescent dyes remain in tissues even after the degradation of EVs [73].

Another method is labelling used protein markers of EVs, such as CD63, which could be conjugated into fluorescent proteins. Reporter imaging using fluorescence or bioluminescence combined with transmembrane proteins could provide information more specific to EVs than direct dye labelling [53].

For clinical applications and deep tissue imaging, radionuclide imaging or MRI are possible, using 111In-oxine, 99mTc-HMPAO and iron oxide NPs.

Some researchers used gold NPs (GNPs) as labelling agents, creating golden EVs with the superior visualization abilities of classical X-ray computed tomography (CT) [13,21,74]. These authors developed a technique for direct and highly efficient uploading of GNPs into EVs, based on glucose-mediated uptake, without affecting EVs' functionality. Subsequently, the golden EVs were tracked with CT and quantitatively analyzed, in order to reveal their tumour targeting, accumulation, and whole-body biodistribution.

In some cases, chemotherapeutic drugs loaded in EVs, such as Dox, are intrinsically fluorescent and used in distribution assessment [29]. The uptake of free Dox or NPs loaded with the drug can be observed at 594 nm using LSM after excitation at 480 nm.

However, accurate tracking of EVs is limited due to the non-specificity of the labelling and retention, or the recirculation of labels after degradation. From the practical point of view, CT or MRI imaging could be more useful for EV tracking compared to fluorescence imaging, because of better resolution and penetration abilities and cost-effectiveness [68,71]. Compared to nuclear imaging, a CT scan allows tracking of EVs for longer periods than MRI. Using CT, but also immunohistochemical staining for human CD63, Cohen [12] tracked golden EVs at 24 h and 48 h after injection to the HNSCC model. Thanks to EV labelling, the authors confirmed that MSC-EVs had higher tumour accumulation compared to A431-EVs, and to synthetic NPs.

Some scientists have also used an in vivo imaging system that combines 2D optical and 3D optical tomography in one platform, known as IVIS imaging [15]. Moreover, tracking EVs can be provided using a different type of microscope, such as LSM [15], SME, or a light microscope, where the accumulation of gold-loaded EVs is observed during histological analysis by dark field microscopy [12].

3.5.5. Modified Extracellular Vesicles for Drug Delivery

Various nano-based drug formulations have been used to improve the therapeutic efficacy of chemical and biomolecular drugs. EVs are easy to be surface modified, which delivers additional functionality to the EVs and is an emerging area in drug delivery research.

Surface-Modified Extracellular Vesicles

On the surface of the EVs' membrane are localized particles which play role in EV protection, tumour targeting, cell adhesion, and uptake, which can be easy to change. Some authors have examined the modification of MSCs to express membrane-binding TRAIL [18,20]. They used MSCs transduced with a lentiviral vector encoding TRAIL to construct MSCT (transfected MSC) which subsequently delivered EVs expressing TRAIL. This nanotechnology can enhance the tumour-targeting effect of TRAIL [20]. Afterwards, the authors prepared a combination of MSCT-EVs (containing TRAIL) with drugs: CTX [20] or SNS032 [18]. The investigators found that the MSCT-EVs system improved the apoptosis index in tumour cells, showed a high inhibitory effect on OSCC, reduced the dosage of free drugs and decreased the side effects of cancer therapy.

Others [15] have transfected EVs with an EBV vector using a Neon electroporator to express a transmembrane protein (EBV Inducted 3 (EBI3) on their membranes, which is abundantly expressed by OSCC cells. As a result, they improved EVs' effectiveness in inhibiting tumour cells. Similarly, the EBV vector was used in NPC to express avb3 integrin subunits on the NPC surface [25]. This integrin binds iRGD, so subsequently EVs were modified to express iRGD, which significantly improved the binding ability of EVs to NPC and the biodistribution of iRGD-EVs.

To sum up, the targeting ability of EVs can be upgraded through appropriate surface modification leading to greater accumulation in tumour cells.

Extracellular Vesicles Combined with pH-Sensitive Peptide for Drug Delivery

It is known that the majority of solid tumours exhibit a pH from 6.5 to 7.4, thus giving the possibility of creating pH-response NPs [75]. The EV membrane can be conjugated with chemotherapy drugs with a hydrazine bond, which is easily disintegrated in an acidic TME, resulting in the quick release of drugs at the tumour site. This method was used by [29] to engineer pH/light sensitive milk-EVs, conjugated to Dox by a pH-cleavable bond. Afterward, the milk-EVs/Dox was used to encapsulate two agents: anthracene endoperoxide derivative (EPT1) and chlorin e6 (Ce6), finally creating EVs@Dox–EPT1 (EV–doxorubicin–anthracene endoperoxide derivative NPs). When the NPs were at the tumour site, Ce6 generated plasmonic heat and accelerated singlet oxygen generation from EPT1 under NIR irradiation. As a result, reliable and tumour site-specific photochemistry was realized in the treatment of OSCC [29].

EV engineering can improve phototherapy techniques and address their limitations. The latest research has focused on incorporating chemotherapeutic agents and photosensitizers or light-absorbing agents into NPs. When these agents are delivered to the tumour site, local irradiation has been shown to kill cancer cells and shrink the tumour.

Extracellular Vesicle Capturing Used in Biomimetic Strategy

The biomimetic strategy is a new technology that extracts the inflammatory cell membrane and uses it to coat nucleic acid or NPs in order to avoid the monitoring of the immune system which prolongs circulation time [76].

This strategy was used by Li [16], who camouflaged chitosan NPs (CAs) with macrophage membranes derived from M-EVs. Chitosan is an important non-viral gene vector that forms a complex with anionic drugs to improve delivery. Firstly, they constructed CAs using the ionic cross-linking method, along with biomimetic nanoparticles coloaded with the miR-144/451a cluster. Next, M-EV coated CAs and, finally, (M-EVs)/CA-miR451a construction were successfully applied for OSCC treatment.

Engineering Extracellular Vesicles by Fusion with Liposome

Another innovation is EV fusion with liposomes, which improved the loading capacity and the targeting capability of EVs. Liposomes are structures that consist of single or multiple concentric lipid bilayers encapsulating an aqueous compartment. They are able to incorporate drugs both within their aqueous core and their lipid bilayers. Fusing the EV membranes with liposomes using the freeze–thaw method creates the possibility of transporting exogenous hydrophobic lipids and hydrophilic cargoes.

Extracellular Vesicle-Coated Metal-Organic Framework Nanoparticles

Metal-organic frameworks (MOFs) are a type of organic–inorganic hybrid compound with one-, two-, or three-dimensional (1D, 2D, 3D) structural topologies, made up of inorganic metal ions/clusters and organic ligands [77]. The result shows that EV-coated MOF NPs are a smart and efficient DDS with an "onboard trigger".

ExomiR-Tracker—A Novel Drug Delivery System

In the reviewed studies, a novel DDS using ExomiR-Tracker [27] was described. ExomiR-Tracker consists of anti-exosomal miR-21 oligonucleotides and anti-exosomal CD63 antibodies creating an anti-CD63-9r/anti-miR complex. Anti-miR oligonucleotides have a sequence complementary to miRs and are often used for their functional inhibition [78]. Anti-miR-21 exhibits specific inhibitory effects on gene expression and, under hypoxic conditions, is upregulated, promoting cell growth and migration [79]. ExomiR-Tracker binds onto the surface of the EVs, leading to incorporation into the cells and the subsequent inhibition of the function of the exosomal miRs in the recipient cells. This strategy allows the use of EVs as natural cargo without isolation and loading [80].

Comparison of Methods for Drug Delivery Systems

DDS preparation is based on chemical methods (viral and non-viral vectors or liposomes) and physical techniques (such as nuclear transfection and electroporation). However, all these methods may cause significant damage to cells, thus their application in vivo is limited [18]. Common viral vectors, such as adenovirus (AV) and retrovirus (RV), are characterized by high-efficiency gene transfection, but there are immunogenicity and biological safety problems. Non-viral vector has become a breakthrough in the research of gene-drug delivery due to advantages such as simple preparation, low toxicity and immunogenicity, but also unlimited size and type of genes [51]. Additionally, non-viral vectors allow the co-delivery of different drug, or the combination of gene therapy with chemotherapy.

Some studies assessed the difference in drug (mTHPC) penetration and efficiency between three types of DDS: conventional liposomes (Foslip®), drug-in-cyclodextrin-in-liposomes (DCL), and EVs [26]. In the Foslip® and DCL methods, the mTHPC is directly loaded in lipid suspension. In contrast, mTHPC-EVs' construction requires the incubation of HUVEC cells in the serum-containing free mTHPC. However, mTHPC aggregates stay inside EVs even after purification and isolation procedures. The assessment of mTHPC loading demonstrated the highest loading capacity in EVs compared to DCL and Foslip® (1.3×10^{-15} g, 0.07×10^{-15} g, 0.05×10^{-15} g, mTHPC per nanovesicle, respectively) which resulted in mTHPC-EVs outperforming other lipid nanovesicles. The total uptake of mTHPC-EVs in the PSCC model was 10 times higher than that for other NPs, so tumours exposed to mTHPC-EVs required a four-times lower light dose to obtain a similar therapeutic effect in photodynamic therapy (PDT) as mTHPC-DCL and Foslip®.

To sum up, investigations confirmed that EVs most effectively improve drug delivery to cancer cells due to their extremely high loading capacity in comparison to other lipid nano-vesicles and allow for a decrease in therapeutic dosage.

3.5.6. Loading of Extracellular Vesicles

The lipid bilayer of EVs protects cargo from degradation in the bloodstream but, unfortunately, makes EV loading challenging.

Several strategies have been proposed and developed for loading material into EVs, e.g., electroporation, sonication, freeze–thaw cycles, and a combination of incubation with permeabilizing agents which have been lipophilically modified (Table S2). Each of these methods has some drawbacks. The disadvantage of electroporation is precipitation and aggregation, leading to an overestimated loading efficiency for EVs [69].

During sonication and incubation, the reorganization and deformation of EVs may occur, which disturbs their integrity [70]. Some researchers consider that charging hydrophobically modified cargo onto EVs is an optimized method. This was used by Deng [14], where cholesterol-modified miR-34a was loaded into EVs of HEK293T cells by co-incubation, without impacting EVs' integrity. The authors found that incubation provides a robust, efficient and highly reproducible method for loading EVs [14,26].

Some authors have used lentiviral vectors [13,17,19,20] or EBV vectors [15]. After transfection of the mother cells, such as MSCs, T cells, fibroblasts, or other epithelial cells, using the miR-encoding vector, it was possible to isolate EVs secreted from the transfected mother cell with overexpression of miR.

A modified calcium chloride-mediated transfection method for loading the miR inhibitor has also been performed [21,81]. This method is used to load miR directly into isolated EVs, instead of transfecting their mother cells.

3.6. Therapeutic Effects of Membrane Vesicle-Based Drug Delivery System for Head and Neck Squamous Cell Carcinoma

EVs have a cross-curricular role in tumor-genesis, cancer progression and immune response by transferring bioactive molecules between the cancer and various cells in the local and distant microenvironments, but are also being used as DDS (Figure 3).

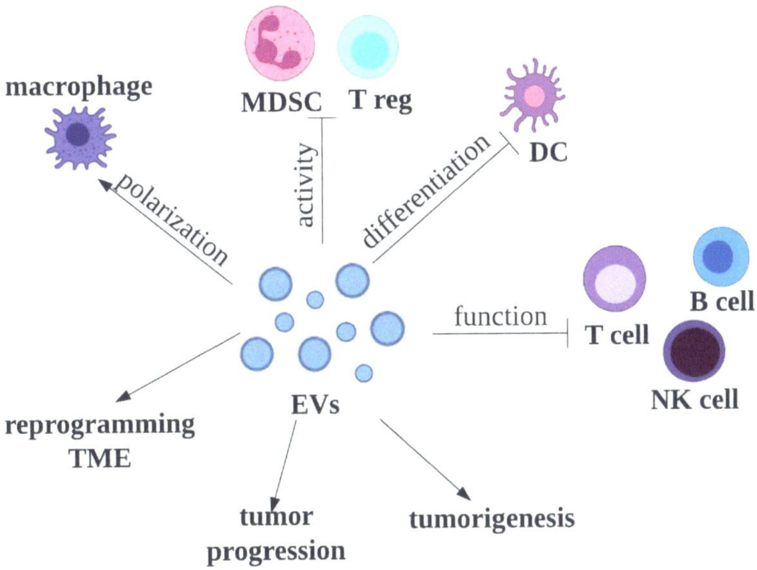

Figure 3. Role of EVs in the tumour microenvironment and impact on the immune system in HNSCC; DC—dendritic cell, MDSC—myeloid-derived suppressor cell, NK—natural killer cell, T reg—T regulatory cell, TME—tumor microenvironment.

3.6.1. Evaluation of Treatment Effectiveness

Cell viability, migration, invasion and wound-healing assay were performed to evaluate DDS efficacy, based on commonly used methods. Cell viability was assessed using the CCK8 Assay Kit. Cell migration and invasion abilities were determined using the Transwell migration assay. To evaluate cell motility, scratch wound healing assays were accomplished and immunofluorescence staining of Ki67 was performed to examine cell proliferation ability. Furthermore, researchers have investigated whether EVs induce apoptosis, which is recognized as a crucial type of cell death, using flow cytometric analysis via annexin V-FITC/PI staining. Chemotherapy effectiveness was revealed by increasing the percentage of apoptotic cells. Moreover, western blotting was performed to confirm the involvement of caspase activity in the EV induced apoptosis, because the activation of caspase pathways is usually involved in apoptosis induction.

3.6.2. Anticancer Agents Derived from Extracellular Vesicles for Head and Neck Squamous Cell Carcinoma Treatment

The following are the first-line chemotherapy drugs for treating HNSCC: paclitaxel (PTX), cisplatin (DDP), doxorubicin (Dox), docetaxel (DTX), Methotrexate and Fluoropyrimidine 5-Fluorouracil (5-FU). Four chemotherapeutics from this group were investigated in the reviewed studies: Dox [29], DTX [13], DDP [21] and 5-FU [28]. Additionally, in one article, Cabazitaxel (CTX), which is mainly used in prostate cancer, was under consideration [20].

The systemic toxicity of commonly used chemotherapeutics to treat HNSCC is a major complication of clinical treatment. It is known that the molecular mechanisms of chemoresistance include the acquisition of stem-cell-like features, epithelial-to-mesenchymal transition (EMT), overexpression of multidrug resistance (MDR) gene-related ATP-binding cassette (ABC) transporters, and activation of DNA repair mechanisms [81]. The responsiveness of cell carcinoma to chemotherapy widely affects prognosis. Moreover, the chemoresistance of cancer cells requires higher drug doses, which increases side effects. Therefore, ways to reduce doses in anti-tumour therapy are being investigated. This can be achieved by combining a chemotherapeutic agent with a chemosensitizer, or by DDSs directly to cancer cells. These obstacles can be overcome by using DDS targeting cancer cells that improve drug accumulation in tumours.

The most common drugs family loaded in EVs are taxane anticancer drugs, such as CTX, PTX and DTX, which bind to tubulin and subsequently suppress microtubule dynamics in cell division, leading to cancer cell death. Moreover, taxol drugs inhibit the apoptosis of cancer cells and promote cell proliferation, inhibiting the phosphorylation of PI3K, Akt and mTOR [63,82–85]. A therapy based on MSCT-EVs loaded with CTX/TRAIL combination was assessed for OSCC treatment [20]. CTX demonstrates antitumor activity superior to that of DTH and is mainly used to treat tumours with resistance to PTX or DTX, due to its poor affinity for P-glycoprotein (P-gp). It adverse effects, poor stability, and poor aqueous solubility impede its clinical applications. The authors compared the anti-tumour effectiveness of CTX-free, free MSCT-EVs and CTX-loaded by MSCT-EVs and observed that MSCT-EVs/CTX were the most effective in killing cancer cells. Finally, they concluded that EVs not only prolong the blood circulation time of CTX and improve its biological activity, but also decrease its toxicity in patients.

The same MSCT-EVs engineered with TRAIL were also used to load SNS032 [18]. SNS032 is known as a new and effective selective CDK9 inhibitor (CDK9—cyclin-dependent kinase 9), responsible for TRAIL resistance of cancer cells. The study demonstrated that SNS032 and TRAIL have a synergistic effect in the treatment of cancer and can both inhibit RNA synthesis and induce apoptosis of cancer cells [9].

The second taxane family member, DTX, was also investigated in HNSCC therapy [13]. DTX resistance of TSCC was modified by EVs loaded with miR-200c. EVs miR-200c decrease chemoresistance for DTX in TSCC. A detailed mechanism for this modification is described in the section below.

Another anticancer drug, Dox, was loaded in milk-EVs to reduce its normal tissue toxicity [29]. Dox cardiotoxicity is a major complication for clinical treatment, thus the researchers engineered special DDS for therapy, i.e., Exo@Dox–EPT1, described above [29]. The EVs derived enhanced the Dox accumulation in tumour tissues and prolonged retention time. The therapeutic result of the free Dox group and EV@Dox–EPT1 were compared with the 808 nm laser irradiation group and it was noted that EV@Dox–EPT1 caused significantly more cytotoxicity in cancer cells under 808 nm laser irradiation than the free Dox group and produced synergistic effects with photochemistry.

Moreover, some authors [28] have revealed that BMEVs showed a synergistic therapeutic effect of 5-FU against OSCC in both in vitro and in vivo studies.

3.6.3. RNA-Based Gene Therapy Delivered by EVs in the HNSCC Treatment

Although more than 30% of HNSCC patients demonstrate a minimal response to anticancer drugs such as cisplatin, the drug is still the first-line chemotherapeutic used for HNSCC patients. Evidence suggests miR dysregulation as one of the mediators of chemoresistance. Therefore, some research has focused on RNA-based gene therapy in HNSCC treatment. Thus, studies have revealed the role of exosomal miR and siRNA in chemotherapeutic resistance.

Extracellular Vesicle Derived miRs

MiRs are short (20–24 nucleotides in length) non-coding RNAs that are involved in the post-transcriptional regulation of gene expression in multicellular organisms by affecting both the stability and translation of mRNAs. In particular, miRs are essential regulators in various cellular processes, including proliferation, apoptosis, autophagy and migration [86,87]. In the reviewed articles, different types of miR loaded into EVs were assessed in HNSCC therapy.

1. MiR-9

MiR-9 was reported as the miR most related to HPV. Some studies noted that HPV + HNSCC cell-derived EVs are rich in miR-9-5p and suggested its positive role in the radiosensitivity of HNSCC cells [88,89]. MiR-9-5p polarizes macrophages into the M1 phenotype producing iNOS, which enhances tumour radiosensitivity [88]. MiR-9 significantly inhibits PPARδ (peroxisome proliferator-activated receptors subtype δ) expression in macrophages, enhancing the sensitization of HNSCC cells to radiation [22].

In summary, the exosomal miR-9 overexpression promotes HNSCC radiosensitivity, and HPV + HNSCC-derived exosomal miR-9 could be a potential treatment strategy for HNSCC.

2 MiR-18a and BART10-5p

Currently, about 15–20% of human cancers are associated with or induced by oncogenic viral factors, which drive oncogenesis mainly through impact on angiogenesis. Virus-associated tumours can be driven by herpes viruses (Kaposi's sarcoma), HPVs (cervical cancer), EBV (nasopharyngeal carcinoma, Burkitt lymphoma, gastric carcinoma), and others. Consequently, investigators have performed research on the relationships between viruses and host miRs.

Some studies used therapy regulation by viral and host miRs to inhibit angiogenesis. Wang [24] performed a study on miR-18a and BART10-5p, one of the miRs of EBV [90]. Both these miRs promote cancer angiogenesis by downregulation of Spry3 expression. Spry3 may have a tumour-suppressor function in NPC [90]. Although two miRs targeted the same gene, they bound different sites of Spry3 and upregulated the protein expression levels of Ras, c-Raf, MEK1/2, mTOR, eIF4E1, Erk1/2, HIF1-a, mmp2, and VEGF. To inhibit NPC angiogenesis, the authors proposed antagomiR-BART10-5p and antagomiR-18a enclosed in iRGD-tagged EVs. They demonstrated that EVs simultaneously containing antagomiR-BART10-5p and antagomiR-18a suppressed the angiogenesis and growth of NPC with higher efficiency than a single treatment. These findings establish a synergistic role between virus and host miRs in the regulation of angiogenesis of virus-associated cancer.

3 MiR-34a

MiR-34a regulates the cell cycle and apoptosis. It has been demonstrated that miR-34a expression levels are low in OSCC tissues and four human OSCC cell lines (HN4, HN6, SCC-9 and CAL27) compared to normal oral tissues [91]. Therefore, the researchers focused on miR-34a delivery into cancer cells [14]. In this study, they observed that miR-34a-EVs led to a significant inhibition of cancer cell proliferation, migration and invasion by downregulation of SATB2 expression (the special AT-rich sequence-binding protein 2). SATB2 modulated the expression of those genes which regulate pluripotency and self-renewal. Overexpression of the SATB2 gene in normal epithelial cells induced transformation, suggesting its role as an oncogene [92]. SATB2 expression in OSCC was associated with metastasis and tumour progression [91].

The study suggests that miR-34a-EVs can be a therapeutic option in HNSCC via targeted inhibition of SATB2.

4 MiR-100-5p and miR-1246

Other investigated miRs were miR-100-5p and miR-1246, which play a role in HNSCC angiogenesis [93,94]. Both in vitro and in vivo studies [18] confirmed that EVs rich in these miRs inhibit cell proliferation and migration but also induce apoptosis by downregulation of several angiogenesis-related factors (such as VEGFA, MMP-9 and ANGPT) and inhibit micro-vascular formation in OSCC tumours.

5 MiR-138

MiR-138 is known to be a tumour suppressor that has been downregulated in OSCCs [95–97] and many other types of HNSCC [98]. The miR-138 target genes play essential roles in cell migration (e.g., ZEB2, HIF-1a), EMT (e.g., TWIST2, EZH2), cell-cycle regulation (e.g., CCND1, CCND3, FOSL1), DNA damage and repair (e.g., H2AX, XRCC1), and senescence (e.g., Sirt1, TERT) [98]. Thus, miR-138 can inhibit proliferation and invasion, induce apoptosis, and enhance the chemosensitivity in many types of cancer.

Some authors have noticed that miR-138 delivered by $\gamma\delta$ TDEVs significantly decreased OSCC cell proliferation and viability, and induced more apoptosis, but also had an immunostimulatory effect on T cells [17]. Therefore, miR-138-EVs are beneficial in OSCC therapy.

6 MiR-144/451a

As described above, in some reviewed studies EVs were loaded with miR-144/451a in complex with chitosan [16] to construct CAs -miR-144/451a. This biomimetic system improved the miR-144/451a cluster effects of miRs on OSCC cells. Their inhibitory function was associated with miR-451a activity which may inhibit the expression of MIF (macrophage migration inhibitory factor) and CAB39 (a key regulator of aseptic 20 kinase). Both are extensively involved in tumorigenesis, promote tumour cell proliferation and differentiation, and inhibit apoptosis [99].

7 MiR-155

MiR-155 is another miR known to be a tumour-promoting factor in many cancers by regulating the BCL6/cyclin D2 axis [100]. This miR leads to the downregulation of FOXO3a (the Forkhead transcription factor O subfamily), which normally acts as a tumour suppressor gene, increases OSCC chemoresistance for DDP, and is directly associated with aggressive progression and poor prognosis in cancers [101,102].

Thus, the researchers hypothesised that the miR-155 inhibitor would be useful in OSCC therapy and noticed that it modulates the level of drug transporter ABCB1 (a drug efflux transporter protein), which is typically involved in chemoresistance in OSCC [21,103]. They observed a significantly lower ABCB1 expression in the xenograft model of OSCC treated with the miR-155 inhibitor, as compared to controls. They also demonstrated downregulation of stemness markers, such as sox2, oct4, nanog, and bmi1, in the group treated with EVs loaded with miR-155 inhibitor, suggesting a possible correlation between stemness phenotype and resistance to DDP in oral cancer.

In conclusion, the downregulation of miR-155 may potentially reverse HNSCC chemoresistance to DDP.

8 MiR-200c

Cui et al. [13] investigated EVs loaded with miR-200c for TSCC therapy [9]. MiR-200c participates in many biological processes, such as the cell cycle [104], steroidogenesis [105], vasculo-genesis [106] and EMT [107], but also sensitizes cancer cells to DTX through the PTEN/Akt pathway [108]. The authors confirmed that EVs could effectively deliver miR-200c to chemo-resistant cells and increase the sensitivity of TSCC cells to DTX [9]. DTX inhibits the development of cancer by affecting microtubules, stops the transition from metaphase to anaphase, and promotes apoptosis [46,49,109–114].

In their revised article, Cui et al. [13] observed that HNSCC cells (human tongue SCC line: HSC-3DR) showed downregulation of miR-200c, which led to decreased apoptosis in tumour cells, and higher migration and invasion associated with EMT and DNA damage. This observation was in line with miR-200c's previously confirmed supportive role in anticancer mechanisms. They concluded that miR-200c decrease is essential for chemoresistance. MiR-200c regulated DTX resistance by targeting TUBB3 (microtubule protein βIII-tubulin) and PPP2R1B (subunit of protein phosphatase 2). Direct transfection of HNSCC cell lines using the miR-200c-encoding lentiviral vector (LV-200c) led to forced overexpression of miR-200c and resulted in higher sensitivity to DTX. miR's role as a chemosensitizer for DTX was also confirmed in vivo by intra-tumour injection of miR-200c-EVs, which significantly suppressed tumour growth in response to DTX treatment.

To summarize, miR-200c derived by EVs decreases HNSCC resistance for DTX.

In conclusion, so far miRs are the most common molecules loaded in EVs for HNSCC therapy. The included studies confirmed miRs' (miR-9, miR–18a, BART10-5p, miR–34a, miR-100-5p, miR-1246, miR-138, miR-144/451a) inhibitory role in HNSCC proliferation, migration and invasion, but increased apoptosis induction. Additionally, some miRs, such as miR-155, miR-200c, and miR-138, improved HNSCC chemosensitivity, and miR-9 increased the radiosensitivity of carcinoma cells. A few miRs, such as miR-144 and miR-451a, additionally had an immunostimulatory effect on T cells.

Extracellular Vesicles-Derived Small Interfering RNA

Small interfering RNA (siRNA), sometimes known as short interfering RNA or silencing RNA, is a molecule similar to miR which is able to regulate the expression of genes by a phenomenon known as RNAi (RNA interference). It inhibits the expression of specific genes with complementary nucleotide sequences by degrading mRNA after transcription, preventing translation.

SiRNA-based technology is a promising strategy, but difficult to apply in clinical practice, because of siRNAs' polyanionic charge, poor stability against serum nuclease degradation, low permeability, immune response induction and toxicity. These traits can be neutralized by placing siRNAs in EVs, which deliver them to targeted cancer cells. This option was assessed by Wang [23], who examined EVs loaded with TRPP2 siRNA complex for the treatment of HNSCC. TRPP2 is a nonselective cation channel markedly increased in HNSCC [54]. TRPP2 enhances metastasis in these cells by regulating EMT. TRPP2 siRNA delivered by EVs to HNSCC cells suppressed TRPP2 protein expression levels, and as a consequence reduced EMT. TRPP2 knockdown significantly decreased ATP-induced Ca2+ release and vimentin and N-cadherin expression levels. Both N-cadherin and vimentin are overproduced in numerous cancers and recognized as prognostic biomarkers in cancero-genesis [115].

A similar strategy was used by others [15] to engineer EVs (octEVs) transferring siRNA to OSCC tumours. Specially prepared EVs along with expression of EBV proteins were loaded with siLCP1–siRNA silencing of LCP1 (lymphocyte cytoplasmic protein 1). LCP1 was recently found to be a regulator of OSCC progression and positively correlates with the primary tumoral size and regional lymph node metastasis [116]. By loading siLCP1 in octEVs, the authors achieved an OSCC tumour-suppressive effect in vitro and in vivo.

Concluding, EVs can protect and deliver siRNA into cancer cells and apply them in clinical practice. SiRNA, by regulation of the gene expression, impacts prognostic biomarkers and inhibits migration and invasion of HNSCC cells.

4. Discussion

In recent years, knowledge of the role of EVs in many inflammatory diseases and cancers has grown rapidly [117,118]. EVs isolated from the plasma of HNSCC patients provide information on tumour status, genetic complexity and immune dysfunction [119], but also on the molecular mechanisms involved in cancer metastasis and resistance to therapy [120–122].

In this article, we have discussed the potential of using membrane vesicle-based drug delivery systems (DDS) in HNSCC therapy. These novel DDS have shown promising advancements in oncology by selectively pointing to cancers, leading to better results and reduced side effects, as well as impacting tumor radio- and chemoresistance [123,124].

EVs offer several advantages, including the ability to protect, stabilize and deliver drugs precisely to the target site. Despite facing biological barriers during transport to tissues, EVs have the inherent ability to overcome this, due to their natural formation [9].

EV administration generates better tolerated and more efficient medicines. The association between the EV's source and its tumour-targeting abilities and biodistribution opens up new ways to devise targeted therapies in order to deliver anti-tumor drugs [69].

EVs may serve as an alternative to cell-based therapeutic approaches. Compared with cell-based therapy, EVs may have a shorter lifetime in circulation. Moreover, EV treatment is associated with controllable cytokine release syndrome, and therefore minimal adverse events, good penetration within the solid tumor, and easy modification [125].

Furthermore, studies confirmed that EVs have direct anti-tumor effects on SCC and stimulate anti-tumour immunity. EVs DDS effectively reverses the multidrug resistance of tumours and improves HNSCC sensitivity for treatment. In many cases, the protection of the loaded molecules by EVs against nucleases and other enzymes in the bloodstream is critical for their use in therapies.

However, despite the growing research in this area, many issues remain incompletely clarified. These include issues necessary for safe administration, such as EVs' pharmacokinetics, biodistribution and proper delivery of effective drug concentrations. EVs have some disadvantages also, relating to their rapid elimination from circulation, high toxicity and lack of targeting specificity, which can be managed by EV modification.

Therapeutic applications of EVs as DDS are limited due to the lack of an ideal EV donor, methods for scalable EV isolation and production, and inefficient drug loading. Moreover, cells produce different types of EVs under different conditions. Due to the heterogeneity of exosomes, recent reports suggest that there is a need to separate exosomes into distinct subpopulations [126]. Thus. scientists are looking for new technologies for the association of a specific marker with an exosome subtype and the exosome subtype with a particular function. Some authors have proposed modern microfluidic and nanotechnological advancements towards isolation and characterization of exosome subpopulations, such as phage display technology, which does not rely on the a priori definition of exosome-related markers, but is based on phage ability in exosome detection [127]. This seems to be a promising tool for the identification and isolation of disease-related exosomes, which is crucial for the effective adoption of exosomes in clinical practice.

Additionally, the development of efficient, sensitive and biocompatible EV labelling and imaging techniques is highly desired. Importantly, although EVs can be nearly non-immunogenic when used autologously, concerns remain about the immunogenicity and toxicity of unnatural DDS.

In HNSCC, the diagnosis of the disease is very often made at a late stage, with the highest mortality [128,129]. Rapid advances in the technology of using EVs as drug carriers make it hopeful that these solutions will be used in the future. The first results are impressive, but there is still a need for further research to integrate such an innovative technique into clinical practice.

Supplementary Materials: The following supporting information can be downloaded at: https://www.mdpi.com/article/10.3390/pharmaceutics15051327/s1, Table S1: The risk of bias included in a systematic review assessed using the OHAT risk of bias.; Table S2: Main data from the included studies.

Author Contributions: Conceptualization, K.D. and K.C.; methodology, K.D.; software, K.C.; validation, K.D. and K.C.; formal analysis, K.C.; investigation, K.D.; resources, K.D.; data curation, K.C.; writing—original draft preparation, K.D.; writing—review and editing, K.D. and K.C.; visualization K.C.; supervision, K.D.; project administration, K.D.; funding acquisition, K.D. All authors have read and agreed to the published version of the manuscript.

Funding: This study was financed by the Centre of Postgraduate Medical Education, grant number 501-1-019-56-22 to K.D. and the APC was funded by the Centre of Postgraduate Medical Education.

Institutional Review Board Statement: Not applicable.

Informed Consent Statement: Not applicable.

Data Availability Statement: Not applicable.

Conflicts of Interest: The authors declare no conflict of interest.

References

1. Johnson, D.E.; Burtness, B.; Leemans, C.R.; Lui, V.W.Y.; Bauman, J.E.; Grandis, J.R. Head and neck squamous cell carcinoma. *Nat. Rev. Dis. Prim.* **2020**, *6*, 92. [CrossRef] [PubMed]
2. Rosenberg, A.J.; Vokes, E.E. Optimizing Treatment De-Escalation in Head and Neck Cancer: Current and Future Perspectives. *Oncologist* **2021**, *26*, 40–48. [CrossRef] [PubMed]
3. Forastiere, A.A.; Zhang, Q.; Weber, R.S.; Maor, M.H.; Goepfert, H.; Pajak, T.F.; Morrison, W.; Glisson, B.; Trotti, A.; Ridge, J.A.; et al. Long-term results of RTOG 91-11: A comparison of three nonsurgical treatment strategies to preserve the larynx in patients with locally advanced larynx cancer. *J. Clin. Oncol.* **2013**, *31*, 845–852. [CrossRef] [PubMed]
4. Elsharkasy, O.M.; Nordin, J.Z.; Hagey, D.W.; de Jong, O.G.; Schiffelers, R.M.; Andaloussi, S.E.; Vader, P. Extracellular vesicles as drug delivery systems: Why and how? *Adv. Drug Deliv. Rev.* **2020**, *159*, 332–343. [CrossRef] [PubMed]
5. Fischbach, C.; Chen, R.; Matsumoto, T.; Schmelzle, T.; Brugge, J.S.; Polverini, P.J.; Mooney, D.J. Engineering tumors with 3D scaffolds. *Nat. Methods* **2007**, *4*, 855–860. [CrossRef] [PubMed]
6. Herrmann, I.K.; Wood, M.J.A.; Fuhrmann, G. Extracellular vesicles as a next-generation drug delivery platform. *Nat. Nanotechnol.* **2021**, *16*, 748–759. [CrossRef]
7. Meng, W.; He, C.; Hao, Y.; Wang, L.; Li, L.; Zhu, G. Prospects and challenges of extracellular vesicle-based drug delivery system: Considering cell source. *Drug Deliv.* **2020**, *27*, 585–598. [CrossRef]
8. Sharma, S.; Masud, M.K.; Kaneti, Y.V.; Rewatkar, P.; Koradia, A.; Hossain, M.S.A.; Yamauchi, Y.; Popat, A.; Salomon, C. Extracellular Vesicle Nanoarchitectonics for Novel Drug Delivery Applications. *Small* **2021**, *17*, e2102220. [CrossRef]
9. Boucherit, N.; Gorvel, L.; Olive, D. 3D Tumor Models and Their Use for the Testing of Immunotherapies. *Front. Immunol.* **2020**, *11*, 603640. [CrossRef]
10. Page, M.J.; Moher, D.; Bossuyt, P.M.; Boutron, I.; Hoffmann, T.C.; Mulrow, C.D.; Shamseer, L.; Tetzlaff, J.M.; Akl, E.A.; Brennan, S.E.; et al. PRISMA 2020 explanation and elaboration: Updated guidance and exemplars for reporting systematic reviews. *BMJ* **2021**, *372*, n160. [CrossRef]
11. Program, N.T. *Handbook for Conducting a Literature-Based Health Assessment Using OHAT Approach for Systematic Review and Evidence Integration*; Office of Health Assessment and Translation (OHAT), Division of the National Toxicology Program, National Institute of Environmental Health Sciences: Durham, NC, USA, 2015; Available online: https://ntpniehsnihgov/ntp/ohat/pubs/handbookjan2015_508pdf (accessed on 31 January 2023).
12. Cohen, O.; Betzer, O.; Elmaliach-Pnini, N.; Motiei, M.; Sadan, T.; Cohen-Berkman, M.; Dagan, O.; Popovtzer, A.; Yosepovich, A.; Barhom, H.; et al. 'Golden' exosomes as delivery vehicles to target tumors and overcome intratumoral barriers: In vivo tracking in a model for head and neck cancer. *Biomater. Sci.* **2021**, *9*, 2103–2114. [CrossRef] [PubMed]
13. Cui, J.; Wang, H.; Zhang, X.; Sun, X.; Zhang, J.; Ma, J. Exosomal miR-200c suppresses chemoresistance of docetaxel in tongue squamous cell carcinoma by suppressing TUBB3 and PPP2R1B. *Aging* **2020**, *12*, 6756–6773. [CrossRef] [PubMed]
14. Deng, W.; Meng, Y.; Wang, B.; Wang, C.X.; Hou, C.X.; Zhu, Q.H.; Tang, Y.T.; Ye, J.H. In vitro experimental study on the formation of microRNA-34a loaded exosomes and their inhibitory effect in oral squamous cell carcinoma. *Cell Cycle* **2022**, *21*, 1775–1783. [CrossRef] [PubMed]
15. Kase, Y.; Uzawa, K.; Wagai, S.; Yoshimura, S.; Yamamoto, J.I.; Toeda, Y.; Okubo, M.; Eizuka, K.; Ando, T.; Nobuchi, T.; et al. Engineered exosomes delivering specific tumor-suppressive RNAi attenuate oral cancer progression. *Sci. Rep.* **2021**, *11*, 5897. [CrossRef]
16. Li, K.; Qiu, Y.; Liu, X.; Huang, F. Biomimetic Nanosystems for the Synergistic Delivery of miR-144/451a for Oral Squamous Cell Carcinoma. *Balk. Med. J.* **2022**, *39*, 178–186. [CrossRef]
17. Li, L.; Lu, S.; Liang, X.; Cao, B.; Wang, S.; Jiang, J.; Luo, H.; He, S.; Lang, J.; Zhu, G. γδTDEs: An Efficient Delivery System for miR-138 with Anti-tumoral and Immunostimulatory Roles on Oral Squamous Cell Carcinoma. *Mol. Ther. Nucleic Acids* **2019**, *14*, 101–113. [CrossRef]
18. Liu, P.; Zhang, Q.; Mi, J.; Wang, S.; Xu, Q.; Zhuang, D.; Chen, W.; Liu, C.; Zhang, L.; Guo, J.; et al. Exosomes derived from stem cells of human deciduous exfoliated teeth inhibit angiogenesis in vivo and in vitro via the transfer of miR-100-5p and miR-1246. *Stem Cell Res. Ther.* **2022**, *13*, 89. [CrossRef]
19. Liu, Y.; Li, H.; Qiu, Y.L.; Li, K.S.; Lu, Y.; Wang, W. Nanoscale biomimetic nano system for the co-delivery of sns032 and tumor necrosis factor related apoptosis inducing ligand to enhance therapeutic efficacy in oral squamous cell carcinoma cell line scc25. *Mater. Express* **2021**, *11*, 1321–1330. [CrossRef]
20. Qiu, Y.L.; Sun, J.M.; Qiu, J.P.; Chen, G.L.; Wang, X.; Mu, Y.X.; Li, K.S.; Wang, W.J. Antitumor Activity of Cabazitaxel and MSC-TRAIL Derived Extracellular Vesicles in Drug-Resistant Oral Squamous Cell Carcinoma. *Cancer Manag. Res.* **2020**, *12*, 10809–10820. [CrossRef]

21. Sayyed, A.A.; Gondaliya, P.; Mali, M.; Pawar, A.; Bhat, P.; Khairnar, A.; Arya, N.; Kalia, K. MiR-155 Inhibitor-Laden Exosomes Reverse Resistance to Cisplatin in a 3D Tumor Spheroid and Xenograft Model of Oral Cancer. *Mol. Pharm.* **2021**, *18*, 3010–3025. [CrossRef]
22. Tong, F.; Mao, X.; Zhang, S.; Xie, H.; Yan, B.; Wang, B.; Sun, J.; Wei, L. HPV + HNSCC-derived exosomal miR-9 induces macrophage M1 polarization and increases tumor radiosensitivity. *Cancer Lett.* **2020**, *478*, 34–44. [CrossRef] [PubMed]
23. Wang, C.; Chen, L.E.I.; Huang, Y.; Li, K.U.N.; Jinye, A.; Fan, T.; Zhao, R.E.N.; Xia, X.; Shen, B.; Du, J.; et al. Exosome-delivered TRPP2 siRNA inhibits the epithelial-mesenchymal transition of FaDu cells. *Oncol. Lett.* **2019**, *17*, 1953–1961. [CrossRef] [PubMed]
24. Wang, J.; Jiang, Q.; Faleti, O.D.; Tsang, C.M.; Zhao, M.; Wu, G.; Tsao, S.W.; Fu, M.; Chen, Y.; Ding, T.; et al. Exosomal Delivery of AntagomiRs Targeting Viral and Cellular MicroRNAs Synergistically Inhibits Cancer Angiogenesis. *Mol. Ther. Nucleic Acids* **2020**, *22*, 153–165. [CrossRef]
25. Wang, X.; Zhang, Y.; Mu, X.; Tu, C.R.; Chung, Y.; Tsao, S.W.; Chan, G.C.F.; Leung, W.H.; Lau, Y.L.; Liu, Y.; et al. Exosomes derived from 3δ -T cells synergize with radiotherapy and preserve antitumor activities against nasopharyngeal carcinoma in immunosuppressive microenvironment. *J. ImmunoTher. Cancer* **2022**, *10*, e003832. [CrossRef]
26. Yakavets, I.; Francois, A.; Lamy, L.; Piffoux, M.; Gazeau, F.; Wilhelm, C.; Zorin, V.; Silva, A.K.A.; Bezdetnaya, L. Effect of stroma on the behavior of temoporfin-loaded lipid nanovesicles inside the stroma-rich head and neck carcinoma spheroids. *J. Nanobiotechnology* **2021**, *19*, 3. [CrossRef] [PubMed]
27. Yamayoshi, A.; Oyama, S.; Kishimoto, Y.; Konishi, R.; Yamamoto, T.; Kobori, A.; Harada, H.; Ashihara, E.; Sugiyama, H.; Murakami, A. Development of antibody–oligonucleotide complexes for targeting exosomal microrna. *Pharmaceutics* **2020**, *12*, 545. [CrossRef]
28. Yang, M.; Luo, Q.; Chen, X.; Chen, F. Bitter melon derived extracellular vesicles enhance the therapeutic effects and reduce the drug resistance of 5-fluorouracil on oral squamous cell carcinoma. *J. Nanobiotechnol.* **2021**, *19*, 259. [CrossRef]
29. Zhang, Q.; Xiao, Q.; Yin, H.; Xia, C.; Pu, Y.; He, Z.; Hu, Q.; Wang, J.; Wang, Y. Milk-exosome based pH/light sensitive drug system to enhance anticancer activity against oral squamous cell carcinoma. *RSC Adv.* **2020**, *10*, 28314–28323. [CrossRef]
30. Bray, F.; Ferlay, J.; Soerjomataram, I.; Siegel, R.L.; Torre, L.A.; Jemal, A. Global cancer statistics 2018: GLOBOCAN estimates of incidence and mortality worldwide for 36 cancers in 185 countries. *CA Cancer J. Clin.* **2018**, *68*, 394–424. [CrossRef]
31. Trivedi, S.; Sun, L.; Aggarwal, C. Immunotherapy for Head and Neck Cancer. *Hematol. Oncol. Clin. N. Am.* **2021**, *35*, 1021–1037. [CrossRef]
32. Jurkiewicz, D.; Dżaman, K.; Rapiejko, P. Laryngeal cancer risk factors. *Pol. Merkur. Lek.* **2006**, *21*, 94–98.
33. Gillison, M.L.; Chaturvedi, A.K.; Lowy, D.R. HPV prophylactic vaccines and the potential prevention of noncervical cancers in both men and women. *Cancer* **2008**, *113*, 3036–3046. [CrossRef] [PubMed]
34. Tsur, N.; Frig, O.; Steinberg-Shemer, O.; Tamary, H.; Kurman, N.; Mizrachi, A.; Popovtzer, A. Characterization of Fanconi Anemia Patients with Head and Neck Squamous Cell Carcinoma: Israel Fanconi Registry. *Isr. Med. Assoc. J.* **2022**, *24*, 491–496. [PubMed]
35. Fang, M.; Huang, W.; Mo, D.; Zhao, W.; Huang, R. Association of Five Snps in Cytotoxic T-Lymphocyte Antigen 4 and Cancer Susceptibility: Evidence from 67 Studies. *Cell Physiol. Biochem.* **2018**, *47*, 414–427. [CrossRef] [PubMed]
36. Wang, Y.; Yang, H.; Duan, G.; Wang, H. The association of the CYP1A1 Ile462Val polymorphism with head and neck cancer risk: Evidence based on a cumulative meta-analysis. *OncoTargets Ther.* **2016**, *9*, 2927–2934. [CrossRef] [PubMed]
37. Wong, I.C.; Ng, Y.K.; Lui, V.W. Cancers of the lung, head and neck on the rise: Perspectives on the genotoxicity of air pollution. *Chin. J. Cancer* **2014**, *33*, 476–480. [CrossRef]
38. Yu, S.S.; Cirillo, N. The molecular markers of cancer stem cells in head and neck tumors. *J. Cell Physiol.* **2020**, *235*, 65–73. [CrossRef]
39. Zhang, Q.; Shi, S.; Yen, Y.; Brown, J.; Ta, J.Q.; Le, A.D. A subpopulation of CD133(+) cancer stem-like cells characterized in human oral squamous cell carcinoma confer resistance to chemotherapy. *Cancer Lett.* **2010**, *289*, 151–160. [CrossRef]
40. Antra; Parashar, P.; Hungyo, H.; Jain, A.; Ahmad, S.; Tandon, V. Unraveling molecular mechanisms of head and neck cancer. *Crit. Rev. Oncol. Hematol.* **2022**, *178*, 103778. [CrossRef]
41. Leon, X.; Garcia, J.; Lopez, M.; Rodriguez, C.; Gutierrez, A.; Quer, M. Risk of onset of second neoplasms and successive neoplasms in patients with a head and neck index tumour. *Acta Otorrinolaringol. Esp.* **2020**, *71*, 9–15. [CrossRef]
42. Osazuwa-Peters, N.; Simpson, M.C.; Zhao, L.; Boakye, E.A.; Olomukoro, S.I.; Deshields, T.; Loux, T.M.; Varvares, M.A.; Schootman, M. Suicide risk among cancer survivors: Head and neck versus other cancers. *Cancer* **2018**, *124*, 4072–4079. [CrossRef]
43. Nayak, S.G.; Pai, M.S.; George, L.S. Quality of life of patients with head and neck cancer: A mixed method study. *J. Cancer Res. Ther.* **2019**, *15*, 638–644. [CrossRef] [PubMed]
44. Bonomo, P.; Paderno, A.; Mattavelli, D.; Zenda, S.; Cavalieri, S.; Bossi, P. Quality Assessment in Supportive Care in Head and Neck Cancer. *Front. Oncol.* **2019**, *9*, 926. [CrossRef] [PubMed]
45. Hutcheson, K.A.; Nurgalieva, Z.; Zhao, H.; Gunn, G.B.; Giordano, S.H.; Bhayani, M.K.; Lewin, J.S.; Lewis, C.M. Two-year prevalence of dysphagia and related outcomes in head and neck cancer survivors: An updated SEER-Medicare analysis. *Head Neck* **2019**, *41*, 479–487. [CrossRef]
46. Fais, S. NK cell-released exosomes: Natural nanobullets against tumors. *Oncoimmunology* **2013**, *2*, e22337. [CrossRef] [PubMed]
47. Pitt, J.M.; Andre, F.; Amigorena, S.; Soria, J.C.; Eggermont, A.; Kroemer, G.; Zitvogel, L. Dendritic cell-derived exosomes for cancer therapy. *J. Clin. Investig.* **2016**, *126*, 1224–1232. [CrossRef] [PubMed]
48. Ventimiglia, L.N.; Alonso, M.A. Biogenesis and Function of T Cell-Derived Exosomes. *Front. Cell Dev. Biol.* **2016**, *4*, 84. [CrossRef]

49. Yoshikawa, T.; Takahara, M.; Tomiyama, M.; Nieda, M.; Maekawa, R.; Nakatsura, T. Large-scale expansion of gammadelta T cells and peptide-specific cytotoxic T cells using zoledronate for adoptive immunotherapy. *Int. J. Oncol.* **2014**, *45*, 1847–1856. [CrossRef]
50. Wang, X.; Xiang, Z.; Liu, Y.; Huang, C.; Pei, Y.; Wang, X.; Zhi, H.; Wong, W.H.; Wei, H.; Ng, I.O.; et al. Exosomes derived from Vdelta2-T cells control Epstein-Barr virus-associated tumors and induce T cell antitumor immunity. *Sci. Transl. Med.* **2020**, *12*, eaaz3426. [CrossRef]
51. Gordon, S.; Martinez, F.O. Alternative activation of macrophages: Mechanism and functions. *Immunity* **2010**, *32*, 593–604. [CrossRef]
52. Liu, J.; Wu, F.; Zhou, H. Macrophage-derived exosomes in cancers: Biogenesis, functions and therapeutic applications. *Immunol. Lett.* **2020**, *227*, 102–108. [CrossRef]
53. Lai, C.P.; Kim, E.Y.; Badr, C.E.; Weissleder, R.; Mempel, T.R.; Tannous, B.A.; Breakefield, X.O. Visualization and tracking of tumour extracellular vesicle delivery and RNA translation using multiplexed reporters. *Nat. Commun.* **2015**, *6*, 7029. [CrossRef] [PubMed]
54. Wu, K.; Shen, B.; Jiang, F.; Xia, L.; Fan, T.; Qin, M.; Yang, L.; Guo, J.; Li, Y.; Zhu, M.; et al. TRPP2 Enhances Metastasis by Regulating Epithelial-Mesenchymal Transition in Laryngeal Squamous Cell Carcinoma. *Cell Physiol. Biochem.* **2016**, *39*, 2203–2215. [CrossRef] [PubMed]
55. Martinez Saez, D.; Sasaki, R.T.; Neves, A.D.; da Silva, M.C. Stem Cells from Human Exfoliated Deciduous Teeth: A Growing Literature. *Cells Tissues Organs* **2016**, *202*, 269–280. [CrossRef]
56. Zhou, J.; Yang, Y.; Wang, W.; Zhang, Y.; Chen, Z.; Hao, C.; Zhang, J. Melanoma-released exosomes directly activate the mitochondrial apoptotic pathway of CD4(+) T cells through their microRNA cargo. *Exp. Cell Res.* **2018**, *371*, 364–371. [CrossRef]
57. Raimondo, S.; Naselli, F.; Fontana, S.; Monteleone, F.; Lo Dico, A.; Saieva, L.; Zito, G.; Flugy, A.; Manno, M.; Di Bella, M.A.; et al. Citrus limon-derived nanovesicles inhibit cancer cell proliferation and suppress CML xenograft growth by inducing TRAIL-mediated cell death. *Oncotarget* **2015**, *6*, 19514–19527. [CrossRef] [PubMed]
58. Kim, K.; Yoo, H.J.; Jung, J.H.; Lee, R.; Hyun, J.K.; Park, J.H.; Na, D.; Yeon, J.H. Cytotoxic Effects of Plant Sap-Derived Extracellular Vesicles on Various Tumor Cell Types. *J. Funct. Biomater.* **2020**, *11*, 22. [CrossRef]
59. Kameli, N.; Dragojlovic-Kerkache, A.; Savelkoul, P.; Stassen, F.R. Plant-Derived Extracellular Vesicles: Current Findings, Challenges, and Future Applications. *Membranes* **2021**, *11*, 411. [CrossRef]
60. Hata, T.; Murakami, K.; Nakatani, H.; Yamamoto, Y.; Matsuda, T.; Aoki, N. Isolation of bovine milk-derived microvesicles carrying mRNAs and microRNAs. *Biochem. Biophys. Res. Commun.* **2010**, *396*, 528–533. [CrossRef]
61. Samuel, M.; Fonseka, P.; Sanwlani, R.; Gangoda, L.; Chee, S.H.; Keerthikumar, S.; Spurling, A.; Chitti, S.V.; Zanker, D.; Ang, C.S.; et al. Oral administration of bovine milk-derived extracellular vesicles induces senescence in the primary tumor but accelerates cancer metastasis. *Nat. Commun.* **2021**, *12*, 3950. [CrossRef]
62. Vader, P.; Mol, E.A.; Pasterkamp, G.; Schiffelers, R.M. Extracellular vesicles for drug delivery. *Adv. Drug Deliv. Rev.* **2016**, *106*, 148–156. [CrossRef] [PubMed]
63. Bahl, A.; Wilson, W.; Ball, J.; Renninson, E.; Dubey, S.; Bravo, A.; Foulstone, E.; Spensley, S.; Bowen, R.; Mansi, J.; et al. Concept: A randomised multicentre trial of first line chemotherapy comparing three weekly cabazitaxel versus weekly paclitaxel in HER2 negative metastatic breast cancer. *Breast* **2022**, *66*, 69–76. [CrossRef] [PubMed]
64. Momen-Heravi, F.; Balaj, L.; Alian, S.; Mantel, P.Y.; Halleck, A.E.; Trachtenberg, A.J.; Soria, C.E.; Oquin, S.; Bonebreak, C.M.; Saracoglu, E.; et al. Current methods for the isolation of extracellular vesicles. *Biol. Chem.* **2013**, *394*, 1253–1262. [CrossRef] [PubMed]
65. Buschmann, D.; Kirchner, B.; Hermann, S.; Marte, M.; Wurmser, C.; Brandes, F.; Kotschote, S.; Bonin, M.; Steinlein, O.K.; Pfaffl, M.W.; et al. Evaluation of serum extracellular vesicle isolation methods for profiling miRNAs by next-generation sequencing. *J. Extracell. Vesicles* **2018**, *7*, 1481321. [CrossRef]
66. Gurunathan, S.; Kang, M.H.; Jeyaraj, M.; Qasim, M.; Kim, J.H. Review of the Isolation, Characterization, Biological Function, and Multifarious Therapeutic Approaches of Exosomes. *Cells* **2019**, *8*, 307. [CrossRef]
67. Noble, J.M.; Roberts, L.M.; Vidavsky, N.; Chiou, A.E.; Fischbach, C.; Paszek, M.J.; Estroff, L.A.; Kourkoutis, L.F. Direct comparison of optical and electron microscopy methods for structural characterization of extracellular vesicles. *J. Struct. Biol.* **2020**, *210*, 107474. [CrossRef]
68. Betzer, O.; Barnoy, E.; Sadan, T.; Elbaz, I.; Braverman, C.; Liu, Z.; Popovtzer, R. Advances in imaging strategies for in vivo tracking of exosomes. *WIREs Nanomed. Nanobiotechnol.* **2020**, *12*, e1594. [CrossRef]
69. Qiao, L.; Hu, S.; Huang, K.; Su, T.; Li, Z.; Vandergriff, A.; Cores, J.; Dinh, P.U.; Allen, T.; Shen, D.; et al. Tumor cell-derived exosomes home to their cells of origin and can be used as Trojan horses to deliver cancer drugs. *Theranostics* **2020**, *10*, 3474–3487. [CrossRef]
70. Smyth, T.; Kullberg, M.; Malik, N.; Smith-Jones, P.; Graner, M.W.; Anchordoquy, T.J. Biodistribution and delivery efficiency of unmodified tumor-derived exosomes. *J. Control. Release* **2015**, *199*, 145–155. [CrossRef]
71. Choi, H.; Lee, D.S. Illuminating the physiology of extracellular vesicles. *Stem Cell Res. Ther.* **2016**, *7*, 55. [CrossRef]
72. Tian, T.; Zhu, Y.L.; Hu, F.H.; Wang, Y.Y.; Huang, N.P.; Xiao, Z.D. Dynamics of exosome internalization and trafficking. *J. Cell Physiol.* **2013**, *228*, 1487–1495. [CrossRef] [PubMed]
73. Lai, C.P.; Mardini, O.; Ericsson, M.; Prabhakar, S.; Maguire, C.; Chen, J.W.; Tannous, B.A.; Breakefield, X.O. Dynamic biodistribution of extracellular vesicles in vivo using a multimodal imaging reporter. *ACS Nano* **2014**, *8*, 483–494. [CrossRef] [PubMed]

74. Perets, N.; Betzer, O.; Shapira, R.; Brenstein, S.; Angel, A.; Sadan, T.; Ashery, U.; Popovtzer, R.; Offen, D. Golden Exosomes Selectively Target Brain Pathologies in Neurodegenerative and Neurodevelopmental Disorders. *Nano Lett.* **2019**, *19*, 3422–3431. [CrossRef] [PubMed]
75. Counihan, J.L.; Grossman, E.A.; Nomura, D.K. Cancer Metabolism: Current Understanding and Therapies. *Chem. Rev.* **2018**, *118*, 6893–6923. [CrossRef] [PubMed]
76. Duan, L.; Xu, L.; Xu, X.; Qin, Z.; Zhou, X.; Xiao, Y.; Liang, Y.; Xia, J. Exosome-mediated delivery of gene vectors for gene therapy. *Nanoscale* **2021**, *13*, 1387–1397. [CrossRef]
77. Kang, Y.; Xu, C.; Meng, L.; Dong, X.; Qi, M.; Jiang, D. Exosome-functionalized magnesium-organic framework-based scaffolds with osteogenic, angiogenic and anti-inflammatory properties for accelerated bone regeneration. *Bioact. Mater.* **2022**, *18*, 26–41. [CrossRef]
78. Miroshnichenko, S.K.; Patutina, O.A.; Burakova, E.A.; Chelobanov, B.P.; Fokina, A.A.; Vlassov, V.V.; Altman, S.; Zenkova, M.A.; Stetsenko, D.A. Mesyl phosphoramidate antisense oligonucleotides as an alternative to phosphorothioates with improved biochemical and biological properties. *Proc. Natl. Acad. Sci. USA* **2019**, *116*, 1229–1234. [CrossRef]
79. Li, L.; Li, C.; Wang, S.; Wang, Z.; Jiang, J.; Wang, W.; Li, X.; Chen, J.; Liu, K.; Li, C.; et al. Exosomes Derived from Hypoxic Oral Squamous Cell Carcinoma Cells Deliver miR-21 to Normoxic Cells to Elicit a Prometastatic Phenotype. *Cancer Res.* **2016**, *76*, 1770–1780. [CrossRef]
80. Yanez-Mo, M.; Siljander, P.R.; Andreu, Z.; Zavec, A.B.; Borras, F.E.; Buzas, E.I.; Buzas, K.; Casal, E.; Cappello, F.; Carvalho, J.; et al. Biological properties of extracellular vesicles and their physiological functions. *J. Extracell. Vesicles* **2015**, *4*, 27066. [CrossRef]
81. Zheng, H.C. The molecular mechanisms of chemoresistance in cancers. *Oncotarget* **2017**, *8*, 59950–59964. [CrossRef]
82. Corn, P.G.; Heath, E.I.; Zurita, A.; Ramesh, N.; Xiao, L.; Sei, E.; Li-Ning-Tapia, E.; Tu, S.M.; Subudhi, S.K.; Wang, J.; et al. Cabazitaxel plus carboplatin for the treatment of men with metastatic castration-resistant prostate cancers: A randomised, open-label, phase 1–2 trial. *Lancet Oncol.* **2019**, *20*, 1432–1443. [CrossRef] [PubMed]
83. Huo, R.; Wang, L.; Liu, P.; Zhao, Y.; Zhang, C.; Bai, B.; Liu, X.; Shi, C.; Wei, S.; Zhang, H. Cabazitaxel-induced autophagy via the PI3K/Akt/mTOR pathway contributes to A549 cell death. *Mol. Med. Rep.* **2016**, *14*, 3013–3020. [CrossRef] [PubMed]
84. Li, Z.; Xuan, Z.; Chen, J.; Song, W.; Zhang, S.; Jin, C.; Zhou, M.; Zheng, S.; Song, P. Inhibiting the NF-kappaB pathway enhances the antitumor effect of cabazitaxel by downregulating Bcl-2 in pancreatic cancer. *Int. J. Oncol.* **2020**, *57*, 161–170. [CrossRef] [PubMed]
85. Vikas; Mehata, A.K.; Suseela, M.N.L.; Behera, C.; Kumari, P.; Mahto, S.K.; Muthu, M.S. Chitosan-alginate nanoparticles of cabazitaxel: Design, dual-receptor targeting and efficacy in lung cancer model. *Int. J. Biol. Macromol.* **2022**, *221*, 874–890. [CrossRef]
86. Di Leva, G.; Garofalo, M.; Croce, C.M. MicroRNAs in cancer. *Annu. Rev. Pathol.* **2014**, *9*, 287–314. [CrossRef]
87. Garzon, R.; Calin, G.A.; Croce, C.M. MicroRNAs in Cancer. *Annu. Rev. Med.* **2009**, *60*, 167–179. [CrossRef]
88. Shi, X.; Shiao, S.L. The role of macrophage phenotype in regulating the response to radiation therapy. *Transl. Res.* **2018**, *191*, 64–80. [CrossRef]
89. Wang, B.; Zhang, S.; Tong, F.; Wang, Y.; Wei, L. HPV(+) HNSCC-derived exosomal miR-9-5p inhibits TGF-beta signaling-mediated fibroblast phenotypic transformation through NOX4. *Cancer Sci.* **2022**, *113*, 1475–1487. [CrossRef]
90. Cai, L.; Ye, Y.; Jiang, Q.; Chen, Y.; Lyu, X.; Li, J.; Wang, S.; Liu, T.; Cai, H.; Yao, K.; et al. Epstein-Barr virus-encoded microRNA BART1 induces tumour metastasis by regulating PTEN-dependent pathways in nasopharyngeal carcinoma. *Nat. Commun.* **2015**, *6*, 7353. [CrossRef]
91. Ge, X.; Gao, J.; Sun, Q.W.; Wang, C.X.; Deng, W.; Mao, G.Y.; Li, H.Q.; Guo, S.S.; Cheng, J.; Wu, Y.N.; et al. MiR-34a inhibits the proliferation, migration, and invasion of oral squamous cell carcinoma by directly targeting SATB2. *J. Cell Physiol.* **2020**, *235*, 4856–4864. [CrossRef]
92. Roy, S.K.; Shrivastava, A.; Srivastav, S.; Shankar, S.; Srivastava, R.K. SATB2 is a novel biomarker and therapeutic target for cancer. *J. Cell Mol. Med.* **2020**, *24*, 11064–11069. [CrossRef]
93. Bai, Y.; Wang, W.; Zhang, Y.; Zhang, F.; Zhang, H. lncRNA MIAT suppression alleviates corneal angiogenesis through regulating miR-1246/ACE. *Cell Cycle* **2019**, *18*, 661–669. [CrossRef]
94. Pakravan, K.; Babashah, S.; Sadeghizadeh, M.; Mowla, S.J.; Mossahebi-Mohammadi, M.; Ataei, F.; Dana, N.; Javan, M. MicroRNA-100 shuttled by mesenchymal stem cell-derived exosomes suppresses in vitro angiogenesis through modulating the mTOR/HIF-1alpha/VEGF signaling axis in breast cancer cells. *Cell Oncol.* **2017**, *40*, 457–470. [CrossRef] [PubMed]
95. Liu, X.; Chen, Z.; Yu, J.; Xia, J.; Zhou, X. MicroRNA profiling and head and neck cancer. *Comp. Funct. Genom.* **2009**, *2009*, 837514. [CrossRef] [PubMed]
96. Manikandan, M.; Rao, A.K.D.M.; Rajkumar, K.S.; Rajaraman, R.; Munirajan, A.K. Altered levels of miR-21, miR-125b-2*, miR-138, miR-155, miR-184, and miR-205 in oral squamous cell carcinoma and association with clinicopathological characteristics. *J. Oral Pathol. Med.* **2015**, *44*, 792–800. [CrossRef] [PubMed]
97. Wong, T.S.; Liu, X.B.; Wong, B.Y.; Ng, R.W.; Yuen, A.P.; Wei, W.I. Mature miR-184 as Potential Oncogenic microRNA of Squamous Cell Carcinoma of Tongue. *Clin. Cancer Res.* **2008**, *14*, 2588–2592. [CrossRef]
98. Jin, Y.; Chen, D.; Cabay, R.J.; Wang, A.; Crowe, D.L.; Zhou, X. Role of microRNA-138 as a potential tumor suppressor in head and neck squamous cell carcinoma. *Int. Rev. Cell Mol. Biol.* **2013**, *303*, 357–385. [CrossRef]

99. Wang, H.M.; Lu, Y.J.; He, L.; Gu, N.J.; Wang, S.Y.; Qiu, X.S.; Wang, E.H.; Wu, G.P. HPV16 E6/E7 promote the translocation and glucose uptake of GLUT1 by PI3K/AKT pathway via relieving miR-451 inhibitory effect on CAB39 in lung cancer cells. *Ther. Adv. Chronic Dis.* **2020**, *11*, 2040622320957143. [CrossRef]
100. Zeng, Q.; Tao, X.; Huang, F.; Wu, T.; Wang, J.; Jiang, X.; Kuang, Z.; Cheng, B. Overexpression of miR-155 promotes the proliferation and invasion of oral squamous carcinoma cells by regulating BCL6/cyclin D2. *Int. J. Mol. Med.* **2016**, *37*, 1274–1280. [CrossRef]
101. Ahn, H.; Kim, H.; Abdul, R.; Kim, Y.; Sim, J.; Choi, D.; Paik, S.S.; Shin, S.J.; Kim, D.H.; Jang, K. Overexpression of Forkhead Box O3a and Its Association with Aggressive Phenotypes and Poor Prognosis in Human Hepatocellular Carcinoma. *Am. J. Clin. Pathol.* **2018**, *149*, 117–127. [CrossRef]
102. Tian, Y.; Qi, P.; Hu, X. Downregulated FOXO3a Associates with Poor Prognosis and Promotes Cell Invasion and Migration via WNT/beta-catenin Signaling in Cervical Carcinoma. *Front. Oncol.* **2020**, *10*, 903. [CrossRef] [PubMed]
103. Ghosh, R.D.; Ghuwalewala, S.; Das, P.; Mandloi, S.; Alam, S.K.; Chakraborty, J.; Sarkar, S.; Chakrabarti, S.; Panda, C.K.; Roychoudhury, S. MicroRNA profiling of cisplatin-resistant oral squamous cell carcinoma cell lines enriched with cancer-stem-cell-like and epithelial-mesenchymal transition-type features. *Sci. Rep.* **2016**, *6*, 23932. [CrossRef] [PubMed]
104. Zheng, R.; Liu, Y.; Zhang, X.; Zhao, P.; Deng, Q. miRNA-200c enhances radiosensitivity of esophageal cancer by cell cycle arrest and targeting P21. *Biomed Pharmacother.* **2017**, *90*, 517–523. [CrossRef] [PubMed]
105. Lu, H.; Zhang, C.; Hu, Y.; Qin, H.; Gu, A.; Li, Y.; Zhang, L.; Li, Z.; Wang, Y. miRNA-200c mediates mono-butyl phthalate-disrupted steroidogenesis by targeting vimentin in Leydig tumor cells and murine adrenocortical tumor cells. *Toxicol. Lett.* **2016**, *241*, 95–102. [CrossRef]
106. Luo, Z.; Wen, G.; Wang, G.; Pu, X.; Ye, S.; Xu, Q.; Wang, W.; Xiao, Q. MicroRNA-200C and -150 play an important role in endothelial cell differentiation and vasculogenesis by targeting transcription repressor ZEB1. *Stem Cells* **2013**, *31*, 1749–1762. [CrossRef]
107. Ma, C.; Ding, Y.C.; Yu, W.; Wang, Q.; Meng, B.; Huang, T. MicroRNA-200c overexpression plays an inhibitory role in human pancreatic cancer stem cells by regulating epithelial-mesenchymal transition. *Minerva Med.* **2015**, *106*, 193–202.
108. Chen, Y.; Sun, Y.; Chen, L.; Xu, X.; Zhang, X.; Wang, B.; Min, L.; Liu, W. miRNA-200c increases the sensitivity of breast cancer cells to doxorubicin through the suppression of E-cadherin-mediated PTEN/Akt signaling. *Mol. Med. Rep.* **2013**, *7*, 1579–1584. [CrossRef]
109. Choi, Y.J.; Lee, K.; Yoon, J.H.; Cho, S.G.; Kim, Y.G.; Jeong, M.; Hwang, H.H.; Lee, S.Y.; Jung, S.E.; Ko, S.G. SH003 and Docetaxel Show Synergistic Anticancer Effects by Inhibiting EGFR Activation in Triple-Negative Breast Cancer. *Biomed Res. Int.* **2022**, *2022*, 3647900. [CrossRef]
110. Feng, B.; Wang, R.; Song, H.Z.; Chen, L.B. MicroRNA-200b reverses chemoresistance of docetaxel-resistant human lung adenocarcinoma cells by targeting E2F3. *Cancer* **2012**, *118*, 3365–3376. [CrossRef]
111. Han, G.; Xu, C.; Yu, D. Mechanisms correlated with chemotherapy resistance in tongue cancers. *J. Cancer Res. Ther.* **2018**, *14*, 1–5. [CrossRef]
112. Jiang, Y.; Huang, W.; Sun, X.; Yang, X.; Wu, Y.; Shi, J.; Zheng, J.; Fan, S.; Liu, J.; Wang, J.; et al. DTX-P7, a peptide-drug conjugate, is highly effective for non-small cell lung cancer. *J. Hematol. Oncol.* **2022**, *15*, 73. [CrossRef] [PubMed]
113. Lee, S.H.; Lee, Y.J. Synergistic anticancer activity of resveratrol in combination with docetaxel in prostate carcinoma cells. *Nutr. Res. Pract.* **2021**, *15*, 12–25. [CrossRef] [PubMed]
114. Zhao, Z.; Wang, H.; Zhang, L.; Mei, X.; Hu, J.; Huang, K. Receptor for advanced glycation end product blockade enhances the chemotherapeutic effect of cisplatin in tongue squamous cell carcinoma by reducing autophagy and modulating the Wnt pathway. *Anti-Cancer Drugs* **2017**, *28*, 187–196. [CrossRef] [PubMed]
115. Natarajan, J.; Chandrashekar, C.; Radhakrishnan, R. Critical biomarkers of epithelial-mesenchymal transition in the head and neck cancers. *J. Cancer Res. Ther.* **2014**, *10*, 512–518. [PubMed]
116. Koide, N.; Kasamatsu, A.; Endo-Sakamoto, Y.; Ishida, S.; Shimizu, T.; Kimura, Y.; Miyamoto, I.; Yoshimura, S.; Shiiba, M.; Tanzawa, H.; et al. Evidence for Critical Role of Lymphocyte Cytosolic Protein 1 in Oral Cancer. *Sci. Rep.* **2017**, *7*, 43379. [CrossRef]
117. Czerwaty, K.; Dzaman, K.; Miechowski, W. Application of Extracellular Vesicles in Allergic Rhinitis: A Systematic Review. *Int. J. Mol. Sci.* **2022**, *24*, 367. [CrossRef]
118. Dzaman, K.; Czerwaty, K. Roles of Exosomes in Chronic Rhinosinusitis: A Systematic Review. *Int. J. Mol. Sci.* **2022**, *23*, 11284. [CrossRef]
119. Hofmann, L.; Ludwig, S.; Vahl, J.M.; Brunner, C.; Hoffmann, T.K.; Theodoraki, M.N. The Emerging Role of Exosomes in Diagnosis, Prognosis, and Therapy in Head and Neck Cancer. *Int. J. Mol. Sci.* **2020**, *21*, 4072. [CrossRef]
120. Mathew, M.; Zade, M.; Mezghani, N.; Patel, R.; Wang, Y.; Momen-Heravi, F. Extracellular Vesicles as Biomarkers in Cancer Immunotherapy. *Cancers* **2020**, *12*, 2825. [CrossRef]
121. Xiao, C.; Song, F.; Zheng, Y.L.; Lv, J.; Wang, Q.F.; Xu, N. Exosomes in Head and Neck Squamous Cell Carcinoma. *Front. Oncol.* **2019**, *9*, 894. [CrossRef]
122. Li, T.; Li, J.; Wang, H.; Zhao, J.; Yan, M.; He, H.; Yu, S. Exosomes: Potential Biomarkers and Functions in Head and Neck Squamous Cell Carcinoma. *Front. Mol. Biosci.* **2022**, *9*, 881794. [CrossRef] [PubMed]
123. Perez-Herrero, E.; Fernandez-Medarde, A. Advanced targeted therapies in cancer: Drug nanocarriers, the future of chemotherapy. *Eur. J. Pharm. Biopharm.* **2015**, *93*, 52–79. [CrossRef] [PubMed]

124. Riley, R.S.; June, C.H.; Langer, R.; Mitchell, M.J. Delivery technologies for cancer immunotherapy. *Nat. Rev. Drug Discov.* **2019**, *18*, 175–196. [CrossRef] [PubMed]
125. Tang, X.J.; Sun, X.Y.; Huang, K.M.; Zhang, L.; Yang, Z.S.; Zou, D.D.; Wang, B.; Warnock, G.L.; Dai, L.J.; Luo, J. Therapeutic potential of CAR-T cell-derived exosomes: A cell-free modality for targeted cancer therapy. *Oncotarget* **2015**, *6*, 44179–44190. [CrossRef]
126. Singh, K.; Nalabotala, R.; Koo, K.M.; Bose, S.; Nayak, R.; Shiddiky, M.J.A. Separation of distinct exosome subpopulations: Isolation and characterization approaches and their associated challenges. *Analyst* **2021**, *146*, 3731–3749. [CrossRef]
127. Maisano, D.; Mimmi, S.; Dattilo, V.; Marino, F.; Gentile, M.; Vecchio, E.; Fiume, G.; Nistico, N.; Aloisio, A.; de Santo, M.P.; et al. A novel phage display based platform for exosome diversity characterization. *Nanoscale* **2022**, *14*, 2998–3003. [CrossRef]
128. Janiak-Kiszka, J.; Nowaczewska, M.; Kazmierczak, W. Oral squamous cell carcinoma—Clinical characteristics, treatment, and outcomes in a single institution retrospective cohort study. *Otolaryngol. Pol.* **2022**, *76*, 12–17. [CrossRef]
129. Przybylski, K.; Majchrzak, E.; Weselik, L.; Golusinski, W. Immunotherapy of head and neck squamous cell carcinoma (HNSCC). Immune checkpoint blockade. *Otolaryngol. Pol.* **2018**, *72*, 10–16. [CrossRef]

pharmaceutics

MDPI

Review

Advances in the Study of Exosomes as Drug Delivery Systems for Bone-Related Diseases

Jiawen Huang [1,†], Yang Xu [1,†], Yuxuan Wang [1], Zhiang Su [2], Tingting Li [3], Sisi Wu [1], Yuheng Mao [1], Shihua Zhang [2,3], Xiquan Weng [1,2,*] and Yu Yuan [1,2,*]

1 Department of Exercise Biochemistry, Guangzhou Sport University, Guangzhou 510500, China
2 School of Exercise and Health, Guangzhou Sport University, Guangzhou 510500, China
3 School of Exercise and Health, Shanghai University of Sport, Shanghai 200438, China
* Correspondence: wengxq@gzsport.edu.cn (X.W.); yuanyumail@126.com (Y.Y.); Tel.: +86-020-3802-4222 (X.W.); +86-020-3802-4623 (Y.Y.)
† These authors contributed equally to this work.

Abstract: Bone-related diseases are major problems and heavy burdens faced by modern society. Current clinical approaches for the treatment of these pathological conditions often lead to complications and have limited therapeutic efficacy. In this context, the development of nanotherapeutic platforms, such as extracellular vesicles, can improve the relevant therapeutic effects. In particular, exosomes are nano-sized, lipid bilayer extracellular vesicles secreted by many cells in mammals. Due to their innate capacity to transport materials—including proteins, lipids, and genes—among cells, as well as their innate attraction to target cells, they are considered to be a crucial medium for cell communication and are involved in a number of biological processes. Exosomes have been used as drug delivery vehicles in recent bone tissue engineering studies, in order to regulate bone homeostasis. However, the precise workings of the exosome regulatory network in maintaining bone homeostasis and its potential for treating bone injury remain unclear. To provide a fresh perspective for the study of exosomes in drug delivery and bone-related diseases, in this paper, we review recent studies on the roles of exosomes for drug delivery in bone homeostasis and bone-related diseases, as well as the composition and characteristics of exosomes and their regulatory roles in bone homeostasis and bone-related diseases, aiming to provide new ideas for the therapeutic application of exosomes in the treatment of bone-related diseases.

Keywords: exosomes; drug delivery vehicles; bone-related diseases

Citation: Huang, J.; Xu, Y.; Wang, Y.; Su, Z.; Li, T.; Wu, S.; Mao, Y.; Zhang, S.; Weng, X.; Yuan, Y. Advances in the Study of Exosomes as Drug Delivery Systems for Bone-Related Diseases. *Pharmaceutics* **2023**, *15*, 220. https://doi.org/10.3390/pharmaceutics15010220

Academic Editor: Augusto Pessina

Received: 25 November 2022
Revised: 30 December 2022
Accepted: 3 January 2023
Published: 9 January 2023

1. Introduction

Bone is one of the most vital organs in the body, and bone cells undergo continuous transformation throughout human life. It has been shown that the occurrence and progression of bone-related diseases are related to the balance of bone formation and bone resorption [1]. Bone-related diseases, such as osteoporosis and osteoarthritis, have become a global public health problem with the increasing aging population [2], the prevalence of obesity, and sedentary lifestyles. Treatment of bone-related diseases requires high doses of oral and intravenous infusion, and excessive drug concentrations in the blood may cause secondary adverse effects in other organs and tissues. In order to prevent reaching blood intoxication levels of various drugs, it is vital to maximize the effective drug concentration distribution at the site of bone lesions. Exosomes are extensively engaged in the regulation of bone formation and bone resorption, according to numerous recently published studies [3,4]. As a part of the drug delivery system (DDS), exosomes have been frequently used in recent years to treat bone-related diseases, due to their good biocompatibility, capacity to traverse biological barriers, and ease of surface modification [5,6]. However, it is still unclear how the exosome regulation network regulates bone homeostasis and whether it can be used to treat bone-related diseases. In this review, along with the pathophysiological process, clinical symptoms, and therapeutic effects related to exosomes, we discuss the functions of exosomes for drug delivery in bone-related diseases.

2. Exosome

Origin and Composition

Over the past decade, researchers have discovered that cells from higher animals and micro-organisms can release extracellular vesicles (EVs), ranging in size from about 40 nm to a few μm [7], including exosomes, microvesicles, and apoptotic blebs [8], and these secreted vesicles belong to a family known as extracellular vesicles. EVs are released by cells under various physiological and pathological circumstances. Exosomes are nanoscale EVs derived from the endocytic pathway—a process by which cells internalize cytoplasm, macromolecules, membranes, and receptors through an endocytic vesicle after a membrane break. Initially, exosomes were found as endocytic vesicles composed of the bilayer membrane of protocells, discovered by Harding et al. [9] and Pan et al. [10]. They have also been found in various body fluids, such as plasma [11], urine [12], cerebrospinal fluid [13], saliva, and amniotic fluid [14], in follow-up studies. Of course, the potential of plant-derived nanovesicles in human health should not be under-estimated [15–17]. Vesicles can carry lipids, proteins, and nucleic acids from donor cells to recipient cells, protect their cargo contents from enzymatic degradation by the internal environment, and promote their intercellular absorption [18], thus realizing material and information exchange between cells [19]. The exosomal membrane is mainly composed of lipids and proteins, including heat-shock proteins (e.g., Hsc70, Hsp70, and Hsp90), membrane transport and fusion proteins (e.g., GTPase, annexin) [20], and proteins involved in multi-vesicle biosynthesis, which enables exosomes to specifically fuse with recipient cells and release their contents [21]. The release of exosomes into the cell requires the following steps: first, endocytic vesicles fuse with early endosomes and initiate cargo sorting. Subsequently, early endosomes develop into late endosomes, which finally rejoin lysosomes. Multivesicular bodies (MVBs), which are produced by some endosomes during the maturation process and are characterized by intraluminal vesicles (ILVs), fuse with the plasma membrane and release ILVs into the extracellular environment to form exosomes [22]. The mechanisms involved in the uptake of exosomes and how their contents enter target cells remain unclear, but what is certain is that the process involves three steps, which are: (1) EVs dock with the recipient cell through specific molecular interactions or non-specific cytokinesis. (2) Upon entry into the recipient cell, the EVs target the nuclear endosome. (3) The internalized EVs release their contents via an endosomal escape pathway. Exosomes range in size from 40 to 150 nm, and their widespread presence in bodily fluids demonstrates their stability in the extracellular environment and exhibits their potential for cell–cell communications [23] (Figure 1). As a result, exosomes are currently key delivery tools for diagnosing and curing tumors and other related diseases in clinical application.

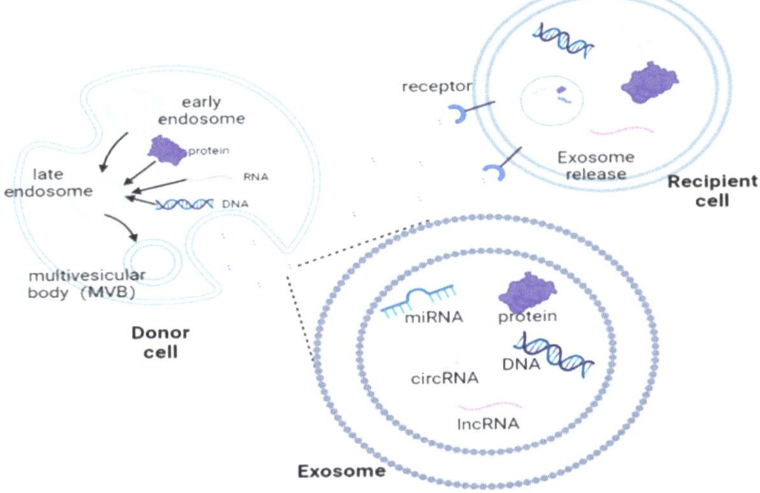

Figure 1. Exosome formation and their role in intercellular communication. Exosomes are formed from endosomes and serve as a link between cells, transporting various biologically active molecules to recipient cells.

3. Exosomes and Drug Delivery Systems

3.1. Advantages of Exosomes as Drug Delivery Vehicles

DDS have evolved in recent years. Liposome- and polymer-based systems have both received extensive study; however, general nanocarriers have limited targeting, poor stability, and are easily phagocytosed by macrophages of the reticuloendothelial system in the liver and spleen [24,25]. In comparison, exosomes are derived from the nanoscale vesicle-like structures of cells with a natural biological origin and complexity. Compared with other systems, exosomes are considered one of the most promising drug delivery carriers, due to their selectivity, safety, stability, and long-distance transport of substances. Exosomes are released into the extracellular space by fusing directly with the recipient cell's plasma membrane and transferred to the target cell by endocytosis and receptor–ligand interactions, delivering the proteins and genetic information contained therein to the target cell, along with bioactive substances [26]. These endogenous drug delivery vehicles are more adaptable to the complex environment in vivo and can successfully deliver drugs to target tissues. While improving drug efficacy, they exhibit low toxicity, low immunogenicity [27], and good biocompatibility [28], opening a new pathway for the transport of genetic and antitumor drugs.

3.2. Exosomes from Different Cells

Exosomes can be produced by almost all cells; however, not all of them can be used to carry drugs. There are strict screening requirements for exosomes that can be employed for drug administration, including surface protein, size, yield, and luminal composition. Exosomes derived from different cells can accurately target illnesses with different drugs to provide specific therapeutic effects. Mesenchymal stem cells (MSCs), immune cells, tumor cells, and certain cell lines are among the most prevalent cell sources. The choice of cell type from which the exosomes are produced is crucial in practical applications, as exosomes inherit numerous traits from their parental cells.

3.2.1. Mesenchymal Stem Cell and Bone Tissue Cells

MSCs are pluripotent stem cells mainly found in bone marrow, adipose tissue, umbilical cord, and other tissues, and are the only cell type that can sustain extensive exosome synthesis [29]. Exosomes derived from MSCs have the capacity to enhance tissue healing, control immunological response, promote cell proliferation, and enhance drug delivery. In comparison to parental cells, they exhibit minimal immunogenicity and low carcinogenic risk [30]. Exosomes derived from bone marrow mesenchymal stem cells (BMSCs) have been discovered to be able to integrate into osteoblasts and boost the expression of osteogenic genes by Qin et al. [31]. According to another study [32], exosomes produced from MSCs could directly and rapidly communicate with chondrocytes through endocytosis, and enhanced the migration of endogenous chondrocytes to defects in vitro and in vivo. Exosomes from human umbilical cord mesenchymal stem cells (UMSCs) have also been shown to successfully block the death of BMSCs in rats with disuse osteoporosis and to prevent osteoporosis through the miR-1263/Mob1/Hippo signaling pathway [33].

It has been established that the transfer of active molecules from cellular sources is essential for bone homeostasis and osteocyte function. Previous studies have revealed a close connection between exosomes and osteocytes [34,35], while recent studies have shown that nearly all osteocytes are able to produce exosomes and have a regulatory function in bone remodeling [36]. The osteogenic process relies on the delivery of exosomes, which are secreted by osteoblast precursors to promote osteogenesis before differentiation into osteoblasts [37]. It has been shown [38] that myostatin-treated osteocyte exosomes drastically down-regulated miR-218 expression. During osteoblast differentiation, miR-218 is induced, which acts to promote the differentiation of undifferentiated bone marrow cells. After being endocytosed by osteoblasts, Runx2 expression may be reduced by the Wnt signaling pathway, which prevents miR-218 from growing. However, there was no obvious change in osteoclast activity after endocytosing these exosomes, indicating that miR-218 may target osteoblasts, rather than osteoclasts, in order to take part in muscle–skeletal communication, or functions as a bone potential therapeutic target for osteoporosis.

It has been found that exosomes are widely involved in the interaction between bone-forming osteoblasts and bone-resorbing osteoclasts. The coordination of these two cells to maintain bone homeostasis under various circumstances can be demonstrated in terms of the exosomal microRNAs (miRNAs) generated by osteoblasts and osteoclasts. When osteoblasts deliver RANKL-containing exosomes to osteoclast precursors, RANKL–RANK signaling is stimulated, promoting the development of osteoclasts. This osteoblast–osteoclast intercellular communication mediated by exosomes may constitute a novel method for bone modeling and remodeling [39]. All of these results indicate the possibility that exosomes derived from MSCs play significant roles in intercellular communication between different types of bone cells.

3.2.2. Immune Cells

Another source from which exosomes can be isolated is immune cells. Exosomes derived from immune cells have immunomodulatory and therapeutic properties, and are crucial for the treatment of cancer. Immune cell-derived exosomes have attracted a lot of interest as a drug delivery platform for effective anticancer therapy, due to their outstanding biocompatibility, low immunogenicity, and high loading capacity [40]. Some researchers have found that the nanovesicles cultured with primary immune cells contain immunoglobulin, which can be used for immunotherapy [41]. Among the various immune cells, neutrophils can respond to inflammation or infection immediately, and are considered to have a dual involvement in both inflammation and malignancy [42]. According to a previous study [43], neutrophil-derived exosomes could eliminate the potential risk of neutrophil phenotype switching from N1 anti-tumoral to N2 pro-tumoral during tumor progression. Xiong et al. [44] have pointed out that M2 macrophage-derived exosomes enriched in miR-5106 could target the salt-inducible-kinase2 (SIK2) and salt-inducible-kinase3 (SIK3) genes to promote the osteogenic differentiation of BMSCs and expedite the healing of fractures. Compared with M2-exosomes, the expression of miR-5106 in M1-exosomes is significantly reduced, suggesting that M1-exosomes may have a stronger osteogenic effect. Numerous studies have demonstrated the value of exosomes derived from various immune cells for therapeutic purposes, as well as the possibility of developing vaccines based on these exosomes.

3.2.3. Tumor Cells

Exosomes derived from tumor cells are particularly crucial in immune regulation, mediating the cross-talk between malignancies and their intended targets to promote metastasis [45]. Han et al. [46] have demonstrated that it is possible to alter the tumor immune microenvironment to increase tumorigenesis, invasion, angiogenesis, and metastatic dissemination. Through the presentation of tumor antigens by exosomes to T-cells by MHC-I molecules on their surface, an immune response against the tumor is triggered. Exosomes are crucial parts of these interactions, according to previous studies [47], which have shown that the recruitment and migration of immune cells to the tumor microenvironment (TME) are regulated by dynamic signals [48]. For instance, exosomes from tumor cells are possible targets for anti-angiogenic therapy, as they are transported to endothelial cells by endocytosis to cause angiogenesis [49]. Tumor cell-derived exosomes facilitate the initial communication between the primary tumor and metastatic sites [50]. Tumor cells in many sites, including those in the prostate, lung, and breast, are prone to bone metastases and have substantial cross-talk with osteocytes in the bone microenvironment [51]. Amphiregulin (AREG) in multiple myeloma-derived exosomes results in the activation of epidermal growth factor receptor (EGFR) ligand in pre-osteoclasts and is involved in multiple myeloma-induced osteoclastogenesis [52]. This demonstrates that exosomes derived from tumor cells play a significant regulatory function in the metastatic process, and are implicated in pathways related to tumor proliferation or inhibition, bringing new research avenues for the development of oncological drugs.

The experiments mentioned above demonstrate the unquestionable potential of exosomes as therapeutic drug carriers. However, additional research is needed to fully comprehend how exosomes from various cells can be used in DDS (Figure 2).

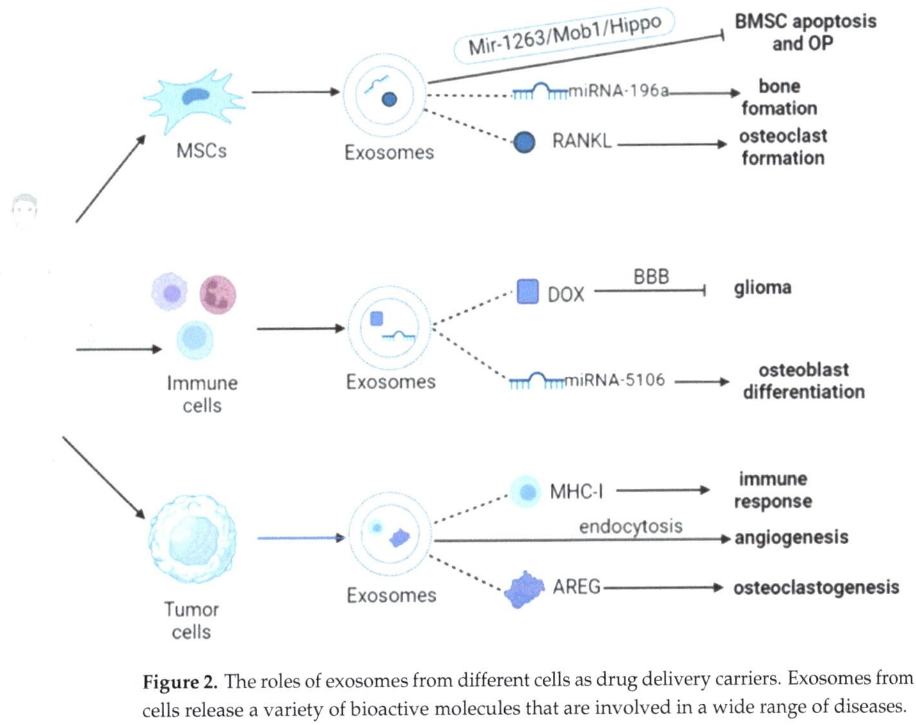

Figure 2. The roles of exosomes from different cells as drug delivery carriers. Exosomes from different cells release a variety of bioactive molecules that are involved in a wide range of diseases.

3.3. Cargo of Exosomes

Various bioactive molecules, including nucleic acids, proteins, lipids, and other small-molecule metabolites, can be carried by exosomes. These may be useful for clinical diagnosis, as they can indicate how blast cells behave and the body's metabolic state under various disease circumstances.

3.3.1. Nucleic Acid

Exosomes can transport different kinds of nucleic acids. In this review, we primarily introduce recent studies on microRNA (miRNA), long non-coding RNA (lncRNA), and circular RNA (circRNA) in relation to bone metabolism. Exosomes can transfer their cargo to target cells and regulate their growth and differentiation, as was previously described. For example, brown adipose-derived exosomes carrying specific miRNAs can influence lipid metabolism by controlling other organs [53]. It has been found [54] that reducing miR-221-3p in exosomes can significantly inhibit chondrocyte proliferation and migration in vitro. By blocking Runx2 and increasing YAP1-mediated MT1DP, exosomes produced from osteoclasts that contain miR-23a-5p may effectively limit osteogenic differentiation [55]. Exosomal miR-141-3p from MDA-PCa-2b cells also promotes osteoblast activity and regulates the bone metastasis microenvironment, which is crucial for the formation of bone metastases and osteogenesis damage in prostate cancer [56]. lncRNAs are involved in the mechanism whereby exosomes regulate bone metabolism. Studies have shown [57] that, in osteoporotic mice, the exosomal lncRNA MALAT secreted by BMSCs can increase osteoblast activity. Furthermore, the exosomal lncRNA RUNX2-AS1, which is released by multiple myeloma cells, can prevent MSCs from differentiating [58]. Accumulating evidence has indicated that circRNAs play multiple functions in the osteogenesis of BMSCs, proving to be a useful target for the therapy of bone diseases. By interacting with miR-210 and miR-335, CircRNA-0127781 may be one of the key regulators of osteoblast differentiation [59]. CircRNA-33287 has been shown to block mir-214-3p, thus enhancing the osteogenic process and activating the establishment of ectopic bone [60]. CircRNA has a circular structure, which is more stable than RNA and difficult to degrade. Although there are currently few studies on how exosomal circRNAs regulate osteogenic differentiation, this structure holds great promise for future research in exosome engineering.

3.3.2. Proteins

Apart from delivering different types of nucleic acids, exosomes can also deliver macromolecules, such as proteins. In the study of Liu et al. [61], exosomes have been found to cross the blood–brain barrier (BBB) and specifically target neurons with enkephalins. In addition to protecting the brain against ischemia-reperfusion injury and reducing the chance of negative effects, this also ensures that adequate enkephalin can reach the brain. It has been reported that exosomes containing the anti-inflammatory protein catalase were successfully administered across the BBB to treat Parkinson's disease [62]. Exosomes carrying the survivin protein, which is a crucial molecule for the detection of cancer, participate in the induction of apoptosis in the TME [63]. Bourdonnay et al. [64] have found that alveolar macrophages (Ams) release exosomes carrying the SOCS1 protein, which alveolar epithelial cells (AECs) may pick up and, thus, limit STAT1 activation and lower inflammatory signals both in vitro and in vivo. As they build up in the bone marrow, antagomir-188—which encourages osteogenic differentiation, inhibits adipogenesis differentiation, and prevents age-related bone loss—is released by CXCR4+ exosome–liposome hybrid NPs [65]. Additionally, research has shown that the PD-L1 antibody-armed exosome vaccination surface can simultaneously prevent PD-1/PD-L1 binding and activate T-cells that are specific to an antigen, in order to treat tumors in a synergistic manner [66].

3.3.3. Other Molecules

At present, exosomes can already deliver a number of chemotherapeutic drugs with greater stability and targeting to target cells. Doxorubicin may be effectively absorbed into breast cancer cells when it is enclosed by exosomes, as has been demonstrated by Tian et al. [67], which considerably improves the drug's therapeutic impact. The therapeutic efficacy of exosomes with paclitaxel formulation against pulmonary metastases has been demonstrated in a Lewis lung carcinoma mouse model [68], revealing the potential of the exosomes as a drug delivery system for the delivery of various chemotherapeutic agents to treatment-resistant cancers. In order to improve the anti-shock function of mice given lipopolysaccharide, Sun et al. [69] have discovered that combining curcumin with exosomes might dramatically increase the anti-inflammatory action of curcumin by enhancing the distribution of curcumin to specific macrophages. Stefano et al. have found that the exosomes possess the ability to carry drugs such as cisplatin [70] and acridine orange [71] into the human body, and can play a key role in the process of tumor metastasis [72].

In summary, exosomes are endogenous carriers of active molecules (e.g., nucleic acids, proteins, cytokines, and drugs), which can communicate with other cells and transfer information to particular target cells [73]. Exosome production by cells is typically elevated in many pathologies [74] and, due to the specificity of their cellular origin, exosomes in the blood can even act as biological markers of diseases.

4. Role of Exosomes as Drug Delivery Systems in Bone-Related Diseases

As mentioned above, the complex membrane composition of exosomes enables them to have high biocompatibility and stability when they function as drug delivery systems. In addition, exosomes have low immunogenicity and strong osmotic pressure in the body [75]. While delivering drugs accurately, they will not activate the body's innate or acquired immune system and, so, the drug discharge reaction after entering cells is significantly reduced. Combining the above advantages, exosomes have the ability to pass through the thick tissue barrier of the body to reach the target, transfer the molecules onto the membrane surface or into the cavity to carry out intercellular signal transmission and, finally, achieve the purpose of regulating the physiological function of the target cell [76]. Therefore, exosomes can be widely used as natural biological carriers in bone-related diseases.

4.1. Role of Exosomes as a Drug Delivery System for Osteoporosis

Osteoporosis is a systemic metabolic disease in which the dynamic balance of bone reconstruction is disrupted due to abnormal bone metabolism in vivo, resulting in altered bone microarchitecture, decreased bone density and quality, increased bone fragility, and fracture susceptibility. In recent research related to DDS, an increasing number of miRNAs, lncRNAs, and other non-coding RNAs (ncRNAs) have been found to play a crucial part in regulating mRNA translation, gene expression, and other processes through signal transmission [77]. ncRNAs have been found to be widely involved in the development and progression of osteoporosis [76,78,79]. With the discovery of ncRNAs in exosomes, the study of the mechanisms by which exosomal ncRNAs regulate bone remodeling and the role of exosomal ncRNAs in the prevention and treatment of osteoporosis is becoming valuable [80].

In the bone microenvironment, miR-27a-3p, miR-150-3p, and miR-196b-5p secreted by BMSCs promoted the expression of Runx2, Osterix, ALP, and osteocalcin, while knockdown of miR-27a-3p and miR-196b-5p increased the expression of osteoclast markers, leading to bone resorption [81,82]. Some scholars have found that BMSC-Exos carrying miR-935 could reduce the signal transducer and activator of transcription 1 (STAT1) level in osteoblasts of ovariectomized (OVX) rats, where the reduction in STAT1 promoted ALP activity and mineralization deposition in osteoblasts. In vivo studies have shown that silencing miR-935 significantly reduced bone mineral density (BMD), trabecular volume (BV/TV), trabecular number (Tb. N), trabecular thickness (Tb. Th), and increased the characterization of femoral trabecular separation (Tb. SP) [83]. Furthermore, lncRNAs also have a regulatory effect on osteogenic differentiation. Knockdown of lncRNA TCONS_00072128 significantly decreased the expression of cysteine proteases 8 (caspase-8) and osteogenic differentiation of BMSCs. In contrast, lncRNA TCONS_00072128 over-expression upgraded the expression of caspase-8 and osteogenic differentiation of BMSCs [84].

Signaling pathways are integral in the action of exosomes secreted by MSCs as vehicles for drug delivery to treat osteoporosis [85]. Researchers have discovered that BMSC-Exos activates the Wnt/β-catenin pathway to promote osteogenic differentiation, due to its being enriched in miR-196a, and delivers it to HFOB1.19 cells to inhibit Dickkopf-1 (Dkk1), a negative regulator of the Wnt/β-catenin pathway [86]. Experiments in mouse models have confirmed that the miR-19b carried by BMSC-Exos could inhibit WWP1 or Smurf2 and increase KLF5 expression through the Wnt/β-catenin signaling pathway, and that activation of the KLF5/β-catenin signaling pathway up-regulates the expression of osteogenic factors (Col I, ALP, and Runx2), and promotes the mineralization process of osteoblasts, thus stimulating osteogenesis [87]. The miR-136-5p carried by BMSC-Exos activates the Wnt/β-catenin pathway by targeting LRP4, and in vitro experiments have found that the delivery of BMSC-Exos-derived miR-136-5p to MC3T3-E1 could promote the proliferation and osteogenic differentiation of MC3T3-E1, thereby promoting osteogenesis [88].

Other tissue-derived stem cells have further impacts, in addition to the modulatory effect of exosomes secreted by BMSCs on osteoporosis. ADMSCs secrete phenotypically characterized miR-146a-containing exosomes, due to the over-expression of miR-146a in diabetic osteoporosis. Exosomes containing miR-146a can reduce the production of inflammatory cytokines in high-glucose-treated osteoclasts and inhibit bone resorption, which had the most effective effect on bone loss in diabetic osteoporotic rats [89]. It has been shown that miR-5106 is highly enriched in macrophage 2-derived exosomes (M2D-Exos), and can be transferred to BMSCs, targeting SIK2 and SIK3 genes to promote osteoblast differentiation [44]. Exosomes derived from human-induced pluripotent stem cells (iPSCs-Exos) effectively stimulated osteogenic differentiation and proliferation in OVX rats, and the effect increased with increasing exosome concentration [90].

Angiogenesis and osteogenesis are closely coupled in the process of bone remodeling. BMSC-Exos carrying miR-29a have been shown to regulate osteogenesis and angiogenesis concurrently, and a large increase in bone mass can be induced through the regulation of miR-29a on angiogenesis by targeting VASH1 [91]. In addition, by acting as an miR-106a sponge, lncRNA H19 transported by exosomes is capable of inhibiting miR-106a. While competitively binding to miR-106a, lncRNA H19 enhances Angpt1-Tie2 signal transduction, increases NO production, and promotes new blood vessel formation and bone mineralization [92]. Another study has indicated that UMSC-Exos does not directly regulate the expression of osteogenic-related genes but, rather, regulates HIF-1α to accelerate bone regeneration by mediating the stimulation of VEGF expression and angiogenic capacity [93].

In summary, exosomes derived from MSCs of different origins have presented unprecedented potential applications in the treatment and intervention of osteoporosis. Secreted exosomes can target receptor cells as part of a drug delivery system or modulate a range of signaling pathways affecting bone formation and bone angiogenesis, thus offering a fresh approach to treating osteoporosis (Figure 3).

4.2. Role of Exosomes as a Drug Delivery System for Fracture

Fractures are the most common physical trauma in humans [94]. It has been estimated that 5–10% of fractures may result in non-union of the fracture, thus adding a longer return to function for patients, causing them a greater financial burden and leading to a waste of medical resources [95]. Fracture healing is a complex physiological process involving the coordinated involvement of multiple cells. A moderate inflammatory response precedes fracture healing, but overactive and persistent inflammation can lead to tissue damage and delay the fracture healing process, while adequate fracture healing can be promoted by suppressing locally over-active immune cells at the fracture site. PD-L1 from exosomes of human umbilical vein endothelial cells (HUVECs) encapsulated in hydrogels promoted tissue formation and healing of fractures in a mouse model of early inflammatory hyperactivity [96].

Recent studies have shown that exosomes play significant roles in the regulation of fracture repair [97]. Based on the continued development of regenerative medicine and bone tissue engineering approaches, MSCs are becoming increasingly promising and attractive as a medium for fracture repair. Recent evidence has suggested that MSC-derived exosomes can provide an effective therapeutic strategy for bone repair [98].

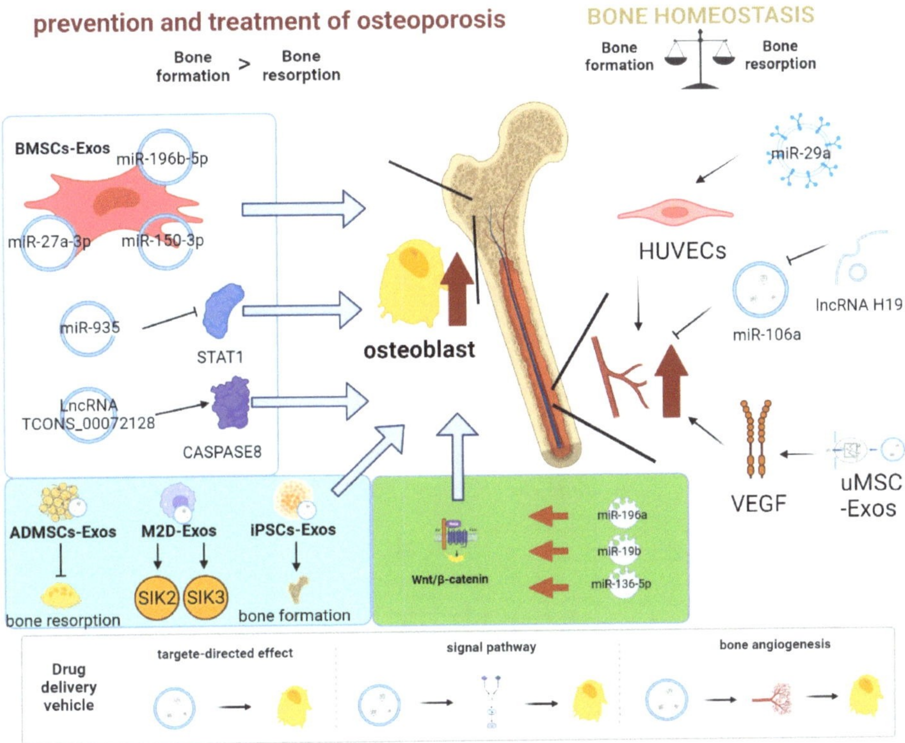

Figure 3. Exosomes act as drug delivery systems in osteoporosis. Exosomes can carry bioactive molecules that act directly on osteoblasts and promote osteoblast proliferation through signaling pathways, while bone angiogenesis also provides a way to prevent osteoporosis.

Numerous studies have shown that exosomes are a new factor of paracrine signaling in BMSCs, playing an important role in tissue repair processes [37]. BMSCs-Exos significantly enhanced the osteogenic differentiation of BMSCs in vitro. Intravenous administration of the MSC–Exo–Aptamer complex in mice has been found to enhance bone mass in OVX rats and accelerate bone healing in a mouse model of femur fracture [99]. Furthermore, in a rat model of non-union, noggin and LDN193189—inhibitors of BMP-2—were used and BMSCs-Exos were found to significantly promote osteogenesis, angiogenesis, and bone healing processes in the rat femur [100]. In a study of BMSC-Exos for the treatment of obesity-induced fractures, miR-467 was found to function as a regulatory molecule for lncRNA H19 and Hoxa10 and to improve fracture healing [101].

The paracrine effect of BMSCs can also be enhanced under hypoxic conditions. It has been demonstrated that BMSCs-Exos under hypoxic (sub-Exos) conditions promote angiogenesis, proliferation, and migration more strongly than exosomes, and that a reduction in the amount of hypoxia-inducible factor 1 (HIF-1α) leads to a substantial decrease in miR-126 in BMSCs and exosomes, thereby eliminating the role of sub-Exos, thus also demonstrating that sub-Exos promotes fracture healing through miR-126 [97].

It has been found that UMSCs not only participate in fracture repair through signaling pathways in addition to BMSCs-Exos, but also promote angiogenesis for fracture healing. By injecting UMSC-Exos into the fracture sites of Sprague Dawley (SD) rats, we have previously observed better bone apposition and continuity of cortical bone; increased protein expression levels of Wnt3a and β-catenin in the Wnt signaling pathway; and significantly higher expression levels of COL-1, OPN, and RUNX2. All of these results demonstrate that UMSC-Exos may be involved in fracture repair in rats through the Wnt signaling pathway [102]. In a rat femur fracture model, it has also been found that UMSC-Exos significantly promoted angiogenesis and bone healing [93]. Additionally, ADSC-Exos function as an immunomodulator in the treatment of bone-related diseases. ADSC-Exos-derived miR-451a has been shown to inhibit macrophage migration inhibitory factor (MIF), which can promote the M1 to M2 polarization of macrophages, inhibit inflammation, and simultaneously accelerate bone healing [103].

In addition, experts have developed a cocktail therapy that simultaneously regulates the balance of M1/M2 macrophages and osteoblasts/osteoclasts, consisting of a natural polymer hyaluronic acid hydrogel, an engineered endothelial cell-derived exosome (EC-ExosmiR-26a-5p), and the IRE-1α inhibitor APY29; their results also showed that the cocktail therapy acts to promote fracture repair [104].

In summary, as a natural biological carrier for drug delivery, exosomes not only can improve fracture healing by promoting osteogenic differentiation through paracrine activation, but also enhance bone healing through signaling pathways and bone angiogenesis. The exosomes secreted by stem cells in a hypoxic environment have a more obvious effect on fracture recovery, which also provides a new idea for promoting fracture healing in the future (Figure 4).

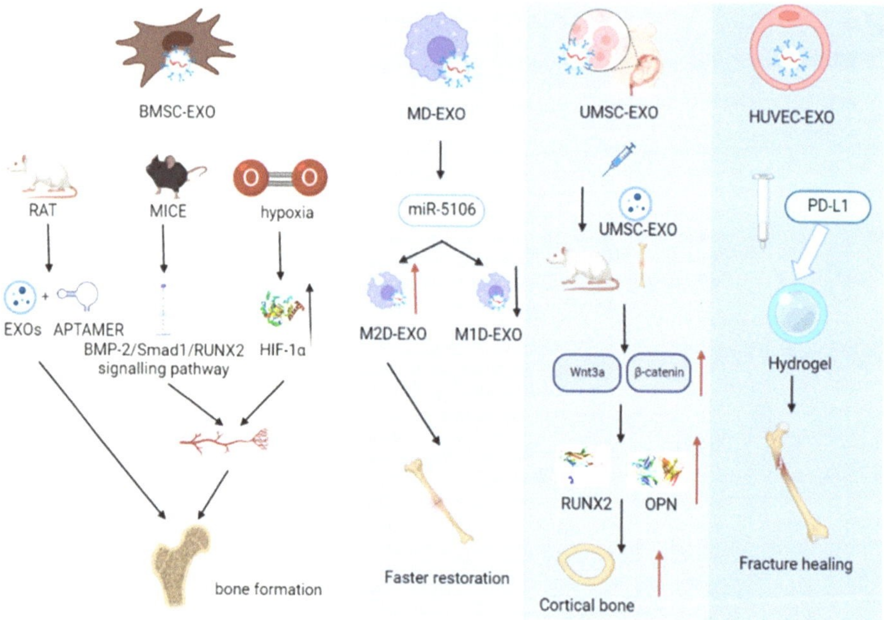

Figure 4. Exosomes act as drug delivery systems in fractures. Exosomes secreted from different stem cells can lead to osteogenic differentiation and promote bone healing.

4.3. Role of Exosomes as Drug Delivery Systems for Osteoarthritis

Osteoarthritis is a prevalent chronic joint disease, characterized by secondary bone hyperplasia and degenerative changes in the articular cartilage. An aging population and more patients with obesity are becoming more prominent with socio-economic development, leading to a gradual rise in the incidence of osteoarthritis [105]. The habits and lifestyles of patients are greatly impacted by osteoarthritis, which significantly interferes with their daily lives. Non-steroidal anti-inflammatory drugs (NSAIDs) are now widely used in medical settings; however, their effects are primarily focused on pain relief, which lessens patient discomfort, rather than cartilage regeneration, eventually resulting in further deterioration of the joints [106]. With the continuous development of regenerative medicine, a large number of studies have found that stem cells can be used to repair tissues or organs, especially stem cell-derived exosomes [106].

Exosomes, as key vehicles for intercellular signal transmission, provide a more advantageous way to evaluate the pathological cells or tissue morphology in osteoarthritis [107]. In addition to promoting angiogenesis, bone remodeling, and chondrocyte proliferation and migration, exosomes can inhibit osteoarthritic chondrocyte apoptosis and reduce cartilage inflammation [107]. Therefore, exosomes derived from BMSCs, adipose mesenchymal stem cells (AMSCs), synovial mesenchymal stem cells (SMSCs), human embryonic stem cells (HESCs), and other types of MSCs can be used as DDS to treat osteoarthritis [108] (Figure 5).

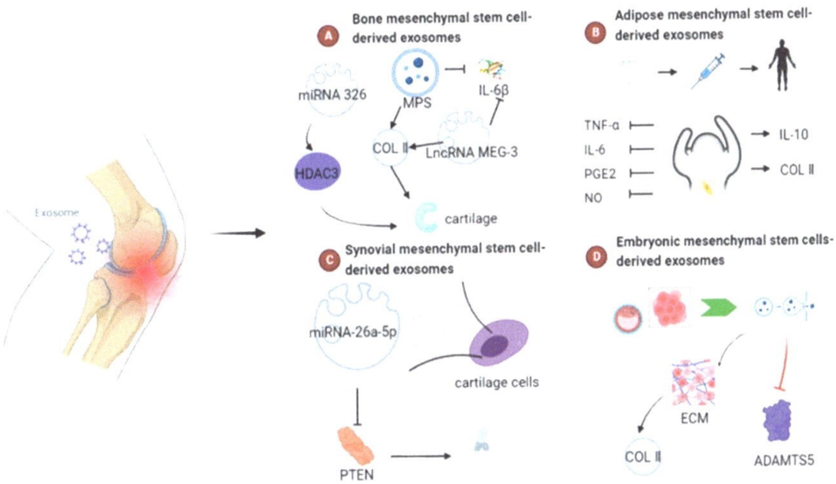

Figure 5. Role of exosomes as drug delivery systems for osteoarthritis. Exosomes derived from different mesenchymal stem cells can be used as DDS to treat osteoarthritis.

4.3.1. Bone Mesenchymal Stem Cell-Derived Exosomes

Using a rat model of osteoarthritis, researchers have found that BMSCs and BMSC-Exos both improved joint cavity and articular cartilage of osteoarthritis rats, alleviated articular cartilage and joint site damages, and restored trabecular bone volume fraction and trabecular bone number in osteoarthritis rats. Additionally, in vitro studies have revealed that BMSC-Exos carrying lncRNA MEG-3 potentially prevent interleukin-1 (IL-1)-induced senescence and apoptosis, while enhancing the production of type II collagen to retain the chondrocyte phenotype [109]. BMSC-Exos have also been found, by He et al. [110], to efficiently stimulate cartilage regeneration and extracellular matrix formation while reducing knee joint discomfort in osteoarthritis rats. Their study also indicated that BMSC-Exos carrying lncRNA MEG-3 has an anti-osteoarthritis targeting effect. Meanwhile, another researcher has discovered that the inhibitory effect of IL-1β on chondrocyte proliferation and migration was dramatically reduced by exosome administration. Exosome pre-treatment considerably reduced the effects of IL-1β on the down-regulation of COL2A1 and ACAN, as well as the up-regulation of matrix metallopeptidase 13 (MMP13) and a disintegrin and metalloproteinase with thrombospondin motifs 5 (ADAMTS5) [110].

In addition to BMSCs-Exos acting in osteoarthritis, the exosomes themselves can act as drug delivery vehicles to deliver miRNAs to chondrocytes and improve the symptoms of osteoarthritis. Exosomal miR-326 generated from BMSCs can target histone deacetylase 3 (HDAC3) and STAT1//NF-kB p65 to prevent chondrocyte and cartilage from pyroptosizing, transfer mir-326 to chondrocytes and cartilage, and reduce the symptoms of osteoarthritis [111]. Studies have suggested that E2F2 is an important member of the E2F family of transcription factors, which are involved in cell proliferation, differentiation, and apoptosis processes [112]. miR-125a-5p has the ability to accelerate chondrocyte migration, and exosomal miR-125a-5p produced by BMSCs enhances chondrocyte migration while inhibiting cartilage degradation by targeting E2F in traumatic osteoarthritis cartilage tissue [113].

Some researchers have also found that TGF-β is an effective inducer of chondrocyte anabolism, and BMSCs-Exos treated with TGFβ3 significantly up-regulated the expression of chondrogenic genes (COL1, COL2B, and ACAN) in osteoarthritis and down-regulated inflammatory marker genes (MMP-13, ADAMTS5, and iNOS), which protected chondrocytes from apoptosis and inhibited macrophage activation; therefore, they presented cartilage-protective and anti-inflammatory properties, preventing the development of osteoarthritis in mice [114]. It is thus reasonable to believe that exosomes derived from BMSCs have promising potential for the development of osteoarthritis treatment through drug delivery.

4.3.2. Adipose Mesenchymal Stem Cell-Derived Exosomes

Regarding the use of regenerative therapies, it has been demonstrated that AMSCs are able to heal damaged cartilage in osteoarthritis due to their chondrogenic potential, capacity for self-renewal, and immunomodulatory properties [115,116]. Therefore, they are considered to be a preferable cell source for osteoarthritis treatment.

Exosomes have been shown to act as a mediator for the paracrine function of AMSCs, which decreased the generation of inflammatory mediators, by Tofino Vian et al. [117]. In a 6-month experiment [118], in which 12 patients (MSC group) were given AMSCs and compared with 12 patients (control group) whose knees were injected with normal saline, the changes in cartilage defects after injection were evaluated by magnetic resonance imaging (MRI). The MRI results indicated that cartilage defects in the MSC group had no significant changes at 6 months, while cartilage defects in the control group increased. For outpatient patients with knee osteoarthritis, intra-articular injections of autologous AMSCs provided acceptable functional improvement and pain relief.

Furthermore, AMSC-Exos boost anti-inflammatory cytokines while lowering the production of inflammatory mediators, among which annexin A1—a component of exosomes—may participate in the anti-inflammatory process. In the chondrocytes in osteoarthritis, exosomes have been shown to reduce inflammatory mediators such as tumor necrosis factor-α (TNF-α), IL-6, prostaglandin E2 (PGE2), and NO [117]. The down-regulation of cyclooxygenase 2 (COX-2) and microsomal prostaglandin E synthase 1 (mPGES-1) can reduce the production of PGE2, and the effect on NO may be contingent on a decrease in the expression of inducible NO synthase. Treatment of osteoarthritis with extracellular vesicles also reduced MMP activity and the expression of MMP-13, while the production of the anti-inflammatory cytokine IL-10 and the expression of col II was markedly increased. These results suggest that exosomes from AMSCs have prospective treatment potential for osteoarthritis.

4.3.3. Synovial Mesenchymal Stem Cell-Derived Exosomes

The synovium is an essential part of the synovial joint, which contributes significantly to the maintenance of articular cartilage homeostasis. Several studies have shown that the number and composition of synovial interstitial-derived exosomes may change in joint diseases, and that exosomes derived from SMSCs may also be used in the treatment of osteoarthritis.

Synovial mesenchymal stem cell-derived exosomes (SMSC-Exos) have been shown [119] to significantly promote cartilage regeneration and inhibit the development of osteoarthritis. SMSC-Exos carrying miR-26a-5p have been shown to inhibit PTEN, thereby suppressing cell apoptosis, inflammation, and improving cartilage damage in osteoarthritis [120]. It also activates the Yes-associated protein by dephosphorylating and reducing extracellular matrix secretion, as well as inducing articular chondrocyte proliferation and migration through Wnt5a and Wnt5b signaling [121].

In a different set of studies, induced pluripotent stem cell-derived-exosomes MSCs (iMSCs-Exos) and SMSC-Exos were injected into the joints in a collagenase-induced osteoarthritis model. The results showed that both iMSC-Exos and SMSC-Exos stimulated the migration and proliferation of chondrocytes, where iMSC-Exos played a stronger role [119].

4.3.4. Other Sources of Mesenchymal Stem Cells

The exosomes secreted from embryonic mesenchymal stem cells have been shown to attenuate the development of osteoarthritis by regulating the balance between the production of cartilage matrix and degeneration. Embryonic stem cells can enhance the expression level of Col II in the cartilage matrix and reduce the expression of ADAMTS5, providing a new target for the development of osteoarthritis drugs and drug delivery systems [122].

Induced pluripotent stem cells (iPSCs) have certain effects on osteoarthritis, as they have the potential to simulate diseases and can be applied to clinical environments [123], being similar to embryonic stem cells in structure, self-regeneration, and specialization [124].

At the same time, the exosomes targeting chondrocytes have been used as carriers to deliver miR-140 to chondrocytes as a new method to treat osteoarthritis. CAP-Exos, which can successfully wrap miR-140 and enter into and distribute miR-140 in chondrocytes in vitro, are created by combining the chondrocyte affinity peptide (CAP) with the lysosomal associated membrane glycoprotein 2b protein on the surface of exosomes. After intra-articular injection, CAP-Exos remain in the joints, compared to unlabeled exosome vesicles, and internal diffusion is negligible. Additionally, CAP-Exos potentially blocked cartilage breakdown protease, transferred miR-140 to the deep cartilage area through thick medium cartilage, and slowed the course of osteoarthritis in a rat model [125].

4.4. *Role of Exosomes as Drug Delivery Systems for Osteosarcoma*

Osteosarcoma, one of the most common primary bone cancers in adolescents, is basically derived from primitive mesenchymal stem cells. The age distribution of osteosarcoma is bimodal, with the first peak occurring at 15–19 years and the second peak occurring at 75–79 years [126]. Notably, males are more frequently affected than females, in general.

Exosomes are essential in tumorigenesis, proliferation, metastasis, anti-apoptosis, immune evasion, and chemotherapy resistance in osteosarcoma [127]. Mesenchymal stem cells communicate with other cells through pathways including EVs. Due to their unique properties, MSCs-derived exosomes (MSC-Exos) can be altered and processed into effective biological carriers, loaded with drugs, transfected with anticancer genes, and employed for targeted therapy of osteosarcoma [128]. Experiments have further demonstrated that the targeting ability of exosomes is due to the chemotaxis of MSC-Exos to osteosarcoma cells by the SDF1-CXCR4 axis [129]. It has been reported that exosomes isolated from MSCs can be used as drug nanocarriers to load the chemotherapeutic drug doxorubicin (DOX), and that the exosome-loaded doxorubicin (Exo-DOX) could be taken up by MG63 cells, thus inducing cell death. Therefore, the modified MSC-Exos can serve as an excellent nanocarrier to target the tumor site and have a better anti-cancer impact [130].

In the area of in vivo drug administration, MSC-Exos offer significant research potential and a wide range of application possibilities, which can lead to novel research techniques and concepts for cancer therapy. However, relevant research is still at the pre-clinical stage, and more fundamental research is required to elucidate the related molecular mechanisms [131].

Exosomes have been shown to regulate the development of osteosarcoma as part of drug delivery, and can positively affect osteosarcoma through signaling pathways such as Wnt/β-catenin, ERK1/2, and JAK2/STAT3. Sha et al. [132] have discovered that Hic-5 could regulate the Wnt/β-catenin signaling pathway through exosomes [133], thereby inhibiting the proliferation of osteosarcoma cells. Exosomal miR-208a derived from the BMSC has been shown to negatively target programmed cell death protein 4 (PDCD4) in order to activate the ERK1/2 signaling pathway, thus promoting the proliferation, migration, and invasion of osteosarcoma cells [127]. It has been reported [134] that lymphocyte cytoplasmic protein 1 (LCP1) in BMSC-Exos promotes the progression of osteosarcoma through the JAK2/STAT3 pathway, suggesting that targeting LCP1 may provide a means to treat osteosarcoma.

Some miRNAs are widely involved in the regulation of osteosarcoma through exosome-based drug delivery systems. By affecting apoptosis-related genes and signaling pathways, including the mitochondrial apoptosis route, the death receptor pathway, and the endoplasmic reticulum system, miRNAs can control the apoptosis of osteosarcoma cells. Exosomes can be viewed as a useful technique for the early diagnosis of osteosarcoma [135], as these aberrant miRNAs can be stored and distributed through exosomes. During the progression of osteosarcoma, miRNAs can be delivered to osteosarcoma cells by exosomes derived from non-tumor cells such as MSCs and AMSCs. It has been observed [136] that miR-206 may be carried by and transported to osteosarcoma cells by BMSC-Exos. Results from both in vitro and in vivo experiments have indicated that BMSC-Exos carrying miR-206 may prevent osteosarcoma cells from proliferating, migrating, and invading, as well as inducing apoptosis in osteosarcoma cells. BMSC-Exos containing miR-206 inhibited the progression of osteosarcoma by targeting transformer 2β (TRA2B) [137]. It has also been shown that synthetic miR-143 introduced into cells was encapsulated and released by exosomes, and miR-143 formed by secreted exosomes was transferred to osteosarcoma cells and prevented the 143B osteosarcoma cell line from migrating.

Moreover, CASC15 is a novel tumor-related lncRNA, the abnormal expression of which has been reported in a variety of tumors, demonstrating that CASC15 is up-regulated in plasma exosomes of patients with osteosarcoma, while CASC15 knockdown can inhibit the progression of osteosarcoma by targeting the miR-338-3p/RAB14 axis. As a possible new therapeutic target for the treatment of osteosarcoma, the exosomal lncRNA LIPR-AS1, which is produced by macrophages, can increase osteosarcoma cell proliferation and invasion while decreasing cell apoptosis [138].

The engineering of AMSCs to secrete miR-101-enriched EVs has been shown to provide effective results. These EVs exert inhibitory effects on cell invasion and migration in vitro once they have been taken up by osteosarcoma cells. Experimental data have supported the function of miR-101 as an osteosarcoma tumor suppressor by down-regulating B-cell lymphoma 6 (BCL6). AMSC-derived miR-101-enriched EVs represent a potential innovative therapy and promising circulating biomarker for metastatic osteosarcoma [139]. These results provide a novel method for the therapy of osteosarcoma, in which exosomes are secreted by other cells and contain specific substances to slow the growth of the disease and exert therapeutic effects on osteosarcoma cells.

Overall, the existing evidence indicates that exosomes, as cellular communication molecules, are very promising for the targeted therapy of osteosarcoma. To date, numerous studies have focused on the role of exosomes derived from MSCs in this context. As exosomes can be derived from a variety of cells, future studies should continue to expand research regarding the source, effectiveness, and specific mechanisms of various exosomes.

5. Conclusions and Future Prospect

Within the last decade, exosomes have been extensively studied as key mediators of intercellular communication. The contents of exosomes, such as lipids, proteins, and genetic material, have shown great potential for the diagnosis and treatment of bone-related diseases. Studies have indicated that exosomes may have advantages as drug carriers, in terms of biocompatibility, stability, and intrinsic targeting, as they have been found to promote angiogenesis, osteoblast differentiation, and bone tissue regeneration through a variety of signaling pathways; however, their use in drug delivery systems is still in its infancy. The majority of research on exosomes is still focused on cellular and animal models and lacks clinical applications. Most experiments with exosomes in animal models are still conducted using tail vein injection; however, the ability of this method to effectively deliver exosomes to the lesion remains to be investigated. Due to the limitations of the production process, the extraction efficiency of exosomes is low. Additionally, some technical, functional, and safety issues regarding exosome-based drug formulations remain unresolved, and there is still a long way to go from laboratory studies to clinical applications.

Nevertheless, it is good to know that, with the rapid expansion of research on exosomes in bone homeostasis, we now have a better understanding of the pathogenesis and treatment of exosomes in bone-related diseases. Exosomal drug delivery methods are anticipated to have greater therapeutic results for a variety of ailments as innovation advances. Likewise, it is anticipated that the miRNA, lncRNA, and proteins carried by exosomes generated from cells related to bone may serve as possible bone markers to assess and identify disorders connected to bone. In addition, in view of the current threat of COVID-19, some people have advocated for the use of extracellular vesicles to treat COVID-19 and even support stem cell therapy and exosome products derived from the umbilical cord, amniotic fluid, and other sources, which they believe can both prevent and treat COVID-19. The wide range of actions of exosomes must be further investigated in the future, in order to provide further possibilities for study in the disciplines of biomedicine and biomaterials, given the significant potential of exosomes for drug delivery in drug therapy.

Author Contributions: Conceptualization, J.H. and Y.X.; writing—original draft preparation, J.H., Y.X., Y.W. and Z.S.; writing—review and editing, J.H., Y.X., S.W., T.L., Y.M. and S.Z.; writing—review and funding acquisition, X.W. and Y.Y. All authors have read and agreed to the published version of the manuscript.

Funding: This work was supported by the National Natural Science Foundation of China (No. 81901430), the Guangdong Provincial Natural Science Foundation of China (No. 2022A1515010379), the Guangdong Provincial Key Laboratory of Physical Activity and Health Promotion (2021B1212040014), and the Innovation Project from Department of Education of Guangdong Province (No. 2021KTSCX055).

Institutional Review Board Statement: Not applicable.

Informed Consent Statement: Not applicable.

Data Availability Statement: Not applicable.

Acknowledgments: We thank Linzhen Rao, Keping Zhang, and Yuting He (Guangzhou Sport University, Guangzhou, China) for their kind help in revising the manuscript.

Conflicts of Interest: The authors declare no conflict of interest.

References

1. Shi, C.; Wu, T.; He, Y.; Zhang, Y.; Fu, D. Recent advances in bone-targeted therapy. *Pharmacol. Ther.* **2020**, *207*, 107473. [CrossRef] [PubMed]
2. Rachner, T.D.; Khosla, S.; Hofbauer, L.C. Osteoporosis: Now and the future. *Lancet* **2011**, *377*, 1276–1287. [CrossRef] [PubMed]
3. Wang, W.; Qiao, S.C.; Wu, X.B.; Sun, B.; Yang, J.G.; Li, X.; Zhang, X.; Qian, S.J.; Gu, Y.X.; Lai, H.C. Circ_0008542 in osteoblast exosomes promotes osteoclast-induced bone resorption through m6A methylation. *Cell Death Dis.* **2021**, *12*, 628. [CrossRef] [PubMed]
4. Zhu, S.; Yao, F.; Qiu, H.; Zhang, G.; Xu, H.; Xu, J. Coupling factors and exosomal packaging microRNAs involved in the regulation of bone remodelling. *Biol. Rev. Camb. Philos. Soc.* **2018**, *93*, 469–480. [CrossRef] [PubMed]
5. Zheng, M.; Huang, M.; Ma, X.; Chen, H.; Gao, X. Harnessing Exosomes for the Development of Brain Drug Delivery Systems. *Bioconjug. Chem.* **2019**, *30*, 994–1005. [CrossRef] [PubMed]
6. Liu, C.; Su, C. Design strategies and application progress of therapeutic exosomes. *Theranostics* **2019**, *9*, 1015–1028. [CrossRef]
7. Logozzi, M.; Di Raimo, R.; Mizzoni, D.; Fais, S. What we know on the potential use of exosomes for nanodelivery. *Semin. Cancer Biol.* **2022**, *86*, 13–25. [CrossRef]
8. Bunggulawa, E.J.; Wang, W.; Yin, T.; Wang, N.; Durkan, C.; Wang, Y.; Wang, G. Recent advancements in the use of exosomes as drug delivery systems. *J. Nanobiotechnol.* **2018**, *16*, 81. [CrossRef]
9. Harding, C.; Heuser, J.; Stahl, P. Receptor-mediated endocytosis of transferrin and recycling of the transferrin receptor in rat reticulocytes. *J. Cell Biol.* **1983**, *97*, 329–339. [CrossRef]
10. Pan, B.T.; Teng, K.; Wu, C.; Adam, M.; Johnstone, R.M. Electron microscopic evidence for externalization of the transferrin receptor in vesicular form in sheep reticulocytes. *J. Cell Biol.* **1985**, *101*, 942–948. [CrossRef]

11. Caby, M.P.; Lankar, D.; Vincendeau-Scherrer, C.; Raposo, G.; Bonnerot, C. Exosomal-like vesicles are present in human blood plasma. *Int. Immunol.* **2005**, *17*, 879–887. [CrossRef]
12. Raj, D.A.; Fiume, I.; Capasso, G.; Pocsfalvi, G. A multiplex quantitative proteomics strategy for protein biomarker studies in urinary exosomes. *Kidney Int.* **2012**, *81*, 1263–1272. [CrossRef] [PubMed]
13. Street, J.M.; Barran, P.E.; Mackay, C.L.; Weidt, S.; Balmforth, C.; Walsh, T.S.; Chalmers, R.T.; Webb, D.J.; Dear, J.W. Identification and proteomic profiling of exosomes in human cerebrospinal fluid. *J. Transl. Med.* **2012**, *10*, 5. [CrossRef]
14. Keller, S.; Ridinger, J.; Rupp, A.K.; Janssen, J.W.; Altevogt, P. Body fluid derived exosomes as a novel template for clinical diagnostics. *J. Transl. Med.* **2011**, *9*, 86. [CrossRef]
15. Logozzi, M.; Di Raimo, R.; Mizzoni, D.; Fais, S. The Potentiality of Plant-Derived Nanovesicles in Human Health-A Comparison with Human Exosomes and Artificial Nanoparticles. *Int. J. Mol. Sci.* **2022**, *23*, 4919. [CrossRef]
16. Logozzi, M.; Di Raimo, R.; Mizzoni, D.; Fais, S. Nanovesicles from Organic Agriculture-Derived Fruits and Vegetables: Characterization and Functional Antioxidant Content. *Int. J. Mol. Sci.* **2021**, *22*, 8170. [CrossRef] [PubMed]
17. Karamanidou, T.; Tsouknidas, A. Plant-Derived Extracellular Vesicles as Therapeutic Nanocarriers. *Int. J. Mol. Sci.* **2021**, *23*, 191. [CrossRef] [PubMed]
18. Ratajczak, J.; Miekus, K.; Kucia, M.; Zhang, J.; Reca, R.; Dvorak, P.; Ratajczak, M.Z. Embryonic stem cell-derived microvesicles reprogram hematopoietic progenitors: Evidence for horizontal transfer of mRNA and protein delivery. *Leukemia* **2006**, *20*, 847–856. [CrossRef] [PubMed]
19. Zaborowski, M.P.; Balaj, L.; Breakefield, X.O.; Lai, C.P. Extracellular Vesicles: Composition, Biological Relevance, and Methods of Study. *Bioscience* **2015**, *65*, 783–797. [CrossRef] [PubMed]
20. Hsu, M.T.; Wang, Y.K.; Tseng, Y.J. Exosomal Proteins and Lipids as Potential Biomarkers for Lung Cancer Diagnosis, Prognosis, and Treatment. *Cancers* **2022**, *14*, 732. [CrossRef]
21. Yang, T.; Martin, P.; Fogarty, B.; Brown, A.; Schurman, K.; Phipps, R.; Yin, V.P.; Lockman, P.; Bai, S. Exosome delivered anticancer drugs across the blood-brain barrier for brain cancer therapy in Danio rerio. *Pharm. Res.* **2015**, *32*, 2003–2014. [CrossRef] [PubMed]
22. Hessvik, N.P.; Llorente, A. Current knowledge on exosome biogenesis and release. *Cell Mol. Life Sci.* **2018**, *75*, 193–208. [CrossRef]
23. Gholizadeh, S.; Shehata Draz, M.; Zarghooni, M.; Sanati-Nezhad, A.; Ghavami, S.; Shafiee, H.; Akbari, M. Microfluidic approaches for isolation, detection, and characterization of extracellular vesicles: Current status and future directions. *Biosens. Bioelectron.* **2017**, *91*, 588–605. [CrossRef] [PubMed]
24. Salvage, J.P.; Thom, C.; Lewis, A.L.; Phillips, G.J.; Lloyd, A.W. Nanoprecipitation of polymeric nanoparticle micelles based on 2-methacryloyloxyethyl phosphorylcholine (MPC) with 2-(diisopropylamino)ethyl methacrylate (DPA), for intracellular delivery applications. *J. Mater. Sci. Mater. Med.* **2015**, *26*, 150. [CrossRef] [PubMed]
25. Peer, D.; Karp, J.M.; Hong, S.; Farokhzad, O.C.; Margalit, R.; Langer, R. Nanocarriers as an emerging platform for cancer therapy. *Nat. Nanotechnol.* **2007**, *2*, 751–760. [CrossRef] [PubMed]
26. Reza-Zaldivar, E.E.; Hernandez-Sapiens, M.A.; Minjarez, B.; Gutierrez-Mercado, Y.K.; Marquez-Aguirre, A.L.; Canales-Aguirre, A.A. Potential Effects of MSC-Derived Exosomes in Neuroplasticity in Alzheimer's Disease. *Front. Cell Neurosci.* **2018**, *12*, 317. [CrossRef] [PubMed]
27. Fais, S.; Logozzi, M.; Lugini, L.; Federici, C.; Azzarito, T.; Zarovni, N.; Chiesi, A. Exosomes: The ideal nanovectors for biodelivery. *Biol. Chem.* **2013**, *394*, 1–15. [CrossRef] [PubMed]
28. Yong, T.; Wang, D.; Li, X.; Yan, Y.; Hu, J.; Gan, L.; Yang, X. Extracellular vesicles for tumor targeting delivery based on five features principle. *J. Control. Release* **2020**, *322*, 555–565. [CrossRef]
29. Yeo, R.W.; Lai, R.C.; Zhang, B.; Tan, S.S.; Yin, Y.; Teh, B.J.; Lim, S.K. Mesenchymal stem cell: An efficient mass producer of exosomes for drug delivery. *Adv. Drug Deliv. Rev.* **2013**, *65*, 336–341. [CrossRef]
30. Rani, S.; Ryan, A.E.; Griffin, M.D.; Ritter, T. Mesenchymal Stem Cell-derived Extracellular Vesicles: Toward Cell-free Therapeutic Applications. *Mol. Ther.* **2015**, *23*, 812–823. [CrossRef]
31. Qin, Y.; Wang, L.; Gao, Z.; Chen, G.; Zhang, C. Bone marrow stromal/stem cell-derived extracellular vesicles regulate osteoblast activity and differentiation in vitro and promote bone regeneration in vivo. *Sci. Rep.* **2016**, *6*, 21961. [CrossRef] [PubMed]
32. Zhang, S.; Chuah, S.J.; Lai, R.C.; Hui, J.H.P.; Lim, S.K.; Toh, W.S. MSC exosomes mediate cartilage repair by enhancing proliferation, attenuating apoptosis and modulating immune reactivity. *Biomaterials* **2018**, *156*, 16–27. [CrossRef] [PubMed]
33. Yang, B.C.; Kuang, M.J.; Kang, J.Y.; Zhao, J.; Ma, J.X.; Ma, X.L. Human umbilical cord mesenchymal stem cell-derived exosomes act via the miR-1263/Mob1/Hippo signaling pathway to prevent apoptosis in disuse osteoporosis. *Biochem. Biophys. Res. Commun.* **2020**, *524*, 883–889. [CrossRef] [PubMed]
34. Helfrich, M.H.; Nesbitt, S.A.; Lakkakorpi, P.T.; Barnes, M.J.; Bodary, S.C.; Shankar, G.; Mason, W.T.; Mendrick, D.L.; Vaananen, H.K.; Horton, M.A. Beta 1 integrins and osteoclast function: Involvement in collagen recognition and bone resorption. *Bone* **1996**, *19*, 317–328. [CrossRef] [PubMed]
35. Crockett, J.C.; Mellis, D.J.; Scott, D.I.; Helfrich, M.H. New knowledge on critical osteoclast formation and activation pathways from study of rare genetic diseases of osteoclasts: Focus on the RANK/RANKL axis. *Osteoporos. Int.* **2011**, *22*, 1–20. [CrossRef]
36. Gao, M.; Gao, W.; Papadimitriou, J.M.; Zhang, C.; Gao, J.; Zheng, M. Exosomes-the enigmatic regulators of bone homeostasis. *Bone Res.* **2018**, *6*, 36. [CrossRef]
37. Furuta, T.; Miyaki, S.; Ishitobi, H.; Ogura, T.; Kato, Y.; Kamei, N.; Miyado, K.; Higashi, Y.; Ochi, M. Mesenchymal Stem Cell-Derived Exosomes Promote Fracture Healing in a Mouse Model. *Stem Cells Transl. Med.* **2016**, *5*, 1620–1630. [CrossRef]

38. Qin, Y.; Peng, Y.; Zhao, W.; Pan, J.; Ksiezak-Reding, H.; Cardozo, C.; Wu, Y.; Divieti Pajevic, P.; Bonewald, L.F.; Bauman, W.A.; et al. Myostatin inhibits osteoblastic differentiation by suppressing osteocyte-derived exosomal microRNA-218: A novel mechanism in muscle-bone communication. *J. Biol. Chem.* **2017**, *292*, 11021–11033. [CrossRef]
39. Deng, L.; Wang, Y.; Peng, Y.; Wu, Y.; Ding, Y.; Jiang, Y.; Shen, Z.; Fu, Q. Osteoblast-derived microvesicles: A novel mechanism for communication between osteoblasts and osteoclasts. *Bone* **2015**, *79*, 37–42. [CrossRef]
40. Zhao, Y.; Liu, T.; Zhou, M. Immune-Cell-Derived Exosomes for Cancer Therapy. *Mol. Pharm.* **2022**, *19*, 3042–3056. [CrossRef]
41. Logozzi, M.; Di Raimo, R.; Properzi, F.; Barca, S.; Angelini, D.F.; Mizzoni, D.; Falchi, M.; Battistini, L.; Fais, S. Nanovesicles released by OKT3 hybridoma express fully active antibodies. *J. Enzym. Inhib. Med. Chem.* **2021**, *36*, 175–182. [CrossRef] [PubMed]
42. Németh, T.; Sperandio, M.; Mócsai, A. Neutrophils as emerging therapeutic targets. *Nat. Rev. Drug Discov.* **2020**, *19*, 253–275. [CrossRef] [PubMed]
43. Wang, J.; Tang, W.; Yang, M.; Yin, Y.; Li, H.; Hu, F.; Tang, L.; Ma, X.; Zhang, Y.; Wang, Y. Inflammatory tumor microenvironment responsive neutrophil exosomes-based drug delivery system for targeted glioma therapy. *Biomaterials* **2021**, *273*, 120784. [CrossRef] [PubMed]
44. Xiong, Y.; Chen, L.; Yan, C.; Zhou, W.; Yu, T.; Sun, Y.; Cao, F.; Xue, H.; Hu, Y.; Chen, D.; et al. M2 Macrophagy-derived exosomal miRNA-5106 induces bone mesenchymal stem cells towards osteoblastic fate by targeting salt-inducible kinase 2 and 3. *J. Nanobiotechnol.* **2020**, *18*, 66. [CrossRef] [PubMed]
45. Rodrigues, G.; Hoshino, A.; Kenific, C.M.; Matei, I.R.; Steiner, L.; Freitas, D.; Kim, H.S.; Oxley, P.R.; Scandariato, I.; Casanova-Salas, I.; et al. Tumour exosomal CEMIP protein promotes cancer cell colonization in brain metastasis. *Nat. Cell Biol.* **2019**, *21*, 1403–1412. [CrossRef] [PubMed]
46. Han, C.; Zhang, C.; Wang, H.; Zhao, L. Exosome-mediated communication between tumor cells and tumor-associated macrophages: Implications for tumor microenvironment. *Oncoimmunology* **2021**, *10*, 1887552. [CrossRef] [PubMed]
47. Fridman, W.H.; Pages, F.; Sautes-Fridman, C.; Galon, J. The immune contexture in human tumours: Impact on clinical outcome. *Nat. Rev. Cancer* **2012**, *12*, 298–306. [CrossRef] [PubMed]
48. Bobrie, A.; Colombo, M.; Raposo, G.; Thery, C. Exosome secretion: Molecular mechanisms and roles in immune responses. *Traffic* **2011**, *12*, 1659–1668. [CrossRef]
49. Ahmadi, M.; Rezaie, J. Tumor cells derived-exosomes as angiogenenic agents: Possible therapeutic implications. *J. Transl. Med.* **2020**, *18*, 249. [CrossRef]
50. Saleem, S.N.; Abdel-Mageed, A.B. Tumor-derived exosomes in oncogenic reprogramming and cancer progression. *Cell Mol. Life Sci.* **2015**, *72*, 1–10. [CrossRef]
51. Li, F.X.; Liu, J.J.; Xu, F.; Lin, X.; Zhong, J.Y.; Wu, F.; Yuan, L.Q. Role of tumor-derived exosomes in bone metastasis. *Oncol. Lett.* **2019**, *18*, 3935–3945. [CrossRef] [PubMed]
52. Raimondo, S.; Saieva, L.; Vicario, E.; Pucci, M.; Toscani, D.; Manno, M.; Raccosta, S.; Giuliani, N.; Alessandro, R. Multiple myeloma-derived exosomes are enriched of amphiregulin (AREG) and activate the epidermal growth factor pathway in the bone microenvironment leading to osteoclastogenesis. *J. Hematol. Oncol.* **2019**, *12*, 2. [CrossRef] [PubMed]
53. Chen, Y.; Pfeifer, A. Brown Fat-Derived Exosomes: Small Vesicles with Big Impact. *Cell Metab.* **2017**, *25*, 759–760. [CrossRef] [PubMed]
54. Wang, R.; Jiang, W.; Zhang, L.; Xie, S.; Zhang, S.; Yuan, S.; Jin, Y.; Zhou, G. Intra-articular delivery of extracellular vesicles secreted by chondrogenic progenitor cells from MRL/MpJ superhealer mice enhances articular cartilage repair in a mouse injury model. *Stem Cell Res. Ther.* **2020**, *11*, 93. [CrossRef] [PubMed]
55. Yang, J.X.; Xie, P.; Li, Y.S.; Wen, T.; Yang, X.C. Osteoclast-derived miR-23a-5p-containing exosomes inhibit osteogenic differentiation by regulating Runx2. *Cell Signal.* **2020**, *70*, 109504. [CrossRef]
56. Ye, Y.; Li, S.L.; Ma, Y.Y.; Diao, Y.J.; Yang, L.; Su, M.Q.; Li, Z.; Ji, Y.; Wang, J.; Lei, L.; et al. Exosomal miR-141-3p regulates osteoblast activity to promote the osteoblastic metastasis of prostate cancer. *Oncotarget* **2017**, *8*, 94834–94849. [CrossRef] [PubMed]
57. Yang, X.; Yang, J.; Lei, P.; Wen, T. LncRNA MALAT1 shuttled by bone marrow-derived mesenchymal stem cells-secreted exosomes alleviates osteoporosis through mediating microRNA-34c/SATB2 axis. *Aging* **2019**, *11*, 8777–8791. [CrossRef]
58. Li, B.; Xu, H.; Han, H.; Song, S.; Zhang, X.; Ouyang, L.; Qian, C.; Hong, Y.; Qiu, Y.; Zhou, W.; et al. Exosome-mediated transfer of lncRUNX2-AS1 from multiple myeloma cells to MSCs contributes to osteogenesis. *Oncogene* **2018**, *37*, 5508–5519. [CrossRef]
59. Zhang, M.; Jia, L.; Zheng, Y. circRNA Expression Profiles in Human Bone Marrow Stem Cells Undergoing Osteoblast Differentiation. *Stem Cell Rev. Rep.* **2019**, *15*, 126–138. [CrossRef] [PubMed]
60. Peng, W.; Zhu, S.; Chen, J.; Wang, J.; Rong, Q.; Chen, S. Hsa_circRNA_33287 promotes the osteogenic differentiation of maxillary sinus membrane stem cells via miR-214-3p/Runx3. *BioMed Pharmacother.* **2019**, *109*, 1709–1717. [CrossRef]
61. Liu, Y.; Fu, N.; Su, J.; Wang, X.; Li, X. Rapid Enkephalin Delivery Using Exosomes to Promote Neurons Recovery in Ischemic Stroke by Inhibiting Neuronal p53/Caspase-3. *BioMed Res. Int.* **2019**, *2019*, 4273290. [CrossRef] [PubMed]
62. Haney, M.J.; Klyachko, N.L.; Zhao, Y.; Gupta, R.; Plotnikova, E.G.; He, Z.; Patel, T.; Piroyan, A.; Sokolsky, M.; Kabanov, A.V.; et al. Exosomes as drug delivery vehicles for Parkinson's disease therapy. *J. Control. Release* **2015**, *207*, 18–30. [CrossRef] [PubMed]
63. Khan, S.; Bennit, H.F.; Wall, N.R. The emerging role of exosomes in survivin secretion. *Histol. Histopathol.* **2015**, *30*, 43–50. [CrossRef] [PubMed]
64. Bourdonnay, E.; Zaslona, Z.; Penke, L.R.; Speth, J.M.; Schneider, D.J.; Przybranowski, S.; Swanson, J.A.; Mancuso, P.; Freeman, C.M.; Curtis, J.L.; et al. Transcellular delivery of vesicular SOCS proteins from macrophages to epithelial cells blunts inflammatory signaling. *J. Exp. Med.* **2015**, *212*, 729–742. [CrossRef]

65. Hu, Y.; Li, X.; Zhang, Q.; Gu, Z.; Luo, Y.; Guo, J.; Wang, X.; Jing, Y.; Chen, X.; Su, J. Exosome-guided bone targeted delivery of Antagomir-188 as an anabolic therapy for bone loss. *Bioact. Mater.* **2021**, *6*, 2905–2913. [CrossRef]
66. Dai, X.; Wang, Z.; Fan, M.; Liu, H.; Yang, X.; Wang, X.; Zhou, X.; Dai, Y.; Zhang, J.; Li, Z. PD-L1 antibodies-armed exosomal vaccine for enhanced cancer immunotherapy by simultaneously in situ activating T cells and blocking PD-1/PD-L1 axis. *Extracell. Vesicle* **2022**, *1*, 100012. [CrossRef]
67. Tian, Y.; Li, S.; Song, J.; Ji, T.; Zhu, M.; Anderson, G.J.; Wei, J.; Nie, G. A doxorubicin delivery platform using engineered natural membrane vesicle exosomes for targeted tumor therapy. *Biomaterials* **2014**, *35*, 2383–2390. [CrossRef] [PubMed]
68. Kim, M.S.; Haney, M.J.; Zhao, Y.; Mahajan, V.; Deygen, I.; Klyachko, N.L.; Inskoe, E.; Piroyan, A.; Sokolsky, M.; Okolie, O.; et al. Development of exosome-encapsulated paclitaxel to overcome MDR in cancer cells. *Nanomedicine* **2016**, *12*, 655–664. [CrossRef]
69. Sun, D.; Zhuang, X.; Xiang, X.; Liu, Y.; Zhang, S.; Liu, C.; Barnes, S.; Grizzle, W.; Miller, D.; Zhang, H.G. A novel nanoparticle drug delivery system: The anti-inflammatory activity of curcumin is enhanced when encapsulated in exosomes. *Mol. Ther.* **2010**, *18*, 1606–1614. [CrossRef]
70. Federici, C.; Petrucci, F.; Caimi, S.; Cesolini, A.; Logozzi, M.; Borghi, M.; D'Ilio, S.; Lugini, L.; Violante, N.; Azzarito, T.; et al. Exosome release and low pH belong to a framework of resistance of human melanoma cells to cisplatin. *PLoS One* **2014**, *9*, e88193. [CrossRef]
71. Iessi, E.; Logozzi, M.; Lugini, L.; Azzarito, T.; Federici, C.; Spugnini, E.P.; Mizzoni, D.; Di Raimo, R.; Angelini, D.F.; Battistini, L.; et al. Acridine Orange/exosomes increase the delivery and the effectiveness of Acridine Orange in human melanoma cells: A new prototype for theranostics of tumors. *J. Enzyme Inhib. Med. Chem.* **2017**, *32*, 648–657. [CrossRef] [PubMed]
72. Zhao, H.; Achreja, A.; Iessi, E.; Logozzi, M.; Mizzoni, D.; Di Raimo, R.; Nagrath, D.; Fais, S. The key role of extracellular vesicles in the metastatic process. *Biochim. Biophys. Acta Rev. Cancer* **2018**, *1869*, 64–77. [CrossRef] [PubMed]
73. Valadi, H.; Ekstrom, K.; Bossios, A.; Sjostrand, M.; Lee, J.J.; Lotvall, J.O. Exosome-mediated transfer of mRNAs and microRNAs is a novel mechanism of genetic exchange between cells. *Nat. Cell Biol.* **2007**, *9*, 654–659. [CrossRef] [PubMed]
74. Hulsmans, M.; Holvoet, P. MicroRNA-containing microvesicles regulating inflammation in association with atherosclerotic disease. *Cardiovasc. Res.* **2013**, *100*, 7–18. [CrossRef] [PubMed]
75. Liang, B.; Burley, G.; Lin, S.; Shi, Y.C. Osteoporosis pathogenesis and treatment: Existing and emerging avenues. *Cell Mol. Biol. Lett.* **2022**, *27*, 72. [CrossRef] [PubMed]
76. Chapurlat, R.D.; Confavreux, C.B. Novel biological markers of bone: From bone metabolism to bone physiology. *Rheumatology* **2016**, *55*, 1714–1725. [CrossRef]
77. Xie, Y.; Chen, Y.; Zhang, L.; Ge, W.; Tang, P. The roles of bone-derived exosomes and exosomal microRNAs in regulating bone remodelling. *J. Cell Mol. Med.* **2017**, *21*, 1033–1041. [CrossRef]
78. Taipaleenmaki, H. Regulation of Bone Metabolism by microRNAs. *Curr. Osteoporos. Rep.* **2018**, *16*, 1–12. [CrossRef]
79. Yuan, Y.; Guo, J.; Zhang, L.; Tong, X.; Zhang, S.; Zhou, X.; Zhang, M.; Chen, X.; Lei, L.; Li, H.; et al. MiR-214 Attenuates the Osteogenic Effects of Mechanical Loading on Osteoblasts. *Int. J. Sports Med.* **2019**, *40*, 931–940. [CrossRef]
80. Wang, Z.; Zhao, Z.; Gao, B.; Zhang, L. Exosome mediated biological functions within skeletal microenvironment. *Front. Bioeng. Biotechnol.* **2022**, *10*, 953916. [CrossRef]
81. Lai, G.; Zhao, R.; Zhuang, W.; Hou, Z.; Yang, Z.; He, P.; Wu, J.; Sang, H. BMSC-derived exosomal miR-27a-3p and miR-196b-5p regulate bone remodeling in ovariectomized rats. *PeerJ* **2022**, *10*, e13744. [CrossRef] [PubMed]
82. Qiu, M.; Zhai, S.; Fu, Q.; Liu, D. Bone Marrow Mesenchymal Stem Cells-Derived Exosomal MicroRNA-150-3p Promotes Osteoblast Proliferation and Differentiation in Osteoporosis. *Hum. Gene. Ther.* **2021**, *32*, 717–729. [CrossRef] [PubMed]
83. Zhang, Y.; Cao, X.; Li, P.; Fan, Y.; Zhang, L.; Ma, X.; Sun, R.; Liu, Y.; Li, W. microRNA-935-modified bone marrow mesenchymal stem cells-derived exosomes enhance osteoblast proliferation and differentiation in osteoporotic rats. *Life Sci.* **2021**, *272*, 119204. [CrossRef]
84. Yang, Y.; Miao, L.; Chang, S.; Zhang, Q.; Yu, L.; He, P.; Zhang, Y.; Fan, W.; Liu, J.; Hao, X. Exosome-Derived LncRNA TCONS_00072128 Mediated Osteogenic Differentiation and Inflammation by Caspase 8 Regulation. *Front. Genet.* **2021**, *12*, 831420. [CrossRef] [PubMed]
85. Rudiansyah, M.; El-Sehrawy, A.A.; Ahmad, I.; Terefe, E.M.; Abdelbasset, W.K.; Bokov, D.O.; Salazar, A.; Rizaev, J.A.; Muthanna, F.M.S.; Shalaby, M.N. Osteoporosis treatment by mesenchymal stromal/stem cells and their exosomes: Emphasis on signaling pathways and mechanisms. *Life Sci.* **2022**, *306*, 120717. [CrossRef] [PubMed]
86. Peng, Z.; Lu, S.; Lou, Z.; Li, Z.; Li, S.; Yang, K.; Li, C. Exosomes from bone marrow mesenchymal stem cells promoted osteogenic differentiation by delivering miR-196a that targeted Dickkopf-1 to activate Wnt/beta-catenin pathway. *Bioengineered* **2021**. *Epub ahead of print*. [CrossRef]
87. Huang, Y.; Xu, Y.; Feng, S.; He, P.; Sheng, B.; Ni, J. miR-19b enhances osteogenic differentiation of mesenchymal stem cells and promotes fracture healing through the WWP1/Smurf2-mediated KLF5/beta-catenin signaling pathway. *Exp. Mol. Med.* **2021**, *53*, 973–985. [CrossRef] [PubMed]
88. Yu, H.; Zhang, J.; Liu, X.; Li, Y. microRNA-136-5p from bone marrow mesenchymal stem cell-derived exosomes facilitates fracture healing by targeting LRP4 to activate the Wnt/beta-catenin pathway. *Bone Jt. Res.* **2021**, *10*, 744–758. [CrossRef] [PubMed]
89. Zhang, L.; Wang, Q.; Su, H.; Cheng, J. Exosomes from Adipose Tissues Derived Mesenchymal Stem Cells Overexpressing MicroRNA-146a Alleviate Diabetic Osteoporosis in Rats. *Cell Mol. Bioeng.* **2022**, *15*, 87–97. [CrossRef] [PubMed]
90. Qi, X.; Zhang, J.; Yuan, H.; Xu, Z.; Li, Q.; Niu, X.; Hu, B.; Wang, Y.; Li, X. Exosomes Secreted by Human-Induced Pluripotent Stem Cell-Derived Mesenchymal Stem Cells Repair Critical-Sized Bone Defects through Enhanced Angiogenesis and Osteogenesis in Osteoporotic Rats. *Int. J. Biol. Sci.* **2016**, *12*, 836–849. [CrossRef] [PubMed]

91. Lu, G.D.; Cheng, P.; Liu, T.; Wang, Z. BMSC-Derived Exosomal miR-29a Promotes Angiogenesis and Osteogenesis. *Front. Cell Dev. Biol.* **2020**, *8*, 608521. [CrossRef] [PubMed]
92. Behera, J.; Kumar, A.; Voor, M.J.; Tyagi, N. Exosomal lncRNA-H19 promotes osteogenesis and angiogenesis through mediating Angpt1/Tie2-NO signaling in CBS-heterozygous mice. *Theranostics* **2021**, *11*, 7715–7734. [CrossRef] [PubMed]
93. Zhang, Y.; Hao, Z.; Wang, P.; Xia, Y.; Wu, J.; Xia, D.; Fang, S.; Xu, S. Exosomes from human umbilical cord mesenchymal stem cells enhance fracture healing through HIF-1alpha-mediated promotion of angiogenesis in a rat model of stabilized fracture. *Cell Prolif.* **2019**, *52*, e12570. [CrossRef] [PubMed]
94. Einhorn, T.A.; Gerstenfeld, L.C. Fracture healing: Mechanisms and interventions. *Nat. Rev. Rheumatol.* **2015**, *11*, 45–54. [CrossRef]
95. van Griensven, M. Preclinical testing of drug delivery systems to bone. *Adv. Drug Deliv. Rev.* **2015**, *94*, 151–164. [CrossRef]
96. Lin, Z.; Xiong, Y.; Meng, W.; Hu, Y.; Chen, L.; Chen, L.; Xue, H.; Panayi, A.C.; Zhou, W.; Sun, Y.; et al. Exosomal PD-L1 induces osteogenic differentiation and promotes fracture healing by acting as an immunosuppressant. *Bioact. Mater.* **2022**, *13*, 300–311. [CrossRef]
97. Liu, W.; Li, L.; Rong, Y.; Qian, D.; Chen, J.; Zhou, Z.; Luo, Y.; Jiang, D.; Cheng, L.; Zhao, S.; et al. Hypoxic mesenchymal stem cell-derived exosomes promote bone fracture healing by the transfer of miR-126. *Acta Biomater.* **2020**, *103*, 196–212. [CrossRef]
98. Irfan, D.; Ahmad, I.; Patra, I.; Margiana, R.; Rasulova, M.T.; Sivaraman, R.; Kandeel, M.; Mohammad, H.J.; Al-Qaim, Z.H.; Jawad, M.A.; et al. Stem cell-derived exosomes in bone healing: Focusing on their role in angiogenesis. *Cytotherapy* **2022**. *Epub ahead of print*. [CrossRef]
99. Luo, Z.W.; Li, F.X.; Liu, Y.W.; Rao, S.S.; Yin, H.; Huang, J.; Chen, C.Y.; Hu, Y.; Zhang, Y.; Tan, Y.J.; et al. Aptamer-functionalized exosomes from bone marrow stromal cells target bone to promote bone regeneration. *Nanoscale* **2019**, *11*, 20884–20892. [CrossRef]
100. Zhang, L.; Jiao, G.; Ren, S.; Zhang, X.; Li, C.; Wu, W.; Wang, H.; Liu, H.; Zhou, H.; Chen, Y. Exosomes from bone marrow mesenchymal stem cells enhance fracture healing through the promotion of osteogenesis and angiogenesis in a rat model of nonunion. *Stem Cell Res. Ther.* **2020**, *11*, 38. [CrossRef]
101. Wang, Y.; Chen, W.; Zhao, L.; Li, Y.; Liu, Z.; Gao, H.; Bai, X.; Wang, B. Obesity regulates miR-467/HoxA10 axis on osteogenic differentiation and fracture healing by BMSC-derived exosome LncRNA H19. *J. Cell Mol. Med.* **2021**, *25*, 1712–1724. [CrossRef] [PubMed]
102. Zhou, J.; Liu, H.X.; Li, S.H.; Gong, Y.S.; Zhou, M.W.; Zhang, J.H.; Zhu, G.Y. Effects of human umbilical cord mesenchymal stem cells-derived exosomes on fracture healing in rats through the Wnt signaling pathway. *Eur. Rev. Med. Pharmacol. Sci.* **2019**, *23*, 4954–4960. [CrossRef] [PubMed]
103. Li, R.; Li, D.; Wang, H.; Chen, K.; Wang, S.; Xu, J.; Ji, P. Exosomes from adipose-derived stem cells regulate M1/M2 macrophage phenotypic polarization to promote bone healing via miR-451a/MIF. *Stem Cell Res. Ther.* **2022**, *13*, 149. [CrossRef] [PubMed]
104. Mi, B.; Chen, L.; Xiong, Y.; Yang, Y.; Panayi, A.C.; Xue, H.; Hu, Y.; Yan, C.; Hu, L.; Xie, X.; et al. Osteoblast/Osteoclast and Immune Cocktail Therapy of an Exosome/Drug Delivery Multifunctional Hydrogel Accelerates Fracture Repair. *ACS Nano* **2022**, *16*, 771–782. [CrossRef] [PubMed]
105. Bijlsma, J.W.; Berenbaum, F.; Lafeber, F.P. Osteoarthritis: An update with relevance for clinical practice. *Lancet* **2011**, *377*, 2115–2126. [CrossRef]
106. Pourakbari, R.; Khodadadi, M.; Aghebati-Maleki, A.; Aghebati-Maleki, L.; Yousefi, M. The potential of exosomes in the therapy of the cartilage and bone complications; emphasis on osteoarthritis. *Life Sci.* **2019**, *236*, 116861. [CrossRef]
107. Fan, W.J.; Liu, D.; Pan, L.Y.; Wang, W.Y.; Ding, Y.L.; Zhang, Y.Y.; Ye, R.X.; Zhou, Y.; An, S.B.; Xiao, W.F. Exosomes in osteoarthritis: Updated insights on pathogenesis, diagnosis, and treatment. Front. *Cell Dev. Biol.* **2022**, *10*, 949690. [CrossRef]
108. Ni, Z.; Zhou, S.; Li, S.; Kuang, L.; Chen, H.; Luo, X.; Ouyang, J.; He, M.; Du, X.; Chen, L. Exosomes: Roles and therapeutic potential in osteoarthritis. *Bone Res.* **2020**, *8*, 25. [CrossRef]
109. Jin, Y.; Xu, M.; Zhu, H.; Dong, C.; Ji, J.; Liu, Y.; Deng, A.; Gu, Z. Therapeutic effects of bone marrow mesenchymal stem cells-derived exosomes on osteoarthritis. *J. Cell Mol. Med.* **2021**, *25*, 9281–9294. [CrossRef]
110. He, L.; He, T.; Xing, J.; Zhou, Q.; Fan, L.; Liu, C.; Chen, Y.; Wu, D.; Tian, Z.; Liu, B.; et al. Bone marrow mesenchymal stem cell-derived exosomes protect cartilage damage and relieve knee osteoarthritis pain in a rat model of osteoarthritis. *Stem Cell Res. Ther.* **2020**, *11*, 276. [CrossRef]
111. Xu, H.; Xu, B. BMSC-Derived Exosomes Ameliorate Osteoarthritis by Inhibiting Pyroptosis of Cartilage via Delivering miR-326 Targeting HDAC3 and STAT1//NF-kappaB p65 to Chondrocytes. *Mediat. Inflamm.* **2021**, *2021*, 9972805. [CrossRef] [PubMed]
112. Kent, L.N.; Leone, G. The broken cycle: E2F dysfunction in cancer. *Nat. Rev. Cancer* **2019**, *19*, 326–338. [CrossRef] [PubMed]
113. Xia, Q.; Wang, Q.; Lin, F.; Wang, J. miR-125a-5p-abundant exosomes derived from mesenchymal stem cells suppress chondrocyte degeneration via targeting E2F2 in traumatic osteoarthritis. *Bioengineered* **2021**, *12*, 11225–11238. [CrossRef] [PubMed]
114. Cosenza, S.; Ruiz, M.; Toupet, K.; Jorgensen, C.; Noel, D. Mesenchymal stem cells derived exosomes and microparticles protect cartilage and bone from degradation in osteoarthritis. *Sci. Rep.* **2017**, *7*, 16214. [CrossRef]
115. Ritter, A.; Friemel, A.; Roth, S.; Kreis, N.N.; Hoock, S.C.; Safdar, B.K.; Fischer, K.; Mollmann, C.; Solbach, C.; Louwen, F.; et al. Subcutaneous and Visceral Adipose-Derived Mesenchymal Stem Cells: Commonality and Diversity. *Cells* **2019**, *8*, 1288. [CrossRef]
116. Damia, E.; Chicharro, D.; Lopez, S.; Cuervo, B.; Rubio, M.; Sopena, J.J.; Vilar, J.M.; Carrillo, J.M. Adipose-Derived Mesenchymal Stem Cells: Are They a Good Therapeutic Strategy for Osteoarthritis? *Int. J. Mol. Sci.* **2018**, *19*, 1926. [CrossRef]

117. Tofino-Vian, M.; Guillen, M.I.; Perez Del Caz, M.D.; Castejon, M.A.; Alcaraz, M.J. Extracellular Vesicles from Adipose-Derived Mesenchymal Stem Cells Downregulate Senescence Features in Osteoarthritic Osteoblasts. *Oxid. Med. Cell Longev.* **2017**, *2017*, 7197598. [CrossRef]
118. Lee, W.S.; Kim, H.J.; Kim, K.I.; Kim, G.B.; Jin, W. Intra-Articular Injection of Autologous Adipose Tissue-Derived Mesenchymal Stem Cells for the Treatment of Knee Osteoarthritis: A Phase IIb, Randomized, Placebo-Controlled Clinical Trial. *Stem Cells Transl. Med.* **2019**, *8*, 504–511. [CrossRef]
119. Zhu, Y.; Wang, Y.; Zhao, B.; Niu, X.; Hu, B.; Li, Q.; Zhang, J.; Ding, J.; Chen, Y.; Wang, Y. Comparison of exosomes secreted by induced pluripotent stem cell-derived mesenchymal stem cells and synovial membrane-derived mesenchymal stem cells for the treatment of osteoarthritis. *Stem Cell Res. Ther.* **2017**, *8*, 64. [CrossRef]
120. Lu, L.; Wang, J.; Fan, A.; Wang, P.; Chen, R.; Lu, L.; Yin, F. Synovial mesenchymal stem cell-derived extracellular vesicles containing microRN555A-26a-5p ameliorate cartilage damage of osteoarthritis. *J. Gene Med.* **2021**, *23*, e3379. [CrossRef]
121. Tao, S.C.; Yuan, T.; Zhang, Y.L.; Yin, W.J.; Guo, S.C.; Zhang, C.Q. Exosomes derived from miR-140-5p-overexpressing human synovial mesenchymal stem cells enhance cartilage tissue regeneration and prevent osteoarthritis of the knee in a rat model. *Theranostics* **2017**, *7*, 180–195. [CrossRef] [PubMed]
122. Wang, Y.; Yu, D.; Liu, Z.; Zhou, F.; Dai, J.; Wu, B.; Zhou, J.; Heng, B.C.; Zou, X.H.; Ouyang, H.; et al. Exosomes from embryonic mesenchymal stem cells alleviate osteoarthritis through balancing synthesis and degradation of cartilage extracellular matrix. *Stem Cell Res. Ther.* **2017**, *8*, 189. [CrossRef] [PubMed]
123. Grskovic, M.; Javaherian, A.; Strulovici, B.; Daley, G.Q. Induced pluripotent stem cells–opportunities for disease modelling and drug discovery. *Nat. Rev. Drug Discov.* **2011**, *10*, 915–929. [CrossRef] [PubMed]
124. Kim, J.; Kang, S.C.; Yoon, N.E.; Kim, Y.; Choi, J.; Park, N.; Jung, H.; Jung, B.H.; Ju, J.H. Metabolomic profiles of induced pluripotent stem cells derived from patients with rheumatoid arthritis and osteoarthritis. *Stem Cell Res. Ther.* **2019**, *10*, 319. [CrossRef] [PubMed]
125. Liang, Y.; Xu, X.; Li, X.; Xiong, J.; Li, B.; Duan, L.; Wang, D.; Xia, J. Chondrocyte-Targeted MicroRNA Delivery by Engineered Exosomes toward a Cell-Free Osteoarthritis Therapy. *ACS Appl. Mater. Interfaces* **2020**, *12*, 36938–36947. [CrossRef]
126. Rickel, K.; Fang, F.; Tao, J. Molecular genetics of osteosarcoma. *Bone* **2017**, *102*, 69–79. [CrossRef]
127. Yang, L.; Huang, X.; Guo, H.; Wang, L.; Yang, W.; Wu, W.; Jing, D.; Shao, Z. Exosomes as Efficient Nanocarriers in Osteosarcoma: Biological Functions and Potential Clinical Applications. *Front. Cell Dev. Biol.* **2021**, *9*, 737314. [CrossRef]
128. Chang, X.; Ma, Z.; Zhu, G.; Lu, Y.; Yang, J. New perspective into mesenchymal stem cells: Molecular mechanisms regulating osteosarcoma. *J. Bone Oncol.* **2021**, *29*, 100372. [CrossRef]
129. Wei, H.; Chen, F.; Chen, J.; Lin, H.; Wang, S.; Wang, Y.; Wu, C.; Lin, J.; Zhong, G. Mesenchymal Stem Cell Derived Exosomes as Nanodrug Carrier of Doxorubicin for Targeted Osteosarcoma Therapy via SDF1-CXCR4 Axis. *Int. J. Nanomed.* **2022**, *17*, 3483–3495. [CrossRef]
130. Wei, H.; Chen, J.; Wang, S.; Fu, F.; Zhu, X.; Wu, C.; Liu, Z.; Zhong, G.; Lin, J. A Nanodrug Consisting Of Doxorubicin And Exosome Derived From Mesenchymal Stem Cells For Osteosarcoma Treatment In Vitro. *Int. J. Nanomed.* **2019**, *14*, 8603–8610. [CrossRef]
131. Fang, Z.; Ding, Y.; Xue, Z.; Li, P.; Li, J.; Li, F. Roles of exosomes as drug delivery systems in cancer immunotherapy: A mini-review. *Discov. Oncol.* **2022**, *13*, 74. [CrossRef] [PubMed]
132. Sha, L.; Ma, D.; Chen, C. Exosome-mediated Hic-5 regulates proliferation and apoptosis of osteosarcoma via Wnt/beta-catenin signal pathway. *Aging* **2020**, *12*, 23598–23608. [CrossRef] [PubMed]
133. Qin, F.; Tang, H.; Zhang, Y.; Zhang, Z.; Huang, P.; Zhu, J. Bone marrow-derived mesenchymal stem cell-derived exosomal microRNA-208a promotes osteosarcoma cell proliferation, migration, and invasion. *J. Cell Physiol.* **2020**, *235*, 4734–4745. [CrossRef] [PubMed]
134. Ge, X.; Liu, W.; Zhao, W.; Feng, S.; Duan, A.; Ji, C.; Shen, K.; Liu, W.; Zhou, J.; Jiang, D.; et al. Exosomal Transfer of LCP1 Promotes Osteosarcoma Cell Tumorigenesis and Metastasis by Activating the JAK2/STAT3 Signaling Pathway. *Mol. Ther. Nucleic. Acids* **2020**, *21*, 900–915. [CrossRef] [PubMed]
135. Cai, X.; Yin, W.; Tang, C.; Lu, Y.; He, Y. Molecular mechanism of microRNAs regulating apoptosis in osteosarcoma. *Mol. Biol. Rep.* **2022**, *49*, 6945–6956. [CrossRef]
136. Zhang, H.; Wang, J.; Ren, T.; Huang, Y.; Liang, X.; Yu, Y.; Wang, W.; Niu, J.; Guo, W. Bone marrow mesenchymal stem cell-derived exosomal miR-206 inhibits osteosarcoma progression by targeting TRA2B. *Cancer Lett.* **2020**, *490*, 54–65. [CrossRef]
137. Shimbo, K.; Miyaki, S.; Ishitobi, H.; Kato, Y.; Kubo, T.; Shimose, S.; Ochi, M. Exosome-formed synthetic microRNA-143 is transferred to osteosarcoma cells and inhibits their migration. *Biochem. Biophys. Res. Commun.* **2014**, *445*, 381–387. [CrossRef]
138. Zhang, H.; Yu, Y.; Wang, J.; Han, Y.; Ren, T.; Huang, Y.; Chen, C.; Huang, Q.; Wang, W.; Niu, J.; et al. Macrophages-derived exosomal lncRNA LIFR-AS1 promotes osteosarcoma cell progression via miR-29a/NFIA axis. *Cancer Cell Int.* **2021**, *21*, 192. [CrossRef]
139. Zhang, K.; Dong, C.; Chen, M.; Yang, T.; Wang, X.; Gao, Y.; Wang, L.; Wen, Y.; Chen, G.; Wang, X.; et al. Extracellular vesicle-mediated delivery of miR-101 inhibits lung metastasis in osteosarcoma. *Theranostics* **2020**, *10*, 411–425. [CrossRef]

pharmaceutics

MDPI

Review

Extracellular Vesicles as Drug Delivery Systems in Organ Transplantation: The Next Frontier

Harry V. M. Spiers [1,2], Lukas K. J. Stadler [1,2], Hugo Smith [1] and Vasilis Kosmoliaptsis [1,2,*]

1 Department of Surgery, University of Cambridge, Addenbrooke's Hospital, Cambridge CB2 0QQ, UK; hs781@cam.ac.uk (H.V.M.S.)
2 NIHR Blood and Transplant Research Unit in Organ Donation and Transplantation, University of Cambridge, Cambridge CB2 0QQ, UK
* Correspondence: vk256@cam.ac.uk

Abstract: Extracellular vesicles are lipid bilayer-delimited nanoparticles excreted into the extracellular space by all cells. They carry a cargo rich in proteins, lipids and DNA, as well as a full complement of RNA species, which they deliver to recipient cells to induce downstream signalling, and they play a key role in many physiological and pathological processes. There is evidence that native and hybrid EVs may be used as effective drug delivery systems, with their intrinsic ability to protect and deliver a functional cargo by utilising endogenous cellular mechanisms making them attractive as therapeutics. Organ transplantation is the gold standard for treatment for suitable patients with end-stage organ failure. However, significant challenges still remain in organ transplantation; prevention of graft rejection requires heavy immunosuppression and the lack of donor organs results in a failure to meet demand, as manifested by growing waiting lists. Pre-clinical studies have demonstrated the ability of EVs to prevent rejection in transplantation and mitigate ischemia reperfusion injury in several disease models. The findings of this work have made clinical translation of EVs possible, with several clinical trials actively recruiting patients. However, there is much to be uncovered, and it is essential to understand the mechanisms behind the therapeutic benefits of EVs. Machine perfusion of isolated organs provides an unparalleled platform for the investigation of EV biology and the testing of the pharmacokinetic and pharmacodynamic properties of EVs. This review classifies EVs and their biogenesis routes, and discusses the isolation and characterisation methods adopted by the international EV research community, before delving into what is known about EVs as drug delivery systems and why organ transplantation represents an ideal platform for their development as drug delivery systems.

Keywords: extracellular vesicles; exosomes; drug delivery systems; ischemia reperfusion injury; allograft rejection; organ transplantation; machine perfusion

Citation: Spiers, H.V.M.; Stadler, L.K.J.; Smith, H.; Kosmoliaptsis, V. Extracellular Vesicles as Drug Delivery Systems in Organ Transplantation: The Next Frontier. *Pharmaceutics* **2023**, *15*, 891. https://doi.org/10.3390/pharmaceutics15030891

Academic Editor: Yong Chen

Received: 23 November 2022
Revised: 22 February 2023
Accepted: 24 February 2023
Published: 9 March 2023

1. Introduction

Extracellular vesicles (EVs) are a heterogeneous group of membrane-derived vesicles released into the extracellular space by cells [1,2]. They play important roles in cell-to-cell communication, functioning as important intermediaries of cell signalling due to their unique biosignatures [3–5], and act as key mediators of many physiological processes [6]. EVs are released from all cell types studied to date, including endothelial cells [7,8], epithelial cells [9] and mesenchymal stem cells [10,11]; hence, they can also be found in a number of biofluids, including blood [12], synovial fluid [13], bile [14], breast milk [15], cerebrospinal fluid [16] and urine [17]. EVs have also been implicated in a number of diseases, including cardiovascular [18–20] and liver diseases [21,22], autoimmune [23] and neurodegenerative conditions [24–26] and cancer [27–30].

EVs are delimited by a lipid bilayer decorated with markers of various biogenesis routes prior to their secretion from the host cell [1]. They measure between 40 nm and

2000 nm, and their further subdivision by size is used to classify the main types of EVs: exosomes, microvesicles and apoptotic bodies (Table 1). Given the heterogeneous sizes and surface marker expressions of these nanoparticles, consensus on specific EV subtype markers remains elusive; therefore, assigning an EV to a specific biogenesis pathway is challenging. The International Society of Extracellular Vesicles (ISEV) has produced guidelines to enable EV researchers to determine the EV population at hand, along with its characteristics and purity [31]. Additional guidance published in the Minimal Information for Studies of EVs 2018 (MISEX2018) provides terminology that can be used to further describe EVs according to their physical characteristics, including size (e.g., small EVs (sEVs) <100 nm or <200 nm and medium/large EVs (m/lEVs) > 200 nm), density, the presence of specific markers (e.g., CD9+ EVs) and the condition (e.g., hypoxic EVs) or cell of origin (e.g., cholangiocyte-derived EVs). [31]

Table 1. Classification of specific extracellular vesicle subtypes. ALIX, ALG-2-interacting protein X; CD, cluster of differentiation; CX3CL1, C-X3-C motif chemokine ligand 1; CXCR4, chemokine receptor type; DNA, deoxyribonucleic acid; GAPDH, glyceraldehyde-3-phosphate dehydrogenase; lncRNA, long non-coding ribonucleic acid; MHC, mass histocompatibility complex; miRNA, micro-ribonucleic acid; mRNA, messenger ribonucleic acid; ROCK, Rho-associated protein kinase; TCR, T cell receptor; TSG101, tumour susceptibility gene 101.

Subtype	Origin	Size (nm)	Alternative Names	Composition	Biological Cargo
Exosomes	Endosome	50–150	Nanovesicles, proteosomes, exosome-like vesicles	*Membrane constituents:* • Tetraspanins (e.g., CD9, CD63, CD81) • Cell adhesion molecules (e.g., integrin) • Cell-type-specific proteins (e.g., CXCR4, TCR, MHC-II) • Lipids (e.g., phosphatidylserine, cholesterol) *Intravesicular components:* • Signal transduction (e.g., Beta-catenin) • Biogenesis factors (ALIX, TSG101, syntenin-1)	Enzymes (e.g., peroxidases), nucleic acids (e.g., miRNAs, mRNA, lncRNA)
Microvesicles	Plasma membrane	150–1000	Microparticles, oncosomes, shedding vesicles, blebbing vesicles	*Membrane constituents:* • Tetraspanins (e.g., CD9, CD63, CD81) • Cell adhesion molecules (e.g., integrin) • Cell-type-specific proteins (e.g., CD14, MHC-II) • Lipids (e.g., phosphatidylethanolamine) *Intravesicular components:* • Signal transduction (e.g., ROCK) • Cytoplasmic material (e.g., GAPDH) • Cytoskeletal microtubules (e.g., actin, tubulin)	Nucleic acids (e.g., miRNAs, mRNA, lncRNA, DNA, histones)

Table 1. *Cont.*

Subtype	Origin	Size (nm)	Alternative Names	Composition	Biological Cargo
Apoptotic bodies	Plasma membrane	500–2000	Apo-EVs	*Membrane constituents:* • Lipids (namely phosphatidylserine) • Cell adhesion molecules (e.g., CX3CL1) *Intravesicular components:* • Signal transduction (e.g., ROCK)	Nucleic acids (including histones, large DNA fragments and some miRNAs), organelles

As the field of targeted drug delivery has expanded, the EV research field has begun to realise the potential of EVs as next-generation drug delivery vehicles. This review provides an overview of the subtypes and biogenesis routes of EVs, as well as methods of EV isolation and characterisation, before delving into the emerging roles of native and bioengineered EVs as drug delivery vehicles and, finally, addressing current real-world applications and challenges, with an emphasis on the field of organ transplantation.

2. Classification and Biogenesis of Extracellular Vesicles

Small EVs—those in the exosomal range of 40–150 nm—represent the smallest EV subtype and are derived by the endosomal pathway (Figure 1). They are generated by invagination of the late endosomal membrane, which is mediated by the endosomal sorting complex required for transport (ESCRT) proteins, including ESCRT-I, known as tumour susceptibility gene 101 (TSG101) [32]. Late endosomal membrane invagination forms intraluminal vesicles (ILVs) in a process orchestrated by ALG-2 interacting protein X (ALIX) after its direct interaction with syntenin-1, a multifunctional adapter protein that is essential for vesicle biogenesis, resulting in a specialised endosomal compartment known as a multivesicular body (MVB) [33]. MVBs fuse with the plasma membrane and exocytose the ILVs as exosomes. Tetraspanins (CD9, CD63, CD81) play a role in directing EV cargo during this process because of their involvement in recycling routes between cellular organelles and the plasma membrane [34,35]. As a result of this complex process, sEVs are enriched in the proteins that mediate their formation, including the ubiquitously expressed syntenin-1, as well as TSG101, ALIX and the variably expressed tetraspanins [1].

Large EVs (lEVs)—or microvesicles—have sizes in the range of 150 nm to 1000 nm, averaging at 250–400 nm [36,37]. Propelled by actomyosin-driven fission into the extracellular space, lEVs result from direct budding from the plasma membrane [38] (Figure 1). lEVs originate from sites of high membrane blebbing [39,40] where a host of factors modulate the deformability and bending of the membrane, including the organisation of the cytoskeleton, lipid composition and membrane fluidity alterations [38]. As a result of this, lEVs have unique lipid characteristics that result in increased uptake by recipient cells [41], such as externalisation of phosphatidylserine phospholipids [42]. Once loaded with cargo, the cone-shaped lipid ceramide promotes membrane bending [43] with the bleb "pinched" free from the cell through acto-myosin contraction [44], a tightly regulated process governed by the Rho family of GTPases [45].

Apoptotic bodies represent the largest EV subpopulation, measuring 1–5 μm. They form during programmed cell death upon disassembly of apoptotic membrane blebs (microtubule spikes [46], apoptodia [47] and beaded apoptodia [48]). These blebs contain carefully packaged cell contents, including organelles and DNA, which are phagocytosed by macrophages after release into the extracellular space [49]. As these vesicles contain numerous cellular components, they express markers that overlap with sEV and lEV populations; therefore, size is a key characteristic for their determination in samples [31].

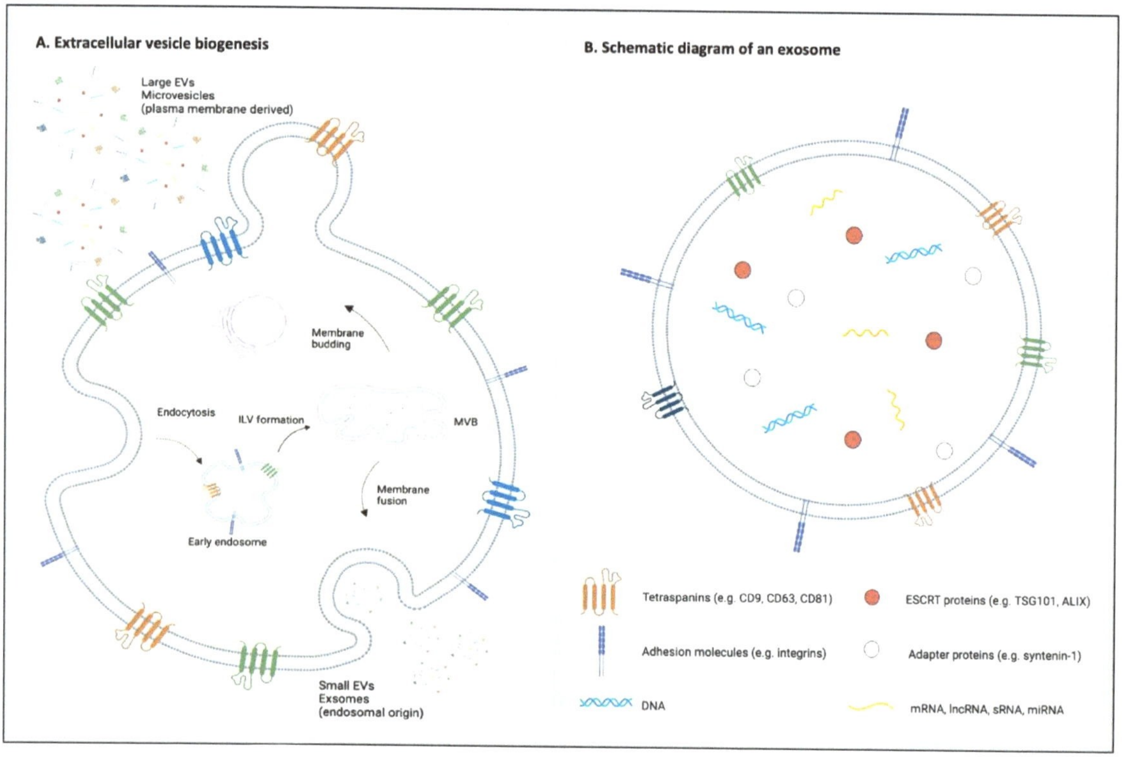

Figure 1. (**A**) Biogenesis of extracellular vesicles (EVs) demonstrating endosomal and membrane-budding pathways. Small EVs (exosomes) are generated through invagination of the cell membrane, which forms intraluminal vesicles (ILVs) that fuse with a multivesicular body (MVB). The MVB fuses with the cell membrane and the small EVs are exocytosed into the extracellular space. Large EVs (microvesicles) form through buddying of the cell membrane, which eventually "pinches" off to form vesicles. (**B**) A schematic of a small EV containing protein, DNA and RNA cargo with surface expression markers in the form of tetraspanins and integrins.

The biogenesis of EVs produces an intraluminal cargo from the parent cell that is protected by their phospholipid membrane, allowing transfer of proteins, lipids, DNA and a full repertoire of RNA species (including mRNA, microRNA (miRNA) and other non-coding RNAs) [1,2]. The ability of EVs to protect a wide variety of nucleic acid species [2], carry these across biological barriers [50–52], utilise endogenous intracellular trafficking mechanisms and trigger a response in recipient cells [53] makes them attractive drug delivery systems for both endogenous and bioengineered compounds.

3. Isolation and Characterisation of Extracellular Vesicles

EVs must be isolated from their respective source samples and other vesicles, after which their size, shape and density can be characterised (Figure 2) [54]. The isolation of EVs from multiple cell sources is well-established, as demonstrated by the transcriptomic atlas of EV RNA from 20 biofluids [55]. However, isolation of specific subspecies remains challenging, given the heterogeneity of EVs in terms of size, density and cargo. Several approaches have been established to isolate EVs, with each requiring a trade-off between purity, EV recovery and the integrity of the isolated vesicle; commonly used methods for EV isolation and purification are outlined in Table 2. As there is no single optimal method of isolation, the choice of technique(s) is based on the downstream application. The ISEV recognises the challenges of EV purification and has issued the following recommendations: EV quantification should be undertaken with at least two methods, including protein amount and particle number. Assessment of transmembrane or glycosylphosphatidylinositol-anchored proteins and membrane-associated cytosolic proteins should then be performed. Contaminants should be evaluated, and images of single EVs obtained using wide-field and close-up assessments should be published [31].

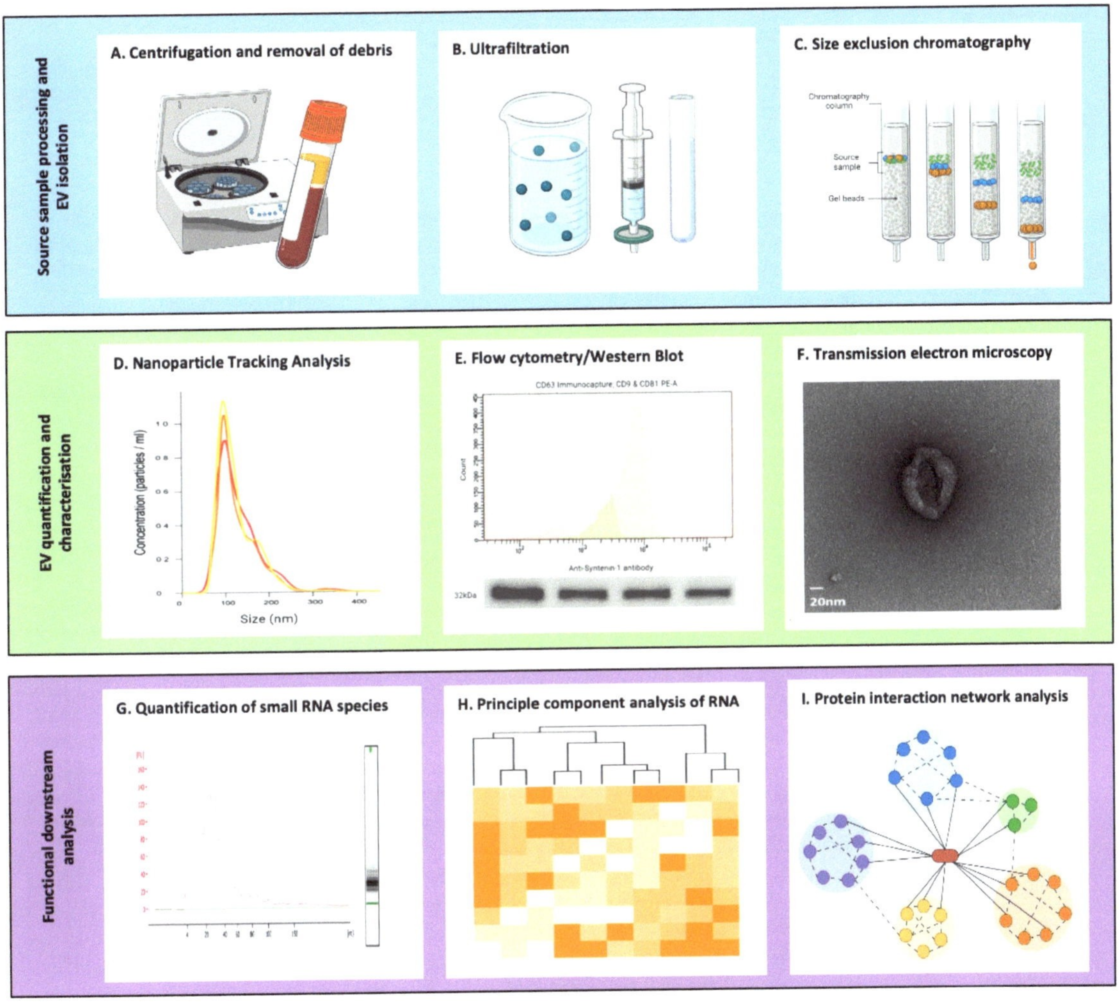

Figure 2. Methods of isolation and characterisation of extracellular vesicles (EVs). (**A**) One example of a source fluid is blood, for which centrifugation can be used to remove cellular debris and isolate serum. (**B**) Ultracentrifugation can be used to remove non-EV particles. (**C**) Size exclusion chromatography separates EVs from a sample based on their movement through a column of gel beads. (**D**) Nanoparticle tracking analysis quantifies the size and concentration of the particles isolated. (**E**) Flow cytometry and Western blotting can be used to confirm the presence of specific EV markers. (**F**) EVs can then be visualised and their morphology confirmed using transmission electron microscopy. (**G**) RNA can be isolated from EVs where smaller RNA species predominate. (**H**) Following next-generation sequencing, principal component analysis can be performed. (**I**) Proteomic analysis of EVs provides insight into the pathways they influence as signalling molecules.

Table 2. Methods of extracellular vesicle isolation.

Methodology	Principle	Advantages	Disadvantages
Ultrafiltration	Biofluid is passed through a porous membrane to filter particles larger than a predetermined size	Time-effective; high yield	Pores blocked with contaminants; contamination (e.g., proteins and RNA); small particles left on pores; EVs damaged by force used
Differential ultracentrifugation	High centrifugal speeds are applied for sufficient time periods to allow individual EVs to travel to the bottom of the tube and accumulate as a pellet; however, the method is less efficient at pelleting smaller/less dense particles	Commonly used; replicable; convenient operation; no sample pre-treatment required	Time-consuming; requires larger volumes of biofluid; unpredictable co-isolation (e.g., lipoproteins); damage to and aggregation and loss of EVs
Density gradient ultracentrifugation	EVs are purified based on their buoyant density by using a medium such as iodixanol and centrifugation	Improved separation of EVs from protein complexes; replicable	Time-consuming; low yield; EV damage; co-isolation of non-EV particles of similar densities
Polymer precipitation	Volume-expanding polymers reduce the solubility of EVs in solution, with isolation following the subsequent low-speed centrifugation	High yield; time-efficient; commercial kits available	Unclear effects of polymers on downstream applications; coprecipitation of proteins with further protein removal kits needed
Size exclusion chromatography	EVs in solution loaded onto a gel bead column, with larger EVs passing around the gel beads and eluting from the column first, whilst smaller particles progress more slowly through the bead matrix and elute later	Vesicle structure and integrity preserved; high purity; reproducible	Time-consuming; post-isolation concentration steps required
Immunoaffinity	Immunocapture utilising beads conjugated with antibodies toward EV surface markers	High sensitivity and specificity; EV subtype separation possible	Expensive; low yield; elution techniques can affect EV integrity

Once isolated, EVs must be characterised to further identify the population present. EV characterisation is a multifaceted process comprising numerous established and emerging techniques, each with their own advantages and disadvantages. Recommendations from the ISEV set out in the MISEV2018 guidelines [31] suggest that contemporary EV studies quantify the sources of EVs in terms of the number of secreting cells, volume of biofluid and mass of tissue (where each is applicable). EV concentration should be assessed according to the total particle number. The typical EV content in the sample should be quantified (commonly by identifying transmembrane or cytosolic proteins) and non-vesicular contaminants tested for following isolation [31]. The size and concentration of EVs in the source sample are assessed using nanoparticle tracking analysis (NTA) and tuneable resistive pulse sensing (TRPS) [56]. NTA involves shining a laser into the sample as it passes under a video capture system and uses dynamic light scattering to calculate size based on the Brownian motion of a particle while calculating concentration by counting the number of particles per frame. TRPS involves driving EVs through a nanopore in an electrolyte fluid cell that is sampled 50,000 times per second using a combination of pressure and voltage, and each particle results in a resistive pulse or "blockage" signal that is detected and measured. The blockade magnitude is directly proportional to the volume of each particle, with the frequency of blockade being directly proportional to the sample concentration. It is also desirable to determine EV morphology, and this can be achieved with microscopy techniques, including transmission electron microscopy (TEM) [57] and cryo-electron microscopy [58]. Techniques employed for EV content include Western blotting for specific EV markers (including the aforementioned syntenin-1, TSG101 and ALIX [1]), flow cytometry [59,60], ExoView [61] and the enzyme-linked immunosorbent assay (ELISA) [62]. Additional high-definition analyses of EV content can be performed using techniques such as mass spectrometry proteomic analysis [63,64] and genomic sequencing for transcriptomic profiling [65].

Reliable and time-efficient EV isolation and characterisation protocols are required for consistent isolation of EVs with therapeutic properties and those that have been bioengineered to function as therapeutic agents. This is not currently the standard, and several issues require addressing to refine the process. Methods to achieve large-volume, high-purity EV isolation that are not expensive, complex or time-consuming and focus on discrimination between specific EV populations during isolation using their distinctive physicochemical or biological properties in order to generate preparations capable of delivering consistent therapeutic effects are essential.

4. Extracellular Vesicles as Therapeutics

EVs can be harnessed therapeutically and the pharmacological classification of EV-based therapeutics depends on the active substance [66]. They can be divided into three main categories: (1) natural EVs, which are native and obtained from genetically engineered cells; (2) hybrid EVs, which are post-modified with drugs or surface ligands; (3) EV-inspired liposomes. In this section, we focus on natural and hybrid EVs, as these are grouped together from a regulatory perspective [66].

4.1. Native EVs as Drug Delivery Systems

The idea of using native EVs for disease therapy, as a sort of "naturally occurring" therapeutic nanoparticle, arose originally from stem cell studies. Several groups investigating the potential therapeutic use of mesenchymal stem cells (MSCs) in the treatment of cardiovascular diseases found that the therapeutic effect of the intervention was not derived from the engrafted cells themselves but rather from their paracrine effectors; in particular, EVs [67–69]. Since those early studies, the use of stem and progenitor cell-derived EVs for the treatment of various diseases has been explored extensively.

Stem cell-derived EVs demonstrate numerous cardioprotective effects, which have made them prime candidates in the treatment of myocardial infarction (MI) and other ischemic events. Studies with animals have shown that EVs promote the survival of heart endothelial cells and cardiomyocytes following ischemic insults through the activation of common survival pathways, such as AKT and ERK [70]. Of particular interest is one recent study that demonstrated the superior effectiveness of the cardiac repair and safety associated with induced pluripotent stem cell (iPSC)-derived EVs compared to the iPSCs themselves [71]. In other studies, EVs have been shown to supress inflammation, decrease oxidative stress and even promote the formation of new blood vessels in animal models of MI [72–74]. EVs that demonstrate cardiovascular effects have been isolated from numerous cellular sources, including the aforementioned MSCs and iPSCs, as well as putative cardiac progenitor cells and even differentiated somatic cells [75–78].

The molecular candidates responsible for the mediation of these EVs' therapeutic effects are most commonly found amongst the miRNA cargo of EVs, which represents the "drug" in this system. For example, extracellular matrix-derived EVs can regulate the acetylation of transcription factor GATA4 via miRNA-199a-3p, thus rescuing the electrical function in bioengineered atria [79]. Similarly, EVs isolated from the cardiosphere were able to ameliorate heart dysfunction in a mouse model of MI by decreasing inflammation and apoptosis via miRNA-146, as well as increasing cardiomyocyte proliferation and promoting angiogenesis [80]. Numerous other miRNAs have been shown to have cardiovascular protective effects in vitro and in animal models, including miRNA-24, miRNA-126, miRNA-181b and miRNA-294-3p [81–83].

Additionally, there are several EV cargo proteins for which roles in mediating therapeutic cardiovascular-protective effects have been demonstrated. Pappalysin-1 is expressed on the surface of EVs from cardiac progenitor cells and has been shown to mediate the pro-survival properties of those EVs through the activation of the IGF-1 receptor and subsequent phosphorylation of its downstream anti-apoptotic effectors AKT and ERK1/2 [84]. Another protein component of EVs with potential therapeutic activity is platelet-derived growth factor D, which has been shown to mediate cardiac regeneration and stimulate angiogenesis in a rat model of acute myocardial infarction [85].

While the therapeutic use of native EVs has so far been most extensively explored in cardiovascular research, there is growing interest in the areas of inflammatory and autoimmune diseases. In the field of dermatology, EVs are starting to garner attention as therapeutics for inflammatory skin diseases; a number of studies have shown that EVs can aid in the process of wound healing, particularly via the molecular actions of miR-21. EVs derived from keratinocytes were shown to promote wound healing by regulating fibroblast function and through stimulation of angiogenesis [86,87]. Similarly, in a recent study of umbilical cord-derived EVs, Liu et al. showed that wound healing could be accelerated by enhancing the proliferation and migration of fibroblasts. [88].

Another area of interest is represented by inflammatory diseases of the central nervous system, an area of the body that is particularly challenging to treat with stem cells due to restricted access via the blood–brain barrier (BBB). EVs, however, have been shown to readily cross the BBB in several studies [89]. In a model of preterm brain injury, EVs from MSCs slowed the signs of inflammation and improved signs of inflammation- induced neuronal degeneration [90]. In a separate study, Clark et al. showed that MSC-derived EVs from the placenta were able to slow disease progression of multiple sclerosis in an animal model of the disease [91].

In light of the proven anti-inflammatory properties of EVs derived from stem cells, their use in the treatment of autoimmune diseases is beginning to be investigated. In one recent example, Cosenza and colleagues isolated EVs from MSCs via ultracentrifugation and first tested their immunosuppressive effects in an in vitro lymphocyte-based assay [92]. They reported reduced T-cell proliferation upon EV exposure, as well as inhibition of plasmablast differentiation of B-cells. Furthermore, in a mouse model of collagen- induced arthritis, the authors found significantly decreased signs of inflammation [92]. Along similar lines, there is significant interest in finding more effective ways of alleviating the systemic symptoms of inflammation in patients with lupus erythematosus. To this end, different research groups have demonstrated the immunosuppressive properties of MSC-derived EVs in models of acute tubular inflammation in the kidney [93], as well as the efficacy of these nanoparticles in promoting cartilage repair in a mouse model of osteochondral defect [94].

Native EVs derived from stem cells and other cell sources have demonstrated clear applicability in the treatment of various pathologies, particularly those with a significant inflammatory component. Advantages over other treatment methods (such as whole cells) include their low immunogenicity (vs. whole cells), their small size (vs. whole cells) and the ease of large-scale production (vs. engineered biomolecules). There are numerous human diseases, however, where a more targeted delivery of the active agent is desirable in order to minimise off-target effects or to deliver a more potent dose with precision.

4.2. Bioengineered Extracellular Vesicles as Therapeutics

The therapeutic efficacy of EVs can be improved synthetically through various strategies; for example, by adding a targeting molecule (antibody, aptamer, etc.) to the EV surface, by loading the nanoparticle with a specific biologically active agent or by extending the time EVs spend in circulation through chemical modifications, creating a so-called "hybrid EV" [95].

One obstacle standing in the way of widespread utilization of EVs in disease therapy is the challenge of ensuring accurate delivery to the site of action while preventing off-target effects. In order to equip EVs with specific targeting molecules, two different strategies have been explored: genetic modification of the producing cell (e.g., specific cell surface receptor expression) and direct chemical modification of the purified EV. One example of the first strategy is the genetic modification of EV-producing cells to express recombinant

EGFR-specific nanobodies with a glycosylphosphatidylinositol (GPI)- anchoring peptide. As EVs carry high levels of GPI, the nanobodies were enriched on the EV surface, which, in turn, equipped the EVs with targeting specificity for EGFR cells [96]. While this method resulted in successful targeting of the EVs toward their intended sites of action, the genetic modification of EV-producing cells may not always be a viable option in future EV therapy due to the time-consuming procedure and the challenges of genetic modification of cells derived from a patient's body fluids.

The strategy of chemically modifying EVs post-purification makes use of the EV membrane composition to specifically attach a targeting moiety with high density and in a controllable manner. One such approach made use of the high levels of phosphatidylserine (PS) in the lipid bilayer of EVs, genetically fusing a targeting peptide to the C1C2 domain of lactadherin, a high-affinity binder of PS [97,98]. Specifically, the group attached an anti-EGFR nanobody to the cell surface of EVs in this manner and found that it resulted in dose-dependent uptake of EVs by $EGFR^+$ cells. Crucially, addition of the fusion peptide did not compromise the integrity or size of the EV, thus further supporting the method's suitability for potential therapeutic uses. Another group made use of the popular click-chemistry—in this case, copper-free azide alkyne cyclo-addition—to furnish MSC-derived EVs with a high affinity integrin $\alpha_v\beta_3$-binding peptide [99]. These bioengineered EVs were able to target the ischaemic region of the brain in a mouse model of artery occlusion. Furthermore, the authors reported reduced inflammatory response in these animals versus control animals treated with non-specific EVs.

As well as their use as mediators of cell targeting, various peptides have also been used to promote internalisation of EVs into target cells. Nakase and co-workers made use of a sulfo-N-ε-maleimidocaproyl-oxysulfosuccinimide ester chemistry to decorate the surface of EVs with an arginine-rich micropinocytosis-inducing peptide. This modification resulted in substantially increased uptake into CHO cells and improved delivery of the EVs' cytotoxic saporin protein cargo [100].

Another area of scientific interest is the modification of the bioactivity of EVs (most commonly by customising the cargo they carry), which would make it possible to adapt their uses to different diseases. One prominent example is the use of EVs as drug delivery vehicles in cancer therapy, whereby engineered EVs would be specifically targeted toward a tumour and deliver a cytotoxic agent. As with the different targeting methods discussed above, loading an EV with a drug or bioactive molecule could be achieved either prior to EV production (i.e., through modification of the cell of origin) or after the EVs have been isolated. Opting for the first approach, Tang at al. incubated their cell line of choice with four different chemotherapeutic agents (including cis-platin and methotrexate) by simply adding those molecules to the cell culture medium for 12 h. Following isolation of the EVs from the cell culture medium via ultracentrifugation, the authors went on to show that they had cytotoxic actions affecting the target cancer cell line [101].

Conversely, EVs can be isolated first then loaded with drugs. Different techniques have been investigated depending on the molecule of choice. In the case of hydrophobic entities or small-molecule drugs, passive diffusion through the EV surrounding lipid bilayer may be possible. Wei et al. isolated EVs from bone marrow MSCs and loaded them with doxorubicin through overnight incubation. Following a dialysis step to ensure removal of free drug, the authors verified the integrity of these modified EVs using NTA and TEM and then tested their activity in a cell proliferation assay. Additionally, they assessed EV cellular uptake using flow cytometry. The authors found high levels of the modified EVs in the target cells, as well as significant growth inhibition [102].

Other methods used to load EVs with anti-cancer agents include sonication, electroporation and treatment with cellular transfection reagents, all of which work by disrupting the vesicle membrane and allow uptake of drug molecules [103]. Examples of their use come from the field of cardiovascular diseases. One group used a custom-made EV transfection reagent—ExoFect—to enrich human peripheral blood-derived EVs with an miRNA-21 inhibitor. This miRNA plays a crucial role in the development of fibrosis after an MI, and use of those modified EVs in a mouse model of MI resulted in significantly reduced fibrosis [104]. In a separate study, Youn et al. employed electroporation to load cardiac progenitor cell-derived EVs with miRNA-322, followed by systemic injection into a mouse model of MI. The intervention resulted in increased angiogenesis and improved recovery in the animals [105].

In sum, EVs clearly have strong potential for widespread use in disease therapy, whether is in their "native" form, exerting anti-inflammatory effects, or as drug delivery vehicles. One possible drawback, however, is the fact that unmodified EVs are subject to rapid circulatory clearance and demonstrate relatively low accumulation in target tissues [106]. The latter issue can be overcome through addition of targeting moieties as described above. In order to address the issue of rapid clearance, EVs can be coated with polyethylene glycol (PEG). PEG is a hydrophilic polymer and has previously been shown to increase the circulation time of nanoparticles [107]. With regard to EVs, it has been reported that PEGylation increases EV circulation time, as well as reducing non-specific interactions with cells [108].

While native, unmodified EVs have shown broad applicability in the pre-clinical treatment of inflammatory diseases, the potential uses of these nanoparticles in the treatment of disease can be significantly expanded through chemical and synthetic modification.

5. Extracellular Vesicles in Organ Transplantation

Given the evidence that native and hybrid EVs are promising drug delivery systems, it is no surprise that these nanoparticles have made their way into clinical practice, being employed for real-world uses as therapeutics in several on-going clinical trials (Table 3). Organ transplantation is the gold standard for treatment for suitable patients with end-stage organ failure. Kidney transplantation, for example, has become a routine procedure because it confers improved length and quality of life in patients, as well as having clear economic benefits [109]. Nevertheless, significant challenges still remain in organ transplantation, including graft rejection requiring extensive immunosuppression and the lack of donor organs available to meet the ever-growing waiting lists [110]. As discussed, the inherent ability of EVs to facilitate the transfer of protein, lipid and RNA payloads to target cells, crossing natural barriers and utilising intrinsic cellular machinery and pathways, makes them an attractive therapeutic vehicle. Additionally, EVs are potentially less immunogenic due to the reduced surface expression of human leucocyte antigens compared to cellular therapies. They are also unable to replicate, which reduces the risk of tumour generation subsequent to their delivery, and their inherent targeting mechanisms reduce off-target effects [53]. These factors make them a promising and realistic clinical drug delivery system for development in organ transplantation, a field associated with unmet needs in terms of donor organ utilisation and long-term graft function whilst also representing a unique platform for the study of EVs and their utilisation as therapeutics.

5.1. Alloimmune Response Modulation

There is increasing evidence that priming and effector mechanisms behind graft rejection are mediated by EVs. Dendritic cells (DCs), important antigen-presenting cells, may be immature or mature and EVs from either population can mediate the opposite effects. In a mouse skin graft model, it appears that immature DC-derived EVs promoted T cell activation without rejection, whilst EVs from mature DCs contrastingly induced effector T cells that led to skin graft rejection [111]. The same group from France characterised immature DC-EVs, which express low levels of ICAM-1, MHC-II, CD89 and CD86 and may mediate suppressive functions [111]. Li et al. went on to demonstrate that EVs from donor-derived immature DCs prolonged graft survival in a mouse model of cardiac transplantation [112]. The proposed effector mechanism involved IL-10 induction, favouring FoxP3 expression in the T cell compartment in addition to reducing interferon-gamma (IFN-y) and IL-17 mRNA. Further studies have corroborated these findings, demonstrating the ability of immature DC derived-EVs to promote short-term graft survival, with the best results obtained when EVs were given alongside immunosuppression or T regulatory cells [112–115]. B cells have been known to secrete EVs [116]; however, it has been shown that they do not secrete them constitutively but rather upon B call activation via appropriate cell signalling [117]. Stimulation of B cells via CD40 and IL-4 results in secretion of an sEV population expressing MHC classes I and II, as well as B cell receptor components and tetraspanins [117]. Relevant to transplantation, sEVs released by activated B cells can be acquired by DCs, which subsequently prime cytotoxic T lymphocytes (CTLs) with the help of CD4+ T cells and natural killer cells; CTLs are known to play an important role in T cell-mediated graft rejection [118].

Table 3. Clinical trials utilising extracellular vesicles as therapeutics that are actively recruiting or completed. [a] Trials currently listed on clinicaltrials.gov; trial names are the same as those found in the clinicaltrials.gov register. EV source is provided where possible, NA indicates that the source was not specified. [b] Where available, EV content has also been added. [c] Trial conclusions have been added where results are available. ANG1, angiopoietin 1; bFGF, basic fibroblast growth factor; CD24, cluster of differentiation marker 24; HGF, hepatocyte growth factor; IL-1B, interleukin-1-beta; NSCLC, non-small cell lung cancer; PDGF-AA, platelet-derived growth factor-AA; siRNA, small interfering ribonucleic acid; TGFb3, transforming growth factor beta-3; TIMP-1 and TIMP-2, tissue inhibitor of matrix metalloproteinases 1 and 2; VEGF, vascular endothelial growth factor; VEGFR, vascular endothelial growth factor receptor.

Number	Name [a]	Condition	EV Source [b]	Location	Phase	NCT Number [c]
			Actively recruiting			
1	Use of Autologous Plasma Rich in Platelets and Extracellular Vesicles in the Surgical Treatment of Chronic Middle Ear Infections	Chronic otitis media	Blood-derived (autologous)	Ljubljana, Slovenia	II/III	NCT04761562
2	Safety Evaluation of Intracoronary Infusion of Extracellular Vesicles in Patients With AMI	Myocardial infarction	Blood-derived	Minnesota, USA	I	NCT04327635
3	Autologous Serum-derived EV for Venous Trophic Lesions Not Responsive to Conventional Treatments (SER-VES-HEAL)	Venous ulcers	Blood-derived (autologous)	Turin, Italy	NA	NCT04652531
4	Bone Marrow Mesenchymal Stem Cell Derived EVs for COVID-19 Moderate-to-Severe Acute Respiratory Distress Syndrome (ARDS): A Phase III Clinical Trial	SARS-CoV-2	Bone marrow MSC-derived (cargo includes VEGFR, VEGF, ANG1, TIMP-1, TIMP-2, IL-1B, PDGF-AA, TGFb3, bFGF, HGF)	Texas, USA	III	NCT05354141
5	Safety and Efficacy of Injection of Human Placenta Mesenchymal Stem Cells Derived Exosomes for Treatment of Complex Anal Fistula	Fistula-in-ano	Human placenta MSC-derived	Tehran, Iran	I/II	NCT05402748
6	Allogenic Mesenchymal Stem Cell Derived Exosome in Patients With Acute Ischemic Stroke	Ischaemic stroke	Allogeneic MSC-derived (cargo enriched for miR-124)	Isfahan, Iran	I/II	NCT03384433

Table 3. *Cont.*

Number	Name [a]	Condition	EV Source [b]	Location	Phase	NCT Number [c]
7	Efficacy and Safety of EXOSOME-MSC Therapy to Reduce Hyper-inflammation In Moderate COVID-19 Patients (EXOMSC-COV19)	SARS-CoV-2	MSC-derived	Indonesia	II/III	NCT05216562
8	A Clinical Study of Mesenchymal Progenitor Cell Exosomes Nebulizer for the Treatment of Pulmonary Infection	Pulmonary infection	Mesenchymal progenitor MSC-derived	Shanghai, China	I/II	NCT04544215
9	Study Investigating the Ability of Plant Exosomes to Deliver Curcumin to Normal and Colon Cancer Tissue	Colon cancer	Plants (cargo of curcumin)	Kentucky, USA	I	NCT01294072
10	Evaluation of the Safety of CD24-Exosomes in Patients With COVID-19 Infection	SARS-CoV-2	CD24-expressing 293-TREx™ cells (EVs enriched for CD24)	Tel Aviv, Israel	I	NCT04747574
11	Clinical Efficacy of Exosome in Degenerative Meniscal Injury (KNEEXO)	Degenerative meniscal injury	MSC-derived	Eskisehir, Turkey	II	NCT05261360
12	The Effect of Stem Cells and Stem Cell Exosomes on Visual Functions in Patients With Retinitis Pigmentosa	Retinitis pigmentosa	Wharton jelly-derived mesenchymal stem cells	Kayseri, Turkey	II/III	NCT05413148
14	Effect of UMSCs Derived Exosomes on Dry Eye in Patients With cGVHD	Dry eye	Umbilical MSC-derived	Guangdong, China	I/II	NCT04213248
15	iExosomes in Treating Participants With Metastatic Pancreas Cancer With KrasG12D Mutation	Pancreatic cancer	MSC-derived (cargo of siRNA against KrasG12D)	Texas, USA	I	NCT03608631
16	Safety and Efficacy of Exosomes Overexpressing CD24 in Two Doses for Patients With Moderate or Severe COVID-19	SARS-CoV-2	CD24-expressing 293-TREx™ cells (EVs enriched for CD24)	Athens, Greece	II	NCT04902183
17	Safety and Effectiveness of Placental Derived Exosomes and Umbilical Cord Mesenchymal Stem Cells in Moderate to Severe Acute Respiratory Distress Syndrome (ARDS) Associated With the Novel Corona Virus Infection (COVID-19)	SARS-CoV-2	Umbilical cord MSC-derived (cargo of unspecified growth factors)	Missouri, USA	I	NCT05387278
18	An Open, Dose-escalation Clinical Study of Chimeric Exosomal Tumor Vaccines for Recurrent or Metastatic Bladder Cancer	Bladder cancer	Chimeric exosomal tumour vaccine	Shanghai, China	I	NCT05559177

Table 3. *Cont.*

Number	Name [a]	Condition	EV Source [b]	Location	Phase	NCT Number [c]
19	A Study of exoASO-STAT6 (CDK-004) in Patients With Advanced Hepatocellular Carcinoma (HCC) and Patients With Liver Metastases From Primary Gastric Cancer and Colorectal Cancer (CRC)	Hepatocellular carcinoma, metastatic gastric and colorectal cancer	Bioengineered (cargo of STAT6 anti-sense oligonucleotide)	California, USA	I	NCT05375604
			Completed			
1	Efficacy of Platelet- and Extracellular Vesicle-rich Plasma in Chronic Postsurgical Temporal Bone Inflammations (PvRP-ear)	Chronic inflammation of temporal bone post-surgery	Blood-derived (autologous)	Ljubljana, Slovenia	NA	NCT04281901
2	Extracellular Vesicle Infusion Treatment for COVID-19 Associated ARDS (EXIT-COVID19)	SARS-CoV-2	Bone marrow MSC-derived	Alabama, USA	II	NCT04493242
3	Safety and Tolerability Study of MSC Exosome Ointment	Psoriasis	MSC-derived (cargo of VEGFR, VEGF, ANG1, TIMP-1, TIMP-2, IL-1B, PDGF-AA, TGFb3, bFGF, HGF)	Singapore	I	NCT05523011
4	A Pilot Clinical Study on Inhalation of Mesenchymal Stem Cells Exosomes Treating Severe Novel Coronavirus Pneumonia	SARS-CoV-2	MSC-derived	Wuhan, China	I	NCT04276987 (conclusion: inhalation of EVs up to a total amount of 2.0×10^9 was feasible and functioned well, with no evidence of prespecified adverse events, immediate clinical instability or dose-relevant toxicity at any of the doses tested. This safety profile was seemingly followed by CT imaging improvement within 7 days)
5	Intra-discal Injection of Platelet-rich Plasma (PRP) Enriched With Exosomes in Chronic Low Back Pain	Chronic lower back pain	Blood derived (autologous)	Uttarakhand, India	I	NCT04849429

Table 3. *Cont.*

Number	Name [a]	Condition	EV Source [b]	Location	Phase	NCT Number [c]
6	Evaluation of Safety and Efficiency of Method of Exosome Inhalation in SARS-CoV-2 Associated Pneumonia (COVID-19EXO)	SARS-CoV-2	MSC-derived	Volga, Russia	I/II	NCT04491240
7	A Tolerance Clinical Study on Aerosol Inhalation of Mesenchymal Stem Cells Exosomes In Healthy Volunteers	Nil	Adipose MSC-derived	Shanghai, China	I	NCT04313647 (conclusion: all volunteers tolerated EV nebulization well, with no serious adverse events observed. The authors suggested that nebulised EVs could be a promising therapeutic strategy in lung injury diseases)
8	Plant Exosomes ± Curcumin to Abrogate Symptoms of Inflammatory Bowel Disease	Inflammatory bowel disease	Plants (cargo of curcumin)	Kentucky, USA	NA	NCT04879810
9	Edible Plant Exosome Ability to Prevent Oral Mucositis Associated With Chemoradiation Treatment of Head and Neck Cancer	Oral mucositis	Grapes	Kentucky, USA	I	NCT01668849
10	Trial of a Vaccination With Tumor Antigen-loaded Dendritic Cell-derived Exosomes (CSET 1437)	Non-small cell lung cancer	Dendritic cell derived (cargo of melanoma-associated antigen)	Villejuif, France	II	NCT01159288 (conclusion: EVs boost the natural killer cell arm of antitumour immunity in patients with advanced NSCLC)

Whist there is evidence of the mechanisms whereby EVs mediate graft rejection, they can also achieve an immunosuppressive effect and promote immune tolerance, a key therapeutic target in transplantation. In a rat model of kidney transplantation, T regulatory (Treg) derived-EVs inhibited T cell proliferation [119]. The EVs secreted by mouse Tregs were shown to have a specific miRNA profile that led to downstream immunosuppressive effects in other immune compartments; miR-150-5p and miR-142-3p were associated with reduced IL-6 secretion by DCs and increased secretion of anti-inflammatory IL-10 whilst suppressing IFN-y secretion by $CD4^+$ T cells [120,121]. The ability of Treg-derived EVs to reduce proliferation of $CD4^+$ T cells and their subsequent secretion of IL-2 and IFN-y has been demonstrated to result from the presence of the ectoenzyme NT5E or CD73, which acts via binding of the adenosine receptor A2aR to facilitate the immunosuppressive effects of Tregs [122–125]. This may translate into prolonged graft survival and effector T-cell proliferation inhibition, as suggested in a renal transplant model of acute rejection. Treg-derived EVs also suppress the proliferation and viability of rejection-mediating CTLs, reducing their ability to produce perforin and IFN-y [126]. This has been applied to a rat model of liver transplantation, where Treg EV-treated rats demonstrated improved short-term survival compared to their non-treated counterparts [126]. These studies highlight the potential therapeutic role of EVs derived from both innate and humoral immune compartments; in this context, EVs may have a role as adjuncts to immunosuppressive therapies. In addition, specific miRNA species, similar to those described above, could be packaged into EVs for delivery as further adjuncts to immunosuppression regimes or even to treat graft rejection. Further work is clearly needed to transfer these promising findings from animal models to clinical practice.

5.2. *Ischemia-Reperfusion Injury*

A major challenge in organ transplantation is ischemia-reperfusion injury (IRI); a tissue injury that occurs when the blood supply to organs is interrupted and then restored [127]. Waiting lists for organ transplantation are growing and the availability of donor organs does not meet the demand [110], leading to an increase in the utilisation of suboptimal (extended criteria or marginal) organs in an attempt to meet needs and reduce waitlist mortality [128,129]. However, marginal organs are more susceptible to ischemia-reperfusion injury (IRI) and an enhanced pathological response to the restoration of oxygenated blood supply, thereby leading to suboptimal graft function [130–132], as well as increased graft immunogenicity [133] and, subsequently, increased rates of allograft rejection [134].

IRI prompts the release of inflammatory mediators and reactive oxygen species, leading to tissue damage, necrosis and release of damage-associated molecular patterns (DAMPs) [135]. DAMP recognition by innate immune cells, such as macrophages, activates the nuclear factor-kappa beta (NF-kB) pathway responsible for transcriptional induction of pro-inflammatory mediators [136]. These include inflammasomes, which control the post-translational proteolytic activation of pro-inflammatory cytokines to orchestrate pyroptosis, a pro-inflammatory form of cell death, which is the ultimate outcome of IRI [136]. NF-kB signalling has been correlated with the release of EVs [137]. Pre-clinical studies have shown that EVs released during IRI are central to immune activation and propagation of inflammation, commonly through interactions with the NF-κB signalling pathway; for example, through upregulation of IL-1B, a potent pro- inflammatory cytokine [138]. There is evidence at the transcriptomic level that human kidneys suffering prolonged delayed graft function post-kidney transplant demonstrate upregulation of NF-kB-mediated signalling pathways [139]. This has been reproduced in a rat model of liver transplantation [140], where mRNA levels of NF-kB pathway mediators, including TNF-alpha, IL-1B and IL-10, were significantly raised during IRI [140], highlighting this inflammatory transcription regulator as a key player in organ IRI.

EVs are a promising therapy for IRI and increasingly studied in pre-clinical models. Human induced pluripotent stem cell (hiPSC)-derived MSC-EVs ameliorated rat kidney IRI through the delivery of specificity protein 1 into target renal cells [141]. More specific mechanisms of IRI have also been targeted by EVs utilising EXPLOR, a novel optogenetically engineered exosome technology. In this study, Kim et al. engineered EVs to deliver super-repressor inhibitor of NF-kB (ExosrIkB), demonstrating significantly improved outcomes in a mouse kidney IRI model [142]. The treated group achieved lower blood levels of urea, creatinine and neutrophil gelatinase-associated lipocalin (a biomarker for renal injury released by renal tubular cells under stress) compared to the naive control group. This was confirmed at the transcriptomic level with reduced gene expression of pro-inflammatory cytokines and adhesion molecule in the treated group [142]. Administration of human cord blood endothelial colony-forming cell (ECFC)- derived EVs protected mice against kidney IRI; exosomes were found to be enriched for miR-86-5p, which inhibits the phosphatase and tensin homolog (PTEN) and enhances Akt phosphorylation [143]. Through these mechanisms, miR-86-5p inhibited hypoxia-induced apoptotic responses, protecting against IRI induced renal injury. Through an alternative mechanism, miR-199a-3p carried by MSC-derived EVs also inhibited apoptosis in a kidney IRI model, this time through downregulation of semaphoring 3A in addition to Akt and ERK pathway activation [144]. Endoplasmic reticulum stress during hypoxia is a known consequence of IRI, leading to misfolding of proteins and cellular dysfunction. miR-199a-5p transfer in bone marrow stem cell-derived sEVs targeted binding immunoglobulin protein to reduce ER stress and restore cellular homeostasis during early reperfusion, mitigating IRI [145].

In the liver, Du et al. demonstrated that MSCs derived from hiPSCs conferred protection against mouse hepatic IRI via activation of sphingosine kinase and the sphingosine-1-phosphage signalling pathway, as well as promoting cell proliferation by the same pathway [146]. The treated group achieved lower alanine and aspartate aminotransferase levels, as well as histological reductions in hepatocyte necrosis and congestion, with increased expression of proliferation markers. In another pre-clinical study, bone marrow-derived DC EVs upregulated anti-inflammatory cytokines TGF-beta, FoxP3 and IL-10, alleviating liver IRI in mice [147]. Activation of Toll-like receptor signalling by DAMPS generated during IRI can induce formation of neutrophil extracellular traps (NETs), the formation of which has been verified as a critical step in liver IRI [148]. Human umbilical cord-derived MSC-EVs are able to transfer functional mitochondria to intrahepatic neutrophils, subsequently maintaining mitochondrial quality through mitochondrial fusion and leading to inhibition of NET formation in a cell culture model of IRI [149]. Steatotic livers are particularly susceptible to IRI and suffer from ferroptosis, a process of iron-dependent cell death [150]. Haem-oxygenase-1 (HO-1) is an antioxidant that can protect cells from oxidative stress; delivery of EVs from bone marrow-derived MSCs overexpressing HO-1 suppressed ferroptosis in a rat model of liver transplant IRI via EV-mediated transfer of miR-29a-3p [151]. miR-29a-3p targeted the iron response element-binding protein 2 (Ireb2), the main regulator of cellular iron homeostasis, leading to a reduction in cellular iron and downregulation of the transferring receptor, preventing further iron uptake by cells [151].

Myocardial IRI has been studied extensively and mechanisms of EV-mediated IRI amelioration that may be translatable to the field of organ transplantation have been highlighted. Rat MSC-derived EVs abolished the production of reactive oxygen species (another mediator of IRI) and improved cardiac function in vitro [152]. They also saw reduced apoptotic activity through autophagy promotion via adenosine monophosphate-activated protein kinase (AMPK) and AKT pathways. In oxygen-glucose deprivation cell culture models, dental pulp-derived MSC-derived EVs containing miR-4732-3p prolonged spontaneous beating, lowered reactive oxygen species and reduced apoptosis in cardiomyocytes [153]. The benefits of miR-4732-3p persisted when the same cells were transplanted into infarcted rat hearts with reduced scar tissue and preserved cardiac function [153]. Villa Del Campo et al. utilised a novel model of human myocardial injury in the form of cryoinjured engineered human myocardium to test the ability of epicardial EVs to promote cardiomyocyte proliferation [154]. The group identified the EV cargos miR-30a, miR-100, miR-27a and miR-30e as the mediators of the observed effect. Although an IRI model was not utilised, these miRNAs demonstrated reductions in apoptosis via Akt and ERK pathway activation, as seen in previously discussed kidney models of IRI. EVs have also been shown to reduce inflammatory cytokines in lung IRI in mice. The reductions in inflammatory cytokines TNF-alpha, IL-1B, IL-6, IL-7 and IL-8 from intratracheal administration of EVs from MSC-EVs, which were coupled with a reduction in lung oedema and lower M1 macrophage polarisation of alveolar macrophages, were suggested to be mediated by transfer of miR-21-5p encapsulated within EVs [155]. Human Wharton jelly mesenchymal stem cell (hWJMSC)-derived EVs have been utilised in the mitigation of lung IRI in a murine lung transplant model with both in vivo and in vitro components [156]. The group were able to achieve significant attenuation of lung dysfunction and injury (reduced oedema, myeloperoxidase levels and neutrophil infiltration) in the group treated with MSC-derived EVs compared to the untreated control group. They further observed significant reductions in proinflammatory cytokines TNF-alpha, IL-17, CXCL1 and HMGB1 [156]. Delving further into the mechanism behind the injury and its treatment, they were able to show downregulation of primary invariant natural killer T cell-produced IL-17 and macrophage-produced TNF-alpha and HMGB1 after IRI cycles [156]. Whilst many studies have focused on mitigating IRI through EV-delivered miRNAs, Cai et al. delivered an miRNA inhibitor packaged into EVs to inhibit the effect of a specific miRNA implicated in IRI [157]. Having identified that miR-206 expression was increased in the bronchoalveolar lavage fluid of patients on days 0 and 1 after lung transplantation, they replicated this finding in a mouse model of IRI resulting from lung transplantation. Delivery of antagomir-206-enriched EVs attenuated lung dysfunction, injury and oedema compared to treatment with EVs alone after murine lung IRI. The enriched EV-treated group also showed decreased expression of pro- inflammatory cytokines and chemokine-ligant-1, a potent chemoattractant for several groups of immune cells that propagate tissue injury [157].

There is clear evidence that EVs (generally derived from stem cells) can be harnessed to attenuate IRI. It is essential that the mechanisms behind their action are understood to allow targeting of specific cellular processes. The specific miRNAs that modulate cellular processes and homeostasis are promising therapeutic targets for future exploration, as are EV-packaged antagonists of cellular miRNAs implicated in IRI. Other biologically active EV cargos mediating their IRI protective effects must be uncovered in order to design appropriate therapeutics. Furthermore, the timing of the delivery of EV-based therapeutics in the treatment of IRI must be explored, with evidence showing that both pre-ischemia and post-reperfusion interventions are possible. Studies are required in human organ systems to understand the mechanisms of IRI and thus enable expansion of therapeutic targeting, as well as to promote clinical translation of EV drug delivery systems.

5.3. Machine Perfusion as a Platform for EV Drug Delivery Systems

Machine perfusion of organs outside the body prior to transplantation has been introduced to mitigate IRI and not only enables graft viability assessment [158,159] but also the delivery of therapeutics for the repair of organs prior to transplantation (Figure 3) [160]. The efficacy of MSC delivery during perfusion to mitigate IRI has been demonstrated in several organ systems [161–163]. Building on the earlier discussion on native EVs as drug delivery systems, EVs from stem cells have also been delivered during organ perfusion with promising results. In a recent study [164], human liver stem cell-derived EVs were delivered with a rat liver model of IRI during normothermic machine perfusion, and attenuation of IRI was demonstrated via improved biochemical markers of liver injury and a histologically assessed reduction in necrosis. A second group from Italy demonstrated the ability of MSC-derived EVs delivered during hypothermic oxygenated perfusion of the kidneys from extended criteria donors to reduce IRI. The treated kidneys demonstrated improved global renal ischemia damage scores, lower apoptotic markers and lower lactate levels [165]. The machine perfusion model provides an ideal platform to test new therapies, such as EV drug delivery systems, with isolated organs. For example, the liver is an ideal organ for the examination of EV therapy, as the vast majority of systemically administered EVs accumulate in the liver [166,167]. EVs can be delivered into the perfusate, directly into the parenchyma itself or even through secretory apparatuses, such as the bile duct in the liver or the ureter in kidneys, providing a variety of delivery methods to implement in trials and optimise. Not only does isolated organ perfusion have the capacity to provide important mechanistic insights concerning EVs, but it is ideal for pharmacological testing [168] and directly translatable to EV drug delivery system assessment. Organ transplantation represents an important clinical field for therapeutic intervention, offering a clear platform enabling simple delivery, rigorous testing and expansion of the use of both native and hybrid EV drug delivery systems.

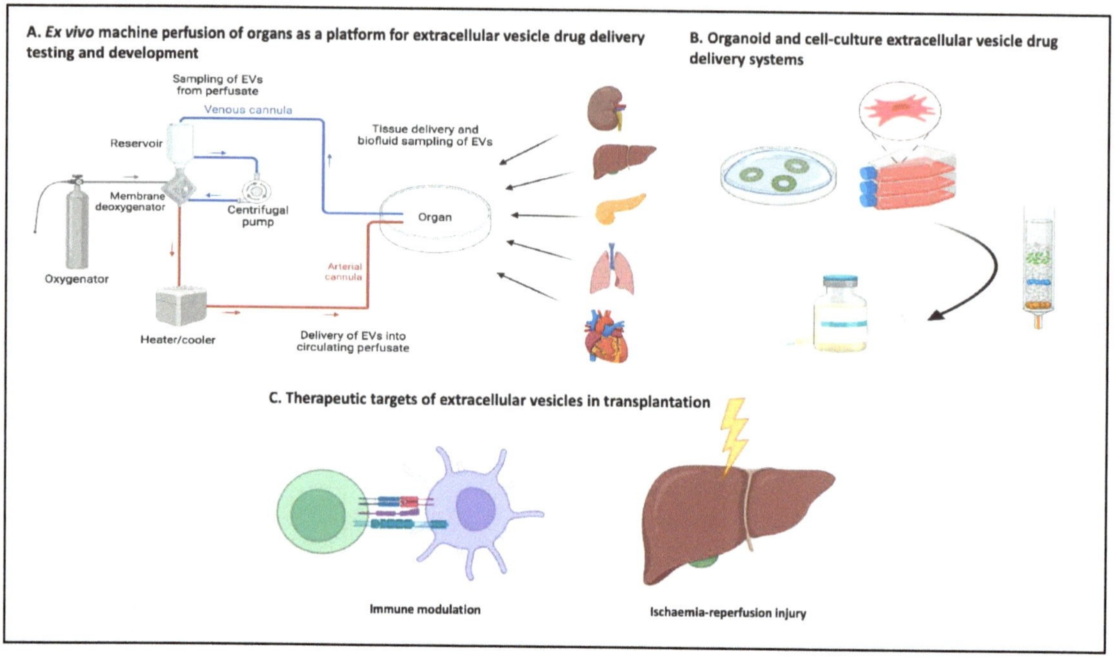

Figure 3. Organ transplantation represents a key area for extracellular vesicle (EV) drug delivery systems. (**A**) Ex vivo machine perfusion of organs provides a platform for EV delivery and allows sampling of organ biofluid post-treatment to monitor response. (**B**) Cell-culture and organoid systems are suitable EV production platforms. (**C**) Delivery of EVs during organ perfusion can modulate the immune system and target ischemia-reperfusion injury.

5.4. Barriers to Clinical Translation

EVs are an attractive drug delivery system because of their ability to reduce the toxic effects that can result from the introduction of a foreign substance into the body. However, larger scale and more specialised clinical translations of EVs remain challenging due to the inherent complexity of the nanoparticles themselves, the heterogeneity in their sizes and natural (batch-to-batch) variations during production, which result in higher intrinsic risks in the production process than for their purely synthetic liposomal counterparts. The production of EV-based drug delivery systems faces several challenges, including a degree of inherent biological variability potentially resulting in product heterogeneity. There are two main areas where this variability may be introduced: firstly, as part of the upstream processing (i.e., inside the cells used to express the desired biological effects) and, secondly, in the downstream processing (i.e., through the manufacturing process itself) [169]. For EVs produced by cells, the culture conditions of the cells strongly influence the product quality—not only in terms of yield but also in terms of composition and subsequent bioactivity [170]. Another important consideration is that EVs are a relatively static product and, except for degradation, they are not expected to change post-harvesting. Therefore, minor changes that could have considerable impact on product quality and activity are more challenging to identify. Ensuring good manufacturing practice is essential and, whilst known process controls from fields such as cell-based therapies could be adapted, the sizes and unique complexity of EVs mean that additional process controls are required. Despite these predicaments, there is significant enthusiasm toward the continuation of the clinical translation of EVs, which has led to a position paper from the ISEV regarding the use of EVs in clinical trials [66]. They build on the current practice followed by manufacturers of biological pharmaceutics, who routinely identify all substances in a drug that exert a particular metabolic, immunological or pharmacological action and are responsible for the drug's biological (therapeutic) effects. If all the therapeutic effects of an EV intended for drug delivery were to be attributed to the loaded molecule and not the EV itself, then the EV would be considered a non-active component; accordingly, it would not be necessary to determine the mechanism of action but only the safety profile of the EV preparation.

Furthermore, the biologically active EVs that can be produced must be understood both in terms of biological cargo and the downstream biological processes they are linked to. Consistent isolation of biologically active sEVs—i.e., exosomes—is extremely challenging due to the lack of specific markers distinguishing them from other sEV species. A recent reassessment of exosome composition in an elegant study utilising high-resolution density gradient fractionation and direct immunoaffinity capture highlighted the presence of annexin A1 and A2, calcium-dependant phospholipid binding proteins, in non-exosomal small to large EVs [1]. Whilst the absence of larger vesicle markers, along with other characteristics, suggests the presence of exosomes, clinical translation requires certainty about the EV subpopulation being used. The ability to isolate single EVs has already been employed clinically, such as in Single Particle Automated Raman Trapping Analysis (SPARTA), which uses EVs as breast cancer biomarkers [171]; further methods of exploring the surface expression of sEVs are needed to identify exosome surface markers. Once identified, the next important step towards clinically translating exosomal subpopulations would be understanding their biological functions. Many studies have utilised a variety of protocols to purify EVs in the exosomal range, but none have allowed reliable association with a function or group of functions. Novel technology, such as phage-based display technology for the identification and isolation of disease-released exosomes, could be used to capture the biological implications of exosome production and release under different conditions [172]. Further progress requires the development of new technologies for the association of a specific marker with an exosome subtype and robust demonstration of a correlation with biological function.

In addition to the barriers outlined above, further research is required before EVs can be routinely used in transplantation. Whilst the mechanisms of graft rejection and IRI have now been explored in depth, there is still a lot to be uncovered and it is essential for the mechanisms behind the therapeutic benefits of EVs to be understood. Modulating the upstream pathways of inflammation, for example, has downstream effects on multiple effector mechanisms that are potentially important in other cellular processes and regulatory mechanisms. Mechanistic insights are essential to ensure the potential inhibition and activation of cellular pathways mediated by EV cargo do not have secondary negative effects unexplored in pre-clinical models thus far.

6. Conclusions and Future Perspectives

There is evidence that native and hybrid EVs may be used as effective drug delivery systems, with their intrinsic ability to protect and deliver a functional cargo by utilising endogenous cellular mechanisms making them attractive as therapeutics. Pre-clinical studies have demonstrated the potential of EVs in preventing rejection in transplantation and mitigating ischemia reperfusion injury in several models. This work has enabled clinical translation of specific (generally stem cell-derived) EV populations and led to several clinical trials actively recruiting patients, the results of which are eagerly awaited. However, EVs' rapid and widespread clinical translation is challenged by the lack of cost-effective, large-scale isolation and characterisation methodologies. The emergence of high-sensitivity characterisation methods is expected to provide important insights into the biology of these powerful nanoparticles, with that improved understanding translating into increased utilisation in clinical practice. Organ transplantation represents an area that has the potential to significantly benefit from EV-based therapeutics. Machine perfusion of isolated organs provides an unparalleled platform for the investigation of EV biology and testing of their pharmacokinetics and pharmacodynamics. The global population of patients with end-stage organ failure, as well as those facing it, will benefit significantly if we can deepen our understanding of thus far unexplained EV-mediated mechanisms and harness EVs' potential as drug delivery systems.

Author Contributions: Conceptualization, H.V.M.S. and V.K.; methodology, H.V.M.S.; investigation, H.V.M.S., L.K.J.S., H.S., V.K; resources, H.V.M.S., L.K.J.S., H.S.; writing—original draft preparation, H.V.M.S., L.K.J.S., H.S.; writing—review and editing, H.V.M.S., V.K.; visualization, H.V.M.S.; supervision, V.K. All authors have read and agreed to the published version of the manuscript.

Funding: The research presented in this manuscript received funding from the National Institute for Health Research Blood and Transplant Research Unit (NIHR BTRU) in Organ Donation and Transplantation at the University of Cambridge in collaboration with Newcastle University and in partnership with NHS Blood and Transplant (NHSBT). We gratefully acknowledge funding from an NIHR Fellowship (PDF-2016-09-065, V.K.) and NIHR Academic Clinical Fellowship (ACF-2020-14-001, H.V.M.S.). V.K. acknowledges funding as a PI Terasaki Scholar. The views expressed are those of the authors and not necessarily those of the National Health Service, the National Institute for Health Research, the Department of Health or National Health Service Blood and Transplant.

Institutional Review Board Statement: Not applicable.

Informed Consent Statement: Not applicable.

Data Availability Statement: No new data were created or analysed in this study. Data sharing is not applicable to this article.

Acknowledgments: No acknowledgements are required for this work.

Conflicts of Interest: The authors have no competing interests to declare.

References

1. Jeppesen, D.K.; Fenix, A.M.; Franklin, J.L.; Higginbotham, J.N.; Zhang, Q.; Zimmerman, L.J.; Liebler, D.C.; Ping, J.; Liu, Q.; Evans, R.; et al. Reassessment of Exosome Composition. *Cell* **2019**, *177*, 428–445.e18. [CrossRef]
2. Valadi, H.; Ekström, K.; Bossios, A.; Sjöstrand, M.; Lee, J.J.; Lötvall, J.O. Exosome-Mediated Transfer of MRNAs and MicroRNAs Is a Novel Mechanism of Genetic Exchange between Cells. *Nat. Cell Biol.* **2007**, *9*, 654–659. [CrossRef]
3. PNAS. Human Tumor Virus Utilizes Exosomes for Intercellular Communication. Available online: https://www.pnas.org/doi/full/10.1073/pnas.1014194107 (accessed on 18 November 2022).
4. Skog, J.; Würdinger, T.; van Rijn, S.; Meijer, D.H.; Gainche, L.; Curry, W.T.; Carter, B.S.; Krichevsky, A.M.; Breakefield, X.O. Glioblastoma Microvesicles Transport RNA and Proteins That Promote Tumour Growth and Provide Diagnostic Biomarkers. *Nat. Cell Biol.* **2008**, *10*, 1470–1476. [CrossRef]
5. Colombo, M.; Raposo, G.; Théry, C. Biogenesis, Secretion, and Intercellular Interactions of Exosomes and Other Extracellular Vesicles. *Annu. Rev. Cell Dev. Biol.* **2014**, *30*, 255–289. Available online: https://www.annualreviews.org/doi/10.1146/annurev-cellbio-101512-122326?url_ver=Z39.88-2003&rfr_id=ori%3Arid%3Acrossref.org&rfr_dat=cr_pub++0pubmed (accessed on 18 November 2022). [CrossRef]
6. Möller, A.; Lobb, R.J. The Evolving Translational Potential of Small Extracellular Vesicles in Cancer. *Nat. Rev. Cancer* **2020**, *20*, 697–709. [CrossRef]
7. Jansen, F.; Yang, X.; Baumann, K.; Przybilla, D.; Schmitz, T.; Flender, A.; Paul, K.; Alhusseiny, A.; Nickenig, G.; Werner, N. Endothelial Microparticles Reduce ICAM-1 Expression in a MicroRNA-222-dependent Mechanism. *J. Cell. Mol. Med.* **2015**, *19*, 2202–2214. Available online: https://onlinelibrary.wiley.com/doi/10.1111/jcmm.12607 (accessed on 18 November 2022). [CrossRef]
8. van Balkom, B.W.M.; de Jong, O.G.; Smits, M.; Brummelman, J.; den Ouden, K.; de Bree, P.M.; van Eijndhoven, M.A.J.; Pegtel, D.M.; Stoorvogel, W.; Würdinger, T.; et al. Endothelial Cells Require MiR-214 to Secrete Exosomes That Suppress Senescence and Induce Angiogenesis in Human and Mouse Endothelial Cells. *Blood* **2013**, *121*, 3997–4006. [CrossRef]
9. Li, X.; Liu, R.; Huang, Z.; Gurley, E.C.; Wang, X.; Wang, J.; He, H.; Yang, H.; Lai, G.; Zhang, L.; et al. Cholangiocyte-Derived Exosomal Long Noncoding RNA H19 Promotes Cholestatic Liver Injury in Mouse and Human. *Hepatology* **2018**, *68*, 599–615. [CrossRef]
10. Sanz-Ros, J.; Romero-García, N.; Mas-Bargues, C.; Monleón, D.; Gordevicius, J.; Brooke, R.T.; Dromant, M.; Díaz, A.; Derevyanko, A.; Guío-Carrión, A.; et al. Small Extracellular Vesicles from Young Adipose-Derived Stem Cells Prevent Frailty, Improve Health Span, and Decrease Epigenetic Age in Old Mice. *Sci. Adv.* **2022**, *8*, eabq2226. [CrossRef]
11. Qin, Y.; Wang, L.; Gao, Z.; Chen, G.; Zhang, C. Bone Marrow Stromal/Stem Cell-Derived Extracellular Vesicles Regulate Osteoblast Activity and Differentiation in vitro and Promote Bone Regeneration in vivo. *Sci. Rep.* **2016**, *6*, 21961. [CrossRef]

12. Yang, T.T.; Liu, C.G.; Gao, S.C.; Zhang, Y.; Wang, P.C. The Serum Exosome Derived MicroRNA-135a, -193b, and -384 Were Potential Alzheimer's Disease Biomarkers. *Biomed. Environ. Sci. BES* **2018**, *31*, 87–96. [CrossRef]
13. Fourcade, O.; Simon, M.-F.; Viodé, C.; Rugani, N.; Leballe, F.; Ragab, A.; Fournié, B.; Sarda, L.; Chap, H. Secretory Phospholipase A2 Generates the Novel Lipid Mediator Lysophosphatidic Acid in Membrane Microvesicles Shed from Activated Cells. *Cell* **1995**, *80*, 919–927. [CrossRef]
14. Ikeda, C.; Haga, H.; Makino, N.; Inuzuka, T.; Kurimoto, A.; Ueda, T.; Matsuda, A.; Kakizaki, Y.; Ishizawa, T.; Kobayashi, T.; et al. Utility of Claudin-3 in Extracellular Vesicles from Human Bile as Biomarkers of Cholangiocarcinoma. *Sci. Rep.* **2021**, *11*, 1195. [CrossRef]
15. Kupsco, A.; Prada, D.; Valvi, D.; Hu, L.; Petersen, M.S.; Coull, B.; Grandjean, P.; Weihe, P.; Baccarelli, A.A. Human Milk Extracellular Vesicle MiRNA Expression and Associations with Maternal Characteristics in a Population-Based Cohort from the Faroe Islands. *Sci. Rep.* **2021**, *11*, 5840. [CrossRef]
16. Spitzer, P.; Mulzer, L.-M.; Oberstein, T.J.; Munoz, L.E.; Lewczuk, P.; Kornhuber, J.; Herrmann, M.; Maler, J.M. Microvesicles from Cerebrospinal Fluid of Patients with Alzheimer's Disease Display Reduced Concentrations of Tau and APP Protein. *Sci. Rep.* **2019**, *9*, 7089. [CrossRef]
17. Sun, I.O.; Lerman, L.O. Urinary Extracellular Vesicles as Biomarkers of Kidney Disease: From Diagnostics to Therapeutics. *Diagnostics* **2020**, *10*, 311. [CrossRef]
18. Liu, J.; Gao, A.; Liu, Y.; Sun, Y.; Zhang, D.; Lin, X.; Hu, C.; Zhu, Y.; Du, Y.; Han, H.; et al. MicroRNA Expression Profiles of Epicardial Adipose Tissue-Derived Exosomes in Patients with Coronary Atherosclerosis. *Rev. Cardiovasc. Med.* **2022**, *23*, 206. [CrossRef]
19. Li, T.; Wang, B.; Ding, H.; Chen, S.; Cheng, W.; Li, Y.; Wu, X.; Wang, L.; Jiang, Y.; Lu, Z.; et al. Effect of Extracellular Vesicles From Multiple Cells on Vascular Smooth Muscle Cells in Atherosclerosis. *Front. Pharmacol.* **2022**, *13*, 1430. [CrossRef]
20. Brown, P.A.; Brown, P.D. Extracellular Vesicles and Atherosclerotic Peripheral Arterial Disease. *Cardiovasc. Pathol.* **2023**, *63*, 107510. [CrossRef]
21. Newman, L.A.; Muller, K.; Rowland, A. Circulating Cell-Specific Extracellular Vesicles as Biomarkers for the Diagnosis and Monitoring of Chronic Liver Diseases. *Cell. Mol. Life Sci.* **2022**, *79*, 232. [CrossRef]
22. Zhang, Y.; Wang, D.; Shen, D.; Luo, Y.; Che, Y.-Q. Identification of Exosomal MiRNAs Associated with the Anthracycline-Induced Liver Injury in Postoperative Breast Cancer Patients by Small RNA Sequencing. *PeerJ* **2020**, *8*, e9021. [CrossRef]
23. Lu, M.; DiBernardo, E.; Parks, E.; Fox, H.; Zheng, S.-Y.; Wayne, E. The Role of Extracellular Vesicles in the Pathogenesis and Treatment of Autoimmune Disorders. *Front. Immunol.* **2021**, *12*, 566299. [CrossRef]
24. Blommer, J.; Pitcher, T.; Mustapic, M.; Eren, E.; Yao, P.J.; Vreones, M.P.; Pucha, K.A.; Dalrymple-Alford, J.; Shoorangiz, R.; Meissner, W.G.; et al. Extracellular Vesicle Biomarkers for Cognitive Impairment in Parkinson's Disease. *Brain* **2023**, *146*, 195–208. [CrossRef]
25. Burgelman, M.; Dujardin, P.; Vandendriessche, C.; Vandenbroucke, R.E. Free Complement and Complement Containing Extracellular Vesicles as Potential Biomarkers for Neuroinflammatory and Neurodegenerative Disorders. *Front. Immunol.* **2022**, *13*, 1055050. [CrossRef]
26. Manna, I.; Quattrone, A.; Benedittis, S.D.; Vescio, B.; Iaccino, E.; Quattrone, A. Exosomal MiRNA as Peripheral Biomarkers in Parkinson's Disease and Progressive Supranuclear Palsy: A Pilot Study. *Park. Relat. Disord.* **2021**, *93*, 77–84. [CrossRef]
27. Lee, Y.-T.; Tran, B.V.; Wang, J.J.; Liang, I.Y.; You, S.; Zhu, Y.; Agopian, V.G.; Tseng, H.-R.; Yang, J.D. The Role of Extracellular Vesicles in Disease Progression and Detection of Hepatocellular Carcinoma. *Cancers* **2021**, *13*, 3076. [CrossRef]
28. Chang, C.-H.; Pauklin, S. Extracellular Vesicles in Pancreatic Cancer Progression and Therapies. *Cell Death Dis.* **2021**, *12*, 973. [CrossRef]
29. Jordan, K.R.; Hall, J.K.; Schedin, T.; Borakove, M.; Xian, J.J.; Dzieciatkowska, M.; Lyons, T.R.; Schedin, P.; Hansen, K.C.; Borges, V.F. Extracellular Vesicles from Young Women's Breast Cancer Patients Drive Increased Invasion of Non-Malignant Cells via the Focal Adhesion Kinase Pathway: A Proteomic Approach. *Breast Cancer Res.* **2020**, *22*, 128. [CrossRef]
30. Lobb, R.J.; Visan, K.S.; Wu, L.-Y.; Norris, E.L.; Hastie, M.L.; Everitt, S.; Yang, I.A.; Bowman, R.V.; Siva, S.; Larsen, J.E.; et al. An Epithelial-to-Mesenchymal Transition Induced Extracellular Vesicle Prognostic Signature in Non-Small Cell Lung Cancer. *Commun. Biol.* **2023**, *6*, 68. [CrossRef]
31. Théry, C.; Witwer, K.W.; Aikawa, E.; Alcaraz, M.J.; Anderson, J.D.; Andriantsitohaina, R.; Antoniou, A.; Arab, T.; Archer, F.; Atkin-Smith, G.K.; et al. Minimal Information for Studies of Extracellular Vesicles 2018 (MISEV2018): A Position Statement of the International Society for Extracellular Vesicles and Update of the MISEV2014 Guidelines. *J. Extracell. Vesicles* **2018**, *7*, 1535750. [CrossRef]
32. Wollert, T.; Hurley, J.H. Molecular Mechanism of Multivesicular Body Biogenesis by ESCRT Complexes. *Nature* **2010**, *464*, 864–869. [CrossRef]
33. Baietti, M.F.; Zhang, Z.; Mortier, E.; Melchior, A.; Degeest, G.; Geeraerts, A.; Ivarsson, Y.; Depoortere, F.; Coomans, C.; Vermeiren, E.; et al. Syndecan–Syntenin–ALIX Regulates the Biogenesis of Exosomes. *Nat. Cell Biol.* **2012**, *14*, 677–685. [CrossRef]
34. Buschow, S.I.; Nolte-'t Hoen, E.N.M.; Van Niel, G.; Pols, M.S.; Ten Broeke, T.; Lauwen, M.; Ossendorp, F.; Melief, C.J.M.; Raposo, G.; Wubbolts, R.; et al. MHC II in Dendritic Cells Is Targeted to Lysosomes or T Cell-Induced Exosomes Via Distinct Multivesicular Body Pathways. *Traffic* **2009**, *10*, 1528–1542. [CrossRef]

35. van Niel, G.; Charrin, S.; Simoes, S.; Romao, M.; Rochin, L.; Saftig, P.; Marks, M.S.; Rubinstein, E.; Raposo, G. The Tetraspanin CD63 Regulates ESCRT-Independent and -Dependent Endosomal Sorting during Melanogenesis. *Dev. Cell* **2011**, *21*, 708–721. [CrossRef]
36. Koifman, N.; Biran, I.; Aharon, A.; Brenner, B.; Talmon, Y. A Direct-Imaging Cryo-EM Study of Shedding Extracellular Vesicles from Leukemic Monocytes. *J. Struct. Biol.* **2017**, *198*, 177–185. [CrossRef]
37. Mathieu, M.; Martin-Jaular, L.; Lavieu, G.; Théry, C. Specificities of Secretion and Uptake of Exosomes and Other Extracellular Vesicles for Cell-to-Cell Communication. *Nat. Cell Biol.* **2019**, *21*, 9–17. [CrossRef]
38. Sedgwick, A.E.; D'Souza-Schorey, C. The Biology of Extracellular Microvesicles. *Traffic* **2018**, *19*, 319–327. [CrossRef]
39. Vizio, D.D.; Morello, M.; Dudley, A.C.; Schow, P.W.; Adam, R.M.; Morley, S.; Mulholland, D.; Rotinen, M.; Hager, M.H.; Insabato, L.; et al. Large Oncosomes in Human Prostate Cancer Tissues and in the Circulation of Mice with Metastatic Disease. *Am. J. Pathol.* **2012**, *181*, 1573–1584. [CrossRef]
40. D'Souza-Schorey, C.; Clancy, J.W. Tumor-Derived Microvesicles: Shedding Light on Novel Microenvironment Modulators and Prospective Cancer Biomarkers. *Genes Dev.* **2012**, *26*, 1287–1299. [CrossRef]
41. Muralidharan-Chari, V.; Clancy, J.W.; Sedgwick, A.; D'Souza-Schorey, C. Microvesicles: Mediators of Extracellular Communication during Cancer Progression. *J. Cell Sci.* **2010**, *123*, 1603–1611. [CrossRef]
42. Wei, X.; Liu, C.; Wang, H.; Wang, L.; Xiao, F.; Guo, Z.; Zhang, H. Surface Phosphatidylserine Is Responsible for the Internalization on Microvesicles Derived from Hypoxia-Induced Human Bone Marrow Mesenchymal Stem Cells into Human Endothelial Cells. *PLoS ONE* **2016**, *11*, e0147360. [CrossRef]
43. Budnik, V.; Ruiz-Cañada, C.; Wendler, F. Extracellular Vesicles Round off Communication in the Nervous System. *Nat. Rev. Neurosci.* **2016**, *17*, 160–172. [CrossRef]
44. Muralidharan-Chari, V.; Clancy, J.; Plou, C.; Romao, M.; Chavrier, P.; Raposo, G.; D'Souza-Schorey, C. ARF6-Regulated Shedding of Tumor Cell-Derived Plasma Membrane Microvesicles. *Curr. Biol.* **2009**, *19*, 1875–1885. [CrossRef]
45. Sedgwick, A.E.; Clancy, J.W.; Olivia Balmert, M.; D'Souza-Schorey, C. Extracellular Microvesicles and Invadopodia Mediate Non-Overlapping Modes of Tumor Cell Invasion. *Sci. Rep.* **2015**, *5*, 14748. [CrossRef]
46. Moss, D.K.; Betin, V.M.; Malesinski, S.D.; Lane, J.D. A Novel Role for Microtubules in Apoptotic Chromatin Dynamics and Cellular Fragmentation. *J. Cell Sci.* **2006**, *119*, 2362–2374. [CrossRef]
47. Poon, I.K.H.; Chiu, Y.-H.; Armstrong, A.J.; Kinchen, J.M.; Juncadella, I.J.; Bayliss, D.A.; Ravichandran, K.S. Unexpected Link between an Antibiotic, Pannexin Channels and Apoptosis. *Nature* **2014**, *507*, 329–334. [CrossRef]
48. Atkin-Smith, G.K.; Tixeira, R.; Paone, S.; Mathivanan, S.; Collins, C.; Liem, M.; Goodall, K.J.; Ravichandran, K.S.; Hulett, M.D.; Poon, I.K.H. A Novel Mechanism of Generating Extracellular Vesicles during Apoptosis via a Beads-on-a-String Membrane Structure. *Nat. Commun.* **2015**, *6*, 7439. [CrossRef]
49. Lane, J.D.; Allan, V.J.; Woodman, P.G. Active Relocation of Chromatin and Endoplasmic Reticulum into Blebs in Late Apoptotic Cells. *J. Cell Sci.* **2005**, *118*, 4059–4071. [CrossRef]
50. Alvarez-Erviti, L.; Seow, Y.; Yin, H.; Betts, C.; Lakhal, S.; Wood, M.J.A. Delivery of SiRNA to the Mouse Brain by Systemic Injection of Targeted Exosomes. *Nat. Biotechnol.* **2011**, *29*, 341–345. [CrossRef]
51. Cooper, J.M.; Wiklander, P.B.O.; Nordin, J.Z.; Al-Shawi, R.; Wood, M.J.; Vithlani, M.; Schapira, A.H.V.; Simons, J.P.; El-Andaloussi, S.; Alvarez-Erviti, L. Systemic Exosomal SiRNA Delivery Reduced Alpha-Synuclein Aggregates in Brains of Transgenic Mice. *Mov. Disord.* **2014**, *29*, 1476–1485. [CrossRef]
52. Liu, Y.; Li, D.; Liu, Z.; Zhou, Y.; Chu, D.; Li, X.; Jiang, X.; Hou, D.; Chen, X.; Chen, Y.; et al. Targeted Exosome-Mediated Delivery of Opioid Receptor Mu SiRNA for the Treatment of Morphine Relapse. *Sci. Rep.* **2015**, *5*, 17543. [CrossRef]
53. Murphy, D.E.; de Jong, O.G.; Brouwer, M.; Wood, M.J.; Lavieu, G.; Schiffelers, R.M.; Vader, P. Extracellular Vesicle-Based Therapeutics: Natural versus Engineered Targeting and Trafficking. *Exp. Mol. Med.* **2019**, *51*, 1–12. [CrossRef]
54. Witwer, K.W.; Buzás, E.I.; Bemis, L.T.; Bora, A.; Lässer, C.; Lötvall, J.; Nolte-'t Hoen, E.N.; Piper, M.G.; Sivaraman, S.; Skog, J.; et al. Standardization of Sample Collection, Isolation and Analysis Methods in Extracellular Vesicle Research. *J. Extracell. Vesicles* **2013**, *2*, 20360. [CrossRef]
55. Hulstaert, E.; Morlion, A.; Cobos, F.A.; Verniers, K.; Nuytens, J.; Eynde, E.V.; Yigit, N.; Anckaert, J.; Geerts, A.; Hindryckx, P.; et al. Charting Extracellular Transcriptomes in The Human Biofluid RNA Atlas. *Cell Rep.* **2020**, *33*, 108552. [CrossRef]
56. Bachurski, D.; Schuldner, M.; Nguyen, P.-H.; Malz, A.; Reiners, K.S.; Grenzi, P.C.; Babatz, F.; Schauss, A.C.; Hansen, H.P.; Hallek, M.; et al. Extracellular Vesicle Measurements with Nanoparticle Tracking Analysis—An Accuracy and Repeatability Comparison between NanoSight NS300 and ZetaView. *J. Extracell. Vesicles* **2019**, *8*, 1596016. [CrossRef]
57. Rikkert, L.G.; Nieuwland, R.; Terstappen, L.W.M.M.; Coumans, F.A.W. Quality of Extracellular Vesicle Images by Transmission Electron Microscopy Is Operator and Protocol Dependent. *J. Extracell. Vesicles* **2019**, *8*, 1555419. [CrossRef]
58. Morandi, M.I.; Busko, P.; Ozer-Partuk, E.; Khan, S.; Zarfati, G.; Elbaz-Alon, Y.; Abou Karam, P.; Napso Shogan, T.; Ginini, L.; Gil, Z.; et al. Extracellular Vesicle Fusion Visualized by Cryo-Electron Microscopy. *PNAS Nexus* **2022**, *1*, pgac156. [CrossRef]
59. Marchisio, M.; Simeone, P.; Bologna, G.; Ercolino, E.; Pierdomenico, L.; Pieragostino, D.; Ventrella, A.; Antonini, F.; Del Zotto, G.; Vergara, D.; et al. Flow Cytometry Analysis of Circulating Extracellular Vesicle Subtypes from Fresh Peripheral Blood Samples. *Int. J. Mol. Sci.* **2020**, *22*, 48. [CrossRef]

60. Maia, J.; Batista, S.; Couto, N.; Gregório, A.C.; Bodo, C.; Elzanowska, J.; Strano Moraes, M.C.; Costa-Silva, B. Employing Flow Cytometry to Extracellular Vesicles Sample Microvolume Analysis and Quality Control. *Front. Cell Dev. Biol.* **2020**, *8*, 593750. [CrossRef]
61. Mizenko, R.R.; Brostoff, T.; Rojalin, T.; Koster, H.J.; Swindell, H.S.; Leiserowitz, G.S.; Wang, A.; Carney, R.P. Tetraspanins Are Unevenly Distributed across Single Extracellular Vesicles and Bias Sensitivity to Multiplexed Cancer Biomarkers. *J. Nanobiotechnol.* **2021**, *19*, 250. [CrossRef]
62. Logozzi, M.; Di Raimo, R.; Mizzoni, D.; Fais, S. Immunocapture-Based ELISA to Characterize and Quantify Exosomes in Both Cell Culture Supernatants and Body Fluids. *Methods Enzymol.* **2020**, *645*, 155–180. [CrossRef]
63. Martínez-Greene, J.A.; Hernández-Ortega, K.; Quiroz-Baez, R.; Resendis-Antonio, O.; Pichardo-Casas, I.; Sinclair, D.A.; Budnik, B.; Hidalgo-Miranda, A.; Uribe-Querol, E.; Ramos-Godínez, M.d.P.; et al. Quantitative Proteomic Analysis of Extracellular Vesicle Subgroups Isolated by an Optimized Method Combining Polymer-based Precipitation and Size Exclusion Chromatography. *J. Extracell. Vesicles* **2021**, *10*, e12087. [CrossRef]
64. Carney, R.P.; Hazari, S.; Colquhoun, M.; Tran, D.; Hwang, B.; Mulligan, M.S.; Bryers, J.D.; Girda, E.; Leiserowitz, G.S.; Smith, Z.J.; et al. Multispectral Optical Tweezers for Biochemical Fingerprinting of CD9-Positive Exosome Subpopulations. *Anal. Chem.* **2017**, *89*, 5357–5363. [CrossRef]
65. Amorim, M.G.; Valieris, R.; Drummond, R.D.; Pizzi, M.P.; Freitas, V.M.; Sinigaglia-Coimbra, R.; Calin, G.A.; Pasqualini, R.; Arap, W.; Silva, I.T.; et al. A Total Transcriptome Profiling Method for Plasma-Derived Extracellular Vesicles: Applications for Liquid Biopsies. *Sci. Rep.* **2017**, *7*, 14395. [CrossRef]
66. Lener, T.; Gimona, M.; Aigner, L.; Börger, V.; Buzas, E.; Camussi, G.; Chaput, N.; Chatterjee, D.; Court, F.A.; Portillo, H.A.D.; et al. Applying Extracellular Vesicles Based Therapeutics in Clinical Trials—An ISEV Position Paper. *J. Extracell. Vesicles* **2015**, *4*, 30087. [CrossRef]
67. Mangi, A.A.; Noiseux, N.; Kong, D.; He, H.; Rezvani, M.; Ingwall, J.S.; Dzau, V.J. Mesenchymal Stem Cells Modified with Akt Prevent Remodeling and Restore Performance of Infarcted Hearts. *Nat. Med.* **2003**, *9*, 1195–1201. [CrossRef]
68. Lai, R.C.; Arslan, F.; Lee, M.M.; Sze, N.S.K.; Choo, A.; Chen, T.S.; Salto-Tellez, M.; Timmers, L.; Lee, C.N.; El Oakley, R.M.; et al. Exosome Secreted by MSC Reduces Myocardial Ischemia/Reperfusion Injury. *Stem Cell Res.* **2010**, *4*, 214–222. [CrossRef]
69. Timmers, L.; Lim, S.K.; Arslan, F.; Armstrong, J.S.; Hoefer, I.E.; Doevendans, P.A.; Piek, J.J.; El Oakley, R.M.; Choo, A.; Lee, C.N.; et al. Reduction of Myocardial Infarct Size by Human Mesenchymal Stem Cell Conditioned Medium. *Stem Cell Res.* **2008**, *1*, 129–137. [CrossRef]
70. Vicencio, J.M.; Yellon, D.M.; Sivaraman, V.; Das, D.; Boi-Doku, C.; Arjun, S.; Zheng, Y.; Riquelme, J.A.; Kearney, J.; Sharma, V.; et al. Plasma Exosomes Protect the Myocardium From Ischemia-Reperfusion Injury. *J. Am. Coll. Cardiol.* **2015**, *65*, 1525–1536. [CrossRef]
71. Adamiak, M.; Cheng, G.; Bobis-Wozowicz, S.; Zhao, L.; Kedracka-Krok, S.; Samanta, A.; Karnas, E.; Xuan, Y.-T.; Skupien-Rabian, B.; Chen, X.; et al. Induced Pluripotent Stem Cell (IPSC)–Derived Extracellular Vesicles Are Safer and More Effective for Cardiac Repair Than IPSCs. *Circ. Res.* **2018**, *122*, 296–309. [CrossRef]
72. Wang, Y.; Zhang, L.; Li, Y.; Chen, L.; Wang, X.; Guo, W.; Zhang, X.; Qin, G.; He, S.; Zimmerman, A.; et al. Exosomes/Microvesicles from Induced Pluripotent Stem Cells Deliver Cardioprotective MiRNAs and Prevent Cardiomyocyte Apoptosis in the Ischemic Myocardium. *Int. J. Cardiol.* **2015**, *192*, 61–69. [CrossRef]
73. Loyer, X.; Zlatanova, I.; Devue, C.; Yin, M.; Howangyin, K.-Y.; Klaihmon, P.; Guerin, C.L.; Kheloufi, M.; Vilar, J.; Zannis, K.; et al. Intra-Cardiac Release of Extracellular Vesicles Shapes Inflammation Following Myocardial Infarction. *Circ. Res.* **2018**, *123*, 100–106. [CrossRef]
74. Timmers, L.; Lim, S.K.; Hoefer, I.E.; Arslan, F.; Lai, R.C.; van Oorschot, A.A.M.; Goumans, M.J.; Strijder, C.; Sze, S.K.; Choo, A.; et al. Human Mesenchymal Stem Cell-Conditioned Medium Improves Cardiac Function Following Myocardial Infarction. *Stem Cell Res.* **2011**, *6*, 206–214. [CrossRef]
75. Barile, L.; Lionetti, V.; Cervio, E.; Matteucci, M.; Gherghiceanu, M.; Popescu, L.M.; Torre, T.; Siclari, F.; Moccetti, T.; Vassalli, G. Extracellular Vesicles from Human Cardiac Progenitor Cells Inhibit Cardiomyocyte Apoptosis and Improve Cardiac Function after Myocardial Infarction. *Cardiovasc. Res.* **2014**, *103*, 530–541. [CrossRef]
76. Kervadec, A.; Bellamy, V.; El Harane, N.; Arakélian, L.; Vanneaux, V.; Cacciapuoti, I.; Nemetalla, H.; Périer, M.-C.; Toeg, H.D.; Richart, A.; et al. Cardiovascular Progenitor–Derived Extracellular Vesicles Recapitulate the Beneficial Effects of Their Parent Cells in the Treatment of Chronic Heart Failure. *J. Heart Lung Transplant.* **2016**, *35*, 795–807. [CrossRef]
77. Liu, H.; Gao, W.; Yuan, J.; Wu, C.; Yao, K.; Zhang, L.; Ma, L.; Zhu, J.; Zou, Y.; Ge, J. Exosomes Derived from Dendritic Cells Improve Cardiac Function via Activation of CD4+ T Lymphocytes after Myocardial Infarction. *J. Mol. Cell. Cardiol.* **2016**, *91*, 123–133. [CrossRef]
78. Ribeiro-Rodrigues, T.M.; Laundos, T.L.; Pereira-Carvalho, R.; Batista-Almeida, D.; Pereira, R.; Coelho-Santos, V.; Silva, A.P.; Fernandes, R.; Zuzarte, M.; Enguita, F.J.; et al. Exosomes Secreted by Cardiomyocytes Subjected to Ischaemia Promote Cardiac Angiogenesis. *Cardiovasc. Res.* **2017**, *113*, 1338–1350. [CrossRef]
79. An, M.; Kwon, K.; Park, J.; Ryu, D.-R.; Shin, J.-A.; Lee Kang, J.; Choi, J.H.; Park, E.-M.; Lee, K.E.; Woo, M.; et al. Extracellular Matrix-Derived Extracellular Vesicles Promote Cardiomyocyte Growth and Electrical Activity in Engineered Cardiac Atria. *Biomaterials* **2017**, *146*, 49–59. [CrossRef]

80. Minghua, W.; Zhijian, G.; Chahua, H.; Qiang, L.; Minxuan, X.; Luqiao, W.; Weifang, Z.; Peng, L.; Biming, Z.; Lingling, Y.; et al. Plasma Exosomes Induced by Remote Ischaemic Preconditioning Attenuate Myocardial Ischaemia/Reperfusion Injury by Transferring MiR-24. *Cell Death Dis.* **2018**, *9*, 320. [CrossRef]
81. Mathiyalagan, P.; Liang, Y.; Kim, D.; Misener, S.; Thorne, T.; Kamide, C.E.; Klyachko, E.; Losordo, D.W.; Hajjar, R.; Sahoo, S. Angiogenic Mechanisms of Human CD34+ Stem Cell Exosomes in the Repair of Ischemic Hindlimb. *Circ. Res.* **2017**, *120*, 1466–1476. [CrossRef]
82. de Couto, G.; Gallet, R.; Cambier, L.; Jaghatspanyan, E.; Makkar, N.; Dawkins, J.F.; Berman, B.P.; Marbán, E. Exosomal MicroRNA Transfer into Macrophages Mediates Cellular Postconditioning de Couto: Exosomal RNA Transfer Modulates Macrophages. *Circulation* **2017**, *136*, 200–214. [CrossRef]
83. Khan, M.; Nickoloff, E.; Abramova, T.; Johnson, J.; Verma, S.K.; Krishnamurthy, P.; Mackie, A.R.; Vaughan, E.; Garikipati, V.N.S.; Benedict, C.; et al. Embryonic Stem Cell–Derived Exosomes Promote Endogenous Repair Mechanisms and Enhance Cardiac Function Following Myocardial Infarction. *Circ. Res.* **2015**, *117*, 52–64. [CrossRef]
84. Barile, L.; Cervio, E.; Lionetti, V.; Milano, G.; Ciullo, A.; Biemmi, V.; Bolis, S.; Altomare, C.; Matteucci, M.; Di Silvestre, D.; et al. Cardioprotection by Cardiac Progenitor Cell-Secreted Exosomes: Role of Pregnancy-Associated Plasma Protein-A. *Cardiovasc. Res.* **2018**, *114*, 992–1005. [CrossRef]
85. Ma, J.; Zhao, Y.; Sun, L.; Sun, X.; Zhao, X.; Sun, X.; Qian, H.; Xu, W.; Zhu, W. Exosomes Derived from Akt-Modified Human Umbilical Cord Mesenchymal Stem Cells Improve Cardiac Regeneration and Promote Angiogenesis via Activating Platelet-Derived Growth Factor D. *Stem Cells Transl. Med.* **2017**, *6*, 51–59. [CrossRef]
86. Li, Q.; Zhao, H.; Chen, W.; Huang, P.; Bi, J. Human Keratinocyte-Derived Microvesicle MiRNA-21 Promotes Skin Wound Healing in Diabetic Rats through Facilitating Fibroblast Function and Angiogenesis. *Int. J. Biochem. Cell Biol.* **2019**, *114*, 105570. [CrossRef]
87. Narauskaité, D.; Vydmantaite, G.; Rusteikaite, J.; Sampath, R.; Rudaityte, A.; Stašyte, G.; Isabel, M.; Calvente, A.; Jekabsone, A. Extracellular Vesicles in Skin Wound Healing. *Pharmaceuticals* **2021**, *14*, 811. [CrossRef]
88. Liu, X.; Li, X.; Wu, G.; Qi, P.; Zhang, Y.; Liu, Z.; Li, X.; Yu, Y.; Ye, X.; Li, Y.; et al. Umbilical Cord Mesenchymal Stem Cell-Derived Small Extracellular Vesicles Deliver MiR-21 to Promote Corneal Epithelial Wound Healing through PTEN/PI3K/Akt Pathway. *Stem Cells Int.* **2022**, *2022*, 1252557. [CrossRef]
89. Ramos-Zaldívar, H.M.; Polakovicova, I.; Salas-Huenuleo, E.; Corvalán, A.H.; Kogan, M.J.; Yefi, C.P.; Andia, M.E. Extracellular Vesicles through the Blood–Brain Barrier: A Review. *Fluids Barriers CNS* **2022**, *19*, 60. [CrossRef]
90. Drommelschmidt, K.; Serdar, M.; Bendix, I.; Herz, J.; Bertling, F.; Prager, S.; Keller, M.; Ludwig, A.-K.; Duhan, V.; Radtke, S.; et al. Mesenchymal Stem Cell-Derived Extracellular Vesicles Ameliorate Inflammation-Induced Preterm Brain Injury. *Brain Behav. Immun.* **2017**, *60*, 220–232. [CrossRef]
91. Clark, K.; Zhang, S.; Barthe, S.; Kumar, P.; Pivetti, C.; Kreutzberg, N.; Reed, C.; Wang, Y.; Paxton, Z.; Farmer, D.; et al. Placental Mesenchymal Stem Cell-Derived Extracellular Vesicles Promote Myelin Regeneration in an Animal Model of Multiple Sclerosis. *Cells* **2019**, *8*, 1497. [CrossRef]
92. Cosenza, S.; Toupet, K.; Maumus, M.; Luz-Crawford, P.; Blanc-Brude, O.; Jorgensen, C.; Noël, D. Mesenchymal Stem Cells-Derived Exosomes Are More Immunosuppressive than Microparticles in Inflammatory Arthritis. *Theranostics* **2018**, *8*, 1399–1410. [CrossRef]
93. Bruno, S.; Grange, C.; Collino, F.; Deregibus, M.C.; Cantaluppi, V.; Biancone, L.; Tetta, C.; Camussi, G. Microvesicles Derived from Mesenchymal Stem Cells Enhance Survival in a Lethal Model of Acute Kidney Injury. *PLoS ONE* **2012**, *7*, e33115. [CrossRef]
94. Zhang, S.; Chu, W.C.; Lai, R.C.; Lim, S.K.; Hui, J.H.P.; Toh, W.S. Exosomes Derived from Human Embryonic Mesenchymal Stem Cells Promote Osteochondral Regeneration. *Osteoarthr. Cartil.* **2016**, *24*, 2135–2140. [CrossRef]
95. Herrmann, I.K.; Wood, M.J.A.; Fuhrmann, G. Extracellular Vesicles as a Next-Generation Drug Delivery Platform. *Nat. Nanotechnol.* **2021**, *16*, 748–759. [CrossRef]
96. Kooijmans, S.A.A.; Aleza, C.G.; Roffler, S.R.; van Solinge, W.W.; Vader, P.; Schiffelers, R.M. Display of GPI-Anchored Anti-EGFR Nanobodies on Extracellular Vesicles Promotes Tumour Cell Targeting. *J. Extracell. Vesicles* **2016**, *5*, 31053. [CrossRef]
97. Kooijmans, S.A.A.; Gitz-Francois, J.J.J.M.; Schiffelers, R.M.; Vader, P. Recombinant Phosphatidylserine-Binding Nanobodies for Targeting of Extracellular Vesicles to Tumor Cells: A Plug-and-Play Approach. *Nanoscale* **2018**, *10*, 2413–2426. [CrossRef]
98. Del Vecchio, K.; Stahelin, R.V. Investigation of the phosphatidylserine binding properties of the lipid biosensor Lactadherin C2 (LactC2), in different membrane environments. *J. Bioenerg. Biomembr.* **2018**, *50*, 1–10. [CrossRef]
99. Tian, T.; Zhang, H.-X.; He, C.-P.; Fan, S.; Zhu, Y.-L.; Qi, C.; Huang, N.-P.; Xiao, Z.-D.; Lu, Z.-H.; Tannous, B.A.; et al. Surface Functionalized Exosomes as Targeted Drug Delivery Vehicles for Cerebral Ischemia Therapy. *Biomaterials* **2018**, *150*, 137–149. [CrossRef]
100. Nakase, I.; Noguchi, K.; Aoki, A.; Takatani-Nakase, T.; Fujii, I.; Futaki, S. Arginine-Rich Cell-Penetrating Peptide-Modified Extracellular Vesicles for Active Macropinocytosis Induction and Efficient Intracellular Delivery. *Sci. Rep.* **2017**, *7*, 1991. [CrossRef]
101. Tang, K.; Zhang, Y.; Zhang, H.; Xu, P.; Liu, J.; Ma, J.; Lv, M.; Li, D.; Katirai, F.; Shen, G.-X.; et al. Delivery of Chemotherapeutic Drugs in Tumour Cell-Derived Microparticles. *Nat. Commun.* **2012**, 3, 1282. [CrossRef]
102. Wei, H.; Chen, J.; Wang, S.; Fu, F.; Zhu, X.; Wu, C.; Liu, Z.; Zhong, G.; Lin, J. A Nanodrug Consisting Of Doxorubicin And Exosome Derived From Mesenchymal Stem Cells For Osteosarcoma Treatment In Vitro. *Int. J. Nanomed.* **2019**, *14*, 8603–8610. [CrossRef]

103. Vader, P.; Mol, E.A.; Pasterkamp, G.; Schiffelers, R.M. Extracellular Vesicles for Drug Delivery. *Adv. Drug Deliv. Rev.* **2016**, *106*, 148–156. [CrossRef]
104. Kang, J.-Y.; Park, H.; Kim, H.; Mun, D.; Park, H.; Yun, N.; Joung, B. Human Peripheral Blood-Derived Exosomes for MicroRNA Delivery. *Int. J. Mol. Med.* **2019**, *43*, 2319–2328. [CrossRef]
105. Youn, S.-W.; Li, Y.; Kim, Y.-M.; Sudhahar, V.; Abdelsaid, K.; Kim, H.W.; Liu, Y.; Fulton, D.J.R.; Ashraf, M.; Tang, Y.; et al. Modification of Cardiac Progenitor Cell-Derived Exosomes by MiR-322 Provides Protection against Myocardial Infarction through Nox2-Dependent Angiogenesis. *Antioxidants* **2019**, *8*, 18. [CrossRef]
106. Wiklander, O.P.B.; Nordin, J.Z.; O'Loughlin, A.; Gustafsson, Y.; Corso, G.; Mäger, I.; Vader, P.; Lee, Y.; Sork, H.; Seow, Y.; et al. Extracellular Vesicle in Vivo Biodistribution Is Determined by Cell Source, Route of Administration and Targeting. *J. Extracell. Vesicles* **2015**, *4*, 26316. [CrossRef]
107. Suk, J.S.; Xu, Q.; Kim, N.; Hanes, J.; Ensign, L.M. PEGylation as a Strategy for Improving Nanoparticle-Based Drug and Gene Delivery. *Adv. Drug Deliv. Rev.* **2016**, *99*, 28–51. [CrossRef]
108. Kooijmans, S.A.A.; Fliervoet, L.A.L.; van der Meel, R.; Fens, M.H.A.M.; Heijnen, H.F.G.; van Bergen en Henegouwen, P.M.P.; Vader, P.; Schiffelers, R.M. PEGylated and Targeted Extracellular Vesicles Display Enhanced Cell Specificity and Circulation Time. *J. Control. Release* **2016**, *224*, 77–85. [CrossRef]
109. Wolfe, R.A.; Ashby, V.B.; Milford, E.L.; Ojo, A.O.; Ettenger, R.E.; Agodoa, L.Y.C.; Held, P.J.; Port, F.K. Comparison of Mortality in All Patients on Dialysis, Patients on Dialysis Awaiting Transplantation, and Recipients of a First Cadaveric Transplant. *N. Engl. J. Med.* **1999**, *341*, 1725–1730. [CrossRef]
110. Annual Activity Report. Available online: https://www.odt.nhs.uk/statistics-and-reports/annual-activity-report/ (accessed on 19 November 2022).
111. Segura, E.; Nicco, C.; Lombard, B.; Véron, P.; Raposo, G.; Batteux, F.; Amigorena, S.; Théry, C. ICAM-1 on Exosomes from Mature Dendritic Cells Is Critical for Efficient Naive T-Cell Priming. *Blood* **2005**, *106*, 216–223. [CrossRef]
112. Li, X.; Li, J.-J.; Yang, J.-Y.; Wang, D.-S.; Zhao, W.; Song, W.-J.; Li, W.-M.; Wang, J.-F.; Han, W.; Zhang, Z.-C.; et al. Tolerance Induction by Exosomes from Immature Dendritic Cells and Rapamycin in a Mouse Cardiac Allograft Model. *PLoS ONE* **2012**, *7*, e44045. [CrossRef]
113. Pang, X.-L.; Wang, Z.-G.; Liu, L.; Feng, Y.-H.; Wang, J.-X.; Xie, H.-C.; Yang, X.-L.; Li, J.-F.; Feng, G.-W. Immature Dendritic Cells Derived Exosomes Promotes Immune Tolerance by Regulating T Cell Differentiation in Renal Transplantation. *Aging* **2019**, *11*, 8911–8924. [CrossRef]
114. Ma, B.; Yang, J.-Y.; Song, W.; Ding, R.; Zhang, Z.; Ji, H.; Zhang, X.; Wang, J.; Yang, X.; Tao, K.; et al. Combining Exosomes Derived from Immature DCs with Donor Antigen-Specific Treg Cells Induces Tolerance in a Rat Liver Allograft Model. *Sci. Rep.* **2016**, *6*, 32971. [CrossRef]
115. Yang, X.; Meng, S.; Jiang, H.; Zhu, C.; Wu, W. Exosomes Derived from Immature Bone Marrow Dendritic Cells Induce Tolerogenicity of Intestinal Transplantation in Rats. *J. Surg. Res.* **2011**, *171*, 826–832. [CrossRef]
116. Raposo, G.; Nijman, H.W.; Stoorvogel, W.; Liejendekker, R.; Harding, C.V.; Melief, C.J.; Geuze, H.J. B Lymphocytes Secrete Antigen-Presenting Vesicles. *J. Exp. Med.* **1996**, *183*, 1161–1172. [CrossRef]
117. Saunderson, S.C.; Schuberth, P.C.; Dunn, A.C.; Miller, L.; Hock, B.D.; MacKay, P.A.; Koch, N.; Jack, R.W.; McLellan, A.D. Induction of Exosome Release in Primary B Cells Stimulated via CD40 and the IL-4 Receptor1. *J. Immunol.* **2008**, *180*, 8146–8152. [CrossRef]
118. Harper, S.J.F.; Ali, J.M.; Wlodek, E.; Negus, M.C.; Harper, I.G.; Chhabra, M.; Qureshi, M.S.; Mallik, M.; Bolton, E.; Bradley, J.A.; et al. CD8 T-Cell Recognition of Acquired Alloantigen Promotes Acute Allograft Rejection. *Proc. Natl. Acad. Sci. USA* **2015**, *112*, 12788–12793. [CrossRef]
119. Aiello, S.; Rocchetta, F.; Longaretti, L.; Faravelli, S.; Todeschini, M.; Cassis, L.; Pezzuto, F.; Tomasoni, S.; Azzollini, N.; Mister, M.; et al. Extracellular Vesicles Derived from T Regulatory Cells Suppress T Cell Proliferation and Prolong Allograft Survival. *Sci. Rep.* **2017**, *7*, 11518. [CrossRef]
120. Tung, S.L.; Fanelli, G.; Matthews, R.I.; Bazoer, J.; Letizia, M.; Vizcay-Barrena, G.; Faruqu, F.N.; Philippeos, C.; Hannen, R.; Al-Jamal, K.T.; et al. Regulatory T Cell Extracellular Vesicles Modify T-Effector Cell Cytokine Production and Protect Against Human Skin Allograft Damage. *Front. Cell Dev. Biol.* **2020**, *8*, 317. [CrossRef]
121. Tung, S.L.; Boardman, D.A.; Sen, M.; Letizia, M.; Peng, Q.; Cianci, N.; Dioni, L.; Carlin, L.M.; Lechler, R.; Bollati, V.; et al. Regulatory T Cell-Derived Extracellular Vesicles Modify Dendritic Cell Function. *Sci. Rep.* **2018**, *8*, 6065. [CrossRef]
122. Deaglio, S.; Dwyer, K.M.; Gao, W.; Friedman, D.; Usheva, A.; Erat, A.; Chen, J.-F.; Enjyoji, K.; Linden, J.; Oukka, M.; et al. Adenosine Generation Catalyzed by CD39 and CD73 Expressed on Regulatory T Cells Mediates Immune Suppression. *J. Exp. Med.* **2007**, *204*, 1257–1265. [CrossRef]
123. Lappas, C.M.; Rieger, J.M.; Linden, J. A2A Adenosine Receptor Induction Inhibits IFN-γ Production in Murine CD4+ T Cells1. *J. Immunol.* **2005**, *174*, 1073–1080. [CrossRef]
124. Romio, M.; Reinbeck, B.; Bongardt, S.; Hüls, S.; Burghoff, S.; Schrader, J. Extracellular Purine Metabolism and Signaling of CD73-Derived Adenosine in Murine Treg and Teff Cells. *Am. J. Physiol. Cell Physiol.* **2011**, *301*, C530–C539. [CrossRef]
125. Smyth, L.A.; Ratnasothy, K.; Tsang, J.Y.S.; Boardman, D.; Warley, A.; Lechler, R.; Lombardi, G. CD73 Expression on Extracellular Vesicles Derived from CD4+CD25+Foxp3+ T Cells Contributes to Their Regulatory Function. *Eur. J. Immunol.* **2013**, *43*, 2430–2440. [CrossRef]

126. Chen, L.; Huang, H.; Zhang, W.; Ding, F.; Fan, Z.; Zeng, Z. Exosomes Derived From T Regulatory Cells Suppress CD8+ Cytotoxic T Lymphocyte Proliferation and Prolong Liver Allograft Survival. *Med. Sci. Monit. Int. Med. J. Exp. Clin. Res.* **2019**, *25*, 4877–4884. [CrossRef]
127. Ponticelli, C. Ischaemia-Reperfusion Injury: A Major Protagonist in Kidney Transplantation. *Nephrol. Dial. Transplant.* **2014**, *29*, 1134–1140. [CrossRef]
128. Hart, A.; Smith, J.M.; Skeans, M.A.; Gustafson, S.K.; Wilk, A.R.; Castro, S.; Foutz, J.; Wainright, J.L.; Snyder, J.J.; Kasiske, B.L.; et al. OPTN/SRTR 2018 Annual Data Report: Kidney. *Am. J. Transplant.* **2020**, *20*, 20–130. [CrossRef]
129. Taylor, R.; Allen, E.; Richards, J.A.; Goh, M.A.; Neuberger, J.; Collett, D.; Pettigrew, G.J. Survival Advantage for Patients Accepting the Offer of a Circulatory Death Liver Transplant. *J. Hepatol.* **2019**, *70*, 855–865. [CrossRef]
130. Ali, J.M.; Davies, S.E.; Brais, R.J.; Randle, L.V.; Klinck, J.R.; Allison, M.E.D.; Chen, Y.; Pasea, L.; Harper, S.F.J.; Pettigrew, G.J. Analysis of Ischemia/Reperfusion Injury in Time-Zero Biopsies Predicts Liver Allograft Outcomes. *Liver Transpl.* **2015**, *21*, 487–499. [CrossRef]
131. Abraham, S.; Furth, E.E. Quantitative Evaluation of Histological Features in "Time-Zero" Liver Allograft Biopsies as Predictors of Rejection or Graft Failure: Receiver-Operating Characteristic Analysis Application. *Hum. Pathol.* **1996**, *27*, 1077–1084. [CrossRef]
132. Zhai, Y.; Petrowsky, H.; Hong, J.C.; Busuttil, R.W.; Kupiec-Weglinski, J.W. Ischaemia–Reperfusion Injury in Liver Transplantation—From Bench to Bedside. *Nat. Rev. Gastroenterol. Hepatol.* **2013**, *10*, 79–89. [CrossRef]
133. Nieuwenhuijs-Moeke, G.J.; Pischke, S.E.; Berger, S.P.; Sanders, J.S.F.; Pol, R.A.; Struys, M.M.R.F.; Ploeg, R.J.; Leuvenink, H.G.D. Ischemia and Reperfusion Injury in Kidney Transplantation: Relevant Mechanisms in Injury and Repair. *J. Clin. Med.* **2020**, *9*, 253. [CrossRef]
134. Zhao, H.; Alam, A.; Soo, A.P.; George, A.J.T.; Ma, D. Ischemia-Reperfusion Injury Reduces Long Term Renal Graft Survival: Mechanism and Beyond. *EBioMedicine* **2018**, *28*, 31–42. [CrossRef]
135. Land, W.G.; Agostinis, P.; Gasser, S.; Garg, A.D.; Linkermann, A. Transplantation and Damage-Associated Molecular Patterns (DAMPs). *Am. J. Transplant.* **2016**, *16*, 3338–3361. [CrossRef]
136. Liu, T.; Zhang, L.; Joo, D.; Sun, S.-C. NF-KB Signaling in Inflammation. *Signal Transduct. Target. Ther.* **2017**, *2*, 17023. [CrossRef]
137. Kato, T.; Miyaki, S.; Ishitobi, H.; Nakamura, Y.; Nakasa, T.; Lotz, M.K.; Ochi, M. Exosomes from IL-1β Stimulated Synovial Fibroblasts Induce Osteoarthritic Changes in Articular Chondrocytes. *Arthritis Res. Ther.* **2014**, *16*, R163. [CrossRef]
138. Budden, C.F.; Gearing, L.J.; Kaiser, R.; Standke, L.; Hertzog, P.J.; Latz, E. Inflammasome-Induced Extracellular Vesicles Harbour Distinct RNA Signatures and Alter Bystander Macrophage Responses. *J. Extracell. Vesicles* **2021**, *10*, e12127. [CrossRef]
139. Ferdinand, J.R.; Hosgood, S.A.; Moore, T.; Ferro, A.; Ward, C.J.; Castro-Dopico, T.; Nicholson, M.L.; Clatworthy, M.R. Cytokine Absorption during Human Kidney Perfusion Reduces Delayed Graft Function–Associated Inflammatory Gene Signature. *Am. J. Transplant.* **2021**, *21*, 2188–2199. [CrossRef]
140. Takahashi, Y.; Ganster, R.W.; Gambotto, A.; Shao, L.; Kaizu, T.; Wu, T.; Yagnik, G.P.; Nakao, A.; Tsoulfas, G.; Ishikawa, T.; et al. Role of NF-KB on Liver Cold Ischemia-Reperfusion Injury. *Am. J. Physiol. Gastrointest. Liver Physiol.* **2002**, *283*, G1175–G1184. [CrossRef]
141. Yuan, X.; Li, D.; Chen, X.; Han, C.; Xu, L.; Huang, T.; Dong, Z.; Zhang, M. Extracellular Vesicles from Human-Induced Pluripotent Stem Cell-Derived Mesenchymal Stromal Cells (HiPSC-MSCs) Protect against Renal Ischemia/Reperfusion Injury via Delivering Specificity Protein (SP1) and Transcriptional Activating of Sphingosine Kinase 1 and Inhibiting Necroptosis. *Cell Death Dis.* **2017**, *8*, 3200. [CrossRef]
142. Kim, S.; Lee, S.A.; Yoon, H.; Kim, M.Y.; Yoo, J.-K.; Ahn, S.-H.; Park, C.H.; Park, J.; Nam, B.Y.; Park, J.T.; et al. Exosome-Based Delivery of Super-Repressor IκBα Ameliorates Kidney Ischemia-Reperfusion Injury. *Kidney Int.* **2021**, *100*, 570–584. [CrossRef]
143. Viñas, J.L.; Burger, D.; Zimpelmann, J.; Haneef, R.; Knoll, W.; Campbell, P.; Gutsol, A.; Carter, A.; Allan, D.S.; Burns, K.D. Transfer of MicroRNA-486-5p from Human Endothelial Colony Forming Cell–Derived Exosomes Reduces Ischemic Kidney Injury. *Kidney Int.* **2016**, *90*, 1238–1250. [CrossRef]
144. Zhu, G.; Pei, L.; Lin, F.; Yin, H.; Li, X.; He, W.; Liu, N.; Gou, X. Exosomes from Human-Bone-Marrow-Derived Mesenchymal Stem Cells Protect against Renal Ischemia/Reperfusion Injury via Transferring MiR-199a-3p. *J. Cell. Physiol.* **2019**, *234*, 23736–23749. [CrossRef]
145. Wang, C.; Zhu, G.; He, W.; Yin, H.; Lin, F.; Gou, X.; Li, X. BMSCs Protect against Renal Ischemia-reperfusion Injury by Secreting Exosomes Loaded with MiR-199a-5p That Target BIP to Inhibit Endoplasmic Reticulum Stress at the Very Early Reperfusion Stages. *FASEB J.* **2019**, *33*, 5440–5456. [CrossRef]
146. Du, Y.; Li, D.; Han, C.; Wu, H.; Xu, L.; Zhang, M.; Zhang, J.; Chen, X. Exosomes from Human-Induced Pluripotent Stem Cell–Derived Mesenchymal Stromal Cells (HiPSC-MSCs) Protect Liver against Hepatic Ischemia/Reperfusion Injury via Activating Sphingosine Kinase and Sphingosine-1-Phosphate Signaling Pathway. *Cell. Physiol. Biochem.* **2017**, *43*, 611–625. [CrossRef]
147. Zheng, L.; Li, Z.; Ling, W.; Zhu, D.; Feng, Z.; Kong, L. Exosomes Derived from Dendritic Cells Attenuate Liver Injury by Modulating the Balance of Treg and Th17 Cells After Ischemia Reperfusion. *Cell. Physiol. Biochem.* **2018**, *46*, 740–756. [CrossRef]
148. Block, H.; Rossaint, J.; Zarbock, A. The Fatal Circle of NETs and NET-Associated DAMPs Contributing to Organ Dysfunction. *Cells* **2022**, *11*, 1919. [CrossRef]
149. Lu, T.; Zhang, J.; Cai, J.; Xiao, J.; Sui, X.; Yuan, X.; Li, R.; Li, Y.; Yao, J.; Lv, G.; et al. Extracellular Vesicles Derived from Mesenchymal Stromal Cells as Nanotherapeutics for Liver Ischaemia–Reperfusion Injury by Transferring Mitochondria to Modulate the Formation of Neutrophil Extracellular Traps. *Biomaterials* **2022**, *284*, 121486. [CrossRef]

150. Yamada, N.; Karasawa, T.; Wakiya, T.; Sadatomo, A.; Ito, H.; Kamata, R.; Watanabe, S.; Komada, T.; Kimura, H.; Sanada, Y.; et al. Iron Overload as a Risk Factor for Hepatic Ischemia-Reperfusion Injury in Liver Transplantation: Potential Role of Ferroptosis. *Am. J. Transplant.* **2020**, *20*, 1606–1618. [CrossRef]
151. Li, X.; Wu, L.; Tian, X.; Zheng, W.; Yuan, M.; Tian, X.; Zuo, H.; Song, H.; Shen, Z. MiR-29a-3p in Exosomes from Heme Oxygenase-1 Modified Bone Marrow Mesenchymal Stem Cells Alleviates Steatotic Liver Ischemia-Reperfusion Injury in Rats by Suppressing Ferroptosis via Iron Responsive Element Binding Protein 2. *Oxidative Med. Cell. Longev.* **2022**, *2022*, e6520789. [CrossRef]
152. Liu, L.; Jin, X.; Hu, C.-F.; Li, R.; Zhou, Z.; Shen, C.-X. Exosomes Derived from Mesenchymal Stem Cells Rescue Myocardial Ischaemia/Reperfusion Injury by Inducing Cardiomyocyte Autophagy Via AMPK and Akt Pathways. *Cell. Physiol. Biochem.* **2017**, *43*, 52–68. [CrossRef]
153. Sánchez-Sánchez, R.; Gómez-Ferrer, M.; Reinal, I.; Buigues, M.; Villanueva-Bádenas, E.; Ontoria-Oviedo, I.; Hernándiz, A.; González-King, H.; Peiró-Molina, E.; Dorronsoro, A.; et al. MiR-4732-3p in Extracellular Vesicles From Mesenchymal Stromal Cells Is Cardioprotective During Myocardial Ischemia. *Front. Cell Dev. Biol.* **2021**, *9*, 734143. [CrossRef]
154. Del Campo, C.V.; Liaw, N.Y.; Gunadasa-Rohling, M.; Matthaei, M.; Braga, L.; Kennedy, T.; Salinas, G.; Voigt, N.; Giacca, M.; Zimmermann, W.-H.; et al. Regenerative Potential of Epicardium-Derived Extracellular Vesicles Mediated by Conserved MiRNA Transfer. *Cardiovasc. Res.* **2022**, *118*, 597–611. [CrossRef]
155. Li, J.W.; Wei, L.; Han, Z.; Chen, Z. Mesenchymal Stromal Cells-Derived Exosomes Alleviate Ischemia/Reperfusion Injury in Mouse Lung by Transporting Anti-Apoptotic MiR-21-5p. *Eur. J. Pharmacol.* **2019**, *852*, 68–76. [CrossRef]
156. Stone, M.L.; Zhao, Y.; Robert Smith, J.; Weiss, M.L.; Kron, I.L.; Laubach, V.E.; Sharma, A.K. Mesenchymal Stromal Cell-Derived Extracellular Vesicles Attenuate Lung Ischemia-Reperfusion Injury and Enhance Reconditioning of Donor Lungs after Circulatory Death. *Respir. Res.* **2017**, *18*, 212. [CrossRef]
157. Cai, J.; Gehrau, R.; Tu, Z.; Leroy, V.; Su, G.; Shang, J.; Mas, V.R.; Emtiazjoo, A.; Pelaez, A.; Atkinson, C.; et al. MicroRNA-206 AntagomiR–enriched Extracellular Vesicles Attenuate Lung Ischemia–reperfusion Injury through CXCL1 Regulation in Alveolar Epithelial Cells. *J. Heart Lung Transplant. Off. Publ. Int. Soc. Heart Transplant.* **2020**, *39*, 1476–1490. [CrossRef]
158. Watson, C.J.E.; Kosmoliaptsis, V.; Pley, C.; Randle, L.; Fear, C.; Crick, K.; Gimson, A.E.; Allison, M.; Upponi, S.; Brais, R.; et al. Observations on the Ex Situ Perfusion of Livers for Transplantation. *Am. J. Transplant.* **2018**, *18*, 2005–2020. [CrossRef]
159. Gaurav, R.; Butler, A.J.; Kosmoliaptsis, V.; Mumford, L.; Fear, C.; Swift, L.; Fedotovs, A.; Upponi, S.; Khwaja, S.; Richards, J.; et al. Liver Transplantation Outcomes From Controlled Circulatory Death Donors: SCS vs. in Situ NRP vs. Ex Situ NMP. *Ann. Surg.* **2022**, *275*, 1156–1164. [CrossRef]
160. Bogensperger, C.; Hofmann, J.; Messner, F.; Resch, T.; Meszaros, A.; Cardini, B.; Weissenbacher, A.; Oberhuber, R.; Troppmair, J.; Öfner, D.; et al. Ex Vivo Mesenchymal Stem Cell Therapy to Regenerate Machine Perfused Organs. *Int. J. Mol. Sci.* **2021**, *22*, 5233. [CrossRef]
161. Thompson, E.R.; Bates, L.; Ibrahim, I.K.; Sewpaul, A.; Stenberg, B.; McNeill, A.; Figueiredo, R.; Girdlestone, T.; Wilkins, G.C.; Wang, L.; et al. Novel Delivery of Cellular Therapy to Reduce Ischemia Reperfusion Injury in Kidney Transplantation. *Am. J. Transplant.* **2021**, *21*, 1402–1414. [CrossRef]
162. Laing, R.W.; Stubblefield, S.; Wallace, L.; Roobrouck, V.D.; Bhogal, R.H.; Schlegel, A.; Boteon, Y.L.; Reynolds, G.M.; Ting, A.E.; Mirza, D.F.; et al. The Delivery of Multipotent Adult Progenitor Cells to Extended Criteria Human Donor Livers Using Normothermic Machine Perfusion. *Front. Immunol.* **2020**, *11*, 1226. [CrossRef]
163. Lee, J.W.; Fang, X.; Gupta, N.; Serikov, V.; Matthay, M.A. Allogeneic Human Mesenchymal Stem Cells for Treatment of E. Coli Endotoxin-Induced Acute Lung Injury in the Ex Vivo Perfused Human Lung. *Proc. Natl. Acad. Sci. USA* **2009**, *106*, 16357–16362. [CrossRef]
164. De Stefano, N.; Navarro-Tableros, V.; Roggio, D.; Calleri, A.; Rigo, F.; David, E.; Gambella, A.; Bassino, D.; Amoroso, A.; Patrono, D.; et al. Human Liver Stem Cell-derived Extracellular Vesicles Reduce Injury in a Model of Normothermic Machine Perfusion of Rat Livers Previously Exposed to a Prolonged Warm Ischemia. *Transpl. Int.* **2021**, *34*, 1607–1617. [CrossRef] [PubMed]
165. Rampino, T.; Gregorini, M.; Germinario, G.; Pattonieri, E.F.; Erasmi, F.; Grignano, M.A.; Bruno, S.; Alomari, E.; Bettati, S.; Asti, A.; et al. Extracellular Vesicles Derived from Mesenchymal Stromal Cells Delivered during Hypothermic Oxygenated Machine Perfusion Repair Ischemic/Reperfusion Damage of Kidneys from Extended Criteria Donors. *Biology* **2022**, *11*, 350. [CrossRef]
166. Charoenviriyakul, C.; Takahashi, Y.; Morishita, M.; Matsumoto, A.; Nishikawa, M.; Takakura, Y. Cell Type-Specific and Common Characteristics of Exosomes Derived from Mouse Cell Lines: Yield, Physicochemical Properties, and Pharmacokinetics. *Eur. J. Pharm. Sci.* **2017**, *96*, 316–322. [CrossRef]
167. Imai, T.; Takahashi, Y.; Nishikawa, M.; Kato, K.; Morishita, M.; Yamashita, T.; Matsumoto, A.; Charoenviriyakul, C.; Takakura, Y. Macrophage-Dependent Clearance of Systemically Administered B16BL6-Derived Exosomes from the Blood Circulation in Mice. *J. Extracell. Vesicles* **2015**, *4*, 26238. [CrossRef] [PubMed]
168. Tingle, S.J.; Thompson, E.R.; Bates, L.; Ibrahim, I.K.; Govaere, O.; Shuttleworth, V.; Wang, L.; Figueiredo, R.; Palmer, J.; Bury, Y.; et al. Pharmacological Testing of Therapeutics Using Normothermic Machine Perfusion: A Pilot Study of 2,4-Dinitrophenol Delivery to Steatotic Human Livers. *Artif. Organs* **2022**, *46*, 2201–2214. [CrossRef]
169. Vulto, A.G.; Jaquez, O.A. The Process Defines the Product: What Really Matters in Biosimilar Design and Production? *Rheumatology* **2017**, *56*, iv14–iv29. [CrossRef]

170. Patel, D.B.; Gray, K.M.; Santharam, Y.; Lamichhane, T.N.; Stroka, K.M.; Jay, S.M. Impact of Cell Culture Parameters on Production and Vascularization Bioactivity of Mesenchymal Stem Cell-Derived Extracellular Vesicles. *Bioeng. Transl. Med.* **2017**, *2*, 170–179. [CrossRef]
171. Penders, J.; Nagelkerke, A.; Cunnane, E.M.; Pedersen, S.V.; Pence, I.J.; Coombes, R.C.; Stevens, M.M. Single Particle Automated Raman Trapping Analysis of Breast Cancer Cell-Derived Extracellular Vesicles as Cancer Biomarkers. *ACS Nano* **2021**, *15*, 18192–18205. [CrossRef]
172. Maisano, D.; Mimmi, S.; Dattilo, V.; Marino, F.; Gentile, M.; Vecchio, E.; Fiume, G.; Nisticò, N.; Aloisio, A.; Santo, M.P.D.; et al. A Novel Phage Display Based Platform for Exosome Diversity Characterization. *Nanoscale* **2022**, *14*, 2998–3003. [CrossRef]

pharmaceutics MDPI

Article

Plant-Derived Extracellular Vesicles as a Delivery Platform for RNA-Based Vaccine: Feasibility Study of an Oral and Intranasal SARS-CoV-2 Vaccine

Margherita A. C. Pomatto [1,2,*], Chiara Gai [1,2], Federica Negro [1], Lucia Massari [1], Maria Chiara Deregibus [2], Cristina Grange [2], Francesco Giuseppe De Rosa [2] and Giovanni Camussi [1,2,*]

1 EvoBiotech s.r.l., 10122 Turin, Italy
2 Department of Medical Science, University of Turin, A.O.U. Città della Salute e della Scienza di Torino, 10126 Turin, Italy
* Correspondence: mpomatto@evobiotech.it (M.A.C.P.); giovanni.camussi@unito.it (G.C.)

Abstract: Plant-derived extracellular vesicles (EVs) may represent a platform for the delivery of RNA-based vaccines, exploiting their natural membrane envelope to protect and deliver nucleic acids. Here, EVs extracted from orange (*Citrus sinensis*) juice (oEVs) were investigated as carriers for oral and intranasal SARS-CoV-2 mRNA vaccine. oEVs were efficiently loaded with different mRNA molecules (coding N, subunit 1 and full S proteins) and the mRNA was protected from degrading stress (including RNase and simulated gastric fluid), delivered to target cells and translated into protein. APC cells stimulated with oEVs loaded with mRNAs induced T lymphocyte activation in vitro. The immunization of mice with oEVs loaded with S1 mRNA via different routes of administration including intramuscular, oral and intranasal stimulated a humoral immune response with production of specific IgM and IgG blocking antibodies and a T cell immune response, as suggested by IFN-γ production by spleen lymphocytes stimulated with S peptide. Oral and intranasal administration also triggered the production of specific IgA, the mucosal barrier in the adaptive immune response. In conclusion, plant-derived EVs represent a useful platform for mRNA-based vaccines administered not only parentally but also orally and intranasally.

Keywords: plant; exosome; extracellular vesicle; delivery; COVID-19; SARS; vaccine; RNA; oral; intranasal

Citation: Pomatto, M.A.C.; Gai, C.; Negro, F.; Massari, L.; Deregibus, M.C.; Grange, C.; De Rosa, F.G.; Camussi, G. Plant-Derived Extracellular Vesicles as a Delivery Platform for RNA-Based Vaccine: Feasibility Study of an Oral and Intranasal SARS-CoV-2 Vaccine. *Pharmaceutics* **2023**, *15*, 974. https://doi.org/10.3390/pharmaceutics15030974

Academic Editor: Yong Chen

Received: 14 February 2023
Revised: 10 March 2023
Accepted: 16 March 2023
Published: 17 March 2023

1. Introduction

Membrane vesicles secreted by cells have been described as a well-preserved evolutionary mechanism involved in communication among cells [1,2]. These vesicles originally described in eukaryotes, including mammalians, were subsequently found to be present in prokaryotes and in plants [3]. Virtually released by any cell type, secreted membrane vesicles are a heterogenous population with a complex structure that reproduces cell complexity at the nanoscale [1,2]. In fact, they are constituted by a lipid bilayer membrane containing several cell constituents that can be shared from the cell of origin with other cell types. This mechanism is the basis for a cell-to-cell mediated transfer of information [1,2,4]. Interestingly, the discovery of a horizontal transfer of vesicle-encapsulated nucleic acids [5–10] protected from enzyme degradation by the vesicle membrane opened up a new field of research that is now rapidly expanding. The term "extracellular vesicles" (EVs) [11] was proposed to include in this heterogenous population membrane vesicles released from multivesicular bodies, also named exosomes, and membrane vesicles originated by budding of plasma membrane, termed microvesicles or ectosomes. Independently of their origin, EVs share a common mechanism of action: the transfer of regulatory transcripts that target genes involved in defined pathways in recipient cells [5–9].

Of interest, the lipid bilayer membrane of EVs guarantees protection of nucleic acid from enzyme degradation, thus preserving the EV cargo [12]. Different reports showed the possibility to engineer EVs with an exogenous nucleic acid using the green fluorescent protein (GFP) mRNA that, once transferred to target cells, was translated into protein [6,7]. Several subsequent studies focused on the exploitation of EVs for drug delivery, with a particular interest in nucleic acids, showing that encapsulated mRNA, non-coding RNA, or DNA can be shared among cells [13]. In addition, strategies to load vesicles with selected membrane proteins have been developed. For instance, a fusion protein interacting with the Endosomal Sorting Complexes Required for Transport (ESCRT) cellular machinery was used to sort a chimeric protein into EVs [14]. The ability of EVs to transfer proteins or nucleic acids to the antigen-presenting cells (APCs) makes them a potential candidate as vaccine carriers [15]. Cells have been engineered to express proteins of SARS-CoV-2 in the EVs to develop a vaccine that induces long-lasting cellular and humoral responses [16]. Bacteria EVs decorated with Spike receptor-binding domain derived from mammalian cell culture were also used to generate anti-viral protein antibodies after intranasal administration [17]. Moreover, a potent SARS-CoV-2 CD8+ T immune response was obtained by generating engineered EVs released by muscle cells [18].

EVs from human cells can be engineered for encapsulating therapeutic agents due to the ability to transfer a great number of biomolecules [19]. However, scalable production of EVs from human cells in GMP conditions is difficult, time-consuming and highly expensive. With respect to human cell-derived EVs, plant-derived EVs may represent a good option for drug delivery because they are non-toxic, are an extractive product that can be produced on a large scale and can be directly manipulated and modified with a wide range of agents [20–24].

In the present study, we evaluated the possible use of edible plant-derived EVs as a delivery platform for mRNA-based vaccines. In fact, due to their resistance, plant-derived EVs represent an ideal natural source for the delivery of drugs such as small interfering RNAs (siRNAs), microRNAs (miRNAs) or poorly soluble natural compounds (e.g., curcumin) [24]. Plant EVs have the advantage, with respect to synthetic nanoparticles, of a high cellular internalization rate, good gastrointestinal stability and low intrinsic immunogenicity [25]. The aim of the present study was to evaluate whether plant-derived EVs were suitable for the delivery of SARS-CoV-2 mRNA as a vaccine via oral and intranasal administration routes. We tested three different SARS-CoV-2 mRNAs coding for full-length surface glycoprotein (FS) (commonly known as S protein), Spike-RBD subunit of S protein (S1) and nucleocapsid phosphoprotein (N). For this purpose, we directly engineered EVs extracted from an easily obtainable liquid source, orange (*Citrus sinensis*) juice, (oEVs) with a proprietary technique and evaluated in vitro the efficiency of mRNA molecules' loading and their protection from degrading stress (RNase enzymes and simulated gastric fluid), the EV delivery of mRNA into target cells, the mRNA translation into protein and the subsequent activation of lymphocyte response. We investigated in vivo the effective production of serum antibodies versus the specific S protein of SARS-CoV-2, the specific immune cell activation and the effect of multiple routes of administration including intramuscular, oral and intranasal routes.

2. Materials and Methods

2.1. *oEV Isolation and Loading*

oEVs were isolated from freshly squeezed orange juice from *Citrus sinensis*, type Tarocco, purchased from a local certified organic producer (Arancebio srl, Francofonte, SR, Italy) in January 2021 and throughout 2022. The orange juice was filtered with a strainer and centrifuged at 4000× *g* for 30 min. The supernatant was ultracentrifuged at 10,000× *g* for 1 h at +4 °C (Optima L-90K ultracentrifuge, rotor 45 Ti, polycarbonate tubes, Beckman Coulter, Milan, Italy). The supernatant was then filtered to reduce the presence of fibers and re-ultracentrifuged at 100,000× *g* for 2 h at +4 °C (Optima L-90K ultracentrifuge, rotor 45 Ti, polycarbonate tubes, Beckman Coulter, Milan, Italy). The pellet was re-suspended in saline solution (NaCl 0.9%, B. Braun, Milan, Italy) added with 1% DMSO (Sigma-Aldrich, Merck, Darmstadt, Germany), filtered with 0.22 filters (Millex, Millipore, Merck, Darmstadt, Germany) for sterilization and stored at −80 °C for further experiments.

mRNA sequences were designed as described in Table 1 and purchased from RiboPro (Oss, The Netherlands). No codon optimization or other mRNA modifications were applied to mRNA sequences. The mRNAs were completed with a 5′UTR designed for high expression, a poly-A tail and a Cap1 with methylation of the first nucleotide to produce a Cap1 structure. After mRNA synthesis, dsRNA was removed to avoid innate immune-mediated translational repression. mRNAs were loaded into oEVs with a proprietary technique described in the patent application WO/2022/152771A1 using cation-based interaction combined with controlled osmotic shock.

Table 1. Selected mRNA sequences from SARS-CoV-2, genomic sequence NC_045512.2.

mRNA Name (Abbreviation)	Gene Symbol (NCBI)	Gene Description	ORF	Nucleotide Position	Nucleotide Number	Reference
N	N	nucleocapsid phosphoprotein	ORF 9	28274–29533	1260 nt	GENE, FASTA
FS	S	surface glycoprotein	ORF 2	21563–25384	3822 nt	GENE, FASTA
S1	S1	surface glycoprotein, Spike-S1-RBD	ORF 2	22518–23186	669 nt	GENE, FASTA

2.2. oEV Characterization

oEVs were analyzed through nanoparticle tracking analysis (NTA) using the NanoSight NS300 system (Malvern Panalytical, Malvern, UK), equipped with NTA 3.4 analytic software. The instrument uses a laser source to inspect the sample and analyzes the Brownian movements of detected particles. The analytic software uses the Stokes–Einstein equation for converting this information into size and concentration parameters. For each sample, oEVs were diluted in a range of 1:200–1:2000 in 1 mL of saline solution (NaCl 0.9%, B. Braun, Milan, Italy) previously filtered with 0.1 μm membranes (Millex, Millipore, Merck, Darmstadt, Germany). Three videos of 30 s duration were recorded and camera levels were set to 15 for all the acquisitions. Settings for NTA post-acquisition were optimized and maintained constant among all samples, and each video was analyzed to measure the mean size and concentration of oEVs.

The morphology and integrity of oEVs were analyzed by transmission electron microscopy (TEM) as previously described [26]. Briefly, oEVs were left to adhere on 200 mesh nickel formvar carbon-coated grids (Electron Microscopy Science, Hatfield, PA, USA) for 20 min. Then, grids were incubated with 2.5% glutaraldehyde plus 2% sucrose. After washing in distilled water, samples were negatively stained with Nano-W and NanoVan (Nanoprobes, Yaphank, NY, USA) and analyzed using a Jeol JEM 1400 Flash electron microscope (Jeol, Tokyo, Japan).

2.3. RNA Extraction and qRT-PCR

Total RNA was extracted from cells and oEVs using a miRNeasy mini kit (Qiagen, Hilden, Germany) following the manufacturer's instructions. RNA was eluted in nuclease-free water (Ambion, Thermo Fisher Scientific, Waltham, MA, USA) and the RNA concentration was assessed by measuring the absorbance at 260 nm with a spectrophotometer (mySPEC, VWR, Radnor, PA, USA). Samples were stored at −80 °C until analysis.

RNA was retro-transcribed to cDNA using a High-Capacity cDNA Reverse Transcription Kit (Thermo Fisher Scientific, Waltham, MA, USA) following the manufacturer's instructions (100 nanograms for cell analysis and 10 μL for oEV analysis). Syn-cel-miR-39 (Qiagen, Hilden, Germany) was added to oEV samples as spike-in during the retro-transcription procedure. For qRT-PCR, each sample was run in triplicate; the primers (Eurofins Genomics, Milan, Italy) are listed in Table S1. For syn-cel-miR-39, the universal primer (Qiagen, Hilden, Germany) was used as the reverse primer. Human ACTB was used as the endogenous control for mRNA incorporation into target cells, whereas cel-mir-39 was used as the endogenous control for mRNA loading into oEVs. cDNA (5 nanograms for cell analysis and 2.5 μL for oEV analysis) was combined with SYBR GREEN PCR Master Mix (Thermo Fisher Scientific, Waltham, MA, USA) as described by the manufacturer's protocol. The Real-Time Thermal Cycler Quant Studio 12k and ExpressionSuite Software 1.0.3 (Thermo Fisher Scientific, Waltham, MA, USA) were used to calculate relative quantification (RQ) values via the $2^{-\Delta\Delta Ct}$ method.

For the generation of standard curves for absolute quantification of mRNAs, each mRNA (S1, FS and N) was spectrophotometrically quantified and 200 ng were reverse transcribed using the High-Capacity cDNA Reverse Transcription Kit (Thermo Fisher Scientific, Waltham, MA, USA). cDNA was serially diluted 1:5 from a starting point of 10 ng to have 11 dilutions. Serial dilutions were run in five replicates using Relative Standard Curve on a 96-well QuantStudio 12K Flex Real-Time PCR system, as described by the manufacturer's protocol (Thermo Fisher Scientific Scientific, Waltham, MA, USA). The calibration curve was used to convert the Ct values of each sample into the corresponding amount of mRNA. The percentage of engineering yield was calculated as follows: (final amount mRNA/oEV)/(starting amount mRNA/oEV). EV loading was repeated in three independent experiments for each mRNA used.

2.4. PCR and Electrophoresis

cDNA was amplified with iProofTM High-Fidelity DNA Polymerase (Biorad, Hercules, CA, USA) following the manufacturer's instructions. The PCR reaction mix was composed of 4 ng cDNA, 500 nM primer (Eurofins Genomics, Milan, Italy), 0.5 μL iProof DNA Polymerase (Biorad, Hercules, CA, USA), 10 μL 5x iProof HF buffer, 1 μL dNTPs, 0.5 μL MgCl2, and nuclease-free water (Thermo Fisher Scientific, Waltham, MA, USA) to reach the reaction volume of 50 μL. The CTR DNA template was amplified with 1.3 kB primers (both provided by the kit) as the internal reaction control. The PCR was performed with VERITI Thermal Cycler (Thermo Fisher Scientific, Waltham, MA, USA), with 30 amplification cycles run. For gel electrophoresis, 15 μL of PCR products was mixed with 3 μL of 6X TriTrack DNA Loading Dye from a GeneRuler 100 bp Plus DNA Ladder Kit (Thermo Fisher Scientific, Waltham, MA, USA). Then, 15 μL of the mix was loaded on a 5% Mini-PROTEAN® TBE Gel (Biorad, Hercules, CA, USA). The electrophoresis cell was filled with 1X TBE buffer (Biorad, Hercules, CA, USA) and the run was performed at 100 V for 45 min. Gels were soaked for 20 min in ethidium bromide (Biorad, Hercules, CA, USA) diluted to 0.5 μg/mL in 1X TBE buffer and subsequently washed in sterile water (B.Braun, Milan, Italy) for 20 min at RT. Images were acquired with a ChemiDoc System (Biorad, Hercules, CA, USA). Data were obtained from three independent experiments.

2.5. Cell Culture

Human macrophages (MV-4-11), human dermal microvascular endothelial cells (HMEC-1) and normal human dermal fibroblasts (NHDF) were obtained from ATCC (Manassas, VA, USA) and cultured following the manufacturer's instructions with, respectively, Iscove's modified Dulbecco's medium (IMDM, ATCC, Manassas, VA, USA), MCDB131 medium (Gibco, Thermo Fisher Scientific, Waltham, MA, USA) and fibroblast growth basal medium (FBM, Lonza, Basel, Switzerland) supplemented with 10% fetal bovine serum (FBS, Life Technologies, Thermo Fisher Scientific, Waltham, MA, USA). Human primary peripheral blood mononuclear cells (PBMC) were isolated from the peripheral blood of healthy donors provided by the Centro Produzione e Validazione Emocomponenti of the A.O.U. Città della Salute e della Scienza di Torino with internal ethical approval. PBMC were isolated via a density gradient using Histopaque®-1077 (Sigma Aldrich, Merck, Darmstadt, Germany), washed with PBS (Thermo Fisher Scientific, Waltham, MA, USA) and plated at a concentration of 2×10^6 cells/mL in a 12-well plate with RPMI 1640 (Euroclone, Milan, Italy) supplemented with 10% FBS (Life Technologies, Thermo Fisher Scientific, Waltham, MA, USA). All cells were incubated at 37 °C with 5% CO_2.

The effect of oEVs on cell viability was evaluated with a MTT Cell Growth Assay Kit following the manufacturer's instructions (Sigma-Aldrich, Merck, Darmstadt, Germany). Briefly, HMEC-1 was plated at a density of 5000 cells/well in 96-well plates (Euroclone, Milan, Italy) and treated with four increasing doses of oEVs (10,000, 50,000, 100,000 and 200,000 particles/cell) diluted in medium (DMEM low glucose with 5% EV-depleted FBS) (Euro-clone, Milan, Italy). The viability measurement was performed after 24 h of treatment, comparing cells cultured with medium, medium plus oEVs or medium plus 50% DMSO as the positive control (Sigma-Aldrich, Merck, Darmstadt, Germany). Data were obtained from three independent experiments.

2.6. mRNA Stress Resistance

To test the resistance to enzyme degradation of mRNAs loaded into oEVs, samples were treated with 0.4 μg/mL Ambion™ RNase A (Invitrogen, Thermo Fisher Scientific, Waltham, MA, USA) and incubated at 37 °C for 30 min as previously described [27]. The reaction was stopped by adding Ambion™ RNase inhibitor (Invitrogen, Thermo Fisher Scientific, Waltham, MA, USA) according to the manufacturer's instructions. Samples were washed by ultracentrifugation at 100,000× g for 2 h at +4 °C using a 10 mL polycarbonate tube (SW 90 Ti rotor, Beckman Coulter Optima L-90 K ultracentrifuge, Beckman Coulter, Milan, Italy) and were resuspended in saline buffer solution for analysis. The resistance to gastrointestinal degradation was investigated as previously described [28]. Briefly, a simulated gastric fluid (SGF) was prepared using 18.5% w/v HCl (pH 2.0), 24 mg/mL of bile extract, pepsin solution (80 mg/mL in 0.1 N of HC_l, pH 2.0) and 4 mg/mL of pancreatin in 0.1 N of N_aHCO_3 (Sigma-Aldrich, Merck, Darmstadt, Germany). Next, 100 μL of each oEV sample was incubated with 1.34 μL of SGF at 37 °C for 60 min. Then, the pH value was adjusted to 6.4 with 1 N N_aHCO_3 to mimic the intestinal solution and incubated for 60 min. Free mRNA was used as a control and the percentage of resistance was defined as the percentage of mRNA remaining after stress treatments in comparison to starting material. Data for each mRNA were obtained from three independent experiments. For experiments with Triton X-100, samples were treated with 1% Triton X-100 (Biorad, Hercules, CA, USA) for 1 h at +4 °C before RNAse treatment and molecular analysis.

2.7. mRNA Incorporation into Target Cells

Human macrophages were plated 60,000 cells/well in 24-well plates (Sarstedt, Milan, Italy) and treated with different stimuli: medium (IMDM plus 10% FBS), or medium plus oEVs, oEV-S1, oEV-FS or oEV-N (1.2×10^{10} oEVs containing 1 μg mRNA/well). As a control, cells were co-incubated or transfected with a similar amount of each mRNA with Lipofectamine® 2000 Reagent (Thermo Fisher Scientific, Waltham, MA, USA) following the manufacturer's instructions. Next, 0.75 μL/well lipofectamine and 1.0 μg/well mRNA were diluted in DMEM low glucose (Euroclone, Milan, Italy), incubated for 5 min at room temperature and added to wells containing medium. After 24 h, cells were harvested and processed for molecular analysis. Data were obtained from three independent experiments.

2.8. Cytofluorometric Analysis of mRNA Translation into Protein

HMEC-1 was plated at 50,000 cells/well in 24-well plates (Sarstedt, Milan, Italy) and treated with different stimuli: medium (MCDB131), or medium plus oEVs, oEV-S1, oEV-FS or oEV-N (1.2×10^{10} oEVs and 1 μg mRNA/well). As the control, cells were transfected with a similar amount of each mRNA using Lipofectamine® 2000 Reagent (Thermo Fisher Scientific, Waltham, MA, USA) following the manufacturer's instructions. Briefly, 0.75 μL/well lipofectamine and 1.0 μg/well mRNA were diluted in DMEM low glucose (Euroclone, Milan, Italy), incubated for 5 min at room temperature and added to each well containing MCDB131 medium plus 10% FBS. Treatment with only lipofectamine reagent was used as the transfection control. After 24 h of treatment, cells were collected and treated using an Inside Perm Kit (Miltenyi Biotec, Bologna, Italy) for the intracellular staining, following the manufacturer's instructions. Briefly, cells were treated with Fix

Inside reagent for 20 min at room temperature, washed with PBS and mixed with anti-N-protein rabbit antibody (1:250, PA1-41098, Invitrogen, Thermo Fisher Scientific, Waltham, MA, USA) or anti-S1-protein mouse antibody (1:100, MA5-38033, Invitrogen, Thermo Fisher Scientific, Waltham, MA, USA) for 1 h at room temperature. After washing, samples were incubated with 5 μg/mL fluorescent secondary antibody anti-mouse (green, A32723, Invitrogen, Thermo Fisher Scientific, Waltham, MA, USA) or anti-rabbit (red, A32740, Invitrogen, Thermo Fisher Scientific, Waltham, MA, USA) for 1 h at room temperature. Finally, samples were washed and resuspended in saline solution for acquisition with CytoFLEX (Beckman Coulter, Milan, Italy) and CytExpert software (v 2.3.0.84, Beckman Coulter, Milan, Italy). Data were obtained from three independent experiments.

2.9. *Confocal Microscopy Analysis of mRNA Translation into Protein*

HMEC-1 were plated at 10,000 cells/well in 8-well chamber slides (Thermo Fisher Scientific, Waltham, MA, USA) and treated with different stimuli: medium (MCDB131), or medium plus oEVs, oEV-S1, oEV-FS or oEV-N using a particle dose of 1.2×10^{10} oEVs/well and 1 μg mRNA/well. As control, the cells were transfected with a similar amount of nude mRNA S1, FS, N. Transfection was performed with Lipofectamine® 2000 Reagent (Thermo Fisher Scientific, Waltham, MA, USA) following the manufacturer's instructions. Briefly, 0.16 μL/well Lipofectamine® 2000 Reagent and 1.0 μg/well mRNA were diluted in DMEM low glucose (Euroclone, Milan, Italy), incubated for 5 min at room temperature and added to each well containing MCDB131 medium plus 10% FBS. Treatment with only Lipofectamine® 2000 Reagent was used as the transfection control.

After 24 h of treatment, cells were washed with PBS, fixed with ice-cold methanol:acetone (1:1), incubated at −20 °C for 10 min and air dried. Then, wells were blocked with PBS with 1% bovine serum albumin (BSA, Sigma-Aldrich, Merck, Darmstadt, Germany) for 30 min at 37 °C, and after washing, were incubated with anti-N-protein rabbit antibody (1:250, PA1-41098, Invitrogen, Thermo Fisher Scientific, Waltham, MA, USA) or anti-S1-protein mouse antibody (1:100, MA5-38033, Invitrogen, Thermo Fisher Scientific, Waltham, MA, USA) for 1 h at RT. After three washes with PBS, samples were incubated with anti-mouse (1:1000, green, A32723, Invitrogen, Thermo Fisher Scientific, Waltham, MA, USA) or anti-rabbit (1:1000, red, A32740, Invitrogen, Thermo Fisher Scientific, Waltham, MA, USA) fluorescent antibodies for 1 h at room temperature, protected from light. After three washes with PBS, samples were incubated with DAPI at 300 nM (Thermo Fisher Scientific, Waltham, MA, USA) for 10 min at room temperature, protected from light. Then, samples were washed three times with PBS and air-dried. One drop of Fluormount Aqueous Mounting Media (Sigma Aldrich, Merck, Darmstadt, Germany) was added to each spot and the glass was covered with a coverslip. Images were acquired with the confocal microscope Axiovert 200M equipped with LSM5 Pascal and analyzed with LSM image browser (Zeiss, Oberkochen, Germany). Data were obtained from three independent experiments.

2.10. *Cytofluorometric Analysis of oEV-GFP*

GFP translation after oEV-mediated delivery was evaluated after 24 h of treatment of HMEC-1 was plated at 30,000 cells/well in 24-well plates (Sarstedt, Milan, Italy) with medium (MCDB131), or medium plus oEVs (1×10^{10} oEVs/well), oEVs loaded with GFP mRNA (oEV-GFP) (1×10^{10} oEVs and 0.83 μg mRNA/well) (OZ Biosciences, Marseilles, France), GFP mRNA or GFP mRNA transfected with lipofectamine. Transfection was performed with Lipofectamine® 2000 Reagent (Thermo Fisher Scientific, Waltham, MA, USA) following the manufacturer's instructions using 1.67 μg/well mRNA. After 24 h, cells were harvested and analyzed.

oEV uptake and GFP delivery were also investigated after RNase and SGF stress. For that purpose, oEVs were previously stained with 1:100 diluted PKH26 fluorescent dye (Sigma-Aldrich, Thermo Fisher Scientific, Waltham, MA, USA) for 30 min at 37 °C and washed by ultracentrifugation at $100{,}000\times g$ for 2 h at +4 °C (SW 90 Ti rotor, Beckman Coulter Optima L-90 K ultracentrifuge, polycarbonate tubes, Beckman Coulter, Milan, Italy).

Stained oEVs were loaded with GFP mRNA (oEV-GFP). oEVs (1.2×10^{10} oEVs/well), oEV-GFP (1.2×10^{10} oEVs and 0.5 μg mRNA/well) and 0.5 μg of free GFP mRNA were subjected to incubation with RNase and SGF and used to treat 20,000 cells/well NHDF in 24-well plates (Sarstedt, Milan, Italy). mRNA was transfected using Lipofectamine® 2000 Reagent (Thermo Fisher Scientific, Waltham, MA, USA) following the manufacturer's instructions.

Data for each mRNA were obtained from three independent experiments. Analysis was performed with CytoFLEX (Beckman Coulter, Milan, Italy) and CytExpert software (v 2.3.0.84, Beckman Coulter, Milan, Italy). Data were obtained from three independent experiments.

2.11. Lymphocytes' Activation In Vitro

Human macrophages plated in 24 well-plates (Sarstedt, Milan, Italy) at a density of 20,000 cells/well were co-incubated with several stimuli: medium (RPMI with 10% FBS), medium plus oEV, oEV-S1, oEV-FS or oEV-N (1.2×10^{10} oEVs and 1 μg /well of mRNA), 2 μg/mL S protein and N protein of SARS-CoV-2 (RP-87706 and RP-87665, Thermo Fisher Scientific, Waltham, MA, USA) and activation beads at 10 μL/well (Dynabeads® Human T-Activator CD3/CD28, Life Technologies, Thermo Fisher Scientific, Waltham, MA, USA). After 5 h, 200,000 PBMC were added to each well, and stimulation with treatments was repeated after 5 days. On day 10 of the experiment, cells were harvested and analyzed.

For cell proliferation analysis, PBMC were labeled with CellTrace™ CFSE dye (Thermo Fisher Scientific, Waltham, MA, USA) following the manufacturer's instructions before incubation with macrophages. At the experiment endpoint, cells were collected and stained with CD4-APC antibody (1:50, 130-113-222, Miltenyi Biotec, Bologna, Italy) using an appropriate isotype.

For marker expression, cells were harvested and stained with CD4-FITC (1:50, MHCD0401, CALTAG Laboratories, Burlingame, CA, USA), CD25-APC-Vio®770, CD69-APC-Vio®770 or HLADR-APC-Vio®770 (1:100, 130-123-469, 130-112-616, 130-111-792, Miltenyi Biotec, Bologna, Italy) with appropriate isotypes.

Antibody staining was performed for 30 min and washed by centrifugation at $500\times g$ for 10 min. Analysis was performed with CytoFLEX (Beckman Coulter, Milan, Italy) and CytExpert software (v 2.3.0.84, Beckman Coulter, Milan, Italy). Data were obtained from three independent experiments.

2.12. Mice Immunization and Sacrifice

The study was conducted according to the National Institute of Health Guidelines for the Care and Use of Laboratory Animals, and approved by the Ethics Committee of the University of Turin and the Italian Ministry of Health (authorization number 514/2021-PR, approved on 12 July 2021). Female BALB/cAnNCrl mice of 6–8 weeks old were purchased from the Department of Molecular Biotechnology and Health Sciences, University of Turin. Behavior and health status were observed daily and weight checked weekly. Immunization was performed by administering empty oEVs and mRNA-loaded oEVs (oEV-S1 or oEV-FS) via intramuscular (IM), oral and intranasal (IN) routes.

For IM and IN administration, animals received one immunization (equivalent to 7.2×10^{11} oEVs containing 60 μg mRNA in 100 μL for IM or 40 μL for IN route of saline solution for each dose) at day 0 and one booster immunization after 3 weeks. For intramuscular administration, treatments were injected into the same hind leg for both doses, whereas for intranasal administration, the dose was pipetted into mice's nostrils. For oral administration, animals received one immunization (equivalent to 1.2×10^{12} oEVs containing 100 μg mRNA in 150 μL of a solution of 1% chitosan for each dose) at day 0 using gavage needle and three booster immunizations after 3 weeks on consecutive days.

Mice were euthanized after 2 weeks from the last booster immunization. The group named oEV-S1 received immunization with S1 mRNA ($n = 6$ for IM, $n = 7$ for IN and $n = 9$ for oral), whereas the group named oEV ($n = 5$ for IM, $n = 7$ for IN and $n = 6$ for oral) received an equivalent dose of unloaded oEV as a negative control. The group named oEV-FS received immunization with FS mRNA ($n = 6$ for IM, $n = 3$ for IN, and $n = 2$ for oral), whereas the group named oEV ($n = 6$ for IM, $n = 4$ for IN and $n = 3$ for oral) received an equivalent dose of unloaded oEV as a negative control.

Immediately after sacrifice, spleens were collected in HBSS (Thermo Scientific, Waltham, MA, USA) and processed for cell isolation. Blood was collected and centrifuged at 3.000× g for 20 min to obtain serum. Sera were stored at −20 °C until use. The bronchoalveolar lavage (BAL) fluid was collected from mice immunized with oEV ($n = 2$) or oEV-S1 ($n = 3$) and stored at −20 °C until use.

Muscle and intestine morphology was evaluated through formalin-fixed paraffin-embedded tissue staining. Paraffin tissue sections (5 μm thick) were routinely stained for microscopic evaluation with H&E (Merck, Darmstadt, Germany) and photographed with an Axioskop microscope (Zeiss, Oberkochen, Germany) equipped with a Canon DS126181 camera (Canon, Tokyo, Japan).

2.13. Antibody Titer Analysis

Specific IgG, IgM, and IgA antibodies against the S protein of SARS-CoV-2 virus in mice serum or BAL samples were detected through enzyme-linked immunosorbent assay (ELISA). For that purpose, Nunc Maxisorp ELISA plates (Thermo Fisher Scientific, Waltham, MA, USA) were coated overnight at 4 °C with 100 μL/well of 1 μg/mL SARS-CoV-2 S1 RBD recombinant protein (RP-87706, Thermo Fisher Scientific, Waltham, MA, USA) diluted in BupH carbonate–bicarbonate buffer (Thermo Scientific, Waltham, MA, USA). After three washes with PBS 1X, plates were blocked with 200 μL/well of PBS 1X–3% bovine serum albumin (BSA, Sigma Aldrich, Merck, Darmstadt, Germany) for 1 h at 37 °C. After five washes with PBS 1X—0.05% Tween20 (Sigma Aldrich, Merck, Darmstadt, Germany), plates were incubated with 100 μL/well of different serial dilutions of samples in duplicate (starting from dilution 1:100). Dilution buffer was also used as a blank: PBS 1X–0.05% Tween20–3% BSA for IgG, PBS 1X–3% BSA–5% FBS for IgM and PBS 1X–0.05% Tween20–3% BSA–5% FBS for IgA. Plates were incubated for 1 h at 37 °C for IgG, 2 h at room temperature for IgA or overnight at 4 °C for IgM. After five washes with PBS 1X–0.05% Tween20, 100 μL/well of secondary antibody was added: goat anti-mouse HRP IgG (1:10.000, 31430, Invitrogen, Thermo Fisher Scientific, Waltham, MA, USA), IgM (1:4.000, 62-6820, Invitrogen, Thermo Fisher Scientific, Waltham, MA, USA) or IgA (1:250, 8850450-88, Invitrogen, Thermo Fisher Scientific, Waltham, MA, USA). After 2 h incubation and five washes with PBS 1X–0.05% Tween20, 100 μL/well of Stabilized Chromogen (TMB, Life Technologies, Thermo Fisher Scientific, Waltham, MA, USA) was added and incubated for 15–30 min at room temperature. The reaction was stopped by adding 100 μL/well of ELISA Stop Solution (Invitrogen, Thermo Fisher Scientific, Waltham, MA, USA). The plates were read at 450 nm using a VICTOR® Nivo™ Plate Reader (PerkinElmer, Milan, Italy) and VICTOR® Nivo™ Control Software (v 4.0.7, PerkinElmer, Milan, Italy). End-point titers were calculated as the last dilution with an optical density ≥ 1.5 blank O.D. value or ≥ 2 blank O.D. value for IgA in BAL samples.

Specificity was evaluated using a competition assay as the percentage of reduction in O.D. value of serum samples (diluted 1:100 for IgM, 1:1000 for IgG and IgA), either control or pre-incubated with 30 μg/mL of SARS-CoV-2 S1 RBD recombinant protein for 1 h at 37 °C.

IgG sensibility was evaluated for the only mouse antibody anti-S protein available, IgG, using serial dilutions of SARS-CoV-2 Spike Protein (RBD) Monoclonal Antibody (MA5-38033, Invitrogen, Thermo Fisher Scientific, Waltham, MA, USA) ranging from 10 to 0.1 ng/mL following IgG protocol.

2.14. Neutralizing Antibody Analysis

A SARS-CoV-2 Neutralizing Antibody ELISA Kit (Invitrogen, Thermo Fisher Scientific, Waltham, MA, USA) was used to detect the level of neutralizing antibodies against SARS-CoV-2 in mice serum following the manufacturer's instructions. Briefly, serum samples were diluted 1:50 with Assay Buffer 1X, and pre-coated plates were washed one time with Wash Buffer 1X. Next, 100 μL of positive control, Assay Buffer 1X (used as a negative control) and pre-diluted serum sample were added to the appropriate wells in duplicate and incubated for 30 min at room temperature. Plates were washed three times and 100 μL of Biotin Conjugate Solution 1X was added to each well. After incubation at room temperature for 30 min, plates were washed three times and 100 μL/well of streptavidin–HRP conjugate solution was added. Then, plates were incubated for 15 min at room temperature and washed three times, and 100 μL/well of substrate solution was added and left for 15 min at room temperature. The reaction was stopped by adding 100 μL/well of Stop Solution and plates were read on a VICTOR® Nivo™ Plate Reader (PerkinElmer, Milan, Italy) using VICTOR® Nivo™ Control Software (v 4.0.7, PerkinElmer, Milan, Italy) at 450 nm, using 620 nm as the reference wavelength. The percentage of neutralization was calculated using the following formula: 1 − (absorbance of unknown sample/absorbance of negative control) × 100.

2.15. Splenocytes' Isolation

Mouse splenocytes were isolated from spleens freshly collected in HBSS (Thermo Fisher Scientific, Waltham, MA, USA). Spleens were disrupted and filtered through a 40 μm cell strainer (PluriSelect, Leipzig, Germany), diluted with PBS (Euroclone, Milan, Italy) and centrifuged at 500× *g* at 4 °C for 5 min. Each pellet was resuspended in 2 mL cold RBC lysis buffer 1X (Thermo Fisher Scientific, Waltham, MA, USA) and incubated on ice for 5 min to lyse red blood cells. The reaction was stopped with 10 mL ice-cold PBS and cells were pelleted at 400× *g* at 4 °C for 5 min and resuspended in RPMI 1640 supplemented with 10% FBS.

2.16. IFN-γ Detection with ELISPOT

Elispot plates (Merck Millipore, Darmstadt, Germany) were activated by adding 15 μL of 35% ethanol to each well, washed twice with PBS, coated with mouse IFN-γ capture antibody (part of Mouse IFN-γ ELISPOT Pair, 551881, BD Bioscience, Eysins, Switzerland) and left overnight at +4 °C. Plates were blocked using RPMI 1640 with 10% FBS for 2 h at room temperature. For each mouse, 3×10^6 fresh splenocytes were plated in each well and re-stimulated with 2 μg/mL S peptide (SARS-CoV-2 S1 RBD recombinant protein, RP-87706, ThermoFisher Scientific, Waltham, MA, USA). For each condition, three technical replicates were performed. Plates were incubated for 44 h at 37 °C with 5% CO_2. Cells were removed and plates were washed twice with deionized water and three times with washing buffer (ELISA wash buffer, Invitrogen, Thermo Fisher Scientific, Waltham, MA, USA). Next, they were incubated with mouse IFN-γ detection antibody for 2 h at room temperature. Then, plates were washed three times with washing buffer and incubated with streptavidin–HRP (557630, BD Bioscience, Eysins, Switzerland) for 1 h at room temperature. Following that, plates were washed four times with washing buffer and twice with PBS, then incubated with substrate solution (AEC substrate set, BD Bioscience, Eysins, Switzerland) for 15 min until spot development. The reaction was stopped by washing with sterile water, and plates were left to air-dry at room temperature in the dark until completely dry. Plate acquisition was performed using an ELISPOT plate reader with ImmunoSpot (S6 Macro M2, ImmunoSpot, Cleveland, OH, USA), and spot counting was performed automatically by ImmunoSpot Software version 7.0.21.0 (ImmunoSpot, Cleveland, OH, USA).

2.17. Cytokine ELISA Analysis

Mouse splenocytes were stimulated with 1 μg/mL of S peptide (SARS-CoV-2 S1 RBD recombinant protein, RP-87706, ThermoFisher Scientific, Waltham, MA, USA), and the supernatant was collected after 24 h, then centrifuged at 1400× *g* × 10 min to remove debris. Quantitative detection of mouse IFN-γ, IL-2, IL-10 and IL-4 levels was performed using a Mouse Th1/Th2 Uncoated ELISA Kit (88-7711-44, Invitrogen, Thermo Fisher Scientific, Waltham, MA, USA) according to the manufacturer's instructions. Briefly, 96-well plates (Corning, Glendale, AZ, USA) were coated with 100 μL/well of capture antibody overnight at 4 °C. After washing, plates were blocked with 200 µL/well of ELISA/ELISPOT Diluent 1X for 1 h at room temperature and washed once with Wash Buffer. Mouse IFN-γ, IL-2, IL-10 and IL-4 standards were reconstituted, and two-fold serial dilutions were performed to produce a standard curve for a total of eight points. Next, 100 µL of samples or ELISA/ELISPOT Diluent as the blank were added to the well in duplicate and incubated for 2 h at room temperature. After washing, 100 µL/well of detection antibody was incubated for 1 h at room temperature. Then, 100 µL/well of Streptavidin-HRP was incubated for 30 min at room temperature and washed five times with Wash Buffer. Following that, 100 µL/well of TMB Solution 1X was incubated for 15 min at room temperature. The reaction was stopped by adding 100 µL/well of Stop Solution and plates were read on a VICTOR® Nivo™ Plate Reader (PerkinElmer, Milan, Italy) using VICTOR® Nivo™ Control Software version 4.0.7 (PerkinElmer, Milan, Italy) at 450 nm, subtracting the 570 nm reference wavelength. Standards curves based on standard O.D. values were used to calculate the cytokine amount (pg/mL) for each sample.

2.18. Cytofluorometric Analysis of Splenocyte-Derived Immune Cells

For ex vivo analysis, mouse splenocytes were stimulated with 1 µg/mL of S peptide (SARS-CoV-2 S1 RBD recombinant protein, RP-87706, ThermoFisher Scientific, Waltham, MA, USA). For marker expression, cells were harvested after 36 h and stained with Viobility Fixable Dye (Miltenyi, Bologna, Italy) and CD3ε-APC (1:50, 130-117-671), CD4-APC-Vio770 (1:50, 130-118-955), CD8-FITC (1:50, 130-122-720), CD69-PE (1:50, 30-115-460), CD3-FITC (1:50, 130-092-962), CD4-VioBlue (1:50, 130-123-208), CD25-PE (1:50, 130-120-696), CD8-FITC (1:50, 130-120-822), CD138-PE (1:50, 130-120-741), CD45R-FITC (1:50, 130-118-323) and appropriate isotypes for each fluorescence (Miltenyi, Bologna, Italy). After staining, cells were washed with PBS, centrifuged at 300× *g* for 10 min and resuspended in PBS for acquisition. For lymphocyte proliferation, cells were stained using a CellTrace™ CFSE cell proliferation kit (Invitrogen, Thermo Fisher Scientific, Waltham, MA, USA) before peptide stimulation in vitro following the manufacturer's instructions. Briefly, 1×10^6 splenocytes were incubated with 1 M CellTrace™ stock solution for 20 min at 37 °C and washed with RPMI 1640 supplemented with 10% FBS. Cells were plated at 1×10^6 cells/mL and stimulated with 1 µg/mL of SARS-CoV-2 S1 RBD recombinant protein (RP-87706, Thermo Fisher Scientific, Waltham, MA, USA). After 5 days, cells were harvested and stained with CD4-APC-Vio770 antibody (1:50, 130-118-955, Miltenyi, Bologna, Italy) and an associated isotype. After staining, cells were washed with PBS, centrifuged at 300× *g* for 10 min and resuspended in PBS for acquisition with a CytoFLEX flow cytometer (Beckman Coulter, Milan, Italy) using CytExpert software (v2.3.0.84, Beckman Coulter, Milan, Italy).

2.19. Biodistribution

Male BALB/cAnNCrl mice were treated with fluorescently labeled oEVs using the IN and oral routes. oEVs were stained using 10 µM of Vybrant™ DiD Cell-Labeling Solution (Thermo Fisher Scientific, Waltham, MA, USA). The same amount of dye (DiD) used for oEV staining was administered as a control to set the background. Treatment was performed with 2×10^{12} oEVs for oral or 1.5×10^{12} oEVs for IN administration in one single dose (n = 5 for stained DiD oEVs, n = 3 for DiD). After 18 h, mice were euthanized and single organs were collected and imaged using an IVIS 200 small animal imaging system (PerkinElmer, Milan, Italy) as previously described [26]. Briefly, the excitation filter was set at 640 nm and the emission filter at 700 nm. The same illumination settings, such as binning factor (4), exposure time (2 s), f/stop (2) and field of views, were used for acquiring all images. The fluorescence signal was normalized to photons per second per centimeter squared per steradian (p/sec/cm^2/sr). Images were acquired and analyzed using Living Image 4.0 software (PerkinElmer, Milan, Italy). The background average photon emission was subtracted from images to normalize the signal. The fluorescence (p/sec/cm^2/sr) was quantified in the region of interest (ROI) drawn freehand. Data were expressed as average radiance ± SD.

2.20. Statistical Analysis

Data were analyzed using GraphPad Prism 6.0 Demo (GraphPad, San Diego, CA, USA). Statistical analyses of three or more groups of data were performed using ANOVA with Dunnett's or Tukey's multiple-comparisons test, as appropriate. A *t*-test was used to compare two groups of data. Values were expressed as their mean ± SD. Statistical significance was established at $p < 0.05$ (* $p < 0.05$, ** $p < 0.01$, *** $p < 0.005$ and **** $p < 0.001$), whereas ns was used to define no statistical significance ($p > 0.05$).

3. Results

3.1. Characterization of oEVs Loaded with SARS-CoV-2 mRNA

To evaluate oEV delivery of mRNA-based vaccine, oEVs were loaded with different mRNA of SARS-CoV-2, coding for: N protein (N), full S protein (FS) and the subunit 1 of S protein (S1) (see Table 1).

Morphology and size analysis by NTA showed that oEVs loaded with mRNA had a biodistribution profile similar to unloaded oEVs. A small increase in size was observed after mRNA loading (Figure 1A,C), with a mean size of 167 ± 10 nm for empty oEVs and 227 ± 24 nm for loaded oEVs. TEM analysis demonstrated an intact membrane of oEV loaded with mRNA, with a round morphology and an electron-dense core (Figure 1B,D) similar to empty oEVs. RNA loading was similar for all three mRNA sequences, showing a comparable increase in RNA ratio with respect to control oEVs (Figure 1E). qRT-PCR analysis demonstrated a statistically significant mRNA loading of oEVs (Figure 1F) with a mean mRNA encapsulation efficiency of 72 ± 11% (Figure 1G) resulting in a loading capacity of 3.51 ± 1.09 ng/10^{11} oEVs (Figure 1H). Additional experiments with the mRNA coding for N protein showed that the co-incubation of oEVs and mRNA was less efficient than oEV loading (Figure S1A) and that the dose of mRNA loadable into oEVs could be increased up to 10 times in terms of total RNA (Figure S1B) and mRNA detected with qRT-PCR (Figure S1C).

Taken together, these data demonstrated that oEVs were efficiently loaded with different mRNA molecules.

3.2. mRNA Loaded into oEVs Was Resistant to Stress

The ability of oEVs to protect mRNA from degradation due to RNase and to simulated gastric fluids (SGF) was evaluated in vitro. RNases are enzymes present in all environmental surfaces and are the main enzymes responsible for RNA degradation (Figure 2A), whereas gastric fluids represent the major stress in the gastrointestinal tract (Figure 2B). The integrity of mRNAs loaded into oEVs and free mRNAs was evaluated after RNase or SGF treatment. As shown in Figure 2C,D, respectively, the RNA amount did not change when mRNA was incorporated into oEVs, whereas free mRNA was significantly reduced after RNase and SGF treatment. Moreover, the analysis of each specific mRNA using qRT-PCR revealed that oEVs protected the mRNA in a statistically significant manner in comparison to free mRNA, with a mean percentage of resistance to stress of 83.3 ± 5.5% after RNase and 86.8 ± 28.0% after SGF for mRNA loaded into oEVs in comparison to 11.9 ± 10.5% after RNase and 54.8 ± 17.5% after SGF for free mRNA (Figure 2E,F). Additional experiments with N mRNA demonstrated that the co-incubation (without engineering) of oEV and mRNA did not protect mRNA from degradation (Figure S1D), confirming the poorer efficiency of the co-incubation technique in oEV loading. The protection was conferred by loading inside oEVs because lipid membrane permeabilization with Triton X-100 reduced the resistance to RNase (Figure S1E,F). These data were also confirmed by PCR experiments showing the disappearance of the mRNA-specific band after RNase (Figure 2G) and SGF (Figure 2H) of free mRNA but not of mRNA loaded into oEVs. Taken together, these data showed that the encapsulation of mRNA into oEVs makes them resistant to degrading conditions, which normally reduce free RNA integrity.

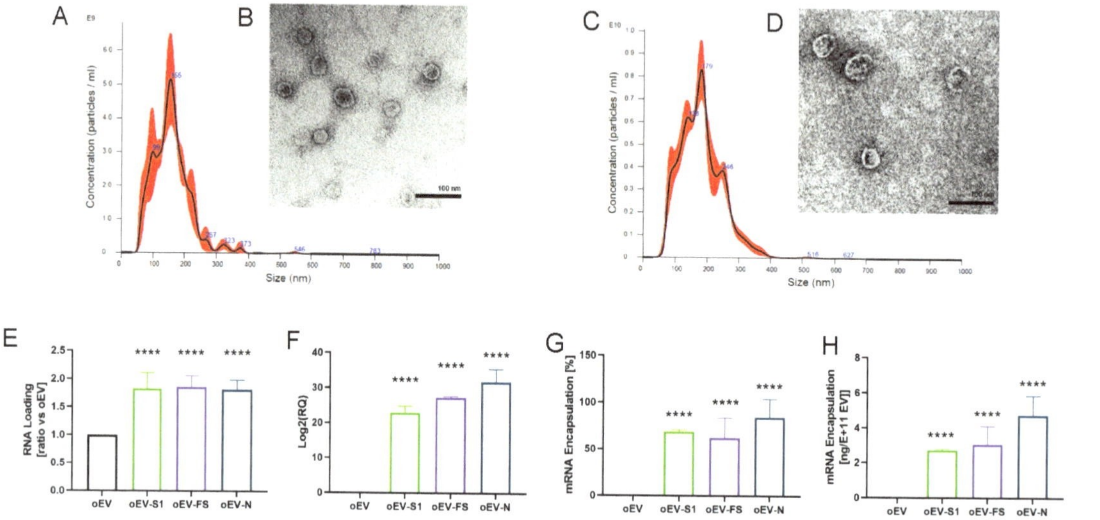

Figure 1. Delivery system characterization. (**A–D**) Representative images of oEVs and oEVs loaded with FS mRNA analyzed with nano-tracking analysis (NTA), and transmission electron microscopy (TEM). NTA of oEV (**A**) and oEV-FS (**C**) and TEM images of oEV (**B**) and oEV-FS (**D**). TEM scale bar 200 nm. (**E**) Total RNA was quantified in oEVs and oEVs loaded with S1, FS and N mRNAs (oEV-S1, oEV-FS, oEV-N) and expressed as ratio versus oEVs. (**F**) mRNA relative quantification was performed using qRT-PCR in oEVs and oEVs loaded with S1, FS and N mRNAs (oEV-S1, oEV-FS, oEV-N). (**G**) Percentage of mRNA encapsulated in oEVs following engineering with S1, FS and N mRNAs (oEV-S1, oEV-FS, oEV-N) in comparison to starting material. (**H**) Quantification of mRNA encapsulated into oEVs expressed as ng/10^{11} EV following engineering with S1, FS and N mRNAs (oEV-S1, oEV-FS, oEV-N). Data are represented as mean ± SD. **** $p < 0.001$.

3.3. *mRNA Was Delivered to Target Cells by oEVs and Translated into Protein*

The effective mRNA delivery to target cells and the translation into protein were evaluated. oEV treatment did not reduce target cells' viability, as shown in Figure S2A. oEVs engineered with all three SARS-CoV-2 mRNA were incubated with macrophages used as APC cells. After 24 h, the delivery of mRNA was analyzed using qRT-PCR technique, showing the incorporation of each specific mRNA in APC. Classical transfection with lipofectamine was used as a control (Figure 3A–C). The mRNA translation into protein was detected by cytofluorimetric analysis (Figure 3D–F) and confirmed by confocal microscopy (Figure 3G), showing the expression of N, S1 and FS proteins in APC when mRNAs were transferred by oEVs or transfected with lipofectamine as the control. Finally, the ability of oEVs to transfer a functional mRNA was confirmed by APC expression of GFP protein 24 h after incorporation of GFP mRNA containing oEVs (Figure 3H,I). Moreover, the uptake of oEVs by target cells and the subsequent GFP expression were preserved after treatment with RNase and SGF (Figure S2B,C).

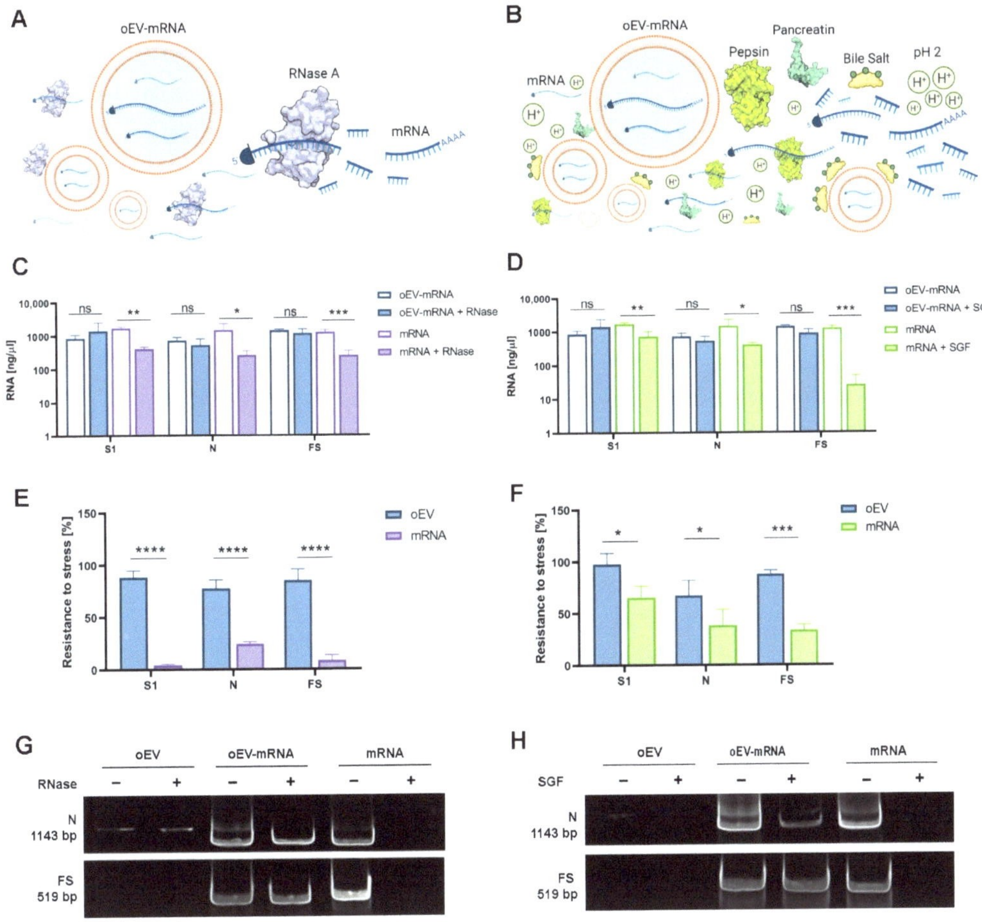

Figure 2. Evaluation of mRNA resistance to stress after loading into oEVs. Free mRNA (mRNA) or mRNA loaded into oEVs (oEV-mRNA) were subjected to two different degrading stresses: RNase A enzyme (**A**) and simulated gastric fluid (SGF) (**B**). The total RNA quantification (expressed as ng/μL) of S1, N, and FS mRNAs was measured when loaded into oEVs or not (free) and compared after treatment with RNase (**C**) or SGF (**D**). The specific resistance of each mRNA (S1, N, and FS) was quantified using qRT-PCR and expressed as the percentage of mRNA remaining after the treatment with RNase (**E**) or SGF (**F**). (**G**,**H**) Representative blots of PCR analysis for N and FS mRNAs in control oEVs (oEV), oEVs loaded with the mRNA (oEV-mRNA) and free mRNA before and after treatment with RNase (**G**) or SGF (**H**). Data are presented as mean ± SD. ns, not statistically significant. $p > 0.05$, * $p < 0.05$, ** $p < 0.01$, *** $p < 0.005$ and **** $p < 0.001$.

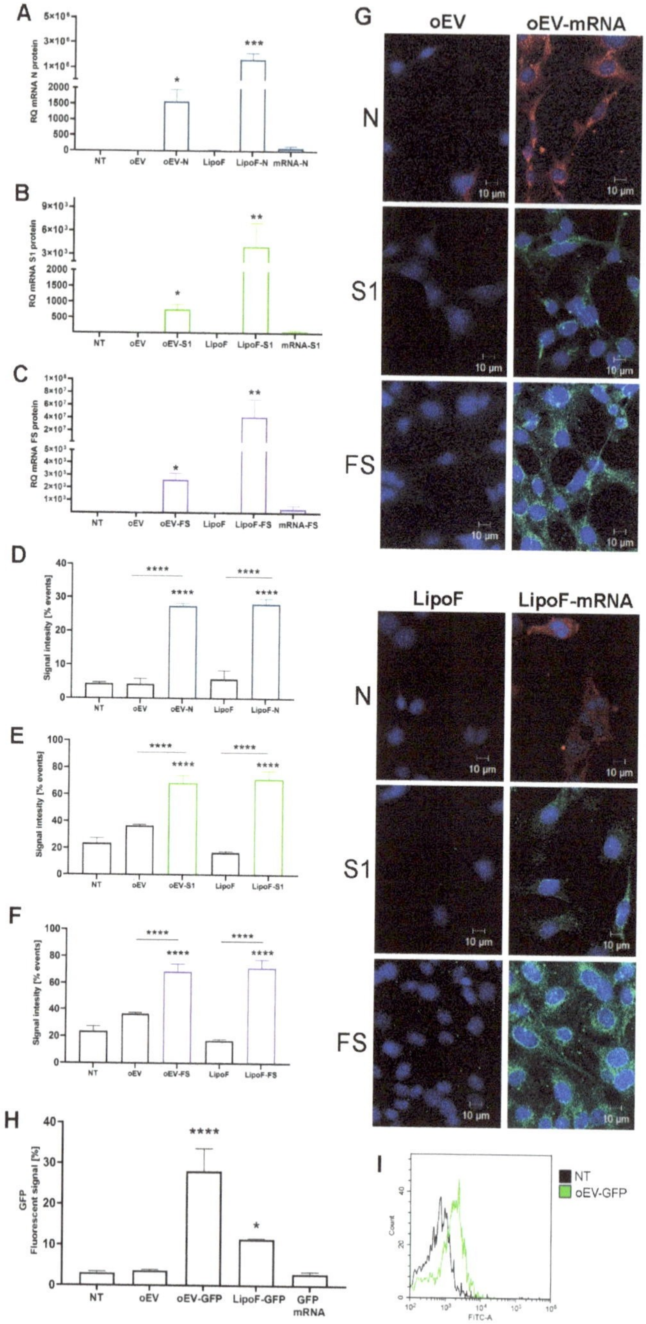

Figure 3. mRNA delivery to target cells and protein translation. Target cells were treated with oEVs loaded with N, S1 and FS mRNAs (oEV-N, oEV-S1, oEV-FS), and the mRNA uptake and translation into protein were evaluated after 24 h. (**A**–**C**) mRNA incorporation (expressed as RQ) was evaluated using

qRT-PCR in comparison to untreated cells (NT) for N (**A**), S1 (**B**) and FS (**C**) mRNA. (**D–F**) The mRNA translation was measured by cytofluorimetric analysis for specific protein N (**D**), S1 (**E**) and FS (**F**) and compared to untreated cells (NT) or specific control oEV (for oEV-mRNA) and LipoF (for LipoF-mRNA). Different controls were used: untreated cells (NT), cells treated with oEVs (oEV), cells transfected with lipofectamine (LipoF) or lipofectamine with mRNA (LipoF-mRNA), and free mRNA. (**G**) Representative images of confocal microscopy of protein translation of N, S1 and FS in target cells after treatment with oEV loaded with mRNAs (oEV-mRNA) or transfected with lipofectamine and mRNA (LipoF-mRNA). As controls, unloaded oEVs (oEV) and transfection reagents (LipoF) were used. Photos are shown as merged images, with the nucleus stained with DAPI (blue) and N protein (red) or S1 and FS proteins (green). (**H**) Target cells were treated with GFP mRNA free (GFP mRNA), transfected with lipofectamine (LipoF-GFP) or loaded into oEVs (oEV-GFP), and fluorescent signal was measured by cytofluorimetric analysis and compared to untreated cells (NT). Treatment with unloaded oEVs (oEV) was used as an additional control. (**I**) Representative histogram showing cytofluorimetric measurement of GFP signal in untreated cells (NT, black line) and cells treated with oEVs loaded with GFP mRNA (oEV-GFP, green line). Data are presented as mean ± SD. * $p < 0.05$, ** $p < 0.01$, *** $p < 0.005$, **** $p < 0.001$.

Together, these experiments demonstrated that oEVs delivered functional mRNA to target cells as it was translated into protein.

3.4. oEV-mRNA Activated Lymphocytes in an In Vitro Model

mRNA-based vaccines imply that the mRNA incorporated into APC is translated into protein and then presented to immune cells, triggering an immune response. To evaluate these steps in vitro, APC cells were co-incubated with oEV-S1, oEV-FS and oEV-N and, after 5 h, PBMC was added. Five days later, APCs were restimulated with the same treatments, and cells were analyzed at day 10 to detect lymphocyte activation, using cytofluorimetric analysis (see treatment scheme in Figure 4A). The treatment with oEVs loaded with all three mRNAs (oEV-S1, oEV-FS and oEV-N) induced a statistically significant activation of lymphocyte CD4+ in comparison to untreated cells (NT) and cells treated with control oEVs. In particular, cell activation was detected as an increase in cell proliferation by CFSE staining (Figure 4B), and a higher expression of activation markers CD25 (Figure 4C), CD69 (Figure 4D) and HLADR (Figure 4E). As positive controls, cells were stimulated with S and N proteins of SARS-CoV-2 and T-Activator CD3/CD28 beads. In conclusion, these data showed the ability of oEVs loaded with specific mRNA to activate an immune response in an in vitro model.

3.5. Mice Immunization via Different Administration Routes Induced Immune Response

To evaluate immunization in vivo, female balb/c mice were treated with oEV-S1 or empty oEV as the negative control, using intramuscular (IM), oral and intranasal (IN) administration as schematized in Figure 5A–C. IM and IN treatments were performed with a dose of 60 μg/mice and repeated after 3 weeks following the classical immunization scheme used for SARS-CoV-2 (Figure 5A,C) [29]. Since the gastrointestinal tract is highly dispersive for drugs, oral treatment was administered by gavage with a dose of 100 μg/mice, and the second administration was repeated for three consecutive days (Figure 5B). No treatments induced suffering in animals, with a weight increase similar to controls and the absence of histological alteration in tissue, suggesting a lack of toxicity (Figure S3). Moreover, the biodistribution following the oral and IN routes was assessed, confirming that oEVs targeted, respectively, the gastrointestinal and the respiratory tract (Figure S4). To assess the treatment immunogenicity, mice were sacrificed at the experiment timepoint and serum and splenocytes were collected to investigate immune stimulation.

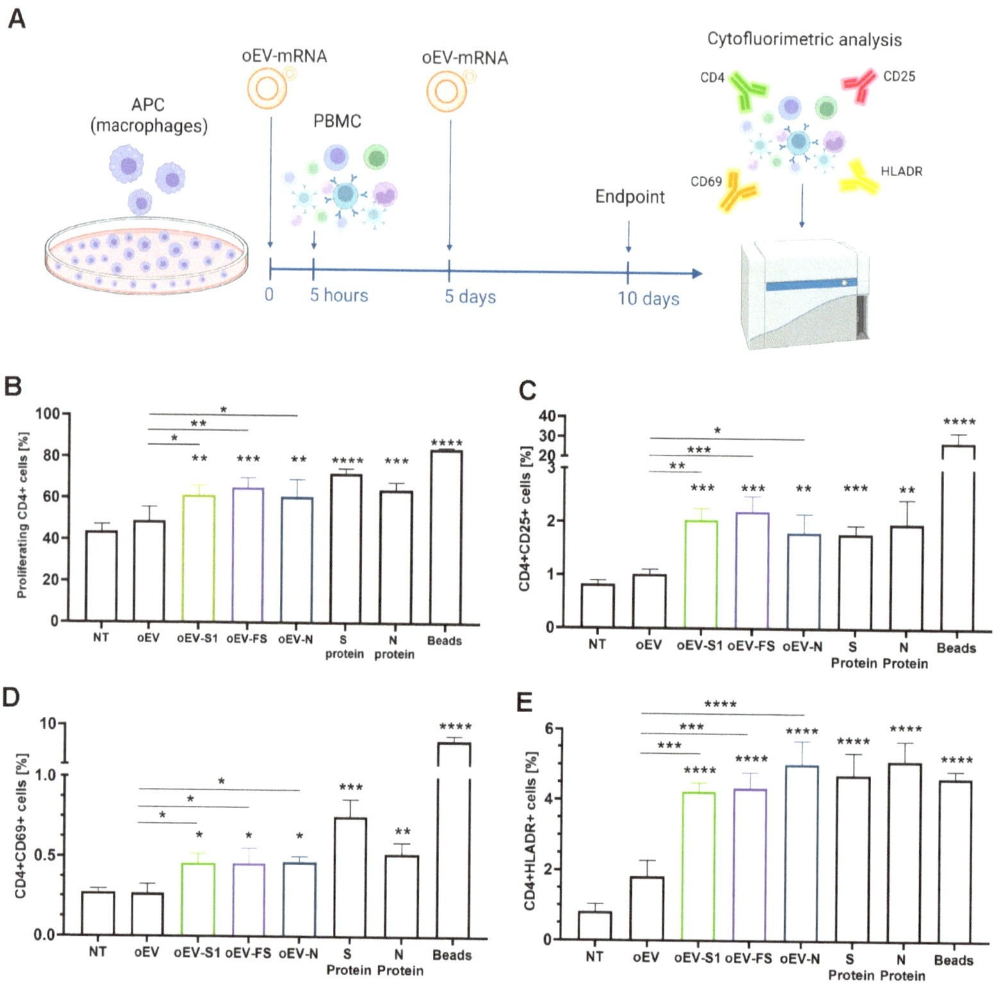

Figure 4. Evaluation of immune cell activation induced by oEV-mRNA using an in vitro model. (**A**) APC cells (macrophages) were treated with oEVs loaded with mRNA (oEV-mRNA) (S1, FS and N), co-incubated with PBMC after 5 h and re-stimulated after 5 days. At the experiment timepoint, cells were harvested and analyzed using a cytofluorimeter. As controls, cells were also untreated (NT), or treated with unloaded oEVs (oEV), S protein, N protein or T-Activator CD3/CD28 beads (Beads). (**B**) CD4+ proliferating cells were quantified as cells positive for CD4+ and CFSE staining. (**C**–**E**) Cells co-expressing CD4 and CD25 (**C**), CD69 (**D**) or HLADR (**E**) in all conditions are shown. Cell positivity is expressed as percentage of events detected. Statistical analysis was performed in comparison to NT treatment, and the oEV-mRNA effect was also compared to oEV treatment. Data are shown as mean ± SD. * $p < 0.05$, ** $p < 0.01$, *** $p < 0.005$, **** $p < 0.001$.

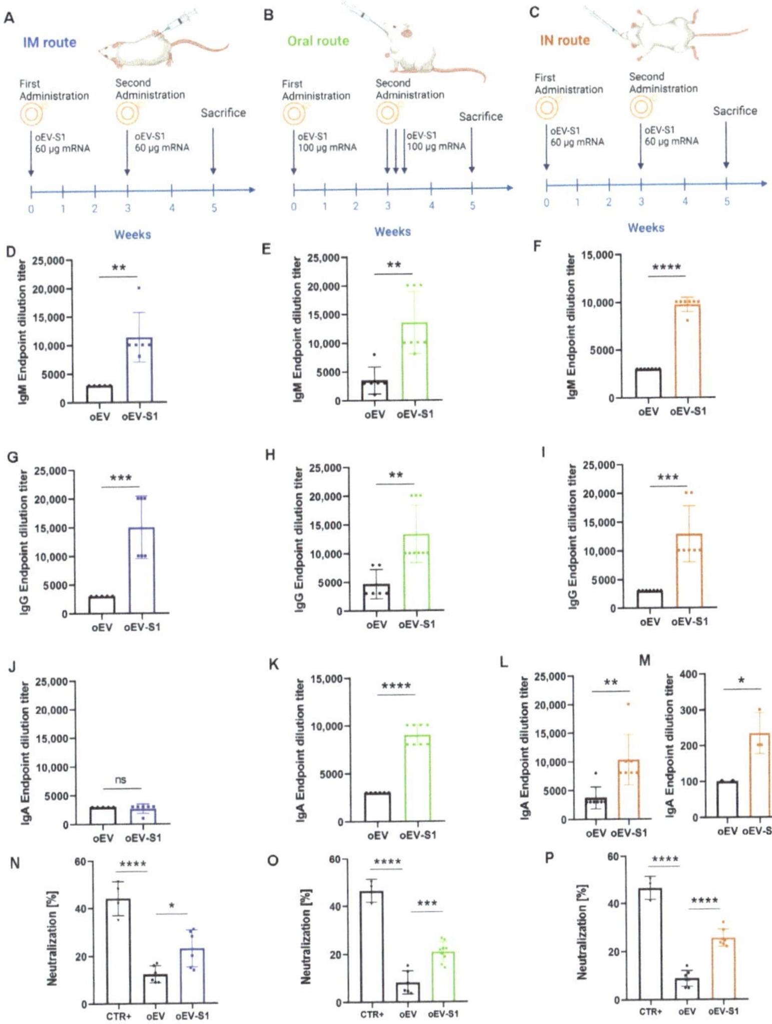

Figure 5. Mice vaccination and antibody detection. Mice were immunized with oEVs loaded with S1 mRNA (oEV-S1) or unloaded oEVs (oEV) via intramuscular (IM) (**A**), oral (**B**) and intranasal (IN) (**C**) routes. As shown, IM and IN immunization included a prime and a booster dose of 60 µg S1 mRNA, whereas oral immunization had a prime dose of 100 µg S1 mRNA and three booster doses in consecutive days. In all treatments, the two administrations were separated by three weeks and mice were sacrificed after five weeks from the first administration for subsequent analysis (see Material and Methods section). (**D–M**) S1-specific antibodies titer was measured by ELISA comparing serum of mice immunized with unloaded oEV or oEV-S1. IgM were analyzed for IM (**D**), oral (**E**) and IN (**F**) administration. IgG titer was determined in IM (**G**), oral (**H**) and IN (**I**) treatment. IgA antibodies were quantified with IM (**J**), oral (**K**) and IN (**L**) routes. (**M**) S1-specific IgA antibodies were also measured in bronchoalveolar lavage (BAL) fluid of IN administration. (**N–P**) Serum-derived neutralizing antibodies were also measured in IM (**N**), oral (**O**) and IN (**P**) administration. The percentage of neutralization induced by oEV-S1 or assay positive control (CTR+) was compared to unloaded oEVs. Data are presented as mean ± SD. ns, not statistically significant.* $p < 0.05$, ** $p < 0.01$, *** $p < 0.005$, **** $p < 0.001$.

Serum SARS-CoV-2-specific antibody titer demonstrated that all three administration routes elicited significant production of specific IgM (Figure 5D–F) and IgG antibodies (Figure 5G–I) in mice immunized with oEV-S1 with respect to mice treated with the unloaded oEVs used as the negative control. Of note, only oral and IN, but not IM, administration elicited a mucosal immune response with the formation of IgA antibodies (Figure 5J–L). For IN administration, the SARS-CoV-2-specific IgA antibody response was also measured in bronchoalveolar lavage (BAL) fluid, showing the presence of specific secretory IgA antibodies following immunization with oEV-S1 (Figure 5M). All antibody assays (IgM, IgG and IgA) were tested for specificity, and the IgG antibody assay was also analyzed for its sensitivity (Figure S5). Additional investigations revealed that serum samples contained neutralizing antibodies specific for SARS-CoV-2 following all three administration routes (Figure 5N–P).

Isolated splenocytes were stimulated with the SARS-CoV-2 S peptide ex vivo to investigate the cell-mediated immune response and verify the activation of Th1 (IFN-γ, IL-2) and Th2 (IL-10, -4). The immunization with oEV-S1 induced specific interferon γ (IFN-γ) secretion in comparison to the vehicle alone (oEV), detected using both ELISPOT assay (Figure 6A–C) and ELISA technique (Figure 6D–F). ELISA measurement of remaining cytokines demonstrated an increase in interleukin-2 (IL-2) in stimulated splenocytes collected by mice immunized with oEV-S1 with respect to oEVs (Figure 6G–I), whereas no enhancement of IL-10 was observed (Figure 6J–L) and IL-4 was not detected.

These findings indicate that vaccination with oEV-S1 using all three administration routes (IM, oral and IN) stimulated cell-mediated immune activation, which is associated with a Th1 cytokine (IL-2 and IFN-γ) rather than Th2 response (IL-10, -4).

Cytofluorimetric analysis of splenocytes upon stimulation with S peptide demonstrated a statistically significant increase in CD4+ lymphocytes following immunization with oEV-S1 in comparison to oEVs alone (Figure 7A), suggesting a specific immune cell activation. Additional investigations showed higher immune cell activation following oral and IN vaccination rather than IM administration. In fact, only mucosal routes (oral and IN), but not IM administration, were able to induce an increase in CD3+CD69+ (Figure 7B) with a higher presence of both CD3+CD4+ and CD3+CD8+ co-expressing CD69+ in mice treated with oEV-S1 in comparison to oEVs alone (Figure 7C,D). Moreover, only immunization with oral and IN routes, but not IM, significantly reduced the expression of regulatory T cell (T reg) CD3+CD25+ (Figure 7E) with a reduction in CD25+ expression in both CD3+CD4+ and CD3+CD8+ (Figure 7F,G). Notably, the presence of specific plasma cell CD138+CD45R− following treatment with oEV-S1 was also detectable after oral and IN but not after IM immunization (Figure 7H) [30]. In conclusion, these data demonstrated that all three administration routes activated a splenic immune cells response (CD4+) but only oral and intranasal immunization were able to induce a higher effect with an increase in specific plasma cells, an increase in CD69+ and reduction in CD25+ co-expression.

In order to also demonstrate in vivo the versatility of oEVs as mRNA carriers, a small number of animals were immunized with oEVs loaded with the bigger mRNA tested during in vitro coding for FS (oEV-FS) and compared to oEVs alone using all three administration routes (IM, oral, and IN). Meanwhile, oEVs efficiently delivered mRNA in vivo, inducing a humoral response with SARS-CoV-2 specific antibody and neutralizing antibodies with all three administration routes (Figure S6). Immune cell stimulation was also confirmed by the increased IFN-γ secretion from splenocytes stimulated with peptide ex vivo (Figure S7). Meanwhile, a change in IL-10 secretion was not observed with oEV-FS in comparison to oEV alone and IL-4 was undetectable, confirming the predominant activation of a Th1 rather than Th2 response (Figure S7). Finally, the splenic immune cell activation was confirmed using FS mRNA, and an increase in CD4+ cell proliferation was induced using all three administration routes (Figure S7).

Taken together, these data demonstrated that oEVs can efficiently deliver multiple SARS-CoV-2 mRNAs in vivo and immunize mice, inducing a specific humoral and cell-mediated immune response.

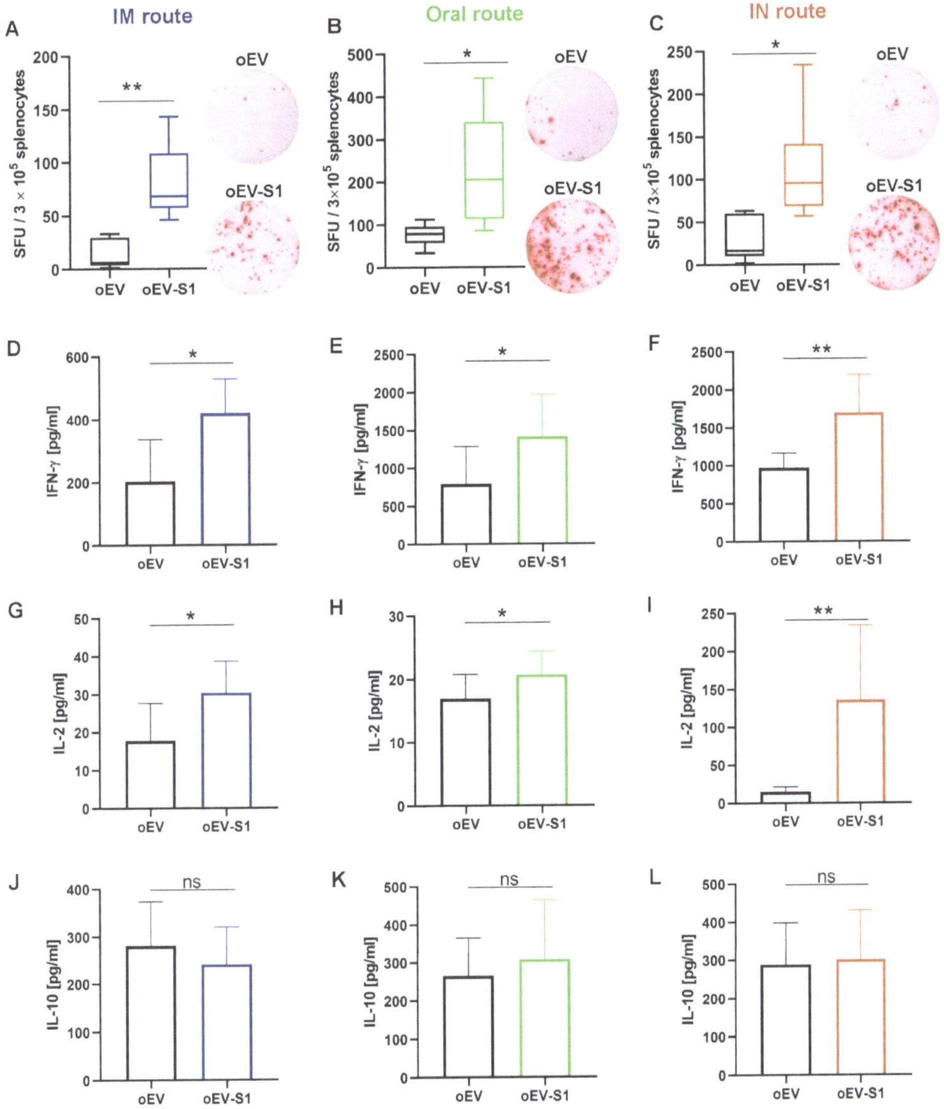

Figure 6. Cytokine secretion from splenocytes isolated from immunized mice via intramuscular (IM), oral and intranasal (IN) routes. (**A–C**) IFN-γ secretion by splenocytes was quantified upon stimulation with SARS-CoV-2 S peptide and expressed as spot-forming units (SFU) per 3×10^5 cells following IM (**A**), oral (**B**) and IN (**C**). Representative spot images for each treatment were also recorded. (**D–L**) ELISA measurement of cytokine secretion by splenocytes after 24 h of stimulation with SARS-CoV-2 S peptide for IFN-γ for IM (**D**), oral (**E**) and IN (**F**) routes; IL-2 for IM (**G**), oral (**H**) and IN (**I**) routes; and IL-10 for IM (**J**), oral (**K**) and IN (**L**) routes, expressed as pg/mL. Statistical analysis was performed comparing splenocytes collected from mice immunized with unloaded oEVs (oEV) and oEVs loaded with S1 mRNA (oEV-S1). Data are expressed as mean ± SD. ns, not statistically significant. $p > 0.05$, * $p < 0.05$, ** $p < 0.01$.

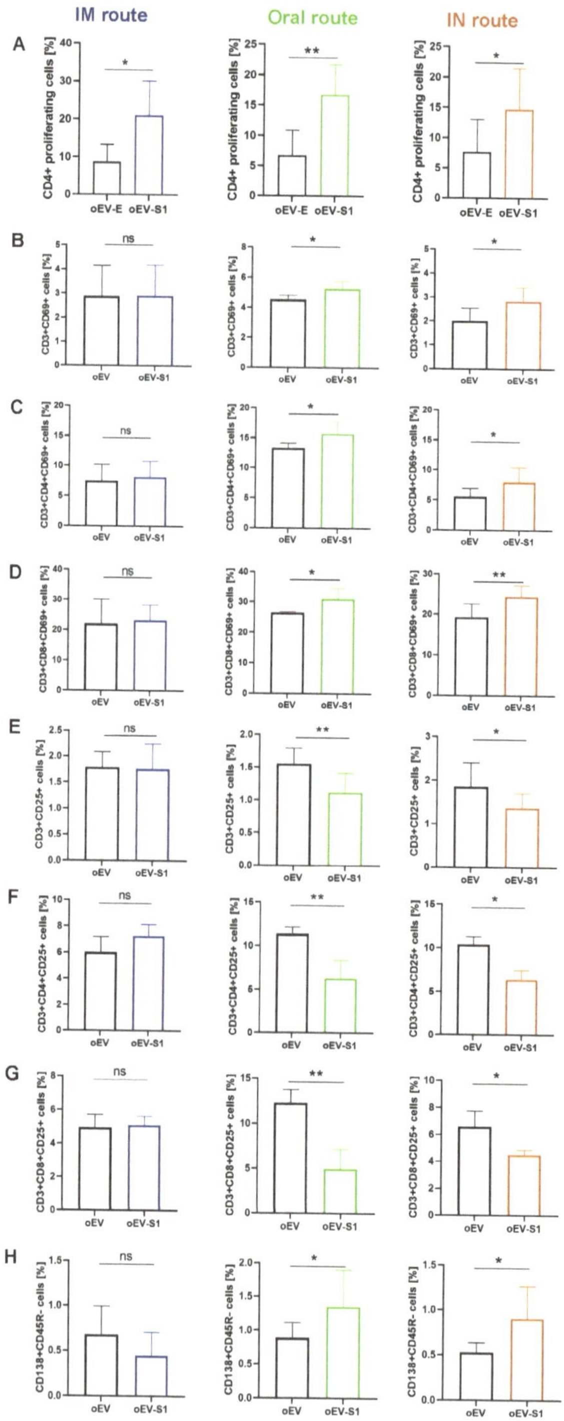

Figure 7. Immune cell activation following peptide stimulation ex vivo. Splenocytes isolated from immunized mice with unloaded oEVs (oEV) or oEVs loaded with S1 mRNA (oEV-S1) were stimulated

with SARS-CoV-2 S peptide and their marker expression was analyzed by cytofluorimetric analysis for all three administration routes (IM, oral and IN). (**A**) CD4+ proliferating cells were quantified as cells positive for CD4+ and CFSE staining. Percentage of cells CD3+CD69+ (**B**), CD3+CD4+ co-expressing CD69+ (**C**), CD3+CD8+ co-expressing CD69+ (**D**), CD3+CD25+ (**E**), CD3+CD4+ co-expressing CD25+ (**F**), CD3+CD8+ co-expressing CD25+ (**G**) and CD138+CD45R− (**H**) are shown. Cell positivity is expressed as percentage of events detected. Statistical analysis compared splenocytes collected from mice immunized with unloaded oEVs (oEV) and oEVs loaded with S1 mRNA (oEV-S1). Data are expressed as mean ± SD. ns, not statistically significant. $p > 0.05$, * $p < 0.05$, ** $p < 0.01$.

4. Discussion

In the present study, we provide a proof of concept that plant-derived EVs may represent a versatile platform for mRNA-based vaccines. Plant-derived EVs are an extractive natural product that may have several advantages with respect to synthetic nanoparticles [31]. The natural membrane envelope facilitates their uptake from target cells, they are not cytotoxic and they protect nucleic acids from enzyme degradation and environmental stress conditions [20–25]. Here, we used EVs purified from orange (*Citrus sinensis*) juice, which were expected to lack toxicity and immunogenicity due to their edible source and oral-induced tolerance. Being a natural product, plant EVs can be purified using a simple extraction process that does not require expensive cell culture conditions, and their ability to transfer a great number of biomolecules makes them a good candidate for drug delivery [19–24]. As a prototype of an mRNA-based vaccine, to evaluate the efficacy of oEVs as a carrier, we selected mRNA coding for SARS-CoV-2 antigens.

In the present study, we demonstrated that oEVs can be efficiently loaded with different mRNA molecules with sizes ranging from 670 to 3820 nt, with a similar encapsulation efficiency and without altering oEVs' integrity. Previous studies on mammalian EVs have shown that membrane vesicles confer stability to nucleic acid from degradation and from low and high pH conditions [32–34]. Here, we demonstrated that mRNA carried by engineered oEVs was highly protected from degradation induced by treatment with RNase enzyme and simulated gastric fluid (SGF) in vitro. Importantly, mRNA conveyed by oEVs was efficiently delivered to target cells and translated into protein. In the target cell, the protein was functional and was able to be presented by APC cells and stimulate a lymphocyte response, detected as the increase in CD4+ proliferating cells and of CD69+, CD25+ and HLADR+ activated cells (Figure 4) [35,36]. These findings suggested the possible efficacy of oEVs as a carrier for mRNA-based vaccines and prompted us to test their effect in mice.

In the vaccine field, the interest in EV-mediated antigen delivery is growing based on the observation that mammalian cells infected with viral pathogens release EVs containing viral constituents able to trigger an immune response [37]. Moreover, EVs carrying S protein have been detected in infected patients, and their potential role in inducing a humoral specific immune response has been suggested [38,39]. Interestingly, compared to soluble antigens, EV-associated antigens were shown to elicit a stronger cytotoxic CD8+ T response [18]. Mammalian cells engineered to express a S and N protein in EVs were shown to efficiently immunize mice after IM injections [16].

Here, we selected the well-studied mRNA coding for subunit S1 of SARS-CoV-2 and demonstrated that IM injection in mice elicited a humoral immune response with the production of specific IgM and IgG against S1 protein, the induction of neutralizing antibodies and a T cell immune response. Splenocytes stimulated with the S peptide exhibited a significant increase in CD4+ proliferating cells upon immunization with oEV-S1 with respect to oEV alone, suggesting that the oEV formulation enables general CD4+ cell activation. The same effect on the increase in CD4+ was also observed in other studies, for instance, Perex et al. [39] when using IN administration of a modified vaccinia virus Ankara (MVA)-based vaccine, and Corbett et al. [29] via IM immunization with mRNA-1273.

In this study, immunization with oEV-S1 stimulated a cell-mediated immune response associated with a Th1 cytokine (IFN-γ, IL-2) rather than a Th2 response (IL-10, IL-4). In fact, we observed an increase in the secretion of IFN-γ and IL-2 from splenocytes stimulated with the S peptide, whereas no difference was detected for IL-10 and IL-4. These data are in accordance with other studies demonstrating the major activation of a Th1 response following vaccination with mRNA coding for the SARS-CoV-2 antigen. Corbett et al. [29] reported that mice vaccinated with mRNA-1273 elicited a predominant Th1 response, detected as production of cytokines IFN-γ, TNF and IL-2 by total CD4 T cells under ex vivo stimulation with SARS-CoV-2 peptide pools. In a study by Zhang et al. [39], the authors showed that splenocytes isolated from mice immunized with SARS-CoV-2 RBD and in vitro re-stimulated with peptide pools covering the SARS-CoV-2 RBD induced a Th1-biased response with a significant increase in IFN-γ and IL-2 secretion, but no differences for Th2 response (IL-6, IL-4) were observed [40]. Moreover, cytokine polarization analysis performed by Sahin et al. [41] on PBMC collected by patients vaccinated with BNT162b1 showed secretion of IFN-γ and IL-2 but most individuals failed to secrete IL-4 [41]. IL-10, instead, was associated with Th2 response in SARS patients [42] and with Th2 response upon vaccination [43].

Since more than 90% of the immune system is located in the gastroenteric tract, we also vaccinated mice via the oral route. Oral immunization induced an effective humoral and cellular immune response, similar to IM administration, indicating efficient protection of mRNA carried by oEVs from gastric degradation in vivo. Indeed, plant EVs are good candidates for oral drug delivery due to their resistance to acidic and basic conditions and to efficient intestinal absorption [7,44,45].

Besides the oral route, another suitable site of administration is represented by the intranasal tract with the presence of many immune cell components able to trigger an immune response, such as macrophages and T- and B-lymphocytes [46]. Here, we observed that an intranasal administration of oEV formulation with S1 mRNA was able to trigger a humoral and cellular immune response similar to oral immunization. The intranasal route for EV-based vaccine was confirmed by a previous report using Salmonella typhimurium EV decorated with the Spike receptor-binding domain derived from mammalian cell culture. In this model, intranasal immunization of the golden Syrian hamster resulted in a high level of serum anti-Spike receptor-binding domain IgG as well as a mucosal response [17]. Wang et al. [47] showed that human lung-derived EVs conjugated with recombinant SARS-CoV-2 receptor-binding domain efficiently immunized mice and reduced inflammation after a challenge with live SARS-CoV-2 in hamsters.

Of interest, both the oral and the intranasal vaccination not only stimulated the specific IgM and IgG antibody production but also the induction of a specific secretory IgA response, a critical component in the mucosal first barrier adaptive immune response [48]. This finding is consistent with the observation that strategies based on mucosal vaccination stimulate IgA secretion in the mucosa [49]. Hassan and colleagues previously showed that an intranasal dose of a chimpanzee adenovirus-vectored vaccine encoding a prefusion stabilized spike protein (ChAd-SARS-CoV-2-S) promoted systemic and mucosal IgA in mice and macaques [50–52]. The study of Popowski et al. [53] reported the vaccination by direct inhalation using nebulization of lyophilized EVs derived from lung or from conditioned medium of HEK 293T cell line previously engineered with the S protein mRNA via electroporation. When compared with liposomes, mRNA-loaded EVs elicited significantly higher production of specific IgG and secretory IgA antibodies, suggesting that EVs are superior to synthetic liposomes as carriers of mRNA-based vaccines [53]. As expected, the biodistribution of oEVs revealed different accumulations when using the intranasal or oral route, showing efficient mRNA delivery and mice immunization in both administration protocols.

Although this did not apply to the intramuscular route, oral and intranasal immunization were shown to also induce increased cell-mediated immune activation. These data are consistent with a previous observation that mucosal vaccine administration can provide not only local but also systemic protection [49,54]. In this study, marker expression of peptide-stimulated splenocytes revealed that oral and IN immunization with oEV-S1 induced an increase in the lymphocyte activation marker CD69+ in comparison with oEV vaccination.

We observed an increase in CD69+ expression on both total CD3+ and CD3+CD4+ and CD3+CD8+. This finding was supported by previous studies that reported the induction of CD8+CD69+ [55] and CD4+CD69+ [56] following vaccination against SARS-CoV-2 [57]. Here, oEV-S1 treatment via the oral and IN routes induced a significant reduction in CD3+, CD3+CD4+, and CD3+CD8+ co-expressing CD25+, a typical marker of regulatory T cell (T reg). CD25 (or the IL-2 receptor α-chain) is considered a key regulator of immune response since its high affinity to IL-2 induces IL-2 deprivation, promoting an important immunosuppressive activity that prevents harmful effects due to immune system hyperstimulation [58]. The inhibitory effects of Tregs on immune response induced post-vaccination have been experimentally demonstrated in different mice models of Treg depletion [58]. T reg depletion was proven to increase vaccine-derived protection in an influenza virus infection model [59] and induced a more durable antibody response to mRNA-COVID-19 vaccination in patients with plasma cell dyscrasia [60]. In this study, mice immunized with oEV-S1 via mucosal routes (oral and IN) also exhibited an increased number of splenic plasma cells in comparison to mice treated with oEV vehicle alone. A similar result was also reported by Gao et al. [61] as an increase in the ratio of CD19−CD138+ plasma cells in total lymphocytes derived from the spleen of mice immunized with RBD9.1 peptide.

Finally, the versatility of oEVs to deliver different immunizing mRNAs was demonstrated using oEVs loaded with FS mRNA in a small number of animals, showing a similar immune response to vaccination with oEV-S1 using all three administration routes (IM, oral, and IN).

5. Conclusions

In conclusion, we successfully demonstrated that EVs derived from edible plants can serve as a carrier for the therapeutic exploitation of nucleic acids. In fact, they confer protection from degradation and allow for efficient delivery to mammalian cells in vitro and in vivo. They may be suitable for the delivery not only of mRNA but also of other nucleic acid molecules, such as siRNA, miRNA, and DNA. In the present study, we demonstrated that mRNA from a viral protein can be loaded in orange-derived EVs, eliciting an immune response with antibody production and immune cell activation. We tested SARS-CoV-2 mRNAs as a proof of concept, but the cargo can be adjusted for targeting different pathogens, paving the way to several applications in the vaccine field. Among administration routes, oral and intranasal represent several advantages as needle-free techniques and were demonstrated to be superior to the IM route, also conferring IgA mucosal protection and increased splenic cell activation. Therefore, edible plant EVs may represent a platform for the delivery of different therapeutic molecules, especially for mucosal absorption.

Supplementary Materials: The following supporting information can be downloaded at: https://www.mdpi.com/article/10.3390/pharmaceutics15030974/s1, Figure S1: oEV loading with an increasing amount of mRNA; Figure S2: Cytotoxicity and uptake of oEV and oEV-GFP in target cells; Figure S3: Mice weight during vaccine treatment via multiple administration routes; Figure S4: Biodistribution of oral and IN administration in vivo; Figure S5: ELISA specificity and sensibility for antibody titer measurement; Figure S6: Antibody production following mice immunization with oEV-FS; Figure S7: Splenic cell activation upon vaccination with oEV-FS; Table S1: Primer sequences used for qRT-PCR and PCR experiments.

Author Contributions: Conceptualization, G.C. and F.G.D.R.; Methodology, M.A.C.P. and C.G. (Chiara Gai); Investigation and Data Curation, M.A.C.P., C.G. (Chiara Gai), F.N., L.M., M.C.D. and C.G. (Cristina Grange); Formal Analysis, M.A.C.P. and C.G. (Chiara Gai); Writing—Original Draft Preparation, M.A.C.P., C.G. (Chiara Gai) and F.N.; Writing—Review and Editing, G.C., C.G. (Cristina Grange) and M.C.D.; Supervision, G.C. and F.G.D.R. All authors have read and agreed to the published version of the manuscript.

Funding: This study was funded by EvoBiotech s.r.l.

Institutional Review Board Statement: The animal study protocol was approved by the Institutional Review Board (or Ethics Committee) of Università degli Studi di Torino (protocol code CC652.163, 12 July 2021).

Informed Consent Statement: Not applicable.

Data Availability Statement: Data are contained within the article.

Acknowledgments: The authors would like to thank Alessandro Scagliotti and Paola Cappello for Elispot acquisition and Federica Antico for technical assistance in tissue histology preparation. Some graphics were created with BioRender.com.

Conflicts of Interest: G.C. currently serves on the Board of Directors, and M.C.D. currently serves as Scientific Advisor at EvoBiotech s.r.l. C.G. (Chiara Gai), F.N., L.M. and M.P. are employees of EvoBiotech s.r.l. C.G. (Chiara Gai), F.G.D.R., G.C., M.C.D. and M.P. are inventors on International Patent Application no. WO/2022/152771A1 entitled "Composition comprising engineered plant-derived extracellular vesicles and use thereof as a vaccine".

References

1. Ratajczak, J.; Wysoczynski, M.; Hayek, F.; Janowska-Wieczorek, A.; Ratajczak, M.Z. Membrane-derived microvesicles: Important and underappreciated mediators of cell-to-cell communication. *Leukemia* **2006**, *20*, 1487–1495. [CrossRef] [PubMed]
2. Raposo, G.; Stoorvogel, W. Extracellular vesicles: Exosomes, microvesicles, and friends. *J. Cell Biol.* **2013**, *200*, 373–383. [CrossRef] [PubMed]
3. Cui, Y.; Gao, J.; He, Y.; Jiang, L. Plant extracellular vesicles. *Protoplasma* **2020**, *257*, 3–12. [CrossRef]
4. Camussi, G.; Deregibus, M.C.; Bruno, S.; Cantaluppi, V.; Biancone, L. Exosomes/microvesicles as a mechanism of cell-to-cell communication. *Kidney Int.* **2010**, *78*, 838–848. [CrossRef] [PubMed]
5. Ratajczak, J.; Miekus, K.; Kucia, M.; Zhang, J.; Reca, R.; Dvorak, P.; Ratajczak, M.Z. Embryonic stem cell-derived microvesicles reprogram hematopoietic progenitors: Evidence for horizontal transfer of mRNA and protein delivery. *Leukemia* **2006**, *20*, 847–885. [CrossRef]
6. Deregibus, M.C.; Cantaluppi, V.; Calogero, R.; Lo Iacono, M.; Tetta, C.; Biancone, L.; Bruno, S.; Bussolati, B.; Camussi, G. Endothelial progenitor cell derived microvesicles activate an angiogenic program in endothelial cells by a horizontal transfer of mRNA. *Blood* **2007**, *110*, 2440–2448. [CrossRef] [PubMed]
7. Aliotta, J.M.; Pereira, M.; Johnson, K.W.; de Paz, N.; Dooner, M.S.; Puente, N.; Ayala, C.; Brilliant, K.; Berz, D.; Lee, D.; et al. Microvesicle entry into marrow cells mediates tissue-specific changes in mRNA by direct delivery of mRNA and induction of transcription. *Exp. Hematol.* **2010**, *38*, 233–245. [CrossRef]
8. Valadi, H.; Ekström, K.; Bossios, A.; Sjöstrand, M.; Lee, J.J.; Lötvall, J.O. Exosome-mediated transfer of mRNAs and microRNAs is a novel mechanism of genetic exchange between cells. *Nat. Cell Biol.* **2007**, *9*, 654–659. [CrossRef]
9. Skog, J.; Würdinger, T.; van Rijn, S.; Meijer, D.H.; Gainche, L.; Sena-Esteves, M.; Curry, W.T.; Carter, B.S.; Krichevsky, A.M.; Breakefield, X.O.; et al. Glioblastoma microvesicles transport RNA and proteins that promote tumour growth and provide diagnostic biomarkers. *Nat. Cell Biol.* **2008**, *10*, 1470–1476. [CrossRef]
10. Quesenberry, P.J.; Aliotta, J.; Deregibus, M.C.; Camussi, G. Role of extracellular RNA-carrying vesicles in cell differentiation and reprogramming. *Stem Cell Res. Ther.* **2015**, *6*, 153. [CrossRef]
11. Gould, S.J.; Raposo, G. As we wait: Coping with an imperfect nomenclature for extracellular vesicles. *J. Extracell. Vesicles* **2013**, *2*, 20389. [CrossRef] [PubMed]
12. Schulz-Siegmund, M.; Aigner, A. Nucleic acid delivery with extracellular vesicles. *Adv. Drug Deliv. Rev.* **2021**, *173*, 89–111. [CrossRef] [PubMed]
13. György, B.; Szabó, T.G.; Pásztói, M.; Pál, Z.; Misják, P.; Aradi, B.; László, V.; Pállinger, E.; Pap, E.; Kittel, A.; et al. Membrane vesicles, current state-of-the-art: Emerging role of extracellular vesicles. *Cell Mol. Life Sci.* **2011**, *68*, 2667–2688. [CrossRef] [PubMed]
14. Desplantes, R.; Lévêque, C.; Muller, B.; Lotierzo, M.; Ferracci, G.; Popoff, M.; Seagar, M.; Mamoun, R.; El Far, O. Affinity biosensors using recombinant native membrane proteins displayed on exosomes: Application to botulinum neurotoxin B receptor. *Sci. Rep.* **2017**, *7*, 1032. [CrossRef]
15. Yoo, K.H.; Thapa, N.; Kim, B.J.; Lee, J.O.; Jang, Y.N.; Chwae, Y.J.; Kim, J. Possibility of exosome based coronavirus disease 2019 vaccine (Review). *Mol. Med. Rep.* **2022**, *25*, 26. [CrossRef]
16. Tsai, S.J.; Atai, N.A.; Cacciottolo, M.; Nice, J.; Salehi, A.; Guo, C.; Sedgwick, A.; Kanagavelu, S.; Gould, S.J. Exosome-mediated mRNA delivery in vivo is safe and can be used to induce SARS-CoV-2 immunity. *J. Biol. Chem.* **2021**, *297*, 101266. [CrossRef]
17. Jiang, L.; Driedonks, T.A.P.; Jong, W.S.P.; Dhakal, S.; Bart van den Berg van Saparoea, H.; Sitaras, I.; Zhou, R.; Caputo, C.; Littlefield, K.; Lowman, M.; et al. A bacterial extracellular vesicle-based intranasal vaccine against SARS-CoV-2 protects against disease and elicits neutralizing antibodies to wild-type and Delta variants. *J. Extracell. Vesicle* **2022**, *11*, e12192. [CrossRef]

18. Ferrantelli, F.; Chiozzini, C.; Manfredi, F.; Leone, P.; Spada, M.; Di Virgilio, A.; Giovannelli, A.; Sanchez, M.; Cara, A.; Michelini, Z.; et al. Strong SARS-CoV-2 N-Specific CD8+ T Immunity Induced by Engineered Extracellular Vesicles Associates with Protection from Lethal Infection in Mice. *Viruses* **2022**, *14*, 329. [CrossRef]
19. Xu, M.; Yang, Q.; Sun, X.; Wang, Y. Recent Advancements in the Loading and Modification of Therapeutic Exosomes. *Front. Bioeng. Biotechnol.* **2020**, *8*, 586130. [CrossRef]
20. Feng, J.; Xiu, Q.; Huang, Y.; Troyer, Z.; Li, B.; Zheng, L. Plant Derived Vesicle-Like Nanoparticles as Promising Biotherapeutic Tools: Present and Future. *Adv. Mater.* **2023**, e2207826. [CrossRef]
21. Jain, N.; Pandey, M.; Sharma, P.; Gupta, G.; Gorain, B.; Dua, K. Recent developments in plant-derived edible nanoparticles as therapeutic nanomedicines. *J. Food Biochem.* **2022**, *46*, e14479. [CrossRef]
22. Bonifacio, B.V.; Silva, P.B.; Ramos, M.A.; Negri, K.M.; Bauab, T.M.; Chorilli, M. Nanotechnology-based drug delivery systems and herbal medicines: A review. *Int. J. Nanomed.* **2014**, *9*, 1–15.
23. Rome, S. Biological properties of plant-derived extracellular vesicles. *Food Funct.* **2019**, *10*, 529–538. [CrossRef] [PubMed]
24. Yang, C.; Zhang, M.; Merlin, D. Advances in plant-derived edible nanoparticle-based lipid nano-drug delivery systems as therapeutic nanomedicines. *J. Mater. Chem. B* **2018**, *6*, 1312–1321. [CrossRef] [PubMed]
25. Pomatto, M.; Gai, C.; Negro, F.; Cedrino, M.; Grange, C.; Ceccotti, E.; Togliatto, G.; Collino, F.; Tapparo, M.; Figliolini, F.; et al. Differential Therapeutic Effect of Extracellular Vesicles Derived by Bone Marrow and Adipose Mesenchymal Stem Cells on Wound Healing of Diabetic Ulcers and Correlation to Their Cargoes. *Int. J. Mol. Sci.* **2021**, *22*, 3851. [CrossRef]
26. Grange, C.; Tapparo, M.; Bruno, S.; Chatterjee, D.; Quesenberry, P.J.; Tetta, C.; Camussi, G. Biodistribution of mesenchymal stem cell-derived extracellular vesicles in a model of acute kidney injury monitored by optical imaging. *Int. J. Mol. Med.* **2014**, *33*, 1055–1063. [CrossRef]
27. Pomatto, M.A.C.; Bussolati, B.; D'Antico, S.; Ghiotto, S.; Tetta, C.; Brizzi, M.F.; Camussi, G. Improved Loading of Plasma-Derived Extracellular Vesicles to Encapsulate Antitumor miRNAs. *Mol. Ther. Methods Clin. Dev.* **2019**, *13*, 133–144. [CrossRef]
28. Zhuang, X.; Deng, Z.B.; Mu, J.; Zhang, L.; Yan, J.; Miller, D.; Feng, W.; McClain, C.J.; Zhang, H.G. Ginger-derived nanoparticles protect against alcohol-induced liver damage. *J. Extracell. Vesicles* **2015**, *4*, 28713. [CrossRef]
29. Corbett, K.S.; Edwards, D.K.; Leist, S.R.; Abiona, O.M.; Boyoglu-Barnum, S.; Gillespie, R.A.; Himansu, S.; Schäfer, A.; Ziwawo, C.T.; DiPiazza, A.T.; et al. SARS-CoV-2 mRNA vaccine design enabled by prototype pathogen preparedness. *Nature* **2020**, *586*, 567–571. [CrossRef]
30. Reddy, S.T.; Ge, X.; Miklos, A.E.; Hughes, R.A.; Kang, S.H.; Hoi, K.H.; Chrysostomou, C.; Hunicke-Smith, S.P.; Iverson, B.L.; Tucker, P.W.; et al. Monoclonal antibodies isolated without screening by analyzing the variable-gene repertoire of plasma cells. *Nat. Biotechnol.* **2010**, *28*, 965–969. [CrossRef]
31. Di Gioia, S.; Hossain, M.N.; Conese, M. Biological properties and therapeutic effects of plant-derived nanovesicles. *Open Med. (Wars)* **2020**, *15*, 1096–1122. [CrossRef] [PubMed]
32. Tetta, C.; Ghigo, E.; Silengo, L.; Deregibus, M.C.; Camussi, G. Extracellular vesicles as an emerging mechanism of cell-to-cell communication. *Endocrine* **2013**, *44*, 11–19. [CrossRef]
33. O'Brien, K.; Breyne, K.; Ughetto, S.; Laurent, L.C.; Breakefield, X.O. RNA delivery by extracellular vesicles in mammalian cells and its applications. *Nat. Rev. Mol. Cell Biol.* **2020**, *21*, 585–606. [CrossRef] [PubMed]
34. Furue, M.; Katz, S.I. Molecules on activated human T-cells. *Am. J. Dermatopathol.* **1988**, *10*, 349–355. [CrossRef]
35. Sala, P.; Tonutti, E. Monitoring clonal expansion in the laboratory. *Clin. Exp. Rheumatol.* **1996**, *14*, S31–S35. [PubMed]
36. Moulin, C.; Crupi, M.J.F.; Ilkow, C.S.; Bell, J.C.; Boulton, S. Extracellular Vesicles and Viruses: Two Intertwined Entities. *Int. J. Mol. Sci.* **2023**, *24*, 1036. [CrossRef]
37. Tertel, T.; Tomić, S.; Đokić, J.; Radojević, D.; Stevanović, D.; Ilić, N.; Giebel, B.; Kosanović, M. Serum-derived extracellular vesicles: Novel biomarkers reflecting the disease severity of COVID-19 patients. *J. Extracell. Vesicles* **2022**, *11*, e12257. [CrossRef]
38. Motallebnezhad, M.; Omraninava, M.; Esmaeili Gouvarchin Ghaleh, H.; Jonaidi-Jafari, N.; Hazrati, A.; Malekpour, K.; Bagheri, Y.; Izadi, M.; Ahmadi, M. Potential therapeutic applications of extracellular vesicles in the immunopathogenesis of COVID-19. *Pathol. Res. Pract.* **2023**, *241*, 154280. [CrossRef]
39. Pérez, P.; Astorgano, D.; Albericio, G.; Flores, S.; Sánchez-Cordón, P.J.; Luczkowiak, J.; Delgado, R.; Casasnovas, J.M.; Esteban, M.; García-Arriaza, J. Intranasal administration of a single dose of MVA-based vaccine candidates against COVID-19 induced local and systemic immune responses and protects mice from a lethal SARS-CoV-2 infection. *Front. Immunol.* **2022**, *13*, 995235. [CrossRef] [PubMed]
40. Zhang, N.N.; Li, X.F.; Deng, Y.Q.; Zhao, H.; Huang, Y.J.; Yang, G.; Huang, W.J.; Gao, P.; Zhou, C.; Zhang, R.R.; et al. A Thermostable MRNA Vaccine against COVID-19. *Cell* **2020**, *182*, 1271–1283. [CrossRef]
41. Sahin, U.; Muik, A.; Derhovanessian, E.; Vogler, I.; Kranz, L.M.; Vormehr, M.; Baum, A.; Pascal, K.; Quandt, J.; Maurus, D.; et al. COVID-19 vaccine BNT162b1 elicits human antibody and TH1 T-cell responses. *Nature* **2020**, *586*, 594–599. [CrossRef] [PubMed]
42. Zhu, M. SARS Immunity and Vaccination. *Cell. Mol. Immunol.* **2004**, *1*, 193–198. [PubMed]
43. Daly, L.M.; Johnson, P.A.; Donnelly, G.; Nicolson, C.; Robertson, J.; Mills, K.H. Innate IL-10 promotes the induction of Th2 responses with plasmid DNA expressing HIV gp120. *Vaccine* **2005**, *23*, 963–974. [CrossRef]
44. Wang, B.; Zhuang, X.; Deng, Z.B.; Jiang, H.; Mu, J.; Wang, Q.; Xiang, X.; Guo, H.; Zhang, L.; Dryden, G.; et al. Targeted drug delivery to intestinal macrophages by bioactive nanovesicles released from grapefruit. *Mol. Ther.* **2014**, *22*, 522–534. [CrossRef] [PubMed]

45. Deng, Z.; Rong, Y.; Teng, Y.; Mu, J.; Zhuang, X.; Tseng, M.; Samykutty, A.; Zhang, L.; Yan, J.; Miller, D.; et al. Broccoli-derived nanoparticle inhibits mouse colitis by activating dendritic cell AMP-activated protein kinase. *Mol. Ther.* **2017**, *25*, 1641–1654. [CrossRef]
46. Lamichhane, A.; Azegami, T.; Kiyono, H. The mucosal immune system for vaccine development. *Vaccine* **2014**, *49*, 6711–6723. [CrossRef] [PubMed]
47. Wang, Z.; Popowski, K.D.; Zhu, D.; de Juan Abad, B.L.; Wang, X.; Liu, M.; Lutz, H.; De Naeyer, N.; DeMarco, C.T.; Denny, T.N.; et al. Exosomes decorated with a recombinant SARS-CoV-2 receptor-binding domain as an inhalable COVID-19 vaccine. *Nat. Biomed. Eng.* **2022**, *6*, 791–805. [CrossRef]
48. Neutra, M.R.; Kozlowski, P.A. Mucosal vaccines: The promise and the challenge. *Nat. Rev. Immunol.* **2006**, *6*, 148–158. [CrossRef]
49. Rudin, A.; Riise, G.C.; Holmgren, J. Antibody responses in the lower respiratory tract and male urogenital tract in humans after nasal and oral vaccination with cholera toxin B subunit. *Infect. Immun.* **1999**, *6*, 2884–2890. [CrossRef]
50. Hassan, A.O.; Kafai, N.M.; Dmitriev, I.P.; Fox, J.M.; Smith, B.K.; Harvey, I.B.; Chen, R.E.; Winkler, E.S.; Wessel, A.W.; Case, J.B.; et al. A Single-Dose Intranasal ChAd Vaccine Protects Upper and Lower Respiratory Tracts against SARS-CoV-2. *Cell* **2020**, *183*, 169–184. [CrossRef]
51. Hassan, A.O.; Shrihari, S.; Gorman, M.J.; Ying, B.; Yuan, D.; Raju, S.; Chen, R.E.; Dmitriev, I.P.; Kashentseva, E.; Adams, L.J.; et al. An intranasal vaccine durably protects against SARS-CoV-2 variants in mice. *Cell Rep.* **2021**, *36*, 109452. [CrossRef] [PubMed]
52. Hassan, A.O.; Feldmann, F.; Zhao, H.; Curiel, D.T.; Okumura, A.; Tang-Huau, T.L.; Case, J.B.; Meade-White, K.; Callison, J.; Chen, R.E.; et al. A single intranasal dose of chimpanzee adenovirus-vectored vaccine protects against SARS-CoV-2 infection in rhesus macaques. *Cell Rep. Med.* **2021**, *2*, 100230. [CrossRef] [PubMed]
53. Popowski, K.D.; Moatti, A.; Scull, G.; Silkstone, D.; Lutz, H.; López de Juan Abad, B.; George, A.; Belcher, E.; Zhu, D.; Mei, X.; et al. Inhalable dry powder mRNA vaccines based on extracellular vesicles. *Matter* **2022**, *5*, 2960–2974. [CrossRef] [PubMed]
54. Kozlowski, P.A.; Williams, S.B.; Lynch, R.M.; Flanigan, T.P.; Patterson, R.R.; Cu-Uvin, S.; Neutra, M.R. Differential induction of mucosal and systemic antibody responses in women after nasal, rectal, or vaginal immunization: Influence of the menstrual cycle. *J. Immunol.* **2002**, *169*, 566–574. [CrossRef]
55. Özbay Kurt, F.G.; Lepper, A.; Gerhards, C.; Roemer, M.; Lasser, S.; Arkhypov, I.; Bitsch, R.; Bugert, P.; Altevogt, P.; Gouttefangeas, C.; et al. Booster dose of mRNA vaccine augments waning T cell and antibody responses against SARS-CoV-2. *Front. Immunol.* **2022**, *13*, 1012526. [CrossRef]
56. Esparcia-Pinedo, L.; Martínez-Fleta, P.; Ropero, N.; Vera-Tomé, P.; Reyburn, H.T.; Casasnovas, J.M.; Rodríguez Frade, J.M.; Valés-Gómez, M.; Vilches, C.; Martín-Gayo, E.; et al. CD4+ T Cell Immune Specificity Changes After Vaccination in Healthy and COVID-19 Convalescent Subjects. *Front. Immunol.* **2022**, *12*, 755891. [CrossRef]
57. Kratzer, B.; Schlax, L.C.; Gattinger, P.; Waidhofer-Söllner, P.; Trapin, D.; Tauber, P.A.; Sehgal, A.N.A.; Körmöczi, U.; Rottal, A.; Feichter, M.; et al. Combined assessment of S- and N-specific IL-2 and IL-13 secretion and CD69 neo-expression for discrimination of post-infection and post-vaccination cellular SARS-CoV-2-specific immune response. *Allergy* **2022**, *77*, 3408–3425. [CrossRef]
58. Batista-Duharte, A.; Pera, A.; Aliño, S.F.; Solana, R. Regulatory T cells and vaccine effectiveness in older adults. Challenges and prospects. *Int. Immunopharmacol.* **2021**, *96*, 107761. [CrossRef]
59. Wen, Z.; Wang, X.; Dong, K.; Zhang, H.; Bu, Z.; Ye, L.; Yang, C. Blockage of regulatory T cells augments induction of protective immune responses by influenza virus-like particles in aged mice. *Microbes Infect.* **2017**, *19*, 626–634. [CrossRef]
60. Terao, T.; Naduka, T.; Ikeda, D.; Fukumoto, A.; Kamura, Y.; Kuzume, A.; Tabata, R.; Tsushima, T.; Miura, D.; Narita, K.; et al. Depletion of CD38-positive regulatory T cells by anti-CD38 monoclonal antibodies induces a durable response to SARS-CoV-2 vaccination in patients with plasma cell dyscrasia. *Br. J. Haematol.* **2022**, *197*, 417–421. [CrossRef]
61. Gao, F.; Huang, J.; Li, T.; Hu, C.; Shen, M.; Mu, S.; Luo, F.; Song, S.; Hao, Y.; Wang, W.; et al. A Highly Conserved Peptide Vaccine Candidate Activates Both Humoral and Cellular Immunity Against SARS-CoV-2 Variant Strains. *Front. Immunol.* **2021**, *12*, 789905. [CrossRef] [PubMed]

MDPI AG
Grosspeteranlage 5
4052 Basel
Switzerland
Tel.: +41 61 683 77 34

Pharmaceutics Editorial Office
E-mail: pharmaceutics@mdpi.com
www.mdpi.com/journal/pharmaceutics

www.ingramcontent.com/pod-product-compliance
Lightning Source LLC
Chambersburg PA
CBHW041432210926
51850CB00013B/3414
* 9 7 8 3 7 2 5 8 2 9 8 3 5 *